KT-171-393

ANESTHESIA and UNCOMMON DISEASES

5th Edition

Edited by

Lee A. Fleisher, MD
Robert D. Dripps Professor and Chair
Department of Anesthesiology and Critical Care
Professor, Department of Medicine
University of Pennsylvania School of Medicine
Philadelphia, Pennsylvannia

LIBRARY TAUNTON AND SOMERSET HOSPITAL

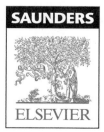

SAUNDERS

ELSEVIER

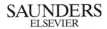

1600 John F. Kennedy Blvd.
Ste 1800
Philadelphia, PA 19103-2899

ANESTHESIA AND UNCOMMON DISEASES
Copyright © 2006, 1998, 1990, 1981, 1973 by Elsevier Inc.

ISBN-13: 978-1-4160-2212-1
ISBN-10: 1-4160-2212-0

All rights reserved. No part of this publication may be reproduced or transmitted in any form or by any means, electronic or mechanical, including photocopying, recording, or any information storage and retrieval system, without permission in writing from the publisher. Permissions may be sought directly from Elsevier's Health Sciences Rights Department in Philadelphia, PA, USA: phone: (+1) 215 239 3804, fax: (+1) 215 239 3805, e-mail: healthpermissions@elsevier.com. You may also complete your request on-line via the Elsevier homepage (http://www.elsevier.com), by selecting 'Customer Support' and then 'Obtaining Permissions'.

Notice

Anesthesiology is an ever-changing field. Standard safety precautions must be followed, but as new research and clinical experience broaden our knowledge, changes in treatment and drug therapy may become necessary or appropriate. Readers are advised to check the most current product information provided by the manufacturer of each drug to be administered to verify the recommended dose, the method and duration of administration, and contraindications. It is the responsibility of the treating physician, relying on experience and knowledge of the patient, to determine dosages and the best treatment for each individual patient. Neither the publisher nor the editor assumes any liability for any injury and/or damage to persons or property arising from this publication.

The Publisher

Library of Congress Cataloging-in-Publication Data
Anesthesia and uncommon diseases. — 5th ed. / editor, Lee A. Fleisher.
    p. ; cm.
  Rev. ed. of: Anesthesia & uncommon diseases / [edited by] Jonathan L. Benumof. 4th ed. c1998.
  ISBN 1-4160-2212-0
  1. Anesthesia—Complications. 2. Rare diseases—Surgery—Complications. 3. Rare diseases
—Pathophysiology. I. Fleisher, Lee A. II. Anesthesia & uncommon diseases.
  [DNLM: 1. Anesthesia. 2. Disease. WO 235 A5791 2006]
  RD87.A54 2006
  617.9'6—dc22

2005047247

Publisher: Natasha Andjelkovic
Developmental Editor: Agnes Byrne
Marketing Manager: Emily M. Christie
Publishing Services Manager: Tina Rebane
Project Manager: Norm Stellander
Design Direction: Steve Stave

Printed in the United States of America

Last digit is the print number: 9 8 7 6 5 4 3 2 1

Working together to grow
libraries in developing countries

www.elsevier.com | www.bookaid.org | www.sabre.org

ELSEVIER   BOOK AID International   Sabre Foundation

This book is dedicated to

My wife, Renee, who is my true partner in life, an outstanding example to our children, and a sounding board.

Two very important teachers from my residency at Yale University, Paul G. Barash and Stanley Rosenbaum. Paul, who was my first Chair, provided me with the encouragement, support, and resources to pursue my interest in the evaluation of the patient with cardiovascular disease undergoing noncardiac surgery. Stanley, who was one of my first attendings, taught me the art and science of caring for patients with complex medical comorbidities and became an important collaborator in my early research efforts. Both of these individuals have remained mentors and became close friends, and their insights have helped me achieve my own goals.

LEE A. FLEISHER

Contributors

DIMITRY BARANOV, MD
Assistant Professor, Department of Anesthesiology and Critical Care, University of Pennsylvania School of Medicine, Philadelphia; Pennsylvania
Neurologic Diseases

SANJAY M. BHANANKER, MD, FRCA
Assistant Professor of Anesthesiology, University of Washington School of Medicine, Seattle, Washington
Burns

RAFAEL CARTAGENA, MD
Assistant Professor, Department of Anesthesiology, University of North Carolina School of Medicine, Chapel Hill, North Carolina; Staff Anesthesiologist, Henrico Doctors Hospital, Richmond, Virginia
Respiratory Diseases

MAURIZIO CEREDA, MD
Clinical Assistant Professor, Department of Anesthesiology and Critical Care, University of Pennsylvania School of Medicine, Philadelphia, Pennsylvania
Renal Diseases

FRANKLYN CLADIS, MD
Assistant Professor of Anesthesia, University of Pittsburgh School of Medicine; Staff Anesthesiologist, Children's Hospital of Pittsburgh, Pittsburgh, Pennsylvania
The Pediatric Patient

BRUCE F. CULLEN, MD
Professor, Department of Anesthesiology, University of Washington School of Medicine, Seattle, Washington
Burns

PETER J. DAVIS, MD
Professor of Anesthesiology, and Pediatrics, University of Pittsburgh School of Medicine; Anesthesiologist-in-Chief, Children's Hospital of Pittsburgh, Pittsburgh, Pennsylvania
The Pediatric Patient

RICHARD P. DUTTON, MD, MBA
Associate Professor, University of Maryland School of Medicine; Director of Trauma Anesthesiology, R. Adams Cowley Shock Trauma Center, University of Maryland Medical System, Baltimore, Maryland
Trauma and Acute Care

NADER M. ENANY, MD
Assistant Professor of Anesthesiology, SUNY Upstate Medical University, Syracuse, New York
Diseases of the Endocrine System

ROBERT A. ERTNER, MD
Department of Anesthesia, Emory University, Atlanta, Georgia
Behavioral and Psychiatric Disorders

GREGORY FISCHER, MD
Instructor, Mount Sinai School of Medicine; Attending Anesthesiologist, Mount Sinai Medical Center, New York, New York
Hematologic Diseases

THOMAS E. GRISSOM, MD, FCCM
Associate Professor, Uniformed Services University of the Health Sciences, Bethesda; Director, Air Force Center for the Sustainment of Trauma and Readiness Skills; R. Adams Cowley Shock Trauma Center, Baltimore, Maryland
Trauma and Acute Care

JIAN HANG, MD, PHD
Assistant Professor, Johns Hopkins University School of Medicine; Attending Physician, Department of Anesthesia, Johns Hopkins Bayview Medical Center, Baltimore, Maryland
The Geriatric Patient

JAMES G. HECKER, PHD, MD
Assistant Professor, Department of Anesthesiology and Critical Care, University of Pennsylvania School of Medicine, Philadelphia, Pennsylvania
Neurologic Diseases

LARS E. HELGESON, MD
Assistant Professor, Department of Anesthesiology,
   Yale University School of Medicine; Attending
   Anesthesiologist, Yale New Haven Hospital,
   New Haven, Connecticut
Obesity and Nutritional Disorders

DAVID L. HEPNER, MD
Assistant Professor of Anesthesia, Harvard Medical
   School; Staff Anesthesiologist, Department of
   Anesthesia, Perioperative and Pain Medicine, and
   Associate Director, Weiner Center for Preoperative
   Evaluation, Brigham and Women's Hospital,
   Boston, Massachusetts
Pregnancy and Complications of Pregnancy

JASON M. HOOVER, BS, MD
Research Associate, Department of Anesthesiology,
   Louisiana State University School of Medicine,
   New Orleans, Louisiana
*Behavioral and Psychiatric Disorders; Patients on Herbal
Medications*

JIRI HORAK, MD
Assistant Professor, Department of Anesthesiology
   and Critical Care, University of Pennsylvania
   School of Medicine, Philadelphia, Pennsylvania
Renal Diseases

JOEL A. KAPLAN, MD
Dean Emeritus and Former Chancellor, and Professor of
   Anesthesiology, University of Louisville School of
   Medicine and Health Science Center, Louisville,
   Kentucky; Clinical Professor of Anesthesiology,
   University of California at San Diego,
   La Jolla, California
Uncommon Cardiac Diseases

ALAN D. KAYE, MD, PhD, DABPM
Professor and Chairman, Department of Anesthesiology,
   and Professor, Department of Pharmacology,
   Louisiana State University School of Medicine,
   New Orleans, Louisiana
*Behavioral and Psychiatric Disorders; Patients on Herbal
Medications*

TOM KELTON, MD
Assistant Instructor, University of Pennsylvania School
   of Medicine; Resident, Department of Anesthesiology,
   Hospital of the University of Pennsylvania,
   Philadelphia, Pennsylvania
Neurologic Diseases

SALIM LAHLOU, MD
Fellow, Regional Anesthesia, Weill Medical College of
   Cornell University, Hospital for Special Surgery,
   New York, New York
Muscle Diseases

RICHARD J. LEVY, MD
Assistant Professor of Anesthesia and Pediatrics,
   University of Pennsylvania School of Medicine;
   Staff Anesthesiologist, Division of Cardiothoracic
   Anesthesia, Children's Hospital of Philadelphia,
   Philadelphia, Pennsylvania
Mitochondrial Diseases

KEITH LITTLEWOOD, MD
Associate Professor of Anesthesiology, University of
   Virginia School of Medicine; Vice-Chair for Education,
   Department of Anesthesiology, University of Virginia
   Health System, Charlottesville, Virginia
Liver Diseases

JAMES J. LYNCH, MD
Assistant Professor, Mayo Clinic College of Medicine,
   Rochester, Minnesota
Congenital Heart Disease

HEATHER MCCLUNG, MD
Assistant Instructor, University of Pennsylvania School
   of Medicine; Resident, Department of Anesthesiology,
   Hospital of the University of Pennsylvania,
   Philadelphia, Pennsylvania
Neurologic Diseases

KATHRYN E. MCGOLDRICK, MD
Professor and Chair, Department of Anesthesiology,
   New York Medical College; Director of Anesthesiology,
   Westchester Medical Center, Valhalla, New York
Eye, Ear, Nose, and Throat Diseases

ALEXANDER MITTNACHT, MD
Assistant Professor of Anesthesiology, Mount Sinai
   School of Medicine; Attending Anesthesiologist,
   Mount Sinai Hospital, New York, New York
Uncommon Cardiac Diseases

STANLEY MURAVCHICK, MD, PhD
Professor of Anesthesiology and Critical Care,
   University of Pennsylvania School of Medicine;
   Staff Anesthesiologist, Hospital of the University of
   Pennsylvania, Philadelphia, Pennsylvania
Mitochondrial Diseases

PATRICK J. NELIGAN, MD
Assistant Professor, Department of Anesthesiology
   and Critical Care, University of Pennsylvania
   School of Medicine; Attending, Hospital of the
   University of Pennsylvania, Philadelphia, Pennsylvania
Renal Diseases; Infectious Diseases and Bioterrorism

EDWARD C. NEMERGUT, MD
Assistant Professor of Anesthesiology and Neurosurgery,
   University of Virginia School of Medicine,
   Charlottesville, Virginia
Liver Diseases

WILLIAM C. OLIVER, JR., MD
Associate Professor, Department of Anesthesiology, Mayo
    Clinic College of Medicine, Rochester, Minnesota
Congenital Heart Disease

ANTHONY N. PASSANNANTE, MD
Associate Professor of Anesthesiology and Residency
    Program Director, University of North Carolina and
    University of North Carolina Hospital,
    Chapel Hill, North Carolina
Respiratory Diseases

DAVID L. REICH, MD
Horace W. Goldsmith Professor and Chair, Department
    of Anesthesiology, The Mount Sinai School of
    Medicine, New York, New York
Uncommon Cardiac Diseases

PETER ROCK, MD, MBA, FCCP, FCCM
Professor of Anesthesiology and Medicine, and Vice-
    Chair, Department of Anesthesiology, University of
    North Carolina School of Medicine,
    Chapel Hill, North Carolina
Respiratory Diseases

MICHAEL F. ROIZEN, MD, PHD
Chair, Department of Anesthesiology, Critical Care
    Medicine and Comprehensive Pain Management,
    Cleveland Clinic Foundation, Cleveland, Ohio
Disease of the Endocrine System

KEITH SCARFO, MS, DO CANDIDATE
College of Osteopathic Medicine,
    Philadelphia, Pennsylvania
Neurologic Diseases

SCOTT SEGAL, MD
Associate Professor of Anesthesia, Harvard Medical
    School; Vice Chairman for Residency Education,
    Brigham and Women's Hospital,
    Boston, Massachusetts
Pregnancy and Complications of Pregnancy

BHAVANI SHANKAR KODALI, MD
Associate Professor, Harvard Medical School; Staff
    Anesthesiologist, Brigham and Women's Hospital,
    Boston, Massachusetts
Pregnancy and Complications of Pregnancy

LINDA SHORE-LESSERSON, MD
Associate Professor of Anesthesia, Mount Sinai School
    of Medicine; Director, Cardiothoracic Anesthesiology,
    Director, CT Anesthesiology Fellowship, and
    Attending Anethesiologist, Mount Sinai Medical
    Center, New York, New York
Hematologic Diseases

FREDERICK E. SIEBER, MD
Associate Professor, Johns Hopkins University School
    of Medicine; Chair and Clinical Director, Department
    of Anesthesia, Johns Hopkins Bayview Medical Center,
    Baltimore, Maryland
The Geriatric Patient

DOREEN SOLIMAN, MD
Assistant Professor of Anesthesia, University of
    Pittsburgh School of Medicine; Staff
    Anesthesiologist, Children's Hospital of Pittsburgh,
    Pittsburgh, Pennsylvania
The Pediatric Patient

PATRICIA B. SUTKER, PHD
Professor, Department of Psychiatry, Louisiana State
    University School of Medicine,
    New Orleans, Louisiana
Behavioral and Psychiatric Disorders

JOHN E. TETZLAFF, MD
Professor of Anesthesiology, Cleveland Clinic Lerner
    College of Medicine of Case Western Reserve
    University; Director, Center for Anesthesiology
    Education, Division of Anesthesiology,
    Critical Care Medicine and Comprehensive Pain
    Management, The Cleveland Clinic Foundation,
    Cleveland, Ohio
Skin and Bone Disorders

MICHAEL K. URBAN, MD, PHD
Associate Professor of Clinical Anesthesia, Director,
    Post-Anesthesia Care Units, Department of
    Anesthesia, Hospital for Special Surgery,
    New York, New York
Muscle Diseases

What are uncommon diseases? The *Oxford English Dictionary* defines "uncommon" as not possessed in common, not commonly (to be) met with, not of ordinary occurrence, unusual, rare. "Rare" has various meanings, such as few in number and widely separated from each other (in space or time), though also including unusual and exceptional. Another synonym for uncommon is "infrequent," the definition of which includes not occurring often, happening rarely, recurring at wide intervals of time. The chapter entitled Respiratory Diseases in this edition aims to review "less common" pulmonary conditions, rather than "uncommon." None of these definitions include quantification.

Why do we need a separate text to help us conduct the anesthetics of illnesses that do not happen often, if that is indeed the case? The simplest answer, congruent with the present obsession with the wisdom of the market, might be that the need has been already proven by the fact that the anesthetic community has bought sufficient copies of the previous four editions of this book to warrant a fifth. Nevertheless, it seems an intriguing question. Are the readers of the book residents studying arcane facts in order to pass certification examinations? Are they investigators searching for relevant questions to research? Are they isolated clinicians faced with the necessity of managing patients with unusual conditions they encounter so infrequently that they do not recall (or never knew) the most relevant facts requisite for providing safe care? Do the many uncommon conditions, even though each might occur infrequently, happen sufficiently often in the aggregate that we would ignore them to the peril of our patients?

To begin to approach this question, we need to consider the practice of medicine and the fact that medicine is a profession. Professions are occupations in which groups of individuals are granted a monopoly by society to learn and apply advanced knowledge in some area for the benefit of that society. The profession has the obligation to transmit that knowledge to others who will join that profession, to develop new knowledge and to maintain standards of practice by self-regulation. There is a moral covenant with society to behave altruistically, that is, for the professional to subsume her or his own personal interests for the benefit of the society. These characteristics

translate into an obligation to provide competent care for all who entrust themselves into our hands, no matter how rare or esoteric their condition may be. In the practice of anesthesiology (and of all of medicine, for that matter), it is not possible for any one individual to know everything necessary to fulfill that responsibility. Thus, we are dependent on rapid access to gain sufficient knowledge to approach that duty.

In the preface to the first edition of *Anesthesia and Uncommon Diseases* (1973), editors Jordan Katz and Leslie B. Kadis stressed their intention to present disease entities whose underlying pathophysiologic processes might profoundly affect normal anesthetic management. They noted that, "In general, the information we wanted to present has never been published." This resulted in "a compendium of what is *and is not* known about unusual diseases as they may or may not relate to anesthesia." The authors expressed the hope that their work would stimulate others to publish their experiences.

The subsequent three decades have seen a remarkable growth and development of knowledge in biomedical science, including anesthesiology and its related disciplines. Many others have indeed published their experiences with conditions covered in editions of this book. This has resulted in understanding the physiology and safe anesthetic management of many of these diseases, so that recommendations for their management can be provided with confidence. It has also been accompanied by recognition of other, not previously recognized, illnesses that have joined the ranks of "uncommon diseases." An example of the former is the present virtually complete understanding of succinylcholine-associated hyperkalemia in certain muscle diseases; an example of the latter is the entire field of mitochondrial diseases, which is the topic of a completely new chapter in this edition.

Anesthesiology has been characterized as hours of boredom interspersed with moments of terror. I would argue strongly that this is an incomplete and misleading characterization, but will not expand on that here. However, as a recovering clinician who spent decades (unsuccessfully) attempting to make every anesthetic as "boring" as possible, I can vouch that terror is indeed an inevitable component of the specialty. Knowledge—technical, experiential, judgmental, didactic—is the most effective deterrent to these vexing episodes, and the best tool to successfully confront them when they occur. This book is a single source of extremely useful and provocative knowledge, for trainees, practitioners and investigators alike. I suspect this is why the previous editions of this book have been so successful, why this updated and much changed edition, with a new editor, new topics, and new contributors, will also be a success, and why we will need further new editions in future.

EDWARD LOWENSTEIN, MD
Henry Isaiah Dorr Professor of Anaesthesia and
Professor of Medical Ethics
Harvard Medial School
Provost, Department of Anesthesia and Critical Care
Massachusetts General Hospital, Boston, Massachusetts

Preface

It was a pleasure to edit the fifth edition of *Anesthesia and Uncommon Diseases,* following the traditions of Dr. Benumof in the fourth edition, and Drs. Katz, Benumof, and Kadis from previous editions. As a resident at Yale New Haven Hospital, the third edition of this book was always an important component of my planning for the next day's anesthetic. Therefore, it was a great honor to be asked to edit this latest edition. In order to both do justice to the previous editions and take this text into the 21st century, the fifth edition of *Anesthesia and Uncommon Diseases* has been revised and restructured. The overall look and feel is different, with a new outline structure and tables. New authors have been invited to offer a new perspective and provide the reader with the latest information. Finally, additional chapters have been included to focus on more recently defined unique disease entities, such as those associated with mitochondrial dysfunction. I am very grateful that an outstanding group of authors agreed to participate in this new edition.

In putting together a multi-author text, numerous people must be acknowledged. I would like to thank my editorial assistant, Kate Musselman, for her outstanding editorial work on the chapters, as well as for managing a diverse group of authors. I would also like to thank Natasha Andjelkovic, my publisher at Elsevier, for her patience and support, and Agnes Byrne, our developmental editor, whose guidance was very valuable.

LEE A. FLEISHER, MD
Editor

Contents

1 Eye, Ear, Nose, and Throat Diseases

Kathryn E. McGoldrick, MD

Many patients presenting for relatively "simple" ophthalmic or otorhinolaryngologic procedures suffer from complex systemic diseases. Although the surgeon may have the luxury of being able to focus on one specific aspect of the patient's condition, the anesthesiologist must be knowledgeable about the ramifications of the entire disease complex and the germane implications for anesthetic management. Issues of safety often are complicated by the logistic necessity for the anesthesiologist to be positioned at a considerable distance from the patient's face, thus preventing immediate access to the airway for certain types of ophthalmic surgery. Additionally, during many laryngologic surgeries the anesthesiologist must share the airway with the surgeon. Moreover, many of these complicated patients undergo surgical procedures that are routinely performed on an ambulatory basis, thereby further challenging the anesthesiologist to provide a rapid, smooth, problem-free recovery.

The focus of this chapter is on several eye as well as ear, nose, and throat (ENT) conditions, many of which are relatively rare. Nonetheless, it behooves the anesthesiologist to understand the complexities involved because failure to do so may be associated with preventable morbidity and mortality.

EYE DISEASES: GENERAL CONSIDERATIONS

Patients with eye conditions are often at the extremes of age, ranging from tiny, fragile infants with retinopathy of prematurity or congenital cataracts to nonagenarians with submacular hemorrhage, and may have extensive associated systemic processes or metabolic diseases.[1] Moreover, the increased longevity characteristic of developed nations has produced a concomitant increase in the longitudinal prevalence of major eye diseases. A study of elderly Medicare beneficiaries followed for 9 years during the 1990s documented a dramatic increase in the prevalence of major chronic eye diseases associated with aging.[2] For example, the prevalence of diabetes mellitus increased from 14.5% at baseline in the study patients to 25.6% nine years later, with diabetic retinopathy among persons with diabetes mellitus increasing from 6.9% to 17.4% of the subset. Primary open-angle glaucoma increased from 4.6% to 13.8%, and the percentage of glaucoma suspects increased from 1.5% to 6.5%. The prevalence of age-related macular degeneration increased from 5.0% to 27.1%. Overall, the proportion of subjects with at least one of these three chronic eye diseases increased impressively from 13.4% to 45.4% of the elderly Medicare population.

Ophthalmic conditions typically involve either the cornea, the lens, the vitreoretinal area, the intraocular pressure–regulating apparatus, or the eye muscles and adnexa. These patients may present for corneal transplantation, cataract extraction, vitrectomy for vitreous hemorrhage, scleral buckling for retinal detachment, trabeculectomy and other glaucoma filtration procedures for glaucoma amelioration, or rectus muscle recession and resection for strabismus, respectively. Conversely, they may require surgery for a condition entirely unrelated to their ocular pathology; nonetheless, their ocular disease per se may present issues for anesthetic management, or the eye pathology may be but one manifestation of a constellation of systemic conditions that constitute a syndrome with major anesthetic implications (Table 1-1).

Other, less common eye defects frequently linked with coexisting diseases include aniridia, colobomas, and optic nerve hypoplasia. *Aniridia,* a developmental abnormality characterized by striking hypoplasia of the iris, is a misnomer, because the iris is not totally absent. The term describes just one facet of a complex developmental disorder that features macular and optic nerve hypoplasia as well as associated cataracts, glaucoma, ectopia lentis, progressive opacification, and nystagmus. At least two types of aniridia have been described. Type I is transmitted in an autosomal dominant fashion; the involved gene is thought to be on chromosome 2. Aniridia type II usually appears sporadically and is associated with an interstitial deletion on the short arm of chromosome 11 (11p13), although rarely a balanced translocation of chromosome 11 may produce familial type II aniridia. In addition to the typical ocular lesions, children with type II aniridia frequently are mentally retarded and have genitourinary anomalies—the ARG triad. Individuals with the chromosome 11 defect and this triad may develop Wilms' tumor[3] and should be followed with regular abdominal examinations and frequent renal ultrasonography at least until they are 4 years old. Chromosomal analysis is indicated in all infants with congenital aniridia.

Coloboma denotes an absence or defect of some ocular tissue, usually resulting from malclosure of the fetal intraocular fissure, or rarely from trauma or disease. Two major types of ocular colobomas are chorioretinal or fundus coloboma and isolated optic nerve coloboma. The typical fundus coloboma is caused by malclosure of the embryonic fissure, resulting in a gap in the retina, retinal pigment epithelium, and choroid. These defects may be unilateral or bilateral and usually produce a visual field defect corresponding to the chorioretinal defect. Although colobomas may occur independent of other abnormalities, they also may be associated with microphthalmos, cyclopia, anencephaly, or other major central nervous system aberrations. They frequently are linked with chromosomal abnormalities, especially the trisomy 13 and 18 syndromes. Colobomas may be seen with the CHARGE (congenital heart disease, choanal atresia, mental retardation, genital hypoplasia, and ear anomalies) syndrome or the VATER (tracheoesophageal fistula, congenital heart disease, and renal anomalies) association. Rarely, isolated colobomas of the optic nerve occur. They may be familial and may be associated with other ocular pathology, as well as with systemic defects including cardiac conditions.

Optic nerve hypoplasia is a developmental defect characterized by deficiency of optic nerve fibers. The anomaly may be unilateral or bilateral, be mild to severe, and be associated with a broad spectrum of ophthalmoscopic findings and clinical manifestations. Visual impairment may range from minimal reduction in acuity[4] to blindness. Strabismus or nystagmus secondary to visual impairment is common. Although optic nerve hypoplasia may occur as an isolated defect in otherwise normal children, the lesion can be associated with aniridia, microphthalmos, coloboma, anencephaly, hydrocephalus, hydranencephaly, and encephalocele. Optic nerve hypoplasia may occur in a syndrome termed *septo-optic dysplasia* or de Morsier's syndrome. There may be coexisting hypothalamic conditions and extremely variable endocrine aberrations.[5,6] An isolated deficiency of growth hormone is most common, but multiple hormonal imbalances, including diabetes insipidus, have been reported. The etiology of optic nerve hypoplasia remains unknown. However, it has been observed to occur with slightly increased frequency in infants of diabetic mothers,[4] and the prenatal use of drugs such as LSD (lysergic acid diethylamide), meperidine, phenytoin, and quinine has been implicated sporadically.

Corneal Pathology and Systemic Disease

A vast spectrum of conditions may be associated with corneal pathology (Table 1-2). Such diverse entities as inflammatory diseases, connective tissue disorders, metabolic diseases, and even skin conditions have been reported in conjunction with corneal abnormalities.[7]

Examples of inflammatory diseases associated with corneal pathology include rheumatoid arthritis, Reiter's syndrome, Behçet's syndrome, and sarcoidosis.

Connective tissues disorders such as ankylosing spondylosis, scleroderma, Sjögren's syndrome, and Wegener's

TABLE 1–1 Ophthalmic Conditions Frequently Associated with Coexisting Diseases	
Aniridia	Macular hypoplasia
Cataracts	Nystagmus
Colobomata	Optic nerve hypoplasia
Corneal dystrophies	Retinal detachment
Ectopia lentis	Retinopathy
Glaucoma	Strabismus

TABLE 1–2 Examples of Systemic Diseases Associated with Corneal Pathology

Connective Tissue Disorders

Ankylosing spondylosis

Scleroderma

Sjögren's syndrome

Wegener's granulomatosis

Inflammatory Diseases

Behçet's syndrome

Reiter's syndrome

Rheumatoid arthritis

Sarcoidosis

Metabolic Diseases

Carbohydrate metabolism disorders

Chronic renal failure

Cystinosis

Gout

Graves' disease

Wilson's disease

Skin Disorders

Erythema multiforme

Pemphigus

granulomatosis have been associated with corneal disturbances.

Metabolic diseases, including cystinosis, disorders of carbohydrate metabolism, gout, hyperlipidemia, and Wilson's disease, have also been linked with corneal pathology. Additionally, such conditions as Graves' hyperthyroid disease, leprosy, chronic renal failure, and tuberculosis may have associated corneal disease. Even skin diseases such as erythema multiforme and pemphigus have corneal manifestations. Finally, mandibulo-oculofacial dyscephaly (Hallermann-Streiff syndrome) is of interest to anesthesiologists because of anticipated difficulty with intubation.

Lens Pathology and Systemic Disease

A cataract is defined as a clouding of the normally clear crystalline lens of the eye. The different types of cataracts include nuclear-sclerotic, cortical, posterior subcapsular, and mixed. Each type has its own location in the lens and risk factors for development, with nuclear-sclerotic cataracts being the most common type of age-related cataract. The leading cause of blindness worldwide, cataracts affect more than 6 million individuals annually.[8] Indeed, cataract surgery is the most frequently performed surgical procedure in the United States with more than 1.5 million operations annually.[9] Over half the population older than age 65 years develop age-related cataracts with related visual disability.[10] Yet, despite extensive research into the pathogenesis and pharmacologic prevention of cataracts, there are no proven means to prevent age-related cataracts.

Although age-related cataracts are the most frequently encountered variety, cataracts may be associated with dermatologic diseases such as incontinentia pigmenti, exogenous substances, genetic diseases, hematologic diseases, infections, and metabolic perturbations (Table 1-3).

TABLE 1–3 Conditions Associated with Cataracts

Aging

Chromosomal Anomalies

Trisomy 13

Trisomy 18

Trisomy 21

Turner's syndrome

Dermatologic Diseases

Incontinentia pigmenti

Exogenous Substances

Alcohol

Ergot

Naphthalene

Parachlorobenzene

Phenothiazines

Metabolic Conditions

Diabetes mellitus

Fabry's disease

Galactosemia

Hypoparathyroidism

Hypothyroidism

Lowe's syndrome

Phenylketonuria

Refsum's disease

Wilson's disease

Xanthomatosis

Infectious Diseases

Herpes

Influenza

Mumps

Polio

Rubella

Toxoplasmosis

Vaccinia

Varicella zoster

Exogenous substances that can trigger cataracts include corticosteroids,[11-13] phenothiazines, naphthalene, ergot, parachlorobenzene, and alcohol.[14] Metabolic conditions associated with cataracts include diabetes mellitus, Fabry's disease, galactosemia, hepatolenticular degeneration (Wilson's disease), hypoparathyroidism, hypothyroidism, phenylketonuria, Refsum's disease, and xanthomatosis. Another metabolic disorder important in the differential diagnosis of congenital cataracts is Lowe's (oculocerebrorenal) syndrome. In this X-linked disorder, cataract is frequently the presenting sign, with other abnormalities appearing later. These anomalies include mental and growth retardation, hypotonia, renal acidosis, aminoaciduria, proteinuria, and renal rickets, requiring calcium and vitamin D therapy.[15,16] Other concomitants include osteoporosis and a distinctive facies (long with frontal bossing). Although lens changes may be seen frequently in heterozygous female children also, affected male children commonly have obvious, dense, bilateral cataracts at birth. They may also be afflicted with associated glaucoma. Interestingly, carrier females in their second decade of life have significantly higher numbers of lens opacities than age-related controls; however, absence of opacities is no guarantee that an individual is not a carrier. Anesthetic management includes careful attention to acid-base balance and to serum levels of calcium and electrolytes. The administration of drugs excreted by the kidney should be observed carefully, and nephrotoxins should be avoided. The patient with osteoporosis should be positioned on the operating table with extreme gentleness.

Infectious causes of cataracts include herpes, influenza, mumps, polio, rubella, toxoplasmosis, vaccinia, and varicella zoster.[17] Chromosomal anomalies associated with cataracts include trisomy 13 (Patau's syndrome), trisomy 18 (Edward's syndrome), and trisomy 21 (Down syndrome). In Patau's and Edward's syndromes, congenital cataracts frequently occur in conjunction with other ocular anomalies, such as coloboma and microphthalmia. Cataracts have also been reported with Turner's syndrome (XO).

An additional type of lens abnormality that can be associated with major systemic disease is *ectopia lentis* (Table 1-4). Displacement of the lens can be classified topographically as subluxation or luxation. Luxation denotes a lens that is dislocated either posteriorly into the vitreous cavity or, less commonly, anteriorly into the anterior chamber. In subluxation, some zonular attachments remain and the lens remains in its plane posterior to the iris, albeit tilted in one direction or another.

The most common cause of lens displacement is trauma, although ectopia lentis may also result from assorted other ocular diseases, such as intraocular tumor, congenital glaucoma, uveitis, aniridia, syphilis, or high myopia. Inherited defects and serious systemic diseases, such as Marfan's syndrome, homocystinuria, Weill-Marchesani

TABLE 1–4   Conditions Associated with Ectopia Lentis
Ocular Conditions
Aniridia
Congenital glaucoma
High myopia
Intraocular tumor
Trauma
Uveitis
Systemic Diseases
Homocystinuria
Hyperlysinemia
Marfan's syndrome
Sulfite oxidase deficiency
Weill-Marchesani syndrome

syndrome, hyperlysinemia, and sulfite oxidase deficiency, are also associated with ectopia lentis. Indeed, lens displacement occurs in approximately 80% of patients with Marfan's syndrome.

Glaucoma and Systemic Disease

Glaucoma is a condition characterized by elevated intraocular pressure (IOP), resulting in impairment of capillary blood flow to the optic nerve and eventual loss of optic nerve tissue and function. Two different anatomic types of glaucoma exist: open-angle or chronic simple glaucoma and closed-angle or acute glaucoma. (Other variations of these processes occur but are not especially germane to anesthetic management. Glaucoma is, in fact, not one disease, but many.)

With open-angle glaucoma, the elevated IOP exists in conjunction with an anatomically patent anterior chamber angle. It is thought that sclerosis of trabecular tissue produces impaired aqueous filtration and drainage. Treatment consists of medication to produce miosis and trabecular stretching. Commonly used eyedrops include epinephrine, echothiophate iodide, timolol, dipivefrin, and betaxolol. Carbonic anhydrase inhibitors such as acetazolamide can also be administered by various routes to reduce IOP by interfering with the production of aqueous humor. All these drugs are systemically absorbed and can, therefore, have anticipated side effects.

It is important to appreciate that maintenance of IOP is determined primarily by the rate of aqueous formation and the rate of aqueous outflow. The most important influence on formation of aqueous humor is the difference in osmotic pressure between aqueous and plasma. This concept is illustrated by the equation:

$$IOP = K[(OPaq - OPpl) + CP]$$

where K = coefficient of outflow, OPaq = osmotic pressure of aqueous humor, OPpl = osmotic pressure of plasma, and CP = capillary pressure. The fact that a small change in solute concentration of plasma can dramatically affect the formation of aqueous humor and hence IOP is the rationale for administering hypertonic solutions, such as mannitol, to reduce IOP.

Fluctuations in aqueous outflow can also markedly change IOP. The primary factor controlling aqueous humor outflow is the diameter of Fontana's spaces, as illustrated by the equation:

$$A = [r^4 \times (Piop - Pv)] \div 8\eta L$$

where A = volume of aqueous outflow per unit of time, r = radius of Fontana's spaces, Piop = IOP, Pv = venous pressure, η = viscosity, and L = length of Fontana's spaces. When the pupil dilates, Fontana's spaces narrow, resistance to outflow is increased, and IOP rises. Because mydriasis is undesirable in both closed- and open-angle glaucoma, miotics such as pilocarpine are applied conjunctivally in patients with glaucoma.

The aforementioned equation describing the volume of aqueous outflow per unit of time clearly underscores that outflow is exquisitely sensitive to fluctuations in venous pressure. Because an elevation in venous pressure results in an increased volume of ocular blood as well as decreased aqueous outflow, it is obvious that considerable increase in IOP occurs with any maneuver that increases venous pressure. Hence, in addition to preoperative instillation of miotics, other anesthetic objectives for the patient with glaucoma include perioperative avoidance of venous congestion and of overhydration. Furthermore, hypotensive episodes are to be avoided because these patients are purportedly vulnerable to retinal vascular thrombosis.

Although glaucoma usually occurs as an isolated disease, it may also be associated with such conditions as Sturge-Weber syndrome, aniridia, mesodermal dysgenesis syndrome, retinopathy of prematurity, Refsum's syndrome, mucopolysaccharidosis, Hurler's syndrome, Stickler's syndrome, Marfan's syndrome, and von Recklinghausen's disease (neurofibromatosis) (Table 1-5). Additionally, ocular trauma, corticosteroid therapy, sarcoidosis, some forms of arthritis associated with uveitis, and pseudoexfoliation syndrome can also be associated with secondary glaucoma.

Primary closed-angle glaucoma is characterized by a shallow anterior chamber and a narrow iridocorneal angle that impedes the egress of aqueous humor from the eye because the trabecular meshwork is covered by the iris (Table 1-6). Relative pupillary block is common in many angle-closure episodes in which iris-lens apposition or synechiae impede the flow of aqueous from the posterior chamber. In the United States, the prevalence of angle-closure glaucoma (ACG) is one tenth as common as open-angle glaucoma. In acute ACG, if the pressure is not reduced promptly, permanent visual loss can ensue as a result of optic nerve damage. It is thought that irreversible optic nerve injury can occur within 24 to 48 hours. Therefore, once the diagnosis of acute ACG has been made, treatment should be instituted immediately. Signs and symptoms include ocular pain (often excruciating), red eye, corneal edema, blurred vision, and a fixed, mid-dilated pupil. Consultation with an ophthalmologist should be sought immediately. Topical pilocarpine 2% is administered to cause miosis and pull the iris taut and away from the trabecular meshwork. A topical β blocker also should be considered. If a prompt reduction in IOP does not ensue, systemic therapy with an agent such as mannitol should be considered, but its potentially adverse hemodynamic effects should be weighed in a patient with cardiovascular disease. If medical therapy is effective in reducing IOP to a safe level and the angle opens, an iridotomy/iridectomy can be performed immediately, or it can be delayed until the corneal edema resolves and the iris becomes less hyperemic (Table 1-7).

TABLE 1–5 Partial Listing of Conditions Associated with Glaucoma	
Ocular Conditions	**Systemic Diseases**
Aniridia	Chromosomal anomalies
Anterior cleavage syndrome	Congenital infection syndromes (TORCH)
Cataracts	Hurler's syndrome
Ectopia lentis	Marfan's syndrome
Hemorrhage	Refsum's disease
Mesodermal dysgenesis	Sarcoidosis
Persistent hyperplastic primary vitreous	Stickler syndrome
Retinopathy of prematurity	Sturge-Weber syndrome
Spherophakia	von Recklinghausen's disease
Trauma	
Tumor	

TABLE 1–6   Anesthetic Objectives for Patients with Glaucoma

Perioperative instillation of miotics to enhance aqueous humor outflow
Avoidance of venous congestion/overhydration
Avoidance of markedly increased venous pressure (e.g., coughing or vomiting)
Avoidance of hypotension that may trigger retinal vascular thrombosis

Retinal Complications of Systemic Disease

Retinal conditions such as vitreous hemorrhage and retinal detachment are most commonly associated with diabetes mellitus and hypertension (Table 1-8). However, collagen disorders and connective tissue diseases, such as systemic lupus erythematosus, scleroderma, polyarteritis nodosa, Marfan's syndrome, and Wagner-Stickler syndrome, are often associated with retinal pathology. Serious retinal complications have been reported with skin conditions such as incontinentia pigmenti. Additionally, such conditions as sickle cell anemia, macroglobulinemia, Tay-Sachs disease, Neimann-Pick syndrome, and hyperlipidemia can result in vitreoretinal disorders. During the past two decades, cytomegalovirus retinitis has been reported in patients with acquired immunodeficiency syndrome. The condition sometimes progresses to cause retinal detachment.

EYE DISEASES: SPECIFIC CONSIDERATIONS

Having provided a brief overview of the broad spectrum of systemic diseases that can be associated with the major types of serious ocular pathology, the focus shifts to specific disease entities and their anesthetic management.

Marfan's Syndrome

Marfan's syndrome is a disorder of connective tissue, involving primarily the cardiovascular, skeletal, and ocular systems. However, the skin, fascia, lungs, skeletal muscle, and adipose tissue may also be affected. The etiology is a mutation in *FBNI,* the gene that encodes fibrillin-1, a major component of extracellular microfibrils, which are the major components of elastic fibers that anchor the dermis, epidermis, and ocular zonules.[18] Connective tissue in this disorder has decreased tensile strength and elasticity. Marfan's syndrome is inherited as an autosomal dominant trait with variable expression.

Ocular manifestations of the syndrome include severe myopia, spontaneous retinal detachments, displaced lenses, and glaucoma. Cardiovascular manifestations include dilation of the ascending aorta and aortic insufficiency. The loss of elastic fibers in the media may also account for dilation of the pulmonary artery and mitral insufficiency resulting from extended chordae tendineae. Myocardial ischemia owing to medial necrosis of coronary arterioles as well as dysrhythmias and conduction disturbances have been well documented. Heart failure and dissecting aortic aneurysms or aortic rupture are not uncommon.

The patients are tall, with long, thin extremities and fingers (arachnodactyly). Joint ligaments are loose, resulting in frequent dislocations of the mandible and hip. Possible cervical spine laxity can also occur. Kyphoscoliosis and pectus excavatum can contribute to restrictive pulmonary disease. Lung cysts have also been described, causing an increased risk of pneumothorax. A narrow, high-arched palate is commonly found.

The early manifestations of Marfan's syndrome may be subtle, and therefore the diagnosis may not yet have been made when the patient comes for initial surgery. The anesthesiologist, however, should have a high index of suspicion when a tall young patient with a heart murmur presents for repair of a spontaneously detached retina. These young patients should have a chest radiograph as

TABLE 1–7   Comparison of Open-Angle Versus Closed-Angle Glaucoma

Open-Angle Glaucoma	Closed-Angle Glaucoma
Anatomically patent anterior chamber angle	Shallow anterior chamber
Trabecular sclerosis	Narrow iridocorneal angle
Ten times more common than closed-angle	Iris covers trabecular meshwork
Painless	Painful
Initially unaccompanied by visual symptoms	Red eye with corneal edema
Can result in blindness if chronically untreated	Blurred vision
	Fixed, dilated pupil
	Can cause irreversible optic nerve injury within 24-48 hours
	Requires emergency treatment

TABLE 1–8 Examples of Conditions Associated with Vitreoretinal Pathology

Diabetes mellitus
Hypertension
Collagen/connective tissue disorders
Marfan's syndrome
Polyarteritis nodosa
Scleroderma
Systemic lupus erythematosus
Wagner-Stickler syndrome
Hyperlipidemia
Human immunodeficiency syndrome
Incontinentia pigmenti
Macroglobulinemia
Neimann-Pick disease
Tay-Sachs disease

well as an electrocardiogram and echocardiogram before surgery. Antibiotics for subacute bacterial endocarditis prophylaxis should be considered, as well as β blockade to mitigate against increases in myocardial contractility and aortic wall tension (dP/dT).

The anesthesiologist should be prepared for a potentially difficult intubation (Table 1-9). Laryngoscopy should be carefully performed to circumvent tissue damage and, especially, to avoid hypertension with its attendant risk of aortic dissection. The patient should be carefully positioned to avoid cervical spine or other joint injuries, including dislocations. The dangers of hypertension in these patients are well known. Clearly, the presence of significant aortic insufficiency warrants that the blood pressure (especially the diastolic pressure) be high enough

TABLE 1–9 Anesthetic Concerns with Marfan's Syndrome

Difficult intubation
Lung cysts
Restrictive pulmonary disease
Dysrhythmias and/or conduction disturbances
Dilation of aorta and pulmonary artery; dissecting/ruptured aortic aneurysms
Aortic and/or mitral insufficiency   Consider antibiotic prophylaxis for subacute bacterial endocarditis.
Myocardial ischemia; heart failure   Consider β blockade.
Propensity to mandibular/cervical/hip dislocation

to provide adequate coronary blood flow but should not be so high as to risk dissection of the aorta. Maintenance of the patient's normal blood pressure is typically a good plan. No single intraoperative anesthetic agent or technique has demonstrated superiority. If pulmonary cysts are present, however, positive-pressure ventilation may lead to pneumothorax.[19] At extubation, one should take care to avoid sudden increases in blood pressure or heart rate. Adequate postoperative pain management is vitally important to avoid the detrimental effects of hypertension and tachycardia.

Graves' Disease

Graves' disease is the most common cause of both pediatric and adult hyperthyroidism. Graves' disease encompasses hyperthyroidism, goiter, pretibial myxedema, and, often but not inevitably, exophthalmos. The condition occurs in conjunction with the production of excess thyroid hormone and affects approximately 3 in 10,000 adults (usually women) typically between 25 and 50 years of age. Graves' ophthalmopathy includes corneal ulcerations and exophthalmos that can be severe. Retro-orbital tissue and the extraocular muscles are infiltrated with lymphocytes, plasma cells, and mucopolysaccharides. The extraocular muscles often are swollen to 5 to 10 times their normal size. If proptosis secondary to infiltrative ophthalmopathy is severe and if muscle function or visual acuity deteriorates, corticosteroid therapy (usually prednisone, 20 to 40 mg/day for adults) is initiated, especially if retrobulbar neuritis develops. Those patients who fail to respond to corticosteroid therapy require surgical intervention. Lateral (Krönlein's) or supraorbital (Naffziger's) decompression is performed.

Graves' disease is thought to be autoimmune in origin, with thyroid-stimulating immunoglobulins directed against thyroid antigens that bind to thyroid-stimulating hormone (TSH) receptors on the thyroid gland. Soft, multinodular, nonmalignant enlargement of the thyroid is typical. There is a strong hereditary component with Graves' disease, and it appears likely that the condition is exacerbated by emotional stress. These patients may have other signs of autoimmune involvement, including myositis and occasionally myasthenia gravis.

Symptoms include weakness, fatigue, weight loss, tremulousness, and increased tolerance to cold. Proptosis, diplopia or blurred vision, photophobia, conjunctival chemosis, and decreased visual acuity may be noted. Cardiac symptoms include a hyperdynamic precordium, tachycardia, and elevated systolic, decreased diastolic, and widened pulse pressures. Atrial fibrillation, palpitations, and dyspnea on exertion may also occur.

The differential diagnosis of Graves' disease includes other causes of hyperthyroidism such as pregnancy that may be associated with the production of an ectopic

TSH-like substance, autoimmune thyroiditis, thyroid adenoma, choriocarcinoma, a TSH-secreting pituitary adenoma, and surreptitious ingestion of triiodothyronine (T_3) or thyroxine (T_4).[20]

The goals of drug therapy in the hyperthyroid patient are to control the major manifestations of the thyrotoxic state and to render the patient euthyroid. The most commonly used agents are the thiourea derivatives propyl-thiouracil (PTU) and methimazole, which act by inhibiting synthesis of thyroid hormone. (PTU may also inhibit the conversion of T_4 to T_3.) Owing to the large glandular storage of hormone, 4 to 8 weeks is usually required to render a patient euthyroid with these drugs. Treatment is typically for several months, after which thyroid reserve and suppressive response to thyroid hormone are reevaluated. The major complication of this therapy is hypothyroidism, and the dosage is usually adjusted to the lowest possible once a euthyroid state is attained.[21] Other side effects encountered in patients taking these antithyroid drugs include leukopenia, which may be therapy limiting, as well as agranulocytosis, hepatitis, rashes, and drug fever. It is thought that β-receptor numbers are increased by hyperthyroidism,[22] and β blockers are used to rapidly control such effects of catecholamine stimulation as tachycardia, tremor, and diaphoresis.[23]

The main areas of concern for the anesthesiologist involve the chronic use of corticosteroids, the possibility of perioperative thyroid storm, and the potential challenge of a difficult intubation, owing to tracheal deviation from a large neck mass[24] (Table 1-10). When surgery is planned for the patient with Graves' disease, it is imperative to determine if the patient is euthyroid because the euthyroid state will diminish the risks of life-threatening thyroid storm and of perioperative cardiovascular complications by more than 90%. Achievement of the euthyroid state is assessed by clinical signs and symptoms, plasma hormone levels, and evidence of gland shrinkage. The patient

TABLE 1–10   Anesthetic Concerns with Graves' Disease

Difficult intubation secondary to tracheal deviation or compression
Side effects of antithyroid drugs, including leukopenia and hepatitis
Effects of chronic steroid consumption
Meticulous intraoperative eye protection and temperature monitoring
Perioperative thyroid storm   Determine euthyroid state.
Associated autoimmune disease(s)
Weakened tracheal rings

should also be evaluated for associated autoimmune diseases. A chest radiograph, lateral neck films, and computed tomography (CT) of the neck and thorax will determine tracheal displacement or compression. If there is a question about the adequacy of the airway or tracheal deviation or compression, an awake fiberoptic intubation is a prudent approach. Additionally, an armored tube or its equivalent is useful if any tracheal rings are weakened. Liberal hydration is advised if the cardiovascular status will permit this intervention. High dose corticosteroid coverage is indicated, and continuous temperature monitoring is essential. Additionally, the eyes must be meticulously protected.

No single anesthetic drug or technique has been proven superior in the management of hyperthyroid patients. However, anticholinergic drugs are not recommended and ketamine should be avoided, even in the patient who has been successfully rendered euthyroid. Sudden thyroid storm secondary to stress or infection is always a possibility, and the clinician must be alert for even mild increases in the patient's temperature or heart rate. Other early signs of thyroid storm include delirium, confusion, mania, or excitement. The differential diagnosis of these symptoms includes malignant hyperthermia, pheochromocytoma crisis, and neuroleptic malignant syndrome. Treatment of thyroid storm is supportive, including infusion of cooled saline solutions, β-blocker therapy, antithyroid drugs, and corticosteroids.

Homocystinuria

Although rare, homocystinuria is generally considered the second most common inborn error of amino acid metabolism, ranking behind only phenylketonuria in frequency. The incidence of phenylketonuria is about 1:25,000,[26] and that of homocystinuria is approximately 1:200,000.[27] An error of sulfur amino acid metabolism, homocystinuria is characterized by the excretion of a large amount of urinary homocystine, which can be detected by the cyanide-nitroprusside test. A host of assorted genetic aberrations may be linked with homocystinuria, but the most common is a deficiency of cystathionine β synthase, with accumulation of methionine and homocystine. The disorder is autosomal recessive. Disease occurs in the homozygote, but the heterozygote is without risk of developing the potentially life-threatening complications of the condition. Although one third of homocystinurics have normal intelligence, most are mentally retarded.

Ectopia lentis occurs in at least 90% of persons with homocystinuria. Frequently there is subluxation of the lens into the anterior chamber, causing pupillary block glaucoma, necessitating surgical correction. Other ocular findings reported in homocystinuria may include pale irides, retinoschisis, retinal detachment, optic atrophy, central retinal artery occlusion, and strabismus.

Owing to abnormal connective tissue, the skeletal findings are similar to those of Marfan's syndrome. Most patients have arachnodactyly, kyphoscoliosis, and sternal deformity. They also may have severe osteoporosis. Kyphoscoliosis and pectus excavatum may be associated with restrictive lung disease.

It is imperative to appreciate that patients with homocystinuria are extremely vulnerable to thrombotic complications associated with high mortality[28] (Table 1-11). Indeed, an untreated homocystinuric patient may have a perioperative mortality rate as high as 50%. Elevated concentrations of homocystine irritate the vascular intima, promoting thrombolic nidus formation and presumably increasing the adhesiveness of platelets.[29] Other possible causes of the thrombotic tendency include increased platelet aggregation, Hageman factor activation, or enhanced platelet consumption as a result of endothelial damage. Patients with homocystinuria are also at risk for hypoglycemic convulsions secondary to hyperinsulinemia. The latter disturbance is thought to be provoked by hypermethioninemia.[30]

Preoperative measures include a low-methionine, high-cystine diet and vitamins B_6 and B_{12} and folic acid to regulate homocystine levels, as well as acetylsalicylic acid and dipyridamole to prevent aberrant platelet function. Besides appropriate dietary and drug therapy, proper perioperative care involves prevention of hypoglycemia and maintenance of adequate circulation. Patients with osteoporosis must be carefully positioned on the operating table. Glucose levels should be monitored perioperatively. Low-flow, hypotensive states must be assiduously avoided. The patients must be kept well hydrated and well perfused.[31] Anesthetic agents are selected that promote high peripheral flow by reducing vascular resistance, that maintain cardiac output, and that foster rapid recovery and early ambulation. Postoperative vascular support stockings that prevent stasis thrombi in leg veins are indicated.

Hemoglobinopathies: Sickle Cell Disease

Hemoglobinopathies are inherited disorders of hemoglobin synthesis. There may be structural derangements of globin polypeptides or, as in thalassemia, abnormal synthesis of globin chains. In hemoglobin (Hb) S, for example, a single amino acid (valine) is substituted for glutamic acid in the β chain. This substitution has no effect on oxygen affinity or molecular stability. Nonetheless, in the setting of low oxygen tension, it causes an intermolecular reaction, producing insoluble structures within the erythrocytes that result in sickling.[32] These atypical red cells lodge in the microcirculation, causing painful vaso-occlusive crises, infarcts, and increased susceptibility to infection. Low oxygen tension and acidic environments are major triggers and determinants of the degree of sickling. Sickled cells are thought to produce a rightward shift ($P_{50} = 31$ mm Hg) of the oxyhemoglobin dissociation curve to enhance oxygen delivery.

Although ophthalmic pathology such as proliferative retinopathy can occur in all varieties of sickling diseases, it is more common in adults with Hb SC or Hb S thalassemia than in those with Hb SS. Proliferative retinopathy usually appears in the third or fourth decades of life and is the result of vascular occlusion. This occlusion of retinal vessels eventually produces ischemia, neovascularization, vitreous hemorrhage, fibrosis, traction, and retinal detachment or atrophy. However, prophylactic laser photocoagulation has been helpful in reducing the incidence of the aforementioned conditions.

The severity of the anemia depends on the amount of Hb S present. In homozygous SS disease, the Hb S content is 85% to 90%, the remainder being Hb F. Sickle cell thalassemia (Hb SF) is characterized by an Hb S content of 67% to 82% and causes somewhat less severe problems. Indeed, patients with Hb SC and Hb S thalassemia typically have a much more benign course than those individuals with Hb SS and usually have only mild anemia and splenomegaly. Heterozygous persons with Hb SA (sickle trait) rarely have serious clinical problems. However, recent literature suggests some increased risk of stroke and pulmonary emboli or infection after the stress of hypothermic, low-flow cardiopulmonary bypass in patients with sickle trait.[33] This purported risk, however, has not been well quantitated.

Sickle cell disease (Hb SS) is an autosomal recessive condition that occurs most frequently in individuals of African ancestry, although the gene for Hb S also occurs in persons with ancestors from areas endemic for falciparum malaria. Eight to 10 percent of American blacks are heterozygous carriers of Hb S; approximately 0.5% of blacks are homozygous for Hb S disease.

Patients with homozygous sickle cell disease have chronic hemolytic anemia (Table 1-12). Organ damage occurs owing to vaso-occlusive ischemia because sickled cells are unable to traverse narrow capillary beds. Additionally, sickled cells have a propensity to adhere to the endothelium and cause release of vasoactive substances. Chronic pulmonary disease gradually progresses as a result of recurrent pulmonary infection and infarction. Eventually, these individuals develop pulmonary hypertension, cardiomegaly, and heart failure, as well as renal failure.

TABLE 1–11 Potential Perioperative Concerns with Homocystinuria

Restrictive lung disease
Positioning-induced fractures associated with osteoporosis
Thrombotic complications
Hypoglycemic convulsions

TABLE 1–12   Perioperative Concerns with Sickle Cell Disease

Anemia
Chronic pulmonary disease
Pulmonary hypertension
Cardiomegaly and heart failure
Renal failure
Extreme vulnerability to dehydration, hypothermia, hypoxia, and acidosis
Hemolytic transfusion reaction resulting from alloimmunization

Multiple problems, including anemia, underlying cardiopulmonary disease, and extreme vulnerability to dehydration, hypothermia, hypoxia, and acidosis place these patients at high perioperative risk. Preoperative management should include correction of anemia. In the past, controversy existed regarding whether these patients should receive a preoperative exchange transfusion with Hb A. Recent data, however, suggest that preoperative transfusion to an Hb level of 10 g/dL, independent of the Hb S percentage, is equally effective in preventing perioperative complications as transfusion designed to establish a level of 10 g/dL *and* an Hb S level below 30%.[34] Controversy also surrounds the issue of the relative risks of transfusion for simple, brief operative procedures in patients who are minimally symptomatic and considered at low risk for intraoperative vaso-occlusive crises. Clearly, all blood transfusion in this setting carries a high risk of hemolytic transfusion reaction owing to alloimmunization from previous exposure.

In terms of intraoperative management, it is important to appreciate that no difference in morbidity or mortality has been shown among assorted anesthetic agents or between regional and general anesthetic techniques.[35] Factors that precipitate sickle crises, such as dehydration, hypoxia, acidosis, infection, hypothermia, and circulatory stasis, should be meticulously prevented. Intraoperative normothermia should be maintained with fluid warmers, breathing circuit humidification, warming blankets, forced-air warmers, and a well-heated operating room. Adequate perioperative volume replacement is critical; aggressive hydration with crystalloid or colloid is indicated except in the presence of congestive heart failure. Supplemental oxygen and mild hyperventilation are desirable to prevent hypoxemia and acidosis. Although pulse oximetry may be valid with Hb S, it is extremely unreliable in the presence of deoxygenated, polymerized Hb S because aggregation of sickled cells interferes with the light-emitting diode. After surgery, oxygen therapy, liberal hydration, and maintenance of normothermia should be continued for a minimum of 24 hours, because crises may occur suddenly postoperatively. Additionally, adequate analgesia, early ambulation, and pulmonary toilet, including incentive spirometry, are important in preventing serious complications. Postoperative pneumonia in this setting can be fatal.

Acquired Immunodeficiency Syndrome

Patients with acquired immunodeficiency syndrome (AIDS) frequently develop cytomegalovirus retinitis,[36] a condition treated by the insertion of a slow-release antiviral drug packet into the vitreous. Occasionally, the retinitis will produce a retinal detachment that requires surgical correction.

Many patients with AIDS are extremely ill with cachexia, anemia, and residual respiratory insufficiency from previous episodes of *Pneumocystis carinii* pneumonia (Table 1-13). In addition to reduced pulmonary reserve, these patients often have limited myocardial reserve as a consequence of the debilitating effects of their underlying disease. The greatest cause of perioperative morbidity and mortality, however, is infection.

A thorough preoperative assessment of the CD_4 (T-helper lymphocyte) cell count, organ function, and volume status is essential. It is mandatory to initiate or continue antibiotic and immune therapy, and organ function must be optimized. Severely debilitated patients may require invasive monitoring, depending to a great degree on the type of surgical procedure being performed, and strict attention must be paid to aseptic technique. Hypoglobulinemia is extremely common in AIDS patients and will reduce drug requirements. Therefore, anesthetic medications must be carefully selected and titrated. Moreover, supplemental oxygen should be provided to prevent perioperative episodes of desaturation. Additionally, these cachectic patients require special precautions to prevent pressure sores. Preemptive pain management may offer protection against additional immune suppression.[37]

It cannot be overemphasized that, because the greatest threat to these patients is infection, strict hygienic practices are critical. Moreover, medical personnel must protect themselves against the hazard of transmission of

TABLE 1–13   Perioperative Concerns with Acquired Immunodeficiency Syndrome

Anemia
Respiratory insufficiency
Reduced myocardial reserve
Vulnerability to infection and pressure sores
Altered drug requirements secondary to hypoglobulinemia
Transmission of HIV or other drug-resistant pathogens

human immunodeficiency virus (HIV) or of other drug-resistant pathogens by scrupulous adherence to universal precautions.

Retinopathy of Prematurity

Although Terry[38] first described the pathologic condition in 1942, the neologism *retrolental fibroplasia* was coined in 1944 by Harry Messenger, a Boston ophthalmologist who was also a Greek and Latin scholar.[39] More recently, however, the term *retinopathy of prematurity* (ROP) has gained widespread acceptance, because it describes the late cicatricial phase of the disease as well as the earlier acute changes.

ROP is usually associated with extremely low-birth-weight (1000-1500 g) preterm infants and "micropremies" (< 750 g) who require oxygen therapy. It is thought that hyperoxia triggers blood vessel constriction in the developing retina, causing areas of peripheral ischemia, poor vascularization, and neovascularization (proliferation of a network of abnormal retinal vessels), which produces fibrosis, scarring, and retinal detachment. Because advances in neonatology have led to 85% survival rates for extremely low-birth-weight infants, it is not surprising that the prevalence of ROP increased in recent decades. Moreover, the assumption that ROP is caused exclusively by excess oxygen in this population is incorrect, because ROP is a disease of multifactorial origin.[40-42] The factors associated with the development of ROP are highly interrelated, but Flynn established that low birth weight was the most significant predictor of risk.[43] Common problems of prematurity include respiratory distress syndrome (which is best managed with a combination of antenatal corticosteroids, postnatal surfactant therapy, and effective ventilation), apnea, bronchopulmonary dysplasia, persistent pulmonary hypertension, patent ductus arteriosus, necrotizing enterocolitis, gastroesophageal reflux, anemia, jaundice, hypoglycemia and hypocalcemia, intraventricular hemorrhage, and ROP (Table 1-14).

Postoperative apnea is the most common problem associated with anesthesia in premature infants.[44] Almost 20% of premature infants can be expected to develop this life-threatening complication, with the greatest risk for infants 50 weeks' postconceptual age (equal to gestational age plus chronologic age) and younger.[45] Apnea may result from prolonged effects of anesthetic agents, a shift of the carbon dioxide response curve, or fatigue of respiratory muscles.[46] Liu and colleagues[46] originally recommended continuous cardiopulmonary monitoring for patients younger than 46 weeks' postconceptual age. However, Kurth and colleagues[47] extended these recommendations to include cardiopulmonary monitoring for infants younger than 60 weeks' postconceptual age for a minimum of 12 apnea-free hours after surgery. Although the incidence of postoperative apnea is inversely related to

TABLE 1–14   Common Problems with Prematurity
Apnea
Respiratory distress syndrome
Bronchopulmonary dysplasia
Patent ductus arteriosus
Persistent pulmonary hypertension
Necrotizing enterocolitis
Anemia
Gastroesophageal reflux
Jaundice
Hypoglycemia/hypocalcemia
Intraventricular hemorrhage
Retinopathy of prematurity

postconceptual age, even full-term infants may occasionally have postoperative apnea.[45] In addition to prematurity as a risk factor, infants with a history of anemia,[48] neonatal apnea spells, respiratory distress syndrome, or pulmonary disease have approximately twice the risk of developing postoperative apnea.

Chronic lung disease, also known as *bronchopulmonary dysplasia,* remains the primary long-term pulmonary complication among premature infants. It is associated with pulmonary hypertension, abnormalities of postnatal alveolarization, and neovascularization.[49] Infants with chronic lung disease have impaired growth[50] and may also have poor long-term cardiopulmonary function, an increased vulnerability to infection,[51] and a markedly increased risk of abnormal neurologic development.[52] An investigation from the University of Chicago, however, reported that administration of nitric oxide to premature infants with respiratory distress syndrome reduced the incidence of chronic lung disease and death.[53]

Bronchopulmonary dysplasia (BPD) is characterized by lack of a widely accepted definition, but many neonatologists define it as a condition requiring supplemental oxygen after 36 weeks' postmenstrual age.[54] Conditions associated with BPD include prematurity, persistent ductus arteriosus, and prolonged ventilation with high inspiratory pressures and oxygen concentrations. Affected patients have abnormalities in lung compliance and airway resistance that may persist for several years. They also have chronic hypercarbia and hypoxemia. Abnormal chest radiographic findings include hyperexpanded lungs, small radiolucent cysts, increased interstitial markings, and peribronchial cuffing. Treatment typically consists of bronchodilators to reduce airway resistance and diuretics to decrease pulmonary edema. Air trapping during assisted ventilation may be minimized by use of a prolonged expiratory time.

TABLE 1–15   Anesthetic Management of Premature Infants

Normothermia critical
Reduced anesthetic requirement
Maintain preductal O_2 saturation at 93% to 95%
Prolonged expiratory time often helpful
Extubate only when infant is vigorous and fully awake
Postoperative cardiopulmonary monitoring for ≥ 12 hours

When premature infants undergo anesthesia and surgery, they must be kept warm, because they defend their core temperature at considerable metabolic cost (Table 1-15). The brown fat cells begin to differentiate at 26 to 30 weeks' gestation and, hence, are absent as a substrate buffer in extremely premature infants.[55] Additionally, infants have a greater surface area per volume compared with adults and will, therefore, tend to lose body heat rapidly in a cold environment. Metabolic acidosis is produced by cold stress. The acidosis causes myocardial depression and hypoxia, which in turn further exacerbates the metabolic acidosis. Warming the operating room (85°F [30°C]) and using warming units may help maintain the infant's body temperature. Warming intravenous and irrigation fluids may also be beneficial. Standard monitoring equipment includes an electrocardiograph, stethoscope, blood pressure monitor, temperature probe, pulse oximeter, and capnograph. A pulse oximeter probe placed in a preductal position on the right hand to reflect the degree of oxygenation in blood flowing to the retina can be compared with one located in a postductal position on the left foot to determine the severity of ductal shunting. Although pulse oximetry findings can be used to diagnose hypoxemia, hyperoxia cannot be detected by pulse oximetry. Maintaining the oxygen saturation at 93% to 95% (preductal) places most premature infants on the steep portion of the oxyhemoglobin dissociation curve and avoids severe hyperoxia.[56] It is important to appreciate that the reported levels of expired carbon dioxide may not accurately reflect $PaCO_2$ if the infant has congenital heart disease or major intrapulmonary shunting. In infants, changes in blood pressure, heart rate, and the intensity of heart sounds are helpful indicators of cardiac function, intravascular volume status, and depth of anesthesia. Hepatic and renal function in premature infants is immature and suboptimal, and their anesthetic requirement is considerably less than that of more mature and more robust infants.

The combination of ventilatory depression from residual anesthetic drugs with immature development of respiratory control centers can cause postoperative hypoventilation and hypoxia as well as apnea. Therefore, these infants must be wide awake and vigorously responsive before they are extubated. When indicated by clinical circumstances,

they should be carefully monitored postoperatively for at least 12 hours for signs of apnea, hypoxia, or bradycardia. The margin of safety for premature infants is narrow. They have minimal pulmonary reserve and rapidly become hypoxic.

Incontinentia Pigmenti

Bloch-Sulzberger syndrome, also known as incontinentia pigmenti, is a rare hereditary disease with dermatologic, neurologic, ocular, dental, and skeletal manifestations (Table 1-16). Inherited via either an autosomal dominant gene or by a sex-linked dominant gene, the condition is observed predominantly in females because it is usually lethal in males.

Skin involvement is typically noted at birth. The dermatopathology begins with inflammatory linear vesicles or bullae that progress to verrucous papillomata and eventually to splashes of pigmentation. By adulthood, however, the aforementioned lesions are replaced by atrophic hypopigmented lesions. Patients are retarded, and spastic paralysis,[57] seizures,[58] microcephaly, hydrocephalus, and cortical atrophy have been reported.

Individuals with incontinentia pigmenti are often blind. In addition to cataracts and strabismus, they may be afflicted with such serious ocular problems as retinitis proliferans and other types of retinopathy,[59-61] chorioretinitis, uveitis, optic nerve atrophy, foveal hypoplasia,[62] and retinal tears or detachments.

Partial anodontia and pegged or conical teeth are characteristic of the condition. Assorted skeletal anomalies are sometimes present.

The major anesthetic concerns involve the teeth and the central nervous system abnormalities. Owing to the dental pathology, airway manipulation must be performed with care. Succinylcholine should be avoided in patients with spastic paralysis, and patients with a high level of spinal cord involvement might theoretically develop autonomic hyperreflexia. No particular anesthetic technique has been recommended for these patients.

Retinitis Pigmentosa

Retinitis pigmentosa consists of a group of diseases, frequently hereditary, marked by progressive loss of retinal

TABLE 1–16   Anesthetic Management of Incontinentia Pigmenti

Control seizures
Careful airway manipulation owing to pegged teeth
Avoid succinylcholine in patients with spastic paralysis
Autonomic hyperreflexia possible with high spinal cord involvement

response, as elicited by electroretinography (ERG). The diseases are characterized by retinal atrophy, attenuation of the retinal vessels, clumping of pigment, and contraction of the field of vision. Retinitis pigmentosa may be transmitted as a dominant, recessive, or X-linked trait and is sometimes associated with other genetic defects.

ERG is a stimulated reflex response study to evaluate a patient for retinitis pigmentosa. The test measures the electrical response of the retina to light stimulation. ERG evaluates the retina and, therefore, should not be equated with visual evoked potential testing, which assesses polysynaptic cortical activity. When ERG is performed in young children, the ophthalmologist may request general anesthesia to enable performance of the test. Although retinitis pigmentosa, absent other genetic abnormalities, does not present any anesthetic challenges related to the patient's medical condition, nonetheless the conditions of the test are unusual and worthy of mention. Similarly, the selection of anesthetic agent is interesting.

ERG is performed in a dark, Faraday cage room with a flashing light source placed over the patient's face. The anesthesiologist frequently must work in cramped quarters, without the usual accoutrements of the operating room, including adequate lighting and a wide range of readily accessible emergency equipment. Additionally, the young patient's face is partially obscured by rather bulky ophthalmologic equipment, and access to the child's airway is less than ideal.

Anesthesia equipment must include a suction apparatus and an immediately available light source. Monitoring should incorporate an electrocardiograph, a pulse oximeter, and an end-tidal carbon dioxide monitor. The airway should be secured with either an endotracheal tube or a laryngeal mask airway.

The choice of anesthetic agents is somewhat traditional rather than truly evidence based. Although ERG is a simple rod-cone reflex response study, anesthetic agents may affect both the amplitude and latency of the ERG responses, thereby distorting the interpretation. Although ketamine is known to cause nystagmus and enhanced electroencephalographic activity, the agent purportedly does not modify ERG responses significantly in rabbits.[63] Indeed, there is a dearth of information available about the effects of anesthetic agents on ERG testing in humans. However, we do know that, in pigs, propofol appears to preserve the photoreceptor response better than thiopental.[64] Furthermore, in dogs, halothane and sevoflurane strongly depress the scotopic threshold response while moderately depressing the b wave and increasing oscillatory potential amplitudes.[65] In rats, photoreceptor and postreceptoral responses recorded under the barbiturate pentobarbital (Nembutal) and the dissociative agent zolazepam (Telazol) differ significantly.[66] Therefore, almost by default, ketamine appears to be the agent of choice for ERG testing in children.

By way of contrast, a brief discussion of visual evoked potentials (VEPs) is indicated. The visual pathway includes the retina, optic nerve, optic chiasm, optic tracts, lateral geniculate nucleus in the thalamus, optic radiation, and occipital visual cortex. Retinal stimulation produces an evoked electrical response in the occipital cortex, which may be altered with impairment of the visual apparatus and associated neural pathways. VEPs are recorded from scalp electrodes positioned over the occipital, parietal, and central areas. They are cortical near-field potentials with long latencies.[67] We have considerably more information about the effects of anesthetic agents on VEPs in humans compared with our meager knowledge in this domain when ERG testing is involved. For example, generally all volatile anesthetics dramatically prolong VEP latency and decrease amplitude in a dose-dependent fashion.[68,69] With intravenous agents, induction doses of thiopental decrease the amplitude and prolong the latency of VEP waves[70] whereas etomidate produces a small increase in latency with no alteration in amplitude.[71] Ketamine has negligible effect on latency but produces a 60% reduction in amplitude.[72] To date, the available data indicate that opioid and ketamine or propofol-based anesthetic techniques, as well as regimens using low-dose volatile anesthetics without nitrous oxide, allow satisfactory intraoperative recordings of VEPs, with the caveat that there may be a high incidence of false-positive or false-negative results.[73]

In summary, because they represent polysynaptic cortical activity, VEPs are exquisitely sensitive to the effects of anesthetic agents and physiologic factors. They are, furthermore, extremely dependent on appropriate stimulation of the retina and may be adversely affected by narcotic-induced pupillary constriction.[74] In contrast, subcortical potentials such as ERG responses, are probably less sensitive to anesthetic effects.

Eye Trauma

Eye trauma may be either penetrating or blunt. Special anesthetic considerations apply in the setting of a penetrating eye injury. Open-eye injuries requiring surgical repair vary in severity from a small corneal leak to a totally disrupted globe with damage to the sclera, cornea, iris, and lens, accompanied by loss of vitreous, choroidal vessel hemorrhage, and retinal detachment. Frequently it is difficult to determine the extent of the injury until after the patient has been anesthetized. However, retrobulbar or peribulbar blocks are not recommended in cases of open globes or extensive ocular trauma in which there is a risk of further disrupting the eye.

It is important to appreciate that any additional damage to the eye that transpires after the initial trauma is not necessarily the result of anesthetic drugs and manipulations. In many instances, for example, the patient may have been crying, coughing, vomiting, rubbing the eye, or squeezing the eyelids closed before anesthesia is induced.[75] These maneuvers are known to increase IOP dramatically. Even a normal blink increases IOP by 10 to 15 mm Hg; forced eyelid closure causes an increase in IOP of more than 70 mm Hg, an effect that may be ameliorated by performing a lid block to prevent lid spasm using the O'Brien technique. Increased IOP also results from other forms of external pressure, such as face mask application and from obstructed breathing or Valsalva maneuvers. Additionally, IOP is increased by succinylcholine and endotracheal intubation, especially if laryngoscopy is difficult or prolonged.

Ideal anesthesia for an eye trauma patient with a full stomach requires preoxygenation via a gently applied face mask followed by a rapid-sequence induction with cricoid pressure and a smooth, gentle laryngoscopy and intubation to ensure a stable IOP (Table 1-17). Experts disagree, however, on the best way to accomplish these goals, particularly the issue of selection of a muscle relaxant to secure the airway in the safest fashion without causing either extrusion of intraocular contents or pulmonary aspiration of gastric contents.

Nondepolarizing neuromuscular blocking agents relax the extraocular muscles and reduce IOP. In general, however, at least 3 minutes must pass before the usual doses of nondepolarizing drugs given in the traditional fashion provide adequate paralysis for endotracheal intubation. During this interval, the unconscious patient's airway is unprotected by a cuffed endotracheal tube and aspiration could occur. Additionally, if paralysis is incomplete, the patient may cough or "buck" on the endotracheal tube, causing an increase in IOP of 40 mm Hg. In contrast, the depolarizing drug succinylcholine provides an opportunity for swift intubation, airway protection, and consistently excellent intubating conditions within 60 seconds. Succinylcholine is rapidly cleared, permitting the patient to return to spontaneous respiration,

which is important if the patient has a difficult airway. Succinylcholine, however, increases IOP by approximately 8 mm Hg. This relatively small increase occurs 1 to 4 minutes after intravenous administration of the drug, and within 7 minutes IOP values return to baseline. Factors contributing to the ocular hypertensive effect of succinylcholine are incompletely understood.

A variety of interventions—including pretreatment with acetazolamide, propranolol, lidocaine,[76] narcotics,[77] clonidine,[78] and nondepolarizing relaxants—have been advocated to prevent succinylcholine-induced increases in IOP. None of these interventions, however, consistently and completely blocks the ocular hypertensive response.[79,80] Therefore, the use of succinylcholine in cases of open globes had traditionally been considered controversial, although this philosophy was based perhaps more on anecdote and "zero tolerance" for a *potential* anesthesia-related complication than on incontrovertible scientific evidence.[81]

If the anesthesiologist elects to use a nondepolarizing agent instead of succinylcholine, the administration of high-dose (400 µg/kg) vecuronium[82] or enlisting the "priming" technique[83] may accelerate the onset of available nondepolarizing muscle relaxants. With priming, approximately one tenth of an intubating dose of muscle relaxant is followed 4 minutes later by an intubating dose. After an additional 90 seconds, intubation may be accomplished. However, the use of large doses of nondepolarizing agents and the priming technique have serious disadvantages, including the risk of aspiration during the interval when the airway is unsecured and the unpredictable onset of sufficient paralysis to permit intubation without coughing. If high doses of such agents as atracurium or mivacurium are used, histamine release can cause untoward side effects, including hemodynamic instability. Large doses (1.2 mg/kg) of rocuronium do not consistently afford conditions for intubation that are as excellent as those provided by succinylcholine. Rapacuronium, the nondepolarizing agent with a rapid onset, showed promise in this setting, but the occurrence of intractable bronchospasm reported after its administration resulted in its removal from markets in the United States.

An acceptable option, unless contraindicated by such conditions as hyperkalemia or a susceptibility to malignant hyperthermia, is to administer succinylcholine after pretreatment with a defasciculating dose of a nondepolarizing relaxant and, if necessary, an appropriate drug to prevent significant increases in blood pressure associated with laryngoscopy. Cases appear in the literature attesting to the apparent safety of using succinylcholine in the open eye/full stomach setting.[84,85]

After intubation is safely and smoothly accomplished, the depth of anesthesia and the extent of muscle relaxation must be adequate to ensure lack of movement and to prevent coughing while the eye is open. This is best

TABLE 1–17 Anesthetic Management of the Open Eye–Full Stomach Situation

Avoid coughing, vomiting, and direct eye pressure.
Ensure adequate anesthetic depth before attempting laryngoscopy.
Administer appropriate adjuvants and neuromuscular blocker before laryngoscopy.
Perform gentle and brief laryngoscopy.
Maintain and monitor intraoperative paralysis.
Maintain stable venous and arterial pressures.
Prevent periextubation bucking and coughing.
Extubate only when patient is fully awake.

determined and followed by assessing the effects of peripheral nerve stimulation with a twitch monitor. Moreover, blood pressure should be carefully maintained within an acceptable range, because choroidal hemorrhage is more likely in open-eye situations when hypertension and increased venous pressure are also present. Prophylactic administration of an antiemetic is recommended to prevent postoperative vomiting. When surgery has been completed and spontaneous respiration has returned and the patient is awake with intact reflexes to prevent aspiration, the endotracheal tube is removed. Intravenous lidocaine (1.5 mg/kg) and a small dose of narcotic may be given before extubation to attenuate periextubation bucking and coughing.

EAR, NOSE, AND THROAT CONSIDERATIONS

Difficulty in managing the airway is a major cause of anesthesia-related morbidity and mortality and when the proposed surgical procedure involves the airway, consummate skill in airway management is required. This is true for a variety of reasons, not the least of which is that the airway may be compromised preoperatively by edema, infection, tumor, or trauma. Moreover, the anesthesiologist and the surgeon often must share the airway in these scenarios. Therefore, effective communication between the anesthesiologist and the surgeon is critical to effect optimal patient outcome.

Sleep Apnea

Sleep patterns disturbed by snoring are thought to occur in approximately 25% of the population.[86] However, most patients who snore do not have apnea or associated episodes of significant hypoxemia. Nonetheless, obstructive sleep apnea (OSA) is a relatively common disorder among middle-aged adults, especially (obese) Americans. Obesity is a critical independent causative/risk factor. The majority of people who have OSA are obese, and the severity of the condition seems to correlate with the patient's neck circumference.[87] In the minority of OSA patients who are nonobese, causative risk factors are craniofacial and orofacial bony abnormalities, nasal obstruction, and hypertrophied tonsils. Young and colleagues[87] reported that the prevalence of OSA associated with hypersomnolence was 2% in women and 4% in men aged 30 to 60 years.

OSA is defined as cessation of air flow for more than 10 seconds despite continuing ventilatory effort, five or more times per hour of sleep, and is usually associated with a decrease in arterial oxygen saturation of more than 4%. Although this review will focus predominantly on OSA, it should be noted for the sake of completeness that the three types of sleep apnea are obstructive, central, and mixed. Central sleep apnea, much rarer than OSA, is also

known as Ondine's curse, an allusion to the mythologic man who was condemned by his rejected lover, a mermaid, to stay awake in order to breathe. Unlike OSA, respiratory efforts temporarily stop in central sleep apnea. Diagnosis is established during polysomnography.

It is generally accepted that many patients with OSA have resultant pathologic daytime sleepiness associated with performance decrements. It has also been well established that patients with *severe* apnea suffer major health consequences as a result of their condition. Yet, it remains somewhat controversial whether patients with less severe forms of this disease incur the same detrimental consequences, owing to methodologic problems and failure to control for confounding factors in many of the relevant investigations. Clearly, the study design with the greatest methodologic rigor for the identification of long-term health consequences of OSA is the prospective, population-based, cohort study.[88] Most clinical research in OSA, however, has used less rigorous research designs, such as case-control, cross-sectional, or case studies that are more susceptible to problems of bias and less able to establish causality between adverse health consequences and OSA. Thus, few absolute conclusions can be drawn at this time about the long-term consequences of *mild to moderate* OSA. However, recently published findings from the Sleep Heart Health Study,[89] the Copenhagen City Heart Study,[90] and others[91] demonstrate a firm association between sleep apnea and systemic hypertension, even after other important patient characteristics, such as age, gender, race, consumption of alcohol, and use of tobacco products are controlled for.

Few definitive data exist to guide perioperative management of patients with OSA (Table 1-18). It is not surprising that many anesthesiologists question whether OSA patients are appropriate candidates for ambulatory surgery. The risks of caring for these challenging patients in the ambulatory venue are further amplified by the unfortunate fact that 80% to 95% of people with OSA are

TABLE 1–18   Anesthetic Management of Patients with Sleep Apnea

Have high index of suspicion with obesity.
Identify and quantify comorbid disease(s).
Perform meticulous airway assessment.
Have low threshold for awake intubation.
Administer sedative-hypnotics and narcotics sparingly.
Use short-acting anesthetic drugs.
Administer multimodal analgesics.
Extubate only when patient is fully awake.
Be able to administer continuous positive airway pressure.
Admit to telemetry ward when indicated.

undiagnosed[92]; they have neither a presumptive clinical and/or a sleep study diagnosis of OSA. This is of concern because these patients may suffer perioperatively from life-threatening desaturation and postoperative airway obstruction. Moreover, serious comorbidities may be present because prolonged apnea results in hypoxemia and hypercarbia, which can lead to increased systemic and pulmonary artery pressures and dysrhythmias. Cor pulmonale, polycythemia, and congestive heart failure may develop.

Sleep apnea occurs when the negative airway pressure that develops during inspiration is greater than the muscular distending pressure, thereby causing airway collapse. Obstruction can occur throughout the upper airway, above, below, or at the level of the uvula.[93,94] Because there is an inverse relationship between obesity and pharyngeal area, the smaller size of the upper airway in the obese patient causes a more negative pressure to develop for the same inspiratory flow.[94,95] Kuna and Sant'Ambrogio have also postulated that there may be a neurologic basis for the disease in that the neural drive to the airway dilator muscles is insufficient or not coordinated appropriately with the drive to the diaphragm.[94] Obstruction can occur during any sleep state but is often noted during rapid eye movement (REM) sleep. Nasal continuous positive airway pressure (CPAP) can ameliorate the situation by keeping the pressure in the upper airway positive, thus acting as a "splint" to maintain airway patency.

The site(s) of obstruction can be determined preoperatively by such techniques as magnetic resonance imaging (MRI), CT, and intraluminal pressure measurements during sleep.[96] Some studies suggest that the major site of obstruction in most patients is at the oropharynx, but obstruction can also occur at the nasopharynx, the hypopharynx, and the epiglottis.[97] Obviously, if the surgery is designed to relieve obstruction at one area but a pathologic process extends to other sites,[98] postoperative obstruction is not only possible but probable, especially when one allows for the edema associated with airway instrumentation.

CPAP devices, at least in the recent past, were often not well tolerated by patients. However, many technologic advances have been made with positive airway pressure devices, making these gadgets more easily tolerated. Additionally, weight loss may improve OSA. Recently, atrial overdrive pacing has shown promising results in patients with central or OSA.[99] Interestingly, French investigators serendipitously observed that some patients who had received a pacemaker with atrial overdrive pacing to reduce the incidence of atrial dysrhythmias reported a reduction in breathing disorders after pacemaker implantation. These cardiologists, therefore, initiated a study to investigate the efficacy of atrial overdrive pacing in the treatment of sleep apnea symptoms in consecutive

patients who required a pacemaker for conventional indications. They found that atrial pacing at a rate 15 beats per minute faster than the mean nocturnal heart rate resulted in a significant reduction in the number of episodes of both central and obstructive apnea.[99] Postulating that enhanced vagal tone may be associated with (central) sleep apnea, the investigators acknowledged, however, that the mechanism of the amelioration of OSA by atrial overdrive pacing is unclear. Moreover, whether these unexpected findings are germane to the sleep apnea patient with normal cardiac function is uncertain. Gottlieb[100] has tantalizingly suggested that a central mechanism affecting both respiratory rhythm and pharyngeal motor neuron activity would offer the most plausible explanation for the reported equivalence in the improvement of central and OSA during atrial overdrive pacing. Do cardiac vagal afferents also inhibit respiration? Perhaps identification of specific neural pathways might also advance efforts to develop pharmacologic treatment for sleep apnea.

A variety of surgical approaches to treating sleep-related airway obstruction are available. They include classic procedures, such as tonsillectomy, that directly enlarge the upper airway, as well as more specialized procedures to accomplish the same objective. Examples of the latter include uvulopalatopharyngoplasty (UPPP), uvulopalatal flap (UPF), uvulopalatopharyngoglossoplasty (UPPGP), laser midline glossectomy (LMG), lingualplasty (LP), inferior sagittal mandibular osteotomy and genioglossal advancement (MOGA), hyoid myotomy (HM) and suspension, and maxillomandibular osteotomy and advancement (MMO). Another approach is to bypass the pharyngeal part of the airway with a tracheotomy.

Although physicians and surgeons have been treating OSA for more than 25 years, a paucity of long-term, standardized results about the efficacy of different therapies are available. One report, however, suggests that at least 50% of patients with sleep apnea syndrome can be managed effectively with one or a combination of therapies. Nasal CPAP, tracheotomy, MMO, and tonsillectomy typically receive high marks for efficacy,[101] and a recent study of UPPP showed positive results that were maintained for a minimum of 1 year.[102] Another study, combining UPPP with genioglossus and hyoid advancement, reported encouraging results in patients with mild and moderate OSA and multilevel obstruction.[103] However, concern about the long-term results of laser-assisted uvulopalatoplasty (LAUP) for the management of OSA was recently voiced.[104] The response has been characterized as varied and unpredictable. It appears that the favorable subjective short-term results of LAUP deteriorated in time. Postoperative polysomnography revealed that LAUP might lead to deterioration of existing apnea. These findings are probably related to velopharyngeal narrowing and progressive palatal fibrosis inflicted by the laser beam.

There is serious and thoughtful ongoing debate about whether OSA patients should undergo surgery as outpatients. Clearly, there is no one-size-fits-all solution.[92] In deciding a management strategy it is important to consider the patient's body mass index and neck circumference, the severity of the OSA, the presence or absence of associated cardiopulmonary disease, the nature of the surgery, and the anticipated postoperative opioid requirement. It seems reasonable to expect that OSA patients without multiple risk factors who are having relatively noninvasive procedures (e.g., carpal tunnel repair, breast biopsy, knee arthroscopy) typically associated with minimal postoperative pain may be candidates for ambulatory status. However, those individuals with multiple risk factors, or those OSA patients having airway surgery, most probably will benefit from a more conservative approach that includes postoperative admission and careful monitoring. It is imperative to appreciate that these patients are exquisitely sensitive to the respiratory depressant effects of opioids. Additionally, the risk of prolonged apnea is increased for as long as 1 week postoperatively.

Is perioperative risk related to the type of anesthesia (general, regional, or monitored anesthesia care) administered? The limited evidence suggests that the type of surgery probably supersedes in importance the selection of anesthetic technique. Certainly, the use of regional anesthesia may not necessarily obviate the need for securing the airway and may even require emergency airway intervention if excessive amounts of sedative-hypnotics or opioids are administered. Regardless of the type of anesthesia selected, sedation should be administered judiciously. Moreover, it is important to be aware that the American Sleep Apnea Association[105] notes that "It may be fitting to monitor sleep apnea patients for several hours after the last doses of anesthesia, longer than non–sleep apnea patients require and possibly through one full natural sleep period."

When confronted with an especially challenging OSA patient requiring general anesthesia, a judicious approach may include awake fiberoptic intubation, administering very low-dose, short-acting narcotics, short-acting muscle relaxants, and a low solubility inhalational agent, and infiltrating the surgical site with a long-acting local anesthetic. Extubation should be performed only when the patient is without residual neuromuscular blockade and fully awake, using a tube changer or catheter, and CPAP should be available postoperatively. These high-risk patients should then be admitted to a telemetry ward or intensive care unit because the challenge of maintaining the airway will extend well into the postoperative period. Respiratory events after surgery in OSA patients may occur at any time.

Anesthetic care of the OSA patient is especially challenging, and few definitive data are available to guide perioperative management. The anesthesiologist should begin by having a high index of suspicion for the diagnosis and then seek to identify and quantify associated comorbidities. The major focus of the anesthesiologist of necessity must be on establishing and maintaining the airway, a challenge that will extend well into the postoperative period, especially if the patient is having surgery involving the oropharyngeal or hypopharyngeal area. Depending on the type of surgery, the anticipated amount of narcotic required postoperatively to manage pain, and the patient's condition, outpatient surgery may not be prudent. The roles that effective communication, monitoring, vigilance, judgment, and contingency planning play cannot be overemphasized.

Recurrent Respiratory Papillomatosis

Recurrent respiratory papillomatosis (RRP) is a disease of viral origin that is caused by human papillomavirus types 6 and 11 (HPV 6 and HPV 11) and is associated with exophytic lesions of the airway that are friable and bleed easily. Although it is a benign disease, RRP has potentially devastating consequences because of its involvement of the airway, the unpredictable clinical course associated with the condition, and the risk of malignant conversion in chronic invasive papillomatosis.

RRP is both the most common benign neoplasm of the larynx among children and the second most frequent cause of childhood hoarseness.[106] The disease is frustrating and often resistant to treatment owing to its tendency to recur and spread throughout the respiratory tract. Although RRP most frequently affects the larynx, the condition can actually involve the entire aerodigestive tract.

The course of the disease is highly variable; some patients undergo spontaneous remission and others experience aggressive papillomatous growth, necessitating multiple surgical procedures over many years. The differential diagnosis of the persistent or progressive stridor and dysphonia associated with RRP in infants includes laryngomalacia, subglottic stenosis, vocal cord paralysis, or a vascular ring (Table 1-19).

In most pediatric series, RRP is typically diagnosed between 2 and 4 years of age, with a delay in correct diagnosis from the time of onset of symptoms averaging about 1 year.[107] The incidence among children in the

TABLE 1–19   Differential Diagnosis of Infantile Progressive Stridor/Dysphonia

Laryngomalacia
Recurrent respiratory papillomatosis
Subglottic stenosis
Vocal cord paralysis
Vascular ring

United States is estimated at 4.3 per 100,000 children, translating into more than 15,000 surgical interventions at a total cost exceeding $100 million annually.[108]

Two distinct forms of RRP are recognized: a juvenile or aggressive form and an adult or less-aggressive form. Adult-onset RRP may reflect either activation of virus present from birth or an infection acquired in adolescence or adulthood. The most common types of human papillomavirus (HPV) identified in the airway are HPV 6 and HPV 11, the same types that cause genital warts. Specific viral subtypes may be correlated with disease severity and clinical course. Children infected with HPV 11, for example, appear to develop greater degrees of airway obstruction at younger ages and have a higher incidence of tracheotomy.[109]

Numerous studies have convincingly linked childhood-onset RRP to mothers with genital HPV infections. Nevertheless, few children exposed to genital warts at birth develop clinical symptoms.[110] Other factors must be operative, such as duration and volume of virus exposure, the behavior of the virus, the presence of local trauma, and patient immunity.

Presenting symptoms include a change in voice, ranging from hoarseness to stridor to aphonia. The stridor can be either inspiratory or biphasic. An associated history of chronic cough and frequent respiratory infections is not uncommon. Children are frequently misdiagnosed initially as having croup, chronic bronchitis, or asthma. Lesions usually are found in the larynx but may also occur on the epiglottis, pharynx, or trachea. The preoperative diagnosis is best made with an extremely small-diameter flexible fiberoptic nasopharyngoscope to more fully establish the extent of airway encroachment.

No single modality has consistently been shown to eradicate RRP. The primary treatment is surgical removal, with a goal of complete obliteration of papillomas and preservation of normal structures. However, in patients in whom anterior or posterior commissure disease or extremely virulent lesions are present, the objective may be revised to subtotal removal with clearing of the airway. It is advisable to "debulk" as much disease as possible, while preventing the complications of subglottic and glottic stenosis, web formation, and diminished airway patency. Whenever possible, tracheostomy is avoided to prevent seeding of papillomas into the distal trachea.

The CO_2 laser has been the favored instrument in the eradication of RRP involving the larynx, pharynx, upper trachea, and nasal and oral cavities. However, large, bulky accumulations of papillomas may require sharp dissection. Adjuvant treatments may include interferon alfa-N1,[111] indole-3-carbinol, acyclovir, ribavirin,[112] retinoic acid, and photodynamic therapy.[113] Clearly, the objective of all interventions is to remove as much disease as feasible without causing potentially scarring permanent damage to underlying mucosa in critical areas. Although the CO_2 laser is the most commonly used laser for laryngeal RRP, the KTP or argon laser could also be used. Papillomas that extend down the tracheobronchial tree often require the use of the KTP laser coupled to a ventilating bronchoscope for removal. Moreover, the recently developed endoscopic microdébrider is showing promise in terms of possibly causing less laryngeal scarring than the CO_2 laser.[114]

The anesthetic management of these patients is often extremely challenging and depends on the site of the lesions, the degree of airway obstruction, and the age of the patient[115] (Table 1-20). The issues are further complicated by the fact that a laser will be used and the anesthesiologist will be sharing the airway with the surgeon. Several approaches should be considered, and each is replete with advantages and disadvantages. A thoughtful risk-benefit analysis is essential. Teamwork and effective communication are critical to optimal outcome. Intraoperative teamwork is enhanced with the availability of video monitors that allow the entire operating room staff to view the surgery as it progresses. Dialogue between the anesthesiologist and the surgeon must continue throughout the procedure, focusing on the current ventilatory status, amount of bleeding, vocal cord motion, concentration of oxygen being administered, and timing of laser use in conjunction with respiration.

The available anesthetic options may be broadly separated into intubation and nonintubation techniques. When the lesions are assumed to be partially obstructing

TABLE 1–20   Anesthetic Options for Recurrent Respiratory Papillomatosis

Intubation Techniques	Nonintubation Techniques
Surgeon gowned and gloved before induction	Same pretreatment and precautions as with intubation
Preoperative dexamethasone	
Slow, gentle inhalation induction with continuous positive airway pressure	Insufflation of volatile agents with spontaneous ventilation
Intubate with smaller than usual, laser-safe endotracheal tube	Total intravenous anesthesia with spontaneous ventilation
Eye protection for patient and staff	Jet ventilation with muscle paralysis
$FiO_2 < 0.3$	
Awake extubation	

the airway, the best approach is a careful, gentle, smooth induction with sevoflurane or halothane, preferably with an intravenous line in place before induction is initiated. Preoperative dexamethasone, 0.5 mg/kg IV, is routinely given. The surgeon should be present in the operating room, and all the requisite equipment to deal with total airway obstruction should be immediately available. Often a jaw thrust combined with positive pressure in the anesthesia circuit will maintain airway patency. Should complete airway obstruction occur, the anesthesiologist may elect to give an appropriate dose of propofol, if indicated, and attempt intubation with a smaller than usual endotracheal tube. If this attempt fails, the surgeon should try using the rigid bronchoscope or, as a last resort, a transtracheal needle should be placed or tracheotomy performed. The anesthesiologist may then choose among several techniques.

If an intubated technique is elected, this approach has the advantage of allowing the anesthesiologist to maintain control of the airway and of ventilation. However, the endotracheal tube increases the risk of airway fire and may impede surgical exposure and access. The smallest possible laser-safe endotracheal tube should be used that permits adequate ventilation. If a cuffed tube is deemed necessary, the cuff should be filled with methylene blue–colorized saline to provide an additional warning if the cuff is perforated.[116] After the airway has been secured with a laser-safe endotracheal tube, the anesthesiologist has the option to administer muscle relaxants. The child's eyes are protected with moist, saline-soaked gauze eye pads placed over the lids. Additionally, all operating room personnel must wear safety glasses and special laser masks with extremely small pores to minimize exposure to the laser plume. The fraction of inspired oxygen (FIO_2) delivered to the patient should be as close to a room air mixture as possible (FIO_2 between 0.26 to 0.3). During resection the surgeon must exercise great care to avoid injuring the anterior commissure, and at least 1 mm of untreated mucosa should be left so that a web does not develop. If the surgeon detects disease in the posterior part of the glottis or in the subglottic region, the endotracheal tube obstructs exposure of these areas to the operative field and an alternative means of anesthesia is selected. Often the surgeon will prefer an apneic technique wherein the endotracheal tube is removed intermittently and surgery is performed while the patient's oxygen saturation is monitored. The endotracheal tube is periodically reinserted as needed. Typically, the lungs are reoxygenated for the same period of time that they were apneic before proceeding with the next "cycle."

Alternatively, a nonintubated technique using spontaneous ventilation with volatile anesthetic agents has been described by several authors.[117,118] The patient is induced in the aforementioned fashion, and maintenance of anesthesia is continued with sevoflurane or halothane that is insufflated into the oropharynx by attaching the fresh gas flow hose to a side port on the suspension laryngoscope. The larynx is anesthetized with topical lidocaine (not to exceed 4 to 5 mg/kg) before proceeding with further surgical intervention. This is not an ideal (or easy) anesthetic technique because the anesthesiologist must deftly balance the anesthetic depth somewhere between too light (triggering laryngospasm) and too deep (causing apnea). Additionally, the operating room environment becomes contaminated, but a vacuum hose is helpful in extracting exhaled gases and virus particles. Total intravenous anesthesia with an infusion of propofol and remifentanil is also appropriate with this nonintubated, spontaneous ventilation technique.[115] The surgeon, however, may complain of too much laryngeal movement with total intravenous anesthesia because patients anesthetized with these agents breathe slowly but very deeply.

Another anesthetic alternative is the use of jet ventilation. Jet ventilation eliminates the potential for an endotracheal tube fire and allows good visualization of the vocal cords and areas distal to them. However, the technique has the risk of barotrauma and may allow transmission of HPV particles into the distal airway. The jet cannula can be positioned either above or below the vocal cords; placement of the cannula proximal to the end of the laryngoscope decreases the risk of possible pneumothorax or pneumomediastinum. With large laryngeal lesions, narrowed airways, and ball-valve lesions, considerable outflow obstruction may develop, leading to increased intrathoracic pressure and pneumothorax. The anesthesiologist must carefully observe chest excursion and ensure that there is unimpeded exhalation. Muscle relaxants are administered to prevent vocal cord motion. Constant communication between anesthesiologist and surgeon about timing of ventilation in relation to surgical manipulation is required. Excessive mucosal drying and gastric distention are other disadvantages of this approach. At the end of the procedure, the trachea is intubated with a standard endotracheal tube.

The trachea is extubated only when the child is fully awake. High humidity and, occasionally, racemic epinephrine are administered postoperatively. The patient is closely monitored for several hours before discharge, and often an overnight stay is advisable, especially if the disease was extensive and the airway was significantly compromised. Continuous pulse oximetry is mandatory and postoperative steroid administration may be helpful.

The scientific community is aggressively working to improve our knowledge about RRP. A national registry of patients with RRP has been formed through the cooperation of the American Society of Pediatric Otolaryngology and the Centers for Disease Control and Prevention.[119] It is expected that this registry will identify patients who are suitable for enrollment in multi-institutional studies of adjuvant therapies and will more sharply define the risk factors for transmission of HPV and the cofactors that determine the virulence of RRP. No doubt future projects will include development of an HPV vaccine and refinements in surgical techniques to minimize laryngeal scarring.

Cystic Hygroma

Cystic hygroma is a rare, multilocular, benign lymphatic malformation, usually involving the deep fascia of the neck, oral cavity, and tongue, although the axilla may also be affected. This type of lymphangioma is capable of massive growth and can be quite disfiguring. Almost all known cases of cystic hygroma have presented by 5 years of age, with most being observed in the neonatal period.[120] In fact, there are cases described in the literature of antenatal diagnosis of cystic hygroma with fetal airway encroachment detected by screening ultrasound. The few infants who survived to delivery were intubated immediately after the head was delivered, with the placenta functioning as an extracorporeal source of oxygenation until the airway was secured.[121,122]

As the tumor grows, it often encroaches on surrounding structures such as the pharynx, tongue, or trachea. Dysphagia and various degrees of airway obstruction are not uncommon. These tumors are not responsive to radiation therapy, and multiple surgical resections are often necessary. Because the tumors are not encapsulated, they easily envelop and grow into surrounding structures, preventing complete excision. The ability of cystic hygromas to elude complete extirpation has led to a recrudescence of injection of sclerosing agents intralesionally as either primary or adjunctive therapy.[123] This approach had been abandoned, but the availability of newer, improved agents has led to better results.

Although sudden enlargement of the tumor can cause a true airway emergency, most commonly the children present for elective resection. Because of mechanical complications, the young child may be malnourished or dehydrated. He or she may also have sleep apnea. Stridor is an ominous sign, suggesting imminent airway decompensation. A chest radiograph should be reviewed for tracheal deviation or mediastinal extension. Although CT or MRI will provide more complete information about the full extent of the lesion, the sedation necessary to obtain such studies may cause airway obstruction—an example of "perfection being the enemy of good."

The patient is given an antisialagogue before anesthesia is administered to minimize secretions that might complicate anesthetic management (Table 1-21). The surgeon is present in the operating room, gowned and gloved, and ready to perform a tracheostomy if necessary. The anesthesiologist must carefully prepare a wide variety of difficult airway equipment in the event of an airway emergency. Clearly, the safest approach in these children is an awake

TABLE 1–21   Anesthetic Management of Cystic Hygroma
Evaluate preoperatively for stridor, tracheal deviation, or mediastinal extension.
Determine optimally tolerated position.
Administer preoperative antisialagogue.
Have surgeon gowned and gloved before induction/intubation.
Apply topical vasoconstrictor to nares.
Know that fiberoptic nasotracheal intubation is often necessary.
Perform extubation with caution.

intubation because a marginally adequate airway while the patient is awake may become totally obstructed during induction when the upper airway muscles relax and the tumor fills the airway. However, because many, if not most, pediatric patients will not tolerate an awake intubation, children with cystic hygroma often undergo a slow, meticulous, titrated inhalation induction of anesthesia with preservation of spontaneous ventilation and application of CPAP. When anesthetic depth is adequate, fiberoptic intubation is performed. Often a large, protruding tongue will make oral intubation impossible, so the nasal route is chosen after administration of an appropriate vasoconstrictor to the nostrils. (If an unsuccessful direct laryngoscopy or an attempt at blind nasal intubation is performed initially, these approaches may trigger bleeding that could hamper subsequent attempts at fiberoptic intubation.) When the surgery is completed, it is helpful to perform direct laryngoscopy because the view may have improved significantly after the resection.[115] This information will prove useful in the event that reintubation is required postoperatively.

If attempts at fiberoptic intubation are unsuccessful, other options include passing a retrograde wire after asking the surgeon to aspirate fluid from the mass (a request that the surgeon may decline to perform owing to concern about recurrence from an incompletely resected, ruptured sac), using a light wand or Bullard laryngoscope, attempting tactile intraoral tube placement, or trying a blind nasal intubation. In the event that these attempts fail and mask ventilation becomes inadequate, a laryngeal mask airway should be inserted. If this fails to open the airway, an emergency surgical airway should be attempted. In the event that the surgeon is unable to expose the trachea, the only remaining option to save the child may be the performance of femoral cardiopulmonary bypass.[115]

Wegener's Granulomatosis

Wegener's granulomatosis (WG) is a systemic disease of unknown etiology characterized by necrotizing granulomas and vasculitis that classically affects the upper and lower airway and the kidneys. Although the etiology remains unestablished, recent interest has focused on the possible role of *Staphylococcus aureus* in the pathophysiology of the disease.[124] WG can have a myriad of head and neck manifestations, including mucosal ulceration of the nose, palate, larynx, and orbit, as well as deafness and subglottic[125] or tracheal stenosis. Ocular disease occurs in 50% to 60% of adults with WG[126] and may include such conditions as necrotizing scleritis with peripheral keratopathy,[127] orbital pseudotumor,[126] and ocular myositis,[126] as well as uveitis, vitreous hemorrhage, and central retinal artery occlusion.[128]

Wegener's granulomatosis often starts with severe rhinorrhea, cough, hemoptysis, pleuritic pain, and deafness. However, it is a truly systemic disease and varies widely in presentation. Indeed, the protean manifestations of WG often produce diagnostic delay. Diagnosis is supported by histopathologic studies showing a vasculitis, parenchymal necrosis, and multinucleate giant cells, but tissue biopsy alone is insufficient to establish the diagnosis of WG. The most specific test is a positive antineutrophil cytoplasmic antibody test (c-ANCA).[129]

WG was once fatal. With the advent, however, of long-term treatment with corticosteroids and cyclophosphamide, affected individuals survive longer, and a broader spectrum of the disease has been observed in recent years. The incidence of subglottic stenosis in WG ranges from 8.5% to 23%.[130] It is a significant cause of morbidity and mortality and typically is unresponsive to systemic chemotherapy. Other treatments have included mechanical subglottic dilation (with or without intratracheal steroid injection) and laser therapy, with variable success. Recently, encouraging results in treating subglottic stenosis have been reported with endoscopic insertion of nitinol stents after dilation of the stenotic segment with bougie dilators.[125] Nitinol is a nickel and titanium alloy that has excellent properties, including biocompatibility, kink resistance, and elasticity, thus resembling the tracheobronchial tree. These metal stents are expandable, serving as an intraluminal support to establish and maintain airway patency. They are usually permanent but can be removed if necessary. For the intervention to be successful, however, the diseased segment must begin at least 1 cm below the vocal cords.

Patients with WG often present for ocular, nasal, or laryngeal surgery. The anesthesiologist must anticipate a host of potential problems (Table 1-22). These challenges include dealing with the side effects of chronic corticosteroid and cyclophosphamide therapy as well as the presence of underlying pulmonary and renal disease. Additionally, midline necrotizing granulomas of the airway may cause obstruction or bleeding at intubation. Some degree of subglottic or tracheal stenosis should also be expected. Chest radiography, CT, or MRI of the airway, arterial blood gas analysis, pulmonary function tests, and

TABLE 1–22 Anesthetic Concerns with Wegener's Granulomatosis
Side effects of steroids and cyclophosphamide
Bleeding induced by airway manipulation
Subglottic stenosis
Tracheal stenosis
Reduced pulmonary reserve
Impaired renal function

determinations of blood urea nitrogen and creatinine levels are helpful guides to optimal anesthetic management.

Acromegaly

Acromegaly is a rare chronic disease of midlife caused by excess secretion of adenohypophyseal growth hormone (GH). (Hypersecretion of GH before epiphyseal closure produces gigantism in younger individuals.) GH acts on a wide variety of tissues, both directly and through release of insulin-like growth factor I (IGF-I), which is released mainly from the liver in response to GH. In addition to stimulating bone and cartilage growth, GH and IGF-I promote protein synthesis and lipolysis while reducing insulin sensitivity and causing sodium retention. Therefore, it is not surprising that acromegaly is characterized by enlargement of the jaw, hands and feet, and soft tissues, as well as diabetes mellitus and hypertension. Severe, chronic hypertension may result in cardiomegaly, left ventricular dysfunction, congestive heart failure, and dysrhythmias. Airway soft tissue overgrowth may produce macroglossia with glossoptosis, vocal cord thickening with hoarseness, and subglottic narrowing. Vocal cord paralysis has also been reported occasionally. Approximately 25% of acromegalics have an enlarged thyroid, which may produce tracheal compression or deviation. Diagnosis is confirmed by elevated 24-hour GH levels in conjunction with increased serum IGF-I levels.

Most pituitary tumors originate in the anterior part of the gland and the overwhelming majority are benign adenomas. Proposed etiologic mechanisms include malfunction of normal growth-regulating genes, abnormal tumor suppressor genes, and changes in genes that control programmed cell death.[131] The prevalence of pituitary tumors is approximately 200 per million of the population,[132] but random autopsy results indicate an incidence as high as 27%,[133] suggesting that the majority of pituitary adenomas are asymptomatic. The most common type of pituitary adenoma causes hyperprolactinemia. Adenomas producing acromegaly and Cushing's disease are more unusual. The annual incidence of acromegaly, for example, is said to be three to eight cases per million.

The primary treatment of acromegaly is surgery, with or without subsequent radiotherapy. However, in the relatively few patients who respond to treatment with dopamine agonists, such as bromocriptine, surgery can be avoided. Somatostatin also inhibits GH release, and long-acting analogues of somatostatin, such as octreotide, may be tried in those who fail to respond to dopamine agonists.[134]

Acromegaly is widely recognized as one of many causes of difficult airway management[135,136] (Table 1-23). Careful preoperative airway assessment is therefore indicated, paying special attention to the possibility of sleep apnea by questioning the patient about any history of loud snoring, frequent nocturnal awakening, and daytime hypersomnolence. It is imperative to appreciate that the risk of death from respiratory failure is threefold greater in acromegaly.[137] Hypertension is common in acromegalics but usually responds to antihypertensive therapy. Myocardial hypertrophy and interstitial fibrosis are also common and may be associated with left ventricular dysfunction. Thus, indicated preoperative studies often include a chest radiograph, electrocardiogram, and echocardiogram, in addition to lateral neck radiographs and CT of the neck.

The pituitary fossa can be approached using the transsphenoidal, transethmoidal, or transcranial route. For all but the largest tumors, the transsphenoidal route is preferred, owing to a lower incidence of associated complications. Otolaryngologists often assist neurosurgeons in performing transsphenoidal hypophysectomy, gaining access to the pituitary fossa using a sublabial or endonasal approach. Hormone replacement, including 100 mg hydrocortisone, is administered intravenously at induction, and prophylactic antibiotics are given. An appropriate vasoconstrictor is applied to the nostrils,

and care must be taken to prevent hypertension or dysrhythmias. Large face masks and long-bladed laryngoscopes should be prepared, and a fiberoptic laryngoscope should be available. Depending on the airway assessment, an awake fiberoptic intubation may be the preferred approach to securing the airway. The intubating laryngeal mask airway has also been used successfully in patients with acromegaly. Equipment for tracheostomy should be immediately available if airway involvement is extensive.

After intubation, the mouth and pharynx should be packed before surgery commences to prevent intraoperative bleeding into the laryngeal area, which may cause postextubation laryngospasm, and into the stomach, which may trigger postoperative nausea and vomiting.

Some surgeons request that a lumbar drain be inserted in patients with major suprasellar tumor extension. The intention is to produce prolapse of the suprasellar part of the tumor into the operative field by injecting 10-mL aliquots of normal saline as needed. Additionally, if the dura is perforated intraoperatively, the lumbar catheter can be left in situ postoperatively to control any leakage of cerebrospinal fluid.[138]

Transsphenoidal surgery is conducted with the patient supine with a moderate degree of head-up tilt. Careful monitoring for venous air embolism is indicated if the head is elevated more than 15 degrees. Other monitoring should include direct arterial blood pressure, electrocardiography, oxygen saturation, and end-tidal carbon dioxide determination. Visual evoked potentials have limited usefulness because they are very sensitive to anesthetic effects. Any anesthetic approach that is compatible with the exigencies of intracranial surgery is acceptable. Regardless of whether an inhalation agent or total intravenous anesthesia is selected, short-acting agents are administered to allow rapid recovery at the end of surgery. Drugs such as propofol, sevoflurane, and remifentanil are excellent agents to accomplish this objective. At the completion of surgery, pharyngeal packs should be removed. When the patient is awake with reflexes intact, extubation should be conducted, taking care not to dislodge nasal packs or stents. Patients should be carefully observed postoperatively for airway patency. Those with sleep apnea should be carefully followed in a monitored unit, because treatment options such as nasal CPAP cannot be applied after transsphenoidal surgery. Narcotics should be administered with special caution to patients with sleep apnea. Hormone replacement with tapered cortisol therapy is critical postoperatively. In addition to anterior pituitary insufficiency, diabetes insipidus may also develop postoperatively, but most borderline cases resolve spontaneously in a few days as posterior lobe function recovers.[138] Other potential complications include cerebrospinal fluid rhinorrhea, meningitis, sinusitis, and cranial nerve palsy.

TABLE 1–23 Perioperative Concerns with Acromegaly

Difficult airway management; suspect sleep apnea

Subglottic narrowing

Tracheal compression or deviation associated with thyroid enlargement

Hypertension
  Cardiomegaly
  Dysrhythmias
  Left ventricular dysfunction
  Congestive heart failure

Diabetes mellitus

Venous air embolism

Postoperative anterior pituitary insufficiency and diabetes insipidus

Postoperative cerebrospinal fluid rhinorrhea, meningitis, sinusitis, and cranial nerve palsy

Ludwig's Angina

Ludwig's angina is a potentially lethal, rapidly expanding cellulitis of the floor of the mouth characterized by brawny induration of the upper neck, usually unaccompanied by obvious fluctuation. Spread of the infection along the deep cervical fascia can result in mediastinitis, mediastinal abscess, jugular vein thrombosis, innominate artery rupture, empyema, pneumothorax, pleural and/or pericardial effusion, subphrenic abscess, necrotizing fasciitis, and mandibular or cervical osteomyelitis. Although the inflammation is typically caused by cellulitis, there can also be a component of gangrenous myositis.[139]

Although one can find mention of the symptoms of this condition in writings dating back to Hippocrates, Ludwig's angina was best described initially in 1836 by its namesake, Karl Friedrich Wilhelm von Ludwig. He described this disease as a rapidly progressive gangrenous cellulitis originating in the region of the submandibular gland that extends by continuity rather than lymphatic spread. During the late 19th and early 20th centuries, Ludwig's angina was commonly considered a complication of administration of local anesthetics used to facilitate extraction of mandibular teeth.[140] It was not until later in the 20th century that the actual pathogenesis of the disease was elucidated. In 1943, Tschiassny[141] clarified the unique role that the floor of the mouth played in the development of the disease. He described how periapical dental abscesses of the second and third mandibular molars penetrate the thin inner cortex of the mandible. Because these roots extend inferior to the mandibular insertion of the mylohyoid muscle, infection of the submandibular space ensues. Owing to communication around the posterior margin of the mylohyoid muscle, rapid involvement of the sublingual space occurs, followed quickly by involvement of the contralateral spaces. The unyielding presence of the mandible, hyoid, and superficial layer of the deep cervical fascia limit tissue expansion as edema develops and progresses. This resistance leads to superior and posterior displacement of the floor of the mouth and the base of the tongue. These patients, therefore, have an open-mouth appearance, with a protruding or elevated tongue, and exhibit marked neck swelling. Soft tissue swelling in the suprahyoid region, combined with lingual displacement and the frequent concomitant of laryngeal edema, can occlude the airway and abruptly asphyxiate the patient.

Although the overwhelming preponderance of cases of Ludwig's angina have an odontogenic origin, other risks include sublingual lacerations, penetrating injuries to the floor of the mouth, sialadenitis, compound mandibular fractures, osteomyelitis of the mandible, otitis media, infected malignancy, and abscesses located under the thyrohyoid membrane.[142] Patients typically present with fever, as well as edema of the tongue, neck, and submandibular region. These symptoms can progress to include dysphagia, inability to handle secretions, dysphonia, trismus, and difficulty breathing. Polymicrobial infections are common. The usual offending organisms include streptococci, staphylococci, and *Bacteroides*.

In the preantibiotic era, Ludwig's angina was associated with mortality rates exceeding 50%. Originally, the extremely sudden manner of death was ascribed to overwhelming sepsis. It was not until the early 20th century that the lethal role of mechanical respiratory obstruction leading to asphyxia was understood.[143] Taffel and Harvey,[144] in 1942, succeeded in reducing mortality to less than 2% by emphasizing early diagnosis and advocating aggressive treatment with wide surgical decompression of the submandibular and sublingual spaces with the patient under local anesthesia. This intervention allowed the elevated base of the tongue to assume an anteroinferior position, thereby preserving the patency of the oropharyngeal airway.

With the increasing availability of antibiotics in the 1940s, a reduction in the incidence of and mortality from Ludwig's angina ensued. Today, aggressive antibiotic therapy in the early stages of the disease has led to a reduced need for surgical decompression and the need for airway intervention (Table 1-24). Patterson and colleagues,[145] for example, reported a series of 20 patients at their institution in whom only 35% required airway control in the form of either tracheotomy or endotracheal intubation. The anticipated need for airway control may differ among groups of patients, with patients who are older and have more comorbidity seeming to be at greater risk for airway obstruction.[146,147] Additionally, patients who are in poorer condition at the time of presentation may well be in danger of imminent airway closure. Clearly, stridor, difficulty managing secretions, anxiety, and cyanosis are late signs of impending obstruction and should serve as indicators of the need for immediate airway intervention.

Airway management may be extremely difficult. Often, preliminary tracheostomy using local anesthesia may be the safest option. Depending on the patient's condition, including the presence or absence of trismus and the ability of the patient to cooperate, other options

TABLE 1–24   Anesthetic Concerns with Ludwig's Angina

Early, aggressive antibiotic therapy may obviate need for airway intervention/surgical decompression.

Older, sicker patients purportedly at increased risk for airway obstruction.

Anticipate difficult airway management.
  Favor awake fiberoptic intubation with an armored tube or tracheostomy—under local anesthesia.

include an awake fiberoptic intubation, or an inhalation induction, preserving spontaneous respiration, followed by intubation with direct laryngoscopy or fiberoptic assistance. If the oropharynx cannot be visualized by CT, a fiberoptic nasotracheal approach is advised. Needless to say, a surgeon should be present and a tracheotomy kit immediately available when the nonsurgical route to establish the airway is selected. Owing to the potential for continued airway swelling after the endotracheal tube is placed, it seems prudent to insert an armored tube to better protect the airway.

CONCLUSION

There has been extraordinary progress in the treatment of many complex ophthalmic and otolaryngologic conditions during the past 25 years. These often complicated patients are presenting for many surgical and diagnostic procedures that did not exist a generation ago. It is essential, therefore, that the anesthesiologist appreciates that few of the conditions presented in this chapter have isolated ophthalmic or ENT pathology. Rather, they frequently are associated with multisystem diseases, and the anesthetic plan must reflect this sobering reality.

Typically, it is inappropriate to insist dogmatically that one anesthetic approach is unequivocally superior to all others in the management of any specific condition, especially the complex entities discussed here. The key to optimal anesthetic management and outcome resides in a comprehensive understanding of the disease process, the surgical requirements, and the effects of our anesthetic agents and techniques on both the individual patient and the proposed surgery.

References

1. McGoldrick KE: Ocular pathology and systemic diseases: Anesthetic implications. In McGoldrick KE (ed): Anesthesia for Ophthalmic and Otolaryngologic Surgery. Philadelphia, WB Saunders, 1992, pp 210-226.
2. Lee PP, Feldman ZW, Ostermann J, et al: Longitudinal prevalence of major eye diseases. Arch Ophthalmol 2003;121:1303-1310.
3. DiGeorge AM, Harley RD: The association of aniridia, Wilms' tumor, and genital abnormalities. Arch Ophthalmol 1966;75:796-798.
4. Petersen RA, Walton DS: Optic nerve hypoplasia with good visual acuity and visual field defects: A study of children of diabetic mothers. Arch Ophthalmol 1977;95:254-258.
5. Skarf B, Hoyt CS: Optic nerve hypoplasia in children: Association with anomalies of the endocrine and central nervous systems. Arch Ophthalmol 1984;102:62-67.
6. Costin G, Murphree AL: Hypothalamic-pituitary function in children with optic nerve hypoplasia. Am J Dis Child 1985;139:249-254.
7. Newlin AC, Sugar J: Corneal and external eye manifestations of systemic disease. In Yanoff M, Duker JS (eds): Ophthalmology, 2nd ed. St. Louis, Mosby, 2004, pp 527-534.
8. Yorston D: A perspective from a surgeon practicing in the developing world. Surv Ophthalmol 2000;45:51-52.
9. Muñoz B, West SK, Rubin GS, et al: Causes of blindness and visual impairment in a population of older Americans: The Salisbury Eye Evaluation study. Arch Ophthalmol 2000;118:819-825.
10. Solomon R, Donnenfeld ED: Recent advances and future frontiers in treating age-related cataracts. JAMA 2003;290:248-251.
11. Jick SS, Vasilakis-Scaramozza C, Maier WC: The risk of cataract among users of inhaled steroids. Epidemiology 2001;12:229-234.
12. Cumming RG, Mitchell P, Leeder SR: Use of inhaled corticosteroids and the risk of cataracts. N Engl J Med 1997;337:8-14.
13. Garbe E, Suissa S, LeLorier J: Association of inhaled corticosteroid use with cataract extraction in elderly patients. JAMA 1998;280:539-543.
14. Cumming RG, Mitchell P: Alcohol, smoking, and cataracts: The Blue Mountain Eye Study. Arch Ophthalmol 1997;115:1296-1303.
15. Richards W, Donnell GN, Wilson WA, et al: The oculocerebrorenal syndrome of Lowe. Am J Dis Child 1965;109:185-203.
16. Morris RC. Renal tubular acidosis: Mechanisms, classification, and implications. N Engl J Med 1969;281:1405.
17. Cotlier E: Congenital varicella cataract. Am J Ophthalmol 1978;86:627-629.
18. Pyeritz RE: The Marfan syndrome. Ann Rev Med 2000;51:481-510.
19. Steward DJ: Manual of Pediatric Anesthesia. New York, Churchill Livingstone, 1979, pp 246-247.
20. Roizen MF: Hyperthyroidism. In Roizen MF, Fleisher LA (eds): Essence of Anesthesia Practice, 2nd ed. Philadelphia, WB Saunders, 2002, p 186.
21. Greer MA: Antithyroid drugs in the treatment of thyrotoxicosis. Thyroid Today 1980;3:1-18.
22. Williams LT, Lefkowitz RJ, Watanabe AM, et al: Thyroid hormone regulation of beta-adrenergic number. J Biol Chem 1977;252:2787-2789.
23. Zonszein J, Santangelo RP, Mackin JF, et al: Propranolol therapy in thyrotoxicosis: A review of 84 patients undergoing surgery. Am J Med 1979;66:411-416.
24. Roizen MF: Anesthetic implications of concurrent diseases. In Miller RD (ed): Anesthesia, 4th ed. New York, Churchill Livingstone, 2000, pp 927-930.
25. Kaplan JA, Cooperman LH: Alarming reactions to ketamine in patients taking thyroid medication treated with propranolol. Anesthesiology 1971;35:229-230.
26. Jervis GA: Phenylpyruvic oligophrenia (phenylketonuria). Res Publ Assoc Res Nerv Ment Dis 1954;33:259.
27. Wyngaarden JB: Homocystinuria. In Beeson PB, McDermott W, Wyngaarden JB (eds): Cecil Textbook of Medicine, 15th ed. Philadelphia, WB Saunders, 1979, p 2028.
28. Brown BR Jr, Walson PD, Taussig LM: Congenital metabolic diseases in pediatric patients: Anesthetic implications. Anesthesiology 1975;43:197.
29. McDonald L, Bray C, Love F, et al: Homocystinuria, thrombosis, and the blood platelets. Lancet 1964;1:745.
30. Holmgren G, Falkmer S, Hambraeus L: Plasma insulin content and glucose tolerance in homocystinuria. Ups J Med Sci 1975;78:215.
31. McGoldrick KE: Anesthetic management of homocystinuria. Anesthesiol Rev 1981;8:42-45.
32. Dean J, Schechter A: Sickle cell anemia: Molecular and cellular basis of therapeutic approaches. N Engl J Med 1978;299:752.
33. Djaiani GN, Cheng DC, Carroll JA, et al: Fast track cardiac anesthesia in patients with sickle cell abnormalities. Anesth Analg 1999;89:598-603.
34. Vichinsky EP, Haberkern CM, Neumayr L, et al: A comparison of conservative and aggressive transfusion regimens in the perioperative management of sickle cell disease. N Engl J Med 1995;333:206-213.
35. McDade WA: Sickle cell disease. In Roizen MF, Fleisher LA (eds): Essence of Anesthesia Practice, 2nd ed. Philadelphia, WB Saunders, 2002, p 302.
36. Skolruk PR, Pomerantz RJ, de la Monte SM., et al: Dual infection of the retina with human immunodeficiency virus type I and cytomegalovirus. Am J Ophthalmol 1989;107:361.
37. Knight PR III: Immune suppression. In Roizen MF, Fleisher LA (eds): Essence of Anesthesia Practice, 2nd ed. Philadelphia, WB Saunders, 2002, p 193.

38. Terry TL: Extreme prematurity and fibroblastic overgrowth of persistent vascular sheath behind each crystalline lens: Preliminary report. Am J Ophthalmol 1942;25:203.

39. Silverman W: Retrolental Fibroplasia: A Modern Parable. New York, Grune & Stratton, 1980.

40. Kinsey VE, Arnold HJ, Kaline RE, et al: Pao₂ levels and retrolental fibroplasia: A report of the Cooperative Study. Pediatrics 1977;60:655.

41. Merritt JC, Sprague DH, Merritt WE: Retrolental fibroplasia: A multifactorial disease. Anesth Analg 1981;60:109.

42. Lucey JF, Dangman B: A reexamination of the role of oxygen in retrolental fibroplasia. Pediatrics 1984;73:82.

43. Flynn JT: Acute proliferative retrolental fibroplasia: Multivariate risk analysis. Trans Am Ophthalmol Soc 1983;81:549.

44. Steward DJ: Preterm infants are more prone to complications following minor surgery than are term infants. Anesthesiology 1982;56:304-306.

45. Tetzlaff JE, Annand DW, Pudimat MA, et al: Postoperative apnea in a full-term infant. Anesthesiology 1988;69:426-428.

46. Liu LMP, Coté CJ, Goudsouzian NG, et al: Life-threatening apnea in infants recovering from anesthesia. Anesthesiology 1983;59:506-510.

47. Kurth CD, Spitzer AR, Broennle AM, et al: Postoperative apnea in preterm infants. Anesthesiology 1987;66:483-488.

48. Welborn LG, Hannallah RS, Luban NLC, et al: Anemia and postoperative apnea in former preterm infants. Anesthesiology 1991;74:1003-1006.

49. Jobe AH, Bancalari E: Bronchopulmonary dysplasia. Am J Respir Crit Care Med 2001;163:1723-1729.

50. Giacoia GP, Venkataraman PS, West-Wilson KI, Faulkneer MJ: Follow-up of school-age children with bronchopulmonary dysplasia. J Pediatr 1997;130:400-408.

51. Groothuis JR, Gutierrez KM, Lauer BA: Respiratory syncytial virus infection in children with bronchopulmonary dysplasia. Pediatrics 1988;82:199-203.

52. Schmidt B, Asztalos EV, Roberts RS, et al: Impact of bronchopulmonary dysplasia, brain injury, and severe retinopathy on the outcome of extremely low-birth-weight infants at 18 months: Results from the trial of indomethacin prophylaxis in preterms. JAMA 2003;289:1124-1129.

53. Schreiber MD, Gin-Mestan K, Marks JD, et al: Inhaled nitric oxide in premature infants with the respiratory distress syndrome. N Engl J Med 2003;349:2099-2107.

54. Martin RJ. Nitric oxide for preemies—Not so fast (editorial). N Engl J Med 2003;349:2157-2159.

55. Schiff D, Stern L, Leduc J: Chemical thermogenesis in newborn infants: Catecholamine excretion and the plasma nonesterified fatty acid response to cold exposure. Pediatrics 1966;37:577-582.

56. Bucher H-U, Fanconi S, Baeckert P, et al: Hyperoxemia in newborn infants: Detection by pulse oximetry. Pediatrics 1989;84:226-230.

57. Shah SN, Gibbs S, Upton CJ, et al: Incontinentia pigmenti associated with cerebral palsy and cerebral leukomalacia: A case report and literature review. Pediatr Dermatol 2003;20:491-494.

58. Hubert JN, Callen JP. Incontinentia pigmenti presenting as seizures. Pediatr Dermatol 2002;19:550-552.

59. Cates CA, Dandekar SS, Flanagan DW, Moore AT: Retinopathy of incontinentia pigmenti: A case report with thirteen years follow-up. Ophthalmic Genet 2003;24:247-252.

60. Goldberg MF: Macular vasculopathy and its evolution in incontinentia pigmenti. Trans Am Ophthalmol Soc 1998;96:55-65.

61. Goldberg MF, Custis PH: Retinal and other manifestations of incontinentia pigmenti (Bloch-Sulzberger syndrome). Ophthalmology 1993;100:1645-1654.

62. Chen SD, Hanson R, Hundal K: Foveal hypoplasia and other ocular signs: A possible case of incontinentia pigmenti? Arch Ophthalmol 2003;121:921.

63. Savovets D. Ketamine: An effective general anesthetic for use in electroretinography. Ann Ophthalmol 1978;10:1510.

64. Tanskanen P, Kylma T, Kommonen B, Karhunen U: Propofol influences the electroretinogram to a lesser degree than thiopentone. Acta Anaesthesiol Scand 1996;40:480-485.

65. Yanase J, Ogawa H: Effects of halothane and sevoflurane on the electroretinogram of dogs. Am J Vet Res 1997;58:904-909.

66. Chaudhary V, Hansen R, Lindgren H, Fulton A: Effects of telazol and nembutal on retinal responses. Doc Ophthalmol 2003;107:45-51.

67. Banoub M, Tetzlaff JE, Schubert A: Pharmacologic and physiologic influences affecting sensory evoked potentials. Anesthesiology 2003;99:716-737.

68. Chi OZ, Field C: Effects of isoflurane on visual evoked potentials in humans. Anesthesiology 1986;65:328-330.

69. Uhl RR, Squires KC, Bruce DL, Starr A: Effect of halothane anesthesia on the human cortical visual evoked response. Anesthesiology 1980;53:273-276.

70. Chi OZ, Ryterbrand S, Field C: Visual evoked potentials during thiopentone-fentanyl-nitrous oxide anaesthesia in humans. Can J Anaesth 1989;36:637-640.

71. Chi OZ, Subramoni J, Jasaitis D: Visual evoked potentials during etomidate administration in humans. Can J Anaesth 1990;37:452-456.

72. Hou WY, Lee WY, Lin SM, et al: The effects of ketamine, propofol and nitrous oxide on visual evoked potentials during fentanyl anesthesia. Ma Tsui Hsueh Tsa Chi Anaesthesiol Sin 1993;31:97-102.

73. Raudzens PA: Intraoperative monitoring of evoked potentials. Ann NY Acad Sci 1982;388:308-326.

74. Chi OZ, McCoy CL, Field C: Effects of fentanyl anesthesia on visual evoked potentials in humans. Anesthesiology 1987;67:827-830.

75. McGoldrick KE: The open globe: Is an alternative to succinylcholine necessary? (editorial). J Clin Anesth 1993;5:1-4.

76. Mahajan RP, Grover VK, Sharma SL, et al: Lidocaine pretreatment in modifying IOP increases. Can J Anaesth 1987;34:41.

77. Sweeney J, Underhill S, Dowd T, Mostafa SM: Modification by fentanyl and alfentanil of the intraocular pressure response to suxamethonium and tracheal intubation. Br J Anaesth 1989;63:688-691.

78. Ghignone M, Noe S, Calvillo O, et al: Effects of clonidine on IOP and perioperative hemodynamics. Anesthesiology 1988;68:707.

79. Miller RD, Way Wl, Hickey RF: Inhibition of succinylcholine-induced increased intraocular pressure by nondepolarizing muscle relaxants. Anesthesiology 1968;29:123-126.

80. Meyers EF, Krupin T, Johnson M, et al: Failure of nondepolarizing neuromuscular blockers to inhibit succinylcholine-induced increased intraocular pressure—a controlled study. Anesthesiology 1978;48:149-151.

81. Vachon CA, Warner DO, Bacon DR: Succinylcholine and the open globe: Tracing the teaching. Anesthesiology 2003;99:220-223.

82. Ginsberg B, Glass PS, Quill T, et al: Onset and duration of neuromuscular blockade following high-dose vecuronium administration. Anesthesiology 1989;71:201-205.

83. Schwarz S, Ilias W, Lackner F, et al: Rapid tracheal intubation with vecuronium: The priming principle. Anesthesiology 1985;62:388-391.

84. Libonati MM, Leahy JJ, Ellison N: Use of succinylcholine in open eye injury. Anesthesiology 1985;62:637-640.

85. Donlon JV Jr: Succinylcholine and open eye injury: II. Anesthesiology 1986;64:525-526.

86. Ostermeier AM, Roizen MF, Hautkappe M, et al: Three sudden postoperative arrests associated with epidural opioids in patients with sleep apnea. Anesth Analg 1997;85:452-460.

87. Young T, Palta M, Dempsey J, et al: The occurrence of sleep-disordered breathing among middle-aged adults. N Engl J Med 1993;328:1230-1235.

88. Piccirillo JF: More information needed about the long-term health consequences of mild to moderate obstructive sleep apnea (editorial). Arch Otolaryngol Head Neck Surg 2001;127:1400-1401.

89. Nieto FJ, Young TB, Lind BK, et al: Association of sleep-disordered breathing, sleep apnea, and hypertension in a large community-based study: Sleep Heart Health Study. JAMA 2000;283:1829-1836.

90. Nymann P, Backer V, Dirksen A, Lange P: Increased diastolic blood pressure associated with obstructive sleep apnea independently of overweight (abstract). Sleep 2000;23:A61.

91. Bixler EO, Vgontzas AN, Lucas T, et al: The association between sleep-disordered breathing and cardiovascular abnormalities (abstract). Sleep 2000;23:A59.

92. Benumof JL: Obstructive sleep apnea in the adult obese patient: Implications for airway management. J Clin Anesth 2001;13:144-156.

93. Hudgel DW: Mechanisms of obstructive sleep apnea. Chest 1992;101:541-549.

94. Kuna ST, Sant'Ambrogio G: Pathophysiology of upper airway closure during sleep. JAMA 1991;266:1384-1389.

95. Beydon L, Hassapopoulos J, Quera MA, et al: Risk factors for oxygen desaturation during sleep after abdominal surgery. Br J Anaesth 1992;69:137-142.

96. Boudewyns AN, DeBacker WA, Van de Heyning PH: Pattern of upper airway obstruction during sleep before and after uvulopalatopharyngoplasty in patients with obstructive sleep apnea. Sleep Med 2001;2: 309-315.

97. Catalfumo FJ, Golz A, Westerman ST, et al: The epiglottis and obstructive sleep apnoea syndrome. J Laryngol Otol 1998;112: 940-943.

98. Farmer WC, Giudici SC: Site of airway collapse in obstructive sleep apnea after uvulopalatopharyngoplasty. Ann Otol Rhinol Laryngol 2000;109:581-584.

99. Garrigue S, Bordier P, Jais P, et al: Benefit of atrial pacing in sleep apnea syndrome. N Engl J Med 2002;346:404-412.

100. Gottlieb DJ: Cardiac pacing—a novel therapy for sleep apnea? (editorial). N Engl J Med 2002;346:444-445.

101. Pirsig W, Verse T: Long-term results in the treatment of obstructive sleep apnea. Eur Arch Otorhinolaryngol 2000;257:570-577.

102. Itasaka Y, Miyazaki S, Tanaka T, et al: Uvulopalatopharyngoplasty for obstructive sleep-related breathing disorders: One-year follow-up. Psychiatry Clin Neurosci 2001;55:261-264.

103. Vilaseca I, Morello A, Montserrat JM, et al: Usefulness of uvulopalatopharyngoplasty with genioglossus and hyoid advancement in the treatment of obstructive sleep apnea. Arch Otolaryngol Head Neck Surg 2002;128:435-440.

104. Finkelstein Y, Stein G, Ophir D, et al: Laser-assisted uvulopalatoplasty for the management of obstructive sleep apnea: Myths and facts. Otolaryngol Head Neck Surg 2002;128:429-434.

105. American Sleep Apnea Association: Sleep apnea and same day surgery. Washington, DC, American Sleep Apnea Association, 1999. Available at www.sleepapnea.org/sameday/html

106. Morgan AH, Zitsch RP: Recurrent respiratory papillomatosis in children: A retrospective study of management and complications. Ear Nose Throat J 1986;65:19-28.

107. Mounts P, Shah KV, Kashima H: Viral etiology of juvenile and adult onset squamous papilloma of the larynx. Proc Natl Acad Sci U S A 1982;79:5425-5429.

108. Derkay CS: Task force on recurrent respiratory papillomas. Arch Otolaryngol Head Neck Surg 1995;121:1386-1391.

109. Rimell FL, Shoemaker DL, Pou AM, et al: Pediatric respiratory papillomatosis: Prognostic role of viral subtyping and cofactors. Laryngoscope 1997;107:915-918.

110. Tenti P, Zappatore R, Migliora P, et al: Perinatal transmission of human papillomavirus from gravidas with latest infections. Obstet Gynecol 1999;93:475-479.

111. Leventhal BG, Kashima HK, Mounts P, et al: Long-term response of recurrent respiratory papillomatosis to treatment with lymphoblastoid interferon alfa-N1. N Engl J Med 1991;325;613.

112. McGlennen RC, Adams GL, Lewis CM, et al: Pilot trial of ribavirin for the treatment of laryngeal papillomatosis. Head Neck 1993;15: 504-512.

113. Shikowitz MJ, Abramson AL, Freeman K, et al: Efficacy of DHE photodynamic therapy for respiratory papillomatosis: Immediate and long-term results. Laryngoscope 1998;108:962-967.

114. Myer CM, Wiliging P, Cotton R: Use of a laryngeal microresector system. Laryngoscope 1999;109:1165-1166.

115. Orr RJ, Elwood T: Special challenging problems in the difficult pediatric airway: Lymphangioma, laryngeal papillomatosis, and subglottic hemangioma. Anesthesiol Clin North Am 1998;16: 869-883.

116. Derkay CS: Recurrent respiratory papillomatosis. Laryngoscope 2001;111:57-69.

117. Benjamin B, Lines V: Endoscopy and anesthesia in non-infective airway obstruction in children. Anaesthesia 1972;27:22-29.

118. Kennedy MG, Chinyanga HM, Steward DJ: Anaesthetic experience using a standard technique for laryngeal surgery in infants and children. Can Anaesth Soc J 1981;28:561.

119. Armstrong LR, Derkay CS, Reeves WC: Initial results from the National Registry for juvenile-onset recurrent respiratory papillomatosis. Arch Otolaryngol Head Neck Surg 1999;125: 743-748.

120. Cohen SR, Thompson JW: Lymphangiomas of the larynx in infants and children: A survey of pediatric lymphangioma. Ann Otol Rhinol Laryngol 1986;127:1.

121. Schulman SR, Jones BR, Slotnick N, et al: Fetal tracheal intubation with intact uteroplacental circulation. Anesth Analg 1993;76:197.

122. Tanaka M, Sato S, Naito H, et al: Anaesthetic management of a neonate with prenatally diagnosed cervical tumor and upper airway obstruction. Can J Anaesth 1994;41:236.

123. Ogita S, Tsuto T, Nakamura K, et al: OK-432 therapy in 64 patients with lymphangioma. J Pediatr Surg 1994;29:784.

124. Popa ER, Tervaert JW: The relation between *Staphylococcus aureus* and Wegener's granulomatosis: Current knowledge and future directions. Intern Med 2003;43:771-780.

125. Watters K, Russell J: Subglottic stenosis in Wegener's granulomatosis and the nitinol stent. Laryngoscope 2003;113:2222-2224.

126. Wardyn KA, Yeinska K, Matuszkiewicz-Rowinska J, Chipczynska M: Pseudotumour orbitae as the initial manifestation in Wegener's granulomatosis in a 7-year-old girl. Clin Rheumatol 2003;22: 472-474.

127. Biswas J, Babu K, Gopal L, et al: Ocular manifestations of Wegener's granulomatosis: Analysis of nine cases. Indian J Ophthalmol 2003;51:217-223.

128. Straatsma BR: Ocular manifestations of Wegener's granulomatosis. Am J Ophthalmol 1957;44:789.

129. Nolle B, Specks U, Luderman J, et al: Anticytoplasmatic autoantibodies: Their immuno-diagnostic value in Wegener's granulomatosis. Ann Intern Med 1989;11:28-40.

130. Langford CA, Sneller MC, Hallahan CW, et al: Clinical features and therapeutic management of subglottic stenosis in patients with Wegener's granulomatosis. Arthritis Rheum 1996;39:1754-1760.

131. Levy A, Hall L, Yeudall WA, Lightman SL: p53 gene mutation in pituitary adenomas: Rare events. Clin Endocrinol 1994;41:809-814.

132. Faglia G, Ambrosi B: Hypothalamic and pituitary tumors: General principles. In Grossman A (ed): *Clinical Endocrinology*. Oxford, Blackwell, 1992, pp 113-122.

133. Burrow GN, Wortzman G, Rewcastle NB, et al: Microadenomas of the pituitary and abnormal sellar tomograms in unselected autopsy series. N Engl J Med 1981;304:156-158.

134. Lamberts SW, Hofland LJ, de Herder WW, et al: Octreotide and related somatostatin analogs in the diagnosis and treatment of pituitary disease and somatostatin receptor scintigraphy. Front Neuroendocrinol 1993;14:27-55.

135. Burn JM: Airway difficulties associated with anaesthesia in acromegaly. Br J Anaesth 1972;44:413-414.

136. Schmitt H, Buchfelder M, Radespiel-Troger M, Fahlbusch R: Difficult intubation in acromegalic patients: Incidence and predictability. Anesthesiology 2000;93:110-114.

137. Murrant NJ, Garland DJ: Respiratory problems in acromegaly. J Laryngol Otol 1990;104:52-55.

138. Smith M, Hirsch NP: Pituitary disease and anaesthesia. Br J Anaesth 2000;85:3-14.

139. Quinn FB Jr: Ludwig angina (commentary). Arch Otolaryngol Head Neck Surg 1999;125:599.

140. Marple BF: Ludwig angina: A review of current airway management. Arch Otolaryngol Head Neck Surg 1999;125:596-598.

141. Tschiassny K: Ludwig's angina: An anatomic study of the lower molar teeth in its pathogenesis. Arch Otolaryngol Head Neck Surg 1943;38:485-496.

142. Penner J: Ludwig's angina. In Roizen MF, Fleisher LA (eds): Essence of Anesthesia Practice, 2nd ed. Philadelphia 2002, p 210.

143. Thomas TT: Ludwig's angina. Ann Surg 1908;47:161, 335.

144. Taffel M, Harvey SC: Ludwig's angina: An analysis of 45 cases. Surgery 1942;11:841-850.

145. Patterson HC, Kelly JH, Strome M: Ludwig's angina: An update. Laryngoscope 1982;92:370-378.

146. Kurien M, Mathew J, Job A, Zachariah N: Ludwig's angina. Clin Otolaryngol 1997;22:263-265.

147. Loughnan TE, Allen DE: Ludwig's angina: The anesthetic management of nine cases. Anaesthesia 1985;40:295.

CHAPTER

2

Uncommon Cardiac Diseases

DAVID L. REICH, MD, ALEXANDER MITTNACHT, MD,
and JOEL A. KAPLAN, MD

The anesthetic management of uncommon cardiovascular disease states differs in no fundamental way from the management of the more familiar problems, since it rests on the same principles of management. These include (1) understanding the disease process and its manifestations in the patient; (2) a thorough understanding of anesthetic and adjuvant drugs, including their cardiovascular effects; (3) the proper use of monitoring; and (4) an understanding of the requirements of the surgical procedure.

Certainly the most common major cardiovascular diseases encountered are atherosclerotic coronary artery disease, degenerative valvular disease, and essentia hypertension. Experience with these disease states has made the anesthesiologist familiar with both the pathophysiology and the management of cardiac patients. Whereas the disease states discussed in this chapter are not often encountered, they can be reduced to familiar patterns of physiology and pathophysiology.

The principle of understanding a disease state and its manifestations in a patient remains the same whether the disease is common or uncommon. An evaluation of the degree of cardiovascular involvement using available clinical and laboratory information is necessary to make a rational assessment of the disease state in each individual patient. A thorough understanding of the cardiovascular effects of the anesthetic and adjuvant drugs to be employed allows the patient to be cared for using a rational anesthetic plan. Advances in cardiovascular pharmacology, anesthetic drugs, and new techniques of circulatory support have provided great flexibility in the management of the patient with impaired cardiovascular function.

The use of hemodynamic monitoring provides the best guide to intraoperative and postoperative treatment of patients with uncommon cardiovascular diseases. Monitoring is certainly no substitute for an understanding of physiology and pharmacology or clinical judgment; rather, the monitoring provides information that facilitates clinical decisions. Because the diseases to be discussed are rarely encountered, extensive knowledge of their pathophysiology, particularly in the anesthetic and surgical setting, is largely lacking, and monitoring helps bridge this gap. An understanding of the requirements of the surgical procedure and good communication with the surgeon are necessary in all operations to anticipate intraoperative problems, but especially in the diseases considered here.

This chapter does not provide an exhaustive list or consideration of all the uncommon diseases that affect the cardiovascular system, although it covers a wide range. No matter how bizarre a disease entity is, it can only affect the cardiovascular system in a limited number of ways. It can affect the myocardium, the coronary arteries, the conduction system, the pulmonary circulation, or valvular function, or it can impair cardiac filling or emptying. Subsections in this chapter follow this basic pattern. Each section is accompanied by tables of uncommon diseases that may produce a cardiomyopathy, coronary artery disease, pulmonary hypertension, or other cardiac disorder, along with various comments and caveats for each disease. This method of presentation provides a reasonable approach to the anesthetic management of uncommon diseases.

CARDIOMYOPATHIES

General Classification

Cardiomyopathies are defined as diseases of the myocardium that are associated with cardiac dysfunction. Cardiomyopathies can be classified in a number of ways. On an etiologic basis they are usually thought of as primary myocardial diseases, in which the basic disease locus is the myocardium itself, or secondary myocardial diseases, in which the myocardial pathology is associated with some systemic disorder. On a pathophysiologic basis, myocardial disease can be broken down into the following categories: dilated (congestive), hypertrophic, and restrictive cardiomyopathy (Fig. 2-1). In 1995, the World Health Organization (WHO) International Society and Cardiology Task Force on the Definition and Classification of Cardiomyopathies developed the currently used clinical classification of cardiomyopathies. The WHO lists a functional classification of cardiomyopathies based on the underlying pathophysiology of cardiac dysfunction and specific cardiomyopathies in which the cardiomyopathy is associated with specific cardiac or systemic disorders (Table 2-1).[1] Unfortunately, there is often not a sharp division among the three categories, and a particular patient may have features suggestive of any or all of them. Dilated cardiomyopathies encompass both inflammatory and noninflammatory forms, and their most prominent clinical feature is myocardial failure manifested as ventricular dilatation, elevated filling pressures, and pulmonary edema. This, for example, is the usual response in cases of severe myocarditis. For the following discussion, the myocarditides will be included with inflammatory dilated cardiomyopathies. The obstructive form of myocardial diseases consists of hypertrophy of the myocardial muscle that may result in impaired filling and obstruction to ventricular outflow. Restrictive cardiomyopathies usually result from an infiltration of the myocardium by fibrous tissue or some other substance that decreases the compliance of the ventricle and impedes filling. They usually present a picture that mimics the physiology of constrictive pericarditis, often coupled with myocardial failure due to loss of muscle mass.

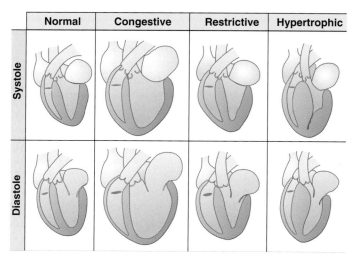

FIGURE 2–1 Illustration of the 50-degree left anterior oblique view of the heart in various cardiomyopathies at end systole and end diastole. *(From Goldman MR, Boucher CA: Value of radionuclide imaging techniques in assessing cardiomyopathy. Am J Cardiol 1980;46:1232. Reproduced with permission.)*

TABLE 2–1   The World Health Organization Classification of Cardiomyopathies

A. Functional classification of cardiomyopathy
  1. Dilated cardiomyopathy
  2. Hypertrophic cardiomyopathy
  3. Restrictive cardiomyopathy
  4. Arrhythmogenic right ventricular cardiomyopathy
  5. Unclassified cardiomyopathies

B. Specific cardiomyopathies
  1. Ischemic cardiomyopathy
  2. Valvular cardiomyopathy
  3. Hypertensive cardiomyopathy
  4. Inflammatory cardiomyopathy
     a. Idiopathic
     b. Autoimmune
     c. Infectious
  5. Metabolic cardiomyopathy
     a. Endocrine
     b. Familial storage diseases and infiltrations
     c. Deficiency
     d. Amyloid
  6. General system disease
     a. Connective tissue disorder
     b. Infiltrations and granulomas
  7. Muscular dystrophies
  8. Neuromuscular disorders
  9. Sensitivity and toxic reactions
  10. Peripartal cardiomyopathy

From Mason JW: Classification of Cardiomyopathies. In Fuster V, Alexander RW, O'Rourke RA (eds): Hurst's The Heart, 11th ed. New York, McGraw-Hill, 2004, p 1883. Reproduced with permission of the McGraw-Hill Companies.

Dilated Cardiomyopathy

Inflammatory (Myocarditis)

Dilated (congestive) cardiomyopathies exist in both inflammatory and noninflammatory forms (Tables 2-2 and 2-3).[2] The inflammatory variety, or myocarditis, is usually the result of infection.[3,4] Myocarditis presents as the clinical picture of fatigue, dyspnea, and palpitations, usually in the first weeks of the infection, progressing to overt congestive heart failure with cardiac dilatation, tachycardia, pulsus alternans, and pulmonary edema. Between 10% and 33% of patients with infectious heart diseases will have electrocardiographic (ECG) evidence of myocardial involvement. Mural thrombi often form in the ventricular cavity and may result in systemic or pulmonary emboli. Supraventricular and ventricular arrhythmias are common. Fortunately, complete recovery from infectious myocarditis is usually the case, but there are exceptions, such as myocarditis associated with diphtheria or Chagas' disease. Occasionally, acute myocarditis may even

progress to a recurrent or chronic form of myocarditis, resulting ultimately in a restrictive type of cardiomyopathy secondary to fibrous replacement of the myocardium.[5] In the bacterial varieties of myocarditis, isolated ECG changes or pericarditis are common and usually benign whereas congestive heart failure is unusual. Diphtheritic myocarditis is generally the worst form of bacterial myocardial involvement, because, in addition to inflammatory changes, its endotoxin is a competitive analog of cytochrome-B and can produce severe myocardial dysfunction.[6] The conduction system is especially affected in diphtheria, producing either right or left bundle branch block, which is associated with a 50% mortality. When complete heart block supervenes, the mortality rate approaches 80% to 100%. Syphilis and leptospirosis represent two examples of myocardial infection by spirochetes.[7] Tertiary syphilis is associated with multiple problems, including arrhythmias, conduction disturbances, and congestive heart failure.

Viral infections manifest themselves primarily with ECG abnormalities, including PR prolongation, QT prolongation, ST and T wave abnormalities, and arrhythmias. However, each viral disease produces slightly different ECG changes, with complete heart block being the most significant. Most of the viral diseases have the potential to progress to congestive heart failure if the viral infection is severe.[8] Especially noteworthy in this regard is coxsackievirus B, which most commonly produces severe viral heart disease. Presenting as fulminating cardiac failure with severe atrioventricular (AV) nodal involvement and respiratory distress, viral myocarditis is common in nursery epidemics of coxsackievirus B infection. Recovery from coxsackievirus B myocarditis is usual, but the condition may have constrictive pericarditis as a sequela. Primary atypical pneumonia has the unusual feature of producing Stokes-Adams attacks secondary to AV node involvement.

Mycotic myocarditis has protean manifestations that depend on the extent of mycotic infiltration of the myocardium and may present as congestive heart failure, pericarditis, ECG abnormalities, or valvular obstruction.

Of the protozoal forms of myocarditis, Chagas' disease, or trypanosomiasis, is the most significant, and it is the most common cause of chronic congestive heart failure in South America. ECG changes of right bundle branch block and arrhythmias occur in 80% of patients. In addition to the typical inflammatory changes in the myocardium that produce chronic congestive failure, a direct neurotoxin from the infecting organism, *Trypanosoma cruzi*, produces degeneration of the conduction system, often causing severe ventricular arrhythmias and heart block with syncope. The onset of atrial fibrillation in these patients is often an ominous prognostic sign.[9]

Helminthic myocardial involvement may produce congestive heart failure, but more commonly symptoms

TABLE 2–2   Inflammatory Cardiomyopathies (Dilated)

Disease Process	Mechanism	Associated Circulatory Problems	Miscellaneous
Bacterial		Arrhythmias, ST-T wave changes	
Diphtherial	Endotoxin competitive analog of cytochrome B	Conduction system, especially BBB Rare, valvular endocarditis	Temporary pacing often required
Typhoid	Inflammatory changes* with fiber degeneration	Arrhythmias Endarteritis, endocarditis, pericarditis, ventricular rupture	
Scarlet fever β-Hemolytic strep	Inflammatory changes	Conduction disturbances and arrhythmias	
Meningococcus	Inflammatory changes and endotoxin, generalized and coronary thrombosis	Disseminated intravascular coagulation Peripheral circulatory collapse (Waterhouse-Friderichsen syndrome)	
Staphylococcus	Sepsis, acute endocarditis		
Brucellosis	Fiber degeneration and granuloma formation	Endocarditis, pericarditis	
Tetanus	Inflammatory changes, cardiotoxin	Severe arrhythmias	Apnea
Melioidosis	Myocardial abscesses		
Spirochetal leptospirosis	Focal hemorrhage and inflammatory changes	Severe arrhythmias Endocarditis and pericarditis	Temporary pacing
Syphilis			
Rickettsial		ECG changes, pericarditis	
Endemic typhus	Inflammatory changes	Arrhythmias	
Epidemic typhus	Symptoms secondary to vasculitis and hypertension	Vasculitis	
Viral			
HIV	Inflammatory changes Myocarditis Neoplastic infiltration	Systolic and diastolic dysfunction Dilated cardiomyopathy and CHF Pericardial effusion Endocarditis Pulmonary hypertension	
Coxsackievirus B	Inflammatory changes	Constrictive pericarditis AV-nodal arrhythmias	
Echovirus	Inflammatory changes	Dysrhythmia	
Mumps	Primary atypical pneumonia—	Heart block	
Influenza	associated Stokes-Adams attacks	Pericarditis	
Infectious mononucleosis	Herpes simplex—associated with intractable shock		
Viral hepatitis	Arbovirus—constrictive pericarditis is reported sequela		
Rubella			
Rubeola			
Rabies			
Varicella			
Lymphocytic Choriomeningitis			
Psittacosis			
Viral encephalitis			
Cytomegalovirus			
Variola			
Herpes zoster			
Mycoses	Usually obstructive symptoms		
Cryptococcosis	Reported CHF		
Blastomycosis			
Actinomycosis		Valvular obstruction	
Coccidiomycosis		Constrictive pericarditis	

	TABLE 2–2 Inflammatory Cardiomyopathies (Dilated)—cont'd			

Disease Process	Mechanism	Associated Circulatory Problems	Miscellaneous
Protozoal			
Trypanosomiasis (Chagas' disease— see text)	Inflammatory changes Neurotoxin of *Trypanosoma cruzi*	Severe arrhythmia secondary to conduction system degeneration Mitral and tricuspid insufficiency secondary to cardiac enlargement	Pacing often required
Sleeping sickness	Inflammatory changes		Unusual manifestations of disease
Toxoplasmosis	Inflammatory changes	Cardiac tamponade	
Leishmaniasis	Inflammatory changes		Unusual manifestations
Balantidiasis			
Helminthic	Inflammatory changes		
Trichinosis	Usually secondary to adult or ova infestation of myocardium or coronary insufficiency secondary to same	Arrhythmias	
Schistosomiasis	Cor pulmonale—secondary pulmonary hypertension		
Filariasis			

*Inflammatory type usually has myofibrillar degeneration, inflammatory cell infiltration, edema.
BBB, bundle branch block; CHF, congestive heart failure; AV, atrioventricular.

are secondary to infestation and obstruction of the coronary or pulmonary arteries by egg, larval, or adult forms of the worm. Trichinosis, for example, produces a myocarditis secondary to an inflammatory response to larvae in the myocardium, even though the larvae themselves disappear from the myocardium after the second week of infestation.

Noninflammatory

The noninflammatory variety of dilated cardiomyopathy also presents as the picture of myocardial failure, but in this case secondary to idiopathic, toxic, degenerative, or infiltrative processes in the myocardium (see Table 2-3).[10,11]

Alcoholic cardiomyopathy is a typical hypokinetic noninflammatory cardiomyopathy, associated with tachycardia and premature ventricular contractions, that progresses to left ventricular failure with incompetent mitral and tricuspid valves. This cardiomyopathy is probably due to a direct toxic effect of ethanol or its metabolite acetaldehyde, which releases and depletes cardiac norepinephrine.[12] Alcohol may also affect excitation-contraction coupling at the subcellular level.[13] In chronic alcoholics, acute ingestion of ethanol produces decreases in contractility, elevations in ventricular end-diastolic pressure, increases in systemic vascular resistance (SVR), and systemic hypertension.[14-16]

Alcoholic cardiomyopathy is classified in three hemodynamic stages. In stage I, cardiac output, ventricular

pressures, and left ventricular end-diastolic volume are normal but the ejection fraction is decreased. In stage II, cardiac output is normal although filling pressures and end-diastolic volume are increased and ejection fraction is decreased. In stage III, cardiac output is decreased, filling pressures and end-diastolic volume are increased, and ejection fraction is severely depressed. In general, all of the noninflammatory forms of dilated cardiomyopathy probably undergo a similar progression.

Doxorubicin (Adriamycin) is an antibiotic with broad-spectrum antineoplastic activities. However, the clinical usefulness of this drug is limited by its cardiotoxicity. Doxorubicin produces dose-related dilated cardiomyopathy. It has been suggested that doxorubicin disrupts myocardial mitochondrial calcium homeostasis. Patients treated with this drug usually have serial evaluations of left ventricular systolic function.[17,18] Dexrazoxane, a free-radical scavenger, may protect the heart from doxorubicin-associated damage.[19]

Pathophysiology

The key hemodynamic features of the dilated cardiomyopathies are elevated filling pressures, failure of myocardial contractile strength, and a marked inverse relationship between afterload and stroke volume.

Both the inflammatory and noninflammatory forms of dilated cardiomyopathies present a picture identical to that of congestive heart failure produced by severe coronary

TABLE 2–3   Noninflammatory Cardiomyopathies (Dilated)

Disease Process	Mechanism	Associated Circulatory Problems	Miscellaneous
Nutritional disorders			
Beriberi	Thiamine deficiency Inflammatory changes	Peripheral AV shunting with low SVR Usually high output failure with decreased SVR, but low output with normal SVR may occur	
Kwashiorkor	Protein deprivation	Degeneration of conduction system	
Metabolic disorders			
Amyloidosis	Amyloid infiltration of myocardium	Associated with restrictive and obstructive forms of cardiomyopathy Valvular lesions Conduction abnormalities	
Pompe's disease Glycogen storage disease type II	α-Glucuronidase deficiency Glycogen accumulation in cardiac muscle	Septal hypertrophy Decreased compliance	
Hurler's syndrome	Accumulation of glycoprotein in coronary tissue and parenchyma of heart	Mitral regurgitation	
Hunter's syndrome	Same	Similar to but milder than Hurler's	
Primary xanthomatosis	Xanthomatosis infiltration of myocardium	Aortic stenosis Advanced coronary artery disease	
Uremia	Multiple metastatic coronary calcifications Hypertension Electrolyte imbalance	Anemia Hypertension Conduction deficits Pericarditis and cardiac tamponade	Most cardiac manifestations dramatically improve after dialysis
Fabry's disease	Abnormal glycolipid metabolism secondary to ceramide trihexosidase with glycolipid infiltration of myocardium	Hypertension Coronary artery disease	
Hematologic diseases			
Leukemia	Leukemic infiltration of myocardium	Arrhythmias Pericarditis	Usually resolves with successful therapy
Sickle cell	Intracoronary thrombosis with ischemic cardiomyopathy	Coronary artery disease Cor pulmonale	
Neurologic disease			
Duchenne's muscular dystrophy	Muscle fiber degeneration with fatty and fibrous replacement	Conduction defects possibly secondary to small vessel coronary artery disease	50% incidence of cardiac involvement
Friedreich's ataxia	Similar to Duchenne's with collagen replacement of degenerating myofibers	Conduction abnormalities ? HOCM	
Roussy-Lévy hereditary polyneuropathy	Similar to Friedreich's ataxia		
Myotonia atrophica	Similar to above	Conduction abnormalities, possibly Stokes-Adams attacks	
Chemical and toxic			
Doxorubicin (see text)			
Zidovudine (see text)			
Ethyl alcohol (see text)	Myofibrillar degeneration secondary to direct toxic effect of ETOH and/or acetaldehyde		
Beer drinker's cardiomyopathy	Probably secondary to the addition of cobalt sulfate to beer with myofibrillar dystrophy and edema	Cyanosis	Acute onset and rapid course

TABLE 2–3   Noninflammatory Cardiomyopathies (Dilated)—cont'd

Disease Process	Mechanism	Associated Circulatory Problems	Miscellaneous
Cobalt intoxication	Similar to beer drinker's cardiomyopathy		CNS symptoms and aspiration pneumonitis are usually the predominant symptoms
Phosphorus	Myofibrillar degeneration secondary to direct toxic effect of phosphorus, which prevents amino acid incorporation into myocardial proteins		Relatively unresponsive to adrenergic agents
Fluoride	Direct myocardial toxin Severe hypocalcemia secondary to fluoride-binding of calcium ion		
Lead	Secondary to nephropathic hypertension Direct toxin	Hypertension	
Scorpion venom	Sympathetic stimulation with secondary myocardial changes		Adrenergic blockade probably indicated
Tick paralysis	?	Toxic myocarditis	
Radiation	Hyalinization and fibrosis due to direct effect of x-radiation	Conduction abnormalities secondary to sclerosis of conduction system Coronary artery disease Constrictive myocarditis and pericarditis	
Miscellaneous and systemic syndromes			
Rejection cardiomyopathy	Lymphocytic infiltration and general rejection phenomena	Arrhythmias and conduction abnormalities	After heart transplantation
Senile cardiomyopathy	Unrelated to coronary artery disease		
Rheumatoid arthritis	Rheumatoid nodular invasion Secondary to coronary arteritis	Mitral and aortic regurgitation Coronary artery disease Constrictive pericarditis	
Marie-Strümpell (ankylosing spondylitis)	Generalized degenerative changes	Aortic regurgitation	
Cogan's syndrome (nonsyphilitic interstitial keratitis)	Fibrinoid necrosis of myocardium	Aortic regurgitation Coronary artery disease	
Noonan's syndrome (male Turner's)	? (No detectable chromosome abnormality)	Pulmonary stenosis Obstructive and nonobstructive cardiomyopathy	
Pseudoxanthoma elasticum (Grönblad-Strandberg)	Connective tissue disorder with myocardial infiltration and fibrosis	Valve abnormality Coronary artery disease	
Trisomy 17-18	Diffuse fibrosis		
Scleroderma of Buschke	Myocardial infiltration with acid mucopolysaccharides		? Viral etiology Self-limited with good prognosis
Wegener's granulomatosis	Panarteritis and myocardial granuloma formation	Mitral stenosis (?) Cardiac tamponade	
Periarteritis nodosa	Panarteritis Changes secondary to hypertension	Conduction abnormalities Coronary artery disease	

Continued

TABLE 2-3   Noninflammatory Cardiomyopathies (Dilated)—cont'd

Disease Process	Mechanism	Associated Circulatory Problems	Miscellaneous
Postpartum cardiomyopathy			
Neoplastic diseases			
Primary mural cardiac tumors		Obstructive symptoms	
Metastases—malignant (especially malignant melanoma)	Mechanical impairment of cardiac function		
Sarcoidosis	Cor pulmonale secondary to pulmonary involvement Sarcoid granuloma leading to ventricular aneurysms	Cor pulmonale ECG abnormalities and conduction disturbances Pericarditis Valvular obstruction	

AV, atrioventricular; SVR, systemic vascular resistance; HOCM, hypertrophic obstructive cardiomyopathy; ETOH, ethanol; CNS, central nervous system.

artery disease, even to the extent that, in some conditions, the process that has produced the cardiomyopathy also involves the coronary arteries. The pathophysiologic considerations are familiar ones. As the ventricular muscle weakens, the ventricle dilates to take advantage of the increased force of contraction that results from increasing myocardial fiber length. As the ventricular radius increases, however, ventricular wall tension rises, increasing both the oxygen consumption of the myocardium and the total internal work of the muscle.

As the myocardium deteriorates further, the cardiac output falls, and a compensatory increase in sympathetic activity occurs to maintain organ perfusion and cardiac output. One feature of the failing myocardium is the loss of its ability to maintain stroke volume in the presence of increased afterload. Figure 2-2 shows that in the failing ventricle the stroke volume falls almost linearly with increases in afterload. The increased sympathetic outflow that accompanies left ventricular failure initiates a vicious cycle of increased resistance to forward flow, decreased stroke volume and cardiac output, and further sympathetic stimulation in an effort to maintain circulatory homeostasis.

Mitral regurgitation is common in severe dilated cardiomyopathies owing to stretching of the mitral annulus (Carpentier type 1) and distortion of the geometry of the chordae tendineae resulting in restriction of leaflet apposition (Carpentier type IIIb).[20] The forward stroke volume improves with afterload reduction, even though there is no increase in ejection fraction. This suggests that reduction of mitral regurgitation is the mechanism of the improvement. Afterload reduction also decreases left ventricular filling pressure, which relieves pulmonary congestion and should preserve coronary perfusion pressure.[21]

The clinical picture of the dilated cardiomyopathies falls into the two familiar categories of "forward" failure and "backward" failure. The features of "forward" failure, such as fatigue, hypotension, and oliguria, are due to decreases in cardiac output with reduced organ perfusion. Reduced perfusion of the kidneys results in activation of the renin-angiotensin-aldosterone system, which increases the effective circulating blood volume through sodium and water retention. "Backward" failure is related to the elevated filling pressures required by the failing ventricles. As the left ventricle dilates, "secondary" mitral regurgitation occurs. The manifestations of left-sided failure include orthopnea, paroxysmal nocturnal dyspnea, and pulmonary edema. The manifestations of right-sided failure include hepatomegaly, jugular venous distention, and peripheral edema.

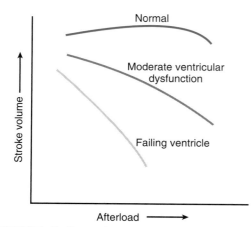

FIGURE 2–2 Stroke volume (SV) as a function of afterload for a normal left ventricle, for a left ventricle with moderate dysfunction, and for a failing left ventricle.

Anesthetic Considerations

ECG monitoring is essential in the management of patients with dilated cardiomyopathies, particularly in those with myocarditis. Ventricular arrhythmias are common, and complete heart block, which can occur from these conditions, requires rapid diagnosis and treatment. The electrocardiogram is also useful in monitoring ischemic changes when coronary artery disease is associated with the cardiomyopathy, as in amyloidosis. Direct intra-arterial blood pressure monitoring during surgery provides continuous blood pressure information and a convenient route for obtaining arterial blood gases. Any dilated cardiomyopathy patient with a severely compromised myocardium who requires anesthesia and surgery should have central venous access for monitoring and vasoactive drug administration. Monitoring right-sided filling pressures is of equal importance in patients with pulmonary hypertension or cor pulmonale. The use of a pulmonary artery catheter (PAC) is much more controversial. The American Society of Anesthesiologists Task Force on Pulmonary Artery Catheterization has published practice guidelines for pulmonary artery catheterization.[22] The indication for PAC placement is dependent on a combination of patient-, surgery-, and practice setting–related factors. Patients with severely decreased cardiac function from dilated cardiomyopathy have significant cardiovascular disease and are considered at increased or high risk. Because there was no evidence-based medicine to support outcome differences, recommendations for PAC monitoring were based on expert opinion at that time. Patients with dilated cardiomyopathy presenting for surgery who have an overall increased- or high-risk score should probably have hemodynamic parameters monitored with a PAC. In addition to measuring right- and left-sided filling pressures, a thermodilution pulmonary artery catheter may be used to obtain cardiac outputs and for the calculation of systemic and pulmonary vascular resistances, which allow for serial evaluation of the patient's hemodynamic status. PAC with fiberoptic oximetry, rapid-response thermistor catheters that calculate right ventricular ejection fraction, and pacing PAC are available. Pacing PAC and external pacemakers provide distinct advantages in managing the patient with myocarditis and associated heart block. Recent evidence seems to provide

further support for clinicians who choose not to use PAC monitoring on the basis of no outcome differences between high-risk surgical patients who were cared for with and without PAC monitoring and goal-directed therapy.[23]

Transesophageal echocardiography (TEE) provides useful data on filling, ventricular function, severity of mitral regurgitation, and the response of the impaired ventricle to anesthetic and surgical manipulations. Recently published guidelines indicate that hemodynamic decompensation is a class I indication for TEE monitoring.[24] With the increased availability of TEE equipment and anesthesiologists trained in its use, this modality will become increasingly important in the perioperative management of patients with cardiomyopathies.

The avoidance of myocardial depression still remains the goal of anesthetic management for patients with dilated cardiomyopathy (Table 2-4), although, paradoxically, β-adrenergic blockade has been associated with improved hemodynamics and improved survival in patients with dilated cardiomyopathy.[25-28] All of the potent volatile anesthetic agents are myocardial depressants, and, for this reason, high concentrations of these agents are probably best avoided in this group of patients. Low doses are usually well tolerated, however. An anesthetic based primarily on a combination of narcotics and sedative-hypnotics (with or without nitrous oxide) can be employed instead. For the patient with severely compromised myocardial function, the synthetic piperidine narcotics (fentanyl, sufentanil, remifentanil, and alfentanil) are useful, because myocardial contractility is not depressed. Chest wall rigidity associated with this technique is treated with muscle relaxants. Bradycardia associated with high-dose narcotic anesthesia may be prevented by the use of pancuronium for muscle relaxation, anticholinergic drugs, or pacing. Pancuronium, however, should be avoided in patients with impaired renal function, which is a common problem in cardiomyopathy patients. For peripheral or lower abdominal surgical procedures, the use of a regional anesthetic technique is a reasonable alternative, provided filling pressures are carefully controlled and the hemodynamic effects of the anesthetic are monitored. One problem is

TABLE 2–4	Treatment Principles of Dilated Cardiomyopathies	
Clinical Problem	Treatment	Relatively Contraindicated
↓ Preload	Volume replacement Positional change	Nodal rhythm High spinal
↓ Heart rate	Atropine Pacemaker	Verapamil
↓ Contractility	Positive inotropes Digoxin	Volatile anesthetics
↑ Afterload	Vasodilators	Phenylephrine Light anesthesia

that regional anesthesia is frequently contraindicated because patients with cardiomyopathies are frequently treated with anticoagulant drugs to prevent embolization of mural thrombi that develop on hypokinetic ventricular wall segments. For shorter procedures, high-dose opioid anesthesia using remifentanil may prove to be advantageous because of the cardiovascular advantages of opioid anesthesia and its extremely short duration of action.

In planning anesthetic management for the patient with dilated cardiomyopathy, associated cardiovascular conditions, such as the presence of coronary artery disease, valvular abnormalities, outflow tract obstruction, and constrictive pericarditis should also be considered. Patients with congestive heart failure often require circulatory support intraoperatively and postoperatively. Inotropic drugs, such as dopamine or dobutamine, have been shown to be effective in low output states and produce modest changes in SVR at lower dosages. In severe failure, more potent drugs such as epinephrine may be required. Phosphodiesterase III inhibitors, such as milrinone, with inotropic and vasodilating properties may improve hemodynamic performance. As noted earlier, stroke volume is inversely related to afterload in the failing ventricle and the reduction of left ventricular afterload with vasodilating drugs such as nitroprusside and nesiritide is also effective in increasing cardiac output. In patients with myocarditis, especially of the viral variety, transvenous or external pacing may be required should heart block occur. Intra-aortic balloon counterpulsation and left ventricular assist devices are further options to be considered in the case of the severely compromised ventricle.

There is a definite increase in the incidence of supraventricular and ventricular arrhythmias in myocarditis and the dilated cardiomyopathies.[29,30] These arrhythmias often require extensive electrophysiologic workup and may be unresponsive to maximal medical therapy. Some patients will present for automatic internal cardioverter-defibrillator implantation. Originally, cardioverting pads were sewn to the epicardial surface via a median sternotomy and the device was implanted in the abdominal wall. The procedure has become markedly less invasive. Presently, the device is implanted in the subcutaneous tissue near the deltopectoral groove and transvenous electrodes are placed in the heart. Intraoperative attempts to elicit arrhythmias are necessary to test the device. Thus, proper ECG monitoring and access to a charged external cardioversion device are important details.

Hypertrophic Cardiomyopathy

Hypertrophic cardiomyopathies usually result from asymmetrical hypertrophy of the basal ventricular septum and occur in either obstructive or nonobstructive forms (Table 2-5). A dynamic pressure gradient in the left ventricular outflow tract (LVOT) is present in the obstructive forms.[31-33] Other conditions can also produce the picture of an obstructive cardiomyopathy such as massive infiltration of the ventricular wall, as in Pompe's disease, where an accumulation of cardiac glycogen in the ventricular wall produces LVOT obstruction. In the following discussion the focus is on the obstructive form.

Hypertrophic obstructive cardiomyopathy (HOCM), asymmetrical septal hypertrophy (ASH), and idiopathic hypertrophic subaortic stenosis (IHSS) are all synonymous terms applied to a form of an idiopathic hypertrophic cardiomyopathy. However, it presents a picture that is typical of the problems encountered in virtually all forms of obstructive cardiomyopathy. The salient anatomic feature of HOCM is hypertrophy of ventricular muscle at the base of the septum in the LVOT. Histologically, this is a disorganized mass of hypertrophied myocardial cells extending from the left ventricular septal wall, often involving the papillary muscles. Intramural ("small vessel") coronary artery disease has been identified in autopsy specimens, especially in areas of myocardial fibrosis. This may represent a congenital component of the disease and probably plays some role in the etiology of myocardial ischemia in these patients.[34]

TABLE 2–5   Cardiomyopathies (Hypertrophic)

Disease Process	Mechanism	Associated Circulatory Problems
Idiopathic concentric hypertrophy	Symmetrical hypertrophy of left ventricle and outflow tract (usually nonobstructive)	
Hypertrophic obstructive cardiomyopathy (IHSS, ASH)	(See text)	
Systemic syndromes		
Glycogen storage disease type II (Pompe's)	Glycogen infiltration of septal walls	Dilated cardiomyopathy
Noonan's syndrome	Left ventricular outflow obstruction	Coronary artery disease
Lentiginosis	Right and left AV-septal hypertrophy	Pulmonary stenosis

IHSS, idiopathic hypertrophic subaortic stenosis; ASH, asymmetrical septal hypertrophy; AV, atrioventricular.

Obstruction of the LVOT is caused by the hypertrophic muscle mass and systolic anterior motion (SAM) of the anterior leaflet of the mitral valve. SAM was thought to be caused by a Venturi effect of the rapidly flowing blood in the LVOT. Recently, echocardiographic data have revealed that excessive anterior mitral valve tissue in combination with a more anterior position of the mitral valve causes the anterior mitral valve leaflet to protrude into the LVOT.[35]

A subaortic pressure gradient is present in symptomatic patients. The outflow tract obstruction can result in hypertrophy of the remainder of the ventricular muscle, secondary to increased pressures in the ventricular chamber. As the ventricle hypertrophies, ventricular compliance decreases and passive filling of the ventricle during diastole is impaired. For this reason, the ventricle becomes increasingly dependent on the presence of atrial contraction to maintain adequate ventricular end-diastolic volume. Occasionally, HOCM is associated with a right ventricular outflow tract obstruction as well.

The determinants of the functional severity of the ventricular obstruction in HOCM are (1) the systolic volume of the ventricle, (2) the force of ventricular contraction, and (3) the transmural pressure distending the outflow tract. Large systolic volumes in the ventricle distend the outflow tract and reduce the obstruction, whereas small systolic volumes narrow the outflow tract and increase the obstruction. When ventricular contractility is high, the outflow tract is narrowed, increasing the obstruction. When aortic pressure is high, there is an increased transmural pressure that distends the left ventricular outflow tract. During periods of hypotension, however, the outflow tract is narrowed. This results in markedly impaired cardiac output and sometimes mitral regurgitation, as the mitral valve becomes the relief point for ventricular pressure.

The current therapeutic options for patients with hypertrophied cardiomyopathy are based on pharmacologic therapy, surgical interventions, percutaneous transluminal septal myocardial ablation, and dual chamber pacing.[36-40] Automatic implantable cardioverter-defibrillators are frequently implanted to treat arrhythmias and to prevent sudden cardiac death.[41,42] The pharmacologic therapy of HOCM has been based on β-blockers. However, it is still not clear if life expectancy is prolonged by this treatment. Verapamil has been used with increasing frequency in patients who do not tolerate β-blockers. Its beneficial effects are likely due to a depression of systolic function and an improvement in diastolic filling and relaxation. In patients whose symptoms are inadequately controlled with β-blockers or verapamil, disopyramide, a type Ia antiarrhythmic agent with negative inotropic and peripheral vasoconstrictive effects, has been used. Amiodarone is increasingly administered to HOCM patients for the control of supraventricular and ventricular arrhythmias.[43]

Most patients with HOCM are treated with only medical therapy. Nevertheless, 5% to 30% of patients with HOCM are candidates for surgical therapy. The surgical intervention in HOCM is myotomy/myomectomy, mitral valve repair/replacement, or valvuloplasty, or a combination of these procedures.[44] The potential complications of surgical correction of the LVOT obstruction include complete heart block and late formation of a ventricular septal defect due to septal infarction. Percutaneous transluminal alcohol septal ablation is performed in the catheterization laboratory but should be restricted to centers with specific experience. At this time it is not regarded as first-line therapy.[45]

Controlled studies did not confirm earlier reports that atrioventricular sequential (DDD) pacing is beneficial for patients with HOCM. Thus, the role of biventricular pacing in subgroups of patients with HOCM has yet to be defined.[46]

Anesthetic Considerations

HOCM had been suggested as a high-risk lesion associated with very high perioperative morbidity in noncardiac surgery.[46a] Based on a retrospective review of perioperative care in 35 patients, it was concluded that the risk of general anesthesia and major noncardiac surgery is low in such patients. However, it was suggested that spinal anesthesia may be relatively contraindicated. Haering and colleagues studied 77 patients with asymmetrical septal hypertrophy who were retrospectively identified from a large database.[46b] Forty percent of patients had one or more adverse perioperative cardiac events, including one patient who had a myocardial infarction and ventricular tachycardia that required emergent cardioversion, whereas the majority of the events were perioperative congestive heart failure. There were no perioperative deaths. Important independent risk factors for adverse outcome in all patients include major surgery and increasing duration of surgery. Unlike the original cohort of patients, type of anesthesia was not an independent risk factor.

Patients with HOCM may be extremely sensitive to small changes in ventricular volume, blood pressure, and heart rate and rhythm. Accordingly, monitoring should be established that allows continuous assessment of these parameters, particularly in patients in whom the obstruction is severe. In patients with HOCM coming to surgery for mitral valve repair/replacement and/ or septal myomectomy, the electrocardiogram, an indwelling arterial catheter (and, in most institutions, a pulmonary artery catheter) are necessary monitors. TEE provides useful data on ventricular function and filling, the severity of LVOT obstruction, and the occurrence of SAM and mitral regurgitation. Assessment of the adequacy of repair requires an experienced echocardiographer.

In patients with HOCM coming for other procedures, the hemodynamic monitors should provide some indication of ventricular volume, force of ventricular contraction, and transmural pressure distending the outflow tract. An indwelling arterial catheter is almost always indicated for beat-to-beat observation of ventricular ejection during major regional or general anesthesia in patients with symptomatic HOCM. Intraoperative echocardiography is the most accurate monitor of ventricular loading conditions and performance in HOCM.

In the anesthetic management of patients with HOCM, special consideration should be given to those features of the surgical procedure and anesthetic drugs that can produce changes in intravascular volume, ventricular contractility, and transmural distending pressure of the outflow tract. Decreased preload, for example, can be produced by blood loss, sympathectomy secondary to spinal or epidural anesthesia, the use of nitroglycerin, or postural changes. Ventricular contractility can be increased by hemodynamic responses to tracheal intubation or surgical stimulation. Transmural distending pressure can be decreased by hypotension secondary to anesthetic drugs, hypovolemia, or positive-pressure ventilation. In addition, patients with HOCM do not tolerate increases in heart rate. Tachycardia decreases systolic ventricular volume and results in a narrowed outflow tract. As noted earlier, the atrial contraction is extremely important to the hypertrophied ventricle. Nodal rhythms should be aggressively treated, using atrial pacing if necessary.

Halothane has major hemodynamic advantages for the anesthetic management of patients with this condition. Halothane decreases heart rate and myocardial contractility, has the least effect of the inhalational anesthetics on SVR, and tends to minimize the severity of the obstruction when volume replacement is adequate. Isoflurane and enflurane cause more peripheral vasodilatation than halothane and are less desirable for this reason. Sevoflurane also decreases SVR to a lesser extent, and thus may be preferable. Agents that release histamine, such as morphine and many benzyl isoquinolinium neuromuscular blockers, are not recommended because of the venodilation they produce. Agents with sympathomimetic side effects (i.e., ketamine and desflurane) are not recommended. High-dose opioid anesthesia causes minimal cardiovascular side effects along with bradycardia and thus may be a useful anesthetic technique in these patients. Preoperative β-blocker and calcium channel blocker therapy should be continued. Intravenous propranolol, esmolol, or verapamil may be administered intraoperatively to improve hemodynamic performance. Table 2-6 summarizes the anesthetic and circulatory management of HOCM.

Anesthesia for Management of Labor and Delivery. Anesthesia for management for labor and delivery in the parturient with HOCM is quite complex. β-Blocker therapy may have been discontinued during pregnancy because of the association with fetal bradycardia and intrauterine growth retardation. Spinal and epidural anesthesia are relatively contraindicated because of the associated vasodilatation. If hypotension occurs during anesthesia, the use of β-agonists such as ephedrine may result in worsening outflow tract obstruction, whereas α-agonists such as phenylephrine could potentially result in uterine vasoconstriction. Nevertheless, the successful management of cesarean section with both general and epidural anesthetics has been reported.[47,48] However, careful titration of anesthetic agents and adequate volume loading (guided by invasive monitoring) is essential to the safe conduct of anesthesia in this clinical setting.

Restrictive Cardiomyopathy

Restrictive cardiomyopathies (i.e., restrictive/obliterative cardiomyopathies) are usually the end stage of myocarditis or of an infiltrative process of the myocardium, such as amyloidosis or hemochromatosis (Table 2-7).

TABLE 2-6   Treatment Principles of Hypertrophic Obstructive Cardiomyopathy

Clinical Problem	Treatment	Relatively Contraindicated
↓ Preload	Volume Phenylephrine	Vasodilators Spinal, epidural
↑ Heart Rate	β-Blockers Verapamil	Ketamine β Agonists
↑ Contractility	Halothane Sevoflurane β-Blockers Disopyramide	Positive inotropes Light anesthesia
↓ Afterload	Phenylephrine	Isoflurane Spinal, epidural

TABLE 2–7   Cardiomyopathies (Restrictive/Obliterative—Including Restrictive Endocarditis)

Disease Process	Mechanism	Associated Circulatory Problems	Miscellaneous
End stage of acute myocarditis	Fibrous replacement of myofibrils		
Metabolic	Amyloid infiltration of myocardium	Valvular malfunction Coronary artery disease	
Amyloidosis Hemochromatosis	Iron deposition and secondary fibrous proliferation	Conduction abnormalities	
Drugs—methysergide (Sansert)	Endocardial fibroelastosis	Valvular stenosis	Similar to changes in carcinoid syndrome
Restrictive endocarditis	Picture very similar to constrictive pericarditis		
Carcinoid	Serotonin-producing carcinoid tumors—but serotonin is apparently not causative agent for fibrosis	Pulmonary stenosis Tricuspid insufficiency and/or stenosis Right-sided heart failure	
Endomyocardial fibrosis	Fibrous obliteration of ventricular cavities	Mitral and tricuspid insufficiency	
Loeffler's disease	Fibrosis of endocardium with decreased myocardial contraction	Subendocardial and papillary muscle degeneration and fibrosis	
Becker's disease	Similar to Loeffler's	Similar to Loeffler's	

When a restrictive cardiomyopathy occurs, it mimics constrictive pericarditis coupled with myocardial dysfunction. Pulsus alternans occurs in both restrictive cardiomyopathies and constrictive pericarditis. Restrictive cardiomyopathies are characterized by impaired ventricular filling and poor ventricular contractility. Cardiac output is maintained in the early stages by elevated filling pressures and an increased heart rate. However, in contrast to constrictive pericarditis, an increase in myocardial contractility to maintain cardiac output is usually not possible. Endocardial fibroelastosis appears similar to restrictive cardiomyopathy in that there is impairment of diastolic ventricular filling but differs in that contractility is not usually impaired.[49]

Anesthetic Considerations

Anesthetic and monitoring considerations in restrictive cardiomyopathies are virtually identical to those of constrictive pericarditis and cardiac tamponade, with the additional feature of poor ventricular function. The combination of a restrictive and a dilated cardiomyopathy results in a more precarious situation than with either condition alone. The reader is referred to the section on constrictive pericarditis for a more detailed discussion of the physiology and management of restrictive ventricular filling and to the section on dilated cardiomyopathy for the management of impaired ventricular function. The anesthetic management must be tailored for whichever feature, restrictive physiology or heart failure, is predominant in a particular patient.

CARDIAC TUMORS

Primary tumors of the heart are unusual. However, the likelihood of encountering a cardiac tumor increases when metastatic tumors of the heart and pericardium are considered. For example, breast and lung cancers metastasize frequently to the heart.[50] Two-dimensional echocardiography and angiography are the major modalities for the preoperative diagnosis of these lesions. Primary cardiac tumors may occur in any chamber or in the pericardium and may arise from any cardiac tissue. Of the benign cardiac tumors, myxoma is the most common, followed by lipoma, papillary fibroelastoma, rhabdomyoma, fibroma, and hemangioma (Table 2-8).[51]

The generally favorable prognosis for patients with benign cardiac tumors is in sharp contrast to the prognosis for those with malignant cardiac tumors. The diagnosis of a malignant primary cardiac tumor is seldom made before extensive local involvement and metastasis have occurred, making curative surgical resection an unlikely event. An aggressive approach including surgery, radiotherapy, and chemotherapy has not significantly altered the poor outlook for these patients.[52]

Benign Cardiac Tumors

Myxomas are most frequently benign tumors. They typically originate from the region adjacent to the fossa ovalis and project into the left atrium. They are usually pedunculated masses that resemble an organized clot on microscopy and may be gelatinous or firm. A left atrial

TABLE 2–8 Primary Neoplasms of the Heart and Pericardium		
Type	No. Cases	Percentage
Benign		
Myxoma	130	29.3
Lipoma	45	10.1
Papillary fibroelastoma	42	9.5
Rhabdomyoma	36	8.1
Fibroma	17	3.8
Hemangioma	15	3.4
Teratoma	14	3.2
Mesothelioma of atrioventricular node	12	2.7
Granular cell tumor	3	0.7
Neurofibroma	3	0.7
Lymphangioma	2	0.5
Subtotal	319	72.0
Malignant		
Angiosarcoma	39	8.8
Rhabdomyosarcoma	26	5.8
Mesothelioma	19	4.2
Fibrosarcoma	14	3.2
Malignant lymphoma	7	1.6
Extraskeletal osteosarcoma	5	1.1
Neurogenic sarcoma	4	0.9
Malignant teratoma	4	0.9
Thymoma	4	0.9
Leiomyosarcoma	1	0.2
Liposarcoma	1	0.2
Synovial sarcoma	1	0.2
Subtotal	125	28.0
Total	444	100.0

Adapted with permission from McAllister HA Jr, Fenoglio JJ Jr: Tumors of the cardiovascular system. *In* Atlas of Tumor Pathology (Fascicle 15). Washington, D.C., Armed Forces Institute of Pathology, 1978.

myxoma may prolapse into the mitral valve during diastole. This prolapsing action results in a ball-valve obstruction to left ventricular inflow that mimics mitral stenosis, and may also cause valvular damage by a "wrecking ball" effect. More friable tumors result in systemic or pulmonary embolization, depending on their location and on the presence of any intracardiac shunts. Cerebral arterial aneurysms are associated with cerebral embolization of myxoma tissue. Pulmonary hypertension may be present due to mitral valve obstruction or regurgitation caused by a left atrial myxoma or pulmonary embolization in the case of a right atrial myxoma. Atrial fibrillation may be present secondary to atrial volume overload. Two-dimensional echocardiography can delineate the location and consistency of these tumors with good precision. Angiography is also valuable but may be complicated by catheter-induced embolization of tumor fragments. Surgical therapy requires careful manipulation of the heart before the institution of cardiopulmonary bypass to avoid embolization and also resection of the base of the tumor (with repair by patching) to prevent recurrence.[53]

Other benign cardiac tumors occur less frequently. In general, intracavitary tumors result in valvular dysfunction or obstruction to flow and tumors localized in the myocardium cause conduction abnormalities and arrhythmias. Papilloma (papillary fibroelastoma) is usually a single villous connective tissue tumor that results in valvular incompetence or coronary ostial obstruction. Cardiac lipoma is an encapsulated collection of mature fat cells. Lipomatous hypertrophy of the interatrial septum is a related disorder that may result in right atrial obstruction. Rhabdomyoma is a tumor of cardiac muscle that occurs in childhood and is associated with tuberous sclerosis. Fibroma is another childhood cardiac tumor.[54]

Malignant Cardiac Tumors

Ten to 25 percent of primary cardiac tumors are malignant, and almost all of these are sarcomas.[55] The curative therapy of sarcomas is based on wide local excision that is not possible in the heart. In addition, the propensity toward early metastasis contributes to the dismal prognosis. Rhabdomyosarcoma may occur in neonates, but most cardiac sarcomas occur in adults. Sarcomas may originate from vascular tissue, cardiac or smooth muscle, and any other cardiac tissue. Palliative surgery may be indicated to relieve symptoms due to mass effects.[56] These tumors respond poorly to radiotherapy and chemotherapy.[57]

Metastatic Tumors Involving the Heart

Breast cancer, lung cancer, lymphomas, and leukemia may all result in cardiac metastases. About one fifth of patients who die of cancer have cardiac metastases. Thus, metastatic cardiac tumors are much more common than primary ones. Myocardial involvement results in congestive heart failure and may be classified as a restrictive cardiomyopathy. Pericardial involvement results in cardiac compression due to tumor mass or tamponade due to effusion. Melanoma is particularly prone to cardiac metastasis.[58]

Cardiac Manifestations of Extracardiac Tumors

Carcinoid is a tumor of neural crest origin that secretes serotonin, bradykinin, and other vasoactive substances. Hepatic carcinoid metastases result in right-sided valvular lesions, presumably from a secretory product that is metabolized in the pulmonary circulation. Recently, serotonin itself has been implicated in the pathogenesis of tricuspid valve dysfunction.[59-61] The end results are thickened valve leaflets that may be stenotic or incompetent, although regurgitation is more common. Even though the tricuspid valve is most commonly involved, this process may involve both right- and left-sided valves.

Pheochromocytoma is a catecholamine-secreting tumor also of neural crest origin. Chronic catecholamine excess has toxic effects on the myocardium that may result in a dilated cardiomyopathy.[62]

Anesthetic Considerations

The presence of a cardiac tumor requires a careful preoperative echocardiographic assessment of cardiac morphology and function. A right-sided tumor (especially myxoma) is a relative contraindication to pulmonary artery catheter insertion because of the risk of embolization, although it may be possible to advance the catheter through the right ventricle after the tumor is resected. The removal of intracardiac tumors is a category II indication for intraoperative TEE monitoring and is particularly useful in the evaluation of the surgical intervention (Fig. 2-3). Left atrial myxomas are well visualized by this technique. However, caution should be exercised in the manipulation of the TEE probe to prevent embolization of friable tumors attached to the posterior wall of the left atrium, because of the proximity of the probe. The management of a left atrial myxoma is similar to that of mitral stenosis. A slow heart rate and high preload should maximize ventricular filling in the presence of an obstructing tumor.

In the absence of a right-sided intracavitary tumor, pulmonary artery catheterization is useful for assessing cardiac function impaired by restrictive cardiomyopathy, pericardial tumor, pericardial effusion, or an obstructive lesion. Avoidance of myocardial depressants, such as the potent volatile agents, and the maintenance of an adequate heart rate are optimal in this scenario. Lower induction doses of ketamine (0.25 to 1.0 mg/kg) or the use of etomidate should minimize hypotension on induction with severely compromised ventricular function.

ISCHEMIC HEART DISEASE

The most important aspects of coronary artery disease remain the same no matter what the etiology of the obstruction of the coronary arteries (Table 2-9). Like coronary artery disease produced by arteriosclerosis, the coronary artery disease produced by an uncommon disease retains the same key clinical features. Physiologic considerations remain essentially the same, as do treatment and anesthetic management.

In the preoperative assessment, the symptoms produced by the coronary artery disease should be determined. The obvious symptoms to look for in the history are angina, the patient's exercise limitations, and symptoms of myocardial failure, such as orthopnea or paroxysmal nocturnal dyspnea. The physical examination retains its importance, especially when quantitative data regarding cardiac involvement are not available. Physical findings such as S3 and S4 heart sounds are important, as are auscultatory signs of uncommon conditions such as cardiac bruits, which might occur in a coronary arteriovenous fistula. If catheterization data are available, the specifics of coronary artery anatomy and ventricular function, such as end-diastolic pressure, ejection fraction, and the presence of wall motion abnormalities, are all useful. Information on ventricular perfusion and function can also be obtained by noninvasive means such as echocardiography and nuclear imaging.[63,64]

After ascertaining the extent of coronary insufficiency, the special aspects of the disease entity producing the coronary insufficiency should be considered. As an example, in ankylosing spondylitis, coronary insufficiency is produced by ostial stenosis, yet valvular problems often coexist and even overshadow the coronary artery disease.[65] In rheumatoid arthritis, however, airway problems may be the most significant part of the anesthetic challenge. Hypertension, which frequently coexists with arteriosclerotic coronary artery disease, is

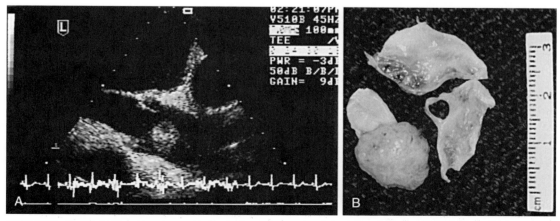

FIGURE 2–3 **A**, Transesophageal image of a mass on the right cusp of the aortic valve. **B**, Photograph of the resected aortic valve (from the same patient) with the tumor attached to the right cusp.

TABLE 2–9 Uncommon Causes of Coronary Artery Disease

I. **Coronary Artery Disease Associated with Cardiomyopathy (Poor Left Ventricular Function)**

  A. Pathologic basis—infiltration of coronary arteries with luminal narrowing

    1. Amyloidosis—valvular stenosis, restrictive cardiomyopathy
    2. Fabry's disease—hypertension
    3. Hurler's syndrome—often associated with valvular malfunction
    4. Hunter's syndrome—often associated with valvular malfunction
    5. Primary xanthomatosis—aortic stenosis
    6. Leukemia—anemia
    7. Pseudoxanthoma elasticum—valve abnormalities

  B. Inflammation of coronary arteries

    1. Rheumatic fever—in acute phase
    2. Rheumatoid arthritis—aortic and mitral regurgitation, constrictive pericarditis
    3. Periarteritis nodosa—hypertension
    4. Systemic lupus erythematosus—hypertension, renal failure, mitral valve malfunction

  C. Embolic or thromboembolic occlusion of coronary arteries

    1. Schistosomiasis
    2. Sickle cell anemia—cor pulmonale depending on length and extent of involvement

  D. Fibrous and hyaline degeneration of coronary arteries

    1. Post transplantation
    2. Radiation
    3. Duchenne's muscular dystrophy
    4. Friedreich's ataxia—? associated with hypertrophic obstructive cardiomyopathy
    5. Roussy-Lévy—hereditary polyneuropathy

  E. Anatomic abnormalities of coronary arteries

    1. Bland-White-Garland syndrome (left coronary artery arising from pulmonary artery)—endocardial fibroelastosis, mitral regurgitation
    2. Ostial stenosis secondary to ankylosing spondylitis—aortic regurgitation

II. **Coronary Artery Disease Usually Associated with Normal Ventricular Function**

  A. Anatomic abnormalities of coronary arteries

    1. Right coronary arising from pulmonary artery
    2. Coronary arteriovenous fistula
    3. Coronary sinus aneurysm
    4. Dissecting aneurysm
    5. Ostial stenosis—bacterial overgrowth syphilitic aortic
    6. Coronary artery trauma—penetrating or nonpenetrating
    7. Spontaneous coronary artery rupture
    8. Kawasaki's disease—coronary artery aneurysm

  B. Embolic or thrombotic occlusion

    1. Coronary emboli
    2. Malaria and/or malarial infested red blood cells
    3. Thrombotic thrombocytopenic purpura
    4. Polycythemia vera

  C. Infections

    1. Miliary tuberculosis—intimal involvement of coronary arteries
    2. Arteritis secondary to salmonella or endemic typhus (associated with active myocarditis)

  D. Infiltration of coronary arteries

    1. Gout – conduction abnormalities, possible valve problems
    2. Homocystinuria

  E. Coronary artery spasm
  F. Cocaine
  G. Miscellaneous

    1. Thromboangiitis obliterans (Buerger's disease)
    2. Takayasu's arteritis

---

also a feature of the coronary artery disease produced by Fabry's disease. Other features to consider are metabolic disturbances that coexist with the coronary artery disease, such as when systemic lupus erythematosus produces both coronary artery disease and renal failure.[66]

Physiology of Coronary Artery Disease and its Modification by Unusual Diseases

The key to the physiology of coronary artery disease is the balance of myocardial oxygen supply and demand (Fig. 2-4). Myocardial oxygen supply depends on many factors, including the heart rate, patency of the coronary arteries, hemoglobin concentration, PaO_2, and the coronary perfusion pressure. The same factors determine supply in uncommon diseases, but the specific manner in which an uncommon disease modifies these factors should be sought. A thorough knowledge of the anatomy of the coronary circulation and how the disease process can affect arterial patency is a useful starting point. This information is usually gained from coronary angiography. In the assessment of the adequacy of coronary perfusion, the viscosity of the blood should be considered, because flow is a function both of the dimensions of the conduit and the nature of the fluid in the system. In disease processes such as thrombotic thrombocytopenic purpura, sickle cell disease, or polycythemia vera, the altered blood viscosity can assume critical importance.[67-70]

Oxygen-carrying capacity must also be considered in certain uncommon disease states. Hemoglobin

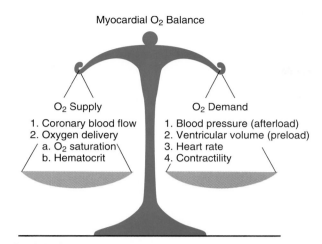

Myocardial O₂ Balance

O₂ Supply
1. Coronary blood flow
2. Oxygen delivery
   a. O₂ saturation
   b. Hematocrit

O₂ Demand
1. Blood pressure (afterload)
2. Ventricular volume (preload)
3. Heart rate
4. Contractility

FIGURE 2–4 Myocardial oxygen supply and demand balance.

concentration is usually not a limiting factor in the supply of oxygen to the myocardium. However, in diseases such as leukemia, anemia may be a prominent feature, and the myocardial oxygen supply may be reduced accordingly. Another example is myocardial ischemia in carbon monoxide poisoning, where the hemoglobin, albeit quantitatively sufficient, cannot carry oxygen. Similarly, the PaO_2 is usually not a limiting factor. But in conditions where coronary artery disease exists concomitantly with cor pulmonale, as in schistosomiasis or sickle-cell disease, the inability to maintain adequate oxygenation may limit the myocardial oxygen supply. In fact, in sickle cell disease, it may be the key feature, because the failure to maintain an adequate PaO_2, secondary to repeated pulmonary infarctions, further increases the tendency of cells containing hemoglobin-S to sickle, compromising myocardial oxygen delivery through "sludging" in the coronary microcirculation.[71]

The major factors determining myocardial oxygen demand include heart rate, ventricular wall tension, and myocardial contractility. Tachycardia and hypertension after tracheal intubation, skin incision, or other noxious stimuli are common causes of increased myocardial oxygen demand during surgery. Additionally, complicating factors of an unusual disease may also produce increases in demand. Increases in rate may occur as a result of tachyarrhythmias secondary to sinoatrial (SA) or AV node involvement in amyloidosis or in Friedreich's ataxia. Increases in wall tension, for example, may occur in severe hypertension associated with systemic lupus erythematosus, periarteritis nodosa, or Fabry's disease. Outflow tract obstruction with increased ventricular work can occur in primary xanthomatosis or in tertiary syphilis; and an increase in the diastolic ventricular radius with increased wall tension can occur in situations such as aortic regurgitation associated with ankylosing spondylitis.

Modern cardiac anesthesia practice should tailor the anesthetic management to the problems posed by the peculiarities of the coronary anatomy. For example, knowledge of the presence of a lesion in the left main coronary artery dictates great care during anesthesia to avoid even modest hypotension or tachycardia. Lesions of the right coronary artery are known to be associated with an increased incidence of atrial arrhythmias and heart block, and steps must be taken either to treat these or to compensate for their cardiovascular effects.

In diseases such as primary xanthomatosis or Hurler's syndrome, the infiltrative process that produces coronary artery disease usually involves the coronary arteries diffusely, but some diseases may have features that can mimic either isolated left main coronary artery disease or right coronary artery disease. The Bland-White-Garland syndrome, which is anomalous origin of the left coronary artery from the pulmonary artery, and coronary ostial stenosis produced by aortic valve prosthesis may both behave as left main coronary artery disease. A similar syndrome could be produced by bacterial overgrowth of the coronary ostia, ankylosing spondylitis, a dissecting aneurysm of the aorta, or Takayasu's arteritis. Right coronary artery disease could be mimicked by the syndrome of the anomalous origin of the right coronary artery from the pulmonary artery or by infiltration of the SA or AV nodes in amyloidosis or Friedreich's ataxia. In small artery arteritis, which occurs in periarteritis nodosa or systemic lupus erythematosus, the small arteries supplying the SA or AV nodes may be involved in the pathologic process, producing ischemia of the conduction system.

In Table 2-9, the uncommon diseases that produce coronary artery disease have been divided into those that produce coronary artery disease associated with good left ventricular function and those associated with poor left ventricular function. In any of these diseases, ventricular function can regress from good to poor. In some conditions, the coronary artery disease progression and ventricular function deterioration occur at the same rate and left ventricular function is eventually severely depressed. In other situations, coronary insufficiency is primary and left ventricular dysfunction eventually occurs after repeated episodes of ischemia and/or thrombosis. Ventricular function must be evaluated by clinical signs and symptoms, echocardiography, nuclear imaging, or cardiac catheterization. The converse is severe arterial disease coupled with relatively good left ventricular function. This is the picture of a cardiomyopathy associated with almost incidental coronary artery disease, as occurs in Hurler's syndrome, amyloidosis, or systemic lupus erythematosus. Most anatomic lesions, such as Kawasaki disease, coronary AV fistula, or coronary insufficiency produced by trauma are usually associated with good left ventricular function. There is a clinical gray zone in which coronary artery disease and poor left ventricular function coexist without either process clearly predominating, such as with tuberculosis and syphilis. These can only be characterized by investigating the extent of involvement of the coronary arteries and the myocardium in the disease process. The following is a more detailed discussion on a few selected disease states that affect the coronary arteries.

Some Uncommon Causes of Ischemic Heart Disease

Coronary Artery Spasm

The luminal narrowing of the coronary arteries secondary to spasm has been associated with angina and myocardial infarction.[72] The mechanism of coronary artery spasm remains unclear. The smooth muscle cells of the coronary artery walls may contract in response to various stimuli. There may be abnormal responses to various vasoactive substances,[73,74] and, in addition, there may be increased α-adrenergic tone.[75] Another theory is that vessels with eccentric atherosclerotic plaques have a segment of disease-free wall that may be a site for vasospasm, which can convert an insignificant obstruction into a critical lesion. Coronary artery vasospasm may respond to nitroglycerin and calcium channel blockers.

Cocaine Abuse

Cocaine can affect the heart in several ways, and the use of cocaine can result in myocardial ischemia, myocardial infarction, and sudden death.[76,77] Cocaine exerts its effects on the heart mainly by two mechanisms: (1) its ability to block sodium channels resulting in a local anesthetic or membrane-stabilizing property and (2) its ability to block the reuptake of norepinephrine resulting in increased sympathetic activity. It is not surprising, therefore, that cocaine, when administered acutely, has been shown to have a biphasic effect on left ventricular function with transient depression followed by a sustained increase in contractility.[78] Cocaine also induces coronary vasospasm and reduced coronary blood flow, while at the same time increasing heart rate and blood pressure. These effects will decrease myocardial oxygen supply and increase myocardial oxygen demand. In addition, cocaine and its metabolites can induce platelets to aggregate and release platelet-derived growth factor that can promote fibrointimal proliferation and accelerated atherosclerosis.[79] Chronic users of cocaine also have an exaggerated response to sympathetic stimuli, which may contribute to the left ventricular hypertrophy frequently observed among chronic users.

Coronary Artery Dissection

When there is separation of the intimal layer from the medial layer of the coronary artery, there may be obstruction of the true coronary artery lumen with subsequent distal myocardial ischemia. Coronary artery dissection may be primary or secondary. Primary coronary artery dissection may occur during coronary artery catheterization or angioplasty and in trauma to the heart. Primary coronary artery dissection may also occur spontaneously. Spontaneous dissection is usually associated with coronary arterial wall eosinophilia and is seen in the postpartum period. Secondary coronary artery dissection is more common and is usually caused by a dissection in the ascending aorta.

Inflammatory Causes

Infectious Causes. Infectious coronary artery arteritis may be secondary to hematogenous spread or secondary to direct extension from infectious processes of adjacent tissue. The infectious process results in thrombosis of the involved artery with myocardial ischemia. Syphilis is one of the most common infectious agents to affect the coronary arteries. Up to 25% of patients with tertiary syphilis have ostial stenosis of their coronary arteries.[80,81]

Noninfectious Causes
Polyarteritis Nodosa. This is a systemic necrotizing vasculitis involving medium and small vessels. Epicardial coronary arteries are involved in the majority of cases of polyarteritis nodosa. After the initial inflammatory response, the coronary artery may dilate to form small berry-like aneurysms that may rupture, producing fatal pericardial tamponade.

Systemic Lupus Erythematosus. The pericardium and myocardium are usually affected in systemic lupus erythematosus (SLE). Patients with SLE, however, may suffer acute myocardial infarction in the absence of atherosclerotic coronary artery disease.[82,83] The hypercoagulable state of SLE, together with a predisposition to premature coronary atherosclerosis, has been implicated. In addition, glucocorticoids used for the treatment of SLE may also predispose these patients to accelerated atherosclerosis.

Kawasaki's Disease (Mucocutaneous Lymph Node Syndrome). This is a disease of childhood. A vasculitis of the coronary vasa vasorum leads to weakened walls of the vessels with subsequent coronary artery aneurysm formation.[84] Thrombosis and myocardial ischemia can also occur. These patients are prone to sudden death from ventricular arrhythmias and occasionally from rupture of a coronary artery aneurysm. Thrombus in the aneurysm may also embolize, causing myocardial ischemia.[85]

Takayasu's Disease. This disease leads to fibrosis and luminal narrowing of the aorta and its branches. The coronary ostia may be involved in this process.[86]

Metabolic Disorders

Homocystinuria. An increased incidence of atherosclerotic disease in patients with high levels of homocysteine is reported.[87] This process may involve intimal proliferation of small coronary vessels and an increased risk of myocardial infarction. Nevertheless, meta-analysis and prospective studies have not consistently confirmed these findings.[88,89]

Congenital Abnormalities of the Coronary Arterial Circulation

Left Coronary Artery Arising from the Pulmonary Artery. This is also known as Bland-White-Garland syndrome. The right coronary arises from the aorta, but the left coronary arises from the pulmonary artery. Flow in the left coronary arterial system is retrograde, with severe hypoperfusion of the left ventricle with myocardial ischemia and infarction. As such, most patients with this disease present in infancy with evidence of heart failure. Untreated patients usually die during infancy. Patients who survive childhood may present with mitral regurgitation from annular dilatation. The goals of medical therapy are to treat congestive heart failure and arrhythmias. The defect can be corrected surgically by primary anastomosis of the left coronary artery to the aorta.[90,91] In older children, a vein graft of the left internal mammary artery may be used to establish anterograde flow in the left coronary arterial system. Improvement in left ventricular function can be expected of surgical survivors if this operation is performed early.[92,93]

Coronary Arteriovenous Fistula. There is an anatomic communication between a coronary artery and a right-sided structure such as the right atrium, right ventricle, or the coronary sinus. The right coronary artery is more frequently affected and is usually connected to the coronary sinus. Most patients are asymptomatic. These patients are at risk for endocarditis, myocardial ischemia, and rupture of the fistulous connection.[94] These fistulas should be corrected surgically.[95]

Anesthetic Considerations

The functional impairment of the myocardium and coronary circulation dictates the extent and type of monitoring to be employed. The selection of ECG leads to monitor is dictated by knowledge of the coronary anatomy. Those diseases in which there is left coronary artery disease are best monitored using precordial leads, such as the V_5 lead. In those diseases with right coronary artery disease, ECG leads used to assess the inferior surface of the heart (leads II, III, or aVF), or the posterior surface (esophageal lead), are preferable.[96-98]

Knowledge of ventricular filling pressures is especially important in diseases associated with poor ventricular function. The use of a pulmonary artery catheter is preferable to central venous pressure monitoring in the assessment of left ventricular function. The etiology of large V waves on the pulmonary capillary wedge pressure waveform that sometimes occur during myocardial ischemia is probably a decrease in diastolic ventricular compliance. However, large V waves did not correlate with other determinants of myocardial ischemia in a study of vascular surgical patients with coronary artery disease.[99]

Two-dimensional TEE is an important monitor of both ventricular function and myocardial ischemia. It can demonstrate regional changes in wall motion that are sensitive signs of myocardial ischemia.[100-102] Urine output is another important parameter and is especially significant in diseases associated with nephropathy, such as long-standing sickle cell disease or systemic lupus.

When severe cardiomyopathy associated with coronary artery disease exists, monitoring cardiac output and SVR is useful in evaluating both the effects of anesthetic drugs and therapeutic interventions. It is quite controversial whether pulmonary artery catheterization is indicated in patients requiring major procedures. In the absence of convincing evidence of outcome benefits associated with pulmonary artery catheterization, decisions regarding this type of monitoring should be made on a case-by-case basis. An indwelling arterial catheter for monitoring arterial blood gases is important, especially when pulmonary disease or cor pulmonale complicates the picture, as in schistosomiasis or sickle cell disease.

One caveat should be noted in the use of intra-arterial monitoring. When peripheral arterial monitoring is used in cases of generalized arteritis, the adequacy of collateral blood flow should be carefully evaluated before cannulation of the peripheral artery. In occlusive diseases, such as Raynaud's disease, Takayasu's arteritis, or Buerger's disease, or in cases of sludging in the microcirculation, as in sickle cell disease, the area distal to the cannulated artery should be checked frequently for signs of arterial insufficiency. Axillary artery catheterization may be preferable.

The anesthetic employed in these conditions should be tailored to the degree of myocardial dysfunction.[103] In cases of pure coronary insufficiency with good left ventricular function, anesthetic management is aimed at decreasing oxygen demand by decreasing myocardial contractility, while preserving oxygen supply by maintaining blood pressure. Techniques commonly employed include the combination of a volatile anesthetic agent with nitrous oxide or use of a nitrous-narcotic technique that employs the intermittent use of vasodilators such as nitroprusside or nitroglycerin for control of hypertension.

When coronary vasospasm is considered, it is important to maintain a relatively high coronary perfusion pressure. Pharmacologic agents such as nitroglycerin and calcium channel blockers may also be used. Patients who are chronic users of cocaine should be considered at high risk for ischemic heart disease and arrhythmias. These patients may respond unpredictably to anesthetic agents and other drugs used in the perioperative period. Ephedrine and other indirect sympathomimetic drugs should be avoided in cocaine users.

In patients with poor ventricular function, the anesthetic technique should maintain hemodynamic stability by avoiding drugs that produce significant degrees of myocardial depression.[104] High-dose opioid techniques or opioid-benzodiazepine combinations have been found to be effective.[105] In periarteritis nodosa or Fabry's disease, hypertension is often associated with poor left ventricular function. In such situations, a vasodilator such as sodium nitroprusside or nitroglycerin can be used to control hypertension rather than a volatile anesthetic. Milrinone and nesiritide are also options. The principles for the management of intraoperative arrhythmias remain the same as for the treatment of arrhythmias in the setting of atherosclerotic coronary artery disease. Regional anesthesia requires monitoring that will allow the appropriate management of associated sympathetic blockade.

PULMONARY HYPERTENSION AND COR PULMONALE

Pulmonary Hypertension

Pulmonary hypertension is defined as an elevation of the mean pulmonary artery pressure above the accepted limit of normal, regardless of the etiology (mean pulmonary artery pressure > 25 mm Hg at rest or > 30 mm Hg during exercise).[106,107]

The normal pulmonary vasculature changes from a high resistance circuit in utero to a lower resistance circuit in the newborn, secondary to several concomitant changes: (1) the relief of hypoxic vasoconstriction that occurs with the first spontaneous breath; (2) the stenting effect of air-filled lungs on the pulmonary vessels, which increases their caliber and decreases their resistance; and (3) the functional closure of the ductus arteriosus, secondary to an increase in the PaO_2. The muscular medial layer of the fetal pulmonary arterioles normally involutes in postnatal life. Assuming there is no severe active vasoconstriction, pulmonary artery pressure remains low, owing to the numerous parallel vascular channels that accept increased blood flow as pulmonary blood volume is increased. For this reason, pressure is not normally increased in the pulmonary circuit, because increased pulmonary blood flow distends the pulmonary vessels, lowering their resistance.

General pathologic conditions that will convert this normally low resistance circuit into a high resistance circuit are summarized by the WHO Diagnostic Classification of Pulmonary Hypertension (Table 2-10). The WHO lists five separate categories of pulmonary hypertension: (1) pulmonary arterial hypertension; (2) pulmonary venous hypertension; (3) pulmonary hypertension with disorders of the respiratory system and/or hypoxemia; (4) pulmonary hypertension caused by chronic thrombotic and/or embolic disease; and (5) pulmonary hypertension caused by disorders affecting the pulmonary vasculature directly.

Increases in capillary or pulmonary venous pressure may be caused by conditions such as left ventricular failure, mitral regurgitation, or mitral stenosis. In addition to the passive increase in pulmonary blood volume, active vasoconstriction also occurs in the pulmonary vascular bed. Hypoxic vasoconstriction induced by ventilation-perfusion mismatching or reflex constriction occurring with the passive stretching of the muscular media of the pulmonary arterioles may be the basis of this phenomenon.[108]

A decrease in pulmonary arterial cross-sectional area results in increased pulmonary vascular resistance, as dictated by Poiseuille's law, which states that resistance to flow is inversely proportional to the fourth power of the radius of the vessels. Very small decrements in a pulmonary cross-sectional area can result in striking increases in resistance. There are a number of causes of decreased pulmonary arterial cross-sectional area. Filarial worms, the eggs of *Schistosoma mansoni,* or multiple small thrombotic emboli are typical of embolic causes of pulmonary hypertension. Primary deposition of fibrin in the pulmonary arterioles and capillaries due to an altered hemostasis with prothrombotic mechanisms, especially increased platelet activation, is another cause of decreased cross-sectional area, and this, in fact, may be the mechanism of primary, or idiopathic, pulmonary hypertension.[109,110] This also may be the cause of the pulmonary arterial hypertension that is rarely associated with the use of oral contraceptives, which are known to increase thrombogenesis.

Pulmonary arterial medial hypertrophy can occur if there is increased flow or pressure in the pulmonary circulation early in life. In this situation, the muscular media of the pulmonary arterioles undergo hypertrophy rather than the normal postnatal involution.[111] As the muscle hypertrophies there is increased reflex contraction in response to the elevations in pulmonary arterial pressure. This raises the pulmonary arterial pressure even higher by further reducing cross-sectional area. If this pulmonary arterial pressure elevation is of long standing, it results in intimal damage to the pulmonary arterioles followed by fibrosis, thrombosis, and sclerosis, with an irreversible decrease in cross-sectional area of the arterial bed, as often occurs in long-standing mitral valve disease or emphysema. Pulmonary hypertension can also be caused by primary vasoconstrictors, such as the seeds of the *Crotalaria* plant, or by hypoxia associated with high-altitude or pulmonary parenchymal disease.[112]

Pulmonary hypertension resulting from increases in pulmonary arterial flow is usually associated with various congenital cardiac lesions, such as atrial septal defect,

TABLE 2–10 Diagnostic Classification of Pulmonary Hypertension	

I. Pulmonary Arterial Hypertension
 	
1.1 Primary pulmonary hypertension
  (a) Sporadic disorder
  (b) Familial disorder
1.2 Related to:
  (a) Collagen vascular disease
  (b) Congenital systemic-to-pulmonary shunts
  (c) Portal hypertension
  (d) Human immunodeficiency virus infection
  (e) Drugs and toxins
    1. Anorexigens
    2. Others
  (f) Persistent pulmonary hypertension of the newborn
  (g) Others
 	
II. Pulmonary Venous Hypertension
 	
2.1 Left-sided atrial or ventricular heart disease
2.2 Left-sided valvular heart disease
2.3 Extrinsic compression of central pulmonary veins
  (a) Fibrosing mediastinitis
  (b) Adenopathy and/or tumors
2.4 Pulmonary veno-occlusive disease
2.5 Others
	III. Pulmonary Hypertension Associated with Disorders of the Respiratory System and/or Hypoxemia
	
	3.1 Chronic obstructive pulmonary disease
	3.2 Interstitial lung disease
	3.3 Sleep-disordered breathing
	3.4 Alveolar hypoventilation disorders
	3.5 Chronic exposure to high altitudes
	3.6 Neonatal lung disease
	3.7 Alveolar-capillary dysplasia
	3.8 Others
	
	IV. Pulmonary Hypertension due to Chronic Thrombotic and/or Embolic Disease
	
	4.1 Thromboembolic obstruction of proximal pulmonary arteries
	4.2 Obstruction of distal pulmonary arteries
	  (a) Pulmonary embolism (thrombus, tumor, ova and/or parasites, foreign material)
	  (b) In-situ thrombosis
	  (c) Sickle cell disease
	
	V. Pulmonary Hypertension due to Disorders Directly Affecting the Pulmonary Vasculature
	
	5.1 Inflammatory conditions
	  (a) Schistosomiasis
	  (b) Sarcoidosis
	  (c) Others
	5.2 Pulmonary capillary hemangiomatosis

From Rubin LJ: Pulmonary hypertension. In Fuster V, Alexander RW, O'Rourke RA (eds): Hurts's The Heart. 11th ed. New York, McGraw-Hill, 2004, p 1579. Reproduced with permission of the McGraw-Hill Companies.

ventricular septal defect, patent ductus arteriosus, or, in adult life, ventricular septal defect occurring after a septal myocardial infarction. Hypoxemia will aggravate this situation. Evidence for this arises from the observation that there is an increased incidence of pulmonary hypertension in infants with congenital left-to-right shunting who are born at high altitudes, compared with similar infants born at sea level. Long-standing increases in flow with intimal damage may result in fibrosis and sclerosis, as noted earlier. An increase in pulmonary arterial pressure in these cases ultimately may result in Eisenmenger's syndrome, in which irreversibly increased pulmonary arterial pressure results in a conversion of left-to-right shunting to right-to-left shunting with the development of tardive cyanosis.

Like systemic arterial hypertension, pulmonary hypertension is characterized by a prolonged asymptomatic period. As pulmonary vascular changes occur, an irreversible decrease in pulmonary cross-sectional area develops and stroke volume becomes fixed as a result of the fixed resistance to flow. As such, cardiac output becomes heart rate dependent. This results in the symptoms of dyspnea, fatigue, syncope, and chest pain. The diagnostic dilemma presented by pulmonary hypertension is in differentiation of primary pulmonary hypertension from secondary pulmonary hypertension. Usually, in secondary pulmonary hypertension, the symptoms of the primary condition are the more prominent and the pulmonary hypertension is of secondary significance. When pulmonary hypertension exists alone, the key feature of its pathophysiology is a fixed cardiac output. Right ventricular hypertrophy commonly occurs in response to pulmonary hypertension, which may progress to right ventricular dilatation and failure.[113]

Cor Pulmonale

Cor pulmonale is usually defined as an alteration in the structure and function of the right ventricle, such as right ventricular hypertrophy, dilation, and failure secondary to pulmonary arterial hypertension that is due to a decrease in the cross-sectional area of the pulmonary bed. This excludes, therefore, right ventricular failure, which occurs after increases in pulmonary arterial pressure secondary to increases in pulmonary blood flow or in pulmonary capillary or venous pressure. Both increases in pulmonary blood flow and passive increases in pulmonary venous and capillary pressure can produce right ventricular failure, but they do not, strictly speaking, produce cor pulmonale. The physiologic considerations in cor pulmonale and in right ventricular failure from other causes are similar. Given this restriction, though, there are still numerous causes of cor pulmonale, including pulmonary parenchymal disease, chronic hypoxia, and primary pulmonary arterial disease.[114]

Cor pulmonale is divided into two types: acute and chronic. Acute cor pulmonale is usually secondary to a massive pulmonary embolus, resulting in a 60% to 70% decrease in the pulmonary cross-sectional area associated with cyanosis and acute respiratory distress. With acute cor pulmonale, there is a rapid increase in right ventricular systolic pressure to 60 to 70 mm Hg, which slowly returns toward normal secondary to displacement of the embolus peripherally, lysis of the embolus, and increases in collateral blood flow. These changes often occur within 2 hours of the onset of symptoms. Massive emboli may be associated with acute right ventricular dilatation and failure, elevated central venous pressure, and cardiogenic shock. Another feature of massive pulmonary embolization is the intense pulmonary vasoconstrictive response.[115,116]

Chronic cor pulmonale presents with a different picture. It is associated with right ventricular hypertrophy and/or dilatation and a change in the normal crescentic shape of the right ventricle to a more ellipsoidal shape. This configuration is consistent with a change from volume work that the right ventricle normally performs, to the pressure work required by a high afterload. Left ventricular dysfunction may occur in association with right ventricular hypertrophy. This dysfunction cannot be related to any obvious changes in the loading conditions of the left ventricle but is probably due to displacement of the interventricular septum. Chronic cor pulmonale is usually superimposed on long-standing pulmonary arterial hypertension that is associated with chronic respiratory disease.[117]

Chronic bronchitis is probably the most common cause of cor pulmonale in adults, and its pathophysiology will be examined as a guide to understanding and managing cor pulmonale from all causes. Initially, the pulmonary vascular resistance in chronic bronchitis is normal or slightly increased because cardiac output increases. Later, there is a further increase in pulmonary vascular resistance or an inappropriately elevated pulmonary vascular resistance for the amount of pulmonary blood flow. Recall that in the normal situation there is a slight decrease in the pulmonary resistance when pulmonary blood flow is increased that is probably secondary to an increase in pulmonary vascular diameter and in flow through collateral channels. In chronic bronchitis, the absolute resistance of the pulmonary circulation may not change, owing to the inability of the resistance vessels to dilate. A progressive loss

of pulmonary parenchyma occurs and, because of dilatation of the terminal bronchioles, there is an increase in pulmonary dead space that causes progressively more severe mismatching of pulmonary ventilation and perfusion. In response to the ventilation-perfusion mismatch, the pulmonary circulation attempts to compensate by decreasing blood flow to the areas of the lung that have hypoxic alveoli. This occurs at the expense of a decrease in pulmonary arteriole cross-sectional area and an elevation in pulmonary arterial pressure.[118]

Long-standing chronic bronchitis results in elevations in pulmonary arterial pressure, with resulting alterations in the structure and function of the right ventricle, such as right ventricular hypertrophy. In any form of respiratory embarrassment, whether it is infection or simply progression of the primary disease, further increases in pulmonary vascular resistance increase pulmonary arterial pressure, and right ventricular failure supervenes. With the onset of respiratory problems in the patient with chronic bronchitis, a number of changes occur that can make pulmonary hypertension more severe and can precipitate right ventricular failure. A respiratory infection produces further abnormalities of the blood gas values, with declines in Pa_{O_2} and elevations in Pa_{CO_2}. Generally the pulmonary artery pressure is directly proportional to the Pa_{CO_2}, though the pulmonary circulation also vasoconstricts in response to hypoxemia. With a fall in Pa_{O_2} there is usually an increase in cardiac output in an effort to maintain oxygen delivery to tissues. This increased blood flow through the lungs may result in further elevations in the pulmonary artery pressure owing to the fixed decreased cross-sectional area of the pulmonary vascular bed. In addition, patients with chronic bronchitis and long-standing hypoxemia often have compensatory polycythemia. The polycythemic blood of the chronic bronchitis produces an increased resistance to flow through the pulmonary circuit because of its increased viscosity, and attempts to increase cardiac output during respiratory compromise simply make the situation worse.

The patient with chronic bronchitis normally has an increase in airway resistance made worse during acute respiratory infection as a result of secretions and edema that further decrease the caliber of the small airways. These patients also have a loss of structural support from degenerative changes in the airways and from a loss of the stenting effect of the pulmonary parenchyma. For these reasons, the patient's small airways tend to collapse during exhalation and there is a rise in airway pressure from this "dynamic compression" phenomenon. In chronic bronchitis and emphysema the decrease in cross-sectional area of the pulmonary vessels results not from fibrotic obliteration of pulmonary capillaries or arterioles but rather from hypertrophy of the muscular media of the pulmonary arterioles. The vessels become compressible but not distensible, so that with exhalation and an increase in intrathoracic pressure, airway compression results in a further increase in pulmonary vascular resistance and an increase in pulmonary arterial pressure. The hypertrophied muscular media prevents the resulting increase in pulmonary arterial pressure from distending the pulmonary vessels and maintaining a normal pulmonary artery pressure. With the onset of respiratory embarrassment in the patient with chronic bronchitis, there are increases in pulmonary artery pressure, afterload, and the work requirement of the right ventricle that may result in right ventricular failure.

A similar pattern may be observed in other forms of pulmonary disease, since the compensatory mechanisms are much the same as in chronic bronchitis. Chronic bronchitis, however, is somewhat more amenable to therapy, because the acute pulmonary changes are often reversible. Relief of hypoxemia, for example, may be expected to afford some amelioration of the pulmonary hypertension. In pulmonary hypertension and cor pulmonale secondary to pulmonary fibrosis, relief of hypoxia probably has little to offer the pulmonary circulation, because the increase in pulmonary vascular resistance is due not to vasoconstriction of muscular pulmonary arterioles but rather to a fibrous obliteration of the pulmonary vascular bed.

Anesthetic Considerations

Monitoring for patients with pulmonary hypertension and cor pulmonale should provide a continuous assessment of pulmonary arterial pressure, right ventricular filling pressure, right ventricular myocardial oxygen supply/demand balance, and some measure of pulmonary function. The electrocardiogram allows for the monitoring of arrhythmias. In the setting of right ventricular hypertrophy where there is an increased possibility of coronary insufficiency, ECG monitoring allows observation of the development of ischemia or acute strain of the right ventricle, seen in the inferior, right precordial, or esophageal ECG leads.

Pulmonary artery pressure monitoring provides an indication of the workload imposed on the right ventricle in cor pulmonale. The pulmonary artery catheter affords the potential for monitoring the pulmonary artery pressure and also for monitoring the central venous pressure as an indication of the right ventricular filling pressure. Most anesthesiologists would choose to use pulmonary arterial monitoring in major surgical procedures associated with significant fluid shifts.

The pulmonary artery catheter can also aid in the distinction between left ventricular failure and respiratory failure. In left ventricular failure an elevated pulmonary artery pressure occurs with an elevated pulmonary capillary wedge pressure, whereas in respiratory failure there is often an elevation of pulmonary artery pressure with a normal pulmonary capillary wedge pressure. The use of the pulmonary artery catheter allows for the determination of cardiac output and pulmonary vascular resistance. It is important to follow the pulmonary artery pressure in this setting because an increase in pulmonary artery pressure is often the cause of acute cor pulmonale and because serial measurements of pulmonary artery pressure and the pulmonary vascular resistance allow the effects of therapeutic interventions to be evaluated.

The right ventricular contractile state and volumes can be estimated by the rapid-response thermistor calculations of right ventricular ejection fraction (RVEF) using specialized pulmonary artery catheters. This device can measure beat-to-beat RVEF but is affected by tricuspid regurgitation and cardiac arrhythmias.

Perioperative TEE is increasingly useful in this patient population owing to the increasing numbers of trained individuals and equipment. Two-dimensional imaging of biventricular function and noninvasive estimates of right ventricular systolic pressure (using the modified Bernoulli equation) are examples of applications of TEE monitoring for patients with pulmonary hypertension.

Pulse oximetry and arterial blood gas sampling are simple ways of assessing pulmonary function. Capnography is not an accurate method of assessing Pa_{CO_2} when significant dead space ventilation is present. The use of an indwelling arterial catheter facilitates arterial blood sampling. Calculation of intrapulmonary venous admixture by using mixed venous blood samples obtained from the pulmonary artery, however, is a more sensitive indicator of pulmonary dysfunction than Pa_{O_2} values alone.

In the anesthetic management of patients with pulmonary hypertension and cor pulmonale, special consideration must be given to the degree of pulmonary hypertension, those factors that improve or worsen it, and the functional state of the right ventricle. For example, if pulmonary hypertension is coexistent with hypoxia in a patient with chronic bronchitis, administration of oxygen may afford significant relief of the pulmonary hypertension. If, however, the pulmonary hypertension is secondary to massive pulmonary fibrotic changes, little relief of pulmonary hypertension would be expected with the administration of oxygen. If the patient has an increase in blood viscosity, as in the polycythemia of chronic hypoxia, moderate hemodilution may be of some benefit in reducing the pulmonary vascular resistance if oxygen delivery can be maintained. When pulmonary hypertension is present without right ventricular failure, potent volatile anesthetics (which are pulmonary vasodilating in higher concentrations) may be the anesthetic drugs of choice. If, with high concentrations of potent volatile anesthetics, however, there is a decrease in hypoxic vasoconstriction, there is a theoretical risk of hypoxemia. Potent volatile agents or ketamine may also be indicated if pulmonary hypertension exists in patients who have pulmonary parenchymal disease with a significant bronchospastic component. In contrast to the volatile anesthetic agents, nitrous oxide might increase pulmonary artery pressure and should be used cautiously in this setting.[119] In addition, factors that predispose to pulmonary vasoconstriction (e.g., hypoxia, hypercarbia, acidosis, hypothermia) should be avoided.[120]

When pulmonary hypertension coexists with cor pulmonale, the anesthetic technique should attempt to preserve right ventricular function. Anesthetic drugs that may have been useful in pulmonary hypertension with preserved right ventricular function are now contraindicated because of their myocardial depressant effects. The primary concern is the maintenance of right ventricular function in the presence of an elevated right ventricular afterload. In this setting, a technique employing an opioid, such as fentanyl, in combination with sedative-hypnotic drugs, such as propofol or midazolam, probably provides the best cardiovascular stability.[121]

Circulatory supportive measures in the setting of right ventricular failure do not differ in theory from measures employed in managing left ventricular failure (Table 2-11). Important concerns are ventricular preload, heart rate, the inotropic state of the ventricle, and ventricular afterload. Right ventricular preload can be assessed by measurement of the central venous pressure. Preload can be augmented by judicious fluid infusion or decreased with a vasodilator, such as nitroglycerin, that primarily affects venous capacitance in low doses. Ventricular preload can also be reduced by initiation of positive-pressure ventilation.

Inotropic support is often required in the setting of right ventricular failure with chronic cor pulmonale. An inotropic agent should be selected only after considering its pulmonary effects, and the effects of the inotropic intervention should be monitored. Just as in left ventricular failure, where the reduction of left ventricular afterload can produce an increase in stroke volume and cardiac output, so in right ventricular failure, reduction in right ventricular afterload can produce similar effects.

Dobutamine or milrinone tend to reduce pulmonary artery pressure and pulmonary vascular resistance and would probably be the inotropic drugs of choice in right ventricular failure without systemic hypotension. If right ventricular perfusion pressures need to be maintained, or when right ventricular contractility is severely impaired, norepinephrine and epinephrine are the preferred catecholamines even in patients with pulmonary hypertension.[122,123] Furthermore, vasopressin is particularly effective for the treatment of systemic hypotension in patients with right ventricular failure. Vasopressin (antidiuretic hormone) is a posterior pituitary hormone that causes dose-dependent vasoconstriction and antidiuretic effects.[124]

Vasodilators that have been found effective in reducing the afterload of the right ventricle include sodium nitroprusside, nitroglycerin, milrinone, adenosine, nifedipine, amlodipine, and prostaglandin E_1.[125,126] Inhaled nitric oxide selectively dilates the pulmonary vasculature and has been used to treat pulmonary hypertension in various clinical settings.[127-129] Prostacyclin acts via specific prostaglandin receptors and has also been shown to reduce pulmonary hypertension.[130] However, the vasodilatation is not selective for the pulmonary vasculature and systemic hypotension may ensue. Various newer prostacyclin analogs, such as epoprostenol, are now given for chronic pulmonary hypertension and may be useful for intraoperative use in the future. One caveat is that inadvertent discontinuation of chronic intravenous epoprostenol therapy may lead to a fatal pulmonary hypertensive crisis. The administration of prostacyclin and milrinone via inhalation has been described as a strategy to reduce systemic side effects.[131] Inhaled prostaglandins are replacing inhaled nitric oxide in some institutions due to cost considerations.

As noted previously, the use of positive-pressure ventilation and positive end-expiratory pressure (PEEP) may produce a decrease in right ventricular preload. Positive-pressure ventilation may produce an increase in pulmonary artery pressure by physically reducing the cross-sectional area of the pulmonary vasculature during the inspiratory phase of ventilation. Before PEEP is instituted it must be remembered that the functional residual capacity is already increased in patients with chronic obstructive pulmonary disease and that the use of PEEP may have little to offer in terms of improving ventilation-perfusion matching.

CONSTRICTIVE PERICARDITIS AND CARDIAC TAMPONADE

Normal Pericardial Function

The pericardium is not essential to life, as is demonstrated from the benign effects of pericardiectomy. However, the pericardium normally provides resistance to overfilling of the ventricles in conditions such as tricuspid regurgitation, mitral regurgitation, or hypervolemic states. The intrapericardial pressure reflects intrapleural pressure and is a determinant of ventricular transmural filling pressure. The pericardium also serves to transmit negative pleural pressure, which maintains venous return to the heart during spontaneous ventilation.[132]

Constrictive Pericarditis

Constrictive pericarditis results from fibrous adhesion of the pericardium to the epicardial surface of the heart (Table 2-12). Its key feature is increased resistance to

TABLE 2–11 Abbreviated Pulmonary Vascular Pharmacopeia

Drug	PAP	PCWP	Q_p	SAP	HR	PVR
α and β Antagonists						
Norepinephrine 0.05-0.5 µg/kg/min	↑	↑ to ↑↑	—	↑↑	NC or ↑	↑
Phenylephrine 0.15-4 µg/kg/min	↑↑	—	↓	↑↑	↓	↑
Epinephrine 0.05-0.5 µg/kg/min	↑	NC or ↓	↑	↑↑	↑	↑
Dopamine 2-10 µg/kg/min	NC or ↑	NC or ↓	↑	NC or ↑	↑	↓
Dobutamine 5-15 µg/kg/min	↑	↓	↑↑	NC or ↑	↑	↓
Isoproterenol 0.015-0.15 µg/kg/min	SL ↓	↓	↑↑	↓	↑↑	↓
Vasopressin 2-8 units/hr	NC or ↑	↑	—†	↑↑	NC or ↓	↑
β Antagonists						
Propranolol 0.5-2.0 mg	—	NC to ↑	NC or ↓	NC or ↓	↓↓	NC or ↑
Esmolol 50-300 µg/kg/min	—	NC to ↑	NC or ↓	NC or ↓	↓↓	NC or ↑
α Antagonists						
Phentolamine 1-3 µg/kg/min	↓	↓	↑	↓	↑	↓
Smooth Muscle Dilators						
Sodium nitroprusside 0.5-3 µg/kg/min	↓	↓	↑↑	↓↓	↑	↓
Nitroglycerin 0.5-5 µg/kg/min	↓↓	↓	NC to ↑	↓	↑	↓
Prostaglandin E_1 0.05-0.1 µg/kg/min	↓↓	↓	↑	↓	↑	↓
Adenosine 50-200 µg/kg/min	↓	↑	↑	NC or ↓	↑ or ↓	↓
Phosphodiesterase III Inhibitors						
Milrinone 0.375-0.75 µg/kg/min	↓	↓	↑	↓	↑	↓
Nitric oxide						
1-80 ppm	↓↓	↑	↑↑	NC	NC	↓↓
Epoprostenol						
(prostacyclin) 2-5 ng/kg/min IV	↓	NC	↑	↓	↑	↓
Iloprost						
(stable prostacycline analog) 10-50 µg via nebulizer	↓↓	NC	↑↑	NC	NC	↓↓

*Data not consistent, either NC, ↑ or ↓, most studies show less increase in PVR with norepinephrine compared with phenylephrine.
†Vasopressin significantly decreases cardiac output.
PAP, pulmonary artery pressure; PCWP, pulmonary capillary wedge pressure; Q_p, pulmonary blood flow; SAP, systemic arterial pressure; HR, heart rate; PVR, pulmonary vascular resistance.
—, data unavailable; SL ↓, slight decrease; NC, no change.

TABLE 2–12   Conditions Producing Constrictive Pericarditis and Cardiac Tamponade

	Associated Cardiac Conditions
Constrictive Pericarditis	
Idiopathic	
Infectious	
Can be sequela of most acute bacterial infections that produce pericarditis	Myocarditis
	Cardiomyopathy
Tularemia	Valve malfunction
Tuberculosis	
Viral—especially arbovirus, coxsackievirus B	
Mycotic	Valvular obstruction
Histoplasmosis	
Coccidioidomycosis	
Neoplastic	
Primary mesothelioma of pericardium	
Secondary to metastases—especially malignant melanoma	
Physical causes	
Radiation	Cardiomyopathy
Post-traumatic	Coronary artery disease
Postsurgical	
Systemic syndromes	
Systemic lupus erythematosus	Cardiomyopathy
	Coronary artery disease
Rheumatoid arthritis	Cardiomyopathy
	Coronary artery disease
	Aortic stenosis
Uremia	Cardiomyopathy
	Cardiac tamponade
Cardiac Tamponade	
Infectious	
Viral—most	Myocarditis
	Cardiomyopathy
	Valve malfunction
Bacterial—especially tuberculosis	
Protozoal	
Amebiasis	
Toxoplasmosis	
Mycotic infection	Valvular obstruction
Collagen disease	
Systemic lupus erythematosus	Cardiomyopathy
	Coronary artery disease
	Constrictive pericarditis
Acute rheumatic fever	
Rheumatoid arthritis	Cardiomyopathy
	Coronary artery disease
	Aortic stenosis
Metabolic disorders	
Uremia	
Myxedema	Low cardiac output
Hemorrhagic diatheses	
Genetic coagulation defects	
Anticoagulants	
Drugs	
Hydralazine	
Procainamide (Pronestyl)	
Phenytoin (Dilantin)	

TABLE 2–12	**Conditions Producing Constrictive Pericarditis and Cardiac Tamponade—cont'd**	
		Associated Cardiac Conditions
Physical causes		
Radiation		Cardiomyopathy
		Coronary artery disease
		Constrictive pericarditis
Trauma (perforation)		
Surgical manipulation		
Intracardiac catheters		
Pacing wires		
Neoplasia		
Primary—mesothelioma, juvenile xanthogranuloma		
Metastatic		
Miscellaneous		
Postmyocardial infarction—ventricular rupture		
Pancreatitis		
Reiter's syndrome		Aortic regurgitation
Behçet's syndrome		
Loeffler's syndrome—endocardial fibroelastosis with eosinophilia		Restrictive cardiomyopathy
Long-standing congestive heart failure		

normal ventricular filling. Constrictive pericarditis is a chronic condition that is usually well tolerated by the patient until the disease is far advanced. Acute cardiac tamponade, in contrast, is a syndrome in which the onset of restrictive symptoms is rapid and dramatic.[133-135]

A number of characteristic hemodynamic features accompany constrictive pericarditis and pericardial tamponade. Rather than the slight respiratory variation in blood pressure seen in normal patients, dramatic respiratory variations in blood pressure (pulsus paradoxus) are present. Kussmaul's sign (jugular venous distention during inspiration) is present. With adequate blood volume, the right atrial pressure in constrictive pericarditis is usually equal to or greater then 15 mm Hg and usually equals the left atrial pressure. The pulmonary artery systolic pressure is usually less than 40 mm Hg, which helps to distinguish constrictive pericarditis from cardiac failure. Both constrictive pericarditis and cardiac tamponade demonstrate a diastolic "pressure plateau" or "equalization of pressures." The right atrial pressure equals the right ventricular end-diastolic pressure, pulmonary artery diastolic pressure, and left atrial pressure. Early in the disease, cardiac output is normal, but with progression the cardiac output falls. Most symptoms are related to this fall in cardiac output or to the elevated venous pressure that develops in response to the decreased cardiac output and restriction of right ventricular filling.

Constrictive pericarditis often resembles a restrictive cardiomyopathy and occasionally presents a diagnostic dilemma. However, in contrast to constrictive pericarditis, cardiac output in a restrictive cardiomyopathy is decreased primarily, left atrial pressure is increased, mean pulmonary artery pressure is increased, and there is no pulsus paradoxus.[136-139]

Because constrictive pericarditis restricts ventricular diastolic filling, normal ventricular end-diastolic volumes are not obtained and stroke volume is decreased. Compensatory mechanisms include an increase in heart rate and contractility, which usually occur secondary to an increase in endogenous catecholamine release. This maintains cardiac output in the presence of the restricted stroke volume until the decrease in ventricular diastolic volume is quite severe. As cardiac output falls there is decreased renal perfusion. This results in increased levels of aldosterone, with a resultant increase in extracellular volume. The increase in extracellular volume increases right ventricular filling pressure, which eventually becomes essential for maintaining ventricular diastolic volume in the presence of severe pericardial constriction.

Cardiac Tamponade

Cardiac tamponade, like constrictive pericarditis, also restricts ventricular diastolic filling, but it is caused by extrinsic compression of the ventricular wall from fluid in the pericardium. Symptoms of cardiac tamponade are usually rapid in onset but depend on the rate and volume of pericardial fluid accumulation. With rapid fluid accumulation in the pericardium, a small volume can produce symptoms.[140] With a more gradual accumulation of fluid, the pericardium stretches, and larger pericardial volumes are tolerated before symptoms occur. Once symptoms begin, however, they proceed rapidly because of the sigmoidal relationship between pressure and volume in the pericardial sac. As the limit of pericardial distensibility is reached, small increases in volume produce dramatic increases in intrapericardial pressure. As such, removal of small volumes of pericardial fluid in a situation of severe cardiac tamponade can produce very dramatic relief of symptoms as a result of a rapid fall in intrapericardial pressure.[141]

The clinical features of cardiac tamponade result from restriction of diastolic ventricular filling and increased pericardial pressure. The increased pericardial pressure is transmitted to the ventricular chamber. This decreases the AV pressure gradient during diastole and impedes ventricular filling. Thus, there is a decrease in the end-diastolic ventricular volume and stroke volume. Increased diastolic ventricular pressure decreases coronary perfusion pressure and also results in early closure of the mitral and tricuspid valves, limiting diastolic flow and reducing ventricular volume. Figure 2-5 provides a diagrammatic summary of the pathophysiology of cardiac tamponade. The compensatory mechanisms in cardiac tamponade are similar to those in constrictive pericarditis. A decrease in cardiac output results in an increase in endogenous catecholamines. The consequent increases in heart rate and contractility help maintain cardiac output in the presence of a decreased stroke volume. Increased contractility increases the ejection fraction, allowing more complete ventricular emptying. Echocardiography will differentiate cardiac tamponade from constrictive pericarditis. Right ventricular and/or right atrial collapse is the echocardiographic hallmark of tamponade.[142]

Cardiac tamponade can be seen in blunt chest trauma when there is rupture of a cardiac chamber. However, the most common cardiac involvement in blunt chest trauma is cardiac contusion. Cardiac contusion may mimic an evolving myocardial infarction, and specific markers for cardiac injury, such as troponin T and troponin I, are increased in both conditions. Blunt chest trauma may also result in tricuspid regurgitation from a ruptured papillary muscle, traumatic ventricular septal defect, and dissection or interruption of the aorta.[143]

Anesthetic Considerations

Monitoring should be aimed at the compensatory mechanisms in constrictive pericarditis and cardiac tamponade. The electrocardiogram should be observed for heart rate and ischemic changes, because the myocardial oxygen supply/demand ratio can be altered by the pathologic process and also by therapeutic interventions. Filling pressures should also be assessed. The decision to use a pulmonary artery catheter or a central venous pressure catheter is based on the following: (1) the state of ventricular function; (2) the surgical procedure; and (3) the postoperative monitoring requirements. Central venous pressure monitoring is indicated in the following instances: (1) if cardiac tamponade is superimposed on an otherwise normal ventricle, as in trauma; (2) if the surgical procedure is only drainage of the tamponade fluid and an exploration of the pericardium in an effort to determine the cause of the tamponade (here the central venous pressure will adequately indicate the relief of cardiac tamponade); and (3) if postoperative monitoring is only aimed at following the potential reaccumulation of pericardial fluid. The central venous pressure is probably more sensitive than the pulmonary capillary wedge pressure in diagnosing reaccumulation of pericardial fluid.

The right ventricle has a very steep Starling curve with a relatively narrow range of filling pressures, which are lower than those of the left ventricle (Fig. 2-6). The filling pressures that would indicate reaccumulation of pericardial fluid are more widely divergent from the normal right ventricular filling pressures than they are from the filling pressures of the left ventricle. Accordingly, monitoring right ventricular filling pressures is a more sensitive indicator of developing tamponade. On the other hand, in chronic cardiac tamponade coupled with a cardiomyopathy, or in constrictive pericarditis of any cause, the pulmonary artery catheter probably provides more useful information. During a pericardiectomy, the pulmonary artery catheter is useful in assessing myocardial depression occurring secondary to cardiac manipulation and in assessing the volume status of the patient. Postoperative monitoring must address both the problems of reaccumulation of pericardial fluid and of the development of overt ventricular failure in patients with an underlying cardiomyopathy. Intra-arterial monitoring is nearly universally indicated in symptomatic constrictive pericarditis and pericardial tamponade.

Two-dimensional echocardiography is well suited to monitoring patients with constrictive pericarditis or tamponade. Intraoperatively, this can be performed with a transesophageal probe. According to the "Practice Guidelines for Perioperative Transesophageal Echocardiography"

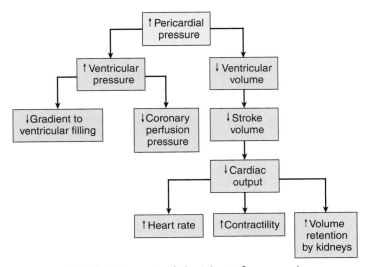

FIGURE 2–5 Schematic of physiology of tamponade.

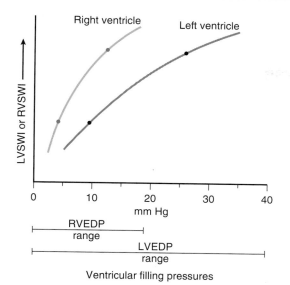

FIGURE 2–6 Right and left ventricular function curves where left or right ventricular stroke work index (LVSWI or RVSWI, respectively) is plotted as a function or right or left ventricular end-diastolic pressure (RVEDP or LVEDP, respectively).

published by the American Society of Anesthesiologists and the Society of Cardiovascular Anesthesiologists, the detection of pericardial effusions or evaluation of pericardial surgery is a category II indication for intraoperative TEE monitoring. The intraoperative evaluation of adequate drainage in patients undergoing pericardial window procedures is classified as a category I indication. Qualitative estimation of the degree of tamponade, localization of effusions, quantitative estimation of ejection fraction, and right- and left-sided preload conditions may be obtained with this technology.

The similar pathophysiology of cardiac tamponade and constrictive pericarditis create similar approaches for circulatory support. Cardiovascular support may be required before definitive therapy in either condition, but especially in cardiac tamponade. Circulatory therapy should be directed toward the three main compensatory mechanisms in these conditions: (1) maintenance of adequate ventricular filling; (2) maintenance of heart rate; and (3) maintenance of myocardial contractility. Intravascular volume maintenance is critical in these conditions, and a decline in filling pressures can result in dramatic decreases in cardiac output. Because an increased heart rate maintains the cardiac output in the presence of a decreased stroke volume, β-agonists are the inotropic drugs of choice because they increase the heart rate and contractility. Direct α-adrenergic agonists such as phenylephrine are contraindicated, because they increase SVR and usually decrease heart rate because of baroreceptor reflexes. With the use of inotropic drugs, such as epinephrine and dopamine, myocardial contractility is also maintained, contributing to homeostasis by increasing ejection fraction.

The first step in the anesthetic management of cardiac tamponade is to assess its severity. The anesthesiologist must decide whether induction of anesthesia can be tolerated. If the patient is tachycardic and hypotensive, with high filling pressures, pericardiocentesis or a pericardial window performed under local anesthesia is probably needed before the induction of general anesthesia. After the partial relief of severe cardiac tamponade, cardiac function should be reassessed. Usually, the hemodynamic situation is markedly improved. In the case of less severe symptoms, it is reasonable to induce general anesthesia using a reduced dosage of intravenous ketamine (0.25 to 1.0 mg/kg) or etomidate. Thiopental and propofol are relatively contraindicated because they may produce dramatic hypotension due to venodilation. High-dose narcotic anesthesia will not depress myocardial contractility, but the associated bradycardia may not be tolerated. The tachycardia associated with the use of pancuronium may be advantageous in maintaining circulatory homeostasis but should be used with caution in patients whose renal function is impaired by prerenal failure.[144-147]

In the presence of restricted ventricular diastolic filling, the initiation of positive-pressure ventilation may severely decrease venous return. When this occurs, intravascular volume must be increased in an effort to increase the ventricular filling pressure. After the relief of tamponade, the physiologic situation tends to revert to normal and further anesthetic requirements will then depend on the degree of cardiac manipulation by the surgeon during exploration of the pericardium (e.g., bleeding from a coronary graft may be the cause of the tamponade).

In constrictive pericarditis the altered physiology remains throughout most of the surgical procedure, whereas in cardiac tamponade the altered physiology is often rapidly relieved by opening the pericardium. The features of anesthetic management are similar to those of unrelieved cardiac tamponade: maintaining the intravascular volume, heart rate, and myocardial contractility. In this setting, similar anesthetic techniques are also used but a number of special problems may arise in the patient who comes to surgery for pericardiectomy. Arrhythmias, often requiring medical therapy, are quite frequent with the dissection of the adherent pericardial sac away from the ventricular epicardial surface. Rapid changes in filling pressures with cardiac manipulation occur. Thus, it is important for the anesthesiologist to be in constant communication with the surgeon concerning the hemodynamic response to the various manipulations of the heart. During pericardiectomy, with frequent episodes of hypotension, it is often difficult to distinguish relative hypovolemia and transient myocardial depression that occur with cardiac manipulation from incipient myocardial failure. Here the pulmonary artery catheter or TEE is particularly useful in distinguishing between hypotension due to hypovolemia and hypotension secondary to myocardial failure.[148]

Pericardiectomy is frequently associated with bleeding and coagulation problems. During the procedure there is a continued oozing of blood from the raw pericardial and epicardial surfaces that often necessitates transfusion. If the patient will not tolerate the severe cardiac manipulation, cardiopulmonary bypass with systemic heparinization is required for circulatory support during the procedure, particularly during the dissection on the posterior cardiac surface. If cardiopulmonary bypass and heparinization are required, then the coagulation problems become very complex. Platelet concentrates, fresh frozen plasma, and cryoprecipitate may be required if the bleeding is massive. These bleeding problems often continue after heparin reversal by protamine. Prophylactic therapy with lysine analog antifibrinolytics (ε-aminocaproic acid or tranexamic acid) or aprotinin should be considered. Even without the use of cardiopulmonary bypass, postoperative mechanical ventilation is probably the safest method of managing the post-pericardiectomy patient with multiple intraoperative problems such as continued bleeding, arrhythmias, and myocardial injury and depression.

UNCOMMON CAUSES OF VALVULAR LESIONS

The normal function of the cardiac valves is to maintain one-way forward flow during the cardiac cycle. Valvular lesions interfere with this function either by producing obstructions to forward flow or by allowing varying degrees of backward flow. This section will consider the pathophysiology of uncommon causes of valvular lesions and how these diseases affect cardiac compensatory mechanisms.

Lesions producing valvular stenosis are usually graded on the basis of valve area, which is normally calculated using echocardiography or by cardiac catheterization (using the Gorlin formula).[149] Flow is also influenced by such factors as blood viscosity and turbulence across the valve. Regurgitant lesions are usually evaluated on an ordinal scale by echocardiography or at angiography, based on the rate of dye clearance. Scales of 1+ through 4+, or estimations of mild, moderate, or severe, are common descriptors.[150-152] Effective regurgitant orifice of the mitral valve can be calculated by echocardiography in many patients, providing a more quantitative estimate of mitral regurgitation.

Rheumatic valvular lesions often exist as isolated defects in a relatively normal cardiovascular system, and they can be present for extended periods without symptoms. In contrast, the uncommon diseases considered here produce valvular lesions that are usually not associated with an otherwise normal circulatory system, because these lesions frequently occur in the setting of cardiomyopathy, pulmonary hypertension, cor pulmonale, or coronary artery disease. The asymptomatic period in rheumatic

lesions is related to the effectiveness of intrinsic cardiovascular compensatory mechanisms, and symptoms begin only when these compensatory mechanisms fail. With the diseases considered in this section, the normal methods of compensation are often severely compromised. Because anesthetic management of valvular lesions is directed at preserving the compensatory mechanisms, it is essential to understand how these diseases interfere with compensation and how anesthetic manipulations interact with them.

Aortic Stenosis (Table 2-13A)

Aortic stenosis results from a narrowing of the aortic valve orifice, with a pressure gradient across this narrow orifice. The obstruction to flow is proportional to the decrease in cross-sectional area of the obstructed outlet. The left ventricle compensates by increasing the transvalvular pressure to maintain flow. The ventricle undergoes concentric hypertrophy in order to force blood across the stenotic valve but suffers a decrease in compliance. As a result of hypertrophy, ventricular wall tension per unit area is decreased but total ventricular oxygen demand is increased because of an increase in left ventricular mass. Another method of compensation for aortic stenosis is an increase in ventricular ejection time that decreases the turbulent flow across the valve, thus decreasing flow resistance and allowing for more complete ventricular emptying.

As ventricular compliance falls, passive filling of the ventricle during diastole is decreased and the ventricle becomes increasingly dependent on atrial augmentation of ventricular diastolic volume. In this setting, the atrial "kick" may contribute as much as 30% to 50% to the left ventricular end-diastolic volume. There is increased intraventricular systolic pressure that virtually eliminates systolic coronary flow. Diastolic subendocardial blood flow also decreases as a result of a lower coronary perfusion pressure. Aortic diastolic pressure must remain high to maintain adequate myocardial blood flow.[153,154]

It should now be considered how an uncommon disease process might affect compensatory mechanisms. First, a disease could potentially interfere with the compensatory mechanism of concentric hypertrophy and increased ventricular contractility. In Pompe's disease, left ventricular hypertrophy occurs but is secondary to massive myocardial glycogen accumulation; and for this reason the ventricular strength is not increased to compensate for the outflow tract obstruction that commonly occurs in this disease. Another example would be amyloidosis in which aortic stenosis is coupled with a restrictive cardiomyopathy. Here, as in Pompe's disease, there is an inability to increase either ventricular muscle mass or contractility. A disease process may also interfere with the critical atrial augmentation of ventricular end-diastolic volume as, for example, in sarcoidosis or Paget's disease. Diseases of this type infiltrate the cardiac conduction system, resulting in

TABLE 2–13A   Uncommon Causes of Valvular Lesions

Disease	Features Affecting Compensatory Mechanisms		Associated Problems
	Atrial Transport and Rhythm	**Contractility and Hypertrophy**	
A. Aortic Stenosis (AS)			
1. Congenital and degenerative diseases			
a. Congenital			
(1) Valvular			
(2) Discrete subvalvular			
(3) Supravalvular			
b. Bicuspid valve			Coarctation of aorta, polycystic kidneys
c. Degenerative			
(1) Senile calcification			
(2) Mönckeberg sclerosis			
2. Infectious diseases			
a. Syphilis		Dilated cardiomyopathy and outflow obstruction	
b. Actinomycosis		Dilated cardiomyopathy and outflow obstruction	
3. Infiltrative diseases			
a. Amyloidosis	Sinoatrial and atrioventricular nodal infiltration	1. Dilated cardiomyopathy 2. Coronary artery disease	
b. Pompe's disease		1. Hypertrophic cardiomyopathy 2. Dilated cardiomyopathy	
c. Fabry's disese		Cardiomyopathy	Hypertension
d. Primary xanthomatosis	Atrial arrhythmias with rapid rate	1. Dilated cardiomyopathy 2. Coronary artery disease	
4. Miscellaneous			
a. Sarcoid	Arrhythmias and inflammation of conduction system	1. Left ventricular dyssynergy with aneurysm 2. Left ventricular infiltration and cardiomyopathy	
b. Endocardial fibroelastosis		1. Restriction of ventricular filling 2. Interference with subendocardial blood flow with decreased oxygen delivery to myocardium	1. Mitral valve malfunction with stenosis producing poor ventricular filling 2. Regurgitation decreasing left ventricular pressure development
c. Methysergide		Restriction of ventricular filling secondary to endocardial fibrosis	Similar to endocardial fibrosis
d. Paget's disease	1. Arrhythmias with loss of atrial kick 2. Complete heart block		Possible mitral stenosis and poor ventricular filling
B. Pulmonary Stenosis (PS)			
1. Congenital			
a. Valvular			
b. Infundibular			
c. Supravalvular with peripheral coarctation			
2. Genetic—Noonan's syndrome		Hypertrophic cardiomyopathy— obstructive and nonobstructive	Aortic regurgitation

Continued

TABLE 2–13A   Uncommon Causes of Valvular Lesions—cont'd

Disease	Features Affecting Compensatory Mechanisms		
	Atrial Transport and Rhythm	**Contractility and Hypertrophy**	**Associated Problems**
3. Infiltrative diseases			
a. Pompe's	Arrhythmias secondary to conduction system infiltration	Dilated cardiomyopathy	Aortic stenosis and outflow tract obstruction
b. Lentiginosis		Massive atrioventricular septal hypertrophy	
c. Sarcoid	Arrhythmias secondary to conduction system involvement	Cardiomyopathy	Cor pulmonale
4. Infectious			
a. Subacute bacterial endocarditis	Heart block		Tricuspid insufficiency
b. Tuberculosis			Pulmonary insufficiency
c. Rheumatic fever	Usually associated with other valvular lesions		
5. Neoplastic			
a. Mediastinal tumors			
b. Primary tumors			
1) Sarcoma	Rhythm or cardiomyopathic complications will depend on extent of wall involvement in the neoplastic process		
2) Myxoma			
c. Malignant carcinoid syndrome		Endocardial fibrosis	1. Pulmonary hypertension 2. Pulmonary regurgitation 3. Tricuspid regurgitation and/or stenosis
6. Physical—extrinsic causes			
a. Aneurysm of ascending aorta or sinus of Valsalva			
b. Constrictive pericarditis		Picture of restrictive cardiomyopathy but usually with good ventricular function	
c. Postsurgical banding			Often associated with other congenital cardiac abnormalities

arrhythmias or heart block with the loss of synchronous atrial contraction. The requirement for elevated ventricular diastolic filling pressure may be compromised in a situation, such as methysergide toxicity, that can produce mitral stenosis coupled with aortic stenosis. This reduces both passive ventricular filling and ventricular filling resulting from atrial contraction.

Diseases that affect the conduction system in addition to producing loss of atrial contraction can also produce tachyarrhythmias, which decrease ventricular ejection time and increase turbulent flow across the valves. Table 2-13A lists causes of aortic stenosis and key features of their pathophysiology that can adversely affect cardiac compensatory mechanisms.

Pulmonic Stenosis (see Table 2-13A)

As in aortic stenosis, the valve area is the critical determinant of transvalvular blood flow. Pulmonic stenosis produces symptoms that are similar to the classic clinical features of aortic stenosis: fatigue, dyspnea, syncope, and angina. The compensatory mechanisms in pulmonic stenosis are similar to those in aortic stenosis. Initially, under the stress of right ventricular outflow obstruction, the right ventricle dilates. However, it eventually undergoes concentric hypertrophy and changes from a crescent-shaped chamber best suited to handle volume loads to an ellipsoidal chamber best suited to handle pressure loads. Second, there is an increase in ejection time, maintained with a slow heart rate. Third, increases in ventricular filling pressure occur as a result of an increase in intravascular volume and a change in the compliance of the right ventricle.

The presence of angina, which occurs occasionally in pulmonic stenosis, should especially be noted. Usually, the right ventricle is a thin-walled chamber with low intraventricular pressures. This normal situation results in a high transmural perfusion pressure and good subendocardial blood flow that limits development of ischemia of the right ventricle. Concentric hypertrophy increases both right ventricular mass and right ventricular pressures, increasing the potential for ischemia of the right ventricle, since right ventricular oxygen requirements are increased and coronary perfusion may be decreased. Cyanosis can occur with severe pulmonic stenosis accompanied by a low, fixed cardiac output. When right ventricular pressure rises, a patent foramen ovale may produce right-to-left interatrial shunting. Usually, isolated pulmonic stenosis is well tolerated for long periods until compensatory mechanisms fail. When a second valvular lesion coexists with pulmonic stenosis, the potential effects of this lesion on compensatory mechanisms should be considered.[155]

Compensatory mechanisms in pulmonic stenosis can be altered in much the same way as in aortic stenosis. Decreases in right ventricular contractility occur in infiltrative diseases of the myocardium, such as Pompe's disease or sarcoidosis. The loss of the atrial "kick" and the development of tachyarrhythmias have the same implications for cardiac function in pulmonic stenosis as in aortic stenosis. In subacute bacterial endocarditis, tricuspid insufficiency may coexist with pulmonic stenosis, producing an impairment of pressure development in the right ventricle, especially when right ventricular failure supervenes. With the increase in right ventricular mass and the increased requirement for oxygen delivery to the right ventricle, the possibility should be considered that oxygen supply might be compromised, as in the coronary artery pathology of Pompe's disease.

Many of these patients are candidates for balloon valvuloplasty of the pulmonary valve. In this procedure, a balloon catheter is placed percutaneously and the tip is guided across the pulmonic valve. The balloon is inflated, tearing the fused leaflets apart.[156] A period of severe hypotension occurs during balloon inflation, and transient loss of consciousness, vomiting, and seizures may occur. Pulmonic regurgitation is invariably produced, but this is usually well tolerated hemodynamically. This procedure has reduced the number of patients presenting for operative valvuloplasty and valve replacement, although there are limited data on the long-term outcome for these patients.[157] In many institutions, anesthesiologists provide monitored care for these patients. Balloon valvuloplasty is also used for selected patients with aortic and mitral stenosis.

Aortic Insufficiency (Table 2-13B)

The primary problem in aortic insufficiency is a decrease in net forward blood flow from the left ventricle from diastolic regurgitation of blood back into the left ventricular chamber. The first question to ask in the setting of aortic insufficiency is whether the condition is acute or chronic, because this is often the main determinant of the degree of compensation. Aortic insufficiency represents an almost pure volume overload of the left ventricular chamber. The left ventricle responds initially with dilation to maximize the effects of increases in fiber length. Acutely, this may result in heart failure, because the increased ventricular diameter increases wall tension and end-diastolic pressure. An acute increase in ventricular volume may also compromise the anchoring of the mitral valve by changing the geometric relationship of the papillary muscles, resulting in mitral regurgitation and pulmonary edema.[158]

In chronic aortic insufficiency, however, a number of compensatory changes minimize the degree of diastolic regurgitation. The first compensatory mechanism is an increase in left ventricular chamber size with eccentric hypertrophy. The left ventricular compliance is increased, which produces an increase in volume at the same filling pressure, thus reducing end-diastolic pressure and wall tension. The increase in ventricular volume allows full use of the Frank-Starling mechanism, whereby the strength of ventricular contraction is increased with increasing fiber length. Ejection fraction is maintained, because both stroke volume and ventricular end-diastolic volume increase together. Despite these compensatory mechanisms, however, a number of studies have shown that ventricular contractility is depressed.[159] Nevertheless, the onset of clinical symptoms of aortic insufficiency does not necessarily correlate with ventricular function status.[160]

In contrast to aortic stenosis, the augmentation of ventricular end-diastolic volume by the atrial contraction is not essential to ventricular compensation in aortic insufficiency. A rapid heart rate seems to be advantageous in aortic insufficiency, because the rapid heart rate in aortic insufficiency reduces the time for diastolic filling and helps prevent diastolic overdistention of the ventricle from regurgitant flow. In aortic insufficiency, the amount of regurgitant flow increases as SVR increases. Thus, the third major compensatory mechanism in aortic insufficiency is the maintenance of a low peripheral resistance, because forward flow in aortic insufficiency is inversely proportional to the SVR.

The increase in chamber size and eccentric hypertrophy, which help maintain cardiac function in aortic insufficiency, can be compromised in such conditions as ankylosing spondylitis in which myocardial fibrosis limits the increase in chamber size to the degree that this disease produces a restrictive picture. Cogan's syndrome produces a generalized cardiomyopathy with coronary artery disease

TABLE 2–13B Uncommon Causes of Valvular Lesions

Disease	Features Affecting Compensatory Mechanism			Associated Cardiovascular Abnormalities
	Left Ventricular Compliance and Contractility	Heart Rate and Rhythm	Vascular Resistance	
A. Aortic Insufficiency				
1. Infiltrative disease				
a. Amyloidosis	Dilated and restrictive cardiomyopathy	Arrhythmias with infiltration of conduction system		1. Coronary artery disease 2. Stenosis or insufficiency of other valves
b. Morquio's c. Scheie's	Usually isolated aortic insufficiency with mild mucopolysaccharidosis			
d. Pseudoxanthoma elasticum	Dilated cardiomyopathy			
2. Infectious disease				
a. Bacterial endocarditis		Complete heart block		Insufficiency of other valves
b. Syphilis	Dilated or restrictive cardiomyopathy	Infiltration of conduction system		1. Aortic stenosis 2. Aortic aneurysm
c. Rheumatic fever				
3. Congenital valve disease				
a. Bicuspid aortic valve				
b. Aneurysm of sinus of Valsalva	Usually intact compensatory mechanisms			
c. Congenital fenestrated cusp				
4. Degenerative				
a. Marfan's	Normal	Normal	Cystic medial necrosis of aorta with dissection	Pulmonic insufficiency
b. Osteogenesis imperfecta	Normal	Normal	Cystic medical necrosis	Mitral regurgitation
5. Inflammatory				
a. Relapsing polychondritis				Mitral regurgitation
b. Systemic lupus erythematosus	Pericarditis and effusion		Hypertension secondary to renal disease	Mitral regurgitation
c. Reiter's syndrome				
d. Rheumatoid arthritis	Congestive cardiomyopathy	Complete heart block		1. Aortic stenosis 2. Mitral stenosis and/or insufficiency 3. Constrictive pericarditis 4. Cardiac tamponade
6. Systemic syndromes				
a. Ankylosing spondylitis		Complete heart block		Aortic dissection
b. Cogan's syndrome	1. Coronary artery disease 2. Dilated cardiomyopathy		Generalized angiitis	
c. Noonan's syndrome	Cardiomyopathy			Pulmonic stenosis
d. Ehlers-Danlos				Spontaneous vascular dissection
7. Miscellaneous causes				
a. Aortic dissection	Interference with compensation depends on cause, e.g., syphilis, Marfan's, traumatic			
b. Methysergide	Endocardial fibrosis—restriction of left ventricular filling			Mitral valve stenosis and/or insufficiency
c. Traumatic rupture	Acute dilatation and failure			

	Features Affecting Compensatory Mechanism			
Disease	Left Ventricular Compliance and Contractility	Heart Rate and Rhythm	Vascular Resistance	Associated Cardiovascular Abnormalities
B. Pulmonic Insufficiency				
1. Congenital				
a. Isolated				
(1) Hypoplastic	Usually tolerated as isolated lesion			
(2) Aplastic				
(3) Bicuspid				
a. Associated with other congenital cardiac lesions	Toleration of pulmonic insufficiency depends on degree of myocardial dysfunction induced by other cardiac lesions			
2. Acquired				
a. Syphilitic aneurysm of pulmonary artery	Dilated cardiomyopathy	Infiltration of conduction system	Luminal narrowing	
b. Rheumatic	Tolerated well in isolation			
c. Bacterial endocarditis		Complete heart block		Endocarditis of other valves
d. Echinococcus cyst	Endocardial fibrosis			Tricuspid valve malfunction
3. Malignant carcinoid syndrome	Endocardial fibrosis			Tricuspid valve malfunction
4. Physical				
a. Traumatic				
b. After valvotomy/valvuloplasty for pulmonic stenosis	Decreased ventricular compliance if right ventricle is hypertrophic from pulmonic stenosis			
5. Functional—secondary to pulmonary hypertension	Ventricular hypertrophy with decreased compliance		Elevated pulmonary resistance due to pulmonary hypertension	1. Chronic obstructive pulmonary disease 2. Mitral stenosis 3. Primary pulmonary hypertension

and can alter the compensatory mechanism by decreasing both the ability of the left ventricle to hypertrophy and that of the coronary arteries to deliver oxygen to the ventricle. Increases in left ventricular compliance could be prevented in situations such as aortic insufficiency produced by methysergide, which produces an endocardial fibrosis and thus decreased ventricular compliance. The usual ability of the left ventricle to maintain the ejection fraction in aortic insufficiency could be compromised by the cardiomyopathy of amyloidosis. The aortic insufficiency produced by acute bacterial endocarditis is occasionally associated with complete heart block, resulting in a slow heart rate with ventricular overdistention and a decrease in cardiac output. Aortic insufficiency due to conditions such as SLE associated with increased peripheral resistance can increase the regurgitant fraction in the presence of the incompetent aortic valve.[161,162]

Pulmonic Insufficiency (see Table 2-13B)

Pulmonic insufficiency usually occurs in the setting of pulmonary hypertension or cor pulmonale but may exist as an isolated lesion, as in acute bacterial endocarditis in intravenous drug users. It may also be iatrogenic, because it frequently is a sequela of pulmonary valvuloplasty procedures. Pulmonic insufficiency is extremely well tolerated for long periods of time. Like aortic insufficiency, it represents a volume overload on the ventricular chamber, but the crescentic right ventricular geometry is such that volume loading is easily handled. Compensatory mechanisms for pulmonic insufficiency are the same as for aortic insufficiency: an increase in right ventricular compliance, rapid heart rate, and low pulmonary vascular resistance. The right ventricle is normally a highly compliant chamber; and with its steep filling pressure-stroke volume curve, it functions very well in the presence of volume increases.

The degree of pulmonic regurgitation is determined by the pulmonary arterial diastolic to right ventricular end-diastolic pressure gradient. For this reason, low pulmonary vascular resistance and low left-sided filling pressure are essential to maintaining forward flow. In general, there is less increase in ventricular end-diastolic volume than in aortic insufficiency. The ejection fraction, however, is not as well maintained in pulmonic insufficiency as it is in aortic insufficiency. With severe pulmonic regurgitation, as in aortic insufficiency, eccentric hypertrophy of the ventricular chamber occurs.[163]

Disease states can interfere with the compensatory mechanisms of the right ventricle in several ways. Diseases that produce pulmonic insufficiency, such as the malignant carcinoid syndrome, also produce an endocardial fibrosis that decreases the ability of the right ventricular chamber to dilate in response to volume loading. Increases in right ventricular afterload increase the regurgitant fraction. This is especially true when pulmonic insufficiency is secondary to pulmonary hypertension. Hypoxemia can increase pulmonary vascular resistance as in the hypoxemia that results from pulmonary vascular dysfunction in carcinoid syndrome. It is unusual for a cardiomyopathy to coexist with isolated pulmonic insufficiency; thus the potential for eccentric hypertrophy is usually left intact. However, syphilis could present a situation in which a cardiomyopathy exists along with pulmonic insufficiency, although this would depend on the extent of syphilitic involvement of the myocardium.

Mitral Stenosis (Table 2-13C)

The primary defect in mitral stenosis is a restriction of normal left ventricular filling across the mitral valve. As in other stenotic lesions, the area of the valve orifice is the key to flow; and, as the orifice gets smaller, turbulent flow increases across the valve and total resistance to flow increases. The important features in compensation of mitral stenosis are (1) increasing the pressure gradient across the valve and (2) prolonging the duration of diastole. The compensatory mechanisms in mitral stenosis include (1) dilation and hypertrophy of the left atrium, (2) increases in atrial filling pressures, and (3) a slow heart rate to allow sufficient time for diastolic flow with minimal turbulence.[164]

Decompensation in rheumatic mitral stenosis usually occurs when there is atrial fibrillation with a rapid ventricular rate. This causes a loss of the atrial contraction and decreased time for ventricular filling, which results in pulmonary vascular engorgement. Thus, altered left ventricular function is usually not the limiting factor in the ability of the heart to compensate for mitral stenosis.[165]

As in other valvular lesions produced by uncommon diseases, coexistent cardiovascular problems that interfere with compensatory mechanisms are very important.

Diseases such as sarcoidosis or amyloidosis can infiltrate ventricular muscle, preventing left ventricular filling by decreasing compliance. Amyloidosis, gout, and sarcoidosis can also affect the conduction system of the heart, resulting in heart block, tachyarrhythmias, or atrial fibrillation.

Tricuspid Stenosis (see Table 2-13C)

Tricuspid stenosis is usually associated with mitral stenosis as a sequela of rheumatic fever. Usually the other valve lesions associated with tricuspid stenosis determine heart function and the tricuspid stenosis often exists as an almost incidental lesion. Isolated tricuspid stenosis is very rare, and the etiology is either carcinoid or congenital. The problems in tricuspid stenosis are similar to those in mitral stenosis. There is a large right atrial to right ventricular diastolic gradient, and flow across the stenotic tricuspid valve is related to valve area.[166,167]

The compensatory mechanisms in tricuspid stenosis are also similar to those in mitral stenosis. An increase in right atrial pressure maintains flow across the stenotic valve, and this is associated with hepatomegaly, jugular venous distention, and peripheral edema. Also, the heart compensates with right atrial dilatation and hypertrophy and increases in the strength of atrial contraction, improving the atrial transport of blood across the stenotic valve. The implications of slow heart rate in tricuspid stenosis are the same as in mitral stenosis. Ventricular contractility is usually well maintained. The onset of atrial fibrillation in tricuspid stenosis is a less crucial event than in mitral stenosis. In tricuspid stenosis it may produce symptoms such as an increase in peripheral edema, whereas in mitral stenosis it results in signs of left-sided failure.[168]

Diseases can interfere with cardiac compensation for tricuspid stenosis in much the same way as they can interfere with cardiac compensation for mitral stenosis. There may be further restriction of right ventricular filling in conditions such as malignant carcinoid syndrome that produce an endocardial fibrosis that reduces right ventricular compliance. Tricuspid stenosis frequently coexists with pulmonic stenosis in the carcinoid syndrome, resulting in a severe restriction of cardiac output.[169]

Mitral Regurgitation (Table 2-13D)

Mitral regurgitation, like aortic regurgitation, results from failure of the affected valve to maintain competence during the cardiac cycle. Mitral regurgitation occurs by one of three basic mechanisms: (1) damage to the valve apparatus itself; (2) inadequacy of the chordae tendineae–papillary muscle support of the valvular apparatus; or (3) left ventricular dilation and stretching of the mitral

TABLE 2–13C Uncommon Causes of Valvular Lesions

Disease	Features Affecting Compensatory Mechanisms			
	Rhythm	Atrial Transport	Left Ventricular Function	Associated Conditions
A. Mitral Stenosis				
1. Inflammatory				
a. Rheumatic fever				
b. Rheumatoid arthritis	Heart block	1. Pericardial constriction 2. Cardiac tamponade	Dilated cardiomyopathy	1. Aortic stenosis and insufficiency 2. Mitral insufficiency
2. Infiltrative				
a. Amyloidosis	1. Heart block 2. Infiltration of conduction system	Atrial dilatation and hypertrophy	Dilated and restrictive cardiomyopathy	Malfunctioning of other valves
b. Sarcoidosis	Infiltration of conductionx system		Dilated cardiomyopathy	1. Pulmonary hypertension 2. Cor pulmonale
c. Gout	Infiltration of conduction system			
3. Miscellaneous				
a. Left atrial myxoma				
b. Parachute mitral valve				
c. Concentric ring of left atrium	Normal compensatory mechanism			
d. Methysergide			Endocardial fibrosis	Mitral insufficiency
e. Wegener's granulomatosis	Arrhythmias secondary to myocardial vasculitis	Myofibrillar degeneration	Dilated cardiomyopathy	
B. Tricuspid Stenosis				
1. Inflammatory				
a. Rheumatic fever	Usually associated with other valvular lesions			
b. Systemic lupus erythematosus	Arrhythmias secondary to pericarditis		1. Coronary artery disease 2. Cardiomyopathy	
2. Fibrotic				
a. Carcinoid syndrome		Fibrosis evolving to hypertrophy and dilatation	1. Pulmonary hypertension with increased right ventricular afterload 2. Endocardial fibrosis	Pulmonic stenosis
b. Endocardial fibroelastosis	Similar to carcinoid syndrome			
c. Methysergide	Similar to carcinoid syndrome			Mitral and aortic valvular adnormality
3. Miscellaneous				
a. Hurler's syndrome	Infiltration of conduction system	Infiltration of atrial wall	Dilated cardiomyopathy	Aortic stenosis
b. Myxoma of right atrium		Usually normal compensatory mechanisms		

valve annulus with a loss of the structural geometry required for valvular closure.[170] Mitral regurgitation represents a volume overload of both the left atrium and the left ventricle, producing as much as a fourfold to fivefold increase in ventricular end-diastolic volume. In mitral regurgitation, ventricular ejection is usually well preserved because of the parallel unloading circuit through the open mitral valve, which allows a rapid reduction of wall tension in the ventricle during systole. However, the volume overload results in an irreversible decrease in contractility. Ironically, mitral regurgitation serves as its own protective afterload reduction system.[171]

Compensatory mechanisms in mitral regurgitation include ventricular dilation, elevations in ventricular

TABLE 2–13D   Uncommon Causes of Valvular Lesions

Disease	Rate	Left Ventricular Function and Compliance	Vascular Resistance	Associated Conditions
A. Mitral Regurgitation (MR)				
1. Conditions producing annular dilatation				
a. Aortic regurgitation		Usually in failure at this stage	Elevated with low output	
b. Left ventricular failure			Usually elevated	
2. Conditions affecting the chordae tendineae and papillary muscles				
a. Myocardial ischemia	Associated arrhythmias, especially bradyarrhythmias	Often poor	Normal or elevated if cardiac output decreased	
b. Chordal rupture				
c. Hypertrophic obstructive cardiomyopathy		Hyperkinetic with low ventricular compliance	Usually elevated	
3. Conditions affecting the valve leaflets				
a. Marfan's syndrome Ehlers-Danlos syndrome Osteogenesis imperfecta		Usually intact—these conditions also affect connective tissue of chordae tendineae		
b. Rheumatic fever				
c. Rheumatoid arthritis	Heart block	Dilated cardiomyopathy		Other associated valve abnormalities
d. Ankylosing spondylitis	Atrioventricular dissociation			Aortic regurgitation
e. Amyloidosis	Sinoatrial and atrioventricular nodal infiltration	Restrictive and dilated cardiomyopathy		Coronary artery disease
f. Gout	Urate deposits in conduction system	Usually normal		Coronary artery disease
B. Tricuspid Regurgitation				
1. Annular dilatation				
a. Right ventricular failure			Often secondary to pulmonary hypertension	
b. Pulmonic insufficiency		Right ventricle in failure or extremely dilated	Often secondary to pulmonary hypertension	
2. Leaflets, chordae, and papillary muscles				
a. Ebstein's anomaly				
b. Acute bacterial endocarditis				
c. Rheumatic fever		Compensation intact		

filling pressure, and the maintenance of low peripheral resistance. As in aortic insufficiency, ventricular dilation allows maximum advantage to be gained from the Frank-Starling mechanism. A low peripheral resistance maintains forward flow, whereas increases in peripheral resistance increase the degree of regurgitant flow through the mitral valve. In mitral regurgitation, the heart benefits from a relatively rapid heart rate, because a slow rate is associated with an increased ventricular diastolic diameter that may distort the mitral valve apparatus even further and result in increased regurgitation, in addition to increasing oxygen demand by an increase in wall tension.

A number of diseases can be cited that interfere with the compensatory mechanisms in mitral regurgitation. When mitral regurgitation is secondary to amyloid infiltration of the mitral valve, ventricular dilatation is compromised by coincident amyloid infiltration of the ventricular myocardium, which restricts ventricular diastolic filling.[172] Amyloid infiltration of the conduction system can cause heart block and bradycardia, resulting in increased mitral regurgitation for reasons noted earlier. In mitral regurgitation associated with left ventricular failure, there is, in addition to poor left ventricular function, an elevation of endogenous catecholamine activity, which increases peripheral vascular resistance to forward flow and regurgitant flow.

Tricuspid Insufficiency (see Table 2-13D)

Tricuspid insufficiency is mechanically similar to mitral insufficiency. The most common cause of tricuspid insufficiency is right ventricular failure.[173] Even in this setting, tricuspid insufficiency is usually well tolerated, just as it is well tolerated when it exists in isolation. Tricuspid insufficiency represents a volume overload of both the right ventricle and the right atrium. But because of the high compliance of the systemic venous system, pressure in the right atrium is usually not so elevated as it is in the left atrium in mitral insufficiency. This remains true until the right ventricle loses its compliance, as it might when faced with a high afterload, as in pulmonary hypertension states.

The main compensatory mechanism in tricuspid insufficiency is adequate filling of the right ventricle. Because the right ventricle is constructed to efficiently handle a volume load, cardiac output is usually maintained. An increase in venous return, that occurs as a result of the negative intrapleural pressure resulting from spontaneous ventilation, helps maintain adequate right ventricular filling even in the presence of tricuspid insufficiency. The main reason tricuspid insufficiency is well tolerated is that it is usually superimposed on a normal right ventricle. Tricuspid insufficiency usually becomes hemodynamically significant when there is coexisting right ventricular failure. In this situation, the loss of integrity of the right ventricular chamber due to the incompetent tricuspid valve results in an increase in regurgitant flow at the expense of forward flow through the pulmonary circulation, decreasing the volume delivered to the left ventricle, with a resulting decrease in cardiac output.

Mitral Valve Prolapse

Mitral valve prolapse is not an uncommon disease per se, with an incidence between 5% and 20% in the general population.[174] However, it does occur in association with uncommon diseases such as HOCM, left atrial myxoma, Wolff-Parkinson-White syndrome, long QT syndrome, Marfan's syndrome, and Ehlers-Danlos syndrome. In mitral valve prolapse, one or both mitral leaflet(s) is(are) displaced into the left atrium during ventricular systole. Complications of mitral valve prolapse include bacterial endocarditis, mitral regurgitation, thromboembolism, arrhythmias (both atrial and ventricular), syncope, and sudden death. The American Heart Association published recommendations for the prevention of bacterial endocarditis in patients with mitral valve prolapse.[175] Patients with suspected mitral valve prolapse and concurrent murmurs of mitral regurgitation should receive endocarditis prophylaxis. Preferably, patients with suspected mitral valve prolapse should undergo echocardiographic evaluation of the mitral valve before any procedure that has an associated risk of bacteremia. Mitral regurgitation documented by Doppler echocardiography, thickening of the mitral valve leaflets or mitral valve apparatus with mitral regurgitation, or exercise-induced mitral regurgitation in patients with mitral valve prolapse is an indication for antibiotic prophylaxis of infectious endocarditis.

Anesthetic Considerations

Perioperative problems will arise from valvular lesions when compensatory mechanisms acutely fail. Monitoring should be selected to give a continuing assessment of the status of these compensatory mechanisms. Certain aspects of monitoring should be considered common to all valvular lesions. The electrocardiogram is essential for monitoring cardiac rhythm and ischemic changes. Filling pressures should certainly be monitored, employing either the pulmonary artery catheter or a central venous pressure catheter, as appropriate to the specific lesion. Blood pressure can best be monitored with an indwelling arterial catheter. In addition, an arterial catheter provides for the monitoring of blood gases, which are important when pulmonary function is compromised. Pulse oximetry is valuable for determining that oxygenation is adequate. TEE is useful for assessing the changes in preload and contractility that result from anesthetic and surgical manipulations. Pulsed-wave Doppler and color flow mapping are useful for determining the flow characteristics of valvular lesions and their response to pharmacologic or surgical manipulations.[176]

In lesions such as aortic or pulmonic stenosis, where high pressure chambers have developed, monitoring of the appropriate ECG lead is mandatory for assessing ischemia.[177,178] Monitoring of rate and rhythm is especially important.[179,180] The reason for aggressive monitoring of filling pressures is clear if it is recalled that lesions, such as mitral stenosis, are exquisitely sensitive to preload.

In tricuspid and pulmonic stenosis, a pulmonary artery catheter may be difficult, if not impossible, to position. However, right-sided filling pressures indicate loading conditions in these lesions and can be monitored with a central venous pressure catheter. If the chest is to be opened in patients in whom it was not possible to pass a pulmonary artery catheter, a pulmonary artery pressure catheter can be inserted under direct vision. A left-sided atrial pressure catheter may also be inserted to follow left-sided filling pressures.

In left-sided valvular lesions, a pulmonary artery catheter is used in many institutions for monitoring both filling pressures and cardiac output. With the pulmonary artery catheter in place, vascular resistances for both the pulmonary and the systemic circulations can be calculated, allowing an assessment of therapeutic interventions, as has been mentioned before. Furthermore, changes in waveforms of the pulmonary capillary wedge pressure or central venous pressure tracings can often indicate increases in regurgitation or the development of regurgitation in situations of ventricular overdistention.

The anesthetic management of valvular lesions must avoid significant depression of contractility, because virtually all valvular lesions depend on good contractility as a major compensatory mechanism. This is especially true if the lesion coexists with a cardiomyopathy in which minor decreases in contractility can result in severe cardiac decompensation. In valvular lesions, a high-dose opioid technique probably represents the least trespass on physiologic reserves. Fentanyl, sufentanil, and remifentanil produce few cardiovascular changes, although bradycardia and chest wall rigidity may occur and postoperative ventilation is often required.[181,182] Rigidity is easily handled by the use of a neuromuscular blocker. Opioid-associated bradycardia may be advantageous in mitral and tricuspid stenotic lesions.

Nitrous oxide is a traditional supplement to narcotic analgesia, but it is a myocardial depressant and has the property of slightly increasing both pulmonary vascular resistance and SVR. This is usually not of great significance, but it may be important in severe regurgitant lesions, when it may increase regurgitant flow.[183,184] Ketamine is probably not an unreasonable anesthetic in regurgitant lesions, owing to its slight sympathetic stimulating properties, but it is contraindicated in stenotic lesions because of the problems associated with tachycardia. Etomidate is an intravenous anesthetic that is well tolerated by patients with valvular lesions.[185] Thiopental and propofol must be administered slowly and titrated to effect if they are to be used safely in patients with valvular disease.[186]

Neuromuscular blockers, when used in valvular lesions, should probably be selected according to their autonomic properties. For example, pancuronium may be useful in aortic or mitral insufficiency owing to the increase in heart rate. In stenotic lesions on the other hand, cisatracurium, rocuronium, and vecuronium will not result in detrimental increases in heart rate.[187,188]

UNCOMMON CAUSES OF ARRHYTHMIAS

Idiopathic Long QT Syndrome

This rare syndrome is usually a familial disorder. The typical patient has a primary prolongation of the QT interval (QTc > 440 ms) and syncopal episodes associated with physical or emotional stress. Congenital deafness is an associated condition.[189,190] In untreated patients, the mortality approaches 5% per year, which is quite remarkable for a population with a median age in the 20s. The severity of the disease is judged by the frequency of syncopal attacks. These attacks may be due to ventricular arrhythmias or sinus node dysfunction. The development of torsades de pointes is especially ominous and may be the terminal event for these patients.[191] Torsades de pointes is a malignant variety of ventricular tachycardia with a rotating QRS axis that is resistant to cardioversion.[192]

The pathogenesis of this syndrome is theorized to be an imbalance of sympathetic innervation. Left stellate ganglion stimulation lowers the threshold for ventricular arrhythmias, whereas right stellate ganglion stimulation is protective against ventricular arrhythmias. Relief of syncope and diminished mortality have been demonstrated in patients receiving β-blockers and those who have had high left thoracic sympathectomies.[193]

Anesthetic Considerations

Whereas the occasional patient will present for high left thoracic sympathectomy and left stellate ganglionectomy, these patients will also present for surgery unrelated to their primary disorder. Because physical stress has been documented as a trigger for syncopal episodes, it would be prudent to maintain β-blockade throughout the perioperative period.

The patient's usual oral dose of β-adrenergic blocker should be given with premedication to allay anxiety. The anesthetic technique should be tailored to minimize sympathetic stimulation. A high-dose opioid anesthetic is appropriate for this purpose and is effective at suppressing catecholamine elevations in response to noxious stimuli. Nitrous oxide causes mild sympathetic stimulation and should be avoided for this reason. Isoflurane and sevoflurane prolong the QT interval, whereas halothane shortens the QT interval.[194] Propofol has been shown to reduce the prolonged QT interval and QT dispersion in patients with idiopathic prolonged QT interval.[195] In especially long procedures, supplemental intravenous doses of a β-blocker or a continuous infusion of esmolol should be used. Droperidol is associated with QT prolongation and should be avoided.

Wolff-Parkinson-White and Lown-Ganong-Levine Syndromes

Wolff-Parkinson-White (WPW) and Lown-Ganong-Levine are preexcitation syndromes that result in supraventricular tachycardias. The presence of accessory anatomic bypass tracts enables the atrial impulse to activate the bundle of His in a shorter interval than it would through the normal AV nodal pathway. If there is an increase in the refractoriness of one of the pathways, then a reentrant tachycardia can be initiated. The electrocardiogram in WPW demonstrates a short PR interval (< 0.12 second), a delta wave (slurring of the R wave upstroke), and a widened QRS complex.[196]

Medications that produce more refractoriness in one pathway than in the other can create a window of functional unidirectional block. This initiates a circle of electrical impulse that results in a rapid ventricular rate. These patients are usually treated with drugs that prolong the refractory period of the AV node, such as β-blockers, verapamil, and digoxin, or drugs that increase the refractory period of the accessory pathway, such as procainamide and amiodarone.[197] However, the response of an individual patient will vary depending on the window of unidirectional block and the different effects the same drug will have on both pathways. For example, verapamil and digoxin may perpetuate the arrhythmias, especially when WPW is associated with atrial fibrillation.[198] A nonpharmacologic approach in the treatment of patients with preexcitation syndromes is catheter ablation of the accessory pathways.[199,200]

Anesthetic Considerations

The current treatment of choice for WPW is ablation of the accessory pathway, which is usually performed in electrophysiologic laboratories.[201,202] Anesthesiologists may be involved in an electrophysiologic diagnostic procedure (for young or uncooperative patients) or surgical ablative procedure.

The procedures often involve periods of programmed electrical stimulation in attempts to provoke the arrhythmias before and after the ablation of the accessory pathway. Antiarrhythmic medications are usually discontinued before the procedure. Thus, the patient presents for an anesthetic in a relatively unprotected state. Premedication is indicated to prevent anxiety that could increase catecholamine levels and precipitate arrhythmias. ECG monitoring should be optimal for the diagnosis of atrial arrhythmias (leads II and V1). In patients undergoing general anesthesia, an esophageal ECG electrode provides the best "noninvasive" atrial complex.

If tachyarrhythmias occur in the setting of an antegrade accessory pathway conduction such as WPW, drugs that prolong conduction time and refractoriness in the AV node should be avoided. Consequently, adenosine, β-blockers, calcium channel blockers, and digoxin are relatively contraindicated in the acute management of tachyarrhythmias in these patients. In the hemodynamically unstable patient, electrical cardioversion is the treatment of choice. If pharmacological treatment is necessary, amiodarone, flecainide, propafenone, or sotalol are the preferred agents; however, effects of these drugs are long lasting and may interfere with procedures and as ablation of the accessory pathways.

If general anesthesia is needed, an opioid-benzodiazepine–based or an opioid-propofol–based anesthetic regimen showed no effect on electrophysiologic parameters of the accessory conduction pathways.[203] Volatile anesthetics increased refractoriness within the accessory and atrioventricular pathways, with halothane having the least effect, followed by isoflurane and enflurane.[204] For patients presenting for ablation of accessory pathways, volatile anesthetics should, therefore, be avoided. For patients with preexcitation syndromes presenting for other procedures, volatile anesthetics may actually be indicated to prevent perioperative tachyarrhythmias.

THE TRANSPLANTED HEART

For the appropriate candidate with end-stage heart disease, heart transplantation has become a widely acceptable treatment modality, both for improving length and quality of life. The first human heart transplantation was performed in the late 1960s, but this practice was discontinued shortly thereafter because of organ rejection and opportunistic infections. Since 1980, with the introduction of more effective immunosuppression and improved survival, the procedure has emerged as a widely acceptable treatment modality for end-stage heart disease.[205] These recipients of heart transplants may present for noncardiac surgery and, therefore, the physiology of the denervated heart and the side effects of the immunosuppressive agents must be considered.

The Denervated Heart

The recipient atrium (which may remain after transplantation) maintains its innervation; however this has no effect on the transplanted heart. Therefore, the transplanted heart is commonly referred to as being denervated. The efferent (to the heart) and afferent (away from the heart) limbs of both the parasympathetic and sympathetic nervous systems are disrupted during cardiac transplantation. This has significant impact on the physiology of the transplanted heart and the response to commonly used pharmacologic agents in the perioperative period. Some degree of sympathetic reinnervation of the transplanted heart has been documented, although this reinnervation is delayed and incomplete.[206,207]

Immunosuppressive Therapy

The main agents used for chronic immunosuppression are calcineurin inhibitors, azathioprine, rapamycins (everolimus/sirolimus), tacrolimus, mycophenolate mofetil, corticosteroids, and azathioprine.[208,209] These drugs may interact with anesthetic agents, and they have side effects with anesthetic implications. Cyclosporine is nephrotoxic and hepatotoxic. Another important side effect associated with the use of cyclosporine is hypertension. Cyclosporine can also lower the seizure threshold. Tacrolimus is nephrotoxic and can lead to diabetes and high blood pressure. Chronic corticosteroid therapy is associated with glucose intolerance and osteoporosis, and azathioprine is toxic to the bone marrow.

Anesthetic Considerations

The physiology and response to pharmacologic agents are very different in the denervated heart. The vagal innervation of the heart is disrupted, and there is a lack of heart rate variability with respiration, vagal maneuvers, and exercise. Cholinesterase inhibitors, such as neostigmine and edrophonium, do not usually produce bradycardia, although there are case reports that link cardiac arrest and bradycardia to neostigmine administration even in the transplanted heart.[210,211] However, the effects on other organ systems (e.g., salivary glands) remain intact, and these drugs must still be used in combination with anticholinergic agents.[212] Similarly, anticholinergic agents, such as atropine, do not increase the heart rate, so that bradycardia is treated with direct-acting agents, such as isoproterenol, or with pacing. A paradoxical response with the development of AV block or sinus arrest after the administration of atropine in patients with transplanted hearts has been reported.[213] Drugs with vagolytic side effects, such as pancuronium, do not produce tachycardia. The denervated sinus and AV nodes have been shown to be supersensitive to adenosine and theophylline.[214]

Sympathetic stimulation can originate from two sources: neuronal or humoral. In the denervated heart, the neuronal input is initially disrupted and only partially restored, but increases in circulating catecholamines will increase heart rate. The Frank-Starling mechanism also aids in preserving the cardiac response to exercise or stress. Because of the denervation, indirect-acting cardiovascular agents have unpredictable effects. The response of the coronary circulation may also be affected.[215,216]

The normal innervated heart responds to an increase in aerobic demand mainly by an increase in heart rate. However, the initial response of the denervated heart to an increased demand is via the Frank-Starling mechanism: increasing stroke volume through preload augmentation. The increase in heart rate via the humoral pathway or circulating catecholamines is delayed. Overall, the response of the denervated heart to exercise or increased metabolic demand is subnormal.[217-219]

Sensory fibers in the heart play an important role in maintaining SVR. With rapid changes in SVR, the denervated heart may not respond appropriately, and these patients tolerate hypovolemia poorly. Sensory fibers in the heart are also important in the manifestations of myocardial ischemia. As such, the patient with a denervated heart may not experience angina, although there are reports to the contrary.

Another factor that must be considered in the anesthetic management of these patients is that the transplanted heart is also predisposed to accelerated coronary artery disease. Fibrous proliferation of the intima of epicardial vessels may result from a chronic rejection process and, within 5 years of transplantation, many patients would have developed significant occlusion of their coronary arteries.[220,221] Therefore, these patients must be evaluated for coronary artery disease.

The immunosuppressive agents also should be considered in the anesthetic plan. Cyclosporine is nephrotoxic and hepatotoxic and, therefore, these organ systems must be evaluated. Corticosteroids predispose patients to osteoporosis and gentle positioning is required. Patients on azathioprine should have an appropriate hematologic workup in the preoperative period.[222,223]

AIDS AND THE HEART

In 2002, there were nearly 900,000 cases of AIDS in the United States according to the Centers for Disease Control and Prevention.[224] The current estimates indicate that more than 40 million people worldwide may be infected with HIV.[225] HIV affects all organ systems, including the cardiovascular system. The heart can be affected by the HIV virus directly, and by opportunistic infections related to the immunocompromised state, malignancies common to the disease, and drug therapy.

Left ventricular diastolic function is affected early in the course of HIV infection. Coudray and colleagues[226] performed an echocardiographic evaluation on 51 HIV-positive patients and compared the results with data obtained from age- and sex-matched controls and found that HIV-positive patients, regardless of the presence of symptomatic disease, had impaired left ventricular diastolic function. The mechanism of this dysfunction is unclear but may be secondary to viral myocarditis, and the clinical significance remains to be determined. In contrast to this diastolic dysfunction early in the course of the infection, systolic dysfunction has been reported late in the course of the disease. This systolic dysfunction may be caused by zidovudine.[227]

Zidovudine is an antiviral agent that inhibits HIV reverse transcriptase. Electron microscopic studies have demonstrated that zidovudine disrupts the mitochondrial apparatus of cardiac muscle.[228,229] Domanski and coworkers, in a randomized prospective study, found that children infected with HIV who were treated with zidovudine had a significant decrease in left ventricular ejection fraction when compared with children infected with HIV who had not received zidovudine.[230] They suggested that left ventricular function should be evaluated by serial examination. Starc and coworkers found that 18% to 39% of children who were diagnosed with AIDS developed cardiac dysfunction within 5 years of follow-up and that cardiac dysfunction was associated with an increased risk of death.[231] The effects of the newer antiviral agents on the heart have not yet been established.

Heart involvement was found in 45% of patients with AIDS in an autopsy study.[232] Pericardial effusion, dilated cardiomyopathy, aortic root dilation and regurgitation, and valvular vegetations were the more frequent findings.[233,234] The pericardium is sometimes affected by opportunistic infections such as cytomegalovirus and by tumors, such as Kaposi's sarcoma and non-Hodgkin's type lymphoma. In addition, an autonomic neuropathy associated with HIV infection has been shown to cause QT prolongation, which may predispose these patients to ventricular arrhythmias.[235]

Anesthetic Considerations

Early in the course of HIV infection there is diastolic dysfunction that is usually clinically insignificant. As the disease progresses, and with prolonged treatment with zidovudine, there is reduction in left ventricular systolic function.[236] Signs and symptoms of left ventricular failure may be masked by concurrent pulmonary disease. An echocardiographic evaluation may provide useful information in this setting. Patients with advanced disease may also have pericardial involvement with pericardial effusion and tamponade.

General anesthesia is considered safe, but drug interactions and their impact on various organ systems and the patients overall physical status should be considered preoperatively. General anesthesia suppresses the immune system, but adverse effects on the disease progress in patients diagnosed with HIV infection or AIDS could not be documented.[237] Regional anesthesia is often the technique of choice, and early concerns about neuraxial anesthesia and the potential spread of infectious material intrathecally could not be confirmed.[238-242]

CONCLUSION

Although the main focus of each of these sections has been on the cardiovascular pathology encountered in uncommon diseases, the clinician should remember that very few of these diseases have isolated cardiovascular pathology. Many of the diseases discussed are severe multisystem

diseases, and an anesthetic plan must also consider the needs of monitoring dictated by other systemic pathology (e.g., measurements of blood sugar in diabetes secondary to hemochromatosis) and the potential untoward effects of drugs in unusual metabolic disturbances (e.g., the use of drugs with histamine-releasing properties such as thiopental or morphine in the malignant carcinoid syndrome).

Certainly, it cannot be proven or stated that one anesthetic technique is absolutely superior to all others in the management of any particular lesion, particularly those due to the unusual conditions discussed here. The key to the proper anesthetic management of any uncommon disease lies in an understanding of the disease process, particularly the compensatory mechanisms involved in maintaining cardiovascular homeostasis, the cardiovascular effects of anesthetic drugs, and the appropriate monitoring of the effects of anesthetic and therapeutic interventions.

References

1. Richardson P, McKenna W, Bristow M, et al: Report of the 1995 World Health Organization/International Society and Federation of Cardiology Task Force on the Definition and Classification of Cardiomyopathies. Circulation 1996;93:841-842.
2. Pinney SP, Mancini DM: Myocarditis and specific cardiomyopathies—endocrine disease and alcohol. In Fuster V, Alexander RW, O'Rourke RA (eds): Hurst's The Heart, 11th ed. New York, McGraw-Hill, 2004, pp 1949-1974.
3. Noutsias M, Pauschinger M, Poller WC, et al: Current insights into the pathogenesis, diagnosis and therapy of inflammatory cardiomyopathy. Heart Fail Monit 2003;3:127-135.
4. Kawai C: From myocarditis to cardiomyopathy: Mechanisms of inflammation and cell death: Learning from the past for the future. Circulation 1999;99:1091-1100.
5. Billingham ME, Tazelaar HD: The morphological progression of viral myocarditis. Postgrad Med J 1986;62:581-584.
6. Loukoushkina EF, Bobko PV, Kolbasova EV: The clinical picture and diagnosis of diphtheritic carditis in children. Eur J Pediatr 1998;157:528-533.
7. Rajiv C, Manjuran RJ, Sudhayakumar N, Haneef M: Cardiovascular involvement in leptospirosis. Indian Heart J 1996;48:691-694.
8. Mason JW: Myocarditis and dilated cardiomyopathy: An inflammatory link. Cardiovasc Res 2003;60:5-10.
9. Higuchi M de L, Benvenuti LA, Martins Reis M, Metzger M: Pathophysiology of the heart in Chagas' disease: Current status and new developments. Cardiovasc Res 2003;60:96-107.
10. Mohan SB, Parker M, Wehbi M, Douglass P: Idiopathic dilated cardiomyopathy: A common but mystifying cause of heart failure. Cleve Clin J Med 2002;69:481-487.
11. Mestroni L, Gilbert EM, Bohlmeyer TJ, Bristow MR: Dilated cardiomyopathies. In Fuster V, Alexander RW, O'Rourke RA (eds): Hurst's The Heart, 11th ed. New York, McGraw-Hill, 2004, pp 1889-1907.
12. Frishman WH, Del Vecchio A, Sanal S, Ismail A: Cardiovascular manifestations of substance abuse: II. Alcohol, amphetamines, heroin, cannabis, and caffeine. Heart Dis 2003;5:253-271.
13. Piano MR, Schertz DW: Alcoholic heart disease: A review. Heart Lung 1994;23:3-17.
14. Piano MR: Alcoholic cardiomyopathy: ncidence, clinical characteristics, and pathophysiology. Chest 2002;121:1638-1650.
15. Spies CD, Sander M, Stangl K: Effects of alcohol on the heart. Curr Opin Crit Care 2001;7:337-343.

16. Bing RJ: Cardiac metabolism: Its contributions to alcoholic heart disease and myocardial disease. Circulation 1978;58:965.

17. Wallace KB: Doxorubicin-induced cardiac mitochondrionopathy. Pharmacol Toxicol 2003;93:105-115.

18. Solem LE, Henry TR, Wallace KB: Disruption of mitochondrial calcium homeostasis following chronic doxorubicin administration. Toxicol Appl Pharmacol 1994;129:214-222.

19. Lipshultz SE, Rifai N, Dalton VM, et al: The effect of dexrazoxane on myocardial injury in doxorubicin-treated children with acute lymphoblastic leukemia. N Engl J Med 2004;351:145-153.

20. Geha AS, El-Zein C, Massad MG: Mitral valve surgery in patients with ischemic and nonischemic dilated cardiomyopathy. Cardiology 2004;101:15-20.

21. Stevenson LW, Bellil D, Grover-McKay M, et al: Effects of afterload reduction on left ventricular volume and mitral regurgitation in severe congestive heart failure secondary to ischemic or idiopathic dilated cardiomyopathy. Am J Cardiol 1987;60:654.

22. American Society of Anesthesiologists Task Force on Pulmonary Artery Catheterization: Practice guidelines for pulmonary artery catheterization: An updated report by the American Society of Anesthesiologists Task Force on Pulmonary Artery Catheterization. Anesthesiology 2003;99:988-1014.

23. Sandham JD, Hull RD, Brant RF, et al: A randomized, controlled trial of the use of pulmonary-artery catheters in high-risk surgical patients. N Engl J Med 2003;348:5-14.

24. Practice guidelines for perioperative transesophageal echocardiography. A report by the American Society of Anesthesiologists and the Society of Cardiovascular Anesthesiologists Task Force on Transesophageal Echocardiography. Anesthesiology 1996;84:986-1006.

25. Waagstein F, Stromblad O, Andersson B, et al: Increased exercise ejection fraction and reversed remodeling after long-term treatment with metoprolol in congestive heart failure: A randomized, stratified, double-blind, placebo-controlled trial in mild to moderate heart failure due to ischemic or idiopathic dilated cardiomyopathy. Eur J Heart Fail 2003;5:679-691.

26. Plank DM, Yatani A, Ritsu H, et al: Calcium dynamics in the failing heart: Restoration by beta-adrenergic receptor blockade. Am J Physiol Heart Circ Physiol 2003;285:H305-H315.

27. Fisher ML, Gottlieb SS, Plotnick GD, et al: Beneficial effects of metoprolol in heart failure associated with coronary artery disease. J Am Coll Cardiol 1994;23:943-950.

28. Erlebacher JA, Bhardwaj M, Suresh A, et al: Beta-blocker treatment of idiopathic and ischemic dilated cardiomyopathy in patients with ejection fractions ≤ = 20%. Am J Cardiol 1993;71:1467-1469.

29. Grimm W, Christ M, Bach J, et al: Noninvasive arrhythmia risk stratification in idiopathic dilated cardiomyopathy: Results of the Marburg Cardiomyopathy Study. Circulation 2003;108:2883-2891.

30. Eckardt L, Haverkamp W, Johna R, et al: Arrhythmias in heart failure: Current concepts of mechanisms and therapy. J Cardiovasc Electrophysiol 2000;11:106-117.

31. Maron BJ: Hypertrophic cardiomyopathy: A systematic review. JAMA 2002;287:1308.

32. Maron BJ, Bonow RO, Cannon RO, et al: Hypertrophic cardiomyopathy: Interrelations of clinical manifestations, pathophysiology, and therapy (in two parts). N Engl J Med 1987;316:780-789, 844-852.

33. Maron BJ, Epstein SE: Hypertrophic cardiomyopathy: A discussion of nomenclature. Am J Cardiol 1079;43:1242.

34. Maron BJ, Wolfson JK, Epstein SE, et al: Intramural ("small vessel") coronary artery disease in hypertrophic cardiomyopathy. J Am Coll Cardiol 1986;8:545-557.

35. Sherrid MV, Chaudhry FA, Swistel DG: Obstructive hypertrophic cardiomyopathy: Echocardiography, pathophysiology, and the continuing evolution of surgery for obstruction. Ann Thorac Surg 2003;75:620.

36. Kovacic JC, Muller D: Hypertrophic cardiomyopathy: State-of-the-art review, with focus on the management of outflow obstruction. Intern Med J 2003;33:521.

37. Yoerger DM, Weyman AE: Hypertrophied obstructive cardiomyopathy: Mechanism of obstruction and response to therapy. Rev Cardiovasc Med 2003;4:199-215.

38. Nishimura RA, Holmes DR: Hypertrophic obstructive cardiomyopathy. N Engl J Med 2004;350:1320-1327.

39. Roberts R, Sigwart U: New concepts in hypertrophic cardiomyopathies: II. Circulation 2001;104:2249-2252.

40. Maron BJ, McKenna WJ, Danielson GK, et al: American College of Cardiology/European Society of Cardiology clinical expert consensus document on hypertrophic cardiomyopathy. A report of the American College of Cardiology Foundation Task Force on Clinical Expert Consensus Documents and the European Society of Cardiology Committee for Practice Guidelines. J Am Coll Cardiol 2003;42:1687-1713.

41. Freedman RA: Use of implantable pacemakers and implantable defibrillators in hypertrophic cardiomyopathy. Curr Opin Cardiol 2001;16:58.

42. Maron BJ, Shen WK, Link MS, Epstein AE: Efficacy of implantable cardioverter-defibrillators for the prevention of sudden death in patients with hypertrophic cardiomyopathy. N Engl J Med 2000;342:365.

43. Sachdev B, Hamid MS, Elliott PM: The prevention of sudden death in hypertrophic cardiomyopathy. Expert Opin Pharmacother 2002;3:499-504.

44. van der Lee C, Kofflard MJ, van Herwerden LA: Sustained improvement after combined anterior mitral leaflet extension and myectomy in hypertrophic obstructive cardiomyopathy. Circulation 2003;108:2088.

45. Gietzen FH, Leuner CJ, Raute-Kreinsen U, et al: Acute and long-term results after transcoronary ablation of septal hypertrophy (TASH): Catheter interventional treatment for hypertrophic obstructive cardiomyopathy. Eur Heart J 1999;20:1342-1354.

46. Maron BJ, Nishimura RA, McKenna WJ, et al: Assessment of permanent dual-chamber pacing as a treatment for drug-refractory symptomatic patients with obstructive hypertrophic cardiomyopathy: A randomized, double-blind, crossover study (M-PATHY). Circulation 1999;99:2927-2933.

46a. Thompson R, Liberthson R, Lowenstein E: Perioperative anesthetic risk of noncardiac surgery in hypertrophic obstructive cardiomyopathy. JAMA 1985;254:2419-2421.

46b. Haering JM, et al: Cardiac risk of noncardiac surgery in patients with asymmetric septal hypertrophy. Anesthesiology 1996;85:254-259.

47. Ishiyama T, Oguchi T, Iijima T, et al: Combined spinal and epidural anesthesia for cesarean section in a patient with hypertrophic obstructive cardiomyopathy. Anesth Analg 2003;96:629-630.

48. Autore C, Brauneis S, Apponi F, et al: Epidural anesthesia for cesarean section in patients with hypertrophic cardiomyopathy: A report of three cases. Anesthesiology 1999;90:1205-1207.

49. Chatterjee K, Alpert J: Constrictive pericarditis and restrictive cardiomyopathy: Similarities and differences. Heart Fail Monit 2003;3:118-126.

50. Sarjeant JM, Butany J, Cusimano RJ: Cancer of the heart: Epidemiology and management of primary tumors and metastases. Am J Cardiovasc Drugs 2003;3:407-421.

51. Reynen K: Frequency of primary tumors of the heart. Am J Cardiol 1996;77:107.

52. Centofanti P, Di Rosa E, Deorsola L, et al: Primary cardiac tumors: Early and late results of surgical treatment in 91 patients. Ann Thorac Surg 1999;68:1236-1241.

53. Bjessmo S, Ivert T: Cardiac myxoma: 40 years' experience in 63 patients. Ann Thorac Surg 1997;63:697-700.

54. Isaacs H Jr: Fetal and neonatal cardiac tumors. Pediatr Cardiol 2004 (April, Epub ahead of print).

55. Blondeau P: Primary cardiac tumors—French studies of 533 cases. Thorac Cardiovasc Surg 1990;38(Suppl 2):192-195.

56. Hoffmeier A, Deiters S, Schmidt C, et al: Radical resection of cardiac sarcoma. Thorac Cardiovasc Surg 2004;52:77-81.

57. Sarjeant JM, Butany J, Cusimano RJ: Cancer of the heart: Epidemiology and management of primary tumors and metastases. Am J Cardiovasc Drugs 2003;3:407-421.

58. Gibbs P, Cebon JS, Calafiore P, Robinson WA: Cardiac metastases from malignant melanoma. Cancer 1999;85:78-84.

59. Moller JE, Connolly HM, Rubin J, et al: Factors associated with progression of carcinoid heart disease. N Engl J Med. 2003;348: 1005-1015.

60. Robiolio PA, Rigolin VA, Wilson JS, et al: Carcinoid heart disease: Correlation of high serotonin levels with valvular abnormalities. Circulation 1995;92:790-795.

61. Jacobsen MB, Nitter-Hauge S, Bryde PE, Hanssen LE: Cardiac manifestations in mid-gut carcinoid disease. Eur Heart J 1995;16: 263-268.

62. Attar MN, Moulik PK, Salem GD, et al: Phaeochromocytoma presenting as dilated cardiomyopathy. Int J Clin Pract 2003;57:547-548.

63. Eagle KA, Berger PB, Calkins H, et al: ACC/AHA Guideline Update for Perioperative Cardiovascular Evaluation for Noncardiac Surgery— Executive Summary: A report of the ACC/AHA task force on practice guidelines (Committee to Update the 1996 Guidelines on Perioperative Cardiovascular Evaluation for Noncardiac Surgery) J Am Coll Cardiol 2002;39:542-553.

64. Park KW: Preoperative cardiology consultation. Anesthesiology 2003;98:754-762.

65. Lautermann D, Braun J: Ankylosing spondylitis—cardiac manifestations. Clin Exp Rheumatol 2002;20(6 Suppl 28):S11-S15.

66. Violi F, Loffredo L, Ferro D: Premature coronary disease in systemic lupus. N Engl J Med 2004;350:1571-1575.

67. Rossi C, Randi ML, Zerbinati P, et al: Acute coronary disease in essential thrombocythemia and polycythemia vera. J Intern Med 1998;244:49-53.

68. Wajima T, Johnson EH: Sudden cardiac death from thrombotic thrombocytopenic purpura. Clin Appl Thromb Hemost 2000;6:108-110.

69. Hoffman JI, Buckberg GD: The myocardial oxygen supply-demand ratio. Am J Cardiol 1978;41:327.

70. Klocke FJ: Coronary blood flow in man. Prog Cardiovasc Dis 1976;19:117-166.

71. Mansi IA, Rosner F: Myocardial infarction in sickle cell disease. J Natl Med Assoc 2002;94:448-452.

72. Kaski JC, Tousoulis D, McFadden E, et al: Variant angina pectoralis. Circulation 1992;85:619-626.

73. Konidala S, Gutterman DD: Coronary vasospasm and the regulation of coronary blood flow. Prog Cardiovasc Dis 2004;46:349-373.

74. Maseri A, Severi S, DeNes M, et al: "Variant" angina: One aspect of a continuous spectrum of vasospastic myocardial ischemia. Am J Cardiol 1978;42:1019-1035.

75. Hillis LD, Braunwald E: Coronary artery spasm. N Engl J Med 1978;299:695-702.

76. Pitts WR, Lange RA, Cigarroa JE, Hillis LD: Cocaine-induced myocardial ischemia and infarction: Pathophysiology, recognition, and management. Prog Cardiovasc Dis 1997;40:65-76.

77. Lange RA, Cigarroa RG, Yancy CW, et al: Cocaine induced coronary artery vasoconstriction. N Engl J Med 1989;321:1557-1562.

78. Stambler BS, Komamura K, Ihara T, Shannon RP: Acute intravenous cocaine causes transient depression followed by enhanced left ventricular function in conscious dogs. Circulation 1993;87:1687-1697.

79. Kugelmass AD, Shannon RP, Yeo EL, Ware JA: Intravenous cocaine induces platelet activation in the conscious dog. Circulation 1995;91:1336-1340.

80. Grigorov V, Goldberg L, Mekel J: Isolated bilateral ostial coronary stenosis with proximal right coronary artery occlusion. Int J Cardiovasc Intervent 2000;3:47-49.

81. Holt S: Syphilitic osteal occlusion. Br Heart J 1977;39:469-470.

82. Asanuma Y, Oeser A, Shintani AK, et al: Premature coronary-artery atherosclerosis in systemic lupus erythematosus. N Engl J Med 2003;349:2407-2415.

83. Ehrenfeld M, Asman A, Shpilberg O, Samra Y: Cardiac tamponade as the presenting manifestation of systemic lupus erythematosus. Am J Med 1989;86:626-627.

84. Parisi Q, Abbate A, Biondi-Zoccai GG, et al: Clinical manifestations of coronary aneurysms in the adult as possible sequelae of Kawasaki disease during infancy. Acta Cardiol 2004;59:5-9.

85. Fulton DR, Newburger JW: Long-term cardiac sequelae of Kawasaki disease. Curr Rheumatol Rep 2000;2:324-329.

86. Malik IS, Harare O, AL-Nahhas A, et al: Takayasu's arteritis: Management of left main stem stenosis. Heart 2003;89:e9.

87. Selhub J, Jacques PF, Bostom AG, et al: Association between plasma homocysteine concentrations and extracranial carotid artery stenosis. N Engl J Med 1995;332:286-291.

88. Cleophas TJ, Hornstra N, van Hoogstraten B, van der Meulen J: Homocysteine, a risk factor for coronary artery disease or not? A meta-analysis. Am J Cardiol 2000;86:1005-1009, A8.

89. Pasceri V, Willerson JT: Homocysteine and coronary heart disease: A review of the current evidence. Semin Interv Cardiol 1999;4:121-128.

90. Turley K, Szarnicki RJ, Flachsbart KD, et al: Aortic implantation is possible in all cases of anomalous origin of the left coronary artery from the pulmonary artery. Ann Thorac Surg 1995;60:84-89.

91. Dodge-Khatami A, Mavroudis C, Backer CL, et al: Anomalous origin of the left coronary artery from the pulmonary artery: Collective review of surgical therapy. Ann Thorac Surg 2002;74:946-955.

92. Schwartz ML, Jonas RA, Colan SD: Anomalous origin of left coronary artery from pulmonary artery: Recovery of left ventricular function after dual coronary repair. J Am Coll Cardiol 1997;30:547-553.

93. Lambert V, Touchot A, Losay J, et al: Midterm results after surgical repair of the anomalous origin of the coronary artery. Circulation 1996;94(9 Suppl):II38-II43.

94. Said SA, el Gamal MI, van der Werf T: Coronary arteriovenous fistulas: Collective review and management of six new cases— changing etiology, presentation, and treatment strategy. Clin Cardiol 1997;20:748-752.

95. Kamiya H, Yasuda T, Nagamine H, et al: Surgical treatment of congenital coronary artery fistulas: 27 years' experience and a review of the literature. J Card Surg 2002;17:173-177.

96. Landesberg G, Mosseri M, Wolf Y, et al: Perioperative myocardial ischemia and infarction: Identification by continuous 12-lead electrocardiogram with online ST-segment monitoring. Anesthesiology 2002;96:264-270.

97. John AD, Fleisher L: Electrocardiography. Int Anesthesiol Clin 2004;42:1-12.

98. London MJ, Kaplan JA: Advances in electrocardiographic monitoring. In Kaplan JA, Reich DL, Konstadt SN (eds): Cardiac Anesthesia, 4th ed. Philadelphia, WB Saunders, 1999, pp 359-400.

99. Haggmark S, Hohner P, Ostman M, et al: Comparison of hemodynamic, electrocardiographic, mechanical, and metabolic indicators of intraoperative myocardial ischemia in vascular surgical patients with coronary artery disease. Anesthesiology 1989;70:19-25.

100. Smith JS, Cahalan MK, Benefiel DJ, et al: Intraoperative detection of myocardial ischemial in high-risk patients: Electrocardiography versus two-dimensional echocardiography. Circulation 1985;72:1015-1021.

101. Ellis JE, Shah MN, Briller JE, et al: A comparison of methods for the detection of myocardial ischemia during noncardiac surgery: Automated ST-segment analysis systems, electrocardiography, and transesophageal echocardiography. Anesth Analg 1992;75:764-772.

102. Comunale ME, Body SC, Ley C, et al: The concordance of intraoperative left ventricular wall-motion abnormalities and electrocardiographic S-T segment changes: Association with outcome after coronary revascularization. Multicenter Study of Perioperative Ischemia (McSPI) Research Group. Anesthesiology 1998;88: 945-954.

103. Kaplan JA, Wynands JE: Anesthesia for myocardial revascularization. In Kaplan JA, Reich DL, Konstadt SN (eds): Cardiac Anesthesia, 4th ed. Philadelphia, WB Saunders, 1999, pp 689-726.

104. Koch CG, Estafanous FG: Anesthesia for coronary artery surgery. Curr Opin Cardiol 1993;8:897-909.

105. Stanley TH, Webster LR: Anesthetic requirements and cardiovascular effects of fentanyl-oxygen and fentanyl-diazepam-oxygen anesthesia in man. Anesth Analg 1978;57:411.

106. Rich S, Dantzker DR, Ayres SM, et al: Primary pulmonary hypertension: A national prospective study. Ann Intern Med 1987;107:216-223.

107. Blaise G, Langleben D, Hubert B: Pulmonary arterial hypertension: Pathophysiology and anesthetic approach. Anesthesiology 2003;99:1415-1432.

108. Peacock AJ: Primary pulmonary hypertension. Thorax 1999;54:1107-1118.

109. Farber HW, Loscalzo J: Prothrombotic mechanisms in primary pulmonary hypertension. J Lab Clin Med 1999;134:561-566.

110. Hassell KL: Altered hemostasis in pulmonary hypertension. Blood Coagul Fibrinolysis 1998;9:107-117.

111. Haworth SG: Pulmonary hypertension in the young. Heart 2002;88:658-664.

112. Gibbs JS: Pulmonary hemodynamics: Implications for high altitude pulmonary edema (HAPE): A review. Adv Exp Med Biol 1999;474:81-91.

113. Rubin LJ: Primary pulmonary hypertension. N Engl J Med 1997;336:111-117.

114. Weitzenblum E: Chronic cor pulmonale. Heart 2003;89:225-230.

115. Stratmann G, Gregory GA: Neurogenic and humoral vasoconstriction in acute pulmonary thromboembolism. Anesth Analg 2003;97:341-354.

116. Smulders YM: Pathophysiology and treatment of haemodynamic instability in acute pulmonary embolism: The pivotal role of pulmonary vasoconstriction. Cardiovasc Res 2000;48:23-33.

117. MacNee W: Pathophysiology of cor pulmonale in chronic obstructive pulmonary disease: I. Am J Respir Crit Care Med 1994;150:833-852.

118. MacNee W: Pathophysiology of cor pulmonale in chronic obstructive pulmonary disease: II. Am J Respir Crit Care Med 1994;150:1158-1168.

119. Tempe D, Mohan JC, Cooper A, et al: Myocardial depressant effect of nitrous oxide after valve surgery. Eur J Anaesthesiol 1994;11:353-358.

120. Blaise G, Langleben D, Hubert B: Pulmonary arterial hypertension: Pathophysiology and anesthetic approach. Anesthesiology 2003;99:1415-1432.

121. Boyd O, Murdoch LJ, Mackay CJ, et al: The cardiovascular changes associated with equipotent anaesthesia with either propofol or isoflurane: Particular emphasis on right ventricular function. Acta Anaesthesiol Scand 1994;38:357-362.

122. Fischer LG, Van Aken H, Burkle H: Management of pulmonary hypertension: Physiological and pharmacological considerations for anesthesiologists. Anesth Analg 2003;96:1603-1616.

123. Kwak YL, Lee CS, Park YH, Hong YW: The effect of phenylephrine and norepinephrine in patients with chronic pulmonary hypertension. Anaesthesia 2002;57:9-14.

124. Gold J, Cullinane S, Chen J, et al: Vasopressin in the treatment of milrinone-induced hypotension in severe heart failure. Am J Cardiol 2000;85:506-508, A11.

125. Murali S, Uretsky BF, Reddy PS, et al: Reversibility of pulmonary hypertension in congestive heart failure patients evaluated for cardiac transplantation: comparative effects of various pharmacologic agents. Am Heart J 1991;122:1375-1381.

126. Nootens M, Schrader B, Kaufmann E, et al: Comparative acute effects of adenosine and prostacyclin in primary pulmonary hypertension. Chest 1995;107:54-57.

127. Steudel W, Hurford WE, Zapol WM: Inhaled nitric oxide: Basic biology and clinical applications. Anesthesiology 1999;91:1090-1121.

128. Mahoney PD, Loh E, Blitz LR, Herrmann HC: Hemodynamic effects of inhaled nitric oxide in women with mitral stenosis and pulmonary hypertension. Am J Cardiol 2001;87:188.

129. Goldman AP, Delius RE, Deanfield JE, Macrae DJ: Nitric oxide is superior to prostacyclin for pulmonary hypertension after cardiac transplantation. Ann Thorac Surg 1995;60:300-305.

130. Hinderliter AL, Willis PW 4th, Barst RJ, et al: Effects of long-term infusion of prostacyclin (epoprostenol) on echocardiographic measures of right ventricular structure and function in primary pulmonary hypertension. Primary Pulmonary Hypertension Study Group. Circulation 1997;95:1479-1486.

131. Haraldsson A, Kieler-Jensen N, Ricksten SE: The additive pulmonary vasodilatory effects of inhaled prostacyclin and inhaled milrinone in postcardiac surgical patients with pulmonary hypertension. Anesth Analg 2001;93:1439-1445.

132. Hoit BD, Faulx MD: Diseases of the pericardium. In Fuster V, Alexander RW, O'Rourke RA (eds): Hurst's The Heart, 11th ed. New York, McGraw-Hill, 2004, pp 1977-2000.

133. Troughton RW, Asher CR, Klein AL: Pericarditis. Lancet 2004;363:717-727.

134. Hancock EW: Constrictive pericarditis. JAMA 1975;232:176.

135. Sagrista-Sauleda J: Pericardial constriction: Uncommon patterns. Heart 2004;90:257-258.

136. Guntheroth WG: Constrictive pericarditis versus restrictive cardiomyopathy. Circulation 1997;95:542-543.

137. Chatterjee K, Alpert J: Constrictive pericarditis and restrictive cardiomyopathy: Similarities and differences. Heart Fail Monit 2003;3:118-126.

138. Field J, Shiroff RA, et al: Limitations in the use of the pulmonary capillary wedge pressure with cardiac tamponade. Chest 1976;70:451.

139. Shabetai R, Fowler NO, et al: The hemodynamics of cardiac tamponade and constrictive pericarditis. Am J Cardiol 1970;26:480.

140. Spodick DH: Acute cardiac tamponade. N Engl J Med 2003;349:684-690.

141. Shabetai R: Pericardial effusion: Haemodynamic spectrum. Heart 2004;90:255-256.

142. Asher CR, Klein AL: Diastolic heart failure: Restrictive cardiomyopathy, constrictive pericarditis, and cardiac tamponade: Clinical and echocardiographic evaluation. Cardiol Rev 2002;10:218-229.

143. Baum V: Anesthetic complications during emergency noncardiac surgery in patients with documented cardiac contusions. J Cardiothorac Vasc Anesth 1991;5:57-60.

144. Aye T, Milne B: Ketamine anesthesia for pericardial window in a patient with pericardial tamponade and severe COPD. Can J Anaesth 2002;49:283-286.

145. Webster JA, Self DD: Anesthesia for pericardial window in a pregnant patient with cardiac tamponade and mediastinal mass. Can J Anaesth 2003;50:815-818.

146. Campione A, Cacchiarelli M, Ghiribelli C, et al: Which treatment in pericardial effusion? J Cardiovasc Surg 2002;43:735-739.

147. Oliver WC Jr, Castro MA, Strickland RA: Uncommon diseases and cardiac anesthesia. In Kaplan JA, Reich DL, Konstadt SN (eds): Cardiac Anesthesia, 4th ed. Philadelphia, WB Saunders, 1999, pp 933-935.

148. Skubas NJ, Beardslee M, Barzilai B, et al: Constrictive pericarditis: Intraoperative hemodynamic and echocardiographic evaluation of cardiac filling dynamics. Anesth Analg 2001;92:1424-1426.

149. Gorlin R, Gorlin SG: Hydraulic formula of the area of stenotic mitral valve, other cardiac valves and central circulatory shunts. Am Heart J 1951;41:1-29.

150. Chen M, Luo H, Miyamoto T, et al: Correlation of echo-Doppler aortic valve regurgitation index with angiographic aortic regurgitation severity. Am J Cardiol 2003;92:634-635.

151. Zoghbi WA, Enriquez-Sarano M, Foster E, et al: Recommendations for evaluation of the severity of native valvular regurgitation with two-dimensional and Doppler echocardiography. J Am Soc Echocardiogr 2003;16:777-802.

152. Quinones MA, Otto CM, Stoddard M, et al: Recommendations for quantification of Doppler echocardiography: A report from the Doppler Quantification Task Force of the Nomenclature and Standards Committee of the American Society of Echocardiography. J Am Soc Echocardiogr 2002;15:167-184.

153. Jackson JM, Thomas SJ: Valvular heart disease. In Kaplan JA, Reich DL, Konstadt SN (eds): Cardiac Anesthesia, 4th ed. Philadelphia, WB Saunders, 1999, pp 727-784.

154. Carabello BA: Clinical practice: Aortic stenosis. N Engl J Med 2002;346:677-682.

155. Almeda FQ, Kavinsky CJ, Pophal SG, Klein LW: Pulmonic valvular stenosis in adults: Diagnosis and treatment. Cathet Cardiovasc Interv 2003;60:546-557.

156. Kern MJ, Bach RG: Hemodynamic rounds series II: Pulmonic balloon valvuloplasty. Cathet Cardiovasc Diagn 1998;44:227-234.

157. Rao PS: Long-term follow-up results after balloon dilatation of pulmonic stenosis, aortic stenosis, and coarctation of the aorta: A review. Prog Cardiovasc Dis 1999;42:59-74.

158. Rahimtoola SH: Aortic valve disease. In Fuster V, Alexander RW, O'Rourke RA (eds): Hurst's The Heart, 11th ed. New York, McGraw-Hill, 2004, pp 1643-1667.

159. Iskandrian AS, Hakki AH, Manno B, et al: Left ventricular function in chronic aortic regurgitation. J Am Coll Cardiol 1983;1:1374-1380.

160. Tarasoutchi F, Grinberg M, Filho JP, et al: Symptoms, left ventricular function, and timing of valve replacement surgery in patients with aortic regurgitation. Am Heart J 1999;138(3 Pt 1):477-485.

161. Jensen-Urstad K, Svenungsson E, de Faire U, et al: Cardiac valvular abnormalities are frequent in systemic lupus erythematosus patients with manifest arterial disease. Lupus 2002;11:744-752.

162. Olearchyk AS: Aortic regurgitation in systemic lupus erythematosus. J Thorac Cardiovasc Surg 1992;103:1026.

163. O'Rourke RA: Tricuspid, pulmonic valve, and multivalvular disease. In Fuster V, Alexander RW, O'Rourke RA (eds): Hurst's The Heart, 11th ed. New York, McGraw-Hill, 2004, pp 1707-1722.

164. Bruce CJ, Nishimura RA: Clinical assessment and management of mitral stenosis. Cardiol Clin 1998;16:375-403.

165. Ross J Jr: Cardiac function and myocardial contractility: A perspective. J Am Coll Cardiol 1983;1:52-62.

166. Waller BF, Howard J, Fess S: Pathology of tricuspid valve stenosis and pure tricuspid regurgitation: I. Clin Cardiol 1995;18:97-102.

167. Keefe JF, Walls J, et al: Isolated tricuspid valvular stenosis. Am J Cardiol 1970;25:252.

168. Morgan JR, Forker AD, et al: Isolated tricuspid stenosis. Circulation 1971;44:729.

169. Moyssakis IE, Rallidis LS, Guida GF, Nihoyannopoulos PI: Incidence and evolution of carcinoid syndrome in the heart. J Heart Valve Dis 1997;6:625-630.

170. Carabello BA: The pathophysiology of mitral regurgitation. J Heart Valve Dis 2000;9:600-608.

171. Rackley CE, Edwards JE, Karp RB: Mitral valve disease. In Hurst JW (ed): The Heart. New York, McGraw-Hill, 1986, pp 754-784.

172. Engelmeier RS, O'Connell JB, Subramanian R: Cardiac amyloidosis presenting as severe mitral regurgitation. Int J Cardiol 1983;4:325-327.

173. Waller BF, Howard J, Fess S: Pathology of tricuspid valve stenosis and pure tricuspid regurgitation: II. Clin Cardiol 1995;18:167-174.

174. Jacobs W, Chamoun A, Stouffer GA: Mitral valve prolapse: A review of the literature. Am J Med Sci 2001;321:401-410.

175. Dajani AS, Taubert KA, Wilson W: Prevention of bacterial endocarditis: Recommendations by the American Heart Association. Circulation 1997;96:358-366.

176. Lambert AS, Miller JP, Merrick SH, et al: Improved evaluation of the location and mechanism of mitral valve regurgitation with a systematic transesophageal echocardiography examination. Anesth Analg 1999;88:1205-1212.

177. Nadell R, DePace NL, Ren J-F, et al: Myocardial oxygen supply/demand ratio in aortic stenosis: Hemodynamic and echocardiographic evaluation of patients with and without angina pectoris. J Am Coll Cardiol 1983;2:258.

178. Rapp AH, Hillis LD, Lange RA, et al: Prevalence of coronary artery disease in patients with aortic stenosis with and without angina pectoris. Am J Cardiol 2001;87:1216-1217.

179. Sorgato A, Faggiano P, Aurigemma GP, et al: Ventricular arrhythmias in adult aortic stenosis: Prevalence, mechanisms, and clinical relevance. Chest 1998;113:482-491.

180. Wolfe RR, Driscoll DJ, Gersony WM, et al: Arrhythmias in patients with valvar aortic stenosis, valvar pulmonary stenosis, and ventricular septal defect: Results of 24-hour ECG monitoring. Circulation 1993;87(2 Suppl):I89-I101.

181. Bovill JG, Warren PJ, Schuller MH: Comparison of fentanyl, sufentanil, and alfentanil anesthesia in patients undergoing valvular heart surgery. Anesth Analg 1984;63:1081.

182. Lehmann A, Boldt J: Remifentanil in cardiac surgery. Anesth Analg 2001;92:557-558.

183. Konstadt SN, Reich DL, Thys DM: Nitrous oxide does not exacerbate pulmonary hypertension or ventricular dysfunction in patients with mitral valvular disease. Can J Anaesth 1990;37:613-617.

184. Schulte-Sasse U, Hess W, Tarnow J: Pulmonary vascular responses to nitrous oxide in patients with normal and high pulmonary vascular resistance. Anesthesiology 1982;57:9.

185. Lindeburg T, Spotoft H, Sorensen MB, et al: Cardiovascular effects of etomidate used for induction and in combination with fentanyl-pancuronium for maintenance of anaesthesia in patients with valvular heart disease. Acta Anaesthesiol Scand 1982;26:205.

186. Myles PS, Buckland MR, Weeks AM, et al: Hemodynamic effects, myocardial ischemia, and timing of tracheal extubation with propofol-based anesthesia for cardiac surgery. Anesth Analg 1997;84:12-19.

187. Hudson RJ, Thomson IR: Pro: The choice of muscle relaxants is important in cardiac surgery. J Cardiothorac Vasc Anesth 1995;9:768-771.

188. Fleming N: Con: The choice of muscle relaxants is not important in cardiac surgery. J Cardiothorac Vasc Anesth 1995;9:772-774.

189. Fraser GR, Froggatt P, James TN: Congenital deafness associated with electrocardiographic abnormalities. Q J Med 1964;33:361.

190. Ocal B, Imamoglu A, Atalay S, et al: Prevalence of idiopathic long QT syndrome in children with congenital deafness. Pediatr Cardiol 1997;18:401-405.

191. Booker PD, Whyte SD, Ladusans EJ: Long QT syndrome and anaesthesia. Br J Anaesth 2003;90:349-366.

192. Moss AJ, Schwartz PJ, Crampton RS, et al: Hereditable malignant arrhythmias: A prospective study of the long QT syndrome. Circulation 1985;71:17.

193. Schwartz PJ, Priori SG, Cerrone M, et al: Left cardiac sympathetic denervation in the management of high-risk patients affected by the long-QT syndrome. Circulation 2004;109:1826-1833.

194. Paventi S, Santevecchi A, Ranieri R: Effects of sevoflurane versus propofol on QT interval. Minerva Anestesiol 2001;67:637-640.

195. Michaloudis D, Kanoupakis E: Propofol reduces idiopathic prolonged QT interval and QT dispersion during implantation of cardioverter defibrillator. Anesth Analg 2003;97:301-302.

196. Oren JW 4th, Beckman KJ, McClelland JH, et al: A functional approach to the preexcitation syndromes. Cardiol Clin 1993;11:121-149.

197. Luedtke SA, Kuhn RJ, McCaffrey FM: Pharmacologic management of supraventricular tachycardias in children: I. Wolff-Parkinson-White and atrioventricular nodal reentry. Ann Pharmacother 1997;31:1227-1243.

198. Gulamhusein S, Do P, Carruthers SG, et al: Acceleration of ventricular response during atrial fibrillation in the Wolff-Parkinson-White syndrome after verapamil. Circulation 1982;65:348.

199. Pappone C, Santinelli V, Manguso F, et al: A randomized study of prophylactic catheter ablation in asymptomatic patients with the Wolff-Parkinson-White syndrome. N Engl J Med 2003;349:1803-1811.

200. Plumb VJ: Catheter ablation of the accessory pathways of the Wolff-Parkinson-White syndrome and its variants. Prog Cardiovasc Dis 1995;37:295-306.

201. Lowes D, Frank G, Klein J, Manz M: Surgical treatment of Wolff-Parkinson-White syndrome. Eur Heart J 1993;14:99-102.

202. Gaita F, Haissaguerre M, Giustetto C, et al: Safety and efficacy of cryoablation of accessory pathways adjacent to the normal conduction system. J Cardiovasc Electrophysiol 2003;14:825-829.

203. Sharpe MD, Dobkowski WB, Murkin JM, et al: Propofol has no direct effect on sinoatrial node function or on normal atrioventricular and accessory pathway conduction in Wolff-Parkinson-White syndrome during alfentanil/midazolam anesthesia. Anesthesiology 1995;82:888-895.

204. Sharpe MD, Dobkowski WB, Murkin JM, et al: The electrophysiologic effects of volatile anesthetics and sufentanil on the normal atrioventricular conduction system and accessory pathways in

Wolff-Parkinson-White syndrome. Anesthesiology 1994;80: 63-70.

205. Taylor DO, Edwards LB, Mohacsi PJ, et al: The registry of the International Society for Heart and Lung Transplantation: Twentieth official adult heart transplant report—2003. J Heart Lung Transplant 2003;22:616-624.

206. Burke MN, McGinn AL, Homans DC, et al: Evidence for functional sympathetic reinnervation of left ventricle and coronary arteries after orthotopic cardiac transplantation in humans. Circulation 1995;91:72-78.

207. Schwaiblmair M, von Scheidt W, Uberfuhr P, et al: Functional significance of cardiac reinnervation in heart transplant recipients. J Heart Lung Transplant 1999;18:838-845.

208. Eisen H, Ross H: Optimizing the immunosuppressive regimen in heart transplantation. J Heart Lung Transplant 2004; 23(5 Suppl):S207-S213.

209. Eisen HJ, Tuzcu EM, Dorent R, et al: Everolimus for the prevention of allograft rejection and vasculopathy in cardiac-transplant recipients. Engl J Med 2003;349:847-858.

210. Backman SB, Fox GS, Stein RD, et al: Neostigmine decreases heart rate in heart transplant patients. Can J Anaesth 1996;43:373-378.

211. Bjerke RJ, Mangione MP: Asystole after intravenous neostigmine in a heart transplant recipient. Can J Anaesth 2001;48:305-307.

212. Smith MI, Ellenbogen KA, Eckberg DL, et al: Subnormal parasympathetic activity after cardiac transplantation. Am J Cardiol 1990;66:1243-1246.

213. Bernheim A, Fatio R, Kiowski W, et al: Atropine often results in complete atrioventricular block or sinus arrest after cardiac transplantation: An unpredictable and dose-independent phenomenon. Transplantation 2004;77:1181-1185.

214. Ellenbogen KA, Thames MD, DiMarco JP, et al: Electrophysiological effects of adenosine on the transplanted human heart. Circulation 1990;81:821-825.

215. Bertrand ME, Lablanche JM, Tilmant M, et al: Complete denervation of the heart to treat severe refractory coronary spasm. Am J Cardiol 1981;47:1375-1377.

216. Aptecar E, Dupouy P, Benvenuti C, et al: Sympathetic stimulation overrides flow-mediated endothelium-dependent epicardial coronary vasodilation in transplant patients. Circulation 1996;94:2542-2550.

217. Auerbach I, Tenenbaum A, Motro M, et al: Attenuated responses of Doppler-derived hemodynamic parameters during supine bicycle exercise in heart transplant recipients. Cardiology 1999;92:204-209.

218. Bengel FM, Ueberfuhr P, Schiepel N, et al: Effect of sympathetic reinnervation on cardiac performance after heart transplantation. N Engl J Med 2001;345:731-738.

219. Cotts WG, Oren RM: Function of the transplanted heart: Unique physiology and therapeutic implications. Am J Med Sci 1997;314: 164-172.

220. Valantine H: Cardiac allograft vasculopathy after heart transplantation: Risk factors and management. J Heart Lung Transplant 2004;23(5 Suppl):S187-S193.

221. Costanzo MR, Naftel DC, Pritzker MR, et al: Heart transplant coronary artery disease detected by coronary angiography: A multi-institutional study of preoperative donor and recipient risk factors. Cardiac Transplant Research Database. J Heart Lung Transplant 1998;17:744-753.

222. Toivonen HJ: Anaesthesia for patients with a transplanted organ. Acta Anaesthesiol Scand 2000;44:812-833.

223. Kostopanagiotou G, Smyrniotis V, Arkadopoulos N, et al: Anesthetic and perioperative management of adult transplant recipients in nontransplant surgery. Anesth Analg 1999;89:613-622.

224. http://www.cdc.gov/hiv/stats.htm

225. UNAIDS Epidemic Update 2003; available at http://www.unaids.org

226. Coudray N, de Zuttere D, Force G, et al: Left ventricular diastolic function in asymptomatic and symptomatic HIV carriers: An echocardiological study. Eur Heart J 1995;16:61-67.

227. Domanski MJ, Sloas MM, Follmann DA, et al: Effect of zidovudine and didanosine treatment on heart function in children infected with human immunodeficiency virus. J Pediatr 1995;127:137-146.

228. Lewis W, Grupp IL, Grupp G, et al: Cardiac dysfunction occurs in the HIV-1 transgenic mouse treated with zidovudine. Lab Invest 2000;80:187-197.

229. Corcuera-Pindado A, Lopez-Bravo A, Martinez-Rodriguez R, et al: Histochemical and ultrastructural changes induced by zidovudine in mitochondria of rat cardiac muscle. Eur J Histochem 1994;34: 311-318.

230. Domanski MJ, Sloas MM, Follmann DA, et al: Effects of zidovudine and didanosine treatment on heart function in children affected with HIV. J Pediatr 1995;127:137-146.

231. Starc TJ, Lipshultz SE, Easley KA, et al: Incidence of cardiac abnormalities in children with human immunodeficiency virus infection: The prospective P2C2 HIV study. J Pediatr 2002;141: 327-334.

232. DeCastro S, Migliau G, Silvestri A, et al: Heart involvement in AIDS: A prospective study during various stages of the disease. Eur Heart J 1992;13:1452-1459.

233. Lipshultz SE: Dilated cardiomyopathy in HIV infected patients. N Engl J Med 1998;339:1153-1155.

234. Kaul S, Fishbein MC, Siegel RJ: Cardiac manifestations of acquired immunodeficiency syndrome: An update. Am Heart J 1991;122: 537-544.

235. Villa A, Foresti V, Confalonieri F: Autonomic neuropathy and prolongation of the QT interval in HIV infection. Clin Autom Res 1995;5:48-52.

236. Griffis CA: Human immunodeficiency virus/acquired immune deficiency syndrome–related drug therapy: Anesthetic implications. CRNA 1999;10:107-116.

237. Balabaud-Pichon V, Steib A: Anesthesia in the HIV positive or AIDS patient. Ann Fr Anesth Reanim 1999;18:509-529.

238. Kuczkowski KM: Human immunodeficiency virus in the parturient. J Clin Anesth 2003;15:224-233.

239. Hughes SC, Dailey PA, Landers D, et al: Parturients infected with human immunodeficiency virus and regional anesthesia: Clinical and immunologic response. Anesthesiology 1995;82:32-37.

240. Kuczkowski KM: Anesthetic considerations for the HIV-infected pregnant patient. Yonsei Med J 2004;45:1-6.

241. Evron S, Glezerman M, Harow E, et al: Human immunodeficiency virus: Anesthetic and obstetric considerations. Anesth Analg 2004;98:503-511.

242. Avidan MS, Jones N, Pozniak AL, et al: The implications of HIV for the anaesthetist and the intensivist. Anaesthesia 2000;55: 344-354.

Congenital Heart Disease

WILLIAM C. OLIVER, JR., MD, and JAMES J. LYNCH, MD

Isolated congenital heart disease (CHD) represents the most common category of birth defects, afflicting approximately 1% of liveborn infants.[1] The incidence of all forms of CHD is 75/1000 live births but 6 to 8/1000 live births when limited to moderate and severe forms.[2,3] From 1940 to 2002 about 1 million individuals with simple congenital heart defects, and half that number each with moderate or complex defects, were born in the United States.[4] The incidence of infants born with severe CHD remains low at 2.5 to 3.0/1000 live births, whereas moderately severe forms of CHD account for another 3/1000 live births.[2] Interestingly, compared with prior studies of CHD, the incidence has been steadily rising by three to nine times, in large measure owing to echocardiography, because earlier studies reflected only patients referred to the major centers for angiography.[2]

Previously, 41% of individuals with CHD died within 1 year of birth and 25% died in the first week of life.[5] Advances in surgery and management of CHD are allowing 85% of these infants and children to reach adulthood[6] with a life expectancy approaching that of the general population. Not only are neonates and infants doing better with treatment, but their preoperative mortality

has decreased. In the not too distant future there will be more adults with CHD than children. It is estimated that in the United States alone, at least 800,000 to 1 million adults currently have CHD.[7,8] The number of affected individuals is growing at an annual rate of 5% per year. Because of the increasing longevity of children, adolescents, and adults with CHD, greater numbers are undergoing noncardiac surgical procedures of both the minor and major variety.[9,10]

The condition of patients with CHD may vary significantly before noncardiac surgery. They may require noncardiac surgery with their CHD totally uncorrected, palliated, or completely corrected. Some individuals may have very mild CHD, requiring relatively little medical attention, whereas others have complex disease that demands significant medical expertise and resources.[2] "Corrective" surgery does not ensure that an individual is "normal" and unaffected by his or her CHD but instead may struggle with a range of problems, such as arrhythmias, congestive heart failure (CHF), and pulmonary hypertension (PAH).[11] Thus, anesthetic management of these persons will be highly individualized and complex, even though the CHD may be the same. Additionally, the crossover of CHD from pediatric to adult places both pediatric and adult anesthesiologists in unique positions, because one may be more familiar with CHD and the other more familiar with adults. This chasm impacts adults with CHD more than pediatric patients, with regard to noncardiac surgery and anesthesia. Patients with CHD who require noncardiac surgery provide a great challenge for anesthesiologists. In the following pages we will describe some of the more common congenital heart defects that an anesthesiologist may encounter in a noncardiac surgical environment from an anatomic, pathophysiologic, and anesthetic perspective.

CLASSIFICATION AND NOMENCLATURE

Defects of CHD are classified in many different ways, each with their own merits, but no one system has been totally satisfactory. From the standpoint of the anesthesiologist caring for these infants, children, and adults, three basic categories are useful from a functional point of view (Table 3-1). The defect will be classified according to increased pulmonary blood flow or decreased pulmonary blood flow. If there is no shunting of blood, the third category is obstruction of blood flow. The clinical representation of this classification is largely CHF or cyanosis. This simple

classification will facilitate formulation of an anesthetic strategy and its delivery.

Presently, there is no unified system of nomenclature for CHD. The terminology and classification suggested by Anderson and colleagues[12] is subsequently modified and used for this chapter. The orientation of the heart in the chest is defined by the direction in which the ventricles are aligned from base to apex (Fig. 3-1). Levocardia is the most common orientation. Because some of these heart defects are also associated with abnormalities of other organ systems, visceral sidedness (situs) is important to note. The cardiovascular, respiratory, and digestive systems acquire asymmetry during a point in embryologic development. Visceral sidedness is characterized as normal (situs solitus), mirror-image (situs inversus), and isomeric or indeterminate (situs ambiguus). Cardiac sidedness is determined by the position of the right atrium (RA), not the direction of the apex of the ventricle. The morphologic RA is normally right sided.[13] Another term, *connection,* is an anatomic term that indicates a direct link between two structures, whereas *drainage* indicates the direction of blood flow. Cardiac morphology is relatively constant compared with the anatomy but is important because it reflects the heart's potential for hemodynamic performance. The morphologic RA is characterized by a large pyramidal appendage and terminal crest (Fig. 3-2). The morphologic left atrium (LA) is very different from the RA in that it does not have a terminal crest or pectinate muscles, and the main body is smooth (Fig. 3-3). The atrioventricular (AV) valves are fibrous tissue flaps that connect ventricles and atria anatomically but separate them electrically. References to right or left AV valve minimize confusion that may occur with tricuspid or

TABLE 3–1   Flow Characteristics of Various Congenital Cardiac Lesions

Increased Pulmonary Blood Flow Lesions

Atrial septal defect
Ventricular septal defect
Patent ductus arteriosus
Endocardial cushion defect (atrioventricular septal defect)
Anomalous pulmonary venous drainage*
Truncus arteriosus*
Single ventricle*
Hypoplastic left heart syndrome

Decreased Pulmonary Blood Flow Lesions

Tetralogy of Fallot
Pulmonary atresia
Tricuspid atresia
Transposition of the great arteries*
Ebstein's anomaly
Eisenmenger's syndrome
Single ventricle*

Obstructive Lesions

Aortic stenosis
Coarctation of the aorta

*Systemic hypoxemia occurs as a result of the mixing of systemic and pulmonary venous returns. Classification as an increased or decreased pulmonary blood flow lesion depends on the absence or presence within the anatomic variation of the obstruction to pulmonary blood flow. Modified from Schwartz AJ, Campbell FW: Pathophysiological approach to congenital heart disease. In Lake CL (ed): Pediatric Cardiac Anesthesia, 3rd ed. Stamford, CT, Appleton & Lange, 1998, p 8.

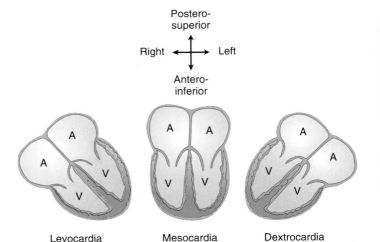

Postero-superior

Right ←——→ Left

Antero-inferior

Levocardia   Mesocardia   Dextrocardia

FIGURE 3–1 The cardiac base-apex axis is independent of cardiac position or sidedness. The three types are shown schematically. A, atrium; V, ventricle. (*Reprinted with permission from Edwards WD: Classification and terminology of cardiovascular anomalies. In Emmanouilides GC, Riemenschneider TA, Allen HD, Gutgesell HP [eds]: Moss and Adams Heart Disease in Infants, Children, and Adolescents: Including the Fetus and Young Adult. Baltimore, Williams & Wilkins, 1995, p 108.*)

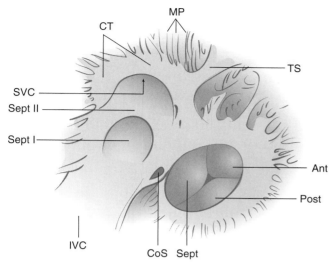

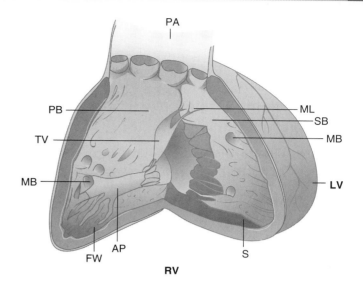

FIGURE 3–2 Interior of right atrium. Ant, anterior; CoS, coronary sinus; CT, crista terminalis (terminal crest); IVC, inferior vena cava; MP, musculi pectinati (pectinate muscles); Post, posterior; Sept, septal; Sept I, septum primum; Sept II, septum secundum; SVC, superior vena cava; TS, tinea sagittalis (sagittal worm); TV, tricuspid valve. *(Reprinted with permission from Van Praagh R: Cardiac anatomy. In Chang E [ed]: Pediatric Cardiac Intensive Care. Baltimore, Williams & Wilkins, 1998, p 4.)*

A

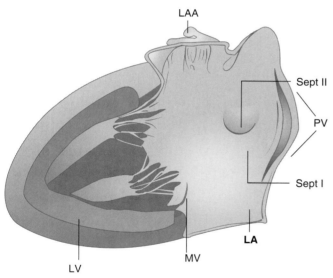

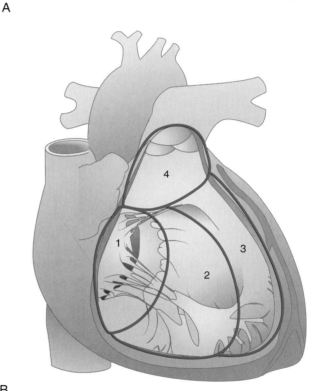

FIGURE 3–3 Interior of LA, left atrium. LAA, left atrial appendage; LV, morphologically left ventricle; MV, mitral valve; PV, pulmonary veins. *(Reprinted with permission from Van Praagh R: Cardiac anatomy. In Chang E [ed]: Pediatric Cardiac Intensive Care. Baltimore, Williams & Wilkins, 1998, p 5.)*

B

FIGURE 3–4 **A,** Interior of RV, right ventricle. AP, anterior papillary muscle; FW, free wall; LV, morphologically left ventricle; MB, moderator band; ML, muscle of Lancisi; PA, pulmonary artery; PB, parietal band; S, septum; SB, septal band; TV, tricuspid valve. **B,** The four main anatomic and developmental components of the right ventricle: (1) atrioventricular canal; (2) sinus; (3) septal band (proximal conus); and (4) parietal band (distal subsemilunar conus). Components 1 and 2 = RV inflow tract. Components 3 and 4 = RV outflow tract. *(Reprinted with permission from Van Praagh R: Cardiac anatomy. In Chang E [ed]: Pediatric Cardiac Intensive Care. Baltimore, Williams & Wilkins, 1998, p 7.)*

mitral valve nomenclature. The morphology of the AV valves typically follows the morphology of the ventricles of entry, not the atria of exit. A morphologic right ventricle is characterized by numerous small papillary muscles arising from the septal and free wall (Fig. 3-4). In contrast, the morphologic left ventricle has two groups of papillary muscles that arise from the free wall of the left ventricle (Fig. 3-5). The positions of the great vessels are generally described in relation to the position of the pulmonary trunk. Normally, the aorta is positioned right and posterior.

In describing the heart, three connections exist: veno-atrial, atrioventricular, and ventriculoatrial. Venoatrial connections include the superior and inferior vena caval veins connecting to the morphologic RA and the pulmonary veins connecting to the morphologic LA. There are four combinations of AV connections: concordant, discordant, univentricular, and ambiguous (Fig. 3-6). Concordant is the normal state, whereas discordant has the RA connected to the left ventricle. If both atria are connected to one ventricle, it is univentricular. The connection to the heart, not the heart itself is defined as univentricular.[13] The ventriculoarterial connections occur in four combinations: concordant, discordant, and double, single, and common outlets (Fig. 3-7). The concordant description is the normal state. Discordant involves a right ventricular origin of the aorta and a left ventricular origin of the pulmonary artery. If both great arteries arise from only one ventricular cavity, it is called double outlet. A single outlet refers to the situation of only one artery arising from a ventricular chamber without another vessel arising at all. A common outlet refers to one vessel that contains both the pulmonary and aorta as undivided roots. More detail regarding the nomenclature complexities of CHD is available.[13]

GENERAL PATHOPHYSIOLOGY PRINCIPLES

Knowledge of the pathophysiology of CHD is important for anesthetic management of these of individuals. Not all defects of CHD include shunting, but an understanding is helpful. Ohm's law (V = IR) is the basic principle of shunt physiology represented as:

Blood flow (Q) = Blood pressure (P)/resistance (R).

With the addition the of Hagen-Poiseuille equation that describes the relationship between flow through a cylinder of constant size and length, a formula can be devised that demonstrates anatomic factors that influence blood flow in CHD:

$$Q \propto P \times D \times 1/R$$

where Q = blood flow, P = pressure gradient, D = diameter, and R = resistance. Another major concept is the relationship between pulmonary vascular resistance (PVR) and systemic vascular resistance (SVR). The equations to calculate these two values are:

PVR = (mean pulmonary artery pressure
        − mean LA pressure)/pulmonary blood flow

SVR = (mean arterial pressure
        − mean RA pressure)/systemic blood flow

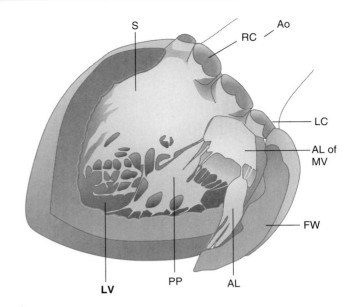

A

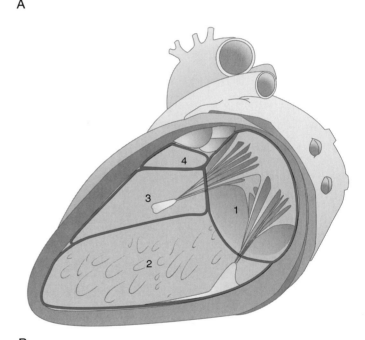

B

FIGURE 3–5 A, Interior of LV, left ventricle. AL, anterolateral (papillary muscle); AL of MV, anterior leaflet of mitral valve; Ao, aorta; FW, free wall; LC, left coronary (ostium); PP, posteromedial papillary (muscle); RC, right coronary (ostium); S, septum. **B,** The four main anatomic and developmental components of the LV: (1) atrioventricular canal; (2) sinus; (3) proximal conus; and (4) distal or subsemilunar conus. Components 1 and 2 = LV inflow tract. Components 1, 3, and 4 = LV outflow tract. *(Reprinted with permission from Van Praagh R: Cardiac anatomy. In Chang E [ed]: Pediatric Cardiac Intensive Care. Baltimore, Williams & Wilkins, 1998. p 9.)*

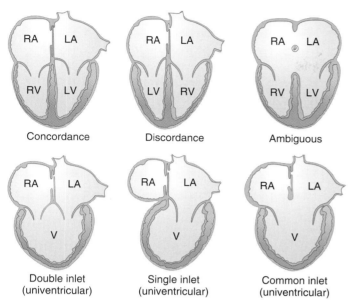

FIGURE 3–6 The possible atrioventricular connections are shown schematically. Concordance is synonymous with the normal state, and discordance is synonymous with ventricular inversion. For either right or left cardiac isomerism, the atrioventricular connection is always ambiguous. There are three possible univentricular forms of connection: double, single, and common inlet. RA, right atrium; RV, right ventricle; LA, left atrium; LV, left ventricle; V, ventricle. *(Reprinted with permission from Edwards WD: Classification and terminology of cardiovascular anomalies. In Emmanouilides GC, Riemenschneider TA, Allen HD, Gutgesell HP [eds]: Moss and Adams Heart Disease in Infants, Children, and Adolescents: Including the Fetus and Young Adult. Baltimore, Williams & Wilkins, 1995, p 121.)*

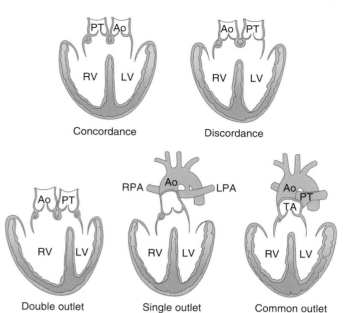

FIGURE 3–7 The possible ventriculoarterial connections are shown schematically. Concordance indicates the normal state, and discordance is synonymous with transposition of the great arteries. There are three other possible connections: double, single, and common outlet. RV, right ventricle; LV, left ventricle; Ao, aorta; RPA, right pulmonary artery; LPA, left pulmonary artery; PT, pulmonary trunk; TA, truncus arteriosus. *(Reprinted with permission from Edwards WD: Classification and terminology of cardiovascular anomalies. In Emmanouilides GC, Riemenschneider TA, Allen HD, Gutgesell HP [eds]: Moss and Adams Heart Disease in Infants, Children, and Adolescents: Including the Fetus and Young Adult. Baltimore, Williams & Wilkins, 1995, p 123.)*

The units for these values are mm Hg/L/min, commonly referred to as *Wood's unit*. PVR is usually below 3 units, whereas the SVR varies between 15 and 30 units.

Pulmonary blood flow can be calculated using the Fick principle with hemoglobin (Hb) concentration, saturations, and oxygen consumptions. Consequently, pulmonary blood flow (Q) is determined by:

$$Q = \frac{\text{oxygen consumption } (V_{O_2})}{\text{Arterial oxygen content (pulmonary vein} - \text{pulmonary artery)}}$$

Many catheterization reports will report the ratio of pulmonary blood flow to systemic blood flow (Q_p/Q_s) to express the degree of shunt. Excessive pulmonary blood flow is more than a Q_p/Q_s of 3. Inadequate pulmonary blood flow is a Q_p/Q_s of less than 1.

In the following pages, various defects of CHD are described concerning anatomy and pathophysiology and important concerns are presented regarding administration of anesthesia to the affected individuals.

NONCARDIAC SURGERY AND CHD

The Mayo clinic reported on 276 patients younger than the age of 50 years with CHD who underwent 480 procedures (surgical or diagnostic) during a 5-year period.[9] Forty-two percent of patients underwent two or more procedures during this interval. The congenital heart defects of the patients are displayed in Table 3-2. Left-to-right shunt was the most common defect found in 56% of the patients, with cyanotic CHD at 25% and obstructive CHD accounting for 17%. The median age at the time of the first procedure was 7 years.[9] The mortality rate (2.6%) was higher than the operative mortality of pediatric patients undergoing cardiac surgery with cardiopulmonary bypass (CPB), which is also the case with mortality for adults (4%) who undergo noncardiac surgery with CHD.[6] Mortality associated with noncardiac surgery in patients with CHD has been reported to be as high as 12% overall and 16% for major procedures.[10]

The challenge in the anesthetic management of patients with CHD corresponds to the multiple facets a particular congenital defect may consist of for each patient. This is supported by the fact that 5.4% of individuals with

TABLE 3–2   Primary Pathophysiologic Finding or Diagnosis in Study Patients with Congenital Heart Disease (N = 276)*

Primary Diagnosis	No. of Patients
Shunt	155
Isolated VSD	58
Patent ductus arteriosus	36
ASD[†]	35
Complete AV septal defect	10
Double-outlet right ventricle	7
Primum ASD and cleft left AV valve	4
Truncus arteriosus	3
Other	2
Cyanotic CHD	68
Single ventricle, excluding heterotaxia	25
Tetralogy of Fallot	15
Pulmonary valve atresia and VSD	10
Complex complete TGA	8
Ebstein's anomaly of the tricuspid valve	5
Simple complete TGA	4
Heterotaxia syndromes	1
Obstructive CHD	48
Pulmonary stenosis[‡]	21
Coarctation syndrome, including interrupted arch	18
Complex TGA	6
Vascular ring	3
Other	5
Congenital aortic regurgitation	1
Congenitally corrected TGA	1
Other anomalies	3

ASD, atrial septal defect; AV, atrioventricular; CHD, congenital heart disease; TGA, transposition of the great arteries; VSD, ventricular septal defect.
*Who underwent a noncardiac surgical procedure between January 1987 and November 1992.
[†]Excluding ostium primum ASD and including partial anomalous pulmonary veins.
[‡]Including subvalvular and supravalvular stenosis.
Reprinted with permission from Warner MA, Lunn RJ, O'Leary PW, Schroeder DR: Outcomes of noncardiac surgical procedures in children and adults with congenital heart disease. Mayo Clin Proc 1998;73:729.

various types of CHD experienced a perioperative complication with their first noncardiac procedure.[9] The incidence more than doubles to 12.9% if the patient is younger than 2 years of age.

The importance of the preoperative assessment and preparation cannot be overestimated. The presence of more severe defects and associated risk factors clearly makes these patients individuals who require the highest degree of care.

Preoperative Assessment and Preparation

For patients with CHD, it is especially important to thoroughly examine prior medical and surgical records to recognize any change in cardiac physiology and identify new or previously existing risk factors. Clearly, prior surgical or catheterization procedures may have resulted in physiologic changes that may impact patient care. A child with hypoplastic left heart syndrome (HLHS) has markedly different anesthetic considerations before and after a Norwood procedure.

Irrespective of whether cyanosis or CHF is present, neurologic, hematologic, renal, and pulmonary systems are profoundly affected.[6] To evaluate the severity of the CHD before surgery, certain characteristics such as arterial saturation less than 75% (cyanosis), Q/P greater than 2, left ventricular outflow tract gradient greater than 50 mm Hg, elevated PVR, and hematocrit (HCT) greater than 60% are established risk factors.[14] Accordingly, medications to treat CHF, inpatient surgical procedures, and higher ASA physical status have been associated with more complications in patients with CHD undergoing noncardiac surgery.[10] PAH is especially important to identify before surgery, because it has been associated with a complication rate of 15%, compared with 4.7% without PAH for patients undergoing noncardiac surgery.[9] Furthermore, differences in the respiratory system and ventilator management accompany the onset of PAH compared with those who do not develop it.[15]

Beyond the expected congenital heart risk factors, it is also important to identify common health disorders such as diabetes, hypertension, renal disease, or extracardiac anomalies that may be overshadowed by the CHD during the preoperative assessment and that are normally expected to increase surgical risk. Extracardiac anomalies are present in 20% to 35% of patients with CHD and tend to be mostly musculoskeletal or involve the central nervous system and renal-urinary system.[3,5] Sixty percent of individuals with extracardiac anomalies and CHD were affected by more than one system, excluding the cardiac anomaly.[16] Table 3-3 includes the most recognized chromosomal abnormalities with extracardiac anomalies to be associated with CHD.[1] Twenty-five percent of extracardiac anomalies exist in those with ventricular septal defect (VSD), tetralogy of Fallot (TOF), patent ductus arteriosus (PDA), complex coarctation, complex VSD, malpositions, and atrial septal defect (ASD). Trisomy 21 accounts for 71% of chromosomal abnormalities in those with CHD. Following trisomy 21, chromosome 22q11, referred to as CATCH, includes cleft palate, abnormal facies, thymic aplasia, cardiac defect, and hypocalcemia.[1] Genetic syndromes associated with CHD have been reviewed.[17]

Musculoskeletal abnormalities must be identified because they may cause obstacles to intubation and ventilation. A high index of suspicion is valuable because symptoms are usually nonspecific. Up to 25% of individuals with CHD may have an extracardiac anomaly involving the airway. Besides musculoskeletal abnormalities, enlarged cardiac or pulmonary vascular structures may

TABLE 3–3 **Chromosomal Causes of Congenital Heart Disease**

Mechanism	Chromosome/Region	Eponym	Characteristic Heart Defect(s)
Tetrasomy	22pter-q11	Cat's-eye syndrome	TAPVR, Persistent left SVC
Trisomy	13	Patau syndrome	VSD, PDA, ASD, dextroposition
	18	Edwards syndrome	VSD, ASD, PDA
	21	Down syndrome	VSD, AVSD, ASD
Monosomy	X	Turner syndrome	LVOT and aorta malformation
Deletion	3p	3p-syndrome	AVSD
	4p	Wolf-Hirschhorn	ASD
	5p	Cri du chat syndrome	Variable (in 30%)
	8 p	8p-syndrome	AVSD
	9p	9p-syndrome	VSD, PDA, PS
Microdeletion	7q11	Williams syndrome	SVAS, PPAS, PS
	17p11.2	Smith-Magenis syndrome	PS, ASD, VSD, AV valve malformation
	17p13.3	Miller-Dieker syndrome	TOF, VSD, PS
	22q11.2	Di George syndrome*	Outflow tract and aortic arch anomalies

ASD, atrial septal defect; AV, atrioventricular; AVSD, atrioventricular septal defect; LVOT, left ventricular outflow tract; PDA, patent ductus arteriosus; PPAS, peripheral pulmonary artery stenosis; PS, pulmonary valve stenosis; SVAS, supravalvar aortic stenosis; TAPVR, PAPVR, total/partial anomalous pulmonary venous return; TOF, tetralogy of Fallot; VSD, ventricular septal defect.
*Related syndromes caused by 22q11 microdeletion: velocardiofacial (Shprintzen) syndrome, conotruncal anomaly-face syndrome.
Reprinted with permission from Brennan P, Young ID: Congenital heart malformation: Aetiology and association. Semin Neonatol 2001;6:18.

threaten airway patency by extrinsic compression in these patients.[18] Careful inspection of the airway in anticipation of tracheal intubation is critical, because respiratory reserve is significantly limited. Obstruction is common with aortic dilation secondary to pulmonary atresia with VSD and major aortopulmonary collaterals and right aortic arch.[19]

It is rare to encounter coronary artery disease in patients with CHD, but chronic myocardial injury may be present in up to 40% of some defects, possibly related to inadequate perfusion for various reasons, but not atherosclerosis. Right-sided myocardial ischemia is more likely in those with right-sided cardiac defects.[14] PDA, coarctation of the aorta, and TOF have been associated with myocardial damage in infancy.[20] Although electrocardiographic (ECG) evidence may be lacking, individuals with CHF are especially at risk for myocardial ischemia.[20] Doppler color flow velocity is a good option to noninvasively assess coronary flow.[21]

Unless surgery is emergent, optimal physical condition is valuable for individuals with CHD. Evidence of worsening CHF with tachypnea or rales should at least delay surgery pending further investigation. However, respiratory abnormalities are often difficult to differentiate from cardiovascular abnormalities with CHD. Wheezing may be evidence of a new pulmonary infection or a manifestation of CHD.

Arrhythmias are common in patients with CHD, especially adolescents and adults.[22] It is important to identify a history of arrhythmias in these patients, because they may be occult or chronic, contributing to a slow hemodynamic deterioration.[23] In adults, Holter monitoring may be recommended to identify occult arrhythmias. Atrial dysrhythmias are especially common since volume loads predispose to dilated atria. The most common arrhythmias to occur in patients with CHD are the intra-atrial reentrant tachycardias (IART). They primarily originate in the RA. Similar to atrial flutter, IART have longer cycle lengths and multiple variations of P wave morphology. Management of these arrhythmias is complicated and has been reviewed.[24] Atrial fibrillation is less common than IART but is as difficult to treat at times, requiring a Maze procedure. Ventricular tachycardia is rare in CHD compared with other arrhythmias, but ventriculotomy may cause electrical instability and ventricular ectopy. Underperfused myocardium due to hypertrophy is predisposed to ventricular dysrhythmias. Sinoatrial node dysfunction and AV conduction abnormalities are also common in CHD, but pacemaker implantation may be challenging.[24] Certain congenital heart defects are more often associated with arrhythmias (Table 3-4). Ebstein's anomaly and corrected transposition of the great arteries (TGA) have a high incidence of accessory AV pathways.[24] In many cases, electrophysiologic sequelae in this population are due to the arrhythmogenic potential of myocardium subjected to septal patches and suture lines in intra-atrial or intraventricular locations, chronic cyanosis, and abnormal volume-pressure physiology.[23,24] Reentrant tachycardias are especially common following certain operations for CHD, such as

TABLE 3–4   Arrhythmias and Commonly Associated Congenital Heart Defects

Arrhythmia	Associated Defects
Tachycardias	
Wolff-Parkinson-White syndrome	Ebstein's anomaly
	"Corrected" transposition
Intra-atrial reentrant tachycardia	Postoperative Mustard
	Postoperative Senning
	Postoperative Fontan
	Other
Atrial fibrillation	Mitral valve disease
	Aortic stenosis
	Single ventricle
Ventricular tachycardia	Tetralogy of Fallot
	Aortic stenosis
	Other
Bradycardias	
SA node dysfunction	Postoperative Mustard
	Postoperative Senning
	Postoperative Fontan
	Other
Congenital AV block	AV septal defects
	"Corrected" transposition
Acquired AV block	VSD closure
	Tetralogy of Fallot repair
	Other

SA, Sinoatrial; AV, atrioventricular; VSD, ventricular septal defect.
Reprinted with permission from Walsh EP: Arrhythmias in patients with congenital heart disease. Cardiac Electrophysiol Rev 2002;6:423.

especially those with cyanotic CHD, where the Hb may reside in the range of 15 to 20 g/dL. The effectiveness of oxygen delivery with an Hb beyond 20 g/dL is unclear. In the neonate or infant for surgery, a Hb of greater than 20 mg/dL may be associated with acidosis or infarction.[27] However, therapeutic phlebotomy is not uniformly recommended.

Hemostasis is an important consideration for surgery, especially since 70% of patients with CHD may have coagulation abnormalities.[28] Excessive bleeding in infants and children may have devastating outcomes. Coagulation derangements may actually be more serious than routine testing can detect. The exact mechanism and pathologic processes responsible for hemostatic abnormalities are not entirely understood, but individuals with CHD are more likely to experience profuse bleeding even with minor surgery.[29] This risk affects both adult and pediatric patients similarly.[27] Medications should be carefully screened to detect the use of warfarin (Coumadin) and aspirin, because these agents may be additive with the abnormalities of coagulation associated with CHD. Certain congenital hemostatic abnormalities such as von Willebrand's disease may be associated with CHD.

In a prospective study of 235 patients younger than the age of 34 years scheduled for cardiac surgery who underwent preoperative evaluation of prothrombin time (PT), activated partial thromboplastin time (APTT), platelet count, thrombin time, and bleeding time, 19% of participants had an abnormality of one laboratory value that was significantly higher than the expected incidence of abnormal coagulation tests in a control population.[30] Seven percent of individuals with CHD had two abnormal coagulation values. Poor cardiac performance, cyanosis, and elevated HCT were associated with the highest incidence of coagulation abnormalities. Goel and coworkers[29] confirmed the hemostatic abnormalities of CHD. Platelet count, PT, APTT, fibrinogen, D-dimer, and factors VII and VIII were obtained on 25 cyanotic and acyanotic children and compared with controls. Twenty-eight percent of both cyanotic and acyanotic individuals had isolated coagulation abnormalities, but 64% of cyanotic patients had more than one coagulation abnormality, as compared with only 20% of acyanotic individuals. Thirty-eight percent of these children with CHD also appeared to be in a state of disseminated intravascular coagulation (DIC), according to D-dimer elevations. A state of accelerated fibrinolysis has been reported by some to be associated with CHD.[31] Platelet function and number have been reported to be abnormal in patients with CHD.[31] Hemostasis is also related to the degree of hypoxia and HCT.[14,28] Cyanotic children are significantly more likely to have evidence of platelet activation than acyanotic ones.[31] Thrombocytopenia has been shown to correlate with arterial saturation.

Age is a factor to consider when evaluating hemostatic considerations, because a large percentage of those

repair of TOF, Mustard or Senning operation, and Fontan procedure. More recently, these procedures have been modified to reduce the likelihood of arrhythmias.

Although neurologic integrity is not at the same risk with noncardiac surgery compared with cardiac surgery, and circulatory arrest in those with CHD, necropsy studies have shown that 2% to 10% of individuals with CHD have central nervous system malformations, increasing the risk of further injury with any subsequent operation.[25] Increased red blood cell mass has also been associated with a higher risk of cerebrovascular injury, often attributed to hyperviscosity of an elevated HCT of cyanotic CHD. In instances of primarily venous, not arterial, thrombosis, the incidence may reach 20% in these patients.[26] Children with polycythemia are at greater risk for thrombosis than adults.[14] Phlebotomy has been recommended by some as a prophylactic measure to reduce the risk of thrombosis but more recently has been associated with an increased risk of stroke, as 50% of patients with cerebrovascular events underwent phlebotomy.[26]

Laboratory evaluation will depend on the congenital heart defect and the complexity of the impending surgery. A recent preoperative Hb concentration is advisable to establish the baseline oxygen delivery needs of patients, with CHD are infants and children. The neonate may be subject to hepatic immaturity, defective clot retraction, DIC, low plasma factor levels, and qualitative platelet dysfunction.[32] As one ages, coagulation profiles change until transitioning to the adult profile (Fig. 3-8). Mean factor prothrombin, VII, IX, and X concentrations remain below adult levels throughout childhood, appearing as prolongation of the APTT and PT.[33] Impaired synthesis of the vitamin K clotting factors is not uncommon in these patients.

Although patients with CHD should have a recent preoperative chest radiograph to compare with a previous chest radiograph, their value is minimal for a majority of pediatric patients. The most important feature is the pattern and degree of pulmonary vascularity. Evidence of interstitial fluid may suggest CHF.

A recent ECG is helpful to establish baseline rhythm, especially in view of the propensity of arrhythmias to occur in both adults and children. The pediatric ECG may be especially difficult to interpret and should be reviewed by a cardiologist.

Premedication

Beyond the normal value of the preoperative visit to relieve anxiety, individuals with CHD generally benefit greatly from premedication. Many of these patients have undergone surgery and may be fearful, and they may also have a higher risk of adjustment problems, such as depression, low self-esteem, and dependence. Consequently,

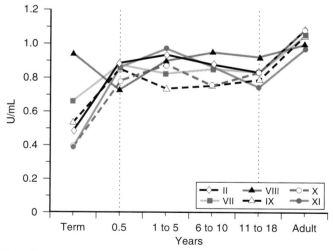

FIGURE 3–8 Development of coagulation factors during childhood. Plasma concentrations of selected contact, vitamin K–dependent, and cofactors of coagulation from term through childhood. It is useful to think of the major changes as occurring in three periods: from birth through the first 6 months of life, from the first year until early adolescence, and during or by the end of adolescence. *(Reprinted with permission from Richardson MW, Allen GA, Monahan PE: Thrombosis in children: Current perspective and distinct challenges. Thromb Haemost 2002;88:900.)*

premedication and a preoperative visit are important for these patients.[34] The age to initiate premedication is unclear, but most agree that infants younger than 6 months of age do not require it.

For many years the goal of premedication was to heavily sedate children to prevent arterial desaturation during induction but not to overly depress the myocardium.[35] A vagolytic agent was included in the premedication to preserve heart rate during induction; however, the move away from halothane for inhalation induction has lessened the need for it. This is advantageous, because its use predisposed to arrhythmias.[35] Although secretions may be slightly greater without a preoperative anticholinergic, there is no evidence of complications without it.[36]

The choices of sedative and analgesic agents for premedication are quite numerous but should be evaluated in terms of the CHD, myocardial function, age, and associated medical conditions. Heavy sedation has been thought to have minimal impact on oxygen saturation, even in cyanotic patients.[37] Recent evidence seems to contradict such a premise. DeBock and colleagues[38] demonstrated a fall of more than 10% in pulse oximeter measurements in 30% of the cyanotic children with premedication consisting of morphine, scopolamine, and barbiturate, whereas acyanotic children experienced a clinically insignificant drop in saturation.

Intramuscular injection is rarely used now, because there are good oral alternatives. Infants between the age of 6 months and 9 months may receive oral pentobarbital (2 to 4 mg/kg). Recently, substitution of oral midazolam (0.75 to 1.0 mg/kg) has proven safe and effective for barbiturate, morphine sulfate, and atropine premedication without a decrease in pulse oximeter derived oxygen saturation (SpO_2). In a comparison between intramuscular injection of morphine and atropine with oral midazolam in children ranging from 1 to 6 years of age scheduled for elective cardiac congenital heart surgery, intramuscular injection led to a significant reduction in saturation, from 84% to 76%, which was absent with oral midazolam.[39] Oral midazolam does not appear to compromise respiratory rate or cardiovascular stability. Because 10% to 30% of children are still not sedated with 1.0 mg/kg of oral midazolam, 1.5 mg/kg of oral midazolam was compared with 1.0 and 0.5 mg/kg in children younger than 2 years of age undergoing congenital heart surgery. Only 4% of those receiving 1.5 mg/kg of midazolam were inadequately sedated.[40] Eight patients of 193 developed hypotension greater than 20% with sedation, but there was no statistically significant difference in the blood pressure or saturation between the infants who received 1.5 mg/kg of midazolam compared with the lower doses.

Oral transmucosal fentanyl citrate has been studied and found to provide adequate sedation in over three fourths of this patient population compared with conventional premedication.[36,41] However, a 38% incidence of vomiting was noted. Lowering the dose of fentanyl to 15 to 20 μg/kg reduced the incidence of nausea and preinduction vomiting to14%,[41] but this technique is not extremely popular.

It is important to carefully observe individuals with CHD for sensitivity to sedatives that may lead to upper airway obstruction, decreases in SpO$_2$, and hypoventilation, especially if PAH is present. PAH can lead to a rapid hemodynamic deterioration on account of a rising PCO$_2$. With CHD, an increase in the PaCO$_2$ from 40 to 45 mmHg raises the mean pulmonary artery pressure from 41 to 47 mm Hg.[42] Increases in PaCO$_2$ were followed with transcutaneous CO$_2$ in patients with CHD with either oral midazolam or intramuscular morphine and scopolamine (Fig. 3-9).[43] Importantly, of the 16 patients with PAH, 9 experienced clinically significant changes in transcutaneous CO$_2$ and oxygen saturation.[43] A similar sensitivity to CO$_2$ has been seen in adults with PAH.[44]

Monitoring

Besides routine monitoring for administration of anesthesia, monitoring for patients with CHD undergoing noncardiac surgery depends on the congenital defect, severity of illness, functional reserve, and surgery.

Indirect blood pressure monitoring is adequate in some cases, because the accuracy of the Dinamap oscillometric monitor compares favorably in both adults and infants with direct intra-arterial measurements, particularly regarding the systolic blood pressure.[45,46] It is necessary to identify any prior operations that involved creating systemic to pulmonary artery shunts that affect the flow

to that extremity. A simple Blalock-Taussig shunt on the left will necessitate blood pressure and pulse oximeter monitoring on the right extremity. In circumstances in which both upper extremities have been affected by shunts, cannulation of a femoral artery is an option. Femoral artery blood pressure monitoring is not associated with more complications than the radial artery in those with CHD, except for neonates who may experience some temporary perfusion abnormalities.[47] Access to arterial blood gas (ABG) analysis with direct arterial monitoring may be desirable and an excellent reason for invasive monitoring.

The need for central venous access and monitoring in patients with CHD depends on the CHD and surgery. Success may be very challenging because of previous operations, chronic vessel occlusion, abnormal anatomy and blood flow, and broad age range. It is difficult to obtain central venous access in about 10% of patients with CHD.[48] Experience is especially important for successful central venous catheter placement with infants weighing less than 5 kg.[49] The incidence of noninfectious complications such as pneumothorax, hemothorax, air embolism, thoracic duct injury, and nerve damage is 1% to 7%, consistent with the challenge of central venous catheter placement.[50,51]

A major concern with central venous catheter placement in patients with CHD is accidental arterial puncture and subsequent large-bore catheter placement. It may cause vascular damage, stroke, airway obstruction, and even death.[52] The incidence of carotid puncture varies from 0% to 23%, depending on the technique and patient's age (Fig. 3-10).[53] A high approach to central venous cannulation in infants and young children will lessen the chance of morbidity. CHD increases the risk of carotid puncture (14.1%) in both adult and pediatric patients compared with others (9.3%). Carotid puncture is also more likely in infants younger than 3 months of age.[54] Although carotid puncture may cause injury, subsequent large catheter insertion causes most of the serious morbidity or mortality.

To minimize this complication when attempting central venous access, an external jugular vein may be substituted for the internal jugular vein. However, success is less than 80% in children[55] and adults. Furthermore, the internal jugular vein is preferred by most for central venous monitoring. The challenge of securing central venous access is especially great in infants younger than 3 months and weighing less than 4 kg,[56] with a success rate below that in adults.[53] Failure rate has varied between 4%[49] and 10%.[48] The relationship of the right internal jugular vein to the carotid artery in children may partially explain the poorer success rate. The position of the right internal jugular vein is not as well defined in children compared with adults and is also more unpredictable in children with CHD than in those without CHD.[57]

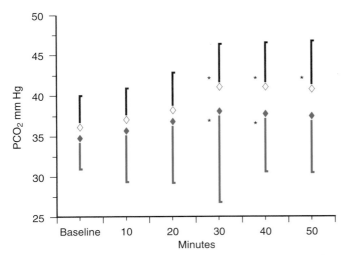

FIGURE 3–9 Changes in transcutaneous PCO$_2$ (mean ± SD) in children with congenital heart disease after premedication with either morphine and scopolamine (*open diamonds*) or midazolam (*closed diamonds*). *$P < .05$ compared with baseline. (*Reprinted with permission from Alswang M, Friesen RH, Bangert P: Effect of preanesthetic medication on carbon dioxide tension in children with congenital heart disease. J Cardiothorac Vasc Anesth 1994;8:416.*)

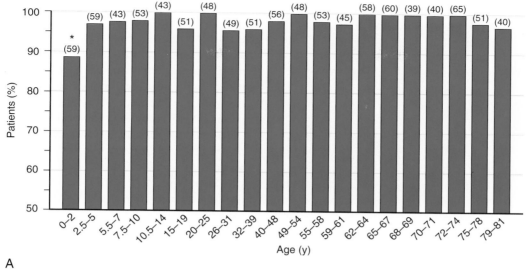

A

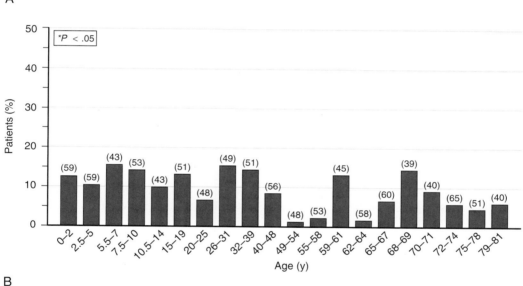

B

FIGURE 3–10 Success rate (**A**) and arterial puncture rate (**B**) as a function of age. Numbers in parentheses indicate the number of patients in each age group. *(Reprinted with permission from Oliver WC, Nuttall GA, Beynen FM, et al: The incidence of artery puncture with central venous cannulation using a modified technique for detection and prevention of arterial cannulation. J Cardiothorac Vasc Anesth 1997;11:853.)*

The right internal jugular vein may be anterior to the carotid artery in 10% to 60% of patients with CHD, depending on the approach to the vein and the position of the head.[57,58] A 45-degree angle with the head and midline will better align the carotid and internal jugular vein to obtain central venous placement.

To facilitate central venous access and avoid complications, ultrasound guidance has been recommended. Ultrasound reduces the number of carotid punctures and increases success rate, especially for less experienced clinicians.[54,58,59] The incidence of carotid puncture in infants and children without ultrasound may be as high as 23%. Ultrasound not only decreased the incidence of carotid puncture but increased the success rate to 100%

in infants younger than 12 months of age, compared with a 77% success rate in highly experienced clinicians using conventional techniques.[54] Ultrasound is also valuable to assess the internal jugular vein. In a series of 500 infants and children with CHD receiving central venous access, the right internal jugular vein was unsuitable for cannulation in 3.2% of patients.[49] Approximately 3% of internal jugular veins may be too small. Table 3-5 displays the recommended length of the central venous catheter for different ages of patients to minimize complications.[60]

Pulse oximetry is a reliable, noninvasive, and continuous method to monitor arterial oxygen saturation (SaO_2) without the necessity for recurrent ABG measurements.[61] However, poor peripheral perfusion or severe oxygen

TABLE 3–5   Recommended Length of Central Venous Catheter (CVC) Insertion in Pediatric Patients Based on Weight

Patient Weight (kg)	Length of CVC Insertion (cm)
2-2.9	4
3-4.9	5
5-6.9	6
7-9.9	7
10-12.9	8
13-19.9	9
20-29.9	10
30-39.9	11
40-49.9	12
50-59.9	13
60-69.9	14
70-79.9	15
≥ 80	16

Reprinted with permission from Andropoulos DB, Bent ST, Skjonsby B, Stayer SA: The optimal length of insertion of central venous catheters for pediatric patients. Anesth Analg 2001;93;885.

desaturation affects its accuracy and reliability.[62,63] Most do not view an SpO_2 of 80% as alarming because efforts to improve oxygenation have usually been initiated before such a saturation is reached. However, patients with CHD are a heterogeneous group with saturations regularly below 90% and not infrequently below 80%. A narrow margin of safety characterizes patients with CHD, so significant declines in SpO_2 may not be tolerated. Adding to the uncertainty, pulse oximeters in patients with CHD tend to overread the SaO_2, delaying the therapeutic response. Moreover, current pulse oximeters may fail to read on average for about one third of the surgery, further complicating patient care decisions.[64]

Masimo Corporation (Laguna Hills, CA) has developed a pulse oximeter that represents a fundamental change in oximetry technology. Signal Extraction Technology (SET) reduces pulse oximeter failure and inaccuracies associated with low perfusion. Recently, in a comparison with Agilent Merlin and the Nellcor N-395, better accuracy and precision in the perioperative period, with saturations below 90% in patients ranging in age from birth to 53 years with CHD undergoing congenital heart repair, were noted.[65] However, accuracy and precision are still lacking for saturations below 70% by all pulse oximeter monitors.

Monitoring arterial oxygen saturation may provide the most complete and accurate information regarding Q_p/Q_s.[66] Anesthesia management of CHD is influenced by Q_p/Q_s to a larger or lesser degree depending on the specific congenital heart anomaly. Excessive pulmonary

flow may lead to hypoperfusion of the systemic circulation, evidenced by metabolic acidosis whereas insufficient pulmonary blood flow may result in severe hypoxia. Although SpO_2 is valuable to assess Q_p/Q_s,[67,68] arterial saturation reaches a certain point where the pulmonary ratio of flow may continue to rise with no ability to be discriminate. Consequently, systemic arterial oxygen saturations do not allow one to specify whether the Q_p/Q_s is 1 or 3, and the arterial saturation will plateau.[66] Acidosis may be the final indication of hypoperfusion from excessive pulmonary blood flow. Thus, systemic venous saturations may provide a better estimate of the pulmonary blood flow ratio (Fig. 3-11).[66] Although better, systemic venous saturation can be two tailed, in that it may be low with a low ratio or low with a high pulmonary blood flow ratio. One needs to measure and observe both the arterial and venous saturations to make the correct therapeutic decision.[66]

Because of the relationship between $PaCO_2$ and PVR, accurate monitoring of $PaCO_2$ is crucial in those with CHD. Even with severe PAH, a degree of PAH is dynamic vasoconstriction and thus reversible.[42] Hypocarbic alkalosis is effective in reducing pulmonary artery pressures in children and infants (Fig. 3-12).[42] End-tidal CO_2 ($ETCO_2$) is routinely used intraoperatively to monitor $PaCO_2$ and has been shown to closely approximate it in most patients. Accuracy of $ETCO_2$ with $PaCO_2$ depends on ventilation-perfusion match, pulmonary blood flow, cardiac output, physiologic dead space, and venous admixture. As a result, significant gradients exist with $ETCO_2$ and $PaCO_2$ in those with cyanotic CHD. $ETCO_2$ commonly underreads $PaCO_2$.[69] The gradient also varies depending on the

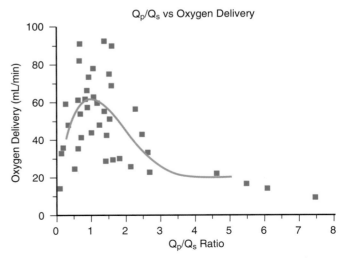

FIGURE 3–11 Systemic oxygen delivery as a function of the Qp/Qs ratio. Superimposed curve represents function generated by nonlinear regression analysis, demonstrating two-tailed function. *(Reprinted with permission from Riordan CJ, Randsbaek F, Storey JH, et al: Balancing pulmonary and systemic arterial flows in parallel circulations: The value of monitoring system venous oxygen saturations. Cardiol Young 1997;7:76.)*

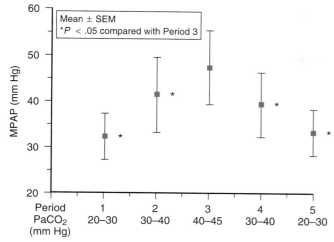

FIGURE 3–12   Values for mean pulmonary artery pressure (MPAP) at physiologic pH and arterial partial pressure of CO_2 (Paco₂) (period 3) compared with values obtained during hypocarbic alkalosis (periods 1, 2, 4, 5). (Reprinted with permission from Morry JP, Lynn AM, Mansfield PB: Effect of pH and Pco₂ on pulmonary and systemic hemodynamics after surgery in children with congenital heart disease and pulmonary hypertension. J Pediatr 1988;113:476.)

congenital defect (Fig. 3-13) because those with acyanotic lesions have less gradient.[69]

Another method used to monitor Paco₂ is transcutaneous CO_2. It has been shown to have a bias of 0.58 mm Hg and precision of 2.1 mm Hg in comparison with Paco₂ in patients undergoing surgery for CHD. Transcutaneous CO_2 is generally only accurate for infants younger than 6 months of age.[70] Accuracy is diminished with poor skin perfusion often present with vasoactive medications.

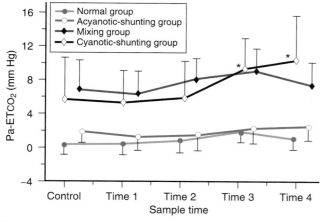

FIGURE 3–13   The mean (±SD) of the arterial to end-tidal CO_2 partial pressure difference (Pa-ETco₂) in the four groups. The Pa-ETco₂ in the cyanotic patients is greater than in the acyanotic patients. There is no statistically significant difference from the control Pa-ETco₂ in the normal, acyanotic-shunting, or mixing groups of patients, but in the cyanotic-shunting group, the Pa-ETco₂ calculated at times 3 and 4 were significantly greater than the values at control, time 1 and time 2. (Reprinted with permission from Lazzell VA, Burrows FA: Stability of the intraoperative arterial to end-tidal carbon dioxide partial pressure difference in children with congenital heart disease. Can J Anaesth 1991;38:862.)

Echocardiography has become routine for all pediatric cardiac surgical procedures and may be helpful in selected noncardiac cases to assess shunt flow or myocardial function. Filling pressures may not correlate with volume measurements, so end-diastolic volume measurements per echocardiography may aid in hemodynamic management. Transesophageal echocardiography is generally tolerated, but 1% to 2% of infants and children may develop airway obstruction. Pulmonary function tests measured before and after placement of the echocardiographic probe reveal minimal changes, even in infants weighing 2 to 5 kg.[71] The hemodynamic effects of transesophageal echocardiography on infants with CHD were found to be minimal as well.[72]

It is problematic in patients with CHD to assess the cardiac output, so they may be susceptible to multiple organ failure. Quantitative measures of cardiac output in conjunction with residual shunts are inaccurate. Doppler echocardiography has not demonstrated agreement with invasive measures of cardiac output. Poor cardiac output can be reflected in mixed venous saturation, base deficit, and serum lactate measurement. Superior vena caval saturation is frequently obtained for cardiac output assessment instead of a true mixed venous blood saturation, but a slight gradient between superior vena caval saturation and mixed venous saturation exists.[73] Even if pulmonary artery catheters were available for determination of cardiac outputs in these patients, markers of tissue perfusion appear more valuable for assessing the patient's status than actual cardiac output.[74]

Additionally, two other important physiologic parameters to monitor include temperature and urine output. Temperature control is crucial, especially in infants and children with CHD, because hypothermia will increase SVR, and if hypothermia leads to shivering, metabolic demand will increase dramatically. The leftward shift of the oxygen-dissociation curve will add to oxygen deficit, because it is more difficult to unload oxygen. The room should be warmed to reduce conductive heat loss and a Bair Hugger® should be utilized.

Ventilation

The manner and degree of ventilation is essential in patients with CHD to stabilize PVR and hemodynamics. Ventilators commonly associated with anesthesia machines do not provide the same degree of gas exchange compared with ventilators used in the intensive care unit, especially in individuals with respiratory failure.[75] The Siemens 300D (Siemens Elema/Maquet, Solna, Sweden) ventilator delivered the greatest mean inspiratory flow at all airway pressures, which is pressure independent in contrast to anesthetic ventilators.[76] Infants with CHD have altered lung compliance and airway resistance, causing them to be very sensitive to changes in ventilation.[77] The presence of PAH further increases the airway resistance, making ventilation even more critical. Children with acyanotic CHD are much more likely to have decreased respiratory compliance than those with cyanotic CHD. Compliance is more related to the pulmonary artery pressure than pulmonary blood flow or shunt direction.

Circulatory Support

Circulatory support for CHD patients undergoing noncardiac surgery may be necessary. The stress of surgery impacts these patients more than others undergoing noncardiac surgery. Stress can manifest as both metabolic and respiratory acidosis and have a prolonged impact.[14] Many patients with CHD have tenuous preoperative ventricular function, so the stress of surgery and anesthesia may diminish ventricular function, potentially causing circulatory failure. Inotropes may be necessary but may cause tachycardia, increased myocardial oxygen consumption, increased SVR, and arrhythmias. Alternatively, milrinone, a relatively new phosphodiesterase inhibitor (PDE), with a rapid onset, stimulates vascular muscle relaxation and myocardial contractility. In one of the few randomized blinded multicenter studies of infants, milrinone was associated with reduced mortality and improved hemodynamics compared with other conventional agents.[78] One must resist the temptation to give excessive fluids to either pediatric or adult patients with CHD to support hemodynamics because it can be catastrophic.[79] Adequate circulatory support is essential to maintain the blood flow of palliative shunts; otherwise, pulmonary perfusion may be reduced significantly, risking further hypoxia and possible shunt thrombosis.[79]

Anesthetic Techniques

There is not one anesthetic technique that can be recommended for patients with CHD, since these individuals vary significantly according to congenital defect and age.[14] A thorough understanding of CHD and the stresses that may accompany surgery are necessary. Anesthetic considerations include shunt flow, myocardial contractility, ventricular dilation or hypertrophy, arrhythmias, PVR, and outflow tract obstruction. Goals should include maintaining shunt flow to provide optimal cardiac output and systemic perfusion, minimizing myocardial depression, and avoiding exacerbating PVR (Table 3-6). The factors that affect PVR are listed in Table 3-6 and are essentially applicable to both children and adults with CHD. In many respects, patients with CHD may behave almost normally; consequently, they may tolerate a conventional anesthetic.[79] In contrast, some patients may have serious functional limitations that require a more complex approach to anesthetic and perioperative management.

Sevoflurane is the agent of choice[22] for inhalation induction of infants and children without CHD because of its low partition coefficient, hemodynamic stability (Fig 3-14A), and its reduced effect on myocardial contractility compared with other volatile agents (see Fig 3-14B).[80] Infants and children with CHD will tolerate sevoflurane concentrations of 8% with significantly less myocardial depression than halothane.[81,82] Because sevoflurane is approximately four times less soluble in blood than halothane, inhalation induction is more rapid with lower inspired concentrations. Ventilation will have minimal effect on the speed of induction with sevoflurane.

TABLE 3-6 Factors Affecting Pulmonary Vascular Resistance (PVR)	
Decrease in PVR	**Increase in PVR**
Increasing PaO_2	Sympathetic stimulation
Hypocarbia	Light anesthesia
Alkalemia	Pain
Minimizing intrathoracic pressure	Acidemia
Spontaneous ventilation	Hypoxia
Normal lung volumes	Hypercarbia
High frequency and jet ventilation	Hypothermia
Avoidance of sympathetic stimulation	Increased intrathoracic pressure
Deep anesthesia	Controlled ventilation
Pharmacologic methods	PEEP
Isoprenaline	Atelectasis
Phosphodiesterase III inhibitors	
Prostaglandin (Pg) infusion (PgE_1 and PgI_2)	
Inhaled nitric oxide	

PEEP, positive end-expiratory pressure.
Reprinted with permission from Lovell AT: Anaesthetic implications of grown-up congenital heart disease. Br J Anaesth 2004;93:131.

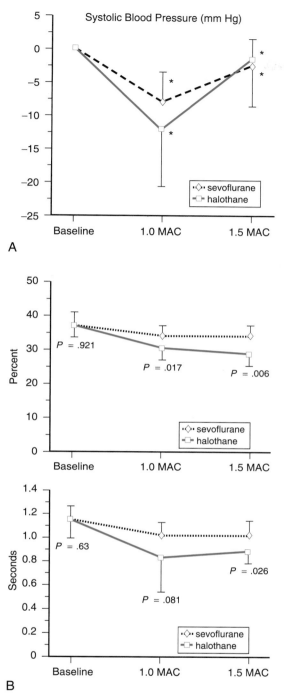

FIGURE 3–14 A, Blood pressure was stable throughout the induction of anesthesia in both groups, children that receive either sevoflurane or halothane. Systolic blood pressure decreased at 1.0 minimal alveolar concentration (MAC) with halothane and sevoflurane, returning to baseline at 1.5 MAC. **B,** Left ventricular shortening fraction (SF; *middle*) and velocity of ventricular circumferential fiber shortening corrected for heart rate (VCFc; *bottom*) decreased with both anesthetic agents. Halothane decreased shortening fraction (two-way analysis of variance with repeated measures; $P = .003$) and VCFc (two-way analysis of variance with repeated measures; $P = .018$) more than sevoflurane. *(Reprinted with permission from Holzman RS, van der Velde ME, Kaus SJ, Body SC, et al: Sevoflurane depresses myocardial contractility less than halothane during induction of anesthesia in children. Anesthesiology 1996;85:1263.)*

The effect of CHD on the uptake and distribution of anesthetic agents involves many factors. A right-to-left shunt will slow inhalation induction, because less anesthetic is absorbed from the lung, and mixing will further dilute blood that is passing to the left, decreasing the arterial concentration of the blood going to the brain, especially the less soluble agent. However, this is rarely problematic. An intravenous induction would be accelerated with a right-to-left shunt. The cyanotic child should be induced with a combination of nitrous oxide and a volatile agent, because it allows for a lower concentration of volatile agent to be given.

Although classically, the left-to-right shunt should promote the speed of inhalation induction, actually the clinical effect is insignificant.[83] Similarly, although intravenous induction should be slowed by a left-to-right shunt, unless the cardiac output is very poor, it is clinically irrelevant. Selection of the anesthetic agent (halothane, isoflurane, fentanyl/midazolam, sevoflurane) does not appear to affect the Qp/Qs ratio in those with left-to-right shunts, as long as the patients were mechanically ventilated at normocapnia and with 100% oxygen (Fig. 3-15).[84] Individuals with single ventricles may be less tolerant of volatile agents. The reactive nature of the pulmonary vasculature will make the behavior of volatile agents unpredictable.

Although isoflurane is not used for inhalation induction in children or adults owing to its pungent smell, it is well suited for anesthetic maintenance compared with halothane. Myocardial function is well preserved during isoflurane administration.[85,86] Isoflurane concentration below 1.0 MAC will provide the same hemodynamic stability that fentanyl (75 µg/kg) and diazepam achieve in those with acyanotic CHD.[87] Similarly, sevoflurane maintains cardiac output and contractility in patients with CHD.[86,88] A prospective study randomizing infants with CHD to either sevoflurane or halothane for inhalation induction for congenital heart surgery found that halothane had twice as many cardiovascular events (hypotension) as sevoflurane ($P = .03$) and a significantly greater lactate level before heparinization than those receiving sevoflurane.[89] The halothane group also had more episodes of bradycardia and emergency drug administration. Equal numbers of cyanotic and acyanotic infants were part of each group. Sevoflurane is associated with a lower incidence of arrhythmias compared with halothane.[86]

Intravenous anesthetics for patients with CHD are the preferred method of anesthetic induction and maintenance, excluding those that require inhalation induction.[90] Many intravenous agents are able to provide safe induction and anesthetic maintenance, but the margin for error with some choices is less.[79]

High-dose narcotic anesthesia has continued to be a popular anesthetic technique for patients with CHD based

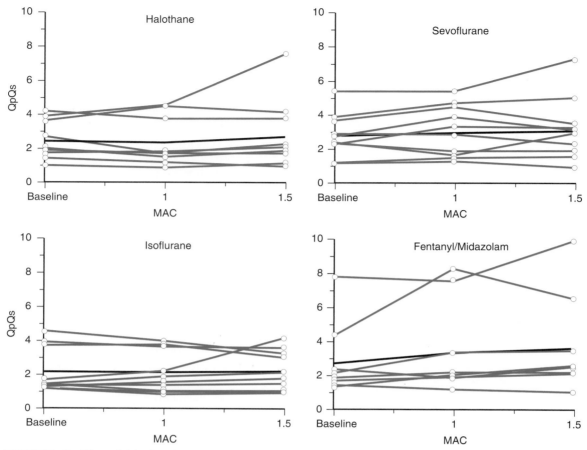

FIGURE 3–15 Individual patient pulmonary-to-systemic blood flow ratio (Qp:Qs) data for each anesthetic (halothane, *n* = 10; sevoflurane, *n* = 11; isoflurane, *n* = 10; and fentanyl/midazolam, n = 9). *Heavy black line* indicates mean value at each anesthetic concentration. *(Reprinted with permission from Laird TH, Stayer SA, Rivenes SM, et al: Pulmonary-to-systemic blood flow ratio effects of sevoflurane, isoflurane, halothane, and fentanyl/midazolam with 100% oxygen in children with congenital heart disease. Soc Pediatr Anesth 2002;95:1204.)*

on the widely held idea of minimizing the hormonally mediated stress response, thereby minimizing pulmonary vascular reactivity and myocardial depression. This was concluded based on a study comparing a narcotic versus volatile agent–based anesthetic for congenital heart surgery. The presence of a metabolic acidosis with halothane was postulated to be the result of failure to attenuate the stress response compared with the narcotic.[91] The relationship between increased perioperative stress response and postoperative complications in newborns undergoing noncardiac operations questions the advisability of a volatile anesthetic in patients with CHD.[92] An opioid anesthetic was associated with a lower perioperative mortality in infants compared with halothane.[91] Fentanyl has remained popular for years in a range of dosages (10 to 150 μg/kg) for induction and maintenance of anesthesia in both pediatric and adult populations with CHD requiring cardiac surgery.[93]

The advantages of fentanyl for patients with CHD include minimal effect on pulmonary and systemic circulations and attenuation of response to intubation

and incision. Fentanyl also attenuates the pulmonary vascular response to suctioning that may cause serious desaturation.[94] In conjunction with midazolam, fentanyl maintains contractility better than most volatile anesthetic agents in these patients.[86] Fentanyl has also been shown to maintain oxygen saturation and hemodynamics as effectively as ketamine in cyanotic CHD.[68] The same has been found concerning sufentanil and flunitrazepam in cyanotic children.[90] Although sufentanil has similar hormonal blocking properties as fentanyl, the hemodynamic predictability is not as good. The addition of a benzodiazepine with fentanyl compared with fentanyl alone in acyanotic infants and children showed better hemodynamic stability, indicating the value of a balanced anesthetic.[87] Shorter-acting agents such as alfentanil have some appeal, especially in noncardiac situations, for use as maintenance anesthetics, but there are some drawbacks.

Recently, the benefit of a narcotic anesthetic has been questioned, because there was no apparent evidence of a relationship between narcotics and outcome in neonates and infants undergoing CPB for cardiac surgery.[95]

Furthermore, the addition of a benzodiazepine did not influence the stress response. It may be that "well compensated" CHD does not require or benefit as much from high-dose narcotic anesthetic technique, but further studies are necessary.[95]

Propofol is a substituted phenol agent that has a rapid onset and short duration of action. The use of propofol for anesthetic maintenance in patients with CHD is not recommended, based on some anecdotal reports of severe fatal metabolic acidosis in children who were critically ill.[96] The occurrence of propofol syndrome that includes metabolic lactic acidosis, myocardial dysfunction, and even death, has been found in critically ill patients, both pediatric and adult.[97,98] In children with CHD undergoing cardiac catheterization, significantly more patients experienced a decrease of more than 20% of the mean arterial pressure (MAP) than those who received ketamine. The SpO_2 in the propofol group fell more than 5% during induction, whereas ketamine was not associated with any reduction in SpO_2.[99] Increased right-to-left shunting may have been responsible, as evidenced consistently during cardiac catheterization of both cyanotic and acyanotic children. Propofol reduces the SVR and hence increases right-to-left shunt, which further reduces pulmonary blood flow in cyanotic patients. Additionally, SaO_2 has fallen as much as 10% in conjunction with decreased pH in cyanotic children.[100] If PVR is high, propofol may exacerbate pulmonary vasoconstriction, increasing ventricular afterload,[101] but does not appear to have any direct effect on PVR.[100] Patients with acyanotic CHD tolerate propofol as long as metabolic acidosis does not become excessive.

Ketamine has been frequently recommended for patients with cyanotic and acyanotic CHD and may be the agent of choice for induction of anesthesia in patients with cyanotic CHD.[102] Its effects are mediated through a centrally activated increase in sympathetic activity. Compared with halothane, it maintains the MAP significantly better in infants with cyanotic CHD.[67,68] In those with CHD undergoing cardiac catheterization, ketamine has been shown to increase HR but causes no change in Qp/Qs.[102] It relaxes bronchial smooth muscle stimulated by endothelin.[103] As well as being superior to isoflurane in those with TOF,[104] ketamine provides excellent analgesia in contrast to propofol, which has no analgesic properties.

Etomidate and thiopental have been used in CHD. Etomidate provides excellent hemodynamic stability in teenagers and adults with CHD.[22] Thiopental has been used for induction in patients with CHD, but myocardial depression and vasodilation cause hemodynamic instability. Careful observation of the pulse oximeter during induction and anesthetic maintenance will help guide dosing to maintain hemodynamics (Fig. 3-16).[68]

Muscle Relaxants

The choice of muscle relaxants for intubation and intraoperative maintenance will rest on the expected duration of the anesthetic, hemodynamics, airway assessment, and other associated medical conditions. The possibility of severe bradycardia with succinylcholine in infants and children limits its usefulness in hemodynamically compromised individuals. There are only a few reasons to use succinylcholine in infants and children with CHD. Pancuronium is a long-acting nondepolarizing neuromuscular blocker that tends to temporarily increase the heart rate and blood pressure through vagolysis, but these effects may be absent in some children with CHD.[105]

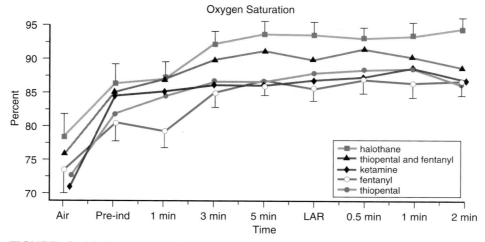

FIGURE 3–16 Oxygen saturations during the period of study for the five groups. Data are mean ± SEM. Time axis: Air = awake control measurements; Pre-Ind = preinduction following preoxygenation; 1 min, 3 min, 5 min = intervals post induction. LAR = laryngoscopy; 0.5 min, 1 min, 2 min = intervals post-intubation. *(Reprinted with permission from Laishley RS, Burrows FA, Lerman J, Roy WL: Effect of anesthetic induction regimens on oxygen saturation in cyanotic congenital heart disease. Anesthesiology 1986;65:675.)*

Muscle relaxants are minimally affected by cyanotic or acyanotic CHD. Shorter-acting neuromuscular blocking agents such as vecuronium, cisatracurium, atracurium, and rocuronium or mivacurium may be selected if the clinical situation calls for it.

ANATOMIC DEFECTS ASSOCIATED WITH INCREASED PULMONARY BLOOD FLOW

Excessive pulmonary blood flow has both cardiac and respiratory consequences. The increased pulmonary blood flow will result in volume overload of the ventricle, causing reduced myocardial function and low cardiac output. Increased pulmonary blood flow will increase left atrial pressure, causing increased pulmonary venous pressures and interstitial edema, ultimately leading to pulmonary vascular disease. The period of time until congenital heart repair occurs is important with respect to onset of pulmonary vascular disease. If repair occurs within 9 months, permanent effects from the defect are unlikely.[106] The period of time before irreversible pulmonary vascular obstructive disease sets in depends on the type of defect and complexity of lesion.

Atrial Septal Defect (ASD)

ASD represents about 30% of all CHD identified in adults. Women are affected two to three times as frequently as men.[8] Nearly 24% of newborns may have a communication between the atria, but only 8% are patent at 1 year of age after spontaneous closure of the defect.[107] Commonly present in low-birth-weight infants, these openings of the atrial septum are rarely associated with clinical symptoms. Those defects with valve openings may be differentiated from those that do not have valves and rarely close spontaneously.

Ostium secundum, ostium primum, patent foramen ovale (PFO), and sinus venosus are the types of ASD classified on the basis of anatomic location of the defect in the atrial septum (Fig. 3-17A). Ostium secundum is located in the area of the fossa ovalis. The ostium primum is located in the lower part of the atrium. The sinus venosus is located high in the atrial septal wall near the junction of the superior vena cava and RA. They occur primarily from excessive resorption of the septum primum or lack of growth of the septum secundum. Anomalous pulmonary venous connections may also be present in 10% of ASD. A PFO is located at the junction of the septum primum and septum secundum. It is not a proper ASD because the foramen ovale exists throughout fetal life and functionally closes as the left atrial pressure exceeds right atrial pressure after birth. In about 25% of people there is no anatomic closure of the foramen ovale, so a communication exists between the RA and LA.

The simple ostium secundum is the most common form of ASD in both the pediatric and adult populations and one of the few defects that may truly manifest first in adulthood. It generally does not close spontaneously but may be unappreciated for years without symptoms. In the future, fewer patients will present with unrecognized ASD because of echocardiography. A murmur

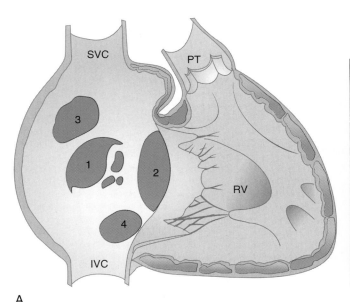
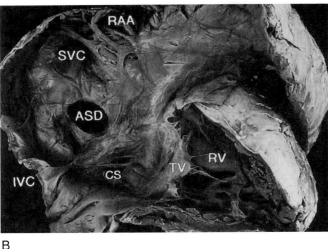

A   B

FIGURE 3–17   A, Atrial septal anatomy. Schematic diagram showing the location of atrial septal defects, numbered in decreasing order of frequency: 1, secundum; 2, primum; 3, sinus venosus; 4, coronary sinus (CS) type. IVC, inferior vena cava; PT, pulmonary trunk; RV, right ventricle; SVC, superior vena cava. **B,** Secundum atrial septal defect (ASD). Right atrial view. SVC, superior vena cava; RAA, right atrial appendage; CS, coronary sinus; IVC, inferior vena cava; TV, tricuspid valve; RV, right ventricle. *(Reprinted with permission from Porter CJ, Feldt RH, Edwards WD, et al: Atrial septal defects. In Emmanouilides GC, Riemenschneider TA, Allen HD, Gutgesell HP [eds]: Moss and Adams Heart Disease in Infants, Children, and Adolescents: Including the Fetus and Young Adult. Baltimore, Williams & Wilkins, 1995, p 688.)*

that was not recognized as pathologic often spurs the diagnosis by the age of 3 to 5 years.[108] Despite its left-to-right nature, severe CHF rarely occurs in the infant on the basis of a solitary ASD. However, it is similarly as rare to see survival past 70 years of age. People with large shunts rarely live to more than 30 to 40 years of age. Ongoing risks for these individuals include paradoxical emboli, bacterial endocarditis, and CHF.

Irrespective of the location of the ASD, the physiologic consequences of this defect are similar. The size of the left-to-right shunt will depend on the size of the defect and the diastolic filling characteristics of the ventricles, with the compliance of the chambers being more important in this respect. Infants will have little left-to-right shunting initially, because PVR is elevated and the right ventricle is hypertrophied (see Fig. 3-17B). Eventually, increased flow to the RA results in volume overload of the right side of the heart, with enlargement of the RA and LA. If the shunt should exceed a Qp/Qs of 1.5, symptoms appear. Dyspnea on exertion will most likely be present by the age of 30 in approximately one third of patients. By age 40, right-sided heart failure with supraventricular tachyarrhythmias may appear in 10% of individuals.[109] Symptoms will progress to severe debilitation with aging.

A large ASD may be associated with a large palpable right ventricular or pulmonary artery impulse. There is wide and fixed splitting of the second heart sound. A systolic ejection flow murmur may be perceived at the left second intercostal space. However, the murmur may be so soft as to be confused with an "innocent" murmur of childhood. Most infants will not have the characteristic murmur. The ECG will frequently reveal a right bundle branch block, as well as right-axis deviation. Atrial tachyarrhythmias are especially common in an adult with an ASD. Atrial fibrillation is the most likely arrhythmia and may precipitate CHF. The chest radiograph may show evidence of increased pulmonary vascularity and PAH reflected by calcification of the pulmonary trunk.[110]

Although an individual with an ASD may be asymptomatic for many years, the systemic hypertension and ischemic heart disease often associated with aging will worsen the compliance of the left ventricle, causing more left-to-right shunt.[110] It is also not uncommon to find mitral insufficiency in 15% of these adult patients. Depending on the type of ASD, the incidence of PAH may vary significantly.[111] Survival with PAH caused by ASD and left-to-right shunt is much longer than primary PAH because the ASD appears to slow progression of pulmonary vasculopathy.

Because PAH occurs and the right ventricle tends to become less compliant with an ASD, eventually, the right ventricle may direct blood from right to left. It is uncommon for an adult with an ASD to develop Eisenmenger's syndrome.[8] Only about 10% of those with large defects of ASD will develop Eisenmenger's syndrome.[111] Patients with Eisenmenger's syndrome who require noncardiac surgery may be receiving some of the medications used to treat primary PAH.[111] Respiratory infections are also common with Eisenmenger's syndrome.

Anesthetic concerns for ASD include excessive pulmonary blood flow, left ventricular dysfunction, especially for adult ASD closure, and paradoxical embolism. Patients with ASD will usually tolerate most anesthetics, unless very severe CHF is present that will require an anesthetic with less myocardial depression. Inhalation or intravenous inductions can be tolerated in most circumstances. Great care should be taken to prevent even small amounts of air, because even a small amount may cause permanent neurologic deficit. For those who have undergone ASD closure as an adult, there remains an increased risk of atrial fibrillation.[34] If Eisenmenger's syndrome is present, refer to the anesthetic considerations of Eisenmenger's syndrome later in the chapter.

Atrioventricular Septal Defects

This group of defects includes the AV septum and valves that result from a failure of the AV septum to develop. Also referred to as "endocardial cushion defects," the two main defects are partial and complete AV septal defects. They represent 4% to 5% of CHD.[5]

The partial defect, accounting for 25% of AV septal defects, includes a primum ASD and a cleft mitral valve.[4] The failure of the septum primum to fuse with the endocardial cushions often results in a large ASD (Fig. 3-18). Symptoms of the partial AV septal defect are more severe than a secundum ASD. CHF may appear as early as infancy with partial AV septal defect. Mitral regurgitation and left-to-right shunting may be severe. A crescendo-decrescendo murmur is heard in the upper lung fields, in association with a holosystolic murmur of mitral regurgitation at the apex. The chest radiograph shows a large heart and may display features consistent with a complete AV septal defect if the left-to-right shunt is large. Normal sinus rhythm is usually present on an electrocardiogram.[110] If the left-to-right shunt is not large, 75% of adult patients will be mildly symptomatic, some asymptomatic for as long as 20 years, but not late in adult life.[112] PAH rarely occurs.

If the shunt is large, surgery to repair the defect is required early in life, with symptomatic relief in over 80% of patients and few complications beyond atrial arrhythmias.[112]

A complete AV septal defect involves not only failure of the septum primum to fuse with the endocardial cushions but also the cushions fail to fuse with each other, resulting in a common AV valve incorporating both atria and ventricles (Fig. 3-19). The common AV valve is usually regurgitant. Figure 3-19A depicts a type A complete AV septal defect. It is the most common type of AV septal defect and is associated with Down syndrome. Nearly 40% of those with Down syndrome have CHD, and 40% will have a complete AV septal defect.[113] Should the valves

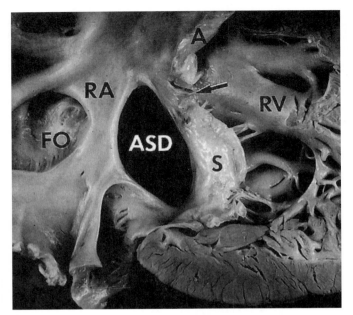

A

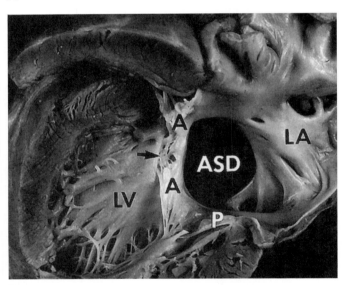

B

FIGURE 3–18 Partial atrioventricular septal defect, with a primum atrial septal defect and a cleft anterior mitral leaflet. **A,** Right ventricular inflow view, showing widened commissure between septal (S) and anterior (A) tricuspid leaflets. **B,** Left ventricular inflow view showing cleft in anterior (A) mitral leaflet with abnormal chordal attachments to midportion of ventricular septum *(arrows)*. ASD, Atrial septal defect; FO, fossa ovalis; LA, left atrium; LV, left ventricle; P, posterior leaflet; RA, right atrium; RV, right ventricle. *(Reprinted with permission from Porter CJ, Feldt RH, Porter CJ, et al: Atrioventricular septal defects. In Emmanouilides GC, Riemenschneider TA, Allen HD, Gutgesell HP [eds]: Moss and Adams Heart Disease in Infants, Children, and Adolescents: Including the Fetus and Young Adult. Baltimore, Williams & Wilkins, 1995, p 708.)*

develop separately instead of forming a common AV valve, the leaflets of both valves will be abnormal and regurgitant (see Fig. 3-19B).

The newborn with complete AV septal defect may have an unremarkable physical examination. The precordium may be hyperdynamic and a systolic murmur may be detected along the left sternal border. The large left-to-right shunt will lead to systemic pressures in both ventricles by 1 year of age and PAH. Frequent respiratory infections and failure to thrive are also characteristic of this defect. Symptoms of CHF, such as poor feeding, poor growth, dyspnea, fatigability, and diaphoresis are common. Cardiomegaly will be present with prominent pulmonary vascular markings consistent with large left-to-right shunts on the chest radiograph (Fig. 3-20). However, normal sinus rhythm is common on the ECG.

Complete repair during infancy is now common, although previously some patients underwent pulmonary artery band and complete repair later. Despite complete repair, 10% to 30% of patients may continue to experience mitral regurgitation, requiring another operation at some point.[114] Anesthetic considerations are similar to the partial AV septal defect, with larger left-to-right shunt and more significant mitral regurgitation.

Ventricular Septal Defect (VSD)

VSD is the most common isolated congenital heart defect, constituting 20% to 33% of all CHD.[2,5] The incidence varies from 1.5 to 3.5 per 1000 term infants.[115] A third of Down syndrome patients will have a VSD.[113] Spontaneous closure may occur in up to half of patients, explaining the lower prevalence of VSD in adults than infants. Extracardiac abnormalities accompany simple VSD in up to 50% of cases.[116] In many instances, repair of the extracardiac anomaly, such as tracheoesophageal fistula, is the reason for the exposure to anesthesia.

Eighty percent of VSDs are perimembranous (infracristal), found in the outflow tract of the left ventricle just beneath the aortic valve (Fig. 3-21). Supracristal or outflow defects account for another 5% to 7% of VSDs. Inlet defects (canal defects) occur in the outflow tract of the right ventricle beneath the pulmonary valve and account for 8% to 11% of VSDs. Inlet defects are also associated with AV septal defects. Muscular defects are often multiple, having the appearance of a "Swiss cheese" defect, and represent 5% to 20% of VSDs.

The size of the VSD will determine the degree of left-to-right shunt.[113] Small to medium defects may limit left-to-right shunt, but a large defect has no resistance to flow and quickly causes volume overload and PAH. A small, moderate, and large VSD has a Qp/Qs ratio of less than 1.5, 1.5 to 2.0, and more than 2.0, respectively.[108] Not all VSDs will require surgical closure but may close spontaneously or simply restrict pulmonary flow as not to affect survival.

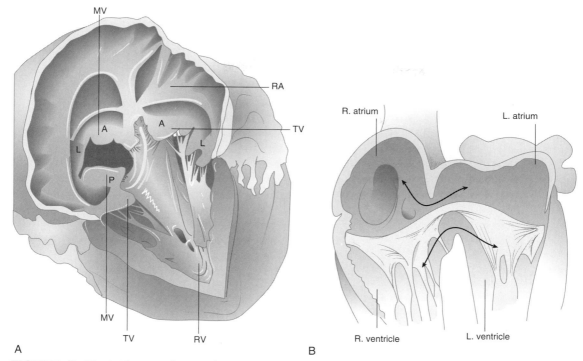

FIGURE 3–19 A, The most frequent form of complete atrioventricular septal defect (type A), originally classified according to division of the anterior bridging leaflet (A) and attachment to the septum. Current interpretation has only the left-sided portion of the anterior leaflet as anterior bridging leaflet, and the right-sided portion is the true anterior tricuspid leaflet. P is the posterior bridging leaflet, and L represents the two lateral leaflets that correspond to posterior mitral and tricuspid leaflets. mitral valve (MV) and tricuspid valve (TV) indicate mitral and tricuspid portions of leaflets, and right atrial (RA) and right ventricular (RV) indicate right atrium and right ventricle respectively. **B,** Schematic four-chamber view of complete atrioventricular (AV) septal defect, showing common valve and atrial and ventricular communications. *(A, reprinted with permission from Porter CJ, Feldt RH, Porter CJ, et al: Atrioventricular septal defects. In Emmanouilides GC, Riemenschneider TA, Allen HD, Gutgesell HP [eds]: Moss and Adams Heart Disease in Infants, Children, and Adolescents: Including the Fetus and Young Adult. Baltimore, Williams & Wilkins, 1995, p 710; B, reprinted with permission from Castaneda AR, Jonas RA, Mayer Jr JE, Hanley FL [eds]: Atrioventricular canal defect. In Cardiac Surgery of the Neonate and Infant, Philadelphia, WB Saunders, 1994, p 168.)*

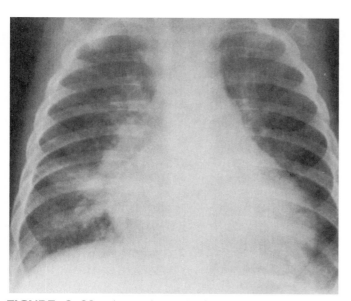

FIGURE 3–20 Chest radiograph of a patient with a complete atrioventricular septal defect showing cardiomegaly and increased pulmonary blood flow. *(Reprinted with permission from Spicer RL: Cardiovascular disease in Down syndrome. Sym Pediatr Cardiol 1984;31:1334.)*

An infant with a VSD will encounter a dynamic shunt flow. Normally after birth, PVR decreases slowly over 2 to 4 weeks to adult levels, which is a protective measure against a rapid increase in pulmonary blood flow and possible pulmonary edema. Left-to-right shunt will increase, contingent on the normal decrease in PVR after birth.[115] If a large VSD is present, within the first 2 weeks to 1 year the infant will develop symptoms of CHF, especially poor feeding. The symptoms will very much resemble the patient with complete AV septal defect. The increased pulmonary blood flow will cause marked ventricular hypertrophy to develop. These infants may develop severe PAH and chronic pulmonary vascular disease even after a year without closure of the VSD.[113] Once pulmonary vascular disease becomes severe, options are restricted for successful treatment.[111] Early diagnosis of a VSD in a newborn is unlikely owing to the normally elevated PVR present at birth and elevated right ventricular pressure that minimize left-to-right shunt. Some patients may never experience a decrease in PVR; consequently, left-to-right shunt may be mild or even reverse. However, by the fourth decade, the right ventricle will have failed.[115]

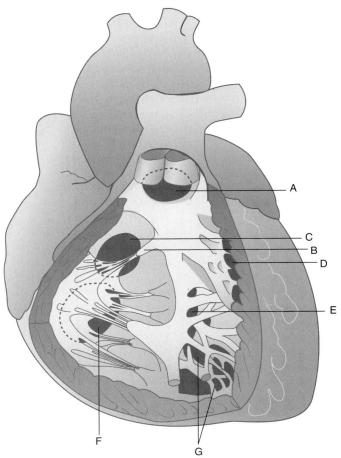

FIGURE 3–21 Anatomic position of defects: A, outlet defect; B, papillary muscle of the conus; C, perimembranous defect; D, marginal muscular defects; E, central muscular defects; F, inlet defect; G, apical muscular defects. *(Reprinted with permission from Graham TP Jr, Gutgesell HP: Ventricular septal defects. In Emmanouilides GC, Riemenschneider TA, Allen HD, Gutgesell HP [eds]: Moss and Adams Heart Disease in Infants, Children, and Adolescents: Including the Fetus and Young Adult. Baltimore, Williams & Wilkins, 1995, p 726.)*

If the right ventricular pressure and PVR decrease as expected in a patient with a VSD, a murmur becomes more prominent and diagnosis of the VSD is more likely.[34] On physical examination, a murmur may be heard only with a small VSD. Moderate defects will usually result in a harsh holosystolic murmur and hyperdynamic precordium owing to increased pulmonary blood flow. The large VSD may appear similar to other VSDs on examination, except sweating and tachypnea are more notable. The chest radiograph shows atrial enlargement, cardiomegaly, and increased pulmonary vascularity. The ECG may reveal ventricular hypertrophy if the VSD is moderate to large.

To prepare for noncardiac surgery in these children with unrepaired lesions, be aware of any extracardiac abnormalies.[116] Although rare, endocarditis is an issue and antibiotics should be administered. If the patient appears in CHF, surgery should be postponed to implement or increase some of the following: digoxin, furosemide, or captopril. Anesthetic management is similar to that for patients with increased pulmonary blood flow. Volatile agents should be used cautiously to avoid exacerbating myocardial depression.

Patent Ductus Arteriosus (PDA)

The transition from fetal circulation after birth requires the functional closure of the ductus arteriosus, which is a communication between the left pulmonary artery and the descending aorta (Fig. 3-22). Functional closure occurs 1 to 4 days after birth.[117] Anatomic closure of the ductus arteriosus is usually complete a month after birth, becoming the ligamentum arteriosum. Although a PDA may exist with other congenital heart defects, an isolated PDA is described here.

An isolated PDA occurs in every 2500 live births,[118] accounting for 10% to 14% of CHD.[5,8,108] It is rare for this anomaly to be missed in infancy or childhood. The incidence of isolated PDA increases as gestational maturity decreases. Approximately 80% of infants weighing less than 1200 g will have a PDA.[108] A PDA can be quite large and can extend from the posterior descending aorta near the origin of the left subclavian artery to the anterior surface of the main pulmonary artery. Various factors,

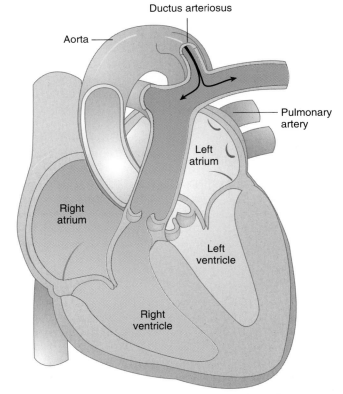

FIGURE 3–22 Patent ductus arteriosus with resultant left-to-right shunting. Some of the blood from the aorta crosses the ductus arteriosus and flows into the pulmonary artery *(arrows)*. *(Reprinted with permission from Brickner ME, Hillis LD, Lange RA: Congenital heart disease in adults. N Engl J Med 2000;342:259.)*

such as hypoxemia, may prevent the normal closure of the ductus arteriosus after birth. A PDA rarely closes spontaneously after infancy.[8] In contrast to premature infants who have a functional problem with the ductus arteriosus, the term infant has an anatomic abnormality whereupon failure to constrict is structural, not functional.

A PDA is associated with left-to-right shunt and excessive pulmonary blood flow. The ductus arteriosus is not structurally identical to other vascular structures, so it has very poor contractile function. If the PDA is large, PVR will determine the degree of left-to-right shunt not the ductus arteriosus. Increased blood flow from PDA to LA may cause additional left-to-right shunting through a PFO, contributing further to left ventricular overload. As the pulmonary artery pressure increases, left-to-right shunting will decrease, but eventually pulmonary vascular changes will become permanent.[109]

If a PDA is small, it may only present problems related to bacterial endocarditis. A larger PDA may remain asymptomatic until childhood or adulthood, whereupon symptoms of fatigue, dyspnea, or palpitations may suddenly appear.[8] Early symptoms include tachypnea, diaphoresis, reduced exercise tolerance, failure to thrive, and recurrent pulmonary infections. PDA may lead to PAH in adulthood. Patients may live until the age of 60, even with CHF and PAH.[111] Mortality with a PDA in adults is 1.8%/year.[119]

A PDA has a characteristic continuous machine murmur, heard mostly at the first or second intercostal space on the left sternal border. Pulses may be bounding, and a widened pulse pressure may be seen with blood pressure monitoring. The ECG is usually unremarkable, except for some evidence of left ventricular hypertrophy if the left-to-right shunt is large. Increased pulmonary vascular markings, as well as an enlarged left atrium and ventricle, may be present on the chest radiograph.

PDA closure in adults is a very challenging operation compared with that in an infant or child.[34] Adults with PDA may be very ill. The PDA may become calcified and/or dilate, making the operation more risky on account of the amount of blood flowing through the PDA.[114]

Beyond the anesthetic considerations of defects with increased pulmonary blood flow, closure of the PDA may be performed through a thoracotomy, percutaneously, or thorascopically. Currently, interventional catheterization is achieving success at placing a Rashkind double umbrella occlusion device to obliterate the PDA and avoid a higher risk operation. Percutaneous measures have been relatively successful, with up to 98% at 1-year follow-up, but unsuccessful in patients weighing more than 5 kg.[120] Percutaneous PDA closure does not require anesthesia and thoracotomy. Residual leaks may occur in 25% of these procedures but are usually clinically insignificant. Thorascopic closure of PDA has also achieved good results with low complications and decreased hospital stay.[118,121] Although good intravenous access is necessary

should excessive blood loss occur with injury to the aorta, noninvasive monitoring is generally acceptable. One-lung ventilation is rarely required and usually not tolerated. Avoiding hyperoxia, especially in the neonatal period, is important to avoid increasing pulmonary blood flow any further. Infants who arrive in the operating room with severe CHF may require ventilation postoperatively.

Anesthesia should include low to moderate doses of fentanyl (25 µg/kg) with a plan for extubation and good analgesia. The diastolic pressure should be observed carefully with a large PDA, because coronary blood flow may suffer if the diastolic pressure is too low, especially because the left ventricular compliance is reduced from the large left-to-right shunt. There is slightly over 10% incidence of ischemic changes in patients with PDA on autopsy.[20] In the premature infant the Hb should not be allowed to drift because of the large amount of fetal Hb present. Anemia will further limit oxygen delivery.

Truncus Arteriosus

Truncus arteriosus is a rare disorder, representing only 1% to 3% of CHD.[122] Nearly three fourths of infants with truncus arteriosus will die by 1 year of age. Truncus arteriosus is caused by a lack of separation of the great vessels *in utero,* so that only one major vessel, the truncal vessel, gives rise to the coronary arteries, aorta, and pulmonary arteries. There is also only one semilunar valve, the truncal valve, that may possess two to seven leaflets, which may be regurgitant in over half the cases. The truncal valve usually overrides both ventricles (80%) or may arise from the right ventricle alone (20%).

Because there are many different presentations, the classification is complex. Classification is based on the position of the main pulmonary artery and whether there is a VSD (type A) or not (type B). There are basically three types of truncus arteriosus, with the fourth type now referred to as pulmonary atresia with VSD. Type Ia, the most common, is present in 50% to 70% of individuals with truncus arteriosus (Fig. 3-23). It is rare to find a truncus arteriosus defect without a VSD.

With truncus arteriosus, the systemic and pulmonary circulations are not separated. The elevated PVR of the infant will initially direct blood systemically; however, as PVR falls, blood is directed to the pulmonary circulation, causing CHF. Ultimately, PVR increases to the degree that obstructive pulmonary vascular disease develops. Without treatment, Eisenmenger's syndrome will occur in about 50% of these people.[111] Some of these patients will develop pulmonary vascular obstruction to the degree that left-to-right shunting will be diminished and symptomatic improvement will occur, allowing survival into adulthood.[110] Occasionally, pulmonary artery stenosis may be present to limit pulmonary blood flow, but severe cyanosis will occur instead.

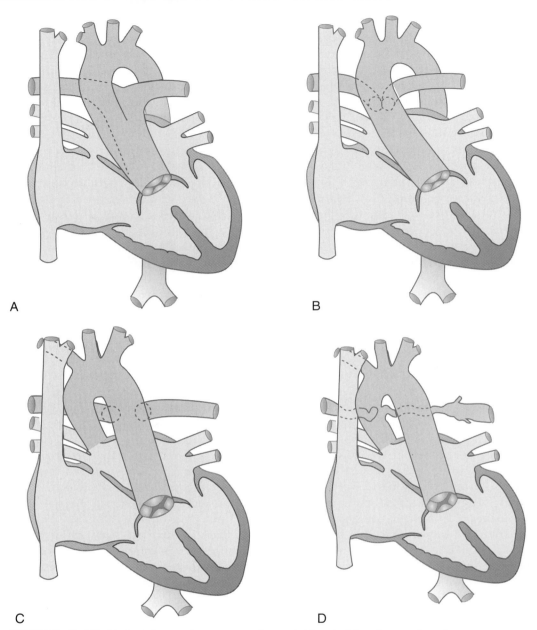

A

B

C

D

FIGURE 3–23 Various forms of truncus arteriosus. **A,** Type I with a short main pulmonary artery segment arising from the leftward, posterior, aspect of the ascending aorta. **B,** Type II with separate origins of the right and left pulmonary arteries arising close to each other on the posterior aspect of the ascending aorta. Note the left-sided aortic arch in **A** and **B. C,** Type III with separate origins of the right and left pulmonary arteries arising far apart from the posterolateral aspect of the ascending aorta. **D,** Type IV, which is more appropriately described as pulmonary atresia and ventricular septal defect; there are separate origins of the right and left pulmonary arteries arising from the descending aorta. Note there is a right-sided aortic arch in **C** and **D.** *(Reprinted with permission from Grifka RG: Cyanotic congenital heart disease with increased pulmonary blood flow. Pediatr Clin North Am 1999;46:413.)*

The infant with truncus arteriosus is critically ill with severe CHF secondary to a high Q_p/Q_s. The infant may be slightly cyanotic at birth, but as the PVR falls, the cyanosis will disappear. These children will rarely present for anything beyond cardiac surgery or catheterization. For patients with type Ia or IIa, it is critical to preserve systemic flow and minimize further pulmonary shunting.

A high-dose fentanyl anesthetic is most commonly used to minimize changes in either pulmonary or systemic circulations. Hyperventilation and high-inspired FIO_2 should be avoided so as to prevent further increasing pulmonary blood flow. Before complete repair at 2 months of age, these infants will receive digoxin, furosemide, and afterload reduction to reduce symptoms of pulmonary overcirculation and pulmonary blood flow.[122] Complete repair will involve creation of a conduit from the right ventricle to the pulmonary artery, closure of the VSD, and creation of a neoaortic valve from the truncal valve (Fig. 3-24). The main reason for improvement in the prognosis for individuals with truncus arteriosus resides in the current strategy of early repair after birth, rather than delaying, which allows the excessive pulmonary blood flow to damage the pulmonary vasculature. Mortality and morbidity is increased if the repair is delayed more than 30 days after birth.[123] Later in life, almost all of these patients will require replacement of the pulmonary conduit, and others may even require repair or replacement of the neoaortic valve.[114] As the infant grows following complete repair, suprasystemic pressures may result in failure of the right ventricle that will require conduit replacement.

Total Anomalous Pulmonary Venous Connection (TAPVC)

This is a very uncommon anomaly, comprising about 1% of CHD. The two forms are partial and total. The partial defect includes pulmonary veins draining to the LA while other veins are draining to other venous connections in the chest. It accounts for only a fourth of anomalous pulmonary venous connections. There are four types of

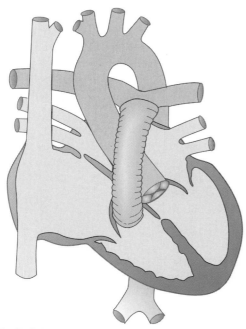

FIGURE 3–24 Repair of truncus arteriosus. The ventricular septal defect has been closed and a valved conduit has been interposed between the right ventricle and the pulmonary artery. Currently, this would typically be a homograft valve. The heart shown has a quadricuspid truncal (now aortic) valve. *(Reprinted with permission from Baum VC: The adult patient with congenital heart disease. J Cardiothorac Vasc Anesth 1996;10:273.)*

TAPVC: supracardiac, cardiac, infradiaphragmatic, and mixed (Fig. 3-25). Some refer to the infradiaphragmatic as intracardiac. Because all the oxygenated blood returns to the RA, an ASD must exist. In the supracardiac and cardiac types of TAPVC with a large ASD the condition resembles an ASD with increased pulmonary blood flow and mixing that leads to less well-oxygenated blood delivered to the systemic circulation and thus cyanosis. The supracardiac type usually drains to the innominate vein and intracardiac type to the coronary sinus. With the infracardiac type, the drainage is usually to the portal vein, but the pulmonary venous flow is obstructed to a degree, resulting in PAH. With all types of TAPVC, the pulmonary veins come together in a confluence behind the heart and then connect to the systemic venous circulation.

Patients with TAPVC may present in many different ways dependent on the pulmonary venous connections, size of the ASD, PVR, pulmonary venous obstruction, and other characteristics. The clinical presentation of TAPVC may vary, but cyanosis is present in all forms. Mild cyanosis and increased pulmonary blood flow from the RA as the PVR falls occur with the supracardiac and cardiac types of TAPVC. Right ventricular overload may occur owing to increased pulmonary blood flow. Surgery is not usually emergent, so medical management is often pursued with digoxin and furosemide. Surgical correction may be undertaken subsequently and electively. In contrast, infradiaphragmatic TAPVC presents with unstable hemodynamics and poor peripheral perfusion, and immediate inotropic support is necessary. Respiratory distress ensues quickly after birth and emergency surgery is necessary to prolong the infant's life. The obstruction to pulmonary venous return is associated with a very poor prognosis.[19] Anesthetic management is reviewed elsewhere.[122,124]

Most patients with TAPVC will die without treatment in the first year.[125] Those who survive for 3 months have a 50% survival rate at 1 year.[125] Some patients have been known to survive to adulthood with TAPVC with a large, nonrestrictive ASD, minimal obstruction to pulmonary venous return, and little pulmonary vascular obstructive disease.[125] If the patient does not have pulmonary venous obstruction, a large ASD is present, and PVR is not excessive, the patient may be approached from an anesthetic standpoint as having an ASD with excessive pulmonary blood flow.

Single Ventricle

The mortality of neonatal congenital heart repair involving two ventricles continues to decline, whereas patients with single-ventricle physiology continue to experience many challenges, accompanied by significant morbidity and mortality. Survival with a single ventricle is only 30% at 1 year after birth, although some individuals may live to adulthood.[126]

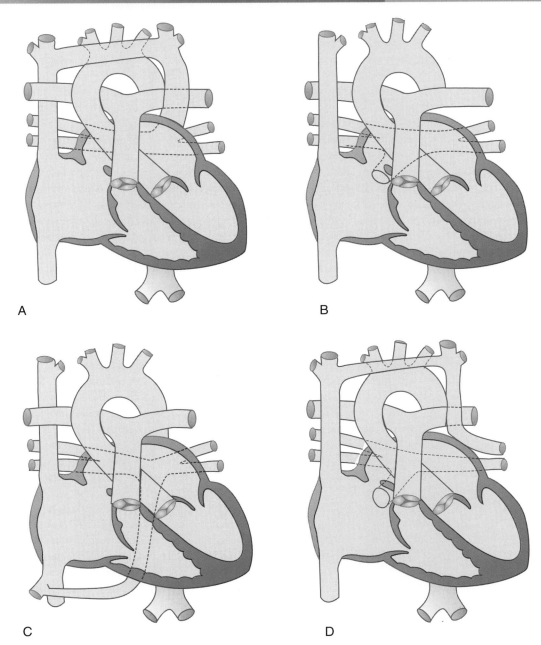

FIGURE 3–25 Four classification of total anomalous pulmonary venous return. **A,** Type I; the four pulmonary veins drain into the vertical vein that enters the innominate vein. **B,** Type II; the pulmonary veins drain into the coronary sinus that enters the right atrium. **C,** Type III; the pulmonary veins join to form a descending vein that courses through the diaphragm and drains into the portal venous system. **D,** Type IV, mixed pulmonary venous return; the two right pulmonary veins and the left lower pulmonary vein drain to the coronary sinus, while the left upper pulmonary vein drains into a vertical vein. Note that in all four there is an atrial septal defect. *(Reprinted with permission from Grifka RG: Cyanotic congenital heart disease with increased pulmonary blood flow. Pediatr Clin North Am 1999;46:419.)*

A wide variety of congenital heart defects are anatomically single-ventricle defects, which account for 1% to 2% of CHD.[126] However, other defects behave as single ventricles because they are unable to properly function as dual ventricle systems, such as HLHS, severe Ebstein's anomaly, tricuspid atresia, and an unbalanced AV septal defect.

The ventricular morphology of two thirds of single ventricle defects is left ventricle. Approximately one fourth of single-ventricle anomalies have morphologic right ventricles. The remaining single-ventricle defects are classified as indeterminate but often are composed of both right and left ventricles. The great vessels appear discordant in

85% of these defects. Both morphology of the ventricle and the relationship of the great arteries are important to note when caring for these patients. Most single ventricles have an atretic AV valve or semilunar valve. Mixing of the systemic and pulmonary venous blood will necessarily occur, producing eventual ventricular overload. Ventricular ejection into either the systemic or pulmonary circulation is dynamic and will depend primarily on SVR and PVR, respectively. Consequently, surgical placement of either a systemic to pulmonary artery shunt or a pulmonary artery band will be required. The age of the patient is also important, because it will influence decisions regarding the care of individuals with the same single ventricle anatomy and physiology.

All current management options for a single-ventricle defect are suboptimal, but a Fontan procedure appears to offer many advantages.[127] The Fontan procedure is based on the principle that the right atrial pressure is capable of providing the force necessary to deliver deoxygenated venous blood to the pulmonary arteries and lungs, so that the well-oxygenated blood may return to the single ventricle without mixing with the deoxygenated venous blood. The solitary ventricle will then become the pump for this well-oxygenated blood to travel systemically, achieving a physiologic circulation without benefit of two ventricles. There have been many modifications of the Fontan operation (Fig. 3-26) since its initial description.

A Fontan operation is performed ideally from 18 months to 4 years of age but is also performed quite frequently during adulthood. The 15-year survival of 60% is the same for those who received a Fontan operation as a child or adult.[127] However, patients who received a Fontan operation as an adult may have different issues to contend with perioperatively and long-term compared with children who

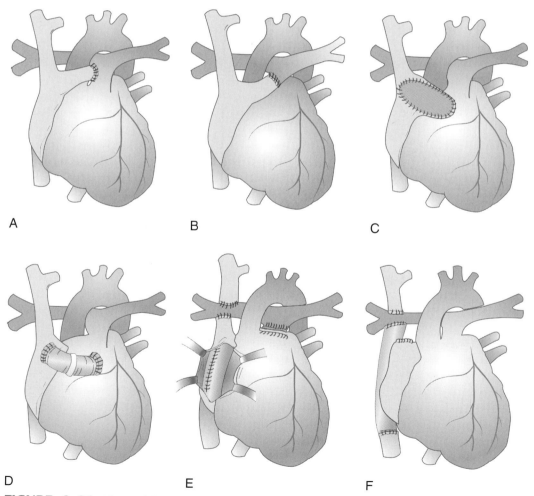

FIGURE 3–26 The modifications of the Fontan procedure. **A,** Direct connection of the right atrial appendage to the side of the main pulmonary artery. **B,** Direct connection of the right atrial appendage of the end of the pulmonary trunk. **C,** Right atrial to right ventricular connection with a pericardial patch. **D,** Right atrial to right ventricular connection with a valved conduit. **E,** Total cavopulmonary anastomosis with an intra-atrial (lateral tunnel) baffle. **F,** Total cavopulmonary anastomosis using an extracardiac conduit. *(Reprinted with permission from Stayer SA, Andropoulos DB, Russell IA: Anesthetic management of the adult patient with congenital heart disease. Anesthesiol Clin North Am 2003;21:666.)*

have undergone the procedure. One major concept that applies to both pediatric and adult patients is the importance of PVR. If PVR is high at the time of surgery, the Fontan operation will fail. However, strict characteristics once thought to be absolutely necessary to consider performing this procedure have been expanded, so that 80% of Fontan procedures are successful. This has been achieved through a variety of measures, but none is more important than the "fenestration" that is made between the atria. Fenestrations have allowed Fontan procedures to be performed in patients not previously considered candidates. The fenestration augments cardiac output at the expense of worse basal oxygenation. It also lessens the risk of complications. Chronic anticoagulation is required.

A patient who has had a Fontan procedure and who requires noncardiac surgery is an anesthetic challenge. Many physiologic changes occur with a Fontan operation. Some of these changes occur rapidly, whereas others may take years to occur. Certain changes are also associated specifically with Fontan procedures done more than 18 years ago that will not be present in more recent Fontan operations. Any history of prior palliative surgery should be noted, because these patients tend to have worse baseline myocardial function.

It is necessary to assess the current functional status of an individual who has had a Fontan operation, irrespective of previous functional class, because ventricular deterioration is inevitable.[127-130] The reason for this gradual circulatory decompensation is not understood. Systolic ventricular function begins to slowly deteriorate at 1 to 5 years but is most discernible after 5 years.[127] The systolic function is more likely to be impaired if the ventricle is a morphologic right ventricle. Functional class and ejection fraction will be excellent during this slow deterioration. Along with reduced systolic function, Doppler echocardiography revealed in 25 patients with CHD that significant systolic incoordination, possibly attributed to the geometry of the muscles resulting from the CHD, was also present in these patients.[130] Even if systolic function is preserved, severe diastolic dysfunction may be present.[130] As the systolic function worsens, AV valve regurgitation may also appear. After 10 years an obvious decline in the functional class is readily apparent.[127] The amount of ventricular dysfunction is directly related to the number of years volume overload was present.

Another challenging characteristic of an individual with a Fontan operation is the propensity for arrhythmia that has become more prevalent as the number of years since surgery increases. Atrial dilation is a major focus, but decreased ventricular function and AV valve insufficiency also play a role in arrhythmogenesis. Arrhythmias are primarily IART,[23] with the most common being atrial flutter.[34] If atrial flutter occurs suddenly, rapid treatment is necessary because CHF may ensue rapidly.[131] Arrhythmias are more likely to occur in those with older-style Fontan operations than individuals with lateral tunnels and cavopulmonary connections.[23] Adults who received a Fontan operation are also more likely to have dysrhythmias. Forty-six percent of adults who underwent a Fontan procedure as adults will have arrhythmias by 10 years.[127] Modifications of the procedure, such as the use of a lateral tunnel, may ameliorate some of the ventricular dysfunction and other associated arrhythmias (Fig. 3-27).[110] Atrial arrhythmias are especially difficult to treat.[23] Twenty percent of survivors will be taking at least one antiarrhythmic medication, excluding digitalis.[131]

Patients who have a Fontan operation tend to be receiving diuretics, afterload-reducing agents, and anticoagulants. Slightly more than half of individuals with a Fontan operation require chronic diuretics. Nearly one third of patients have had a thrombotic episode after the procedure, with biochemical evidence of thrombosis

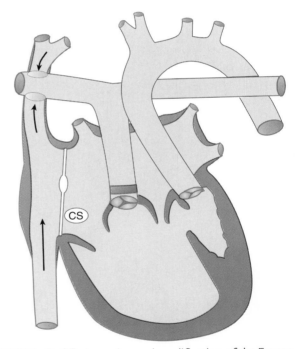

FIGURE 3–27 Lateral tunnel modification of the Fontan operation in a heart with single ventricle. After resection of the native atrial septum, an intra-atrial baffle directs inferior vena caval return through the right atrium. The superior vena cava has been transected and both ends anastomosed to the right pulmonary artery. A hole has been placed in the baffle material to allow decompression of the right atrium if necessary. This may close spontaneously or may be closed by an intravascularly placed device in the catheterization laboratory, or a pursestring suture may be placed around it (the "adjustable atrial septal defect") for later elective closure. The pulmonary artery has been ligated proximally. The coronary sinus (CS) has been incorporated into the low-pressure neo-left atrium, which will result in minor arterial desaturation. It can be appreciated that the cephalad-superior vena cava/right pulmonary artery anastomosis represents a bidirectional Glenn shunt. *(Reprinted with permission from Baum VC: The adult patient with congenital heart disease. J Cardiothorac Vasc Anesth 1996;10:272.)*

present long after surgery.[132] Beyond the well-recognized risk of perioperative thrombotic complications, long-term coagulation changes reveal a lowered protein C and S value compared with age-matched controls but no difference in antithrombin levels.[132] Fifty percent of Fontan patients have elevated levels of factor VIII.

Protein-losing enteropathy (PLE) is a major risk factor for anesthesia in patients who have had a Fontan procedure. It occurs in 10% of patients, characterized by significant peripheral edema, low serum albumin, hypomagnesemia, and hypocalcemia.[34,131] The immune system is depressed, making these patients susceptible to respiratory tract infections. Especially important is that induction of anesthesia in these individuals has been noted to be a significant risk, with hemodynamic instability and even cardiovascular collapse not uncommon. Furthermore, several major classes of anesthetic agents, as well as other medications, are affected by the hypoalbuminemia. Any patient with PLE who requires surgery deserves special care to assess his or her current metabolic, protein, and hemodynamic status as well as their recent condition.

Anesthetic management of a patient who has had a Fontan operation has special considerations. The right atrial pressure must be adequate to maintain good cardiac output. Previous right atrial filling pressures should be noted. The right atrial pressure also reflects ventricular function, AV valve sufficiency and function, PVR, and pulmonary artery size.[131] There is a gradient between the RA and the LA that is partially fixed, due to the lungs, that determines the cardiac output. If PVR increases, the gradient between the RA and LA increases and the likelihood of poor cardiac output and systemic oxygen delivery increases; consequently, it is essential to minimize PVR. Parameters that are important to achieve to minimize PVR include hypocarbia, alkalosis, decreased intrathoracic pressures, normothermia, and minimal PEEP. Positive-pressure ventilation inhibits pulmonary blood flow, diminishes cardiac output, and increases PVR, whereas negative pressure does the opposite.[133] Afterload reduction may be used to reduce PVR and increase cardiac output. Inhaled nitric oxide (20 ppm) is beneficial in patients with a Fontan operation who have increased PVR and increased transpulmonary gradient because there is no change in systemic blood pressure, as can be caused by some pulmonary vasodilators.[134] The response to nitric oxide is rapid, or the individual may be a nonresponder. Nitric oxide may be instrumental in restoring oxygenation without hemodynamic consequences.[134]

Hypoplastic Left Heart Syndrome (HLHS)

Before 1970 HLHS was considered fatal. It is the fourth most common congenital anomaly requiring neonatal surgery,[135] making up 7% of CHD.[3] Today, treatment involves either a heart transplant or a staged repair ending

in a Fontan procedure to separate the pulmonary and systemic circulations. The anesthesiologist must understand the anatomic and physiologic issues to provide anesthesia to these patients for a noncardiac operation.

HLHS includes aortic valve atresia, hypoplasia of the ascending and arch of the aorta, and atresia or stenosis of the mitral valve. The apex of the heart is formed almost entirely by the right ventricle (Fig. 3-28), while the left ventricle is nonfunctional. Pulmonary and systemic venous blood will mix in the RA. Systemic perfusion, especially coronary perfusion, will be supplied by the PDA. Excessive pulmonary blood flow will diminish systemic perfusion, leading to coronary hypoperfusion and shock. The mixed venous saturation is an excellent modality to detect anaerobic metabolism, especially if it is less than 30%. As long as PVR remains high, the infant will appear cyanotic, but systemic perfusion will be adequate.

If a heart transplant is not performed for HLHS, ductal flow cannot continue to supply the systemic metabolic needs of the infant. A Norwood procedure is performed to create unobstructed systemic and coronary perfusion but also to ensure a stable source of pulmonary blood flow (Fig. 3-29).

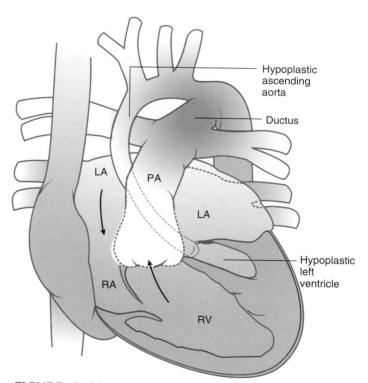

FIGURE 3–28 Native anatomy in hypoplastic left heart syndrome (HLHS). Note the hypoplastic left ventricle, aortic valve atresia, and diminutive ascending aorta. Systemic blood flow is propelled by the right ventricle (RV) via the pulmonary artery (PA), and ductus arteriosus. Pulmonary venous return enters the right side of the heart through a foramen ovale or an atrial septal defect. LA, left atrium; RA, right atrium. *(Reprinted with permission from Nicolson SC, Steven JM, Jobes DR: Hypoplastic left heart syndrome. In Lake CL [ed]: Pediatric Cardiac Anesthesia. Stamford, CT, Appleton & Lange, 1998, p 338.)*

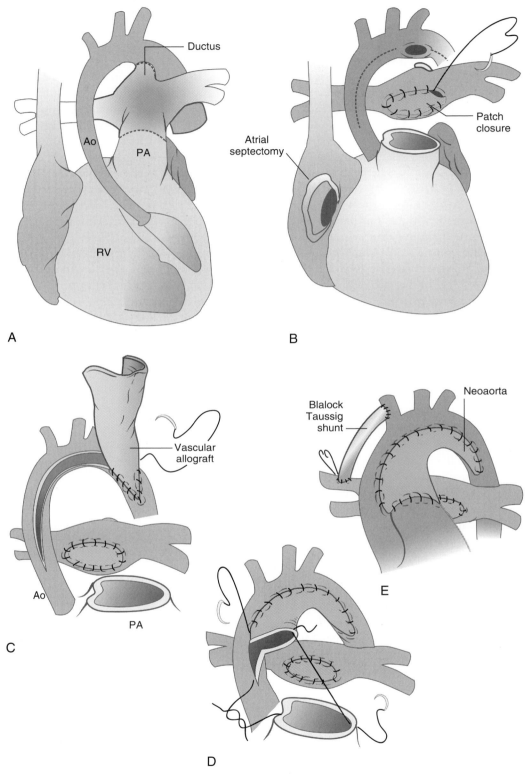

FIGURE 3–29 Norwood procedure. **A,** *Dotted lines* indicate transection points of the main pulmonary artery (PA) and ductus arteriosus. **B,** Atrial septectomy to avoid pulmonary venous hypertension. Patch closure of distal main PA. Longitudinal incision in aorta extending beyond ductus arteriosus, which has been divided and ligated. **C** and **D.** Construction of neoaorta using the proximal main PA, ascending aorta (Ao), and vascular allograft. **E,** Pulmonary blood flow supplied by a right modified Blalock-Taussig shunt connecting the right subclavian artery to the right PA. *(Reprinted with permission from Nicolson SC, Steven JM, Jobes DR: Hypoplastic left heart syndrome. In Lake CL [ed]: Pediatric Cardiac Anesthesia. Stamford, CT, Appleton & Lange, 1998, p 342.)*

A neoaorta is fashioned from the pulmonary artery and a shunt placed between the aorta and pulmonary artery to regulate pulmonary blood flow. Currently a Blalock-Taussig shunt is included in the "modified Norwood."[19] Owing to advancements of the Norwood procedure, 85% to 94% of infants survive to a bidirectional cavopulmonary anastomosis[136] and 40% to 60% of infants will survive to be evaluated for a Fontan procedure.[137]

Within a year of a Norwood procedure, a bidirectional cavopulmonary anastomosis or hemi-Fontan procedure is performed. With a hemi-Fontan procedure all pulmonary blood flow arises exclusively from the superior vena cava (Fig. 3-30). The pulmonary veins deliver well-oxygenated blood to the single atrium while the inferior vena cava instead delivers desaturated blood to the single atrium, resulting in blood with a saturation of 85% for systemic delivery.[138] The hemi-Fontan procedure reduces the stress on the pulmonary vessels and PVR to handle the entire cardiac output; instead, the cardiac output is maintained by pulmonary venous blood derived from the superior vena cava and by deoxygenated blood derived from the inferior vena cava. It is the staging of the repair of HLHS that improved 5-year survival to 70%.[139] With improved survival there are more opportunities for these infants to undergo noncardiac surgery. After bidirectional cavopulmonary anastomosis or a hemi-Fontan procedure, a modified Fontan operation completes the staged repair of HLHS. The 10-year survival has still only reached 50% or less for patients with HLHS.[135]

Anesthetic management for noncardiac surgery will depend on the stage of repair. Anesthesia for a Norwood procedure has been reviewed.[140] Fentanyl was associated with a more stable intraoperative course than halothane. Following a Norwood procedure but before the hemi-Fontan procedure, it is important to effectively balance systemic and pulmonary blood flow during a noncardiac operation. A Qp/Qs ratio maintained near 1.0 should provide optimal pulmonary, and especially systemic, perfusion. Two factors that will influence outcome the most in patients after a Norwood procedure include ventricular function and flow across the shunt.[141] Inhalation or intravenous induction may be used, depending on the ventricular function. Maintenance anesthesia should consist of a low-dose volatile agent and narcotics. Fentanyl will help stabilize systemic and pulmonary blood flows. PaO_2 and SpO_2 should be followed carefully but will not always accurately reflect the balance between pulmonary and systemic flows. A broader range of inspired oxygen concentrations and PcO_2 is tolerated once there has been more time elapsed since the Norwood procedure.

After a bidirectional Glenn or hemi-Fontan operation, inhalation induction is tolerated quite well by infants and children. The PVR should not be allowed to increase, but it does not have to be low for a bidirectional Glenn or hemi-Fontan operation, in contrast to the

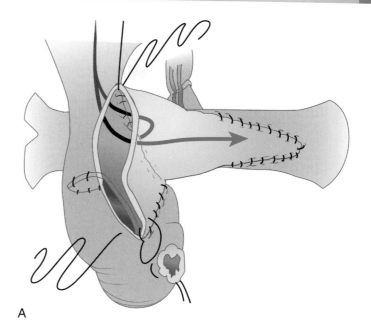

A

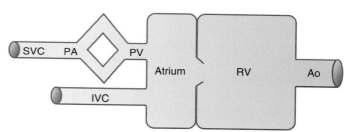

B

FIGURE 3–30 **A,** Hemi-Fontan. The superior vena cava is associated with the augmented pulmonary arteries, and a dam is positioned to separate the common atrium from the caval-pulmonary anastomosis. **B,** Schematic illustration of the blood flow pattern in children after hemi-Fontan operation. Pulmonary blood flow is derived exclusively from superior vena cava (SVC) drainage flowing directly through the pulmonary bed. Venous return is split nearly equally between SVC flow that passes through the pulmonary circulation (PA and PV) entering the common atrium and inferior vena cava (IVC) blood that enters the atrium directly. The single ventricle (RV) need only supply sufficient flow to perfuse the systemic circulation; thus the volume load is equivalent to a normal systemic ventricle. Ao, aorta. *(Reprinted with permission from Nicolson SC, Steven JM, Kurth CD, et al: Anesthesia for noncardiac surgery in infants with hypoplastic left heart syndrome following hemi-Fontan operation. J Cardiothoracic Vasc Anesth 1994;8:335.)*

modified Fontan procedure. Right atrial filling pressures must be maintained, especially if PVR is slightly elevated, because with adequate filling pressures the inferior vena cava can support the cardiac output.[138] Tidal volumes must be below normal even though moderate hypocarbia is desirable. If ventilation does not result in oxygen saturations at least as good as in the preoperative period, ventilation parameters should be reviewed. Regional block is recommended for analgesia to avoid significant respiratory depression associated with systemic narcotics.

ANATOMIC DEFECTS ASSOCIATED WITH DECREASED PULMONARY BLOOD FLOW

Patients with cyanotic CHD may desaturate severely. In most cases, infants with cyanotic CHD do not survive very long without surgical intervention. The two most common defects of cyanotic CHD are TOF and Eisenmenger's syndrome.[142]

Tetralogy of Fallot (TOF)

TOF is the most common form of cyanotic CHD after 1 year of age, accounting for 10% of all CHD.[109] It is also the most common cyanotic defect encountered in adults.[110] Without surgery, a majority of patients die in childhood. Twenty-five percent will survive to adolescence without surgery but face a mortality rate of 6.4% per year.[110] Only 3% will survive until the age of 40.

TOF contains four main characteristics, although the essence of the defect has been argued for many years without resolution: a nonrestrictive VSD, obstruction of the right ventricular outflow tract with or without supravalvular pulmonary stenosis, right ventricular hypertrophy, and an overriding aorta (Fig. 3-31). There is a range of morphology, anatomy, signs, symptoms, and pathophysiologic consequences related primarily to the degree of pulmonary blood flow obstruction.[143] A feature that is consistently present with TOF is right ventricular

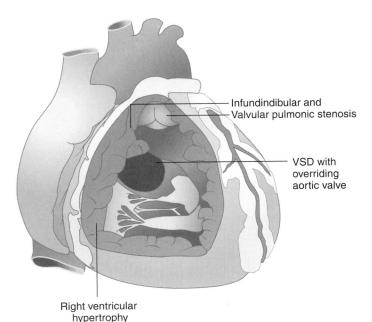

FIGURE 3–31 The interior of the right ventricle, showing the characteristic defects of tetralogy of Fallot: pulmonic stenosis, ventricular septal defect (VSD), overriding aorta, and right ventricular hypertrophy. *(Reprinted with permission from Stayer SA, Andropoulos DB, Russell IA: Anesthetic management of the adult patient with congenital heart disease. Anesthesiol Clin North Am 2003;21:663.)*

Labels in figure: Infundindibular and Valvular pulmonic stenosis; VSD with overriding aortic valve; Right ventricular hypertrophy

infundibular narrowing. Until the infundibulum becomes more active and pulmonary blood flow becomes obstructed by closure of PDA, 25% of infants with TOF are acyanotic. However, pulmonary blood flow may be obstructed at levels other than the infundibulum. The pulmonary valve is stenotic in three fourths of individuals and absent in 2% to 6%.[144]

Obstructed pulmonary blood flow at the level of the infundibulum with a VSD causes a right-to-left shunt that is largely fixed. However, changes in PVR and SVR can alter the amount of right-to-left shunt enough to precipitate "tet" spells. These episodes are profound states of cyanosis associated with increased right-to-left shunt, primarily occurring in infants 2 to 3 months of age that can progress to unconsciousness. These hypercyanotic spells are not limited only to TOF but occur in other cyanotic CHD. Treatment includes maneuvers to lessen the right-to-left shunt, such as increasing SVR or decreasing PVR. "Tet" spells may also be initiated by infundibular spasm in response to sympathetic stimulation or β-adrenergic medications. Adequate filling pressures and volume status are imperative in these patients, because hypovolemia may increase sympathetic stimulation or further reduce oxygen delivery, which may result in acidosis and, consequently, increase PVR, further exacerbating the right-to-left shunt. "Tet" spells are infrequent or absent by the age of 2 to 3 years and very rarely occur in children or adolescents. They do not occur in adults.[142]

Some patients with TOF may be palliated with a modified Blalock-Taussig shunt (Fig. 3-32) until complete repair is warranted.[143] Although most patients will be repaired during infancy, adults also may undergo complete repair of TOF,[145] most commonly between the ages of 13 to 43 years. Surgical mortality is higher in adults (2.5% to 8.5%) than infants (<3.0%).[142] Furthermore, actuarial survival is less the older the patient is at the time of surgery.[146] Older patients often have previously undergone aortopulmonary shunts or have significant aortopulmonary collaterals that increase the difficulty of a complete repair. Once repaired, survival rates range from 80% to 94% over 20 years[34] and 80% of patients are symptom free.[147] Reoperation is necessary in less than 10% of patients.

Patients who require noncardiac surgery after TOF repair have several risk factors that need to be carefully monitored. These individuals have an increased risk of arrhythmias and sudden death, even though they have undergone repair.[23,142,147] On Holter monitoring, arrhythmias are detected in 40% to 50% of individuals after repair of TOF. Scarring from the atriotomy or ventriculotomy may contribute to this risk of arrhythmias. Atrial flutter or fibrillation is far more common than ventricular arrhythmias, especially because the age of repair is greater. These rhythm disturbances may cause considerable morbidity.[23] It has not been possible to identify which patients are at increased risk of sudden death after repair

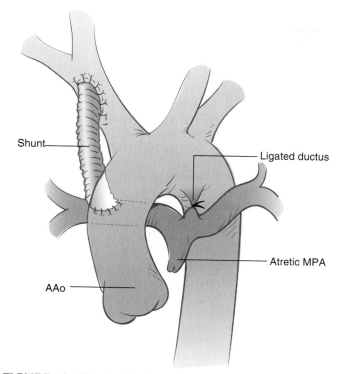

FIGURE 3–32 Modified Blalock-Taussig shunt. Note the atretic main pulmonary artery (MPA) and the ligated ductus arteriosus (ductus). A Gore-Tex tube graft (shunt) is sewn side-to-side between the innominate artery and the right pulmonary artery. Size of the tube graft (3.5 mm, 4.0 mm, or 5.0 mm) is chosen at surgery depending on patient size and caliber of pulmonary artery. Some surgeons perform the shunt through a median sternotomy, and others choose a lateral thoracotomy; cardiopulmonary bypass is usually not required. AAo, ascending aorta. *(Reprinted with permission from Waldman JD, Wernly JA: Cyanotic congenital heart disease with decreased pulmonary blood flow in children. Pediatric Clin North Am 1999;46:388.)*

of TOF. It is not uncommon to see polymorphic ventricular ectopy by Holter monitoring in patients with TOF. Inducible VT is noted in 15% to 30% of patients.[23]

Before anesthesia, a patient who underwent TOF repair should be evaluated for evidence of pulmonary regurgitation. The right ventricle may dilate and develop worsening function and left ventricular failure with pulmonary regurgitation. However, the need for pulmonary valve replacement is not absolute with pulmonary regurgitation, because it may be tolerated well for years.[34] It is now questionable whether complete relief of the right ventricular to pulmonary artery gradient is even necessary at the time of repair, because significant infundibular resection is needed to accomplish it, and more than a third of patients at long-term follow-up have been identified with pulmonary regurgitation.[148] Obstruction of the right ventricular outflow tract is not uncommon and is the most common reason for reoperation. Assessment of the ventricular function is vital before any anesthetic because the function may deteriorate. However, if the repair is

good, then the patient should be in condition to tolerate most operations.[147]

These patients may have a greater risk of developing myocardial ischemia during noncardiac surgery. Anomalous coronary arteries are present in 10% of those with TOF.[142] Thirty-five percent of infants with TOF have evidence of myocardial ischemia.[20]

Anesthetic management of infants with TOF will primarily occur in the catheterization laboratory or during a palliative or complete repair and has been reviewed.[149] Anesthetic induction can be achieved with ketamine, administered intramuscularly or intravenously with relative safety if ventilation is maintained. Ketamine has not been found to increase PVR in these patients[150] or precipitate "tet" spells.[102] It is effective at maintaining the SVR,[110] yet does not significantly alter Q_p/Q_s.[102] Ketamine provides superior hemodynamic control compared with isoflurane in infants with TOF, not just during induction but with anesthetic maintenance as well.[104] Fewer children and infants with TOF required inotropic support with ketamine than isoflurane before CPB.

An inhalation induction may also be safely performed in patients with TOF,[67] but the blood pressure must be carefully observed to avoid a decrease in SVR that may increase the right-to-left shunt. In general, anesthetic induction will improve peripheral saturation in those with cyanotic CHD.[67,68] Fentanyl (10 to 25 μg/kg) and a very low inspired concentration of volatile agent is recommended for anesthesia maintenance in those with TOF.

Opioids offer several advantages, such as circulatory stability for anesthetic management of TOF,[87,94] but benefit from the addition of other agents.[90] When flunitrazepam was added to a sufentanil-based anesthetic for infants and children undergoing complete repair of TOF, plasma levels of norepinephrine were suppressed more fully compared with the administration of sufentanil alone. Furthermore, the response to stimulation was not suppressed as well with opioids alone compared with opioids and benzodiazepines.[90]

If a patient is evaluated with TOF and absent pulmonary valve, extreme airway obstruction is a risk, secondary to the very large pulmonary arteries that lie on the bronchi.[144] Bronchomalacia is also a real concern. Any signs of respiratory infection should be carefully followed up, because the risk of these infections is significant.

Complete repair of TOF has not been achieved in some individuals. Poor pulmonary blood flow may have been remedied by aortopulmonary shunts that improved symptoms (Fig. 3-33). These adults tend to have a less severe form of TOF. Although cyanotic, they have developed significant aortopulmonary collaterals that increased pulmonary blood flow. They may experience some dyspnea and limited exercise tolerance. Without complete repair, they have erythrocytosis, hyperviscosity, abnormal hemostasis, cerebral abscesses, or stroke and endocarditis.[142]

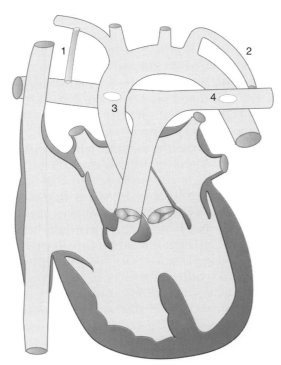

FIGURE 3–33   Palliative aortopulmonary anastomoses. The anastomoses shown on this figure of a heart with tetralogy of Fallot represent the following: 1, modified Blalock-Taussig; 2, classic Blalock-Taussig; 3, Waterston (Waterston-Cooley); 4, Potts. *(Reprinted with permission from Baum VC: The adult patient with congenital heart disease. J Cardiothorac Vasc Anesth 1996;10:270.)*

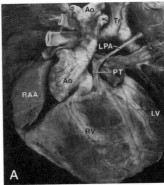
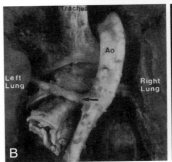
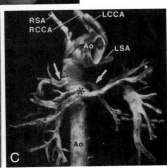

FIGURE 3–34   Pulmonary atresia and ventricular septal defect. **A,** Anterior view of unopened specimen from an 18-year old shows dextroposed aorta (Ao), right aortic arch, and severely hypoplastic pulmonary trunk (PT) and left pulmonary artery (LPA). **B,** Posterior view of mediastinal structures from a 4-year old with pulmonary situs inversus, right aortic arch, and right atrial isomerism shows origin of large systemic collateral artery *(arrow)* to left lung from descending thoracic aorta. **C,** Anterior view of right aortic arch from an 8-year old shows mirror-image brachiocephalic branching, aberrant retroesophageal left subclavian artery (LSA), and origin of two small collateral arteries *(arrows)* and one large trifurcating collateral artery (*). LCCA, left common carotid artery; LV, left ventricle; RAA, right atrial appendage; RCCA, right common carotid artery; RSA, right subclavian artery; RV, right ventricle; Tr, trachea; TV, tricuspid valve. *(Reprinted with permission from Mair DD, Edwards WD, Julsrud PR, et al: Pulmonary atresia and ventricular septal defect. In Emmanouilides GC, Riemenschneider TA, Allen HD, Gutgesell HP [eds]: Moss and Adams Heart Disease in Infants, Children, and Adolescents: Including the Fetus and Young Adult. Baltimore, Williams & Wilkins, 1995, p 985.)*

Hemoptysis is possible and may be severe.[145] Severe volume overload resulting in CHF is also present in many of these individuals. Management of these patients from an anesthetic point of view should strive to maintain SVR, and fentanyl and ketamine accomplish this effectively.

Pulmonary Atresia with VSD

Pulmonary atresia with VSD makes up 2% of CHD. It is the most severe form of TOF, differentiated by pulmonary valve atresia and variable size and distribution of the pulmonary artery tree. The pulmonary arteries are much more abnormal than in TOF. The complex pulmonary anatomy sometimes relegates the patient to life-long chronic cyanosis. However, advances in surgical techniques have increased the number of patients capable of complete repair.

The central pulmonary arteries of pulmonary atresia have no anatomic connection with the right ventricle (Fig. 3-34A). In most cases the pulmonary trunk is little more than a cord or is altogether missing. If the right and left pulmonary arteries communicate, they are described as confluent. The blood supply to the lungs is largely derived from collateral vessels originating from the descending aorta or other systemic sources such as a PDA. The collateral vessels from the aorta follow the distribution of the pulmonary arterial branches to the lungs. The collateral vessels may travel to the lung segments alone or connect at some point with the pulmonary arterial vessels traveling to the same segments of the lung (see Fig. 3-34B). The complexity of the pulmonary artery and collateral circulation to the lung results in many clinical scenarios for affected persons (see Fig. 3-34C). The pulmonary blood supply is so variable and complex, whereas the intracardiac structure is straightforward. The pulmonary arteries may be quite hypoplastic, making complete surgical correction difficult or impossible. The VSD is nonrestrictive and connects morphologically distinct right and left ventricles.

At birth these infants become very cyanotic, especially on PDA closure, or slightly cyanotic if significant collateral vessels are present. Eventually, patients will outgrow their collateral supply to become more cyanotic and require intervention. A number of operations, usually three, will be needed to centralize the complex pulmonary blood supply, referred to as "unifocalization."[151] Unifocalization means that the central pulmonary arteries are confluent and continuous with all distal pulmonary arterioles. During the process of reaching unifocalization, these patients may appear for noncardiac procedures with various amounts of pulmonary blood flow.

To reach complete repair, the central arteries cannot be hypoplastic, or right ventricular failure would ensue. Most frequently, a staged operation is performed, when appropriate, with placement of a conduit from the right ventricle to the pulmonary arteries, followed by closure of the VSD.[151] The right ventricular-pulmonary artery conduit stimulates more pulmonary artery growth than aortopulmonary shunts. A single-stage complete repair for infants has been shown to achieve early cardiovascular physiologic normalization and avoid multiple operations.[152] It may also reduce the chance of obstructive pulmonary vascular disease that can occur with aortopulmonary collaterals.[152] The long-term results appear good with this one-stage approach, but additional studies will be necessary to validate it.[19]

As most patients with pulmonary atresia and VSD age, additional shunts or complete repair will be necessary. Those who have received complete repair will eventually require replacement of the right ventricle to pulmonary artery conduits later in life. These patients should be carefully evaluated for current and previous information regarding pulmonary artery distribution, cyanosis, and relative exercise tolerance. Anesthesia management is similar to those with TOF.

An important condition genetically transmitted that is associated with pulmonary atresia and VSD is the velocardiofacial syndrome. It is the second most common genetic condition associated with CHD. Velocardiofacial syndrome has many otolaryngologic manifestations, immune dysfunction, airway abnormalities, and reactive pulmonary airways. There is a propensity for chronic lung infections.[153] The anesthesiologist should be prepared for the possibility of severe bronchospasm.[152,154]

Transposition of the Great Arteries (TGA)

TGA constitutes 5% to 7% of CHD.[3,5] It is the most frequent cyanotic defect.[5] The morphologic right ventricle gives rise to the aorta, and the morphologic left ventricle gives rise to the pulmonary artery (Fig. 3-35). Without treatment, 95% of infants will die before 1 year of age. The operation of choice now is the arterial switch procedure. It is associated with low mortality, and patients should have a normal life expectancy. In contrast to many other congenital anomalies, additional cardiac surgery is unlikely. Extracardiac anomalies are rarely present with TGA.[34]

TGA is usually designated with D or L. The "D" indicates that the aorta is anterior and to the right of the

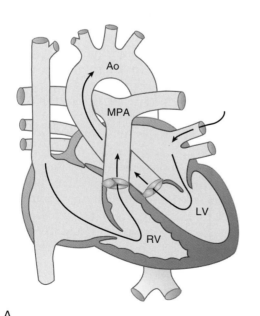 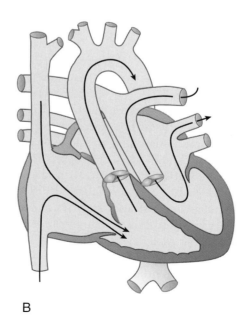

A   B

FIGURE 3–35 Normal heart (**A**) and a heart with transposition of the great arteries (TGA) (**B**). Note the right ventricle (RV) is in continuity with the main pulmonary artery (MPA), while the left ventricle (LV) is in continuity with the aorta (Ao). In the heart with TGA, the RV is in continuity with the Ao, and the LV is in continuity with the MPA. *(Reprinted with permission from Grifka RG: Cyanotic congenital heart disease with increased pulmonary blood flow. Pediatr Clin North Am 1999;46:407.)*

pulmonary artery, whereas "L" indicates the aorta is anterior and to the left of the pulmonary artery. TGA rarely contains an ASD or VSD but often has a large PDA. If there is AV discordance, the defect is referred to as a "corrected" TGA and it behaves in a physiologically normal manner.

TGA classically has parallel pulmonary and systemic circulations that result in severe cyanosis, which is made worse by the subsequent reduction in PVR that follows birth and the ensuing increased pulmonary blood flow that will ultimately cause pulmonary vascular disease. Without associated defects, the ductus arteriosus and PFO must provide communication between atria. Atrial communication generates improved oxygen saturation but may cause CHF. However, a small shunt such as an ASD or VSD may be associated with slightly better mortality than in those patients with severe cyanosis and no communication.

Infants with a restrictive ASD or obstructed aortic arch are severely cyanotic and have a poor prognosis with TGA. A communication may be required for viability, so a balloon septostomy is performed to increase oxygenation. Because the left atrial pressure is usually higher than the right atrial pressure, shunting will be in the direction of left to right. Most cases of TGA have an intact ventricular septum, but for those patients who have a VSD, cyanosis is mild but pulmonary blood flow is large. These individuals are prone to CHF and are often cyanotic and tachypneic. Early in their life they lead fairly normal lives, but myocardial function is depressed in contrast to normal hearts. A chest radiograph may frequently demonstrate an enlarged heart.[142] Although an anesthesiologist may interact with a patient who has TGA in the catheterization suite, contact will be minimal unless to provide anesthesia for the arterial switch.[155]

Although the arterial switch is currently utilized for most TGA infants, prior to its advent there were several surgical options to correct TGA. The Senning operation uses atrial native tissue to redirect blood from the RA to the left ventricle, whereas the Mustard procedure uses an intra-atrial baffle to direct systemic blood to the left ventricle (Fig. 3-36).[110] The Rastelli procedure connects the pulmonary artery with RV and the LV with the aorta. Individuals who underwent a Senning, Mustard, or Rastelli procedure are likely to require an anesthetic for additional cardiac or noncardiac procedures. Long-term survival approaches 50% at 30 years.

The primary problem with correction of TGA with a Senning or Mustard, procedure is right ventricular failure, because it supports the systemic circulation. The right ventricle remains the primary pump for systemic circulation, so eventually tricuspid regurgitation and right ventricular failure develop. Pulmonary obstructions may also occur in some instances. Besides gradual onset of circulatory failure, these patients have an increased risk for severe atrial dysrhythmias.[142] They may

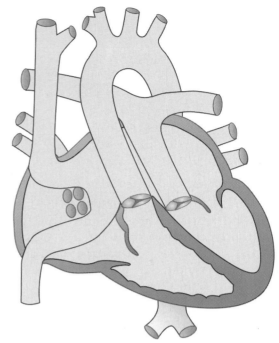

FIGURE 3–36 Mustard operation. An intra-atrial baffle has been placed to redirect vena caval return posterior to the baffle to the left ventricle. The pulmonary veins enter to the right of the baffle; thus, pulmonary venous return is to the right atrium and then to the aorta. A Senning operation uses native atrial tissue to redirect blood flow, accomplishing the same result. *(Reprinted with permission from Baum VC: The adult patient with congenital heart disease. J Cardiothorac Vasc Anesth 1996;10:271.)*

be present in 30% of cases[23] and are primarily reentry tachycardias attributed to trauma of the sinus node and atrial scarring.[23] Only 50% of individuals have sinus rhythm 20 years after surgery.[34] Ventricular arrhythmias are much less common than atrial arrhythmias and are rarely responsible for death. Another benefit of the arterial switch is the preservation of ventricular function compared with other operations for TGA.[34]

Patients with "corrected" transposition are functionally normal with respect to the pulmonary and circulatory circulation. It represents less than 1% of CHD. Median survival is approximately 45 years. Blood will be well oxygenated without surgical intervention, but they are not immune to right ventricular failure in adulthood because the systemic pump is a morphologic right ventricle.[34] Evidence of dysrhythmias and AV valve regurgitation should be sought before any surgery and anesthesia.[118]

Tricuspid Atresia (TA)

TA represents about 3% of CHD but is the third most common cause of cyanotic CHD. It is defined as complete agenesis of the tricuspid valve without any direct communication between the RA and the right ventricle (Fig. 3-37). An ASD or VSD is almost always present. In 70% of cases (type I), there is ventriculoarterial concordance. There are

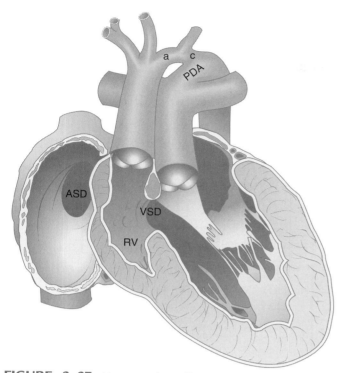

FIGURE 3–37 Heart specimen illustrating a common variant of tricuspid atresia type IIc: D-transposition of the great arteries associated with coarctation of the aorta (c), hypoplasia of the aortic arch (a), patent ductus arteriosus (PDA), small ventricular septal defect (VSD), and hypoplasia of the right ventricle (RV). Note the adequate atrial septal defect (ASD). *(Reprinted with permission from Rosenthal A, Dick M: Tricuspid atresia. In Emmanouilides GC, Riemenschneider TA, Allen HD, Gutgesell HP [eds]: Moss and Adams Heart Disease in Infants, Children, and Adolescents: Including the Fetus and Young Adult. Baltimore, Williams & Wilkins, 1995, p 904.)*

three subgroups of type of TA based on the presence of a VSD and pulmonary stenosis (Fig. 3-38). Type Ib is the most common form of TA with a small VSD and pulmonary stenosis. TA is also uniformly associated with other cardiac anomalies that result in a variety of pulmonary blood flows and clinical manifestations. Extracardiac anomalies are present in 20% of those with TA.

Presentation at infancy will depend on whether pulmonary blood flow is reduced (cyanosis) or excessive (CHF). Excessive pulmonary blood flow is less common. A degree of cyanosis is still likely with excessive pulmonary blood flow, because significant mixing of systemic and pulmonary venous return is unavoidable. The size of the communication between the right and left sides of the heart also influences the degree of cyanosis. Factors that determine the physiology of TA are listed in Figure 3-39. Hypoxic spells similar to "tet spells" may occur in infancy and can cause profound cyanosis.

Treatment in these infants is primarily surgical, with either an operation to increase pulmonary blood flow (shunt) or to decrease pulmonary blood flow (pulmonary artery band). Some type of surgical intervention is almost always required before 1 year of age. It is possible to achieve balanced pulmonary and systemic flows without intervention, with survival into the second decade. However, ventricular function will likely deteriorate, progressing to CHF. Brain abscesses and strokes are more common in these infants.

Anesthetic management of infants with TA for noncardiac procedures is challenging. Profound cyanosis may impair noninvasive monitoring of oxygen saturation.[65] Nitrous oxide and sevoflurane may be used for a gentle

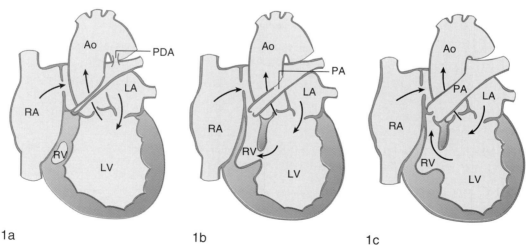

1a   1b   1c

FIGURE 3–38 Type I: Tricuspid atresia without transposition of the great arteries. Type Ia: Pulmonary blood flow depends on a patent ductus arteriosus or bronchial collaterals because of pulmonary atresia. Type Ib: Restrictive pulmonary blood flow due to a small ventricular septal defect (VSD), small right ventricular cavity, and infundibular pulmonary stenosis. Type Ic: Normal or increased pulmonary blood flow due to a large VSD and an adequate pulmonary outflow tract. *(Reprinted with permission from Lowe DA, Stayer SA, Rehman MA: Abnormalities of the atrioventricular valves. In Lake CL [ed]: Pediatric Cardiac Anesthesia. Stamford, CT, Appleton & Lange, 1998, p 409.)*

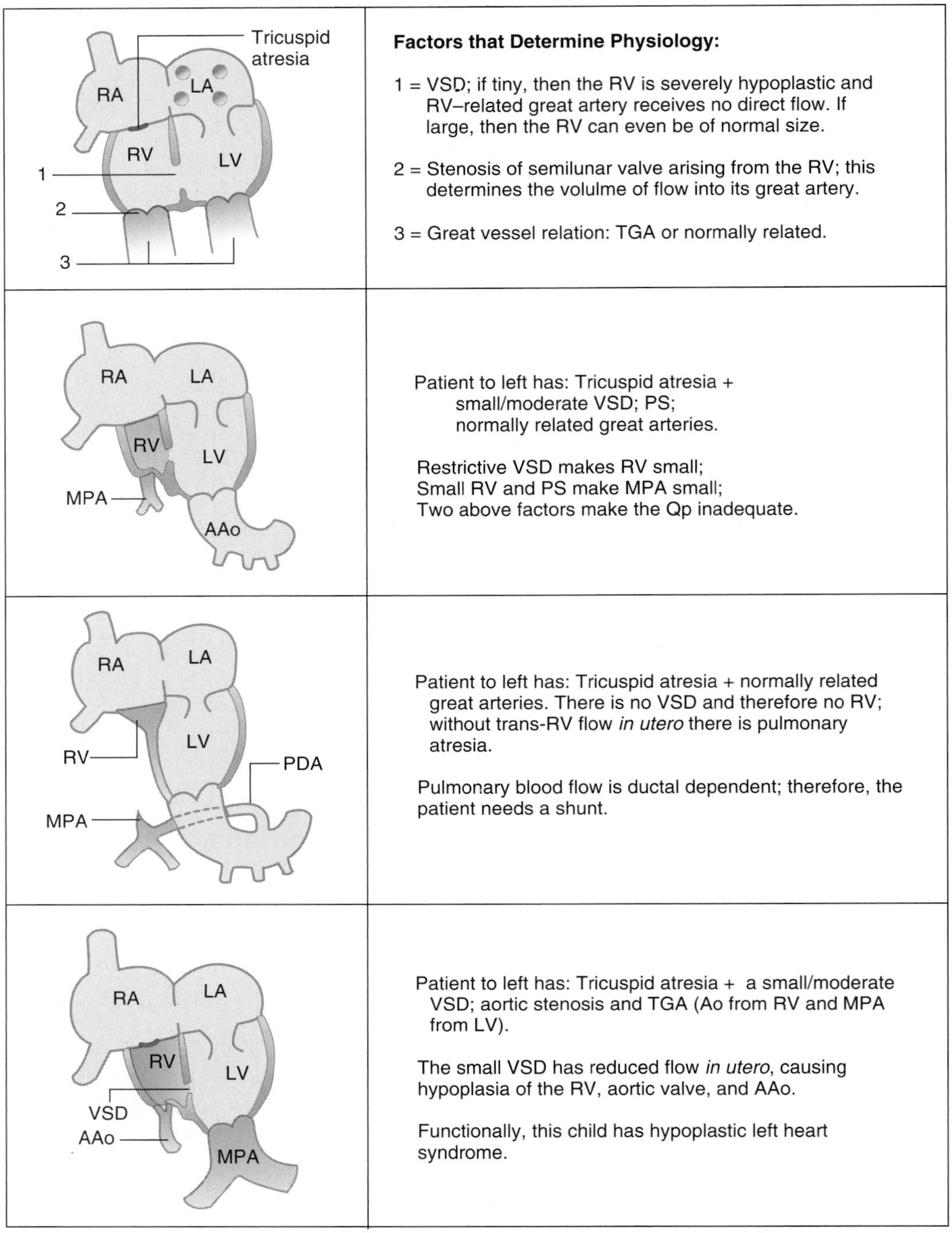

FIGURE 3–39 Tricuspid atresia: physiology and common variations. Ventricular septal defect (VSD), right ventricle (RV), left atrium (LA), right atrium (RA), transposition of the great arteries (TGA), pulmonary stenosis (PS), main pulmonary artery (MPA), pulmonary blood flow (Q$_P$), aorta (Ao), ascending aorta (AAo). *(Reprinted with permission from Waldman JD, Wernly JA: Cyanotic congenital heart disease with decreased pulmonary blood flow in children. Pediatr Clin North Am 1999;46:393.)*

inhalation induction followed by a change to a narcotic-based anesthetic once intravenous access is established. The MAP must be kept up to maintain shunt patency. Although fluid deficits accumulate preoperatively, careful rehydration is necessary.

TA is the classic indication for a Fontan procedure.[156] It is usually performed between 2 and 15 years of age,

if indicated.[156] Some of these patients may have undergone a superior cavopulmonary anastomosis before a Fontan procedure. This anastomosis involves end-to-side (bidirectional Glenn) or atrial dam (hemi-Fontan) to connect to the right pulmonary artery (see Fig. 3-30).[118] To complete the Fontan operation, an anastomosis of the inferior vena cava to the pulmonary artery will be necessary.

Ebstein's Anomaly

Ebstein's anomaly represents 0.5% of patients with CHD.[3] They range from severely ill neonates to asymptomatic adults later in life.[157-159] The mortality for infants may reach 20% in the first year. The mean age of death is approximately 20 years, with 15% alive at 60 years.[159]

Ebstein's anomaly includes an abnormal tricuspid valve and "atrialized" right ventricle that results in a poorly functioning right ventricle. Eighty percent of patients with Ebstein's anomaly will have an ASD or PFO.[142] Cyanosis is present in about half of these individuals.[158] VSD, pulmonary stenosis or atresia, and mitral valve abnormalities may accompany Ebstein's anomaly.

The main pathology of Ebstein's anomaly is derived from a tricuspid valve that is displaced downward toward the right ventricle, causing abnormalities of the septal and posterior leaflets of the valve. The level of valve displacement will largely determine the extent of valvular dysfunction and thus the degree of right ventricular dysfunction. Displacement of the valve also affects the leaflets (Fig. 3-40). The posterior and septal leaflets are actually displaced below the "true" annulus into the right ventricle, with a large amount of "atrialized" right ventricle between the tricuspid valve annulus and the attachments of the leaflets (Fig. 3-41). The anterior and posterior leaflets are very adherent to the endocardium. The anterior leaflet is usually malformed, large, and sail like. The posterior leaflet is usually tethered.

The "atrialized" ventricle is thin and dilated, much like the atrium. The extent of "atrialized" right ventricle present indicates the hemodynamic capabilities.[160] There are also fewer cells in the Ebstein's right ventricle than are found in a normal right ventricle, which contributes to ventricular dilation in addition to the significant tricuspid regurgitation. The left ventricle may also be poorly contractile, along with mitral valve prolapse.[160] Functional class is an excellent gauge of the severity of Ebstein's anomaly before administering an anesthetic for a noncardiac procedure.

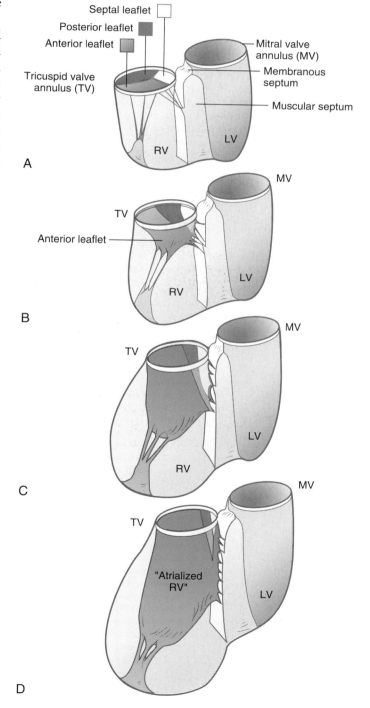

FIGURE 3–40 Ebstein's anomaly of the tricuspid valve. **A,** Normal anatomy, as would be seen in a subxiphoid four-chamber view, on echocardiogram. The mitral valve ring is more cephalad than the tricuspid ring, elevated by the membranous portion of the interventricular septum. The muscular septum separates the left ventricle (LV) and right ventricle (RV) cavities. **B,** Mild displacement of the septal and posterior leaflets that are tethered by fibrous chords to the septum. The anterior leaflet compensates by elongating and coapting downward within the RV cavity, creating a difference between tricuspid valve closure point and annulus. The valve itself is mildly regurgitant. This patient may be picked up incidentally as an asymptomatic child or adult. **C,** Moderate-to-severe downward displacement and tethering of two tricuspid valve leaflets. This valve is quite regurgitant, and there may be compromise of cardiac output. **D,** Because of right-to-left shunting through the associated atrial septal defect (ASD) and reduced pulmonary blood flow from functional as well as anatomic obstruction, this child would present as displaced down into the RV apex, the atrialized portion of the RV comprises most of the RV cavity, and there is probably secondary/associated pulmonary atresia. This child may well die in utero from cardiac output inadequate to sustain life. *(Reprinted with permission from Waldman JD, Wernly JA: Cyanotic congenital heart disease with decreased pulmonary blood flow in children. Pediatr Clin North Am 1999;46:403.)*

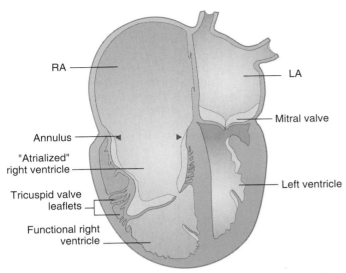

FIGURE 3–41 Anatomy of the anomaly of the tricuspid valve as seen in Ebstein's anomaly. RA, right atrium; LA, left atrium. *(Reprinted with permission from Spitaels SEC: Ebstein's anomaly of the tricuspid valve complexities and strategies. Cardiol Clin 2002;20:432.)*

once right ventricular function begins to weaken further. Frequently, these infants will not survive surgery.[143]

The most common *presenting* symptoms of Ebstein's anomaly are exertional dyspnea (71%), exertional palpitations (37%), and cyanosis (30%).[158] However, the clinical presentation of Ebstein's anomaly varies greatly. Older children may present with a murmur, and adolescents may be diagnosed with the onset of arrhythmias.[142] If the tricuspid valve is minimally displaced, tricuspid regurgitation may actually be mild enough to go unrecognized until adulthood. In fact, the diagnosis may be made by accident with few, if any, symptoms.[142] Older patients primarily complain of fatigue and dyspnea on exertion.[160] If the right ventricular function deteriorates enough, cyanosis may emerge during adulthood. Jugular venous distention is not common until the end because the RA is massively dilated (Fig. 3-43).

A chest radiograph may reveal extreme cardiomegaly in a neonate. In a mild case, the chest radiograph may be almost normal. However, 60% of chest radiographs will show the heart to be enlarged, secondary to right atrial dilation. The electrocardiogram will show evidence of right bundle branch block or right atrial enlargement in over 50% of cases.[158,159] Twenty-five percent of patients with Ebstein's anomaly will have Wolff-Parkinson-White syndrome, often evident by electrocardiography.[34] Invasive diagnostic measures such as cardiac catheterization are rarely necessary to confirm or diagnose Ebstein's anomaly any longer, because echocardiography is usually diagnostic.[159]

The anatomic relationship of the right ventricle in Ebstein's anomaly causes blood to be poorly directed to the pulmonary arteries. Consequently, the right ventricle

Slightly less than 7% of those with Ebstein's anomaly present in infancy, whereas others may even arrive as stillbirths. An infant with Ebstein's anomaly is very cyanotic owing to a large right-to-left shunt. Because of the "atrialized" right ventricle and corresponding poor ventricular function, tricuspid regurgitation is more severe, further raising the right atrial pressure beyond the left atrial pressure, and hence worsening cyanosis. Cyanosis from a right-to-left shunt adversely affects survival (Fig. 3-42).[158] If a child survives the neonatal period, cyanosis may resolve as the infant ages and PVR is lowered. However, cyanosis may recur

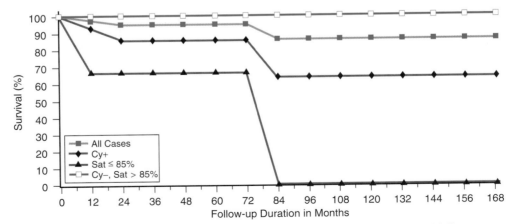

FIGURE 3–42 Survival curve for 46 patients with Ebstein's anomaly on medical follow-up and survival pattern according to presence of cyanosis and aortic oxygen saturation. Survival curves for (■) all 46 patients on medical follow-up, (◆) patients having cyanosis (Cy+), (▲) patients with arterial oxygen saturation 85% or less (Sat = ↑ 85%) and (□) patients without cyanosis and patients with arterial oxygen saturation above 85% (Cy−, Sat > 85%). *(Reprinted with permission from Jaiswal PK, Balakrishnan KG, Saha A, et al: Clinical profile and natural history of Ebstein's anomaly of tricuspid valve. Int J Cardiol 1994;46:117.)*

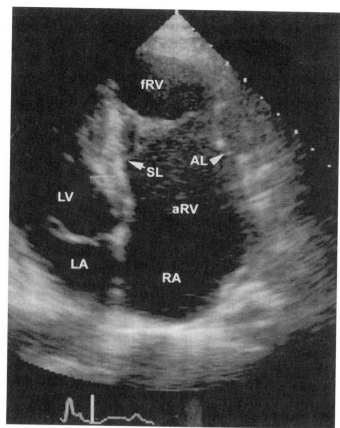

FIGURE 3–43 Transthoracic echocardiogram. Parasternal four-chamber view shows a dilated right atrium (RA) and the atrialized right ventricle (aRV). The functional right ventricle (fRV) is small. The septal leaflet (SL) is completely adherent. The anterior leaflet (AL) has distal focal attachments to the ventricular wall, with a tongue of tissue completing the valvar ring at the junction of the inlet and trabecular components of the right ventricle. *(Reprinted with permission from Spitaels SEC: Ebstein's anomaly of the tricuspid valve complexities and strategies. Cardiol Clin 2002;20:434.)*

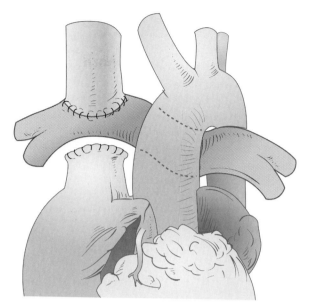

Bidirectional Glenn Shunt

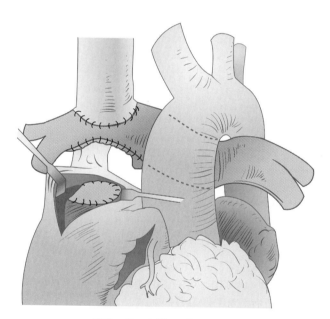

Bidirectional Glenn Shunt
Intra-atrial patch

FIGURE 3–44 Two surgical techniques used to construct bidirectional superior cavopulmonary connections. *(Reprinted with permission from Bradley SM, Mosca RS, Hennein HA, et al: Bidirectional superior cavopulmonary connection in young infants. Circulation 1996;94(Suppl II):II-6.)*

may only be capable of delivering blood flow from the inferior vena cava to the pulmonary artery. To solve this problem, a bidirectional Glenn operation is performed (Fig. 3-44). It connects the superior vena cava to the superior aspect of the right pulmonary artery, from which blood from the superior vena cava travels to the pulmonary artery, bypassing the right ventricle. It is referred to as a "one and a half repair." It is a breakthrough in managing cyanotic CHD because it permits greater pulmonary blood flow without overloading the ventricle.[161] The right ventricle is already overloaded from tricuspid regurgitation.[110] The expectation with a bidirectional Glenn operation is that patients will maintain an SpO_2 of 80% to 85% temporarily.[162] This operation is usually part of a staged procedure in infants younger than 6 months old. Before placement of a bidirectional Glenn operation, the cyanotic infant most likely underwent placement of an arterial shunt to improve pulmonary blood flow. However, patients

have had a bidirectional Glenn procedure successfully performed when younger than age 2 months as the primary operation with good results.[152] Thrombosis is a great concern with a bidirectional Glenn operation, noted in up to 7% of infants. It produces severe morbidity and even mortality.

Replacement of the tricuspid valve occurs less often, owing to the success of tricuspid valve repair.[160] Repair is performed in 60% to 80% of patients with good long-term survival.[157,163] The tricuspid valve is a more difficult valve to repair than other valves and more likely to result in complications postoperatively. Tricuspid valve repair involves plication of the free wall of the "atrialized" right ventricle, posterior tricuspid annuloplasty, and right atrial reduction. The repair is based on the construction of a monocusp valve fashioned by the use of the anterior leaflet of the tricuspid valve. If tricuspid valve repair is not possible, the valve is excised and replaced with a prosthetic one. At 1-year follow-up, 92% of patients with tricuspid repair were in NYHA class I or II and the heart size had even regressed in some.[157]

Anesthesia for patients with Ebstein's anomaly depends to a large degree on the clinical manifestations. The anatomic variation of the tricuspid valve and degree of valvular displacement, right-to-left shunt, right and left ventricular dysfunction, and occurrence of tachy-arrhythmias are instrumental in assessing the status in those with Ebstein's anomaly. Once symptoms appear, the hemodynamics are usually more tenuous and arrhythmias a greater likelihood.[159] The right ventricular dysfunction makes these patients especially high risk for anesthesia. The right ventricular dysfunction is worsened by the tricuspid regurgitation. Any negative influence on the right ventricle may precipitate low cardiac output and right-sided heart failure, especially because these patients are prone to poor cardiac output, worsening of right-to-left shunt, and serious dysrhythmias. Similarly, poor left ventricular function is an especially ominous feature before anesthesia.[159] Loss of the atrial kick can abruptly worsen a tenuous hemodynamic status. If the patient is especially ill, an intravenous induction with ketamine and fentanyl is recommended. Ketamine is especially useful in patients with severe illness and unstable hemodynamics.

One must be very observant in Ebstein's anomaly patients during the perioperative period for the occurrence of arrhythmias. Supraventricular arrhythmias are known to occur in 25% to 30% of individuals and are frequently associated with reentry arrhythmias, such as Wolff-Parkinson-White syndrome.[158,142] Wolff-Parkinson-White syndrome is especially common in patients with Ebstein's anomaly, in part because of the way the right atrium becomes incorporated into the ventricle, bypassing the annulus fibrosis of the tricuspid valve. Wolff-Parkinson-White syndrome may be found in approximately 25% of Ebstein's anomalies.[34] Electrophysiologic testing may be warranted in certain patients before anesthesia. Patients with Ebstein's anomaly may respond poorly to classic treatment for supraventricular arrhythmias like verapamil, especially if the arrhythmia is a reentrant type. Atrial fibrillation in association with Wolff-Parkinson-White syndrome can degenerate rapidly into ventricular fibrillation.

Ventricular arrhythmias are especially malignant and fatal in this defect.[157] It is important to review the chronic antiarrhythmic medications that the patient may be receiving. Even following tricuspid valve repair, ventricular fibrillation is still a major concern, because surgery does not alleviate the risk of lethal ventricular dysrhythmias. Radiofrequency ablation has been less successful in treating arrhythmias associated with Ebstein's anomaly than the general population.[142]

Eisenmenger's Syndrome

Ten-year survival is approximately 80%.[142] The median survival is to the mid 30s,[79] with a mean age of death of 25 ± 12 years, which is actually better than once believed. Survival greatly exceeds primary PAH. There seems to be something about the congenital heart defect that is protective compared to the patient who develops primary PAH.

Patients with Eisenmenger's syndrome began with CHD characterized by a left-to-right shunt with corresponding excessive pulmonary blood flow. The most common defects associated with Eisenmenger's syndrome are listed in Table 3-7. An isolated VSD is by far the most common cause.[164] Over a period of time excessive pulmonary blood flow causes hypertrophy of the pulmonary vascular tree. Initially, only the pulmonary artery pressure rises and the PVR remains normal. As the medial hypertrophy of the pulmonary vessels occurs and the pulmonary artery pressure rises, the changes are still reversible. Eventually, the pulmonary vasculature is obliterated by the arteritis and thrombosis, which leads to the rise in PVR. The progression of the PVR is the final irreversible step that ultimately leads to a reversal of shunt direction, right to left.

Although the disease process begins early in life, symptoms of severe cyanosis and fatigue may not appear until late childhood or even adulthood. Erythrocytosis is common. Hemoptysis, palpitations, edema, and syncope are also common. Palpitations, present in almost 80% of patients,[164] are often due to atrial fibrillation. Syncope is important to note because it is associated with a worse prognosis. Central cyanosis, clubbing, and a right ventricular heave are some of the more prominent physical findings. It is helpful to know the extent of pulmonary vascular disease derived from cardiac catheterization. Pulmonary vascular disease is much more advanced in patients with Eisenmenger's syndrome than in other patients.[164] The degree of pulmonary vascular obstruction is the key to prognosis.

Hemodynamic data are important to know regarding any anesthetic for these individuals. The mean right atrial pressure is surprisingly normal in most, but the left atrial pressure is often elevated. If the right atrial pressure is more than 8 mm Hg, the prognosis is worse.[164] The mean pulmonary artery pressure has been found to be

TABLE 3–7 **Distribution of Various Defects in 201 Patients of Eisenmenger's Syndrome**

Diagnosis	Frequency	Percentage	Male	Female
VSD	67	33.33	35	32
ASD	60	29.85	30	30
PDA	29	14.43	13	16
VSD + ASD	4	1.99	1	3
VSD + PDA	6	2.98	4	2
ASD + PDA	1	0.49	1	0
Shunt lesion and aortic stenosis	3	1.49	0	3
Shunt lesion + mitral stenosis	1	0.49	0	1
Shunt lesion + coarctation of aorta	3	1.49	0	3
DORV, VSD, PAH	8	3.98	1	7
D-TGA VSD	3	1.49	1	2
Primum ASD	4	1.99	2	2
Complete atrioventricular septal defect	3	1.49	1	2
Single atrium	2	0.98	1	1
Sinus venosus ASD	2	0.98	1	1
Aortopulmonary window	3	1.49	1	1
L-TGA VSD	1	0.49	0	1
TAPVC	1	0.49	0	1
Total	201	100.00	92	109

ASD, atrial septal defect; DORV, double outlet right ventricle; D-TGA, dextro-transposition of great arteries; L-TGA, levo-transposition of great arteries; PAH, pulmonary arterial hypertension; PDA, patent ductus arteriosus; TAPVC, total anomalous pulmonary venous connection; VSD, ventricular septal defect.
Reprinted with permission from Saha A, Balakrishnan KG, Jaiswal PK, et al: Prognosis for patients with Eisenmenger syndrome of various aetiology. Int J Cardiol 1994;45:201.

68 ± 15 mm Hg, in conjunction with an aortic pressure of 80 ± 13 mm Hg.

Surgical procedures in these patients are associated with a high morbidity and mortality, even for relatively minor procedures.[165] Anesthesia considerations are important to minimize the risk for these patients. Meticulous attention must be paid to these patients to achieve good outcomes.

If the Hb is above 21 g/dL, then some have recommended prophylactic phlebotomy. More recently, Ammash and associates[165] found a higher mortality associated with those who had undergone prophylactic phlebotomy. Excessive Hb levels may contribute to excessive thrombosis, as well as bleeding. Although these patients are dependent on higher levels of Hb for adequate oxygen delivery to the tissues, the viscosity of the blood may actually reduce oxygen delivery at some point.

Although general anesthetics are usually performed for surgery, regional anesthesia has been more recently accepted.[79] Overall, patients with Eisenmenger's syndrome are highly preload dependent. Fluid shifts and hypovolemia are poorly tolerated. Because of the preoperative fast, intravascular volume depletion is common. It is important to maintain SVR. Decreases in SVR will exacerbate right-to-left shunting, will worsen cyanosis, and have been associated with sudden cardiovascular collapse.[79] Increases in SVR may exacerbate ventricular function but are generally better tolerated than decreases in SVR. Blood loss and volume depletion should be minimized. Central venous monitoring and arterial cannulation are highly recommended in these patients. The right atrial pressure may not always reflect an increase in PVR. One should strive to avoid situations that will increase the PVR, such as hypercarbia, PEEP, acidosis, and increased intrathoracic pressure. Because the PVR is fixed to a large extent, patients will not adjust rapidly to volume changes and hemodynamic changes. The pulse oximeter can be very helpful in determining the overall direction of shunting in these patients and may be the best method available to monitor PVR. Most selective pulmonary vasodilators will have little effect on the PVR in Eisenmenger's syndrome, although prostacyclin (epoprostenol) has demonstrated some benefit. One must be very careful to avoid paradoxical embolism, taking all the precautions.

OBSTRUCTION OF BLOOD FLOW

If obstruction to either aortic or pulmonary valves occurs, then ventricular hypertrophy will likely ensue by childhood. Although these conditions are not complex, they occur very frequently and can have serious consequences.

COARCTATION OF THE AORTA

Coarctation of the aorta is a discrete narrowing of the proximal thoracic aorta just opposite the insertion of the ductus arteriosus (juxtaductal), which, although a simple anatomic defect, has many different presentations (Fig. 3-45). It appears in 6% to 8% of those with CHD.[3] Without treatment, coarctation carries significant morbidity and mortality, with a 25% mortality rate at 20 years, 50% at 30 years, and 75% at 50 years.[110,166] The mean age of death without surgery for coarctation is 35 years,[34] which is more than a 50% reduction compared with a normal life span.

Coarctation of the aorta is associated with many other congenital anomalies, and only about a fourth of coarctations occur as isolated defects.[167] An example is the finding of coarctation in 25% of aortic stenosis and bicuspid aortic valve.[168] When coarctation exists with other congenital heart defects, it is referred to as a "complex coarctation." Besides the association with cardiac defects, coarctation of the aorta is also more likely to be present with extracardiac anomalies such as Turner's syndrome, and other extra cardiac anomalies most commonly found in the musculoskeletal, gastrointestinal, or respiratory systems.[3,16] In a large series from Johns Hopkins Hospital over a 30-year period, Turner's syndrome was the most common noncardiac congenital anomaly associated with coarctation.[169] Head and neck abnormalities are also common with coarctation. The importance of these associations resides in the potential for abnormalities of the airway.

The hemodynamics associated with coarctation of the aorta vary greatly. Cardiogenic shock and acidosis may be present in the newborn, because the entire cardiac output must traverse the obstruction. The newborn is less likely to be able to adapt rapidly to the severe obstruction to left ventricular flow. If collaterals or other defects are present, the obstruction to left ventricular outflow may be less severe. Nearly 75% of infants with coarctation and symptoms of CHF died without treatment, primarily due to the effect of coarctation on myocardial function.[167] Because the coarctation is usually before the ductus arteriosus, a neonate will tolerate it better if prostaglandin therapy is instituted to maintain the patency of the ductus arteriosus.

Infants are most likely to present with tachypnea and CHF in almost 50% of cases.[169] Others may develop chronic CHF over the ensuing months after birth. The heart will compensate for outflow obstruction with left

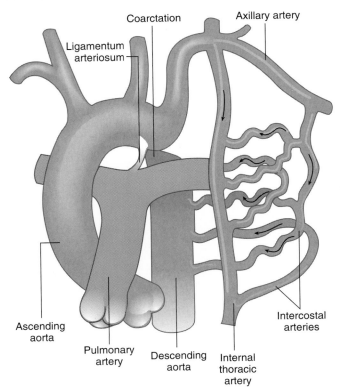

FIGURE 3–45 Coarctation of the aorta. Coarctation causes severe obstruction of blood flow in the descending thoracic aorta. The descending aorta and its branches are perfused by collateral channels from the axillary and internal thoracic arteries through the intercostal arteries *(arrows)*. *(Reprinted with permission from Brickner ME, Hillis LD, Lange RA: Congenital heart disease in adults: I. N Engl J Med 2000;342:261.)*

ventricular hypertrophy. Children usually present asymptomatically, with the unexpected discovery of hypertension. Gradients between the left ventricular outflow tract and distal blood pressure may exceed 80 mm Hg. The gradient is at the systolic, not diastolic, blood pressure, so the pulse pressure is widened with a coarctation. Commonly, the difference will be in the upper versus lower extremities. Pulses below the coarctation will be diminished and delayed in timing compared with other pulses. The diagnosis will be made with routine physical examination that identifies discrepancies in the blood pressures in the arms and legs. The child with long-standing coarctation will often have evidence of left ventricular hypertrophy on the electrocardiogram and rib notching on the chest radiograph. However, 25% may have a normal electrocardiogram.[167] These patients have developed collaterals from the intercostals and subclavian arteries.

Patients normally become surgical candidates by the age of 3 to 5 years. Surgical repair has been discussed previously.[169] Surgical approaches include resection of the coarctation with an end-to-end anastomosis, subclavian flap aortoplasty, or aortoplasty with homograft or synthetic material (Fig. 3-46). Surgical repair in adults is

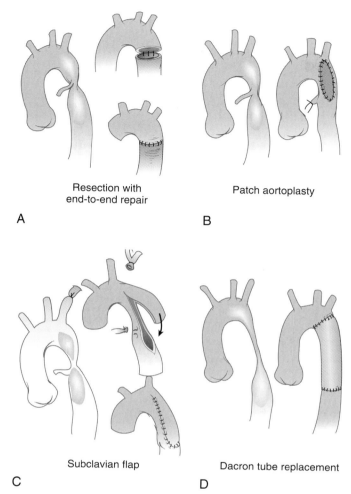

Resection with end-to-end repair

A

Patch aortoplasty

B

Subclavian flap

C

Dacron tube replacement

D

FIGURE 3–46 Surgical techniques for repair of coarctation. Illustrated are the several methods of surgical repair for coarctation of the aorta. **A,** Resection with end-to-end repair, the standard repair for patients beyond age 1. **B,** Patch aortoplasty, seldom used for primary repair because of a 5% (or higher) risk of late patch aneurysm but still used for recurrent coarctation. **C,** Subclavian flap, used primarily up to age 2. **D,** Dacron tube replacement, best when the coarctation segment is long. *(Reprinted with permission from Webb GD, Harrison DA, Connelly MS: Challenges posed by the adult patient with congenital heart disease. Adv Intern Med 1996;41:448.)*

more difficult because the aorta is more sclerotic, aneurysms of the intercostal arteries are more common, and cardiovascular disease may be present.[34] Surgery for re-coarctation (0.5% to 4%) is much less common than in the past, when it was 8%.[118,167] Surgery for re-coarctation still affects 16% of neonates who undergo repair for coarctation.[169] Surgical technique for correction of the coarctation can increase the risk of restenosis. It is more likely to occur 6 years after surgery.[169]

Balloon angioplasty is less invasive and is a viable alternative to surgery for coarctation of the aorta. Both surgery and angioplasty are recognized to leave a persistent gradient of 20 mm Hg or less that may cause problems in the future. Balloon angioplasty has been successful in

79% of children who developed restenosis after their initial surgery and 82% successful with "native" coarctation of the aorta.[170] Restenosis after balloon angioplasty is below 20%, except for infants without previous surgery, who develop restenosis with angioplasty in 71% of cases.[170] Awareness of this is important because a severe gradient may be present to affect hemodynamics during noncardiac surgery.[171]

Anesthetic management[172] has been reviewed for repair of coarctation. It is important to note the chance of worsening myocardial ischemia in an infant with coarctation of the aorta and CHF. Histopathologic examination has demonstrated evidence of myocardial ischemia in nearly 40% of infants, with coarctation of the aorta probably related to poor coronary perfusion and hypertrophied myocardium. Chronic ischemia may impact myocardial function, especially during noncardiac surgery.[20]

If the patient has undergone previous coarctation, comprehensive evaluation of the blood pressure in the extremities is warranted to identify any residual gradient.[118] Although children who undergo surgery will be normotensive after repair, 50% of adults will have persistent hypertension after repair[8] and will carry the same cardiovascular risk as anyone with hypertension and coronary artery disease.[110]

Congenital Aortic Stenosis

Congenital aortic stenosis accounts for 3% to 6% of CHD.[34] The prevalence of a bicuspid aortic valve may be 1% to 2%, with many cases "clinically silent." Congenital bicuspid aortic stenosis is one of the most common congenital malformations of the heart. PDA and coarctation of the aorta occur commonly with congenital aortic stenosis.

Normally, the aortic valve has a surface area of 2 cm^2/m^2. Obstruction to left ventricular outflow may occur through different abnormalities: valvular (70%), subvalvular, and supravalvular aortic stenosis (Fig. 3-47). Infants and children with aortic stenosis have thickened and rigid valve tissue with various levels of commissural separation. Typically, the valve is bicuspid. As a consequence of the hemodynamically significant flow across the valve, the infant or child will develop concentric hypertrophy. This hypertrophied myocardium is at risk for coronary blood imbalances, as the demand is outstripped by the supply, especially in the subendocardial area. The pressure gradient across the valve is not a linear relationship, but is proportional to the square of the flow. So as the flow doubles, the gradient quadruples. A peak systolic gradient of 60 mm Hg in concert with a normal cardiac output results in a valve area of 0.5 cm^2, which is considered critical obstruction. Left ventricular end-diastolic pressure is also frequently elevated. It should be noted that myocardial blood supply may be compromised, despite normal anatomic patency of the coronary arteries.[168]

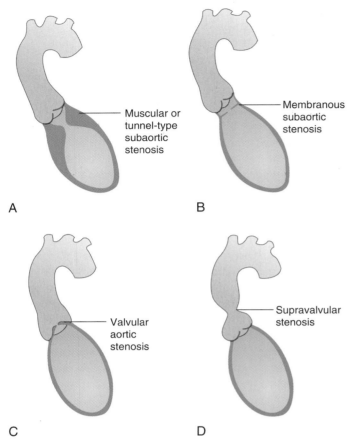

FIGURE 3–47 Types of congenital aortic stenosis. **A,** Fibromuscular or tunnel-type of subaortic stenosis with obstruction to left ventricular emptying by muscular overgrowth of the entire outflow tract. **B,** Membranous subaortic stenosis in which a membrane is present 1 to 2 cm below the aortic valve orifice obstructing ventricular outflow. **C,** Thickened, domed, fused leaflets of congenital valvular stenosis. **D,** The "hourglass" narrowing of the supravalvular aorta producing supravalvular stenosis. *(Reprinted with permission from Rosen DA, Rosen KR: Anomalies of the aortic arch and valve. In Lake CL [ed]: Pediatric Cardiac Anesthesia. Stamford, CT, Appleton & Lange, 1998, p 432.)*

Congenital aortic stenosis in children may be associated with a severe obstruction that may appear essentially asymptomatic yet in other cases may manifest significant symptoms with a less dramatic gradient. Although severe aortic stenosis can be fatal during the neonatal period, most patients (84%) actually survive 15 years, although the long-term prognosis is largely unknown.[173]

Exertional fatigue may be the most common symptom, but many children will grow up without any knowledge of their condition. Under stress there is the possibility of sudden death. There is a harsh systolic crescendo-decrescendo murmur frequently present at the base of the heart. The electrocardiogram and chest radiograph may be normal despite the presence of severe aortic stenosis. Cardiac catheterization is rarely needed today to establish the site and severity of obstruction to the left ventricle. One cannot accurately follow the progression of aortic stenosis and left ventricular obstruction through such measures as electrocardiography, physical findings, or chest radiography, so echocardiographic Doppler ultrasound evaluations are required.

Management of congenital aortic stenosis may follow percutaneous balloon valvuloplasty or surgically performed aortic valvuloplasty. The surgical options include closed transventricular valvotomy, open valvotomy with inflow occlusion, or open valvotomy with extracorporeal circulation.

Most children with aortic regurgitation as well as outflow obstruction are receiving a Ross procedure.[19] A Ross procedure substitutes the aortic valve with a pulmonary autograft and places a pulmonary or aortic homograft between the right ventricle and the main pulmonary artery. Although many patients have impaired myocardium due to the aortic valve disease, the Ross is now being used in complex congenital heart operations. The 20-year assessment of these pulmonary autografts appears excellent so far, with few complications.[174] The Ross procedure avoids the need for anticoagulation in children and allows continued growth. The actuarial survival at 16 years was 74%.[175] The adult with aortic stenosis will frequently need a valve replacement.[34]

One needs to know that even if the infant has had an intervention for aortic stenosis, one may later anesthetize a patient with the possibility of restenosis, aortic regurgitation, and especially sudden death.[173] Moreover, almost all children will require some type of re-intervention following surgery in the ensuing 10 years.[173] In many of these children, aortic valve replacement may be necessary. The replacement of the aortic valve with the patient's own pulmonary valve has been reported with early short-term success[175] and offers the patient an option that continues to be evaluated but appears very promising.

Many pediatric patients with aortic stenosis are not in CHF and therefore may not require the high-dose narcotic anesthetic. It is important that the patients do not become profoundly hypovolemic, or severe reduction in blood pressure may result in myocardial ischemia to the hypertrophied myocardium. Inhalation induction may be tolerated unless there is severe CHF, whereupon intramuscular ketamine may be the ideal choice, with high-dose fentanyl after intravenous access is obtained. Severe bradycardia or tachycardia may not be tolerated very long.

CONCLUSION

Because of advancements in surgery and medical management there are more individuals of all ages surviving longer with CHD. This has resulted in many patients requiring the same noncardiac operations as others who do not have CHD. These patients can do well with noncardiac surgery, but special consideration needs to be given to the native CHD, surgical interventions, and functional capacity.

The aim is to obtain as much information as possible on the condition of the individual to develop the optimal anesthetic plan individualized for this particular patient to provide an anesthetic that will be safe and effective despite the great variation in age and physical condition.

References

1. Brennan P, Young ID: Congenital heart malformations: Aetiology and associations. Semin Neonatol 2001;6:17-25.
2. Hoffman JI, Kaplan S: The incidence of congenital heart disease. J Am Coll Cardiol 2002;39:1890-1900.
3. Report of the New England Regional Infant Cardiac Program. Pediatrics 1980;65:375-461.
4. Hoffman JI, Kaplan S, Liberthson RR: Prevalence of congenital heart disease. Am Heart J 2004;147:425-439.
5. Feldt RH, Avasthey P, Yoshimasu F, et al: Incidence of congenital heart disease in children born to residents of Olmsted County, Minnesota, 1950-1969. Mayo Clin Proc 1971;46:794-799.
6. Mott AR, Fraser CD Jr, McKenzie ED, et al: Perioperative care of the adult with congenital heart disease in a free-standing tertiary pediatric facility. Pediatr Cardiol 2002;23:624-630.
7. Warnes CA, Liberthson R, Danielson GK, et al: Task force 1: The changing profile of congenital heart disease in adult life. J Am Coll Cardiol 2001;37:1170-1175.
8. Brickner ME, Hillis LD, Lange RA: Congenital heart disease in adults: I. N Engl J Med 2000;342:256-263.
9. Warner MA, Lunn RJ, O'Leary PW, et al: Outcomes of noncardiac surgical procedures in children and adults with congenital heart disease. Mayo Perioperative Outcomes Group. Mayo Clin Proc 1998;73:728-734.
10. Hennein HA, Mendeloff EN, Cilley RE, et al: Predictors of postoperative outcome after general surgical procedures in patients with congenital heart disease. J Pediatr Surg 1994;29:866-870.
11. Morris CD, Menashe VD: 25-year mortality after surgical repair of congenital heart defect in childhood: A population-based cohort study. JAMA 1991;266:3447-3452.
12. Anderson RH, Becker AE, Freedom RM, et al: Sequential segmental analysis of congenital heart disease. Pediatr Cardiol 1984;5:281-287.
13. Edwards WD: Classification and terminology of cardiovascular anomalies. In Emmanouilides GC, Riemenschneider TA, Allen HD, Gutgesell HP (eds): Moss and Adams Heart Disease in Infants, Children, and Adolescents: Including the Fetus and Young Adult. Baltimore, Williams & Wilkins, 1995, pp 106-131.
14. Burrows FA: Anaesthetic management of the child with congenital heart disease for non-cardiac surgery. Can J Anaesth 1992;39:R60-R70.
15. Schindler MB, Bohn DJ, Bryan AC, et al: Increased respiratory system resistance and bronchial smooth muscle hypertrophy in children with acute postoperative pulmonary hypertension. Am J Respir Crit Care Med 1995;152:1347-1352.
16. Greenwood RD, Rosenthal A, Parisi L, et al: Extracardiac abnormalities in infants with congenital heart disease. Pediatrics 1975;55:485-492.
17. Gelb BD: Genetic basis of syndromes associated with congenital heart disease. Curr Opin Cardiol 2001;16:188-194.
18. Kussman BD, Geva T, McGowan FX: Cardiovascular causes of airway compression. Paediatr Anaesth 2004;14:60-74.
19. Corno AF: Surgery for congenital heart disease. Curr Opin Cardiol 2000;15:238-243.
20. Tawes RL Jr, Berry CL, Aberdeen E, et al: Myocardial ischemia in infants: Its role in three common congenital cardiac anomalies. Ann Thorac Surg 1969;8:383-390.
21. Harada K, Yasuoka K, Tamura M, et al: Coronary flow reserve assessment by Doppler echocardiography in children with and without congenital heart defect: Comparison with invasive technique. J Am Soc Echocardiogr 2002;15:1121-1126.
22. Andropoulos DB, Stayer SA, Skjonsby BS, et al: Anesthetic and perioperative outcome of teenagers and adults with congenital heart disease. J Cardiothorac Vasc Anesth 2002;16:731-736.
23. Collins KK, Dubin AM: Detecting and diagnosing arrhythmias in adults with congenital heart disease. Curr Cardiol Rep 2003;5:331-335.
24. Walsh EP: Arrhythmias in patients with congenital heart disease. Card Electrophysiol Rev 2002;6:422-430.
25. Fallon P, Aparicio JM, Elliott MJ, et al: Incidence of neurological complications of surgery for congenital heart disease. Arch Dis Child 1995;72:418-422.
26. Ammash N, Warnes CA: Cerebrovascular events in adult patients with cyanotic congenital heart disease. J Am Coll Cardiol 1996;28:768-772.
27. Tempe DK, Virmani S: Coagulation abnormalities in patients with cyanotic congenital heart disease. J Cardiothorac Vasc Anesth 2002;16:752-765.
28. Suarez CR, Menendez CE, Griffin AJ, et al: Cyanotic congenital heart disease in children: Hemostatic disorders and relevance of molecular markers of hemostasis. Semin Thromb Hemost 1984;10:285-289.
29. Goel M, Shome DK, Singh ZN, et al: Haemostatic changes in children with cyanotic and acyanotic congenital heart disease. Indian Heart J 2000;52:559-563.
30. Colon-Otero G, Gilchrist GS, Holcomb GR, et al: Preoperative evaluation of hemostasis in patients with congenital heart disease. Mayo Clin Proc 1987;62:379-385.
31. Levin E, Wu J, Devine DV, et al: Hemostatic parameters and platelet activation marker expression in cyanotic and acyanotic pediatric patients undergoing cardiac surgery in the presence of tranexamic acid. Thromb Haemost 2000;83:54-59.
32. Kern FH, Morana NJ, Sears JJ, et al: Coagulation defects in neonates during cardiopulmonary bypass. Ann Thorac Surg 1992;54:541-546.
33. Richardson MW, Allen GA, Monahan PE: Thrombosis in children: Current perspective and distinct challenges. Thromb Haemost 2002;88:900-911.
34. Webb GD, Harrison DA, Connelly MS: Challenges posed by the adult patient with congenital heart disease. Adv Intern Med 1996;41:437-495.
35. Seelye ER: Anaesthesia for children with congenital heart disease. Anaesth Intens Care 1973;1:512-516.
36. Goldstein-Dresner MC, Davis PJ, Kretchman E, et al: Double-blind comparison of oral transmucosal fentanyl citrate with oral meperidine, diazepam, and atropine as preanesthetic medication in children with congenital heart disease. Anesthesiology 1991;74:28-33.
37. Stow PJ, Burrows FA, Lerman J, et al: Arterial oxygen saturation following premedication in children with cyanotic congenital heart disease. Can J Anaesth 1988;35:63-66.
38. DeBock TL, Davis PJ, Tome J, et al: Effect of premedication on arterial oxygen saturation in children with congenital heart disease. J Cardiothorac Anesth 1990;4:425-429.
39. Levine MF, Hartley EJ, Macpherson BA, et al: Oral midazolam premedication for children with congenital cyanotic heart disease undergoing cardiac surgery: A comparative study. Can J Anaesth 1993;40:934-938.
40. Masue T, Shimonaka H, Fukao I, et al: Oral high-dose midazolam premedication for infants and children undergoing cardiovascular surgery. Paediatr Anaesth 2003;13:662-667.
41. Friesen RH, Carpenter E, Madigan CK, et al: Oral transmucosal fentanyl citrate for preanaesthetic medication of paediatric cardiac surgery patients. Paediatr Anaesth 1995;5:29-33.
42. Morray JP, Lynn AM, Mansfield PB: Effect of pH and P_{CO_2} on pulmonary and systemic hemodynamics after surgery in children with congenital heart disease and pulmonary hypertension. J Pediatr 1988;113:474-479.
43. Alswang M, Friesen RH, Bangert P: Effect of preanesthetic medication on carbon dioxide tension in children with congenital heart disease. J Cardiothorac Vasc Anesth 1994;8:415-419.
44. Fullerton DA, Kirson LE, St Cyr JA, et al: Influence of hydrogen ion concentration versus carbon dioxide tension on pulmonary vascular resistance after cardiac operation. J Thorac Cardiovasc Surg 1993;106:528-536.
45. Nystrom E, Reid KH, Bennett R, et al: A comparison of two automated indirect arterial blood pressure meters: With recordings from a radial arterial catheter in anesthetized surgical patients. Anesthesiology 1985;62:526-530.

46. Scott WA: Haemodynamic monitoring: Measurement of systemic blood pressure. Can Anaesth Soc J 1985;32:294-298.

47. Glenski JA, Beynen FM, Brady J: A prospective evaluation of femoral artery monitoring in pediatric patients. Anesthesiology 1987;66:227-229.

48. Denys BG, Uretsky BF: Anatomical variations of internal jugular vein location: Impact on central venous access. Crit Care Med 1991;19:1516-1519.

49. Mitto P, Barankay A, Spath P, et al: Central venous catheterization in infants and children with congenital heart diseases: Experiences with 500 consecutive catheter placements. Pediatr Cardiol 1992;13:14-19.

50. Eisenhauer ED, Derveloy RJ, Hastings PR: Prospective evaluation of central venous pressure (CVP) catheters in a large city-county hospital. Ann Surg 1982;196:560-564.

51. Sitzmann JV, Townsend TR, Siler MC, et al: Septic and technical complications of central venous catheterization: A prospective study of 200 consecutive patients. Ann Surg 1985;202:766-770.

52. Milo S, Sawaed S, Adler Z, et al: Misplaced arterial catheter in an infant causes intraoperative death. J Cardiothorac Vasc Anesth 1992;6:101-104.

53. Oliver WC Jr, Nuttall GA, Beynen FM, et al: The incidence of artery puncture with central venous cannulation using a modified technique for detection and prevention of arterial cannulation. J Cardiothorac Vasc Anesth 1997;11:851-855.

54. Verghese ST, McGill WA, Patel RI, et al: Ultrasound-guided internal jugular venous cannulation in infants: A prospective comparison with the traditional palpation method. Anesthesiology 1999;91:71-77.

55. Nicolson SC, Sweeney MF, Moore RA, et al: Comparison of internal and external jugular cannulation of the central circulation in the pediatric patient. Crit Care Med 1985;13:747-749.

56. Hayashi Y, Uchida O, Takaki O, et al: Internal jugular vein catheterization in infants undergoing cardiovascular surgery: An analysis of the factors influencing successful catheterization. Anesth Analg 1992;74:688-693.

57. Mallinson C, Bennett J, Hodgson P, et al: Position of the internal jugular vein in children: A study of the anatomy using ultrasonography. Paediatr Anaesth 1999;9:111-114.

58. Alderson PJ, Burrows FA, Stemp LI, et al: Use of ultrasound to evaluate internal jugular vein anatomy and to facilitate central venous cannulation in paediatric patients. Br J Anaesth 1993;70:145-148.

59. Asheim P, Mostad U, Aadahl P: Ultrasound-guided central venous cannulation in infants and children. Acta Anaesthesiol Scand 2002;46:390-392.

60. Andropoulos DB, Bent ST, Skjonsby B, et al: The optimal length of insertion of central venous catheters for pediatric patients. Anesth Analg 2001;93:883-886.

61. Wahr JA, Tremper KK, Diab M: Pulse oximetry. Respir Care Clin North Am 1995;1:77-105.

62. Schmitt HJ, Schuetz WH, Proeschel PA, et al: Accuracy of pulse oximetry in children with cyanotic congenital heart disease. J Cardiothorac Vasc Anesth 1993;7:61-65.

63. Carter BG, Carlin JB, Tibballs J, et al: Accuracy of two pulse oximeters at low arterial hemoglobin-oxygen saturation. Crit Care Med 1998;26:1128-1133.

64. Freund PR, Overand PT, Cooper J, et al: A prospective study of intraoperative pulse oximetry failure. J Clin Monit 1991;7:253-258.

65. Oliver WC Jr, Belau MM, Barnes RD, et al: Accuracy and precision of Masimo SET, Agilent Merlin, and Nellcor N-395 pulse oximeters in patients undergoing cardiopulmonary bypass for congenital heart defects. Anesth Analg 2003;96:141A.

66. Riordan CJ, Locher JP Jr, Santamore WP, et al: Monitoring systemic venous oxygen saturations in the hypoplastic left heart syndrome. Ann Thorac Surg 1997;63:835-837.

67. Greeley WJ, Bushman GA, Davis DP, et al: Comparative effects of halothane and ketamine on systemic arterial oxygen saturation in children with cyanotic heart disease. Anesthesiology 1986;65:666-668.

68. Laishley RS, Burrows FA, Lerman J, et al: Effect of anesthetic induction regimens on oxygen saturation in cyanotic congenital heart disease. Anesthesiology 1986;65:673-677.

69. Lazzell VA, Burrows FA: Stability of the intraoperative arterial to end-tidal carbon dioxide partial pressure difference in children with congenital heart disease. Can J Anaesth 1991;38:859-865.

70. Tobias JD, Wilson WR Jr, Meyer DJ: Transcutaneous monitoring of carbon dioxide tension after cardiothoracic surgery in infants and children. Anesth Analg 1999;88:531-534.

71. Andropoulos DB, Ayres NA, Stayer SA, et al: The effect of transesophageal echocardiography on ventilation in small infants undergoing cardiac surgery. Anesth Analg 2000;90:47-49.

72. Andropoulos DB, Stayer SA, Bent ST, et al: The effects of transesophageal echocardiography on hemodynamic variables in small infants undergoing cardiac surgery. J Cardiothorac Vasc Anesth 2000;14:133-135.

73. Rasanen J, Peltola K, Leijala M: Superior vena caval and mixed venous oxyhemoglobin saturations in children recovering from open heart surgery. J Clin Monit 1992;8:44-49.

74. Duke T, Butt W, South M, et al: Early markers of major adverse events in children after cardiac operations. J Thorac Cardiovasc Surg 1997;114:1042-1052.

75. Marks JD, Schapera A, Kraemer RW, et al: Pressure and flow limitations of anesthesia ventilators. Anesthesiology 1989;71:403-408.

76. Stayer SA, Andropoulos DB, Bent ST, et al: Volume ventilation of infants with congenital heart disease: A comparison of Drager, NAD 6000 and Siemens, Servo 900C ventilators. Anesth Analg 2001;92:76-79.

77. Bancalari E, Jesse MJ, Gelband H, et al: Lung mechanics in congenital heart disease with increased and decreased pulmonary blood flow. J Pediatr 1977;90:192-195.

78. Hoffman TM, Wernovsky G, Atz AM, et al: Prophylactic intravenous use of milrinone after cardiac operation in pediatrics (PRIMACORP) study. Prophylactic Intravenous Use of Milrinone After Cardiac Operation in Pediatrics. Am Heart J 2002;143:15-21.

79. Lovell AT: Anaesthetic implications of grown-up congenital heart disease. Br J Anaesth 2004;93:129-139.

80. Holzman RS, van der Velde ME, Kaus SJ, et al: Sevoflurane depresses myocardial contractility less than halothane during induction of anesthesia in children. Anesthesiology 1996;85:1260-1267.

81. Knobelsdorff GV, Schmitt-Ott S, Haun C, et al: The effects of sevoflurane versus halothane on systemic hemodynamics during induction for congenital heart disease in infants. Anesthesiology 1998;89:A1257.

82. Krane EJ, Su JY: Comparison of the effects of halothane on newborn and adult rabbit myocardium. Anesth Analg 1987;66:1240-1244.

83. Tanner GE, Angers DG, Barash PG, et al: Effect of left-to-right, mixed left-to-right, and right-to-left shunts on inhalational anesthetic induction in children: A computer model. Anesth Analg 1985;64:101-107.

84. Laird TH, Stayer SA, Rivenes SM, et al: Pulmonary-to-systemic blood flow ratio effects of sevoflurane, isoflurane, halothane, and fentanyl/midazolam with 100% oxygen in children with congenital heart disease. Anesth Analg 2002;95:1200-1206.

85. Wolf WJ, Neal MB, Peterson MD: The hemodynamic and cardiovascular effects of isoflurane and halothane anesthesia in children. Anesthesiology 1986;64:328-333.

86. Rivenes SM, Lewin MB, Stayer SA, et al: Cardiovascular effects of sevoflurane, isoflurane, halothane, and fentanyl-midazolam in children with congenital heart disease: An echocardiographic study of myocardial contractility and hemodynamics. Anesthesiology 2001;94:223-229.

87. Morgan P, Lynn AM, Parrot C, et al: Hemodynamic and metabolic effects of two anesthetic techniques in children undergoing surgical repair of acyanotic congenital heart disease. Anesth Analg 1987;66:1028-1030.

88. Glenski JA, Friesen RH, Berglund NL, et al: Comparison of the hemodynamic and echocardiographic effects of sufentanil, fentanyl, isoflurane, and halothane for pediatric cardiovascular surgery. J Cardiothorac Anesth 1988;2:147-155.

89. Russell IA, Miller Hance WC, Gregory G, et al: The safety and efficacy of sevoflurane anesthesia in infants and children with congenital heart disease. Anesth Analg 2001;92:1152-1158.

90. Barankay A, Richter JA, Henze R, et al: Total intravenous anesthesia for infants and children undergoing correction of tetralogy of Fallot: Sufentanil versus sufentanil-flunitrazepam technique. J Cardiothorac Vasc Anesth 1992;6:185-189.

91. Anand KJ, Hickey PR: Halothane-morphine compared with high-dose sufentanil for anesthesia and postoperative analgesia in neonatal cardiac surgery. N Engl J Med 1992;326:1-9.

92. Anand KJ, Sippell WG, Aynsley-Green A: Randomised trial of fentanyl anaesthesia in preterm babies undergoing surgery: Effects on the stress response [erratum appears in Lancet 1987 Jan 24;1(8526):234]. Lancet 1987;1:62-66.

93. Hickey PR, Hansen DD, Wessel DL, et al: Pulmonary and systemic hemodynamic responses to fentanyl in infants. Anesth Analg 1985;64:483-486.

94. Hickey PR, Hansen DD, Wessel DL, et al: Blunting of stress responses in the pulmonary circulation of infants by fentanyl. Anesth Analg 1985;64:1137-1142.

95. Gruber EM, Laussen PC, Casta A, et al: Stress response in infants undergoing cardiac surgery: A randomized study of fentanyl bolus, fentanyl infusion, and fentanyl-midazolam infusion. Anesth Analg 2001;92:882-890.

96. Parke TJ, Stevens JE, Rice AS, et al: Metabolic acidosis and fatal myocardial failure after propofol infusion in children: Five case reports. BMJ 1992;305:613-616.

97. Perrier ND, Baerga-Varela Y, Murray MJ: Death related to propofol use in an adult patient. Crit Care Med 2000;28:3071-3074.

98. Burow BK, Johnson ME, Packer DL: Metabolic acidosis associated with propofol in the absence of other causative factors. Anesthesiology 2004;101:239-241.

99. Lebovic S, Reich DL, Steinberg LG, et al: Comparison of propofol versus ketamine for anesthesia in pediatric patients undergoing cardiac catheterization. Anesth Analg 1992;74:490-494.

100. Williams GD, Jones TK, Hanson KA, et al: The hemodynamic effects of propofol in children with congenital heart disease. Anesth Analg 1999;89:1411-1416.

101. Kondo U, Kim SO, Nakayama M, et al: Pulmonary vascular effects of propofol at baseline, during elevated vasomotor tone, and in response to sympathetic alpha- and beta-adrenoreceptor activation. Anesthesiology 2001;94:815-823.

102. Morray JP, Lynn AM, Stamm SJ, et al: Hemodynamic effects of ketamine in children with congenital heart disease. Anesth Analg 1984;63:895-899.

103. Sato T, Matsuki A, Zsigmond EK, et al: Ketamine relaxes airway smooth muscle contracted by endothelin. Anesth Analg 1997;84:900-906.

104. Tugrul M, Camci E, Pembeci K, et al: Ketamine infusion versus isoflurane for the maintenance of anesthesia in the prebypass period in children with tetralogy of Fallot. J Cardiothorac Vasc Anesth 2000;14:557-561.

105. Maunuksela EL, Gattiker RI: Use of pancuronium in children with congenital heart disease. Anesth Analg 1981;60:798-801.

106. Haworth SG: Pulmonary hypertension in the young. Heart 2002;88:658-664.

107. Fukazawa M, Fukushige J, Ueda K: Atrial septal defects in neonates with reference to spontaneous closure. Am Heart J 1988;116:123-127.

108. Driscoll DJ: Left-to-right shunt lesions. Pediatr Clin North Am 1999;46:355-368.

109. Therrien J, Webb G: Clinical update on adults with congenital heart disease. Lancet 2003;362:1305-1313.

110. Baum VC: The adult patient with congenital heart disease. J Cardiothorac Vasc Anesth 1996;10:261-282.

111. Granton JT, Rabinovitch M: Pulmonary arterial hypertension in congenital heart disease. Cardiol Clin 2002;20:441-457.

112. Hynes JK, Tajik AJ, Seward JB, et al: Partial atrioventricular canal defect in adults. Circulation 1982;66:284-287.

113. Spicer RL: Cardiovascular disease in Down syndrome. Pediatr Clin North Am 1984;31:1331-1343.

114. Stayer SA, Andropoulos DB, Russell IA: Anesthetic management of the adult patient with congenital heart disease. Anesthesiol Clin North Am 2003;21:653-673.

115. Graham TP Jr, Gutgesell HP: Ventricular septal defects. In Emmanouilides GC, Riemenschneider TA, Allen HD, Gutgesell HP (eds): Moss and Adams Heart Disease in Infants, Children, and Adolescence: Including the Fetus and Young Adult. Baltimore, Williams & Wilkins, 1995, pp 724-725.

116. Hardin JT, Muskett AD, Canter CE, et al: Primary surgical closure of large ventricular septal defects in small infants. Ann Thorac Surg 1992;53:397-401.

117. Reller MD, Colasurdo MA, Rice MJ, et al: The timing of spontaneous closure of the ductus arteriosus in infants with respiratory distress syndrome. Am J Cardiol 1990;66:75-78.

118. Galli KK, Myers LB, Nicolson SC: Anesthesia for adult patients with congenital heart disease undergoing noncardiac surgery. Int Anesthesiol Clin 2001;39:43-71.

119. Harrison DA, Benson LN, Lazzam C, et al: Percutaneous catheter closure of the persistently patent ductus arteriosus in the adult. Am J Cardiol 1996;77:1094-1097.

120. Hofbeck M, Bartolomaeus G, Buheitel G, et al: Safety and efficacy of interventional occlusion of patent ductus arteriosus with detachable coils: A multicentre experience. Eur J Pediatr 2000;159:331-337.

121. Laborde F, Noirhomme P, Karam J, et al: A new video-assisted thoracoscopic surgical technique for interruption of patient ductus arteriosus in infants and children. J Thorac Cardiovasc Surg 1993;105:278-280.

122. Grifka RG: Cyanotic congenital heart disease with increased pulmonary blood flow. Pediatr Clin North Am 1999;46:405-425.

123. Hanley FL, Heinemann MK, Jonas RA, et al: Repair of truncus arteriosus in the neonate. J Thorac Cardiovasc Surg 1993;105:1047-1056.

124. Lake CL: Anomalies of the systemic and pulmonary venous returns. In Lake CL: Pediatric Cardiac Anesthesia. Stamford, CT, Appleton & Lange, 1998, pp 358-363.

125. Rodriguez-Collado J, Attie F, Zabal C, et al: Total anomalous pulmonary venous connection in adults: Long-term follow-up. J Thorac Cardiovasc Surg 1992;103:877-880.

126. Hager A, Kaemmerer H, Eicken A, et al: Long-term survival of patients with univentricular heart not treated surgically. J Thorac Cardiovasc Surg 2002;123:1214-1217.

127. Veldtman GR, Nishimoto A, Siu S, et al: The Fontan procedure in adults. Heart 2001;86:330-335.

128. Gentles TL, Gauvreau K, Mayer JE Jr, et al: Functional outcome after the Fontan operation: Factors influencing late morbidity. J Thorac Cardiovasc Surg 1997;114:392-403.

129. Gentles TL, Mayer JE Jr, Gauvreau K, et al: Fontan operation in five hundred consecutive patients: Factors influencing early and late outcome. J Thorac Cardiovasc Surg 1997;114:376-391.

130. Penny DJ, Rigby ML, Redington AN: Abnormal patterns of intraventricular flow and diastolic filling after the Fontan operation: Evidence for incoordinate ventricular wall motion. Br Heart J 1991;66:375-378.

131. Driscoll DJ, Offord KP, Feldt RH, et al: Five- to fifteen-year follow-up after Fontan operation. Circulation 1992;85:469-496.

132. Rauch R, Ries M, Hofbeck M, et al: Hemostatic changes following the modified Fontan operation (total cavopulmonary connection). Thromb Haemost 2000;83:678-682.

133. Penny DJ, Hayek Z, Redington AN: The effects of positive and negative extrathoracic pressure ventilation on pulmonary blood flow after the total cavopulmonary shunt procedure. Int J Cardiol 1991;30:128-130.

134. Goldman AP, Delius RE, Deanfield JE, et al: Pharmacological control of pulmonary blood flow with inhaled nitric oxide after the fenestrated Fontan operation. Circulation 1996;94:1.

135. Mahle WT, Spray TL, Wernovsky G, et al: Survival after reconstructive surgery for hypoplastic left heart syndrome: A 15-year experience from a single institution. Circulation 2000;102:III136-III141.

136. Forbess JM, Cook N, Roth SJ, et al: Ten-year institutional experience with palliative surgery for hypoplastic left heart syndrome: Risk factors related to stage I mortality. Circulation 1995;92:II262-II266.

137. Bailey LL, Gundry SR: Hypoplastic left heart syndrome. Pediatr Clin North Am 1990;37:137-150.

138. Nicolson SC, Steven JM, Kurth CD, et al: Anesthesia for noncardiac surgery in infants with hypoplastic left heart syndrome following hemi-Fontan operation. J Cardiothorac Vasc Anesth 1994;8:334-336.

139. Goldberg CS, Gomez CA: Hypoplastic left heart syndrome: New developments and current controversies. Semin Neonatol 2003;8: 461-468.

140. Hansen DD, Hickey PR: Anesthesia for hypoplastic left heart syndrome: Use of high-dose fentanyl in 30 neonates. Anesth Analg 1986;65:127-132.

141. Laussen PC: Neonates with congenital heart disease. Curr Opin Pediatr 2001;13:220-226.

142. Brickner ME, Hillis LD, Lang RA: Congenital heart disease in adults: II. N Engl J Med 2000;342:334-342.

143. Waldman JD, Wernly JA: Cyanotic congenital heart disease with decreased pulmonary blood flow in children. Pediatr Clin North Am 1999;46:385-404.

144. Stayer SA, Shetty S, Andropoulos DB: Perioperative management of tetralogy of Fallot with absent pulmonary valve. Paediatr Anaesth 2002;12:705-711.

145. Rammohan M, Airan B, Bhan A, et al: Total correction of tetralogy of Fallot in adults—surgical experience. Int J Cardiol 1998;63: 121-128.

146. Murphy JG, Gersh BJ, Mair DD, et al: Long-term outcome in patients undergoing surgical repair of tetralogy of Fallot. N Engl J Med 1993;329:593-599.

147. John S, John C, Bashi VV, et al: Tetralogy of Fallot: Intracardiac repair in 840 subjects. Cardiovasc Surg 1993;1:285-290.

148. Oechslin EN, Harrison DA, Harris L, et al: Reoperation in adults with repair of tetralogy of Fallot: Indications and outcomes. J Thorac Cardiovasc Surg 1999;118:245-251.

149. Samuelson PN, Lell WA: Tetralogy of Fallot. In Lake CL: Pediatric Cardiac Anesthesia. Stamford, CT, Appleton & Lange, 1998, pp 307-308.

150. Hickey PR, Hansen DD, Cramolini GM, et al: Pulmonary and systemic hemodynamic responses to ketamine in infants with normal and elevated pulmonary vascular resistance. Anesthesiology 1985;62:287-293.

151. Millikan JS, Puga FJ, Danielson GK, et al: Staged surgical repair of pulmonary atresia, ventricular septal defect, and hypoplastic, confluent pulmonary arteries. J Thorac Cardiovasc Surg 1986;91:818-825.

152. Reddy VM, Liddicoat JR, Hanley FL: Midline one-stage complete unifocalization and repair of pulmonary atresia with ventricular septal defect and major aortopulmonary collaterals. J Thorac Cardiovasc Surg 1995;109:832-844.

153. Shprintzen RJ: Velocardiofacial syndrome. Otolaryngol Clin North Am 2000;33:1217-1240.

154. Oliver WC Jr, Murray MJ, Raimundo HS, et al: The use of halothane to treat severe bronchospasm after a unifocalization procedure. J Cardiothorac Vasc Anesth 1995;9:177-180.

155. DiNardo JA: Transposition of the great vessels. In Lake CL: Pediatric Cardiac Anesthesia. Stamford, CT, Appleton & Lange, 1998, pp 320-322.

156. Gale AW, Danielson GK, McGoon DC, et al: Fontan procedure for tricuspid atresia. Circulation 1980;62:91-96.

157. Danielson GK, Fuster V: Surgical repair of Ebstein's anomaly. Ann Surg 1982;196:499-504.

158. Jaiswal PK, Balakrishnan KG, Saha A, et al: Clinical profile and natural history of Ebstein's anomaly of tricuspid valve. Int J Cardiol 1994;46:113-119.

159. Spitaels SE: Ebstein's anomaly of the tricuspid valve complexities and strategies. Cardiol Clin 2002;20:431-439.

160. Danielson GK: Ebstein's anomaly: Editorial comments and personal observations. Ann Thorac Surg 1982;34:396-400.

161. Kawashima Y, Kitamura S, Matsuda H, et al: Total cavopulmonary shunt operation in complex cardiac anomalies: A new operation. J Thorac Cardiovasc Surg 1984;87:74-81.

162. Bradley SM, Mosca RS, Hennein HA, et al: Bidirectional superior cavopulmonary connection in young infants. Circulation 1996;94: II5-II11.

163. Danielson GK, Driscoll DJ, Mair DD, et al: Operative treatment of Ebstein's anomaly. J Thorac Cardiovasc Surg 1992;104:1195-1202.

164. Saha A, Balakrishnan KG, Jaiswal PK, et al: Prognosis for patients with Eisenmenger syndrome of various aetiology. Int J Cardiol 1994;45:199-207.

165. Ammash NM, Connolly HM, Abel MD, et al: Noncardiac surgery in Eisenmenger syndrome. J Am Coll Cardiol 1999;33:222-227.

166. Campbell M: Natural history of coarctation of the aorta. Br Heart J 1970;32:633-640.

167. Tawes RL Jr, Aberdeen E, Waterston DJ, et al: Coarctation of the aorta in infants and children: A review of 333 operative cases, including 179 infants. Circulation 1969;39:I173-I184.

168. Tawes RL Jr, Berry CL, Aberdeen E: Congenital bicuspid aortic valves associated with coarctation of the aorta in children. Br Heart J 1969;31:127-128.

169. Zehr KJ, Gillinov AM, Redmond JM, et al: Repair of coarctation of the aorta in neonates and infants: A thirty-year experience. Ann Thorac Surg 1995;59:33-41.

170. Doyle TP, Hellenbrand WE: The role of cardiac catheterization in the evaluation and treatment of neonates with congenital heart disease. Semin Perinatol 1993;17:122-134.

171. Kimball TR, Reynolds JM, Mays WA, et al: Persistent hyperdynamic cardiovascular state at rest and during exercise in children after successful repair of coarctation of the aorta. J Am Coll Cardiol 1994;24:194-200.

172. Beynen FM, Tarhan S: Anesthesia for surgical repair of heart defects in children. In Tarhan S (ed): Cardiovascular Anesthesia and Postoperative Care. Chicago, Year Book Medical, 1989, pp 116-118.

173. Gaynor JW, Bull C, Sullivan ID, et al: Late outcome of survivors of intervention for neonatal aortic valve stenosis. Ann Thorac Surg 1995;60:122-125.

174. Marino BS, Wernovsky G, Rychik J, et al: Early results of the Ross procedure in simple and complex left heart disease. Circulation 1999;100:II162-II166.

175. Gerosa G, McKay R, Ross DN: Replacement of the aortic valve or root with a pulmonary autograft in children. Ann Thorac Surg 1991;51:424-429.

4 Respiratory Diseases

RAFAEL CARTAGENA, MD, ANTHONY N. PASSANNANTE, MD, and
PETER ROCK, MD, MBA

A thorough knowledge of pulmonary anatomy and physiology is of paramount importance to the practicing anesthesiologist. Familiarity with common clinical conditions such as chronic obstructive lung disease (COPD) and asthma is presumed. In this chapter we present a comprehensive review of less common pulmonary conditions, organized in an anatomic manner, and discuss, in order, the pulmonary vasculature, conditions that obstruct the airways, the pulmonary interstitium, and conditions extrinsic to the lungs that affect pulmonary function, such as severe arthritic disorders. We then move to a discussion of drug-induced lung injury and conclude by discussing rare infectious pulmonary diseases, including severe acute respiratory syndrome (SARS).

Many of the conditions discussed in this chapter are severe, and some are difficult to diagnose. Patients with pulmonary disease may present with varied symptoms, including productive or nonproductive cough, fever, shortness of breath, chest pain, and decreased exercise tolerance. In most circumstances, patients who have these conditions will already be under the care of an internist or pulmonary specialist. In many cases, the evaluation necessary to arrive at an accurate diagnosis will be comprehensive and includes a detailed history and physical examination, a chest radiograph, and pulmonary function tests (PFTs), including spirometry, diffusing capacity, and lung volume determination, and perhaps even arterial blood gas (ABG) analysis. For some conditions bronchoscopy and biopsy will have been performed, and others require echocardiography or cardiac catheterization for diagnostic certainty. For urgent or emergent surgery, the gravity of the clinical situation often precludes additional diagnostic assessment. For elective surgery, preoperative evaluation should include a review of these diagnostic studies and a determination as to whether the clinical condition of the patient has changed in a substantial way. If a diagnosis has already been established, there is no evidence to suggest that repetition of a test such as spirometry and lung volume determination, which is the gold standard for the presence or absence of pulmonary disease but a poor predictor of who will go on to develop a pulmonary complication after surgery, is indicated before proceeding to surgery.[1] If a diagnosis has not been established in a patient who has symptoms consistent with one of the diseases discussed in this chapter, pulmonary consultation should be obtained preoperatively, because the patient's pulmonary disorder may well be a more pressing concern than an elective surgical procedure.

Unfortunately, pulmonary complications are common after many surgical procedures, particularly those involving the upper abdomen or thorax.[2-4] Preexisting lung disease, smoking, anesthetic time in excess of 180 minutes, and advanced age are also risk factors for pulmonary complications.[4,5] There is no standard definition of exactly what constitutes a pulmonary complication, but the most important complications are those that cause significant morbidity, such as postoperative pneumonia, or postoperative respiratory failure. Because all of the disorders discussed in this chapter constitute preexisting lung disease, patients with these disorders who come to the operating room are at increased risk of postoperative pulmonary complications. Effective preoperative and intraoperative treatments for the individual diseases are discussed in the main body of this chapter. In the postoperative period aggressive treatment with mechanical measures such as incentive spirometry has been shown to minimize the frequency of the occurrence of pulmonary complications.[6,7]

DISEASES OF THE PULMONARY CIRCULATION

Pulmonary Arteriovenous Fistulas

Pulmonary arteriovenous (AV) fistulas are abnormal communications between the arterial and venous pulmonary circulation that result in shunting of blood from right to left without traversing the pulmonary capillary network. This shunt results in a decreased fraction of the pulmonary circulation participating in gas exchange, mixing of oxygenated and deoxygenated blood, and, as a consequence, a reduction in Pao_2. Many patients with pulmonary AV fistulas are asymptomatic, but associated signs and possible symptoms consistent with chronic hypoxemia are possible (Table 4-1).

There are several known causes of pulmonary AV fistula formation (Table 4-2). Many pulmonary AV fistulas are the result of congenital malformations and may be

TABLE 4–1   Signs and Symptoms of Arteriovenous Fistula

Shortness of breath
Dyspnea with exertion
Bloody sputum
Cyanosis
Clubbing
Bruit
Low arterial oxygen saturation
Polycythemia
Abnormal vasculature or nodules on chest radiograph

TABLE 4–2   Causes of Pulmonary Arteriovenous Fistulas

Congenital
Hereditary hemorrhagic telangiectasia (Rendu-Osler-Weber syndrome)
Chest trauma
Cavopulmonary shunting*
Hepatic cirrhosis
Pulmonary hypertension

*First stage of a Fontan repair for single ventricle physiology, generally performed at 4 to 6 months of age. A cavopulmonary shunt is constructed and directs superior vena caval blood flow to the confluent pulmonary arteries.

associated with hereditary hemorrhagic telangiectasia (Osler-Weber-Rendu syndrome).[8] Hereditary hemorrhagic telangiectasia is transmitted in an autosomal dominant pattern and most commonly seen in middle-aged women, although diagnosis in early childhood is possible. Patients with this syndrome are more likely to have multiple fistulas and more severe symptoms.

Patients with pulmonary AV fistula are at risk for rupture of fistula with resulting hemothorax and hemoptysis, which are potentially life threatening. Thrombus formation within the fistula may also occur, with the potential for embolization of clot to the brain, resulting in symptoms such as stroke or seizures. Embolization of other organ systems is also a possibility. If the thrombus becomes infected, septic emboli and potential abscess formation may result.

Surgical intervention in the management of pulmonary AV fistulas becomes necessary when cardiac symptoms are more pronounced, significant respiratory symptoms are present, room air desaturation develops, or complications such as emboli with central nervous system (CNS) manifestations have occurred. Surgical preoperative evaluation requires chest computed tomography (CT) and pulmonary arteriography to localize the lesion. Pulmonary lobectomy, segmentectomy, or wedge resection via thoracotomy or video-assisted thoracoscopic surgery (VATS) are the most commonly performed surgical procedures. Embolization procedures are gaining wider acceptance and can be utilized preoperatively in the event of hemorrhage or as stand-alone therapy.[9]

Anesthetic evaluation focuses on the degree of shunt and hypoxemia. Analysis of an arterial blood gas sample will provide much of this information. Review of the pulmonary angiogram will reveal the size of the lesion and whether multiple fistulas are present. A significant fistula in the nonoperative lung may compromise arterial oxygenation if one-lung ventilation is required for surgical exposure. Efforts to minimize flow through a pulmonary AV fistula will revolve around avoiding increased pulmonary vascular resistance and elevated levels of positive end-expiratory pressure (PEEP).

Intraoperative management frequently requires one-lung ventilation to optimize surgical exposure. A double-lumen endotracheal tube (ETT) provides the added benefit of isolating the nonoperative lung and airways from any bleeding, which may occur during a potentially bloody resection. The risk of significant bleeding is decreased if the lesion has been embolized before resection. Large-bore intravenous access is recommended in the event significant hemorrhage occurs. An arterial catheter is also indicated to monitor oxygenation and guide resuscitative efforts. An important anesthetic goal is to minimize flow through the pulmonary AV fistula. AV fistulas do not have capillary beds and have lower resistance to blood flow than normal pulmonary vasculature. It is important to avoid a general increase in pulmonary vascular resistance (PVR), because this will increase flow through the AV fistula. Similarly, minimizing the use of PEEP will minimize increases in PVR and help minimize blood flow through the pulmonary AV fistula. Because of the risk of paradoxical emboli passing through the fistula, extra caution must be taken to avoid injection of any air or particulate debris into the venous system, because such debris may bypass the pulmonary capillary bed and gain access into systemic arteries where end-organ embolization can occur. Preoperative evaluation should include assessment of neurologic function to rule out prior embolic stroke, and postoperative evaluation should include a neurologic check as well, to look for perioperative CNS embolization.

Wegener's Granulomatosis

Wegener's granulomatosis (WG) is a rare disorder characterized by necrotizing giant cell granulomatosis of the upper respiratory tract and lung, widespread necrotizing vasculitis, and focal glomerulonephritis. WG may also affect the cardiovascular, neurologic, and gastrointestinal systems.[10] Although the etiology of WG is unknown, an autoimmune disorder is suspected. A typical patient is in the fourth or fifth decade, and men are twice as likely to have WG as women. Symptoms associated with WG are vague, and diagnosis can be elusive (Table 4-3). Biopsy of a lesion is necessary to make the diagnosis.

If the disease process advances, there is the potential for significant respiratory and renal compromise, as well as hearing and vision loss (Table 4-4). Cardiac involvement is uncommon, although pericarditis, coronary arteritis, valvular involvement, and left ventricular hypertrophy have been reported. Current therapy with cyclophosphamide, corticosteroids, methotrexate, or azathioprine yields very good results, with long-term remission occurring in the majority of patients.

Preoperative assessment is directed toward evaluating any of the potential complications of WG that the patient

TABLE 4–3   Common Signs and Symptoms of Wegener's Granulomatosis
Hematuria
Shortness of breath
Wheezing
Hemoptysis
Bloody sputum
Cough
Chest pain or pleuritis
Sinusitis
Ulcers or lesions around the nose
Weight loss
Weakness
Fever
Joint pain

may have acquired, with renal and pulmonary insufficiency being the most common. Blood urea nitrogen and creatinine levels will provide adequate insight into the patient's renal function. A pulmonary flow-volume loop may be indicated if the patient is suspected of having tracheal stenosis and, by providing information about the dynamic changes in tracheal caliber, can supplement static radiographic images. WG may cause either obstructive or restrictive lung disease, which can be severe. Spirometry or other PFTs can help determine the severity of such disease. Bronchoscopy and a neck and chest CT may be necessary to fully evaluate subglottic stenosis and provide an indication of what size ETT can be placed safely.

Several aspects of WG may complicate management of the patient's airway. A significant amount of granulation tissue is likely to be present in and around the nose and nasopharynx. Insertion of a nasotracheal tube or nasal airway may be impossible or traumatic with attendant hemorrhage and is best avoided. Additionally, lesions on the epiglottis or oropharynx may inhibit direct laryngoscopy, despite a normal airway examination. Once the vocal cords have been visualized, the ETT may be difficult to place,

TABLE 4–4   Complications of Wegener's Granulomatosis
Chronic renal insufficiency or renal failure
Hearing loss
Tracheal stenosis
Pulmonary insufficiency
Functional nasal deformities
Vision loss

owing to subglottic stenosis, and may require multiple laryngoscopies. If the patient is receiving corticosteroids at the time of surgery, stress dosing should be considered. In view of these concerns, it is best to proceed with a conservative plan for managing the airway in this population, with immediate availability of difficult airway equipment, multiple sizes of ETTs, and the means to obtain a surgical airway. If the patient is known to have significant tracheal or bronchial stenosis, care should be taken to prevent air-trapping and auto-PEEP by allowing sufficient time for exhalation.

Lymphomatoid Granulomatosis

Lymphomatoid granulomatosis (LYG), also known as angiocentric lymphoma, is a rare lymphoproliferative disease that is angiodestructive and frequently progresses to lymphoma. LYG mimics WG clinically and radiographically, although recent advances have identified it as a malignant B-cell lymphoma associated with immunosuppression and Epstein-Barr virus (EBV). Diagnosis requires histologic evaluation of a biopsy specimen. It was recently categorized as a lymphoma, although if diagnosed early (grade I angiocentric immunoproliferative lesions) it is considered benign, although premalignant.[11] Typically, it presents in the fifth or sixth decade, affecting males twice as often as females. The etiology of LYG is unknown, although the incidence of LYG in patient populations with immune dysfunction, such as human immunodeficiency virus (HIV) infection and organ transplant recipients, is significantly increased when compared with the general population. Based on this observation, speculation that LYG may result from an opportunistic infection has now been confirmed through laboratory investigation.

The disease process primarily involves the lungs, although the skin, kidneys, and central nervous system can also be affected. Signs and symptoms resulting from LYG are numerous, with an emphasis on the pulmonary system, and include an increased risk of pneumonia (Table 4-5). Unlike WG, glomerulonephritis is not part of this clinical picture. LYG is frequently fatal, with 60% to 90% mortality at 5 years, although a small number of patients may undergo spontaneous recovery and complete remission. The cause of death is usually related to extensive destruction of the lungs and resulting respiratory failure.[12] Corticosteroids are the treatment of choice, resulting in relief of symptoms such as fever, cough, chest pain, weight loss, and sinusitis. If not diagnosed in the premalignant phase, and if the disease has progressed to lymphoma, chemotherapy is necessary. The combination of cyclophosphamide, doxorubicin, and vincristine and prednisone (CHOP) is often used. Radiation therapy may be indicated for localized disease. More recently, immunomodulation with interferon alfa-2b has played a role in treatment.

TABLE 4–5   Clinical Manifestations of Lymphomatoid Granulomatosis
Hemoptysis
Cough
Dyspnea
Chest pain
Pneumothorax
Pleural effusions
Atelectasis
Fever and weight loss
Hepatomegaly
Erythema
Mononeuritis multiplex
Peripheral sensory neuropathy

In preparation for anesthesia, evaluation of the patient's pulmonary function is the primary concern. Chest radiography may reveal bilateral nodules, cavitations, pleural effusions, or pneumothorax. In the presence of advanced disease, ABG analysis and spirometry help define the extent of the patient's respiratory compromise and parenchymal destruction. A thorough preoperative neurologic evaluation is advised because of the high incidence of peripheral neuropathy. Toxicities related to any chemotherapeutic agents the patient may have received should also be considered. The CHOP protocol's toxicities include peripheral neuropathy, cardiomyopathy, and myelosuppression.

Several issues should be considered when planning an anesthetic for a patient with LYG. The presence or potential for peripheral neuropathy in this patient population may deter many anesthesiologists from utilizing regional techniques (i.e., for fear that any subsequent neurologic dysfunction will be assigned to the regional anesthetic technique). However, the choice of anesthetic must be based on a consideration of risks and benefits, and there is no evidence that regional anesthesia worsens LYG. Respiratory compromise increases the risk of hypoxia under general anesthesia or if the patient hypoventilates secondary to sedating medications used for premedication or for monitored anesthesia care. If general anesthesia is chosen, the potential need for postoperative intubation and respiratory support should be addressed with the patient. The need for postoperative mechanical ventilation is more likely in cases of advanced disease with extensive destruction of lung tissue, pleural effusions, or pneumothorax. There is no clear answer to which anesthetic technique is superior, and the approach should be tailored to the individual's comorbidities and surgical procedure. Long-term corticosteroid therapy in this population may result in adrenal suppression, and stress doses of corticosteroids should be considered.

Churg-Strauss Syndrome

Churg-Strauss syndrome (CSS), also known as allergic granulomatosis, is a rare systemic vasculitis that may affect multiple organ systems, particularly the lungs. Diagnosis requires the presence of at least four of the six following criteria: bronchospasm, eosinophil count greater than 10%, neuropathy (poly or mono), nonfixed pulmonary infiltrates, paranasal sinus abnormalities, and extravascular eosinophils (Table 4-6).[13] Patients frequently present in the fifth or sixth decade and may have a long-standing history of asthma. Both genders are affected equally. Cardiac involvement occurs later in the course and is the major cause of death. CNS manifestations such as cerebral infarcts, subarachnoid hemorrhage, and optic neuritis are common. CSS is treated with corticosteroids, which generally results in dramatic improvement or resolution of symptoms. The length of required therapy is proportional to the severity of symptoms and may be as long as 1 year.

Elective surgery should be postponed if management of bronchospasm has not been optimized. Involvement of other organ systems may necessitate neurologic and renal evaluations. Cardiac evaluation may require testing such as echocardiography to assess myocardial function if the patient has congestive heart failure or endocarditis. Preoperative assessment should include a chest radiograph and PFTs. Chest radiography may reveal multiple small pulmonary nodules or diffuse interstitial disease. Pleural effusions are noted in up to 30% of CSS patients. Spirometry typically demonstrates an obstructive pattern, although restrictive disease may also occur. A decrease in diffusion capacity may be observed from a loss of alveolar capillary surface area.

Intraoperative management should include principles applied to all asthmatics to minimize airway reactivity. If possible, avoidance of airway instrumentation and positive-pressure ventilation is desirable. A prolonged expiratory phase may be needed in patients with more advanced obstructive disease if positive-pressure ventilation is utilized, and preoperative spirometry will provide guidance in this area. β-Blockers should be avoided, if possible, because of the risk of bronchospasm and exacerbation of congestive heart failure (CHF). If needed for control of ischemic heart disease, selective β_1-adrenergic agents, preferably short acting, should be used. Perioperative corticosteroids should be considered because of the risk of adrenal suppression from long-term corticosteroid therapy.

Primary Pulmonary Hypertension

Primary pulmonary hypertension (PPH) is an idiopathic disease and is a diagnosis of exclusion (Table 4-7). The prevalence of PPH is thought to be approximately 1:1 million, with women being twice as likely as men to present with the disease. Some cases appear to be genetically linked.[14] Overall, PPH is more severe and aggressive than secondary pulmonary hypertension. Vascular remodeling, an alteration in pulmonary vascular tone, and a loss of cross-sectional pulmonary arterial area are responsible for the increase in pulmonary vascular resistance seen in this disease. Dyspnea is the most common presenting symptom, and syncope is a particularly poor prognostic sign. Right-to-left shunting may occur in the 30% of patients with a patent foramen ovale (PFO). Death typically results from hypoxia, a further increase in pulmonary artery pressures (PAP), and eventually right ventricular failure.[15]

Historically, treatment for PPH relied on oxygen and calcium channel blockers in an effort to decrease pulmonary vascular resistance (PVR) (Table 4-8). In addition, warfarin (Coumadin) is used to reduce the risk of thromboembolism resulting from the enhanced platelet activity seen in PPH. Pulmonary embolism or primary pulmonary vascular thrombosis is poorly tolerated in this patient population. Diuretics and digoxin are also employed when right

TABLE 4-6   Clinical Manifestations of Churg-Strauss Syndrome

Sinusitis
Nasal polyps
Pulmonary infiltrates
Diffuse interstitial lung disease (rare)
Hemoptysis
Pleural effusions
Cutaneous nodules and rashes
Hypertension
Glomerulonephritis
Coronary vasculitis
Endocarditis
Congestive heart failure
Peripheral neuropathy
Mononeuritis multiplex
Cerebral infarct
Subarachnoid hemorrhage
Optic neuritis

TABLE 4-7   Symptoms and Signs of Primary Pulmonary Hypertension

Dyspnea
Fatigue
Syncope or pre-syncope
Angina
Peripheral edema and other signs of right-sided heart failure
Cyanosis

TABLE 4–8   Current Therapies for Primary Pulmonary Hypertension

Therapy	Advantages	Disadvantages
Nitric oxide	Pulmonary circulation selective vasodilation; increases Pao_2	Possible formation of toxic byproducts; prolonged bleeding times; expensive
Prostaglandins (epoprostenol, treprostinil, iloprost)	Potent vasodilation; inhibits platelet aggregation and smooth muscle cell proliferation	Not selective for pulmonary circulation; systemic hypotension; headaches; expensive; requires continuous infusion or inhalation
Phosphodiesterase-5 inhibitors (dipyridamole, sildenafil)	Possible synergy with nitric oxide therapy	
Endothelin receptor antagonist (Bosentan)	Recently approved by FDA	Limited data available
Calcium channel blockers	High efficacy; inexpensive	Less effective in severe cases; negative inotropic effects can worsen right ventricular failure
Oxygen	Directly reduces pulmonary vascular resistance in cases of hypoxia	None
Coumadin	Improved long-term survival; decreases risk of intrapulmonary thrombosis	Increased bleeding risk
Magnesium	Vasodilation through blockage of Ca^{2+} channels; enhance nitric oxide synthase activity; releases prostaglandin I	Risk of magnesium toxicity: weakness, sedation, ECG changes

ventricular failure ensues. More recently, promising results have been achieved with prostaglandins (PGI_2, PGE_1; alprostadil) and nitric oxide to induce pulmonary vasodilation with minimal systemic effects. These may be used separately or in combination.[14] Currently, prostacyclins must be delivered by continuous intravenous infusion owing to their short half-life. Nitric oxide is delivered by inhalation and requires a tank and delivery system. Phosphodiesterase-5 inhibitors such as sildenafil and dipyridamole potentiate the pulmonary vasodilation resulting from nitric oxide and can be used separately or in a combined fashion.[14] Unfortunately, cost and unwieldy delivery systems have limited the use of these therapies to the short term or the most severe of cases. New approaches to delivering PGI_2 are under development, including the inhaled, subcutaneous, and oral routes. Another new agent is bosentan, an oral endothelin receptor antagonist that is thought to inhibit smooth muscle vasoconstriction and proliferation and has been approved by the U.S. Food and Drug Administration (FDA) to treat PPH.[14]

Preoperative studies focus on the severity of the patient's pulmonary hypertension, the degree of hypoxia, and the effects of these on the heart (Table 4-9). ABG analysis will elucidate the level of hypoxia and acidemia, both of which exacerbate pulmonary hypertension. A chest radiograph may reveal enlarged main pulmonary arteries or an enlarged heart due to right ventricular hypertrophy

or right atrial dilation. An electrocardiogram may also reveal changes consistent with pulmonary hypertension (e.g., right atrial enlargement), as well as the presence of abnormal cardiac rhythm (e.g., atrial fibrillation). Sinus rhythm is essential to adequate right ventricular filling. Preoperative echocardiography is helpful in determining the extent of right ventricular hypertrophy and function, right atrial enlargement, pulmonic or tricuspid valve dysfunction, and patency of the foramen ovale. Pulmonary systolic

TABLE 4–9   Suggested Preoperative Studies to Assess Pulmonary Hypertension

Study	Possible Significant Findings
Arterial blood gas analysis	Level of hypoxemia and acidosis; assess relative value of supplemental oxygen
Chest radiograph	Enlarged pulmonary arterial root; enlarged right heart
Electrocardiography	Dysrhythmias; signs of right-sided heart strain
Echocardiography	Assess right ventricle function and hypertrophy; valvular dysfunction and right atrial enlargement; patency of foramen ovale; estimate pulmonary artery pressure

pressures may be estimated by Doppler techniques. A more reliable method of measuring pulmonary pressures, gauging response to therapies, and detecting a patent foramen orale is right-sided heart catheterization. This procedure should only be considered if other studies have not provided an adequate assessment of disease severity and is not typically needed for preanesthetic evaluation. If the patient is being treated with digoxin, serum potassium and digoxin levels should be measured.

It is essential to keep the high morbidity and mortality of this disease in mind when preparing to deliver an anesthetic to a PPH patient and not assume the risk of perioperative complications is low even if the patient is undergoing a "minor" procedure. Regional anesthetic techniques do not preclude the need for invasive monitoring and vasoactive therapy. Each patient's needs should be considered individually. All medications being used to treat the patient's PPH and resulting right-sided heart failure should be continued in the perioperative period. Warfarin will need to be discontinued and replaced with a heparin infusion preoperatively. The risk of a thromboembolic event and the possibility of a right-to-left shunt justify a preoperative hospital admission to administer heparin. Sedation must be carefully titrated; oversedation may lead to hypoxia, whereas not adequately addressing a patient's anxiety may also cause a rise in PVR.

Intraoperative management should emphasize maintenance of cardiac output and systemic blood pressure while minimizing further increases in pulmonary artery pressures and the risk of right ventricular failure. Invasive monitors, used selectively, including an arterial catheter, pulmonary artery catheter, and transesophageal echocardiography, may be helpful in the management of these patients. These invasive monitors allow for sampling of arterial blood, pharmacologic manipulation of pulmonary artery pressures and cardiac output, and detection of right ventricular failure, while maintaining adequate ventricular preload. Many different anesthetic techniques have been used successfully in patients with PPH. Regional, epidural, and general anesthesia with controlled ventilation are all reasonable options. Spinal anesthesia may result in a significant reduction in systemic vascular resistance and may precipitate a drop in preload with no change in pulmonary vascular pressures. This may result in inadequate coronary flow to perfuse the right side of the heart, with consequent right ventricular ischemia and failure. Drugs commonly used in the provision of anesthesia are safe in patients with PPH. An exception is nitrous oxide, which has been implicated in raising PVR in several studies. Another exception is ketamine, which has sympathomimetic properties and may cause unintended increases in pulmonary vascular resistance.

In the event that an increase in PVR does occur, every effort must be made to avoid right ventricular ischemia and possible right ventricular failure. Helpful maneuvers include hyperventilation and maximizing PaO_2 to decrease PVR. Inhaled drugs such as nitric oxide, 20 to 40 ppm, and prostacyclin (inhaled; IV) can selectively decrease pulmonary artery pressure with minimal decreases in systemic blood pressure. Milrinone and amrinone are excellent choices when a decrease in PVR and increase in cardiac contractility is desired, although a decrease in systemic vascular resistance will also occur. Dobutamine will increase contractility and may decrease PVR. In the event that an increase in systolic blood pressure is desired to avoid right ventricular ischemia, norepinephrine may have a slight advantage over phenylephrine.[16]

OBSTRUCTIVE DISEASE

Cystic Fibrosis

Cystic fibrosis (CF) is a genetic disease that follows an autosomal-recessive pattern and that affects chloride channels. With an incidence of 1:2000 to 1:4500 in whites, CF is one of the more common inherited conditions. It results in a significant reduction in life expectancy and quality of life. The responsible gene is found on the long arm of chromosome 7 and codes for a protein known as cystic fibrosis transmembrane conductance regulator (CFTR), which functions as a chloride channel. This defect decreases the water content of various secretions throughout the body resulting in increased viscosity. CF is a universally fatal disease, although advances in therapy have resulted in significant gains in quality of life and longevity. There are a wide variety of clinical manifestations seen in CF (Table 4-10).

Pulmonary manifestations result from the inability to clear thickened and inspissated mucus from the airways. This causes airway obstruction and impaired defense against bacterial infection, which results in the majority of deaths related to CF. Recurrent bacterial infections result in dilation of the conducting airways leading to bronchiectasis.[17] Although CF is a chronic progressive disease, the extent of current pulmonary infection fluctuates, creating significant daily variability in a patient's pulmonary function. Eventually as the disease progresses, there is destruction of parenchyma and conduction airways. Loss of pulmonary arterial cross-sectional area results in pulmonary hypertension. Chronic hypoxemia also develops.

Patients with more advanced disease may develop spontaneous pneumothorax. The etiology of pneumothorax is unknown but presumably involves rupture of subpleural blebs through the visceral pleura. This becomes more likely in advanced disease. Over a lifetime, the incidence of pneumothorax may be as high as 20% in adult CF patients. Application of positive-pressure ventilation can increase the risk of spontaneous pneumothorax. In the event of pneumothorax, surgical pleurodesis

TABLE 4–10   Clinical Manifestations of Cystic Fibrosis

Sign or Symptom	Cause
Nasal sinusitis and polyps	Abnormal mucus production and secretion; chronic infections
Chronic bronchitis	Hypersecretion of viscid mucus and impaired host defenses
Obstructive pulmonary disease	Due to chronic pulmonary infections and airway plugging from excessive mucus secretion
Pneumothorax	Rupture of subpleural blebs through the visceral pleura
Failure to thrive	Chronic infection and malabsorption
Recurrent pancreatitis	Obstruction of pancreatic ducts with viscous exocrine secretions
Gastroesophageal reflux disease	Unknown
Maldigestion	Biochemically abnormal intestinal mucins impair absorption of specific nutrients; abnormal bile secretion and absorption
Fat-soluble vitamin deficiencies	Abnormal bile secretion and absorption
Obstructive azoospermia	Atretic or absent vas deferens
Salt-loss syndromes	Inability to create hypotonic sweat

is the treatment of choice for CF patients who have a low anesthetic risk; higher-risk patients frequently receive talc pleurodesis as a safer, yet less effective, alternative.[18]

The chronic hypoxia seen in this population causes an increase in pulmonary vascular resistance and pulmonary hypertension. Ventilation-perfusion inequality results in hypoxemia. Loss of pulmonary arteriole cross-sectional area causes increased pulmonary vascular resistance and pulmonary hypertension, which is exacerbated by chronic hypoxemia. The severity of pulmonary hypertension correlates with the severity of CF. Chronic pulmonary vasoconstriction (from hypoxia) results in a muscularization of the pulmonary arterial vascular tree, which results in cor pulmonale, although the initial enlargement of the right ventricle is considered a beneficial adaptation to the increased resistance to pulmonary blood flow. The only therapy effective in treating pulmonary hypertension and improving right ventricular performance in this population is oxygen.[19]

The primary gastrointestinal manifestation of CF is malabsorption and steatorrhea due to pancreatic dysfunction from obstruction of pancreatic ducts with viscous exocrine secretions. Malnutrition and deficiencies of fat-soluble vitamins such as vitamin K can increase the

patient's risk of bleeding if this issue is not addressed. Glucose intolerance due to pancreatic dysfunction (impaired endocrine function) is also common and may require insulin therapy. An increased incidence of gastroesophageal reflux disease (GERD) has also been reported in this population.[20]

Preparation for anesthesia should focus on evaluation of the patient's pulmonary status. Significant deterioration due to increased respiratory secretions or infection can be seen in a patient from one day to the next. Surgery should be postponed, if possible, unless the patient is at a baseline level of health. Preoperative testing should include a recent chest radiograph to diagnose pneumothorax, pneumonic processes, or bullous disease. In one series of patients with CF, 16% had an asymptomatic pneumothorax. Thus, chest radiography is essential in these patients.[18] Coagulation studies such as prothrombin time and partial thromboplastin time can provide information regarding coagulopathy resulting from vitamin K deficiency or general malnutrition. Sedating premedications should be given only if absolutely necessary, owing to the risk of exacerbating the preexisting respiratory compromise, and then under close observation with administration of supplemental oxygen to minimize the risk of desaturation. All CF patients should be questioned regarding symptoms consistent with GERD. If present, appropriate premedications and aspiration precautions such as a rapid-sequence induction should be considered although CF patients may desaturate rapidly when apneic.

Choice of anesthetic technique will be primarily determined by the scheduled procedure, although regional techniques offer some advantages. Avoidance of airway instrumentation will decrease the risk of bronchospasm and aspiration. Avoiding positive-pressure ventilation will decrease the incidence of perioperative pneumothorax formation. If a long-acting or continuous regional technique is chosen, postoperative opioid requirements will decrease. The risk of postoperative respiratory insufficiency may be less with regional anesthetic techniques, although this has not been rigorously studied.

The plan for general anesthesia should take into account the increased risk of aspiration (from GERD) and bronchospasm. The likelihood of chronic sinusitis and the presence of paranasal sinus polyps are reasons to avoid nasal instrumentation, if possible. A rapid-sequence induction proceeded by nonparticulate antacids and H_2 antagonists may help minimize the likelihood and consequences of pulmonary aspiration of gastric contents. However, use of rapid-sequence induction may result in uncontrolled systemic and pulmonary hemodynamics, and its use must balance airway risks with the risk of cardiovascular instability. Positive-pressure ventilation is usually preferable to spontaneous ventilation in advanced cases of CF, owing to the risk of respiratory fatigue and marginal tidal volumes. CF is an obstructive process, and prolonged expiratory times may be necessary, as will humidification of inspired gases and minimization of peak airway pressures to reduce the risk of barotrauma and pneumothorax. Low respiratory rates and smaller than usual tidal volumes may be necessary. Nitrous oxide should be used with caution because of the increased risk of pneumothorax formation with positive-pressure ventilation, as well as the likely presence of multiple blebs.

INFILTRATIVE AND INTERSTITIAL DISEASES

Bronchiolitis Obliterans Organizing Pneumonia

Bronchiolitis obliterans organizing pneumonia (BOOP) is an inflammatory lung disease of unknown etiology. It has been associated with bone marrow transplantation, although there is a very low incidence of BOOP in this population.[21] BOOP has not been conclusively determined to be more than an incidental finding. It results from the formation of granulation tissue, which obstructs the lumens of small airways and extends into the alveoli. The formation of the granulation tissue is associated with connective tissue proliferation, fibrinous exudates, and inflammation of alveolar and airway walls. These changes yield a clinical picture that presents as a flu-like illness with cough and dyspnea. BOOP shares many characteristics of idiopathic pulmonary fibrosis, with the most significant difference being the reversibility of the fibrinous changes in BOOP owing to the preservation of lung architecture.[21]

Corticosteroids are commonly used, although some cases resolve spontaneously. Typically, therapy lasts for 1 year with resolution of symptoms by the end of the third month of treatment. Symptoms may recur, particularly if the course of corticosteroids is not completed. Other agents such as erythromycin and cyclophosphamide have been used as treatment, although their efficacy is not well established. In the event that cyclophosphamide has been used, the risk of leukopenia and, more rarely, thrombocytopenia or anemia should be kept in mind.

Radiologic evaluation is consistent with an organizing pneumonia with patchy consolidation in a diffuse peripheral distribution. Effusions are a rare finding. Spirometry typically demonstrates a restrictive pattern, although it is possible to find an obstructive component. Decreased diffusion capacity and an increased alveolar-arterial oxygen gradient are common. Definitive diagnosis requires lung biopsy, typically performed thoracoscopically.

Because of the high success rate in treating BOOP and the fact that dramatic improvement is typically seen after a few weeks of therapy with prednisone, it is unlikely that many patients will present for surgery with respiratory compromise. These factors also suggest that it may be prudent to defer all but the most emergent surgery in patients just beginning treatment for BOOP. A review of recent radiographs and spirometry, along with a history and physical examination, will typically provide enough information as to whether the patient's pulmonary function has been optimized for elective procedures. In the event surgery is emergent and cannot be postponed, the primary anesthetic issues relate to ventilator management. As in other restrictive lung diseases, high peak pressures may occur with positive-pressure ventilation unless appropriate reductions in tidal volume are made. Rapid arterial hypoxemia can occur with apnea. The use of low levels of PEEP will improve functional residual capacity and assist in maintaining Pa_{O_2}. Continuation of PEEP or continuous positive airway pressure in the postoperative period may be necessary to maintain functional residual capacity.

Idiopathic Pulmonary Hemosiderosis

Idiopathic pulmonary hemosiderosis (IPH) is a rare disorder of unknown etiology characterized by diffuse alveolar hemorrhage and is a diagnosis of exclusion. The disease is primarily seen in infants and children. There is an association with cow's milk hypersensitivity, celiac disease, autoimmune hemolytic anemia, and several other autoimmune disorders, such as lupus, periarteritis nodosa, and WG, which suggests an immunologic basis for IPH, but no firm relationship has been established. Clinically, IPH is similar to the immune-mediated alveolar hemorrhage seen in syndromes such as Goodpasture's syndrome (see later) and WG, although extrapulmonary involvement is not present as it is in these disorders. Hemoptysis, anemia, and pulmonary infiltrates on chest radiograph are the common presenting signs and symptoms. The clinical course of IPH is variable with some reports of spontaneous remission. Other patients will die suddenly of severe alveolar hemorrhage or more gradually from respiratory insufficiency within 3 years of initial presentation. As a result of recurrent hemorrhage, pulmonary fibrosis with restrictive lung disease and eventually pulmonary hypertension and cor pulmonale will ensue (Table 4-11).

Corticosteroids are the cornerstone of therapy for IPH. Although the long-term efficacy of corticosteroid therapy for IPH is unclear, it is still the best option currently available. Long-term, if not lifelong, therapy is usually required, and complications arising from corticosteroid therapy are a concern, which leads physicians to minimize doses. This increases the risk of recurrence. Treatments with plasmapheresis, azathioprine, and cyclophosphamide have been attempted with some success, but these therapies are generally reserved for patients refractory to corticosteroid therapy. Definitive therapy is offered by double-lung transplantation, although there is a case report of recurrence of IPH 40 months after transplantation.[22]

TABLE 4–11　Sequelae of Idiopathic Pulmonary Hemosiderosis

	Etiology
Recurrent hemoptysis	Active alveolar bleeding; very young children may not be able to expectorate heme
Anemia	Chronic iron deficiency anemia related to sequestration of hemosiderin within alveolar macrophages
Pulmonary fibrosis	Scar tissue and clot formation at the sites of alveolar hemorrhage
Restrictive lung disease	Pulmonary fibrosis
Pulmonary hypertension	Obstruction of pulmonary blood flow in interstitial fibrosis
Cor pulmonale	Pulmonary fibrosis and hypertension

Evaluation of ongoing alveolar hemorrhage and quantification of the extent of any fibrotic changes is essential to preoperative assessment. The presence of dyspnea or hemoptysis provides a starting point. Gas exchange is impaired by ongoing alveolar hemorrhage, and there is an increased need for transfusion in the perioperative period owing to the acute and chronic loss of red blood cells. It is prudent to postpone elective surgery until active alveolar hemorrhage resolves. Evaluating recent chest radiographs for bilateral alveolar infiltrates or new or changing infiltrates will help identify ongoing alveolar hemorrhage. These infiltrates usually resolve 1 to 2 weeks after the bleeding has stopped. Honeycombing may be observed if pulmonary fibrosis has developed. Preoperative spirometry is recommended, because a restrictive pattern develops over the course of the disease. If active bleeding is present, the diffusion capacity will be artificially elevated, owing to absorption by intra-alveolar hemoglobin. Anemia frequently develops from ongoing alveolar hemorrhage, and measuring the amount of serum hemoglobin is essential.

If intubation is part of the anesthetic plan, the largest possible ETT should be placed to facilitate bronchoscopy, if needed, and adequate pulmonary toilet. As with other restrictive processes, higher airway pressures will occur unless a decreased tidal volume is selected. The risk of pneumothorax is increased. Corticosteroids or other therapies for IPH should be continued throughout the perioperative period.

Chronic Eosinophilic Pneumonia

Chronic eosinophilic pneumonia (CEP) is a rare disorder of unknown etiology characterized by subacute respiratory symptoms caused by infiltration of the alveoli and interstitium by an eosinophil-rich inflammatory process.

For the diagnosis to be made, there must be no identifiable cause for the pneumonia such as infection or sarcoidosis. CEP is more likely to occur in women and is frequently preceded by the development of adult-onset asthma. Common presenting symptoms include constitutional complaints such as night sweats, weight loss, fevers, and a cough. Progression to dyspnea may occur if not treated. Chest radiographs may show dense peripheral infiltrates, which have been described as a "photographic negative of pulmonary edema."[23] Spirometry in a symptomatic untreated patient typically reveals a restrictive pattern. Diffusion capacity is reduced. If bronchospasm is also present, the picture may be mixed with a reversible obstructive component.

Corticosteroids are used in the treatment of CEP and are very effective. Improvement of symptoms is frequently seen in 1 to 3 days, with radiographic resolution occurring over several months. Unfortunately, recurrence is common once corticosteroid therapy is discontinued, and thus treatment may be needed for life. CEP patients with concurrent asthma seem to have a lower recurrence rate. It has been suggested that this may be due to the use of inhalation corticosteroids as part of the management of asthma in this population.[24] Because of the effectiveness of corticosteroid therapy, the prognosis for CEP is excellent.

If at all possible, surgery should be delayed until CEP patients have received corticosteroid therapy and experienced resolution of symptoms. Typically, 7 to 14 days are needed for complete resolution. In the event of emergency surgery, the pathophysiologic alterations seen in CEP are similar to those of any other pneumonia. Fever may result in reduced intravascular volume and an increased metabolic rate. Fluid resuscitation to restore euvolemia before induction will decrease the risk of hemodynamic instability. The increased metabolic rate and increased shunt fraction due to perfusion of inflamed alveoli will increase the speed of desaturation on induction if apnea developes. Excellent preoxygenation and expeditious securing of the airway is therefore essential. Intraoperative ventilator management must be individualized with an effort to minimize airway pressures while delivering adequate volumes. If an obstructive component is present, bronchodilator therapy may be helpful and expiratory times may need to be prolonged. PEEP should be used with caution, because it may divert blood flow from ventilated alveoli and increase the shunt fraction. Adrenal suppression may exist, because many of these patients are receiving long-term corticosteroid therapy and the use of perioperative corticosteroid dosing should be considered.

Goodpasture's Syndrome

Goodpasture's syndrome (GS) is an autoimmune disorder that affects the lungs and the kidneys. It is caused by circulating anti–glomerular basement membrane (anti-GBM) antibodies that bind to the vascular basement membrane in the lung and kidneys, resulting in an autoimmune reaction. The end result is rapidly progressing glomerulonephritis that is frequently accompanied by vasculitis and pulmonary hemorrhage. The incidence is approximately 1:100,000, with both genders being affected equally. Genetic factors are thought to increase the likelihood of developing GS, although environmental factors such as smoking, infection, inhalation injury, volume overload, and exposure to high concentrations of oxygen increase the odds that pulmonary hemorrhage will occur.[25,26] The genetic component of GS is poorly defined. However, there is increased occurrence (88%) of HLA-DR2 in patients with anti-GBM disease compared with controls (30%). There is also an increased incidence of disease in twins, siblings, and cousins of those with GS. Inheritance of certain allelic variants of immunoglobulin heavy chain also increases susceptibility to anti-GBM disease.[26] Onset of the disease is dramatic, with sudden hemoptysis, dyspnea, and renal failure (Table 4-12). New-onset hypertension may also be part of the presentation. Renal biopsy is necessary to make the diagnosis and distinguish GS from collagen vascular diseases such as WG.

Because of the sudden onset and severity of the disease, initial treatment frequently requires hemodialysis and mechanical ventilation. If the patient survives the acute phase, high-dose corticosteroids and cyclophosphamide induce immunosuppression and plasmapheresis is used to clear anti-GBM antibodies and complement. Therapy usually lasts 3 to 6 months, with resolution of symptoms occurring within the first 2 months. End-stage renal disease is a common complication of the disease, and renal transplantation may be necessary. Early diagnosis and treatment has a strong correlation with better outcomes.

If at all possible, surgery should be delayed until medical management is underway and pulmonary involvement has resolved. In all likelihood, some renal insufficiency, if not failure, will still be present. Preoperative evaluation should include blood urea nitrogen and creatinine determinations and urinalysis to assess renal function. The patient's symptoms and medical condition at the time of operation will dictate the extent of the required pulmonary evaluation. This may include a chest radiograph, ABG analysis, spirometry, and diffusing capacity to quantify the extent and significance of pulmonary hemorrhage.[27] If pulmonary involvement is ongoing, hypoxemia and a restrictive defect on spirometry are common. A chest radiograph in a typical patient shows diffuse bilateral alveolar infiltrates from the pulmonary hemorrhage. Microcytic anemia from ongoing hemorrhage is also typical.

Oxygenation is the primary challenge of the anesthetic management of patients who have active GS. With ongoing alveolar hemorrhage, patients will not only have impaired gas exchange at the alveolar level but will most likely be anemic. These will contribute to decreased oxygen delivery to the tissues. Exposure of the lungs to an increased oxygen tension and high airway pressures may exacerbate alveolar hemorrhage. These stresses, along with overly aggressive fluid resuscitation, should be avoided in all patients with GS to minimize the risk of further anti-GBM–mediated lung injury. An intra-arterial catheter is indicated when caring for patients with anything more than mild disease. For major operations in patients with significant pulmonary impairment, placement of a pulmonary artery catheter or transesophageal echocardiography may be helpful in guiding resuscitation and hemodynamic management. When selecting anesthetic agents and other medications, renal function must be considered, and any potentially nephrotoxic drugs should be avoided. Dosing of medications that rely on renal excretion should be altered based on the patient's creatine clearance.

Pulmonary Alveolar Proteinosis

Pulmonary alveolar proteinosis (PAP) is a rare disorder characterized by accumulation of a lipoprotein-rich substance in the alveoli. There appear to be three distinct forms of PAP. Congenital PAP, which presents in infancy, is caused by mutations in the genes coding for surfactant proteins. There is a defect in surfactant-associated protein B (SP-B), which results in accumulation of surfactant-like material in alveoli.[28] The secondary form involves decreased alveolar macrophage activity, either functional impairment or decreased number, which may be related to immunosuppression, myeloid disorders, and hematologic malignancies, infection, or inhalation of noxious fumes. There is also an idiopathic categorization, which does not fit into either of the above categories and accounts for 90% of the cases.[29] Idiopathic PAP is thought to be due to reduced clearance of surfactant. The proteinaceous material found in the lungs of patients with PAP is surfactant. Patients typically present with gradual onset of cough and worsening dyspnea with exertion. Chest pain, fever, and hemoptysis may also be present. Patients may also

TABLE 4–12 Symptoms and Signs Seen in Goodpasture's Syndrome

Dyspnea
Fatigue and weakness
Hematuria
Oliguria
Hemoptysis
Anemia
Hypertension
Azotemia
Proteinuria

have clubbing, cyanosis, and rales. Definitive diagnosis of PAP requires transbronchial or open-lung biopsy. The clinical course of PAP is variable. Some patients have spontaneous improvement or remission; others experience persistent but stable symptoms. The other possible clinical course is steady progression of the disease with worsening hypoxia and increased risk of infection.

Chest radiographs typically have bilateral perihilar infiltrates extending into the periphery in a "butterfly" or "bat wing" distribution suggestive of pulmonary edema.[30] The appearance of the chest radiograph may be out of proportion to the severity of the symptoms the patient is experiencing. High-resolution CT findings tend to more closely correlate with the clinical picture. PFTs frequently reveal a mild restrictive pattern with a severe reduction in diffusing capacity. ABG analysis demonstrates hypoxemia and an increased alveolar-arterial gradient due to interpulmonary shunting.[29]

Therapy for congenital PAP is supportive, with lung transplantation being the only definitive therapy currently available. Secondary PAP will typically resolve with treatment of the underlying disorder. Whole-lung lavage, also known as bronchopulmonary lavage (BPL), has been used in the treatment of acquired PAP for 40 years and is still the current standard of care. More recently there have been reports of lobar lavage through fiberoptic bronchoscopes in the treatment of PAP.[31] This latter approach is very time consuming and uncomfortable for the patient and may be most useful in patients who cannot tolerate whole-lung lavage or the required general anesthetic.

A patient with moderate to severe disability due to PAP should be evaluated for the need for BPL before any elective surgical procedure. Caring for patients receiving BPL is significantly easier if the contralateral lung has been recently lavaged, because this will dramatically improve oxygenation during one-lung ventilation, which is required to perform the procedure. Preoperative testing should be directed by the patient's level of dyspnea, baseline oxygen saturation, and time since the last BPL was performed. In patients with more severe symptoms, preoperative ABG analysis or measurement of room air resting arterial saturation analysis is indicated. Chest radiography is unlikely to be useful in evaluating the extent of disease.

BPL requires a general anesthetic and placement of a double-lumen ETT. A rapid decrease in oxygen saturation on induction is common, making excellent preoxygenation and expedient placement of the double-lumen ETT critical. An intra-arterial catheter is useful in monitoring the patient's oxygenation and hemodynamic response to the procedure. Confirmation of correct positioning of the ETT by fiberoptic visualization is appropriate. Testing for leaks that would allow contamination of the ventilated lung by spillage of lavage fluid is essential. Then the nonventilated lung is lavaged repeatedly with saline while the ipsilateral chest wall is mechanically percussed. The procedure is repeated until the drained saline is nearly clear, indicating removal of the majority of the lipoproteinaceous material. The fluid used for the lavage should be warmed to decrease the risk of hypothermia; additionally, the volume of the drainage as well as the presence of bubbles should be closely monitored to ensure isolation of the contralateral lung. Oxygenation may improve during the instillation of fluid as alveolar pressure increases. This results in decreased perfusion to the lavaged lung (which is not being ventilated) and thus improves overall ventilation-perfusion matching. Hypoxia is most likely to occur during the drainage phases of the procedure, when an increase in intrapulmonary shunting occurs due to the dramatic drop in alveolar pressure. Significant hemodynamic changes can also occur during the infusion of the saline into the lung. Hypotension, as well as an increase in central venous pressure and pulmonary capillary wedge pressure, is not unusual. Use of transesophageal echocardiography has suggested that these changes were due to impaired venous return to the left side of the heart.[32] Presumably, saline infusion compresses alveolar capillaries, increasing pulmonary vascular resistance and resulting in an increase in central venous pressure, while also causing decreased left-sided heart output owing to decreased blood flow to the left ventricle. In some cases the contralateral lung can be lavaged during the same anesthetic, although it is not uncommon to wait several days between treatments. BPL may result in improvement lasting 12 to 18 months before it is again required.

Sarcoidosis

Sarcoidosis is a chronic granulomatous disease of unknown etiology that can involve almost any organ system. The diagnosis is usually made in the first half of adult life, with an occurrence in the United States of 20 to 50 per 100,000, with a higher incidence in African-Americans, people of Northern European decent, and females. The annual mortality rate of a patient with sarcoid is low but is increased by symptomatic cardiac[33] or neurologic[34] involvement. The initial presentation of sarcoid will vary depending on the organ systems affected. Frequently, abnormal chest radiographs in asymptomatic individuals raise suspicion. The lesions responsible for sarcoidosis are noncaseating granulomas, which may spontaneously resolve or proceed to fibrosis.

The vast majority of sarcoid patients have pulmonary involvement. Many are asymptomatic, whereas others will have nonspecific complaints such as chest pain, dyspnea, and nonproductive cough. Radiographic abnormalities progress from bilateral hilar adenopathy to diffuse pulmonary infiltration, and, in severe cases, pulmonary fibrosis. PFTs frequently demonstrate restrictive disease with decreased volumes and diffusion capacity. In some cases an obstructive pattern may also be present owing to airway narrowing. In more advanced cases ABG analysis reveals hypoxemia and an increased alveolar-arterial gradient. Cardiac symptoms occur in a significant number of sarcoid patients. Some are the result of myocardial granulomas, and others are secondary to respiratory system disease. Possible findings include conduction abnormalities (complete heart block, bundle branch block, or first-degree AV block), ventricular arrhythmias, congestive heart failure, pericarditis, supraventricular tachycardia, ventricular aneurysms, and sudden death.[33]

Neurologic findings in sarcoid are uncommon, although all of the nervous system is at risk. Possible manifestations of neurologic involvement include seizures, progressive dementia, diabetes insipidus, hydrocephalus, and acute mononeuropathy. Facial nerve neuropathy is the most common of the neurologic lesions and usually has a benign course.[34]

There is also the potential for airway involvement. This occurs in approximately 5% of patients with sarcoidosis.[35] Symptoms may include dyspnea, dysphagia, throat pain, hoarseness, a weak voice, or stridor. Most lesions are supraglottic and involve the epiglottis, aryepiglottic folds, and arytenoids.[36] These lesions may result in airway compromise and, rarely, the need for tracheostomy. Vocal cord paralysis has also been reported and is due to recurrent laryngeal neuropathy caused by sarcoid mediastinal lymphadenopathy.[37] Encountering a pregnant patient with a history of sarcoid is not unusual, because sarcoid occurs with an increased frequency in women of childbearing age. However, in general, pregnancy tends to improve sarcoid-related symptoms. This is presumably owing to increased cortisol levels during pregnancy.[38]

Corticosteroids are often required to treat sarcoid. Systemic corticosteroids appear to improve or shorten the length of most symptoms related to sarcoidosis. Owing to the relapsing and remitting nature of the disease it is difficult to verify the efficacy of this treatment. As is often the case, early diagnosis and treatment appears to improve the likelihood of successful treatment. Radiation therapy and immunosuppressants such as cyclophosphamide and azathioprine may also be used as treatment. Serial chest radiographs, PFTs, and serum angiotensin-converting enzyme (ACE) levels can be used to follow the progress of a patient. Serum ACE appears to be synthesized within sarcoid granulomas. High levels are associated with more severe pulmonary infiltration, and lower levels are seen with disease inactivity. Trends within a given patient are more important than the absolute level of ACE. Cardiac rhythm abnormalities can occur as a result of sarcoid heart disease and may necessitate placement of a pacemaker or implantable cardiac defibrillator, as well as other treatment for arrhythmias, cardiomyopathy, and heart failure.

Preparation for anesthesia in a patient with a history of sarcoidosis should focus on the airway and pulmonary function, as well as a on review of other organ systems known to have been affected in that particular patient. A review of recent chest radiographs along with PFTs is recommended. If a history of significant dyspnea is present, an ABG analysis is warranted. Screening for airway involvement can be accomplished by inquiring about dysphagia, hoarseness, or throat pain. If suspected, an evaluation by indirect laryngoscopy and, if necessary, head and neck CT will provide the necessary anatomic data. Swelling of supraglottic structures may increase the difficulty of intubation and increase the risk of postoperative respiratory compromise. Delaying surgery to allow for adequate corticosteroid therapy may be appropriate. Other preoperative testing is guided by the patient's history and may include electrocardiography and echocardiography if cardiac involvement or advanced pulmonary fibrosis is present. All ongoing cardiac therapy should be continued perioperatively. Because of the sporadic nature of neurologic symptoms, a thorough neurologic examination is advisable during preoperative evaluation to help differentiate between existing deficits and those resulting from anesthetic interventions, surgery, or positioning for surgery. Renal involvement also occurs, making review of recent electrolyte and renal function data advisable.

Intraoperative management of an asymptomatic patient should be uneventful and require little change in the anesthetic plan when compared with a healthy individual undergoing the same procedure. The presence of significant restrictive lung disease will require altered ventilator management and consideration of the need for postoperative ventilatory support. An intra-arterial catheter will be helpful in managing oxygenation and ventilation and allows close observation and early detection of any hemodynamic instability. In caring for patients with significant pulmonary fibrosis, placement of a pulmonary artery catheter or use of transesophageal echocardiography may help guide resuscitation and hemodynamic management. Sarcoid patients with an implantable cardiac defibrillator may need to have these devices inactivated for fear of interference from electrocautery units, although modern units are less susceptible to this issue. In this event, defibrillator pads should be placed during the period of inactivation to allow for external pacing and defibrillation, if needed. Airway management will be dictated by the preoperative evaluation; awake fiberoptic intubation or elective tracheostomy may occasionally be necessary. Continuation of corticosteroid therapy with consideration of stress-dosing is encouraged.

Systemic Lupus Erythematosus

Systemic lupus erythematosus (SLE) is a connective tissue disease resulting from autoantibodies directed at cellular nuclei antigens found in multiple organ systems. The cause of SLE is unknown. SLE can occur in anyone but most commonly afflicts women of childbearing age. Its incidence is estimated at 40 per 100,000 in North America.

Arthritis is the most common clinical manifestation of SLE. Other common signs and symptoms include cutaneous lesions such as butterfly malar erythema, Raynaud's phenomenon, oral ulcers, and recurrent noninfectious pharyngitis. Anemia, thrombocytopenia, leukopenia, and an increased incidence of thrombus formation are all possible hematologic sequelae. Renal involvement, in the form of glomerulonephritis, has a highly variable course. Neurologic findings include cognitive dysfunction, migraine-like headaches, and seizures. Pericarditis, small pericardial effusions, valvular abnormalities, and endocarditis represent the majority of the cardiac manifestations of SLE. Congestive heart failure may occur but is typically not the result of cardiomyopathy.[39] Treatment is typically directed at specific symptoms. Examples include nonsteroidal anti-inflammatory drugs (NSAIDs) for arthritic pain, glucocorticoids for anemia and thrombocytopenia, anticonvulsants for seizures, anticoagulants for thrombosis, and dialysis for end-stage renal disease. Other treatments may include plasmapheresis, azathioprine, and cyclophosphamide.

Pulmonary manifestations of SLE are numerous (Table 4-13). These conditions are the direct result of autoantibody reactions in the lung vasculature, lung parenchyma, and pleura. Histopathologic findings include alveolar wall damage, inflammatory cell infiltration, hemorrhage, and hyaline membranes. Some of these manifestations are thought to occur primarily in SLE patients with antiphospholipid antibodies. The presence of these antibodies is referred to as antiphospholipid syndrome (APS), with 50% of cases of APS being in patients with SLE although only a minority of SLE patients have APS.[40] The primary defect in APS is recurrent arterial and venous thrombosis,[41] although there is an association with pulmonary hypertension and diffuse alveolar hemorrhage. Alveolar hemorrhage and pulmonary hypertension are particularly dire manifestations and predict a higher mortality.[42]

Preoperative testing should be directed toward the affected organ systems. Many SLE patients have mild disease and require little deviation from the routine perioperative evaluation and care required for a given operation. A review of serum creatinine and blood urea nitrogen levels is reasonable to rule out any occult renal involvement. Pulmonary evaluation may include chest radiography, ABG analysis, and PFTs if current symptoms and history suggest pleuropulmonary involvement. A restrictive pattern is frequently seen on PFTs, although if bronchiolitis is present there will be obstruction as well. The diffusing capacity is reduced when interstitial disease is present. Diffusing capacity is normal when corrected for diminished lung volumes if respiratory muscle dysfunction is the sole cause of underlying restrictive lung disease.[43] Patients with significant pulmonary involvement may require postoperative ventilation. Ventilator management should be tailored to their specific disease process: diaphragmatic weakness or interstitial fibrosis. During the perioperative period it must be kept in mind that patients with APS are at increased risk of thrombosis, and appropriate precautions must be taken. Perioperative corticosteroid dosing may be required for patients with adrenal insufficiency due to chronic corticosteroid administration.

TABLE 4–13 Pulmonary Manifestations of Systemic Lupus Erythematosus

Finding	Comment
Primary Manifestations	
Lupus pneumonitis	Mimics acute infectious pneumonia
Diffuse alveolar hemorrhage	Rare; may be associated with APS
Lupus pleuritis	Pleurisy and pleural effusion are common in SLE
Interstitial pneumonia	Includes lymphocytic and BOOP variants
Pulmonary hypertension	Resembles PPH; associated with APS
Bronchiolitis	Rare and unexplained
Chronic interstitial lung disease	Resembles idiopathic pulmonary fibrosis
Secondary Manifestations	
Pulmonary Embolism	Due to recurrent thrombosis associated with APS
Respiratory muscle dysfunction	Subsegmental atelectasis; elevated diaphragm "Shrinking lung syndrome"

APS, antiphospholipid syndrome; BOOP, bronchiolitis obliterans organizing pneumonia; PPH, primary pulmonary hypertension. Data from references 40 to 42.

Idiopathic Pulmonary Fibrosis

Idiopathic pulmonary fibrosis (IPF), also referred to as cryptogenic fibrosing alveolitis, is an interstitial lung disease of uncertain etiology. It is a progressive illness with a median survival time of 3 to 4 years. This rare condition has a prevalence rate of about 5 per 100,000 and is more common in current or former smokers. A typical patient is a middle-aged man. Diagnosis is based on the presence of the histologic pattern of usual interstitial pneumonia and exclusion of other causes of this histologic pattern. Extrapulmonary involvement does not occur. The presentation is insidious and typically involves dyspnea and a nonproductive cough. Physical examination frequently reveals fine crackles at the lung bases, expanding upward as the disease progresses. Clubbing, cyanosis, peripheral edema, and cor pulmonale are later findings. There must be a restrictive pattern on spirometry and radiologic changes on chest radiograph or high-resolution CT consistent with the diagnosis.[44]

There is also an increased incidence of pulmonary malignancy in IPF patients. Unfortunately, it is unclear if resection of these lesions adds to life expectancy in this population.[45] There is no effective treatment currently available, although therapy with corticosteroid and cytotoxic agents is frequently attempted. There are currently many novel therapies in development intended to block fibrogenic pathways that may be of benefit (Table 4-14).[46] Lung transplantation is the only therapeutic option available for IPF. Although thought to be effective, there is still only a 49% survival rate 5 years post transplantation.[47]

IPF patients presenting for surgery will typically be tachypneic and cyanotic and will appear to be in poor health. Preoperative evaluation should include a review of recent spirometry and other PFTs. A decrease in lung volumes with a reduction in diffusion capacity is expected. Ventilation-perfusion inequality and impaired diffusion result in hypoxemia. In patients with advanced disease, echocardiography may reveal pulmonary hypertension and cor pulmonale. There appears to be a very high incidence of GERD in IPF patients.[48] It is appropriate to consider premedicants to reduce gastric volume and acidity, as well as an anesthetic technique to minimize the risk of pulmonary aspiration of gastric contents. An aspiration event in such a patient could easily be fatal. Placement of an intra-arterial catheter is advised for all but the most vigorous of these patients undergoing minor surgery.

Patients with IPF are most likely to present to the operating room for lung biopsy to establish the diagnosis, for lung transplant in a curative effort, or for resection of a pulmonary neoplasm. These procedures commonly require one-lung ventilation, a challenge in patients with advanced disease. Placement of a double-lumen ETT will provide the added ability to provide passive oxygenation to the nonventilated lung in an effort to minimize hypoxemia.

Acute Respiratory Distress Syndrome

Acute respiratory distress syndrome (ARDS) is a severe form of acute lung injury that occurs as a result of an underlying illness or lung injury. It may occur in as many as 10 to 20 per 100,000 individuals.[49] Several disorders have been implicated as risk factors for developing ARDS, some through direct lung injury, others by a systemic inflammatory response (Table 4-15). The underlying lesion is injury to the alveolar-capillary membrane and increased alveolar-capillary permeability. Proteinaceous edema fluid accumulates in the alveoli, resulting in impaired oxygenation and poorly compliant (stiff) lungs. ARDS develops acutely over a 1- to 2-day period. If a patient is alert and spontaneously ventilating, anxiety and dyspnea will be the earliest signs. As inflammatory changes occur, tachypnea and increased work of breathing will be noted. Mechanical ventilation is required to maintain oxygenation. Chest radiographs typically reveal diffuse bilateral alveolar infiltrates very similar to the findings of pulmonary edema. There is no laboratory test to diagnose ARDS. As a clinical diagnosis, criteria for diagnosing ARDS are acute onset of respiratory distress requiring intubation and mechanical ventilation; a PaO_2/FIO_2 ratio of less than 200, a chest radiograph with bilateral infiltrates suggestive of pulmonary edema, and no evidence of CHF or, if measured, a pulmonary artery wedge pressure less than 18 mm Hg.[50] ARDS has a high mortality rate, which is in the range of 35% to 40%. Patients who do survive generally return to a pulmonary function near their baseline. If a defect does remain it is likely to be a restrictive defect or decreased diffusion capacity, and more disabling sequelae are possible.[51]

Intraoperative management of ARDS is an extension of the care the patient is receiving in the intensive care unit. Many patients will have a severe underlying injury or illness, which will also require significant attention in the perioperative period. The approach to ventilator management plays a significant role in the mortality rate

TABLE 4–14 Experimental Idiopathic Pulmonary Fibrosis Therapies	
Interferon-γ 1b	Inhibition of fibroblast proliferation and collagen synthesis
Pirfenidone	Inhibits synthesis of collagen and tumor necrosis factor-α
Acetylcysteine	Stimulates glutathione synthesis

Data from Selman M, Thannickal VJ, Pardo DA, et al: Idiopathic pulmonary fibrosis: Pathogenesis and therapeutic approaches. Drugs 2004;64:405-430.

TABLE 4–15 Clinical Disorders Associated with ARDS	
Direct Lung Injury	**Indirect Lung Injury**
Aspiration of gastric contents	Sepsis
Inhalation of toxic fumes	Major trauma
Near-drowning	Reperfusion injury
Pulmonary contusions	Massive transfusion
Diffuse pulmonary infection	Drug overdose

Data from Hudson LD, Steinberg KP: Acute respiratory distress syndrome: Clinical features, management, and outcome. In Fishman AP, et al (eds): Fishman's Pulmonary Diseases and Disorders. New York, McGraw-Hill, 1998, p 2550.

from ARDS. Instituting low tidal volume ventilation on the order of 4 to 6 mL/kg (predicted body weight) and maintaining plateau pressures of less than 30 cm H_2O were found to reduce the mortality from ARDS by almost 20%.[52] This approach may result in hypercapnia and respiratory acidosis, which can be treated with sodium bicarbonate. There are currently no data to suggest a particular level of respiratory acidosis, which is dangerous.[53] There is no clear evidence to support that pressure-cycled ventilation is superior to volume-cycled ventilation. Administration of PEEP is necessary and results in recruitment of alveoli and better ventilation-perfusion matching. There is no set level of PEEP that has been shown to be superior.[54] Other maneuvers such as sigh breaths and periodic rotation of the patient to the prone position may result in improved oxygenation but are not associated with an improvement in outcomes. Invasive monitors will frequently be in place when the patient arrives in the operating room; if not, an intra-arterial catheter should be inserted. For procedures involving major fluid shifts, placement of a pulmonary artery catheter or use of transesophageal echocardiography may be helpful in guiding resuscitation and avoiding overzealous fluid administration, which might adversely impact the patient's respiratory status. Colloids such as albumin and hetastarch offer no advantage over crystalloid solutions because impaired alveolar-capillary membranes allow both classes of fluid to reach the extravascular space.

Pulmonary Histiocytosis X

Pulmonary histiocytosis X (PHX) is also called pulmonary Langerhans cell granulomatosis and is an uncommon interstitial lung disease that has an association with cigarette smoking. Related disorders are Hand-Schüller-Christian disease and Letterer-Siwe disease. The primary defect appears to be the pathologic accumulation of Langerhans cells around bronchioles and the pulmonary vasculature, leading to the formation of granulomas and fibrosis. Most PHX patients present in early adulthood and have a history of cigarette smoking; there is equal representation of men and women. Presenting symptoms are nonspecific and include nonproductive cough, dyspnea, fatigue, fever, and weight loss (Table 4-16). The presence of reticulonodular infiltrates, of upper and middle lobe cysts, and of stellate nodules with sparing of the costophrenic angle on chest radiography is highly suggestive of PHX. Diagnosis is confirmed by bronchoalveolar lavage (BAL) or biopsy. Results of spirometry in this population may yield an obstructive, restrictive, mixed, or normal pattern. A decrease in diffusion capacity appears to be the most consistent finding. Physical limitation in this population is frequently out of proportion to the results of spirometry, and the presence of pulmonary hypertension may play a significant role in contributing to diminished exercise capacity.

TABLE 4–16   Comorbidities Related to or Caused by Pulmonary Histiocytosis X

Symptom	Notes
Spontaneous pneumothorax	May be recurrent
Hemoptysis secondary to aspergillosis	Rare
Primary lung tumors	Causative relationship is unclear
Secondary pulmonary hypertension	Common, may result in cor pulmonale
Central diabetes insipidus	Occurs with central nervous system involvement
Cystic bone lesions	Cause bone pain and pathologic fractures

In advanced disease, pulmonary artery pressures in the range of 60 mm Hg are not unusual.[55]

The course of PHX is unpredictable. Improvement or complete remission may occur spontaneously or as the result of smoking cessation. A minority of patients progress to pulmonary fibrosis. Age (older than 26 years), an FEV_1/FVC ratio less than 0.66, and a right ventricular/total lung capacity ratio greater than 0.33 have been suggested as predictors of advanced disease and increased mortality.[56] Corticosteroids and chemotherapeutic agents are utilized in attempts to treat PHX, but the disease is frequently refractory to treatment. Lung transplantation has been performed with success, although there are reports of recurrence of PHX in the transplanted lungs of patients who had extrapulmonary involvement and resumed smoking.[57]

Patients who are in remission or have only mild symptoms do not require special preoperative evaluation or intraoperative management beyond that warranted by the scheduled procedure. In cases in which more advanced disease is present, a review of results of PFTs and ABG analysis and an evaluation of pulmonary pressures by echocardiography or direct measurement are advisable. Based on these results, intraoperative management should be tailored to avoid increases in pulmonary artery pressure. Placement of a pulmonary artery catheter may be necessary to help achieve this goal. The risk of pneumothorax in this population warrants an effort to minimize peak airway pressures. If diabetes insipidus is present, treatment with desmopressin should be continued in the perioperative period. The potential for pathologic fractures due to cystic bone lesions requires special attention to positioning and padding of the patient. As in all cases where pulmonary disability exists preoperatively, the potential for postoperative ventilatory support should be factored into the anesthetic plan and discussed in advance with the patient.

Lymphangioleiomyomatosis

Lymphangioleiomyomatosis (LAM) is a rare progressive interstitial lung disease of unknown origin that frequently leads to deteriorating lung function and death secondary to respiratory failure. The disease occurs in women of reproductive age and is exacerbated by pregnancy. It also occurs in males and females with tuberous sclerosis. The condition results from the proliferation of interstitial smooth muscle and formation of cysts, which obliterate the airways. Complaints of dyspnea are the typical presenting symptom. Individuals with LAM develop hyperinflated lungs with an increased total lung capacity. They also develop an obstructive pattern on spirometry. Spontaneous pneumothorax due to cyst rupture is common. Obstruction and eventual rupture of the thoracic duct, resulting in chylothorax, is another manifestation of the disease. Hemoptysis may occur but is uncommon. Chest radiographs are normal appearing early in the disease but resemble those of end-stage emphysema in advanced disease. Reticulonodular opacities may also be seen. An obstructive or occasionally a mixed pattern is present on spirometry, along with a significant decrease in diffusion capacity. Exercise capacity will be severely decreased owing to ventilation-perfusion inequality and increased work of breathing.[58] ABG analysis typically reveals a decrease in PO_2 and PCO_2 although pH is normal.[59]

Estrogen is suspected of playing a role in the development of LAM. This notion arises from the almost exclusive occurrence of the disease in women of childbearing age, its exacerbation by pregnancy, and the presence of estrogen receptors on biopsy tissue. Effective treatment of LAM is difficult. Corticosteroids are ineffective. Modalities aimed at blocking the effects of estrogen have been somewhat more successful. These approaches include oophorectomy, progesterone, and tamoxifen. Lung transplantation is offered to patients with advanced disease, although this is frequently complicated by disease-associated problems such as pleural adhesions, postoperative chylothorax, pneumothorax, and recurrent LAM.[60]

Preoperative evaluation should include a review of recent PFTs and chest radiographs, as well as ABG analysis in advanced cases. Elective surgery should be postponed until after significant chylothorax, if present, can be drained and chest tubes inserted to resolve existing pneumothoraces. Recurrent leakage of lymph results in an impaired immune response and nutritional wasting, which increase the patient's risk of perioperative complications and should be addressed before surgery by enteral or parenteral nutritional support. For patients with advanced disease, ventilator management should be similar to that used for a patient with severe emphysema, including prolonged expiratory times and avoidance of high inspiratory pressures. Postoperative ventilatory support may be required if the patient has severe underlying disease and is undergoing major or extensive surgery.

Placement of an intra-arterial catheter is helpful in obtaining serial ABGs to guide ventilator management.

ARTHRITIC DISEASES CREATING UPPER AIRWAY AND RESPIRATORY PROBLEMS

Ankylosing Spondylitis

Ankylosing spondylitis (AkS) is a chronic inflammatory process of unknown etiology that primarily deforms the axial skeleton, resulting in fusion. The disease is predominately diagnosed in young adults, with men more likely to be affected than women. Prevalence in the United States is in the range of 1 in 1000. There does appear to be a genetic component to AkS, because most affected individuals are HLA-B27 positive.

Owing to chronic inflammatory changes that occur at the ligamentous insertions onto bone, the vertebrae begin to grow into each other, forming outgrowths known as syndesmophytes. These changes result in the appearance of a "bamboo spine" in radiologic evaluation and decreased mobility of the spine. This process generally begins in the sacral and lumbar regions, with cervical involvement occurring much later in the disease course. Extraskeletal manifestations of AkS may occur, particularly peripheral joint manifestations, although they are for the most part uncommon. These include aortic insufficiency, cardiac conduction abnormalities, iritis, upper lobe fibrobullous disease, and pleural effusions. If fibrobullous disease does develop, the risk of aspergilloma and hemoptysis is very high.[61]

Involvement of the sternocostal, costovertebral, and thoracic spine results in decreased mobility of the thoracic cage and a restrictive ventilatory pattern. Although decreased exercise tolerance is common in AkS, it is thought to be due to deconditioning as opposed to a primary pulmonary defect.[62] The limitation in thoracic cage movement is almost totally compensated for by increased diaphragmatic excursion.[63] As the disease progresses, decreased exercise tolerance also is caused by the restrictive lung process.

Historically, treatment for AkS was symptom based and relied on NSAIDs and physical therapy to reduce back pain and stiffness. Using NSAIDs for long-term therapy poses an increased risk of peptic ulcers and gastritis in this population. For this reason, COX-2 inhibitors have been increasingly utilized as an alternative. The recent controversy regarding the cardiovascular safety of COX-2 inhibitors, suggests careful consideration of the risks and benefits of such therapy. Sulfasalazine, methotrexate, and corticosteroids are used in severe cases. The FDA has granted approval for the use of tumor necrosis factor-α inhibitors in the treatment of AkS. This promising new treatment may be the first therapy that will increase range of motion in AkS patients.

A patient with advanced AkS presents a significant challenge to the anesthesiologist. Frequently these patients will present for orthopedic procedures on the hips and knees. Preoperative evaluation should include radiographs of the lower and cervical spine to assess the extent of fusion. Caution should be exercised when instrumenting the airway because of involvement of the cervical spine. Decreased range of motion and poor mouth opening can make direct laryngoscopy difficult, and excess force applied to the neck can result in cervical fracture. Atlantoaxial subluxation is also present in a subset of these patients.[64] If advanced disease is present, an alternative approach to airway management, such as LMA placement or awake fiberoptic intubation, is recommended. Neuraxial anesthesia is very challenging in AkS patients. The ossification of spinal ligaments significantly narrows or closes altogether the intervertebral space and prevents optimal positioning. Alternatives that have been reported to be successful include a lateral approach to spinal placement[65] and placement of caudal catheters.[66]

Intraoperative management must include special attention to positioning owing to the inflexibility of the patient's spine. Diaphragmatic function should be optimized during spontaneous ventilation because of the presence of a restrictive thoracic cage. This can be accomplished by avoiding the Trendelenburg position and using large ETTs when possible. Interscalene blocks, which can result in short-term ipsilateral diaphragmatic paralysis, should be avoided. Higher peak pressures may occur with positive-pressure ventilation and are expected. Adequate ventilation during laparoscopic surgery may not be possible and hypercarbia may develop. If not excessive, it can be tolerated until the end of the procedure. Strictest extubation criteria should be observed in this population, because their heavy reliance on diaphragmatic function increases their risk of postoperative respiratory insufficiency and emergent reintubation carries a significant risk of morbidity and failure.

Kyphosis and Scoliosis

Scoliosis is a lateral and rotational deformity of the spine that also results in deformity of the rib cage. Kyphosis is an exaggerated anterior flexion of the spine resulting in a rounded or hunchbacked appearance. These disorders are frequently seen together and are referred to as kyphoscoliosis. The vast majority of cases can be classified as idiopathic, congenital, or neuromuscular. The idiopathic form is the most common and is more likely to occur in women than men. Corrective surgery is performed for scoliosis when spine angulation, also known as the Cobb angle, exceeds 50% in the thoracic or 40% in the lumbar spine.[67]

Preoperative assessment should focus on any cardiovascular, respiratory, or neurologic impairment related to the deformity. The frequent presence of restrictive lung disease is the result of a narrowed chest cavity. Although patient history will provide significant insight into the level of disability, PFTs and ABG analysis are crucial in evaluating the extent of restriction and hypoxemia. This information will guide decisions regarding postoperative ventilatory support. PFTs are likely to demonstrate a reduced vital capacity and total lung capacity, as well as a normal residual volume. Hypoxemia results from ventilation-perfusion inequality. Patients may also hypoventilate. Cor pulmonale resulting from chronic hypoxemia and pulmonary hypertension may be present in advanced cases. These concerns make electrocardiography, echocardiography, and, in some situations, an exercise stress test reasonable components of preoperative testing. A history and physical examination is sufficient to evaluate the patient's neurologic status. It is important to document any preexisting neurologic deficits so as to differentiate between baseline deficits and those resulting from surgery. This is also helpful in minimizing further injury secondary to positioning or airway management. Corrective spine surgery is the procedure that is most likely to bring these patients to the operating room. There are many variations to such procedures, including anterior, posterior, and combined approaches, as well as lumbar and/or thoracic level repairs. A combined anterior and posterior approach under a single anesthetic has a higher rate of major complications when compared with a staged procedure and is best avoided if at all possible.[68] Many elements of the anesthetic plan, such as positioning and the need for one-lung ventilation, will be dictated by the specific procedure.

Despite differences in the types of spine surgery there are several concerns that apply to all. These procedures frequently involve significant blood loss, possible one-lung ventilation, and the need for deliberate hypotension. The patients have underlying pulmonary restrictive disease. All of these factors make arterial line placement and ABG analysis critical to effective perioperative management. The presence of restrictive lung disease combined with prone or lateral positioning can make oxygenation and ventilation with acceptable peak airway pressures challenging. The use of an anesthesia machine or ventilator capable of pressure control ventilation may be helpful. Based on the level of preoperative disability, the need for postoperative ventilation should be discussed with the patient and family. Of note, adequate oxygenation during one-lung ventilation for anterior thoracic approaches may be difficult. Placement of a double-lumen ETT instead of a bronchial blocker offers the advantage of delivering passive oxygenation to the nonventilated lung. However, such tubes have a disadvantage, which is the need to switch to a single-lumen ETT at the end of the procedure if postoperative ventilation is required. Improvement in the patient's pulmonary function does not occur immediately after surgery, and if any improvement does occur it may take a few months to several years depending on the procedure.[69] Large-bore venous access, central or otherwise, is needed to ensure rapid replacement of intraoperative blood loss. Central venous pressure monitoring is of limited usefulness in these procedures owing to the effects of positioning on the values obtained and to the possible presence of pulmonary hypertension and cor pulmonale, which reduces the value of central venous pressure monitoring in determining the adequacy of intravascular volume. Transesophageal echocardiography is a reasonable choice to monitor intravascular volume status and cardiac contractility if the patient's position allows and if it is available.

Spinal cord monitoring such as somatosensory evoked potentials (SSEPs) and, to a lesser extent, motor evoked potentials (MEPs) are frequently utilized to detect direct trauma or vascular compromise to the spinal cord. Data obtained by transesophageal echocardiography and $S\overline{v}O_2$ monitoring suggest that spinal cord ischemia that results from distraction of the spine is the result of both direct compression of the spinal cord as well as decreased cardiac output and blood pressure caused by compression of vena cava or the heart.[70] Intraoperative neurologic monitoring has become the standard of care for procedures involving significant distraction of the spine. Patient temperature, pH, and adequate blood pressure must all be maintained within narrow limits to maximize the effectiveness of SSEP monitoring. There is a great deal of debate regarding which anesthetic agents are preferred when SSEP monitoring is used. The literature is frequently contradictory, and institutional preferences vary greatly, although propofol infusions and nitrous oxide are popular. It does appear that the single most important factor is administration of a stable anesthetic with minimal bolus dosing and close communication with the individual monitoring the evoked potentials. The use of MEP monitoring would clearly prevent the use of neuromuscular blockade during the procedure.

DRUG-INDUCED LUNG INJURY

Bleomycin Toxicity

Bleomycin is an antineoplastic antibiotic used in combination chemotherapy for a number of malignancies, including Hodgkin's lymphoma, Wilms' tumor, and testicular cancer. Although effective in treating bacterial and fungal infections, it is not used for these purposes because of its cytotoxicity. The appeal of utilizing bleomycin in combination chemotherapy protocols is that it does not have a myelosuppressive effect. This avoids adding to the bone marrow toxicity common to other antineoplastic agents. Unfortunately, bleomycin carries the risk of inducing pulmonary toxicity, which can result in pulmonary fibrosis and can be life threatening. The risk of a patient developing pulmonary toxicity due to bleomycin therapy appears to be related to several factors. Total dose received has been shown to relate to the extent

of pulmonary toxicity in animals, but this relationship is less clear in humans and there is no consensus on a cumulative dose that acts as a threshold for increased risk, although more than 300,000 IU has been suggested.[71] Some studies have suggested intravascular administration as a risk factor when compared with intramuscular dosing.[72] Chest irradiation in conjunction with bleomycin therapy appears to increase the risk of bleomycin-induced pulmonary fibrosis, as does advanced age, a history of smoking, and treatment with other chemotherapeutic agents that have pulmonary toxicities, such as busulfan, carmustine, semustine, and lomustine. Impaired renal function increases the risk of toxicity by reducing the elimination of bleomycin from the body.

Pulmonary toxicity due to bleomycin results in pulmonary fibrosis, similar to what is seen in IPF. Patients will usually present with a nonproductive cough accompanied by dyspnea. Chest radiographs initially reveal bibasilar infiltrates, but as the process continues the radiograph will take on a "honeycomb lung" appearance. PFTs will have a restrictive pattern in symptomatic patients but are of little predictive value in asymptomatic patients who have been exposed to bleomycin.

When evaluating a patient for anesthesia who has received bleomycin, focused questioning regarding their pulmonary function, presence of symptoms such as a dry cough, dyspnea, or decreased exercise tolerance, and presence of risk factors such as large cumulative dose, chest radiation, or smoking is essential. If the patient denies symptoms, chest radiographs, PFTs, and ABG analysis are not likely to be useful. Symptomatic patients require testing to quantify their disability, plan appropriate perioperative care, and determine the need for postoperative ventilatory support.

A landmark study by Goldiner and colleagues has guided the anesthetic management of bleomycin patients for 25 years. This study implicated hyperoxia and fluid overload as factors that increase the risk of perioperative pulmonary morbidity and mortality in patients who have received bleomycin in the past.[73] Although there have been subsequent studies that question these guidelines, there is no reason to believe that providing a higher FIO_2 than what is needed to maintain adequate oxygenation is of any benefit to these patients. The one exception to this is during preoxygenation, which is relatively brief, before induction of general anesthesia.[72] In cases in which adequate oxygenation does require an FIO_2 greater than 30%, the use of PEEP is advisable, because it may facilitate oxygen action without necessitating higher levels of FIO_2. Fluid therapy should be conservative, with the goal of maintaining adequate intravascular volume and avoiding excess fluid administration. There is no evidence to support the use of colloid instead of crystalloid in this population. For operations in which significant blood loss or significant fluid shifts are expected, intra-arterial and central venous catheters are recommended. There is no clear answer as to how long after completion of therapy with bleomycin a patient continues to be at risk for pulmonary fibrosis, although minimizing FIO_2 for an interval of 1 to 2 years would seem prudent.

In patients with documented pulmonary bleomycin toxicity, higher than normal peak pressures are expected with positive-pressure ventilation, although this may be necessary for adequate oxygenation and ventilation. Strict extubation criteria should be observed, because the patients are at increased risk of postoperative pulmonary complications; and the use of sedating medications, which decrease respiratory effort, should be minimized postoperatively. If the surgery permits, the use of regional techniques with minimal sedation and opioids may be helpful. Good postoperative pulmonary toilet, including deep breathing and coughing, must be encouraged in an attempt to minimize the occurrence of postoperative pulmonary complications.

INFECTIOUS DISEASES

Severe Acute Respiratory Syndrome (SARS)

Severe acute respiratory syndrome (SARS) is a highly infectious disease thought to be transmitted by a coronavirus (SARS-CoV). It results in atypical pneumonia, which may progress to respiratory distress syndrome. Recognition of this syndrome occurred in 2002, with the initial cases occurring in Southeast Asia. During 2003 SARS had made its way to North America, with hundreds of cases occurring in the Ontario province of Canada. All told there were over 8000 reported cases of SARS worldwide, resulting in over 700 deaths. There is no way of knowing if, when, or where another outbreak may occur, but familiarity with the syndrome and how to contain the spread is the responsibility of all health care professionals.

SARS is capable of infecting otherwise healthy individuals by contact or droplet spread, which may be person to person or indirectly through contact with contaminated surfaces, because the coronavirus can live in the environment for 24 to 48 hours. The virus enters the body through mucosal surfaces in the respiratory tract and eyes. The incubation period is 2 to 7 days. Presenting symptoms are vague and include high fever, dry cough, malaise, myalgia, and shortness of breath, which typically progresses to pneumonia and in severe cases to ventilator-dependent respiratory distress syndrome. Diagnosis is based on clinical and epidemiologic data, because there is no laboratory test available to reliably detect infection early in the clinical course.[74] Treatment of infected patients is primarily supportive and similar to that of any other atypical pneumonia. None of the currently available antiviral drugs has been shown to be effective against SARS-CoV.

The majority of the anesthesiologist's contact with SARS patients will occur during airway management for patients in respiratory distress. Because the anesthesiologist will be in close proximity to the patient's upper airway, there is a high risk of exposure to the virus. Full contact precautions, including wearing disposable fluid-resistant gowns, goggles, face shields, double gloving, hand washing, and use of N95 (or equivalent) masks that have been fit tested, are advised.[75] Standard surgical face masks and gowns are completely inadequate. It is just as important to wear correct protective equipment as it is to remove and dispose of it in a way that will not contaminate the wearer or others. Some institutions have taken the added precaution of using personal protection systems (PPS) for personnel involved in high-risk procedures with SARS patients. These PPS units consist of belt-mounted powered air purifiers with HEPA filters and a lightweight headpiece. Use of this equipment requires training as well as adequate time to put it on. The noise generated by the system makes communication difficult.[75,76] Attention must also be directed to avoiding contamination of anesthesia workstations and equipment. This includes placing high-efficiency filters on the inspiratory and expiratory limbs of ventilators and anesthesia machines. Providers must be mindful of everything they touch or that comes into contact with the patient and have these materials appropriately cleaned or disposed of. Maintaining a separate clean and a separate dirty work area may be helpful in this regard.[76]

Echinococcal Disease of the Lung

Echinococcal or hydatid disease occurs when a human is infected with *Echinococcus granulosus,* which is a canine tapeworm. The eggs of the worm are passed in the feces of infested dogs. Humans acquire the infection by unintentionally ingesting the eggs. Larvae then migrate to the liver, with some eventually arriving in the lungs and other tissues. The parasites then mature to form hydatid cysts. The lung forms a protective granulomatous layer around the cyst, which over time becomes fibrotic. It is estimated that hydatid cysts grow 1 to 2 cm a year.[77] Due to the fecal-oral transmission, this disease is more common in children than adults. Overall it is rare in North America but common in other parts of the world. These cysts are frequently asymptomatic, and pulmonary cysts are often detected on routine chest radiographs. The most likely symptoms are cough, dyspnea, or chest pain. Rupture of a cyst can occur spontaneously or on surgical manipulation. This may result in an anaphylactic reaction or spread the disease to other organs. For this reason transthoracic needle aspiration should never be attempted. Chest radiographs will reveal a cystic lesion, which may be rather large, accompanied by an area of pneumonitis or atelectasis. There is no effective medical treatment for hydatid cyst of the lung, and surgical removal is the preferred therapeutic option.

Patients with small asymptomatic cysts do not require any preoperative evaluations beyond the routine. Larger cysts may result in respiratory compromise, typically presenting as dyspnea. Spirometry may reveal decreased volumes due to the space-occupying lesion. Respiratory acidosis and hypoxemia may also be present. In advanced disease, there is the possibility that the patient may not tolerate surgery and anesthesia. In these very rare circumstances, removal of the cyst has been performed under thoracic epidural anesthesia with success.[78] For patients considered reasonable candidates for general anesthesia, one-lung ventilation may be requested to optimize surgical exposure for resection of the cyst. Isolation of the contralateral lung field has the added benefit of decreasing the risk of contamination should the cyst rupture during surgery. In cases in which there is only unilateral disease, there is little reason for the patient to have difficulty tolerating one-lung ventilation, as the unaffected side is primarily responsible for gas exchange if the cyst is clinically significant. An arterial catheter is appropriate when one-lung ventilation is planned. Close communication between surgeon and anesthesiologist during drainage and delivery of the cyst is essential to avoid spillage. In the event of contamination, anaphylaxis may occur and the anesthesiologist should be prepared for this by having large-bore intravenous access, as well as immediate availability of epinephrine, diphenhydramine, and corticosteroids.

CONCLUSION

We have reviewed a heterogeneous panoply of rare pulmonary conditions. Clinical interactions with patients with these disorders may range from a simple excisional biopsy in a patient with asymptomatic pulmonary sarcoid, to a hip replacement in a patient with ankylosing spondylitis, to a double-lung transplant for a patient with end-stage cystic fibrosis. The spectrum of possible procedures therefore extends from the routine to the extraordinarily complicated. Successful management of patients with these disorders is often challenging in both the conceptual and technical realms. An understanding of the pathophysiology and treatment of the uncommon pulmonary disorder will allow the anesthesiologist to anticipate likely clinical problems and tailor anesthetic management to minimize the chance of intraoperative and postoperative complications.

References

1. Lawrence VA, Dhanda R, Hilsenbeck SG, Page CP: Risk of pulmonary complications after elective abdominal surgery. Chest 1996;110: 744-750.

2. Ferguson MK: Preoperative assessment of pulmonary risk. Chest 1999;115(5 Suppl):58S-63S.

3. Passannante AN, Rock P: When should pulmonary function tests be performed preoperatively? In Fleisher LA: Evidence-Based Practice of Anesthesiology. Philadelphia, WB Saunders, 2004.

4. Rock P, Passannante AN: Assessment: Pulmonary. Anesthesiol Clin North Am 2004;22:77-91.

5. Wightman JA: A prospective survey of the incidence of postoperative pulmonary complications. Br J Surg 1968;55:85-91.

6. Celli BR: What is the value of preoperative pulmonary function testing? Med Clin North Am 1993;77:309-325.

7. Stock MC, Downs JB, Gauer PK, et al: Prevention of postoperative pulmonary complications with CPAP, incentive spirometry, and conservative therapy. Chest 1985;87:151-157.

8. Dines DE, Arms RA, Bernatz PE, Gomes MR: Pulmonary arteriovenous fistulas. Mayo Clin Proc 1974;49:460-465.

9. Litzler PY, Douvrin F, Bouchart F, et al: Combined endovascular and video-assisted thoracoscopic procedure for treatment of a ruptured pulmonary arteriovenous fistula: Case report and review of the literature. J Thorac Cardiovasc Surg 2003;126:1204-1207.

10. Lake CL: Anesthesia and Wegener's granulomatosis: Case report and review of the literature. Anesth Analg 1978;57:353-359.

11. Pietra GG, Salhany KE: Lymphoproliferative disorders. In Fishman AP, et al (eds): Fishman's Pulmonary Diseases and Disorders. New York, McGraw-Hill, 1998, pp 1870-1872.

12. Katzenstein AL, Carrington CB, Liebow AA: Lymphomatoid granulomatosis: A clinicopathologic study of 152 cases. Cancer 1979;43:360-373.

13. Masi AT, Hunder GG, Lie JT, et al: The American College of Rheumatology 1990 criteria for the classification of Churg-Strauss syndrome (allergic granulomatosis and angiitis). Arthritis Rheum 1990;33:1094-1100.

14. Blaise G, Langleben D, Hubert B: Pulmonary arterial hypertension: Pathophysiology and anesthetic approach. Anesthesiology 2003;99:1415-1432.

15. Fischer LG, Van Aken H, Burkle H: Management of pulmonary hypertension: Physiological and pharmacological considerations for anesthesiologists. Anesth Analg 2003;96:1603-1616.

16. Kwak YL, Lee CS, Park YH, Hong YW: The effect of phenylephrine and norepinephrine in patients with chronic pulmonary hypertension. Anaesthesia 2002;57:9-14.

17. Gibson RL, Burns JL, Ramsey BW: Pathophysiology and management of pulmonary infections in cystic fibrosis. Am J Respir Crit Care Med 2003;168:918-951.

18. Flume PA: Pneumothorax in cystic fibrosis. Chest 2003;123:217-221.

19. Bright-Thomas RJ, Webb AK: The heart in cystic fibrosis. J R Soc Med, 2002;95(Suppl 41):2-10.

20. Scott RB, O'Loughlin EV, Gall DG: Gastroesophageal reflux in patients with cystic fibrosis. J Pediatr 1985;106:223-227.

21. Epler GR: Bronchiolitis obliterans organizing pneumonia. Arch Intern Med 2001;161(2):158-164.

22. Calabrese F, Giacometti C, Rea F, et al: Recurrence of idiopathic pulmonary hemosiderosis in a young adult patient after bilateral single-lung transplantation. Transplantation 2002;74:1643-1645.

23. Carrington CB, Addington WW, Goff AM, et al: Chronic eosinophilic pneumonia. N Engl J Med 1969;280:787-798.

24. Marchand E, Etienne-Mastroianni B, Chanez P, et al: Idiopathic chronic eosinophilic pneumonia and asthma: How do they influence each other? Eur Respir J 2003;22:8-13.

25. Turner AN, Rees AJ: Goodpasture's disease and Alport's syndrome. Annu Rev Med 1996;47:377-386.

26. Kelly PT, Haponik EF: Goodpasture syndrome: Molecular and clinical advances. Medicine (Baltimore) 1994;73:171-185.

27. Ewan PW, Jones HA, Rhodes CG, Hughes JM: Detection of intrapulmonary hemorrhage with carbon monoxide uptake: Application in Goodpasture's syndrome. N Engl J Med 1976;295: 1391-1396.

28. Nogee LM, de Mello DE, Dehner LP, Colten HR: Brief report: Deficiency of pulmonary surfactant protein B in congenital alveolar proteinosis. N Engl J Med 1993;328:406-410.

29. Trapnell BC, Whitsett JA, Nakata K: Pulmonary alveolar proteinosis. N Engl J Med 2003;349:2527-2539.
30. Mazzone P, Thomassen MJ, Kavuru M: Our new understanding of pulmonary alveolar proteinosis: What an internist needs to know. Cleve Clin J Med 2001;68:977-978, 981-982, 984-985 passim.
31. Cheng SL, Chang HT, Lau HP, et al: Pulmonary alveolar proteinosis: Treatment by bronchofiberscopic lobar lavage. Chest 2002;122: 1480-1485.
32. Swenson JD, Astle KL, Bailey PL: Reduction in left ventricular filling during bronchopulmonary lavage demonstrated by transesophageal echocardiography. Anesth Analg 1995;81: 634-637.
33. Shammas RL, Movahed A: Sarcoidosis of the heart. Clin Cardiol 1993;16:462-472.
34. Heck AW, Phillips LH 2nd: Sarcoidosis and the nervous system. Neurol Clin 1989;7:641-654.
35. Wills MH, Harris MM: An unusual airway complication with sarcoidosis. Anesthesiology 1987;66:554-555.
36. Neel HB 3rd, McDonald TJ: Laryngeal sarcoidosis: Report of 13 patients. Ann Otol Rhinol Laryngol 1982;91(4 pt 1): 359-362.
37. Jaffe R, Bogomolski-Yahalom V, Kramer MR: Vocal cord paralysis as the presenting symptom of sarcoidosis. Respir Med 1994;88: 633-636.
38. Euliano TY, White SE, Aleixo L: Sarcoidosis in a pregnant woman. J Clin Anesth 1997;9:78-86.
39. Mills JA: Systemic lupus erythematosus. N Engl J Med 1994;330: 1871-1879.
40. Menon G, Allt-Graham J: Anaesthetic implications of the anti-cardiolipin antibody syndrome. Br J Anaesth 1993;70:587-590.
41. Glueck HI, Kant KS, Weiss MA, et al: Thrombosis in systemic lupus erythematosus: Relation to the presence of circulating anticoagulants. Arch Intern Med 1985;145:1389-1395.
42. Orens JB, Martinez FJ, Lynch JP 3rd: Pleuropulmonary manifestations of systemic lupus erythematosus. Rheum Dis Clin North Am 1994;20:159-193.
43. Chick TW, DeHoratius RJ, Skipper BE, Messner RP: Pulmonary dysfunction in systemic lupus erythematosus without pulmonary symptoms. J Rheumatol 1976;3:262-268.
44. American Thoracic Society: Idiopathic pulmonary fibrosis: Diagnosis and treatment. International consensus statement. American Thoracic Society (ATS), and the European Respiratory Society (ERS). Am J Respir Crit Care Med 2000;161(2 pt 1):646-664.
45. Fujimoto T, Okazaki T, Matsukura T, et al: Operation for lung cancer in patients with idiopathic pulmonary fibrosis: Surgical contraindication? Ann Thorac Surg 2003;76:1674-1678; discussion 1679.
46. Selman M, Thannickal VJ, Pardo A, et al: Idiopathic pulmonary fibrosis: Pathogenesis and therapeutic approaches. Drugs 2004;64: 405-430.
47. Thabut G, Mal H, Castier Y, et al: Survival benefit of lung transplantation for patients with idiopathic pulmonary fibrosis. J Thorac Cardiovasc Surg 2003;126:469-475.
48. Raghu G: The role of gastroesophageal reflux in idiopathic pulmonary fibrosis. Am J Med 2003;115(Suppl 3A):60S-64S.
49. Goss CH, Brower RG, Hudson LD, Rubenfeld GD: Incidence of acute lung injury in the United States. Crit Care Med 2003;31: 1607-1611.
50. Bernard GR, Artigas A, Brigham KL, et al: The American-European Consensus Conference on ARDS: Definitions, mechanisms, relevant outcomes, and clinical trial coordination. Am J Respir Crit Care Med 1994;149(3 pt 1):818-824.
51. Herridge MS, Cheung AM, Tansey CM, et al: One-year outcomes in survivors of the acute respiratory distress syndrome. N Engl J Med 2003;348:683-693.
52. Ventilation with lower tidal volumes as compared with traditional tidal volumes for acute lung injury and the acute respiratory distress syndrome. The Acute Respiratory Distress Syndrome Network. N Engl J Med 2000;342:1301-1308.
53. Moloney ED, Griffiths MJ: Protective ventilation of patients with acute respiratory distress syndrome. Br J Anaesth 2004;92: 261-270.
54. Brower RG, Lanken PN, MacIntyre N, et al: Higher versus lower positive end-expiratory pressures in patients with the acute respiratory distress syndrome. N Engl J Med 2004;351: 327-336.
55. Fartoukh M, Humbert M, Capron F, et al: Severe pulmonary hypertension in histiocytosis X. Am J Respir Crit Care Med 2000;161:216-223.
56. Delobbe A, Durieu J, Duhamel A, Wallaert B: Determinants of survival in pulmonary Langerhans' cell granulomatosis (histiocytosis X). Groupe d'Etude en Pathologie Interstitielle de la Societe de Pathologie Thoracique du Nord. Eur Respir J 1996;9: 2002-2006.
57. Etienne B, Bertocchi M, Gamondes JP, et al: Relapsing pulmonary Langerhans cell histiocytosis after lung transplantation. Am J Respir Crit Care Med 1998;157:288-291.
58. Carrington CB, Cugell DW, Gaensler EA, et al: Lymphangioleiomyomatosis: Physiologic-pathologic-radiologic correlations. Am Rev Respir Dis 1977;116:977-995.
59. Corrin B, Liebow AA, Friedman PJ: Pulmonary lymphangiomyomatosis: A review. Am J Pathol 1975;79: 348-382.
60. Boehler A, Speich R, Russi EW, Weder W: Lung transplantation for lymphangioleiomyomatosis. N Engl J Med 1996;335: 1275-1280.
61. Rosenow E, Strimlan CV, Muhm JR, Ferguson RH: Pleuropulmonary manifestations of ankylosing spondylitis. Mayo Clin Proc 1977;52: 641-649.
62. Carter R, Riantawan P, Banham SW, Sturrock RD: An investigation of factors limiting aerobic capacity in patients with ankylosing spondylitis. Respir Med 1999;93:700-708.
63. Grimby G, Fugl-Meyer AR, Blomstrand A: Partitioning of the contributions of rib cage and abdomen to ventilation in ankylosing spondylitis. Thorax 1974;29:179-184.
64. Ramos-Remus C, Gomez-Vargas A, Guzman-Guzman JL, et al: Frequency of atlantoaxial subluxation and neurologic involvement in patients with ankylosing spondylitis. J Rheumatol 1995;22: 2120-2125.
65. Kumar CM, Mehta M: Ankylosing spondylitis: Lateral approach to spinal anaesthesia for lower limb surgery. Can J Anaesth 1995;42: 73-76.
66. DeBoard JW, Ghia JN, Guilford WB: Caudal anesthesia in a patient with ankylosing spondylitis for hip surgery. Anesthesiology 1981;54:164-166.
67. Winkler M, Marker E, Hetz H: The peri-operative management of major orthopaedic procedures. Anaesthesia 1998;53(Suppl 2): 37-41.
68. McDonnell MF, Glassman SD, Dimar JR 2nd, et al: Perioperative complications of anterior procedures on the spine. J Bone Joint Surg Am 1996;78:839-847.
69. Raw DA, Beattie JK, Hunter JM: Anaesthesia for spinal surgery in adults. Br J Anaesth 2003;91:886-904.
70. Bernard JM, Le Penven-Henninger C, Passuti N: Sudden decreases in mixed venous oxygen saturation during posterior spinal fusion. Anesth Analg 1995;80:1038-1041.
71. O'Sullivan JM, Huddart RA, Norman AR, et al: Predicting the risk of bleomycin lung toxicity in patients with germ-cell tumours. Ann Oncol 2003;14:91-96.
72. Waid-Jones MI, Coursin DB: Perioperative considerations for patients treated with bleomycin. Chest 1991;99:993-999.

73. Goldiner PL, Carlon GC, Cvitkovic E, et al: Factors influencing postoperative morbidity and mortality in patients treated with bleomycin. BMJ 1978;1: 1664-1667.

74. Centers for Disease Control and Prevention: Severe acute respiratory syndrome (SARS). Available at http://www.cdc.gov/ncidod/sars/clinicalguidance.htm, 2004.

75. Kamming D, Gardam M, Chung F: Anaesthesia and SARS. Br J Anaesth 2003;90:715-718.

76. Peng PW, Wong DT, Bevan D, Gardam M: Infection control and anesthesia: Lessons learned from the Toronto SARS outbreak. Can J Anaesth 2003;50:989-997.

77. Balikian JP, Mudarris FF: Hydatid disease of the lungs: A roentgenologic study of 50 cases. Am J Roentgenol Radium Ther Nucl Med 1974;122:692-707.

78. Dyer RA, Gordon PC, De Groot KM, et al: Excision of a giant hydatid cyst of the lung under thoracic epidural anaesthesia. Anaesth Intensive Care 2001;29:181-184.

CHAPTER

5 Liver Diseases

KEITH LITTLEWOOD, MD, and EDWARD C. NEMERGUT, MD

The liver plays a crucial role in many of the homeostatic processes of the body and, as a result, is affected by countless disease processes and physiologic abnormalities. Conversely, the dysfunctional liver can profoundly affect the function and reserve of multiple organ systems in the surgical patient. With the added complexities of perioperative stressors, a rational approach to the anesthetic management of patients with liver disease may seem a daunting task.

Fortunately, an understanding of (1) normal hepatic structure and function, (2) the acute and chronic responses of the liver to various types of injury, and (3) the behavior of the healthy or diseased liver during perioperative events allows a fairly straightforward approach to management issues. With these commonalities in mind, in the following sections we first discuss pertinent normal hepatic anatomy and physiology. Within this framework, representative individual disease processes are then examined and, finally, anesthetic management is addressed.

NORMAL HEPATIC ANATOMY

A complete review of normal liver structure and function is beyond the scope of this discussion. The intricacies of current concepts in hepatic function and disease can be found in standard reference texts.[1,2] The goal here is to concisely present aspects of hepatic anatomy and physiology with implications for perioperative care of the patient with liver disease. Points of emphasis are (1) the dual blood supply of systemic blood via the hepatic artery and portal venous blood from the splanchnic circulation; (2) histologic arrangement of hepatocytes, including the unique hepatic sinusoids and the resulting blood-hepatocyte interface; and (3) isolation of biliary and blood compartments with regulation of enterohepatic circulation.

The liver is the largest parenchymal organ in the human body, representing approximately 2% of total body weight in the adult. Blood flow to the liver is normally

100 mL/ 100 g of tissue per minute, or 25% to 30% of the resting cardiac output. The liver is well situated to many of its metabolic functions by its interposition between the splanchnic and systemic venous systems. A critical result of this arrangement, however, is that approximately 75% of the blood supply to the liver is delivered by the portal vein. This blood is partially deoxygenated as a result of oxygen extraction by the splanchnic organs. After coursing through capillary beds of the stomach, pancreas, spleen, and intestines, portal venous blood does contain high concentrations of nutrients, as well as secreted and ingested exogenous substances. Under normal circumstances this portal blood provides 35% to 50% of the oxygen delivered to the liver. The well-oxygenated blood of the hepatic artery delivers the remaining 50% to 65% of oxygen, despite representing only 25% of the liver's blood supply. Portal venous flow is dependent on the normal variations in splanchnic blood flow as regulated by the arterioles and capillary flow of the splanchnic bed. Hepatic artery blood flow demonstrates autoregulatory changes in response to blood pressure, as well as to portal blood flow and sinusoidal oxygen levels.

Understanding liver structure can be difficult because of different nomenclatures regarding both its gross and its microscopic anatomy. The liver may be thought of as comprising two major lobes, the right and left, as roughly divided by the falciform ligament. These lobes can be further subdivided into the eight segments of Couinaud (Fig. 5-1). Based conceptually on separate vascular and biliary branches, this classification belies the common "crossover" of these structures, especially hepatic veins, between segments.

From a surgical perspective, segments may be resected for the purpose of excision of pathological lesions or, more recently, living-directed donation for transplantation. When draining hepatic veins or portions of the biliary tree for remaining segments are removed, the remaining segments will be subject to venous congestion and/or biliary leakage. In the case of resection for transplantation, if nonresected tissue contains significant arterial and portal vein supply for resected tissue the latter will demonstrate areas of ischemia after transplant owing to the loss of this blood supply.

The older classic concept of the basic hepatic histologic structure is that of the hepatic lobule (Fig. 5-2). This model is that of a polygon, typically a hexagon, with branches of the portal triad (hepatic artery, portal vein,

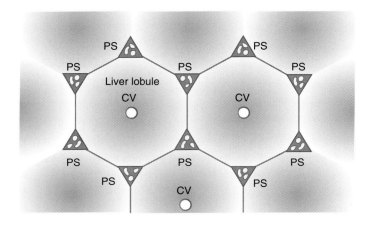

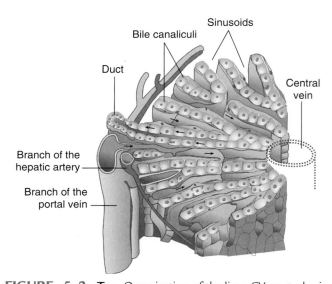

FIGURE 5-2 **Top,** Organization of the liver. CV, central vein; PS, portal space containing branches of bile duct, portal vein, and hepatic artery. **Bottom,** Arrangement of plates of liver cells, sinusoids, and bile ducts in a liver lobule, showing centripetal flow of blood in sinusoids to central vein and centrifugal flow of bile in bile canaliculi to bile ducts. *(Reproduced with permission from Ganong WF: Review of Medical Physiology, 21st ed. New York, McGraw-Hill, 2003.)*

FIGURE 5-1 Anatomic relationships of hepatic segments and their vascular structures.

and bile duct) at the vertices. A central vein (technically a venule) marks the central axis of the lobule. Mixed arterial and portal blood flows from the vessels at each vertex, via the sinusoids, to the common central vein. The sinusoids are formed by one-cell thick plates of hepatocytes and lined with endothelial cells. These sinusoids differ from normal capillaries because of the mixture of portal venous and arterial blood by which they are supplied. They also lack a basement membrane, and their endothelium has fenestrations typically ranging in size from 50 to 200 nm. These fenestrations and the low sinusoidal pressure allow a multitude of solutes, including macromolecules, to enter the perisinusoidal space of Disse. Here, molecules are in direct contact with the microvilli of the hepatocyte's basolateral membrane. There is evidence that the fenestrations are modified by contractile components along their circumference, thus offering some regulation of the movement of large molecules between the sinusoidal blood and the space of Disse. The hepatocyte also has specialized canalicular membrane portions with distinct microvilli. In combination with the adjacent hepatocyte, this specialized area forms the wall of the bile canaliculi, its isolation completed by tight intercellular junctions. Intracellular actin and myosin filaments along the canalicular channel are presumed to promote drainage of bile into the canals of Hering and subsequently into the interlobar bile ducts.

The alternative histologic perspective is the acinus model. The venule, which was considered to be central in the lobule model, is now the peripheral structure. This places the portal triad structures centrally, with concentric zones radiating out to the draining venule. The zones are numbered from 1 to 3 with progression to the vein. Conceptually, these zones reflect decreasing oxygen content in the sinusoidal blood and decreasing concentrations of nutrients (and toxins) arriving from the gut. Although less easily visualized histologically, the zones of the acinar model correlate with differential enzyme concentrations, metabolic activities, and degree of cellular damage caused by a variety of agents and situations. Figure 5-3 diagrams the perspectives and nomenclature of the lobular and acinar models.

Although hepatocytes make up about 80% of the liver, a host of other cells are found in the liver. Two of the many nonparenchymal cells of the liver deserve mention. *Kupffer cells* are members of the monocyte-phagocyte system (macrophage derived) and typically reside on the luminal aspect of sinusoidal endothelial cells. Their phagocytic and inflammatory responses are important in several of the disease processes to be discussed. *Stellate cells* (Ito cells) are found in the space of Disse and, in health, store lipids and vitamin A. In the fibrogenic response to injury, however, the stellate cells undergo transformation to fibroblasts and produce collagen, which is an early step in the "capillarization" of the sinusoids, with loss of fenestrations and

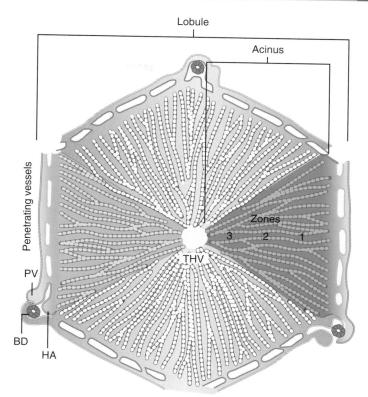

FIGURE 5–3 Microscopic liver architecture depicted schematically. The classic hexagonal lobule is centered around a central vein (terminal hepatic venule), with portal tracts at three of its apices. The triangular acinus has as its base the penetrating vessels, which extend from portal veins and hepatic arteries to penetrate the parenchyma. The apex is formed by the terminal hepatic vein. Zones 1, 2, and 3 represent metabolic regions increasingly distant from the blood supply. *(Reproduced, with permission from Crawford JM: The liver and the biliary tract. In Cotran RS, Kumar V, Collins T (eds): Robbins Pathologic Basis of Disease, 6th ed. Philadelphia, WB Saunders, 1999, p 846.)*

creation of a pseudo–basement membrane. This is believed to be a fundamental step in the development of hepatic fibrosis and cirrhosis, to be discussed below.

FUNCTIONS OF THE LIVER IN HEALTH

Carbohydrate Metabolism

The liver routinely provides the body's widely varying energy requirements under the modulation of neural and endocrine regulators. Complex interacting systems of energy storage and utilization are required to compensate for asynchronous periods of nutritional ingestion and energy demand. Figure 5-4 presents a simplified diagram of carbohydrate and lipid metabolism in the hepatocyte.

Many cells of the body are glucose dependent (e.g., erythrocytes, renal medulla, and retina) or glucose preferential (e.g., brain). Maintenance of blood glucose levels is accomplished by glycogenolysis or gluconeogenesis, depending on nutritional circumstances. Glycogenolysis,

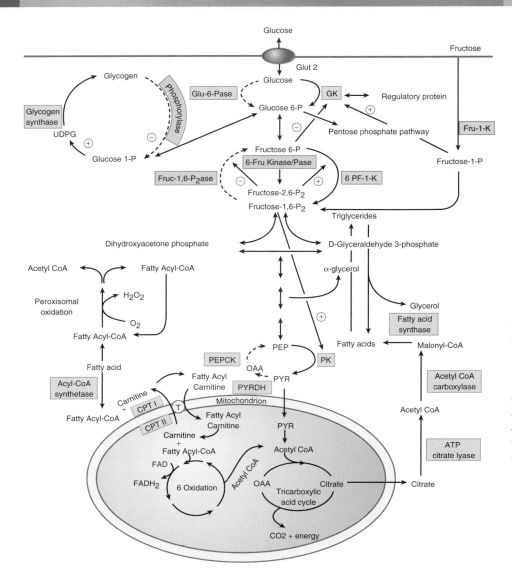

FIGURE 5–4 Hepatic carbohydrate and lipid metabolism. Gluconeogenic pathways are identified by *dashed lines*. GK, glucokinase; Glu-6-Pase, glucose-6-phosphatase; 6-Fru Kinase/Pase, 6-phosphofructo-2-kinase/fructose-2,6-bisphosphatase; Fructose 6-P, fructose-6-phosphate; 6 PF-1-K, 6-phosphofructo-1-kinase; Fruc-1,6-P2 ase, fructose-1,6-biphosphatase; PK, pyruvate kinase; PEPCK, phosphoenol pyruvate carboxykinase; CPT, carnitine palmitoyltransferase; Glut 2, glucose transporter 2; T, carnitine:acylcarnitine transferase; PEP, phosphoenol pyruvate; FAD, flavine adenine dinucleotide; PYR, pyruvate; OAA, oxaloacetate; UDPG, uridine diphosphate glucose. *(Reproduced, with permission from Stolz A: Liver physiology and metabolic function. In Feldman M, Friedman LS, Sleisenger MH (eds): Sleisenger & Fordtran's Gastrointestinal and Liver Disease, 7th ed. Philadelphia, WB Saunders, 2002, p 1204.)*

promoted by epinephrine and glucagon, is the process by which glucose is eventually released from stored glycogen. The liver and skeletal muscle contain the vast majority of the body's glycogen. Glucose-6-phosphatase in the liver is capable of converting glucose-6-phospate (cleaved from glycogen by glycogen phosphorylase) to glucose for release into the blood. Muscle, however, lacks glucose-6-phosphatase, and thus its glycogen is destined for utilization in the myocyte. Glycogen stores in the adult liver during fasting are capable of providing adequate glucose levels for 24 to 48 hours, representing 250 to 500 mg of glucose. It is interesting to note that during this period of fasting, the brain will initiate transition from glucose dependency to ketone metabolism and thus sustain itself while markedly decreasing the body's daily glucose utilization. Gluconeogenesis is the creation of glucose from lactate, pyruvate, and amino acids, themselves the

products of anaerobic and catabolic metabolism. It is stimulated with the depletion of glycogen stores.

The liver can rapidly switch from glycogen breakdown to formation, depending on the nutritional circumstances and energy requirements of the moment. This is because the enzyme systems involved in glycogen creation (glycogen synthase) and breakdown (glycogen phosphorylase) are activated and deactivated by their phosphorylation state as modulated by the presence of glucose, glucose-6-phosphate, and endocrine mediators. In this way, proglycogen and macroglycogen are immediately available as a glucose source when needed, or as a depository for storage of excess glucose.

Disruption of carbohydrate homeostasis can be a manifestation of liver dysfunction. Acute liver injury (e.g., viral hepatitis) is often associated with mild hypoglycemia despite normal or depressed insulin levels. Postulated mechanisms for this abnormality include partial depletion of glycogen reserves, decreased gluconeogenesis, ineffective glycogen repletion after dietary carbohydrate intake, and decreased glucagon promotion of glycogenolysis. Hypoglycemia can be pronounced in the alcoholic despite apparently minimal hepatic decompensation. This occurs because ethanol itself cannot be used in gluconeogenesis and, further, its metabolism can critically reduce the availability of pyruvate for gluconeogenesis. In fulminant hepatic failure of any cause, hypoglycemia can be life threatening.

Glucose intolerance, conversely, is often observed in chronic liver disease, especially cirrhosis. Although insulin levels may actually be elevated because of decreased hepatic clearance, peripheral receptors are decreased in number. Additionally, receptor binding characteristics and activity may be altered. Hepatocytes may also be isolated from the usual concentrated levels of portal pancreatic insulin release because of portosystemic shunting. Skeletal muscle in the cirrhotic patient demonstrates decreased glycogen stores and impaired uptake of glucose, thought to be an effect of increased serum free fatty acids. This decreased uptake by muscle amplifies hyperglycemia in the fed state.

The liver processes other carbohydrates, some of which will be discussed in the context of metabolic abnormalities. Fructose, which is mentioned here because of its seemingly universal presence in the modern western diet from fructose corn syrup derivatives, and the impact of fructose intolerance, is discussed later. Fructose is converted to fructose-1-phosphate (fru-1-P) in the liver, which in turn increases glucokinase activity. Fru-1-P cannot directly enter the gluconeogenic pathway, but its metabolites (glyceraldehyde-3-phosphate and dihydroxylacetone) can enter the glycolytic pathway, be converted to fructose-1, 6-P_2 for gluconeogenesis or glycolysis, or serve as glycerol building blocks for phospholipids and triglycerols. Finally, fructose is more readily incorporated into fatty acid synthesis than is glucose, having bypassed early steps and regulations of this process.

Lipid Metabolism and Transport

Fatty acids provide the most efficient energy source for both intrahepatic and extrahepatic storage and utilization. The liver's central role in lipid metabolism, beyond utilization, involves regulated conversion of excess carbohydrates to fatty acids, esterification of free fatty acids to form triglycerides for transport and storage, and synthesis of transport proteins. In normal circumstances, the liver takes up a relatively fixed amount of free (nonesterified) fatty acids regardless of dietary intake. This provides the major energy source for hepatocytes. The nutritional state determines the subsequent balance between synthesis and esterification of fatty acids in the fed state versus oxidation in the fasting state.

Hepatic steatosis ("fatty liver") refers to abnormal accumulation of predominately triglycerides with fatty acids in hepatocytes. Steatosis occurs when triglyceride production exceeds secretion into the plasma (usually after incorporation into very low density lipoproteins). Abnormalities of either production and/or secretion can thus be responsible for fatty liver. Previously defined in terms of weight percentage (greater than 5%) or number of hepatocytes affected (greater than 30% in a lobule), the diagnosis is now also grossly correlated to findings of noninvasive imaging. Some conditions associated with steatosis that are considered later include obesity, alcohol ingestion, pregnancy, nonalcoholic steatohepatitis, and certain drug toxicities.

Cholesterol is not a direct energy source but serves as a structural unit of membranes and is a precursor for steroid production. Most cholesterol is synthesized in the liver and, in combination with dietary cholesterol, is either secreted in the bile, incorporated into lipoproteins for plasma transport, or converted to bile acids. Figure 5-5 provides an overview of lipoprotein metabolism and transport.

Protein Synthesis

With the exception of immunoglobulins, the liver produces the vast majority of proteins found in plasma. These include most of the proteins of coagulation, plasma-binding proteins involved in transport (e.g., albumin, transferrin, lipoprotein, and haptoglobin), and acute phase reactants. This wide variety of proteins share many common synthetic pathways but have distinguishing characteristics of substrate, modulation, and kinetics that explain the clinically variable response to injury and disease. For example, those clotting factors dependent on vitamin K for post-translational modification can be affected by its nutritional intake or absorption, while inflammatory mediators stimulate acute-phase reactants. Serum albumin levels reflect not only production from available amino acids but also volume of distribution, abnormal losses (e.g., ascites, pleural effusion, or proteinuria), and regulators responding to parameters such as serum oncotic pressure. Those altered protein levels, which are actually reflections of liver disease, will develop after variable periods, dependent on the synthetic rates and plasma half-times of the particular proteins.

Thus, although it is generally true that serum protein levels will be decreased with liver dysfunction, the specific laboratory abnormality and time frame (i.e., hours or days in the case of coagulation factors versus weeks in the case of albumin) are important diagnostic clues in liver disease.

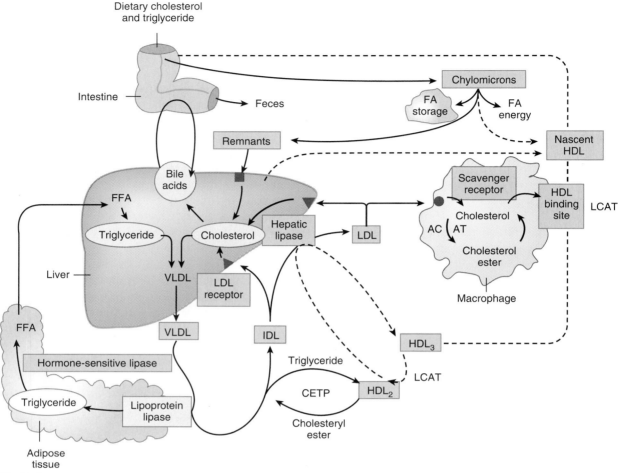

FIGURE 5–5 Lipoprotein metabolism. FFA, free fatty acids; ACAT, acylcholesterol acyltransferase; CETP, cholesteryl ester transfer protein; LCAT, lecithin-cholesterol acyltransferase; FA, fatty acids; LDL, low-density lipoproteins; HDL, high-density lipoproteins; VLDL, very-low-density lipoproteins. *(Reproduced, with permission from Stolz A: Liver physiology and metabolic function. In Feldman M, Friedman LS, Sleisenger MH (eds): Sleisenger & Fordtran's Gastrointestinal and Liver Disease, 7th ed. Philadelphia, WB Saunders, 2002, p 1211.)*

Detoxification and Transformation

The liver is the major site in which both xenobiotics and endogenous substances undergo detoxification and/or transformation. These changes usually generate less active and more hydrophilic compounds. There are notable exceptions in which transformation actually renders substances toxic. This is discussed in the section on hepatotoxins that follows. The pathways involved are categorized into three phases. Phase 1 metabolism alters the molecule by reactions (usually involving the cytochrome P450 enzyme system) such as oxidation, reduction, and hydrolysis. Phase 2 metabolism conjugates the parent molecule or its metabolite with a polar molecule such as acetate, amino acid, sulfate, or glutathione, and thus further enhances water solubility. The more recently defined phase 3 elimination is an energy-dependent excretion. A particular molecule may undergo any or all of these processes. Changes in the pathway(s) utilized may occur as dictated by substrate concentrations, enzyme induction, disease, and nutritional status.

Bilirubin Metabolism

Bilirubin is a tetrapyrrole produced from the breakdown of heme at the rate of about 250 mg/day in the normal adult. About two thirds comes from hemoglobin of senescent erythrocytes processed by the reticuloendothelial system, and the remainder mostly from non-hemoglobin hemoproteins such as cytochrome P450 enzymes. The turnover of myoglobin is slow enough that its substantial hemoprotein content does not contribute significantly to bilirubin production. Heme is first converted to biliverdin by heme oxygenase and then to bilirubin by biliverdin reductase. This unconjugated bilirubin, which is water insoluble and neurotoxic at sufficiently high levels, is bound to albumin and transported to the hepatocyte.

Here it is conjugated with glucuronic acid by uridine diphosphatase-glucuronyl-transferase to form bilirubin monoglucuronide and diglucuronide. After secretion into canaliculi, bilirubin is incorporated into bile and remains unchanged through the gallbladder and most of the small intestine. In the terminal ileum and colon, hydrolysis by bacterial enzymes produces urobilinogen, which is reabsorbed, and re-excreted predominately in bile with a small fraction filtered by the kidney into the urine.

THE INJURED LIVER

Cellular Responses in Injury and Disease

As mentioned earlier, the liver can suffer injury from a variety of processes, both primary to the organ (e.g., viral hepatitis) and secondary (e.g., right-sided heart failure or metastatic cancer). Regardless of the multitude of causes, however, a few general categories of cellular consequences are typically observed.

Hepatitis is simply liver injury associated with the incursion of inflammatory cells. Depending on the type of hepatitis, hepatocyte injury may stimulate the inflammatory response (e.g., toxic injury) or be secondary to it.

Degeneration is defined in terms of microscopic findings. Foamy degeneration occurs with ineffective biliary excretion, whereas ballooning degeneration is found in toxic and immunologically mediated injury. Steatosis specifically represents accumulation of fat droplets in the cell. Multiple small accumulations are seen in microvesicular steatosis (as seen in the acute fatty liver of pregnancy), whereas macrovesicular steatosis is defined as a large nucleus-displacing droplet (as seen in obese and diabetic patients).

Necrosis can occur after a variety of injuries. Necrosis demonstrates poorly stained cells with lysed nuclei, frequently exhibiting zonal distributions. Centrilobular necrosis is a common pattern in which the most severe damage immediately surrounds the central vein. This is characteristic of toxins and ischemic injury, the latter presumably reflecting the decreasing oxygen content of the sinusoidal blood as it flows to the terminal venule, whereas the toxic pattern may reflect not only relative hypoxia but also regions of high metabolic activity and biotransformation. Periportal necrosis, conversely, is exceedingly unusual but may be found in preeclamptic patients for unknown reasons. With most injuries, a variety of necrotic and inflammatory patterns are seen. Focal necrosis denotes scattered necrosis within lobules, whereas more severe bridging necrosis spans adjacent lobules. More severe still are submassive necrosis and massive necrosis in which entire lobules or most of the liver are affected, respectively. *Apoptosis,* the energy-dependent deconstruction of cells with an attenuated inflammatory response and salvage of cell components that can be reutilized,

will not be discussed here. The conditions and regulators that influence apoptosis in the liver are being elucidated.[3,4] Whether the balance between necrosis and apoptosis can be predicted or even manipulated clinically remains to be seen.

Regeneration and *fibrosis* represent two different outcomes in the liver's attempt to replace lost or extinct liver units. The liver, since at least the ancient Greek myth of Prometheus, has a deserved reputation for its unparalleled ability to regenerate. When its connective tissue framework is left intact the liver can, as demonstrated in living directed liver donors and recipients, actually re-form itself from less than half of its original size. Similarly, the liver that has suffered submassive and even massive necrosis may subsequently recover essentially normal structure, except for minor abnormalities of bile ductules and parenchymal arrangement. Stimulating factors thus far identified in the human include epidermal growth factor, transforming growth factor, and hepatocyte growth factor.

Fibrosis is a very different consequence of injury response. It is generally irreversible and will compromise function to at least some extent. Fibrosis results from the deposition of collagen within the space of Disse, around portal tracts, or around the central vein by transformed stellate cells (see previous description of anatomy). Previously healthy hepatocytes are eventually replaced with connective tissue. *Cirrhosis* is the term applied to nodules of regenerating hepatocytes within such scar tissue, reflecting the impact of disruption of the normal connective framework before or during regeneration. This architectural disruption results in increased resistance to hepatic blood flow with eventual portal hypertension and decreased functional mass with impairment of metabolic and excretory function. Box 5-1 outlines causes of hepatic fibrosis and cirrhosis with representative causes. Obviously, cirrhosis and fibrosis represent the consequences of a wide range of diseases. In the western world, about 90% of cirrhosis of known etiology is related to alcoholic liver disease, viral hepatitis, or biliary disease. Approximately 10% of cases are of unknown etiology and termed *cryptogenic cirrhosis.*

Laboratory Manifestations of Hepatobiliary Dysfunction

The multiple functions of the liver and its vulnerability to a variety of extrahepatic abnormalities have already been emphasized and are relevant to the discussion of laboratory evaluation. Most commonly used tests have significant limitations of sensitivity and specificity and are capable of assessing very narrow aspects of hepatic function. The concept of a single test or even a panel of tests that represent a measure of hepatic reserve or "liver function tests" is therefore flawed. Different patterns of abnormalities do, however, often correlate with the instigating clinical presentation and allow further targeted investigation.

BOX 5–1   Etiologies of Hepatic Fibrosis and Cirrhosis

Medications	Chronic hepatitis (B, C, and D)	Hereditary tyrosinemia
α-Methyldopa	Cytomegalovirus	Ornithine transcarbamylase
Amiodarone	Echinococcosis	Porphyrias
Isoniazid	Schistosomiasis	Tyrosinosis
Methotrexate	Syphilis (tertiary and congenital)	Wilson's disease
Nitrofurantoin	Metabolic and genetic disorders	Wolman's disease
Oral contraceptives	α₁-Antitrypsin deficiency	Autoimmune chronic hepatitis
Sulfa antibiotics	Abetalipoproteinemia	Biliary obstruction (chronic)
Vitamin A	Alagille syndrome	Budd-Chiari syndrome (including
Toxins	Biliary atresia	Veno-occlusive subset)
Alcohol	Familial intrahepatic cholestasis	Cystic fibrosis
Arsenic	(Byler's disease) types 1, 2, and 3	Idiopathic portal hypertension
Carbon tetrachloride	Fanconi's syndrome	Jejunoileal bypass
Chlordecone	Fructose intolerance	Nonalcoholic steatohepatitis
Methylene diamine	Galactosemia	Primary biliary cirrhosis
Pyrrolizidine alkaloids	Gaucher's disease	Primary sclerosing cholangitis
Infection	Glycogen storage disease	Right-sided heart failure and tricuspid
Brucellosis	Hemochromatosis	regurgitation (chronic)
Capillariasis	Hereditary fructose intolerance	Sarcoidosis

Tests commonly selected to evaluate liver disease are summarized in typical pathologic patterns in Table 5-1. The tests can be broadly divided into two categories, those that reflect liver injury as opposed to those that actually depend on the function of the liver. The markers of direct injury include released hepatic enzymes. Synthetic function can be reflected in protein levels and clotting times, whereas dye clearance and drug transformation can be used to investigate blood flow and metabolic capacity.

Tests That Reflect Hepatic Clearance

Ammonia. The liver normally clears ammonia from the blood and converts it to urea for renal excretion. With severe liver dysfunction and/or portosystemic shunting, ammonia levels may be elevated. Although commonly used in the evaluation of possible hepatic encephalopathy, ammonia levels correlate poorly with the severity of clinical presentation.

TABLE 5–1   Characteristic Biochemical Markers in Liver Disease

Etiologies and Laboratory Results*	Hepatocellular Necrosis			Biliary Obstruction		Chronic Infiltration
	Toxin or Ischemia	Viral	Alcohol	Complete†	Partial	
Aminotransferases	50-100×	5-50×	2-5×	NL to 5×	NL to 5×	1-3×
Alkaline phosphatase	1-3×	1-3×	1-10×	2-20×	2-20×	NL to 20×
Bilirubin	1-5×	1-30×	1-30×	1-30×	1-5×	NL to 5×
Prothrombin time	Prolonged. Minimal or no improvement with vitamin K			Often prolonged. May improve with parenteral vitamin K		Normal
Albumin	Decreased in chronic disease			Often normal; may be decreased		Usually normal
Illustrative disorders	Shock liver, acetaminophen toxicity	Hepatitis A or B		Pancreatic Cancer	Hilar tumor, sclerosing cholangitis	Sarcoid, metastatic carcinoma

* ×, times elevation from normal; NL, normal
†Acute onset of complete biliary obstruction may result in massive elevations in aminotransferases that are transient and in the range of 20 to 50 times normal.
Modified from Davern TJ, Scharschmidt B: Biochemical liver tests. In Feldman M, Friedman LS, Sleisenger MH (eds): Sleisenger & Fordtran's Gastrointestinal and Liver Disease, 7th ed. Philadelphia, Elsevier, WB Saunders, p 1231.

Bilirubin. As discussed with normal metabolism, bilirubin is a product of heme breakdown. It exists in conjugated (water soluble) and unconjugated (lipid soluble) forms, which are reported imprecisely as the direct and indirect fractions, respectively. Serum bilirubin is usually less than 1 mg/dL and unconjugated. Elevated serum levels occur in most significant liver disease. With primary biliary cirrhosis, alcoholic hepatitis, and fulminant failure the degree of elevation correlates with prognosis. The appearance of conjugated bilirubin in the blood is thought to be from hepatocyte reflux but does not discriminate between obstructive and parenchymal causes. Other causes of elevated bilirubin include Gilbert's syndrome; increased production in situations such as hemolysis, ineffective erythropoiesis, or hematoma resorption; and inherited disorders of bilirubin transport.

Tests That Reflect Synthetic Function

Albumin. Albumin is synthesized only in the liver, typically at a rate of 100 to 200 mg/kg/day in the adult, and under normal circumstances the plasma half-life is 3 weeks. Abnormalities are poorly specific for liver disease, however, because many factors affect its production and turnover. Nutritional state, plasma osmotic pressure, and thyroid levels, for example, all affect the rate of albumin production. Increased albumin losses as seen in nephrotic syndrome, burns, and protein-wasting enteropathies also affect the balance between production and loss of albumin. Hypoalbuminemia can be helpful in assessing chronic liver disease when nonhepatic causes are excluded. Its prolonged half-life means that measured changes are slow to develop and slow to revert to normal in relation to the causative process's onset and resolution.

Prothrombin Time. Prothrombin time (PT) determinations depend on serum concentrations of fibrinogen, prothrombin, and factors V, VII, and IX, all of which are products of the liver. Furthermore, the half-life of these factors is short enough (less than 24 hours) that the PT changes rapidly. An abnormal PT can result from reduced factor synthesis (as seen in vitamin K deficiency, liver failure, and warfarin therapy) or increased factor loss (as seen in disseminated intravascular coagulation).

Vitamin K deserves special mention in the context of the PT. Prothrombin and factors VII, IX, and X undergo post-translational carboxylation of glutamic acid residues that is necessary for activity and requires vitamin K as a cofactor. Deficiency of vitamin K or antagonism of this process by warfarin is thus understood to alter the PT. Additionally, in the jaundiced patient, a favorable response to parenteral vitamin K implies that intake or absorption of vitamin K is abnormal, as opposed to a nonresponse, which implies that parenchymal disease is at least in part the basis for abnormality (see Table 5-1).

Serum Enzyme Tests

Alkaline Phosphatase. Hepatic alkaline phosphatase (AP) is concentrated in the canalicular hepatocyte membrane and bile duct epithelial cells, and increased production and release appear to cause the elevated AP levels seen in cholestasis. However, AP exists in normal tissues throughout the body as well as in extrahepatic neoplasms. A further diagnostic issue arises from the fact that states of increased metabolic activity are associated with increased AP activity in the affected tissue. For these reasons, young adults with rapid bone growth and gravid patients with placental production routinely have elevated AP levels.

AP levels as high as three times normal occur in many liver diseases and are often diagnostic. More pronounced elevations suggest infiltrative processes or biliary obstruction, the latter of which can be either intrahepatic (e.g., tumor) or extrahepatic. Diagnostically, if the entire biliary tree is not obstructed then the unaffected portion of the liver can often maintain bilirubin within normal ranges, but AP will be markedly elevated.

γ-Glutamyl Transpeptidase. γ-Glutamyl transpeptidase (GGTP) has a tissue distribution similar to alkaline phosphatase except that it has low concentrations in bone. Thus, GGTP may be helpful in discriminating the source of AP elevations. GGTP can also be quite sensitive to the ingestion of alcohol and drugs, including several anticonvulsants. The variability of this phenomenon, however, makes GGTP a suggestive but unreliable indicator of alcohol ingestion.

Aminotransaminases. Aspartate aminotransferase (AST, also known as SGOT [serum glutamic oxaloacetic transaminase]) and alanine aminotransferase (ALT, also known as SGPT [serum glutamic pyruvic transaminase]) are participants in gluconeogenesis. Both enzymes are plentiful in the cytosol of the hepatocyte, while an AST isozyme is present in the mitochondria as well. AST is also found in a variety of tissues including heart, brain, and skeletal muscle; ALT is more specific to the liver. These enzymes are elevated in many forms of liver disease, presumably as a result of leakage from damaged cells. Substantial hepatic necrosis as found in chemical and ischemic injury appears to be particularly associated with elevation of these enzymes. Nonspecific AST elevations can be seen with injury to skeletal or cardiac muscle, so ALT levels should be evaluated as well. Notably, advanced cirrhosis can exist without significant elevations if active cell injury is absent or minimal at the time of evaluation.

The relative increases in AST and ALT (the AST/ALT ratio) can be useful in supporting a diagnosis of alcohol injury (AST/ALT > 2) versus most other acute liver injuries (AST/ALT ≤ 1), although cirrhosis is also associated with AST/ALT > 1. Absolute levels can be diagnostic when extreme, and helpful when moderately elevated, as depicted in Table 5-1.

Lactate Dehydrogenase. Because of its presence in tissues throughout the body, lactate dehydrogenase (LDH) usually offers little diagnostic discrimination beyond that of aminotransaminases. LDH does, however, demonstrate a short-lived but exceptionally high elevation in ischemic injury, and a moderate but sustained elevation in some malignancies.

DISEASES AND DYSFUNCTION OF THE LIVER

Liver dysfunction has been categorized in a variety of ways. Clinical presentation (e.g., jaundice), etiology (e.g., viral hepatitis), circumstances (e.g., postoperative liver dysfunction), time frame, and/or severity (e.g., subfulminant liver failure) are commonly used descriptors. None of these approaches is complete. For example, acute liver failure may have an infectious or toxic etiology, whereas viral hepatitis may result in abrupt severe liver dysfunction or proceed along a chronic subclinical course. The discussion to follow will first address representative individual causes of liver dysfunction and then relevant situations that can be the common outcome of several disease processes (e.g., cirrhosis and acute liver failure).

Etiology of Liver Dysfunction

Viral Hepatitis

Although there are a vast number of viruses that have the capacity to produce hepatitis (Table 5-2), there are only five viruses that produce liver disease as their primary clinical manifestation.[5] Each of the five hepatitis viruses has been designated with a letter (e.g., hepatitis A virus,

TABLE 5–2   Uncommon Causes of Viral Hepatitis

Virus	Vaccine Available
Epstein-Barr virus (EBV)	No
Cytomegalovirus (CMV)	No
Herpesvirus, type 1	In development
Herpesvirus, type 2	In development
Coxsackievirus, type B	No
Echoviruses	No
Adenovirus	Yes—for certain subtypes, limited to military use
Yellow fever virus	Yes
Varicella zoster virus	Yes
Measles	Yes

hepatitis B virus) according to their clinical manifestations (Table 5-3). It is important to remember that although each virus infects the liver, the viruses have different biochemical, biologic, and clinical characteristics. Indeed, the viruses do not form a formal phylogenetic family and are not related to one another per se. Although infection with each virus can be associated with significant morbidity and mortality, infection with any virus may result in an anicteric illness and may not be diagnosed as hepatitis.[6]

Hepatitis A. The hepatitis A virus (HAV) is a 27- to 32-nm nonenveloped virus with a 7.5-kb genome of single-stranded RNA. HAV is the only member of the genus *Hepatovirus* in the viral family Picornaviridae. HAV is almost always transmitted via the fecal-oral route through the ingestion of contaminated food or drink. After ingestion, the virus is absorbed through the small bowel and transported via the portal blood flow to the liver.[7] The virus replicates in the liver and is then shed into the blood or, more commonly, through the bile and into the stool. Viral shedding begins as early as the second week of infection and consequently may occur before the patient experiences any clinical signs or symptoms of hepatitis (see later). Viral shedding may continue until 2 weeks after the onset of jaundice. Although the virus is shed into the stool in high titers, titers of virus in the blood remain low during the short (1-2 week) viremic phase.[8] As such, transmission of HAV by blood transfusion is extremely rare, although transmission from a single donor has been reported.[9,10] The virus has also been transmitted to hemophiliacs with contaminated factor VIII concentrates.[11]

After an incubation of 15 to 50 days, patients may experience the acute onset of systemic complaints, including fever, malaise, nausea, vomiting, and abdominal pain. Patients may also note the appearance of dark urine and jaundice. Mild hepatic enlargement and tenderness is noted in approximately 85% of patients, with splenomegaly noted in 15% of patients or less.[12] Coagulopathy, encephalopathy, and renal failure are rare in the setting of acute HAV infection.[12,13] HAV is normally a self-limited illness with complete recovery noted in most patients in less than 2 months; however, serious complications can occur.[14] Underlying liver disease is associated with increases in the risk of fulminant hepatic failure with HAV superinfection.[15,16] Chronic hepatitis does not occur, but an atypical relapsing course has been described in both children and adults.[17]

Diagnosis is normally confirmed by serologic testing. Anti-HAV IgM is detectable in the serum approximately 3 weeks after exposure. Early diagnosis is also possible with the detection of HAV in stool using electron microscopy or the detection of viral RNA; however, both of these methods are impractical. Although 75% of adult patients with HAV have obvious clinical manifestations, up to 70% of infections in children younger than age 6 years are

TABLE 5–3	Characteristics of Human Hepatitis Viruses				
Virus	**Hepatitis A**	**Hepatitis B**	**Hepatitis C**	**Hepatitis D**	**Hepatitis E**
Virus Family	Picornaviridae	Hepadnaviridae	Flaviviridae	Viroid	Calciviridae
Genome	ssRNA	Partially dsDNA	SsRNA	ssRNA	ssRNA
Transmission					
Fecal-oral	Yes	No	No	No	Yes
Sexual	No	Yes	Rare	Rare	No
Blood/ Percutaneous	Rare	Yes	Yes	Yes	No
Incubation Period	15-50 days	4-26 wk	2-26 wk	3-7 wk	15-60 days
Immunity	IgG anti-HAV	IgG HBsAb	Unknown	IgG HBsAb	IgG anti-HEV
Chronic Hepatitis	No	Yes	Yes	Yes	No
Fulminant Failure	<1%	<1%	Rare	2%-10%	1% (30% in pregnancy)
Cirrhosis	No	Yes	Yes	Yes	No

Adapted from Ryder SD, Beckingham IJ: ABC of diseases of liver, pancreas, and biliary system: Acute hepatitis: BMJ 2001;322:151-153; and Berenguer M, Wright T: Viral hepatitis. In Feldman M, Friedman L, Sleisenger M (eds): Sleisenger & Fordtran's Gastrointestinal and Liver Diseases, 7th ed. Philadelphia, WB Saunders, 2002.

totally asymptomatic.[18] When one considers the combination of the developing bowel habits of young children with their capacity to act as asymptomatic carriers, it should come as no surprise that young children are considered the principal reservoir for the virus.

HAV infections occur throughout the world but are clearly more common in developing countries with poor sanitation. In the United States, the incidence of HAV infection is 9 to 10 per 100,000, with an overall seroprevalence of 30%. Two highly effective vaccines has been available in the United States since 1996.[18] The vaccines have been recommended for children[19] and adults[18] with chronic liver disease. Anesthesiologists and all health care providers should consider immunization. In the event of possible transmission of HAV to a health care provider, a single dose of 0.02 mL/kg immune globulin is highly effective in preventing infection if given within 14 days of exposure.[18]

Hepatitis B. The hepatitis B virus (HBV) is a 42-nm enveloped virus with 3.2-kb genome of partially double-stranded DNA. HBV is a member of the viral family Hepadnaviridae. Worldwide, more than 400 million people are chronically infected by HBV.[20,21] Unlike HAV, HBV is primarily transmitted by blood, blood products, and sexual contact. Perinatal infection can occur and there is evidence that infection can occur across mucous membranes by semen, saliva, and breast milk.[22] Intravenous drug abuse (IVDA) remains a major mode of HBV transmission[23] and outbreaks among intravenous drug abusers are frequently reported.[24] Nosocomial transmission has been reported through the use of multidose vials of

local anesthetics.[25] Acupuncture has been linked to occasional outbreaks of HBV.[26] Fortunately, transfusion-related HBV infection is a rare event, as HBV screening of donated blood and appropriate screening of donors has been routine for almost 2 decades.[21] Nevertheless, it is estimated that 1:50,000 to 1:63,000 transfused units transmits HBV.[27]

In the United States, Canada, Europe, and Australia sexual transmission is the most important mode of HBV infection.[28,29] Both heterosexual and homosexual activities can transmit HBV, but heterosexual activity accounts for the majority of HBV infections. Prostitutes, their clients, and individuals with many sexual partners are at an increased risk of HBV infection. The risk of heterosexual transmission is greater when the infected person is female than when the infected person is male.[5] In endemic regions like China and sub-Saharan Africa, most infections occur neonatally or in early childhood,[21] and sexual transmission is less important.

After parenteral exposure, there is a long asymptomatic incubation period with a range of 4 to 26 weeks (average, 6 to 8). During this incubation period, infected hepatocytes synthesize and secrete large quantities of noninfective hepatitis B surface antigen (HBsAg). Consequently, HBsAg is detectable before the onset of signs and symptoms of hepatitis. Hepatitis B DNA (HBV-DNA) is detectable in the serum by polymerase chain reaction (PCR) shortly after HBsAg and indicates active viral replication. HBeAg, another important indicator of active viral replication, is also detectable at this time. Continued expression of HBeAg is an important biochemical predictor of progression to chronic hepatitis (see later). IgM to hepatitis core antigen

(HBc), a viral protein not detected in the serum, can be detected in the serum shortly before the onset of acute illness. IgM anti-HBc is gradually replaced by IgG anti-HBc over several months. IgG anti-HBs does not appear until after the resolution of jaundice and clinical symptoms and after the disappearance of HBsAg. During this "core window" after the disappearance of HBsAg and before the appearance of anti-HBs, IgM anti-HBc (and IgM anti-HBe, if available) are the only laboratory markers of HBV infection.

Of the approximately 325,000 new infections in the United States each year, approximately 60% of patients will develop subclinical disease without jaundice and completely recover. Twenty-five percent of infected patients will develop acute hepatitis characterized by fever, nausea, vomiting, anorexia, abdominal pain, and jaundice. Almost all patients who develop acute hepatitis will completely recover; however, approximately 1% of patients will develop fulminant hepatic failure and will die without liver transplantation. Five to 10 percent of patients will become "healthy carriers" of the disease. These individuals do not normally manifest signs or symptoms of hepatitis but are able to transmit the disease to others. Less than 5% of patients infected with HBV will develop a persistent infection characterized by mild but persistent elevation of serum transaminases for months to years. Most patients with persistent infection will ultimately recover; however, 20% to 30% will go on to develop chronic hepatitis and cirrhosis. There is evidence that patients who develop chronic hepatitis may have a defective immune response.[30-32] HBV cirrhosis is a significant risk factor for hepatocellular carcinoma, and approximately 10% of patients with HBV cirrhosis will go on to develop hepatocellular carcinoma.

Unlike HAV, HBV infection tends to be more severe in younger patients. In neonates and children younger than 1 year of age, the risk of an infection becoming chronic is 90%. For children aged 1 to 5 years, the risk of chronic infection is 30%. For children older than the age 5, the risk of chronic infection approaches that of adults.[21,33] It has been postulated that transplacental passage of HBeAg from an infected mother to the fetus induces immune tolerance in the neonate.[34]

Highly effective HBV vaccines have been available for almost 20 years. In 1991, the CDC recommended universal childhood vaccination against HBV in the United States. Broad-based vaccination initiatives have been effective in reducing the incidence of HBV infection in Alaska[35] and reducing the incidence of hepatocellular carcinoma in Taiwan.[36] Before HBV vaccination was widespread, the incidence of anti-HBs among anesthesiologists was greater than fourfold higher than that of the general population.[37] As such, the practice of anesthesiology is an independent risk factor for the development of HBV.[38,39] All anesthesiologists should be vaccinated against HBV.

In the event of possible transmission of HBV to a nonimmunized individual (such as from an accidental needle stick), passive immunization with hepatitis B immune globulin (HBIG) is available. Current recommendations are to administer HBIG in a dose of 0.05 to 0.07 mL/kg immediately after exposure. A second dose 30 days after exposure may further reduce the risk of HBV infection. If HBIG is not given within 7 days of infection, antiviral treatment should be considered.

Most antiviral therapy in HBV is directed toward the treatment of chronically infected patients.[40] Therapy with interferon alfa has proven effective in the elimination HBeAg in patients chronically infected with HBV.[41,42] Therapy normally consists of a 16-week course of either 5 mU daily or 10 mU three times a week. Lamivudine, a nucleoside analog, is available orally for HBV.[43] Long-term treatment with lamivudine has been shown to reduce fibrosis and necrosis in patients with chronic HBV infections.[44]

Despite these impressive results, there is evidence of emerging lamivudine-resistant mutants.[45] Adefovir dipivoxil, another nucleoside analog, is also effective.[46] Adefovir seems to have efficacy against lamivudine-resistant mutants.[47]

Hepatitis D (Delta Agent). Hepatitis D virus (HDV) is a 35-nm viroid with a 1.7-kb genome of single-stranded RNA. The viroid is enveloped with HBsAg and requires co-infection with HBV for HDV infection and replication. Delta agent was first noted in 1977,[48] and its unique structure was described in 1986.[49] Like HBV, HDV is transmitted parenterally. Intravenous drug abuse remains the most common mode of transmission in North America, Europe, and Australia.[50-52] Sexual transmission of HDV can occur[53] but may be less efficient than HBV. Perinatal infection of HDV is rare.

HDV infection can occur in two settings.[54] In *acute co-infection,* HDV infection occurs at the same time as acute HBV infection. This normally happens when a patient has been exposed to blood or serum from a patient harboring both infections. *Superinfection* can occur when a patient with a persistent HBV infection or chronic hepatitis becomes infected with HDV. Co-infection with HBV and HDV results in a more severe course of acute hepatitis and increased risk (3% to 4%) of fulminant hepatic failure. Nevertheless, approximately 90% of co-infected patients go on to complete recovery and develop immunity.

Secondary to defective immunity (see earlier), patients with chronic HBV infection provide the ideal host for HDV superinfection. Approximately 10% of patients superinfected with HDV will go on to fulminant hepatic failure that rapidly progresses to death. Most of the remaining 90% of patients will go on to develop an accelerated cirrhotic picture.[55] A small percentage of patients will recover and develop consequent immunity.

The diagnosis of HDV infection is normally made by the detection of IgM anti-HDV. IgM anti-HDV is not normally detectable in patient serum until the onset of acute hepatitis and jaundice. It is possible to detect HDV antigen (HDVAg) in patient serum before the onset of hepatitis during the late incubation period; however, HDVAg is present only transiently and hence testing may be unreliable. HDV-RNA is the earliest marker of infection and can be detected by PCR, but this is rarely used establish HDV infection.

There is no specific treatment for HDV. Because HDV infection is only possible in the case of HBV infection, and vaccination reliably prevents HBV infection, vaccination against HBV remains the best method to prevent HDV infection.

Hepatitis C. The hepatitis C virus (HCV) is a 55-nm enveloped virus with 9.4-kb genome of single-stranded RNA. HCV is the only member of the genus *Hepacivirus* in the viral family Flaviviridae. Worldwide, more than 170 million people are chronically infected with HCV.[56] HCV was not identified until 1989.[57] Like HBV, HCV is primarily transmitted by blood, blood products, and sexual contact. The two biggest risk factors for HCV infection are intravenous drug abuse (IVDA) and blood transfusion prior to 1990.[58,59] Indeed, HCV has been identified as the etiologic agent in over 85% of all cases of post-transfusion non-A, non-B hepatitis before 1991.[5] Since routine screening for anti-HCV and blood donor risk factor assessment by most blood donor centers in 1991, transfusion-related infection of HCV is a rare event.[58,59] It is estimated that 1 in 103,000 transfused units transmits HCV.[27]

Consequently, IVDA has emerged as the principal risk factor in the North America, Europe, and Australia.[60] Perinatal transmission is rare and occurs exclusively from mothers who are HCV RNA positive at the time of delivery.[61,62] Perinatal transmission may be more common if co-infection with the human immunodeficiency virus (HIV) exists.[63] It is unclear whether birth by Cesarean-section increases or decreases the risk of perinatal transmission.[61,64-66] Breast feeding appears to pose little risk to the infant.[67,68] As noted earlier, sexual transmission of HCV is possible; however, transmission is significantly less efficient than for HBV. Nevertheless, prostitutes and their clients, men who have sex with other men, and individuals with multiple sexual partners are at increased risk for HCV infection. There is some suggestion that co-infection with HIV[69] or herpes simplex virus type 2[58] may increase the likelihood of HCV infection. Although the virus is present in saliva of chronically infected persons,[70] transmission through casual contact seems an unusual means of transmission.[71] Patient-to-patient transmission has occurred during colonoscopy,[72] and patients have been infected during surgery.[73] In one hospital,

an anesthesia assistant became infected from a patient and subsequently spread the infection to five other patients.[74]

In contrast to HBV, HCV has a high rate of progression to chronic disease and eventual cirrhosis. After infection, HCV has a long incubation period that ranges from 2 to 26 weeks (average, 7 to 8 weeks).[56] Of the approximately 175,000 persons infected in the United States each year, 75% will develop subclinical disease. The remaining 25% develop a symptomatic disease characterized by fever, nausea, vomiting, abdominal pain, anorexia, and jaundice. Approximately 1% of patients with symptomatic disease will develop fulminant hepatic failure that rapidly progresses to death without transplantation. Almost 80% of all patients infected with HCV will go on to develop chronic hepatitis characterized by mild, episodic elevations in transaminases and occasional jaundice.[56] More than 25% of patients with chronic hepatitis will go on to develop cirrhosis. HCV cirrhosis is a significant risk factor for hepatocellular carcinoma, with an estimated risk of 1% to 4% per year.[56,75]

The detection of antibodies against HCV is both sensitive and specific for HCV infection. Newer, third-generation enzyme immunoassays can detect antibodies within 4 to 10 weeks of infection.[75] Unlike HBV, PCR to detect HCV-RNA is commonly utilized in clinical practice to determine viral load. Viral load has been determined to be a significant predictor of the efficacy of antiviral therapy.[76] In addition, the detection of HCV-RNA is the most sensitive and specific test of HCV infection.[77] There is significant controversy regarding the use of liver biopsy in HCV infection.[78-81]

There are a variety of treatment regimens available for HCV. Standard interferon three times a week for 24 to 48 weeks was approved for use in 1990 and has been successful in the treatment of HCV infection.[75] Interferon alfa (alfa-2a or 2b), 3 MU three times a week for 24 to 48 weeks, has shown response rates as high as 40%[76] and seems to be more effective than standard interferon. Pegylated interferons have been used to treat HCV since the late 1990s and have shown superior results when compared with interferon alfa.[82] When pegylated interferons are combined with ribavirin, studies have shown response rates as high as 88% in certain patient groups.[83,84]

There is no vaccine available for HCV. Hence, avoiding exposure best prevents infection. For anesthesiologists and other health care professionals, the observation of universal precautions is critical. Prophylaxis after an accidental exposure is not currently recommended. There are no randomized, controlled studies examining the efficacy of therapy in acute HCV infection; however, one study showed that after treatment with interferon alfa-2b for 24 weeks, 43 of 44 patients did not have detectable HCV-RNA.[85]

Hepatitis E. The hepatitis E virus (HEV) is a 32-nm nonenveloped virus with 7.5-kb genome of single-stranded RNA.

HEV was discovered in 1983 and is part of the alpha-super group of viruses. Some virologists place HEV in the Caliciviridae family of viruses. HEV is responsible for the majority of cases of what was previously called enterically transmitted non-A, non-B hepatitis (ET-NANBH).[86] Like HAV, HEV is almost always transmitted via the fecal-oral route through the ingestion of contaminated food or drink. During epidemics, the most common mode of transmission is the ingestion of fecally contaminated water.[87] Compared with HAV, there is a low rate of person-to-person transmission of household contacts. Nosocomial infection has been reported.[88]

After ingestion, the virus is absorbed through the small bowel and transported via the portal blood flow to the liver. After an incubation period of 15 to 60 days (average, 35 to 42) a preicteric phase characterized by fever and malaise is reported by 95% to 100% of patients. An icteric phase characterized by abdominal pain, nausea, vomiting, anorexia, and jaundice follows shortly after. Symptoms normally resolve in less than 6 weeks, although the fulminant hepatic failure is a rare but reported complication. A characteristic feature of HEV is the high incidence of progression to fulminant hepatic failure in pregnant women. If contracted in the third trimester, HEV mortality may exceed 20%.

The diagnosis of HEV is normally made by exclusion after travel to an endemic area (South and Central America, Southeast Asia including China, India, and Africa). Nevertheless, assays to detect both IgM anti-HEV and IgG anti-HEV are commercially available. PCR can be utilized to detect HEV-RNA; however, this is almost always done only for research purposes.

Currently, there is no vaccine available for HEV. The administration of immune globulin from endemic areas has not decreased infection rates during epidemics.[89] As such, it seems unlikely that the use of immune globulin would be of no particular use in the event of an exposure in a nonendemic area such as North America or Europe. Health care providers should utilize universal precautions when dealing with patients with suspected HEV infections. Obviously, pregnant women should avoid any kind of exposure to HEV.

Hepatitis G. Hepatitis G virus (HGV) was first described in the serum of a patient with non-A, non-B, non-C hepatitis.[90] HGV and so-called GB viruses have been described.[91] HGV/GB are detectable in a substantial proportion of blood donors.[92] HGV and GB have a genomic sequence similar to HCV. Despite its genetic similarity to HCV, it does not appear that HGV/GB causes liver disease.[93] Indeed, the initial patient was later found to have HCV. Probably the most interesting aspect of HGV/GB study is that patients co-infected with HIV and HGV/GB seem to enjoy prolonged survival.[94]

Hydatid Cyst Disease

Hydatid cyst disease is caused by an infection of the animal tapeworm *Echinococcus*. Like all tapeworms, *Echinococcus* lives in the small bowel of definitive hosts. Definitive hosts include carnivorous animals such as dogs, wolves, and other canines. Tapeworm-infected canines pass eggs in their feces, which contaminate the environment. Sheep, cattle, and humans become intermediate hosts when they ingest the eggs by eating contaminated foodstuffs. Infected domestic dogs remain the most important vector for transmission of hydatid disease.[95,96]

Once the eggs are ingested, gastric acid and digestive pancreatic enzymes dissolve the egg's external shell. The larvae then penetrate the bowel wall, enter the portal circulation, and are carried to the liver. Approximately 70% of the larvae remain in the liver, with 20% infecting the lungs, although other organs, including the brain,[97] spinal cord,[98,99] kidney,[100] and heart[101] can be infected. In the liver, *Echinococcus* has virtually no symptoms until the cysts become very large. Although pain is the most common complaint, a large cyst may cause obstructive jaundice, cholangitis, pancreatitis, or portal hypertension.[95,96] Blunt trauma may cause cyst rupture.[102] Diagnosis is normally made by serologic testing after abdominal imaging reveals hepatic cysts. An eosinophilia may also be present.

The treatment of large hydatid cysts is surgical, and the anesthesiologist is likely to encounter patients scheduled for cyst drainage. The surgical approach may be attempted by laparoscopy,[103] laparotomy, or thoracotomy if a subdiaphragmatic cyst is present. There are multiple case reports of an anaphylactic reaction to hydatid fluid during surgical excision.[104-106] Preoperative steroids and antihistamines[107] should be considered.

Genetic Causes of Liver Disease

Alagille Syndrome (Arteriohepatic Dysplasia). Alagille syndrome (AGS) is a rare inherited disorder characterized by the progressive loss of the intralobular bile ducts and narrowing of extrahepatic bile ducts.[108] It is the most common form of familial intrahepatic cholestasis, and over 90% of patients experience chronic cholestasis.[108,109] The disease has an autosomal dominant pattern of inheritance, and over 70% of patients have a mutation in the jagged 1 (*JAG1*) gene on the short arm of chromosome 20.[109] AGS has an incidence of approximately 1:100,000 live births.

Most patients present with jaundice, clay-colored stools and other symptoms of mild cholestasis during the neonatal period. Patients might also present with rapidly progressive, fulminant hepatic failure. The disease is slowly progressive, and treatment is generally supportive. Approximately 15% of patients will require transplantation.[110] A Kasai procedure may provide patients with some relief; however, a previous

Kasai increases perioperative mortality if the patient should require hepatic transplantation.[110]

Although the primary manifestation of AGS is cholestasis, AGS is of particular interest to anesthesiologists secondary to the high morbidity of its associated conditions. Over 90% of patients with AGS have congenital heart disease. Approximately 67% of patients have uncomplicated peripheral pulmonic stenosis; however, the remaining 33% have more serious defects, including tetralogy of Fallot (16%), patent ductus arteriosus (5%), ventricular septal defect (4%), and atrial septal defect (4%). The presence of significant cardiovascular disease is associated with increased perioperative mortality during liver transplantation.[110] So-called "butterfly vertebrae" resulting from clefting abnormalities are present in as many as 85% of patients.[108,111] Patients are described as having a characteristic facies, and as many as 90% of patients have ophthalmologic abnormalities, commonly anterior chamber defects such as posterior embryotoxon.[108,111] Patients have a characteristic short stature, and resistance to growth hormone has been described.[112]

A meticulous preoperative evaluation of patients with AGS is critical for perioperative planning and optimization of care. Careful attention must be given to associated conditions, with particular attention to each patient's cardiac,[113] hepatic, renal, and orthopedic disease.[114] In some patients, a vitamin K deficiency develops secondary to malabsorption. If blood loss is possible, preoperative clotting studies may be indicated. Severe postoperative cholestasis has been reported in patients with AGS.[115]

α_1-Antitrypsin Deficiency. α_1-Antitrypsin deficiency is the most common metabolic disease affecting the liver. The disease is most common among white Europeans, in whom the incidence of disease may be as high as 1:1500 persons.[116] The disease is somewhat less common among North American and Australian whites, in whom the incidence approaches 1:2000 persons. The incidence among African, Asian, and Hispanic individuals is very low. The precise geographic distribution of the disease is critically dependent on the specific genotype.

α_1-Antitrypsin is a potent serine protease inhibitor synthesized in the liver and secreted into the blood. As it circulates, it binds to and promotes the degradation of serine proteases produced throughout the body. One of the most important proteases inhibited by α_1-antitrypsin is elastase. Indeed, α_1-antitrypsin is responsible for more than 90% of all the serum antielastase activity and is principally involved in the degradation of alveolar elastase. Once bound to its protease target, the α_1-antitrypsin: protease complex binds to a receptor on hepatocytes and is removed from the circulation.[117]

The α_1-antitrypsin gene has been localized to chromosome 14 and is part of the SERPIN (*Serine Protease*

*In*hibitor) supergene. This gene cluster also encodes for corticosteroid binding globulin, C1 inhibitor, and antithrombin III.[116] At least 17 different mutant alleles of α_1-antitrypsin have been described; however, two mutations account for the majority of disease. Individuals homozygous for the more common S mutation (Glu264Val) have a 40% decrease in serum α_1-antitrypsin concentration.[118] The S mutation is more common among Southern Europeans, with peak incidences recorded in the Iberian peninsula.[116] Individuals homozygous for the more serious Z mutation (Glu342Lys) have an 85% decrease in serum α_1-antitrypsin concentration.[118] Unlike the S mutation, the Z mutation is more common among Northern and Western Europeans, with peak incidences in northern France, the United Kingdom, and Scandanavia.[116] In general, the S mutation only produces clinically significant disease when it is combined with the Z mutation (SZ genotype).

The low serum protein concentrations observed in individuals with α_1-antitrypsin deficiency do not occur secondary to defective protein synthesis but rather to ineffective processing and secretion.[119,120] These ineffective processes leave the hepatocyte with large quantities of defective protein that accumulate in the cell. Defective processing is particularly severe in the Z mutation, where processing errors lead to the formation of long polymers of Z– α_1-antitrypsin.[119] In both mutations, the excess of defective α_1-antitrypsin is visible under light microscopy as large cytoplasmic inclusions. Stores of excessive defective protein ultimately can interfere with normal hepatic function.[121]

The abnormal accumulation of defective protein leads to hepatocyte death and eventual cirrhosis. In general, the severity of hepatic disease is closely associated with the amount of accumulated protein. Liver disease does not occur in individuals with unusual mutations of α_1-antitrypsin that do not result in the accumulation of defective protein the hepatocyte. There is significant variation in clinical presentation and age at onset among patients with α_1-antitrypsin deficiency, even among individuals with the same genotype. It has been suggested that the variation in the age at onset of liver disease is due to variations in the rate of synthesis between individuals.[122] Indeed, the appearance of jaundice in infants with ZZ α_1-antitrypsin deficiency may reflect a chronic infection resulting in increased synthesis of defective protein.[123] Regardless, the appearance of jaundice during the neonatal period is a poor prognostic sign. Although α_1-antitrypsin deficiency has a number of other manifestations, it is well accepted that liver disease has the greatest effect on survival.

The other primary clinical manifestations of individuals with α_1-antitrypsin deficiency occur secondary to the absence of normal protease inhibition. The most obvious manifestation of disease secondary to the lack of normal protease inhibition occurs in the lung, as patients with α_1-antitrypsin deficiency suffer from the early onset of panlobular emphysema. All individuals experience an age-related decline in the forced expiratory volume in 1 second (FEV_1) after age 30; however, this decline is accelerated by α_1-antitrypsin deficiency. This acceleration is further exacerbated by tobacco smoke, which can double the rate of decline.[124]

The diagnosis of α_1-antitrypsin deficiency is made by the measurement of serum α_1-antitrypsin concentration. The genotype is confirmed by protein electrophoresis. There is no specific therapy for α_1-antitrypsin deficiency, and liver transplantation may be required.

Cystic Fibrosis. Cystic fibrosis (CF) is the single most common lethal inherited disease among white populations, with an incidence of approximately 1:3300 persons in the United States. CF was one of the first genetic diseases to be characterized. The gene for CF, the cystic fibrosis transmembrane conductance regulator *(CFTR),* resides on chromosome 7. Presence of the gene results in defective cellular chloride conductance. Although the principal manifestation of CF is pulmonary with associated viscid secretions, atelectasis, emphysema, and chronic infections with mucoid chronic infection with *Pseudomonas aeruginosa,* hepatic abnormalities may complicate 20% of cases. Portal hypertension and eventual hepatic cirrhosis may complicate up to 10% of all CF cases and represent the second most common cause of death after respiratory failure. As the median age of CF increases secondary to a reduction in mortality, there has been concern that the incidence of liver disease would increase.

Although pathologic elevation of liver enzymes is frequently observed in infants, most patients do not progress to childhood or adult cirrhosis.[125] Nevertheless, it is clear that certain genotypes are clearly associated with liver dysfunction and an increased incidence of cirrhosis.[126] There is also an increased incidence of liver disease in patients with certain major histocompatibility complex genotypes,[127] male gender, coexisting liver disease, and poor nutrition (especially fatty acid deficiency). Major liver disease is rarely noted in the absence of pancreatic insufficiency.

When hepatic disease advances to cirrhosis, it normally presents during the first decade of life. Portal hypertension is usually manifested by splenomegaly, hypersplenism with thrombocytopenia, and ascites.[128] Bleeding of esophageal varices is also noted in some patients. Transjugular intrahepatic portosystemic shunting (TIPS) has been used with success in children and adolescents with refractory esophageal bleeding.[129,130] In severe cases, liver transplantation has been performed.[131,132] The anesthesiologist should be aware that the metabolism of certain drugs[133] may be increased in CF secondary to increased hepatic drug clearance.[134]

Galactosemia. Galactosemia is an inherited deficiency of the enzyme galactose-1-phosphate uridyltransferase. Galactose-1-phosphate uridyltransferase catalyzes the conversion of galactose-1-phosphate to UDP-galactose, and deficiency leads to the abnormal accumulation of galactose-1-phosphate in cells. The enzyme is normally present in liver and erythrocytes. Galactosemia is an extremely rare disorder with an incidence of approximately 1:60,000 births. Galactose-1-phosphate is directly toxic to cells, and accumulation is most notable in the kidney, liver, and brain.

Breast milk contains lactose, a disaccharide consisting of glucose and galactose. As newborn infants receive up to 20% of their caloric intake in the form of lactose, infants with galactosemia rapidly accumulate galactose-1-phosphate. Routine newborn screening normally makes the diagnosis of galactosemia. If the diagnosis is not made, the accumulation of galactose-1-phosphate can ultimately lead to cataracts, severe mental retardation, and cirrhosis. Treatment involves the avoidance of lactose in the diet; however, patients treated appropriately still develop long-term complications, including cognitive impairment, cataracts, speech abnormalities, and primary ovarian failure.[135,136] Infants born with galactosemia have an increased incidence of *Escherichia coli* neonatal sepsis that normally precedes the diagnosis of galactosemia.[137] Without treatment, the disease is generally fatal, although case reports of adult patients presenting decompensated cirrhosis exist.[138] *Galactokinase deficiency,* another inherited disorder of galactose metabolism, is less common than galactosemia and generally has a milder course.[139]

Galactosemia may present the anesthesiologist with several unique challenges. Newly diagnosed newborns who have been treated for a short time may have elevated clotting times and be prone to bleeding. Some patients may have hemolysis, and preoperative evaluation of hemoglobin may be valuable in any jaundiced patient. Finally, albuminuria may cause an osmotic diuresis, and, consequently, urine volume may be a poor indicator of intravascular volume.

Glycogen Storage Diseases. Glycogen is the principal storage form for glucose in the human body. It is composed of long chains of glucose joined together by α-1,4 linkages. The chains intermittently branch by α-1,6 linkages to form long, tree-like strands of stored glucose. Glycogen stands as a ready reserve for glucose in times of metabolic need. Glycogen metabolism principally occurs in skeletal muscle and liver. Skeletal muscle glycogen provides exercising muscles with a ready source of fuel while hepatic glycogen serves to maintain plasma glucose during fast. The glycogen storage disorders compromise a family of 10 different diseases. Each disease is characterized by an enzyme deficiency in glycogen metabolism. Only glycogen storage disorders type I, III, and IV are associated with severe hepatic disease. The characteristics of the glycogen storage disorders are summarized in Table 5-4.

The perioperative management of any patient with a glycogen storage disorder requires meticulous care and planning. Obviously, the blood glucose level should be carefully monitored in any patient with a type I or III glycogen storage disorder. NPO guidelines should be followed, and patients may require preadmission for the intravenous administration of glucose-containing fluids. Case reports of successful anesthetic management of patients with a type I glycogen storage disease have been reported.[140-142] Patient-controlled sedation with propofol during spinal anesthesia has also been successfully employed.[143] Patients with a type III glycogen storage disease may pose a special challenge to anesthesiologists secondary to muscle disease.[144] Liver transplantation has been used to treat type I, III, and IV glycogen storage diseases,[145] but cardiomyopathy may persist in type IV secondary to cardiac amylopectin deposition.[146]

Hereditary Fructose Intolerance. Hereditary fructose intolerance (HFI) is an inherited deficiency of the enzyme fructose-1,6-bisphosphate aldolase (aldolase B). Aldolase B catalyzes the conversion of fructose-1,6-bisphosphate to two triose phosphates, dihydroxyacetone phosphate and glyceraldehyde-3-phosphate. Deficiency leads to the abnormal accumulation of fructose-1-phosphate and initiates severe symptoms when patients are exposed to fructose. The enzyme is normally present in liver, kidney, and small bowel. HFI is an extremely rare disorder, with an incidence of approximately 1:23,000 births, almost three times that of galactosemia.

When patients consume fructose or sucrose (a disaccharide consisting of glucose and fructose), the acute presentation of abdominal pain, malaise, hypoglycemia, nausea, and vomiting is often noted. Continued ingestion of fructose yields jaundice, hepatomegaly, and renal dysfunction.[147] Persistent fructose consumption results in fulminant hepatic failure. Treatment consists of the

TABLE 5–4 Glycogen Storage Disorders

Disease	Enzyme Deficiency	Main Clinical Features	Liver Disease	Treatment	Notes
Type Ia (von Gierke's disease)	Glucose-6-phosphatase	Profound hypoglycemia Growth failure Metabolic acidosis Hyperlipidemia Renal failure (by second decade of life) Diagnosis in infancy	Hepatomegaly (normal spleen) Hepatic adenomas (by second decade of life) Occasional hepatocellular carcinoma	Portal diversion shunting Glucose supplementation (cornstarch, nocturnal glucose infusion) Liver transplantation	Type Ib (10% of type I disease) also associated with neutropenia and neutrophil dysfunction
Type IIIa (Cori-Forbe's disease)	Liver and muscle debranching enzyme	Profound hypoglycemia Growth failure Progressive muscle weakness with activity Muscle atrophy More tolerant to fasting than type I Diagnosis in infancy	Hepatomegaly (normal spleen) Hepatic adenomas (less common than type I) Rare hepatocellular carcinoma	High-protein, low-carbohydrate diet Glucose supplementation (cornstarch, nocturnal glucose infusion) rarely necessary	Type IIIb (15% of type III) has normal muscle debranching enzyme and no muscular symptoms Generally improves with age
Type IV (Andersen's disease)	Branching enzyme	Failure to thrive Abdominal distention Miscellaneous gastrointestinal complaints Cardiomyopathy Hypoglycemia rare Diagnosis in infancy	Hepatosplenomegaly Progressive macronodular cirrhosis Hepatic failure	Death without liver transplantation	Rare

avoidance of fructose and sucrose in the diet. Unlike galactosemia, patients are normally without symptoms if fructose is avoided, and intellectual development is unimpaired. Some investigators believe that HFI is underdiagnosed, and formal testing yields the diagnosis among patients with unexplained, chronic abdominal pain.[148] Secondary to an almost complete absence of dietary sucrose, patients with HFI have an excellent dentition.[149] Obviously, oral medications containing sucrose or fructose should be avoided in patients with HFI.

Hereditary Hemochromatosis. Hereditary hemochromatosis is an autosomal recessive disease characterized by an inappropriately high degree of iron absorption. In the past, it had been theorized that the disorder occurred due to alcohol abuse and was merely a secondary nutritional disorder; however, the gene was later found to reside on the short arm of chromosome 6, closely linked to the genes encoding for human leukocyte antigen (HLA).[150,151] It was not until 1996 that the gene responsible for hemochromatosis *(HFE)* was discovered, allowing for formal genetic testing and diagnosis.[152] There are a variety of conditions, both acquired and idiopathic, that can be characterized by excessive total body iron (Table 5-5). In many cases, these diseases mimic hereditary hemochromatosis and may be superficially indistinguishable in their clinical manifestations. Nevertheless, it is universally accepted that hereditary hemochromatosis refers specifically to increased iron absorption secondary to *HFE*-related genetic mutations.

As specific *HFE* mutations are identified and investigated, it has become increasingly clear that hereditary hemochromatosis represents a spectrum of clinical disease. Indeed, some homozygotes may manifest disease without a substantial increase in iron stores[153] whereas others do not manifest clinical symptoms in any appreciable way. In addition, although *HFE* is equally distributed between the sexes, clinical disease is two to eight times more common in men than women. It has become increasingly popular to classify patients with hereditary hemochromatosis into four groups: (1) genetic predisposition without abnormalities, (2) iron overload without symptoms, (3) iron overload with early symptoms, and (4) iron overload with end organ damage.[154] It is clear that other factors, genetic and environmental,[155] influence the development of clinical disease. Indeed, the early observation of the link between hereditary hemochromatosis, cirrhosis, and alcohol abuse may be explained by the fact that alcohol further increases the absorption of iron.[156]

The normal adult has a total body iron content of 3 to 5 g. Most iron is recycled through the phagocytosis of senescent erythrocytes and only 1 to 2 mg of iron is normally lost each day.[157] Obviously, losses may be greater among menstruating women and in the case of acute or chronic blood loss. Consequently, dietary iron absorption

TABLE 5–5 Iron Overload Conditions
Primary Iron Overload
Hereditary hemochromatosis
Non–*HFE*-related
Juvenile hemochromatosis
Transferrin receptor-2 mutations
Ferroportin-1 mutations
African iron overload
Secondary Iron Overload
Red blood cell transfusions
Iron loading anemias
Thalassemia major
Sideroblastic anemia
Chronic hemolytic anemia
Aplastic anemia
Pyruvate kinase deficiency
Long-term dialysis
Chronic liver disease
Hepatitis B
Hepatitis C
Alcoholic liver disease
Nonalcoholic steatohepatitis
Portocaval shunting

Adapted from Harrison SA, Bacon BR: Hereditary hemochromatosis: Update for 2003. J Hepatol 2003;38:S14-S23.

is tightly regulated with the amount absorbed paralleling the body's needs. In hereditary hemochromatosis, regulatory processes fail.[155,158] This results in an abnormal increase in dietary iron absorption with iron deposition in the skin, heart, pancreas, joints, and liver.

Hereditary hemochromatosis is surprisingly common. In some white European populations, 10% to 12% of people are heterozygous carriers of the disease.[159] The incidence of homozygous hereditary hemochromatosis ranges between 1:100 to 1:400 in white persons of European descent.[160,161]

Primary presentation of symptomatic hereditary hemochromatosis is becoming rare. Most patients are asymptomatic and report for evaluation and genetic testing after a family member develops the disease. Nevertheless, most symptomatic patients present in the fifth or sixth decade of life. The liver is the first organ to be affected in hemochromatosis, and hepatomegaly is noted in nearly 100% patients. The most common presenting symptoms include generalized weakness, malaise, arthralgias, abdominal pain, and impotence (in men).[162] Physical examination may reveal hepatomegaly and, in advanced cases, signs and symptoms of cirrhosis including ascites and jaundice. Diabetes mellitus, secondary to pancreatic iron deposition, may also occur, although it is rare in the absence of cirrhosis. Iron deposition in skin may give patients a bronze coloration. Indeed, hemochromatosis has been referred to as "bronze diabetes." Iron deposition in the heart can lead to fibrotic changes and most commonly to a restrictive cardiomyopathy. An increase in fatal and nonfatal arrhythmias is also noted. An arthropathy, especially of the hands, is noted in about 50% of patients but does not commonly present before age 50.

As iron accumulates in the liver, significant hepatocyte damage occurs. The fundamental disease mechanism results from direct iron toxicity and the consequent increase in iron-generated free radical production.[163-166] The increased oxidative stress results in lipid peroxidation,[165,166] mitochondrial injury,[154] and impaired calcium homeostasis.[164,165] This results in an inflammatory response, fibrin deposition, and ultimately hepatic cirrhosis. Further oxidative stress may result in DNA damage and an increased risk of hepatocellular carcinoma.[164] Hepatocellular carcinoma is the most common cause of death in hereditary hemochromatosis and the risk is 200 times greater than the general population.[167] Complications arising from cirrhosis and congestive heart failure are other common causes of death.

Once the diagnosis of hereditary hemochromatosis is made, treatment with phlebotomy and reduction of alcohol and dietary iron intake should be initiated. The goal of therapy is to not make the patient iron deficient or anemic.[154] Thus, careful monitoring of hemoglobin, iron levels, ferritin, and transferrin saturation should guide therapy. Although phlebotomy and careful monitoring of dietary intake effectively reduce iron stores, therapy does not reverse cirrhosis nor totally eliminate the risk of hepatocellular carcinoma. This is especially true among patients first diagnosed at a more advanced age. As such, early diagnosis and treatment, ideally before the onset of symptoms, is critical. Liver transplantation may represent the only treatment in advanced disease or in cases of hepatocellular carcinoma; however, many studies reveal decreased survival in transplanted patients with hereditary hemochromatosis compared with other indications.[168]

Hereditary Tyrosinemia Type 1 (HT1). There are four known deficiencies in the catabolism of tyrosine: alkaptonuria and tyrosinemia types 1, 2, and 3. Only tyrosinemia type 1 is associated with liver disease. HT1 is an inherited deficiency of the enzyme fumarylacetoacetate hydrolase (FAH). The enzyme catalyzes the final step in phenylalanine and tyrosine catabolism, the conversion of fumarylacetoacetate to acetoacetate and fumarate. FAH deficiency leads to the abnormal accumulation of "upstream" tyrosine metabolites fumarylacetoacetate (FAA) and maleylacetoacetate (MAA). Both FAA and MAA are converted to two toxic products, succinyl acetoacetate (SAA) and succinylacetone (SA). SAA and SA have been shown to interfere with DNA ligase activity,[169] reduce blood and liver stores of glutathione,[170] and interfere with heme metabolism. These effects combine to decrease the body's ability to deal with oxidative stress and directly result in mutagenic damage and chromosomal breakage.[171] Initially, liver biopsy reveals steatohepatitis; however, this advances to fibrosis and cirrhosis.

HT1 is an extremely rare disorder with an incidence of approximately 1:100,000 births; however, the incidence may be higher in northern Europe (1:8000) and in Quebec, Canada (1:1846).[172,173] Essentially two forms of the disease exist, an acute form and a chronic form. In the acute form, patients present with symptoms of severe hepatic dysfunction during the first 6 months of life. Liver biopsy reveals steatohepatitis that advances to fibrosis and micronodular cirrhosis with bile duct proliferation. In general, the acute form is rapidly fatal within the first year of life without hepatic transplantation.

The chronic form of HT1 presents more slowly than the acute form, with patients rarely seeking medical care before the age of 1 year. The progress of hepatic dysfunction tends to occur more slowly, and patients develop other symptoms, including nephropathy, rickets, and serious neurologic problems.[174] Secondary to continued DNA damage, a substantial risk of hepatocellular carcinoma exists. Liver biopsy reveals less cholestasis than the acute form; however, macro- and micronodular cirrhosis are eventually noted. Liver transplantation is normally indicated within the first decade of life; however, recent advances in the understanding and treatment[175] of HT1 offer some hope.[176] Patients may develop hypertrophic cardiomyopathy. Anemia and thrombocytosis may be observed. Clotting studies may be prolonged.

There is no specific information regarding anesthetic care in patients with HT1; however, preoperative assessment of cardiac, hepatic, metabolic, and hematologic function should be considered if possible.

Lysosomal Storage Diseases. Lysosomal storage diseases are a heterogenous group of diseases resulting from different defects in lysosomal function. Each disease normally reflects a lysosomal enzyme deficiency and a consequent inability to metabolize various biomolecules. Most diseases follow an autosomal recessive pattern of inheritance. Of the more than 30 well-classified diseases, only a small number result in hepatic disease and impairment.

Mucopolysaccharidoses. Each mucopolysaccharidosis (MPS) results from the deficiency of an enzyme responsible for glycosaminoglycan (GAG) metabolism. GAGs are complex, long-chain carbohydrates that are normally linked to proteins to form proteoglycans. Proteoglycans are common constituents of connective tissue.

MPS I results from the deficiency of α-L-iduronidase. At least three phenotypes exist: (1) MPS IH (Hurler's disease) has an acute course characterized by hepatosplenomegaly, mental retardation, and death normally occurring in the first decade; (2) MPS IS (Scheie's disease) has a less severe course characterized by hepatosplenomegaly after the age of 5 and normal life span without mental retardation; and (3) MPS IH/S follows an intermediate course. In all diseases, hepatosplenomegaly can be massive and the diseases can cause profound skeletal dysplasia.[177] Myocardial, coronary, and valvular heart disease are commonly observed.[177] Corneal "clouding" is an expected complication, and patients may present for corneal transplant. Patients frequently require surgical intervention for orthopedic abnormalities. A stiff neck, large tongue, and tonsillar hypertrophy may make intubation difficult.[178,179] Copious airway secretions may be treated with anticholinergics. Fiberoptic intubation through a laryngeal mask airway (LMA) has been reported and may represent a useful technique, especially in children.[180] Patients should be considered at risk for airway obstruction and postobstructive pulmonary edema.[181] Failure of epidural anesthesia has been reported and may be related to the accumulation of GAGs in the epidural space.[182] Perioperative antibiotics may be indicated in patients with valvular disease.

MPS II (Hunter's disease) results from the deficiency of iduronate sulfatase and has an X-linked recessive pattern of inheritance. Both a severe infantile and mild juvenile form of the disease exist. In addition to massive hepatosplenomegaly, GAGs accumulate in the head and neck and patients have a short neck and large tongue. Unlike MPS I, corneal disease is rare. Nevertheless, endotracheal intubation can be difficult[178,179] and acute airway obstruction has been reported.[183] Failure of the LMA to secure the airway in a patient with MPS II has been reported[184]; however, fiberoptic intubation through an LMA has also been reported and may represent a useful technique in children.[180] Sleep apnea and postobstructive pulmonary edema have been reported.[181]

MPS VII (Sly syndrome) results from the deficiency of β-glucuronidase and has an autosomal recessive pattern of inheritance. At least four phenotypes exist.[185] The neonatal form of the disease presents as hydrops fetalis and is uniformly fatal.[186] An infantile form presents as hepatosplenomegaly, jaundice, and inguinal and umbilical hernias. It is rapidly progressive and has a poor prognosis. A second infantile form also presents as hepatosplenomegaly but seems to have a milder course.[187] The adult form of MPS VII presents in adolescence and is not normally complicated by hepatic involvement. Patients may have cardiac involvement with mitral and/or aortic insufficiency. Acute aortic dissection has been reported. Secondary to the accumulation of GAGs in the head and neck, patients with MPS VII may also be difficult to intubate; however, this has not been specifically reported with MPS VII. Intraoperative complete heart block has been observed.[188] Patients with aortic or mitral insufficiency may require perioperative antibiotic prophylaxis.

Lipid Storage Disorders. Each of the lipid storage disorders results from the deficiency of an enzyme responsible for lipid metabolism. The lipid storage disorders include Fabry's disease (FD), Gaucher's disease (GD), and Niemann-Pick disease (NPD). Only GD and NPD have hepatic manifestations and are discussed here.

Gaucher's disease results from the deficiency of acid β-glucosidase and has an autosomal recessive pattern of inheritance. GD is the most common lysosomal storage disease. Three phenotypes have been described.[189,190] The adult type (GD type 1) represents 99% of cases and has a variable onset. It is characterized by thrombocytopenia,[191] anemia, and hepatosplenomegaly. Bone pain is a common complaint, and pathologic fractures can occur. Although hepatosplenomegaly may be the most prominent feature, most morbidity occurs secondary to bone pain. Intelligence is normal, and neurologic symptoms are rare. The availability of placental and now recombinant glucocerebrosidase has improved morbidity in many patients and can result in a decrease in liver volume.[191,192] Improvement in blood coagulation abnormalities has also been described.[193] Adult GD has a carrier rate of approximately 1:18 among Ashkenazi Jews and an annual incidence of approximately 1:1000 live births in the United States.[189]

The accumulation of glycosphingolipids in the head and neck may make endotracheal intubation difficult, and patients may require a smaller than predicted endotracheal tube. Patients should be considered at risk for upper airway obstruction.[194,195] A small mouth may make LMA insertion difficult.[194] Preoperative evaluation should include a baseline hemoglobin and platelet count, because patients are at risk for anemia and thrombocytopenia. Spinal anesthesia has been used with success.[196]

Infantile GD (GD type 2) is characterized by hepatosplenomegaly and severe developmental delay. Stridor and laryngospasm are frequent complications. The disease progresses rapidly, and death occurs before age 2. Juvenile GD (GD type 3) is characterized by ataxia, hepatosplenomegaly, and mental retardation. The typical onset occurs during childhood and patients normally die before age 15. Juvenile GD has a peak incidence in the Swedish Norrbotten population, with an incidence of 1:50,000 persons. Gastroesophageal reflux and chronic aspiration can complicate both types 2 and 3 GD. As in type 1 GD, the airway management of patients with types 2 and 3 may be difficult and patients are at risk for postoperative respiratory compromise.[197] Regional anesthesia has been used with success and should be considered.

Niemann-Pick disease results from the deficiency of sphingomyelinase and has an autosomal recessive pattern of inheritance. At least six phenotypes of NPD have been described; however, three forms make up the majority of cases.[198] Infantile neuropathic NPD (NPD type A) normally presents before 6 months of age and is characterized by hepatosplenomegaly, lymphadenopathy, seizures, and mental retardation. A progressive loss of intellectual capacity and motor function is noted secondary to increased deposition of sphingomyelin in the central nervous system.

Non-neuronopathic NPD (NPD type B) has a variable age of presentation and a more heterogenous expression. Nevertheless, most patients are diagnosed in childhood with hepatosplenomegaly. Unlike type A, patients with type B NPD are neurologically intact and systemic deposition of sphingomyelin is more prominent. Hepatic cirrhosis may develop and portal hypertension and ascites can complicate patient disease. Many type B patients develop pulmonary disease characterized by severe diffusion limitations. Such patients may have low PaO$_2$ and develop cor pulmonale and right ventricular failure in the second decade of life.

Patients with type C NPD actually have a deficiency in cholesterol transport that leads to a disease that is phenotypically similar to type A and B NPD.[199] Patients with type C disease present with prolonged neonatal jaundice. Hepatosplenomegaly is less severe than in types A and B, and patients normally undergo slowly progressive neurodegeneration.

Airway management may be more difficult in patients with NPD.[200] Pulmonary disease may complicate perioperative care, especially in individuals with type B disease. Liver transplantation has successfully reduced some of the clinical manifestations in patients with type A and B NPD; however, morbidity and mortality of liver transplantation may be extremely high secondary to pulmonary and neurologic disease.[201,202]

Other Lysosomal Storage Diseases

Mannosidosis results from the deficiency of α-mannosidase.[203] An infantile form of the disease is characterized by progressive mental retardation and hepatosplenomegaly. Cataracts and corneal clouding may also be observed. An adult form has a delayed onset and allows for longer survival. A small mouth and a large tongue may make intubation difficult. Death normally occurs before age 5. An autosomal recessive pattern of inheritance is noted in this extremely rare disease.

Wolman's disease results from the deficiency of acid lipase and is characterized by the deposition of cholesterol esters throughout the body.[204] Hepatosplenomegaly and eventual cirrhosis are among the more prominent manifestations; however, pulmonary disease with a high alveolar diffusion gradient may be severe. Adrenal calcification is a unique feature. Neonatal survival is impossible without total parental nutrition, and death occurs within the first year of life. Bone marrow transplantation has been successfully utilized to treat Wolman's disease.[205] There is no specific information regarding anesthesia in patients with Wolman's disease.

Porphyria. The porphyrias make up a family of inherited diseases resulting from deficiencies in one or more of the enzymes required for heme synthesis. The enzymatic deficit results in the accumulation of "upstream" metabolites and consequent symptoms (Fig. 5-6). As more than 75% of heme synthesis takes place in the bone marrow, porphyrias are associated with variable hepatic disease. Traditionally, porphyrias are generally divided into erythropoietic or hepatic types, depending on whether the excess production of metabolic intermediates takes place in the liver or in the bone marrow. Porphyrias can be further divided into those with neurovisceral symptoms (acute porphyrias) and those characterized by photosensitivity and cutaneous symptoms (cutaneous porphyrias). Table 5-6 summarizes the characteristics of the various porphyrias.[206]

Acute intermittent porphyria (AIP) is the most common type of porphyria, with a prevalence of about 1:10,000 to 1:20,000 people. Secondary to the disease's ability to cause neuronal damage, the incidence of AIP among patients with psychiatric disorders may be as high as 1:500.[207,208] AIP may be considered the prototype for all acute porphyrias, as the presentation of all acute porphyrias is similar with specific diagnosis requiring laboratory analysis.

In AIP, patients suffer a deficiency of PBG deaminase activity. Because a complete deficiency would be incompatible with life, most patients have approximately 50% of normal PBG deaminase activity. The deficiency results

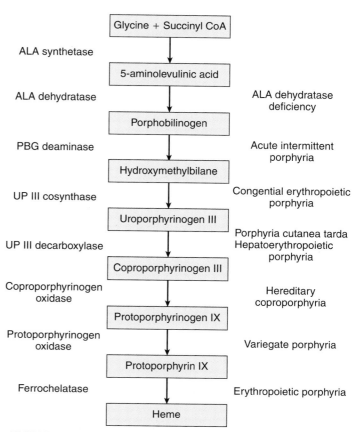

FIGURE 5–6 Heme synthesis and the enzymatic defects of porphyria.

TABLE 5-6 The Porphyrias

Disease	Enzyme Defect	Autosomal Inheritance	Site of Expression	Notes
Acute Porphyrias				
ALA dehydratase deficiency	ALA dehydratase	Recessive	Liver	Very rare
Acute intermittent porphyria (AIP)	PBG deaminase	Dominant	Liver	Most common acute porphyria
Hereditary coproporphyria	Coproporphyrinogen oxidase	Dominant	Liver	Similar to AIP
Variegate porphyria	Protoporphyrinogen oxidase	Dominant	Liver	Common in South Africa
Cutaneous Porphyrias				
Porphyria cutanea tarda	Uroporphyrinogen III decarboxylase	Dominant	Liver	Most common porphyria
Hepatoerythropoietic porphyria	Uroporphyrinogen III decarboxylase	Recessive	Liver, erythropoietic	Similar to CEP
Erythropoietic protoporphyria	Ferrochelatase	Dominant	Liver, erythropoietic	Mild hemolysis Gallstones Occasional liver disease
Congenital erythropoietic porphyria (CEP)	Uroporphyrinogen III cosynthase	Recessive	Erythropoietic	Splenomegaly Hemolysis

in an increase in cellular 5-aminolevulinic acid (ALA). Most patients are generally asymptomatic until some event stimulates the production of ALA. The deficiency of PBG deaminase activity results in relative ALA overproduction and consequent symptoms. Precipitating factors that lead to an acute exacerbation include (1) stimulation of ALA synthetase production in the liver; (2) endocrine factors including the female reproductive cycle; (3) fasting, especially in combination with alcohol intake; (4) induction of hepatic cytochrome P450 that leads to ALA synthetase production through a reduction in inhibitory heme; and (5) emotional stress, including surgery and chronic illness.[206] Clinical onset occurs most often after puberty and is more common in women, likely secondary to the effects of hormones and corticosteroids on the liver.

An acute attack is normally heralded by the presence of colicky abdominal pain, nausea, and vomiting, followed by the appearance of dark urine.[209] Patients may also complain of diarrhea or constipation. Classically, neurologic symptoms follow the onset of visceral complaints and may be highly variable. Patients may experience seizures, peripheral neuropathy, and cranial nerve deficits. They may become psychotic. Hyponatremia may be observed secondary to the syndrome of inappropriate antidiuretic hormone release (SIADH).

The cornerstone of treatment in AIP, as all acute porphyrias, includes the recognition and avoidance of precipitating factors. Once precipitating factors have been eliminated, glucose therapy (400 g/day) and/or heme arginate (3 mg/kg/day for 3 days) may be instituted.[206] Glucose and heme arginate work to decrease ALA

synthetase activity and have been found to reduce the urinary excretion of ALA and shorten the length of an acute attack.

In the patient with a history of acute porphyria, optimal perioperative care includes careful planning and communication between surgeons, anesthesiologists, and internists. Presurgical admission for intravenous hydration with glucose-containing fluids is an important step in the patient with a history of acute attacks. A large carbohydrate load may suppress the synthesis of ALA synthetase and may be beneficial.[210] The selection of appropriate anesthetics and analgesics is important, because many drugs frequently used in anesthesia have the capacity to induce ALA synthetase and cytochrome P450.[211,212] Table 5-7 summarizes the safety of various drugs frequently used in anesthesia. Many otherwise asymptomatic patients with AIP (or any acute porphyria) may present for anesthesia with a misdiagnosed "surgical" abdomen. Patients should be kept warm, because cold-induced stress may precipitate an acute crisis. Regional anesthesia has been used with success.[213]

Liver transplantation has been used successfully to cure AIP.[214] Attempts to treat other porphyrias with liver transplantation have met with mixed success.[215-219]

Wilson's Disease (Hepatolenticular Degeneration). Wilson's disease (WD) is an autosomal recessive disease that results in the abnormal accumulation of copper in the liver, kidney, and central nervous system. WD is one of the oldest diseases to be recognized as familial, being first described by Kinnear Wilson in 1912 as a progressive

TABLE 5–7	Porphyria and the Safety Anesthetics	
Generally Considered Safe	**Unclear**	**Generally Considered Unsafe**
Intravenous Agents		
Midazolam	Ketamine	Barbiturates
Lorazepam	Diazepam	Etomidate
Propofol		
Inhaled Agents		
Nitrous Oxide	Isoflurane	Enflurane
Desflurane	Halothane	
Analgesics		
Fentanyl	Alfentanil	
Morphine	Sufentanil	
Muscle Relaxants		
Succinylcholine	Atracurium	
Vecuronium	Pancuronium	
Local Anesthetics		
Bupivacaine	Lidocaine	
Procaine		
Various		
Atenolol		Glucocorticoids
Atropine		Hydralazine
Droperidol		
Labetalol		
Neostigmine		

Adapted from Jensen NF, Fiddler DS, Striepe V: Anesthetic considerations in porphyrias. Anesth Analg 1995;80:591-599; and Stevens JJ, Kneeshaw JD: Mitral valve replacement in a patient with acute intermittent porphyria. Anesth Analg 1996;82:416-418.

disease characterized by hepatic cirrhosis and softening of the lenticular nucleus.[220] Over the past century, WD has changed from a universally fatal familial disease to a treatable disease with multiple therapeutic options. WD is present in all populations and has an incidence of approximately 1:30,000 persons. The gene responsible has been located in chromosome 13. The disease is more common among Jewish eastern Europeans and certain Asian populations.[221]

Copper is an essential metal required for the normal function of a variety of enzymes including lysyl oxidase, superoxide dismutase, tyrosinase, and monoamine oxidase.[222,223] Copper metabolism is a complex process.[224] Briefly, copper is absorbed from the small intestine and bound to albumin. Over 90% of copper-bound albumin is taken up by the liver.[223] In the liver, copper binds to apo-ceruloplasmin to form ceruloplasmin. It is noteworthy that the incorporation of copper into apo-ceruloplasmin is an ATP-dependent process. Saturated with six molecules of copper, ceruloplasmin is released into the blood. Ceruloplasmin is also an acute phase reactant, with increased levels found in various inflammatory conditions. Throughout the body, copper is taken up by cells and delivered to its target enzymes after binding to various thiol-rich metallochaperones.[225]

The only physiologic means of copper excretion is through the bile. In WD, patients lose the ability to effectively mobilize copper for biliary excretion.[226] This defect leads to increased serum levels of copper. High levels of copper induce metallochaperone production. As metallochaperones are able to sequester copper in a nontoxic form, patients normally remain asymptomatic until copper supply overwhelms the absorptive power of metallochaperones. Ceruloplasmin levels are low in patients with WD, as they are in patients with liver cirrhosis of any cause.[227]

The presentation of WD varies widely. In general, patients present with symptoms of liver disease before the onset of neurologic symptoms.[228] Normally, WD presents in children and young adults with nonspecific symptoms including nausea, vomiting, and abdominal pain. Patients may give a history of mild, intermittent jaundice, and some patients may present with hepatomegaly or hepatosplenomegaly. WD may also present as fulminant hepatic failure[229,230] or an incidental, asymptomatic elevation of serum transaminases. WD can imitate a variety of liver diseases, including autoimmune hepatitis. WD should be considered in the differential diagnosis of established liver disease, even in the preschool-aged child.[231]

Most patients present with the neurologic manifestations of WD in adulthood. Pseudosclerosis is noted, and patients present with parkinsonian features or rigid dystonia. The classically described lenticular degeneration of WD tends to present in childhood and is more often associated with dystonia. Children are often described as having a "sardonic smile." The clinical hallmark of WD is the presence of a Kayser-Fleischer ring, a yellow-brown ring around the cornea. The Kayser-Fleischer ring is caused by copper deposition in Descemet's membrane. The ring is best demonstrated under slit lamp examination; however, the ring may be plainly visible. The Kayser-Fleischer ring is present in over 98% of patients with neurologic manifestations of WD and over 80% of patients with WD.[223] Approximately 30% of patients with WD will have psychiatric symptoms. The most common symptoms include depression and irritability; however, patients may present with frank catatonia.[232,233]

The diagnosis of WD requires a high index of suspicion, because the presentation is similar to many causes of cirrhosis. Indeed, WD may underlie coexisting liver disease. In general, the diagnosis should be considered in any patient younger than 40 with the signs and symptoms of hepatic dysfunction, especially in cirrhotic patients with unexplained central nervous system dysfunction. As noted earlier, the presence of a Kayser-Fleischer ring and a low serum ceruloplasmin level virtually seals the diagnosis. In patients with normal ceruloplasmin levels, high urinary copper and high copper on liver biopsy may support the diagnosis.

D-Penicillamine is considered the gold standard in the medical treatment of WD. D-Penicillamine is capable of reversing the hepatic, neurologic, and psychiatric manifestations of WD. Penicillamine therapy is not likely to be effective in patients with fulminant failure, dystonia, or severe lenticular degeneration. Adverse reactions to penicillamine including rashes, lymphadenopathy, and a lupus-like syndrome. Life-threatening thrombocytopenia[234] or leukopenia[235] is uncommon. Because penicillamine has an anti-pyridoxine effect, pyridoxine should be supplemented. Trientine may be effective in penicillamine-sensitive patients.[236] Zinc, which may induce more metallochaperone production, is also effective.[237]

Liver transplantation may be required in cases of fulminant failure and will reverse the hepatic manifestations of WD.[238,239] Improvement of neurologic symptoms has been inconsistently reported.[238,240]

Anesthesia in patients with WD should include a careful preoperative assessment with regard to the multiple organ systems that can be affected. A preoperative platelet count should be obtained in any patient taking penicillamine. Because metoclopramide may exacerbate a patient's extrapyramidal symptoms, it should be avoided. Droperidol, promethazine, and prochlorperazine should also be avoided because they may aggravate preexisting movement disorders.

Drug-Associated and Other Toxic Liver Disease

The central circulatory position and metabolic roles of the liver have already been discussed, but once again deserve mention from the perspective of toxic injury. The liver receives high concentrations of ingested compounds by portal blood flow from the splanchnic bed. Hepatocytes in turn take up such compounds and subject them to the metabolic processes discussed previously with detoxification and biotransformation. An exhaustive list of naturally occurring substances, manufactured chemicals, and pharmacologic agents has been implicated in liver disease, with pharmaceuticals being the most common. Table 5-8 is intended to provide examples of the types of damage caused by representative agents but is in no way a

TABLE 5–8   Types of Toxic Hepatic Injury

Hepatocellular Damage	Representative Agents
Microvesicular fatty change	Tetracycline, salicylates, yellow phosphorus, ethanol
Macrovesicular fatty change	Ethanol, methotrexate, amiodarone
Centrilobular necrosis	Bromobenzene, carbon tetrachloride, acetaminophen, halothane, rifampin
Diffuse or massive necrosis	Halothane, isoniazid, acetaminophen, methyldopa, trinitrotoluene, *Amanita phalloides* (mushroom) toxin
Hepatitis, acute and chronic	Methyldopa, isoniazid, nitrofurantoin, phenytoin, oxyphenisatin
Fibrosis-cirrhosis	Ethanol, methotrexate, amiodarone, most drugs that cause chronic hepatitis
Granuloma formation	Sulfonamides, methyldopa, quinidine, phenylbutazone, hydralazine, allopurinol
Cholestasis (with or without hepatocellular injury)	Chlorpromazine, anabolic steroids, erythromycin estolate, oral arsenicals contraceptives, organic arsenicals

Reproduced, with permission from Crawford JM: The liver and the biliary tract. In Cotran RS, Kumar V, Collins T (eds): Robbins Pathologic Basis of Disease, 6th ed. Philadelphia, WB Saunders, 1999, p 869.

complete listing. Clinical manifestations range from minor asymptomatic biochemical changes to cholestatic signs and symptoms to massive liver necrosis, depending not only on the agent but also on the patient's pre-exposure condition, concurrent disease, and extent of exposure. *Toxic injury can thus be included in virtually every differential diagnosis in the patient with liver disease.*

Several distinctions are important in considering toxic liver disease. One issue concerns the type of toxicity of a substance. Although certain chemicals enter the body in toxic form, injury in most cases results from metabolites that, ironically, are usually the result of hepatic transformation. Another categorization of toxins is based on the consistency with which they cause disease. Intrinsic hepatotoxins consistently produce damage in a dose-dependent manner in otherwise healthy patients, most often with a short latency. *Amanita* mushrooms and trichlorethane are examples of intrinsic hepatotoxins. Idiosyncratic hepatotoxin exposure, in contrast, produces liver disease infrequently and to a variable severity after a variable latent period. The idiosyncratic pattern can obviously be extremely challenging diagnostically. Some idiosyncratic hepatotoxins produce mild symptoms or asymptomatic biochemical changes with routine exposure (e.g., isoniazid and halothane) but can cause severe liver disease in susceptible individuals and/or certain circumstances. Additionally, under certain conditions, even intrinsic hepatotoxins can produce variable injury in exposures otherwise considered safe (e.g., acetaminophen in the patient with alcoholic hepatic injury).

Inhalational Anesthetics. Hepatic injury associated with the administration of inhalational anesthetic agents is, of course, especially important to the anesthesiologist. Halothane was introduced into practice in 1956, and was found to be rarely associated with hepatic necrosis. It is now accepted that halothane actually produces at least two types of hepatotoxicity. In up to 20% of adults who receive a halothane anesthetic, patients will have a milder effect with slight increases in aminotransferases and variable clinical complaints of fever, nausea, and malaise. Somewhere in the range of 1 in 7,000 to 35,000 patients, depending on risk factors, will have fulminant hepatic necrosis that has been termed *halothane hepatitis.* Transaminases and bilirubin levels are elevated, and the patient is jaundiced and often encephalopathic. The classic histologic examination reveals hepatitis with centrilobular necrosis; zonal, bridging, and panlobular necrosis have been described. Risk factors include age (very rare in childhood), gender (twice as common in women), repeated exposure within 3 months (as much as a 15-fold increase), and perhaps a history consistent with the milder postoperative hepatotoxic symptoms listed earlier. The mortality rate has been reported to be 10% to 50%, although recovery is typically complete in survivors.

Halothane hepatitis is a model for idiosyncratic hepatotoxicity, and thus its mechanisms have been extensively investigated. A variety of observations including increased risk from re-exposure and the often-reported fever, rash, arthralgias, and eosinophilia led to research that has supported the theory of an immunologic basis for halothane hepatitis. Cytochrome P4502E1 metabolizes halothane to trifluoroacetyl chloride. This reactive molecule was initially investigated as a direct hepatotoxin. The current immunogenic theory, however, focuses on its acetylation of endoplasmic reticulum proteins. These trifluoroacetylated (TFA) proteins, in turn, are thought to serve as neoantigens that elicit an antibody response to both the altered proteins and native hepatocyte proteins in susceptible patients. Corroborating evidence includes the detection of TFA proteins in patients with a history of halothane exposure as well as antibodies to the TFA hapten (and carrier protein components) in patients with actual halothane hepatitis. Further support can be found in reports of cross sensitization to methoxyflurane and perhaps enflurane by prior halothane exposure. Additionally, while as much as 20% of absorbed halothane may be metabolized, newer agents undergo orders of magnitude less biodegradation (approximate values: enflurane 2% to 3%, sevoflurane 1% to 2%, isoflurane 0.2%, and desflurane 0.02%) and in correlated fashion are believed to be rarely or never the cause of hepatitis.

Ischemic Liver Injury

The manifestations of ischemic injury to the liver have been labeled as hepatic infarction, shock liver, centrilobular necrosis, and, most commonly, the inaccurate term *ischemic hepatitis.* As might be expected, hypotension and/or hypoxemia are the usual precipitating factors and result from a variety of processes ranging from obvious situations such as cardiac dysfunction, intraoperative events, and trauma, to less intuitive causes such as obstructive sleep apnea and heat stroke.

Diagnosis relies on identification of an offending episode and typical biochemical response. LDH usually shows very high elevations both in terms of absolute values and relative to transaminase elevations. Biopsy is not typically required but, when performed, demonstrates widespread necrosis of the central lobule with minimal inflammation. Severity ranges from subclinical biochemical changes to fulminant failure. Treatment is supportive with correction of instigating processes.

Liver Function in the Geriatric Patient

The liver exhibits functional and structural changes with aging. Decreased liver weight with fibrosis and proportionally decreased blood flow has been described. Functionally, reduced regenerative capacity, altered response to endocrine stimulation, and altered drug metabolism are relevant to the perioperative physician.[241] Overall function is relatively resilient to these changes, however. There is a paucity and conflict of data regarding the impact of age on risk in the geriatric patient undergoing anesthesia. For example, one series of patients in the 1980s undergoing portosystemic procedures showed better mortality in patients who were 55 and younger,[242] although differences in disease severities and comorbidities were either pronounced or not described. General survival of cirrhotics with bleeding varices in different eras have correlated with Child-Pugh classification but not age.[20,243] There is little evidence that age is an important perioperative risk factor compared with actual hepatic function.

Biliary Cirrhosis

Biliary cirrhosis is simply cirrhosis caused by biliary obstruction of any type, regardless of location in the biliary tree. Primary biliary disease is a defined as immunogenic disease of the intrahepatic bile ducts. Secondary biliary cirrhosis occurs with prolonged obstruction from mechanical causes, sclerosing cholangitis, and diseases that promote cholestasis such as biliary atresia and cystic fibrosis.

Primary Biliary Cirrhosis. Primary biliary cirrhosis (PBC) is an autoimmune disease commonly occurring with other autoimmune diseases (e.g., rheumatoid arthritis, CREST syndrome, pernicious anemia, and sicca complex). In the modern era, PBC is often diagnosed before actual cirrhotic changes and the name has thus become something of a misnomer. PBC follows a progression through four stages. It is first characterized by periductular inflammation and interlobular duct injury with granuloma formation, and then reactive ductular proliferation with cholestasis. Following this, there is decreasing inflammation but development of septal fibrosis and architectural disruption with worsening cholestasis. Finally, cirrhosis occurs with obliteration of normal bile ducts, continued inflammation, and cholestasis.

PBC has a 10:1 predilection for females, usually of middle age. Although it has been found in populations throughout the world, PBC is more prevalent and increasing in incidence in western countries. Alkaline phosphatase elevations and symptoms of fatigue and pruritus are typical but nonspecific early in the disease. Diagnosis is based on antimitochondrial antibodies with confirmatory liver biopsy. A variety of autoantibodies may be present, especially rheumatoid factor, anti-smooth muscle, and thyroid specific; these may occur without obvious coexisting disease. Advanced disease leads to the portal hypertension and liver failure of end-stage cirrhosis.

Liver failure typically occurs 5 to 10 years after diagnosis. Prognostic models appear to be more accurate than in many types of progressive liver disease and are helpful in considering the appropriate time for consideration of liver transplantation. Immunosuppressive drugs have had limited success in controlling the progression of PBC. Ursodeoxycholic acid (UDCA, a hydrophilic bile acid) has been shown to increase survival time without transplantation in PBC patients.[244] A report from a multicenter trial, however, did not find this benefit. These patients, who were allowed to continue UDCA or switch from placebo to UDCA on completion of the trial, did not experience significant improvement of transplant-free survival.[245] UDCA currently remains a standard treatment for PBC, but further evaluation through large-scale studies is anticipated.[246]

Secondary Biliary Cirrhosis. Prolonged biliary obstruction, whether intrahepatic or extrahepatic (also known as extrinsic or mechanical obstruction), can lead to cirrhosis regardless of etiology. Obviously, a multitude of diseases can cause secondary biliary cirrhosis. Primary sclerosing cholangitis is the most common cause of secondary intrahepatic cholestasis but is still less common than PBC. In infancy and early childhood, cholestatic syndromes associated with atresia of intrahepatic and/or extrahepatic ducts often demonstrate rapid progression to fibrosis. Even when relief of obstruction is possible, this progression is not reliably halted. Adults more typically suffer from extrahepatic cholestasis such as chronic pancreatitis with stricture, pancreatic cancer, and choledocholithiasis.

Presentation and diagnosis depend on the instigating process, but jaundice and pruritus are often present. Alkaline phosphatase is typically highly elevated both absolutely (greater than four times normal) and relative to other liver panel abnormalities. Treatment involves diagnosis and treatment of the cause of cholestasis. Extrahepatic obstruction is often successfully relieved by surgical or endoscopic procedures. Intrahepatic obstruction is more problematic with limited curative options. Biliary atresia is an example. In this disease of infants in which initially normal bile ducts are obliterated in the first 3 months of life, most children will not survive to their first birthday without treatment. The Kasai procedure (hepatoportoenterostomy), in which a hilar core is opened so as to allow the cut bile ducts to drain unobstructed, can delay cirrhosis until the age of 3 to 4 years. Biliary atresia, however, remains the most common reason for liver transplantation in younger children.

Pregnancy-Associated Liver Disease

One to 3 percent of gravid patients can be expected to have liver test abnormalities at some point during their pregnancy. Patients with preexisting liver disease may experience deterioration during pregnancy, and pregnant patients can develop coincident liver disease. This section will focus on liver processes uniquely associated with pregnancy.

Most biochemical tests remain within the normal ranges of the general population during pregnancy. Exceptions include alkaline phosphatase and albumin. Alkaline phosphatase production by the placenta causes elevations in early pregnancy, eventually reaching levels that are three to four times normal nongravid values. Although albumin production is thought to be normal in pregnancy, increased blood volumes result in serum albumin decreases of about 1 g/dL.

Intrahepatic Cholestasis of Pregnancy (IHCP). IHCP occurs commonly in pregnancy, with great variation between populations. Its cause is unknown, but associated factors include a personal or family history of IHCP and history of cholestasis with oral contraceptives. Onset is usually in the third trimester, typically with symptoms of pruritus, nausea, and in some cases abdominal pain. Jaundice occurs in about one fourth of patients, typically weeks after the onset of pruritus. Alkaline phosphatase is usually elevated beyond the normal increases of pregnancy, and transaminases are usually normal but may occasionally be slightly elevated. In those rare cases in which liver biopsy is performed, histologic findings are usually limited to cholestasis without inflammatory or necrotic changes.

IHCP usually has minimal maternal impact; resolution of symptoms and laboratory abnormalities is typically complete within a month of delivery. The incidence of premature delivery and perhaps perinatal mortality is increased. Treatment includes observation of mother and fetus, ursodeoxycholic acid, which decreases pruritus and may slow IHCP progression, and prophylactic administration of vitamin K to compensate for cholestatic malabsorption.

Preeclampsia and Eclampsia. Preeclampsia occurs in up to 10% of pregnancies in general. Preeclampsia is the triad of hypertension (greater than 140/90 mm Hg), proteinuria (greater than 300 mg/24 hr), and edema, usually occurring in the late second or third trimester that cannot be attributed to other causes. Eclampsia occurs when seizures are superimposed upon preeclampsia, which happens in about 0.3% of preeclamptic patients. The pathophysiology of preeclampsia is thus far undefined, although theories abound. Popular proposed mechanisms often overlap and include endothelial cell injury, abnormal spiral artery development with compromised placental perfusion, thromboxane imbalance with prostacyclin, intravascular volume contraction, and abnormal renal function. Recent attention has focused on disruption of endothelial production of nitric oxide, prostacyclin, and tissue plasminogen activator. This approach emphasizes the change in vascular tone as well as coagulation changes.

Serum transaminases ranging from several times normal to as high as 100 times normal are found in nearly 25% of preeclamptics and 90% of those with eclampsia. Symptoms include epigastric or right upper quadrant discomfort. Complications that are believed to be associated with preeclampsia and eclampsia are hepatic rupture and/or infarction, fulminant hepatic failure, and subcapsular hematoma. Biopsy has demonstrated periportal fibrin deposition and areas of necrosis. Treatment is delivery, after which rapid normalization of laboratory values is typical. This decision is relatively straightforward when the fetus has an adequate maturity profile to ensure viability with delivery but problematic earlier in pregnancy. Delay in delivery entails risk of progression of preeclampsia but is believed to confer improved outcome on the fetus.

HELLP Syndrome. The syndrome of hemolysis, elevated liver enzymes, and low platelets occurs in late pregnancy and usually with at least some of the signs of preeclampsia. Moderate transaminase elevations and thrombocytopenia are defining conditions of HELLP. Microangiopathic hemolysis is thought to be related to fibrin deposition; it produces schistocytes and fragment cells on peripheral smear, elevated serum LDH, and decreased hemoglobin. Biopsy, although rarely required, reveals periportal or focal necrosis and sinusoidal fibrin deposition with hemorrhage.

Maternal complications of HELLP include seizures (eclampsia), placental abruption, and disseminated intravascular coagulation. Fetal complications include prematurity, intrauterine growth retardation, and increased perinatal mortality as high as 30% in some earlier series. Treatment, as with preeclampsia, is delivery. Liver transaminases typically normalize within 1 week, whereas platelet counts continue to decline for 24 to 48 hours post partum and eventually normalize in 2 weeks.

Hepatic Infarction or Rupture. Hepatic rupture is thought to occur in about 1 in 200,000 pregnancies, most often in association with preeclampsia or eclampsia, less often with acute fatty liver of pregnancy or HELLP syndrome, and extremely rarely without associated hepatic disease. Clinically, infarction or rupture presents as acute abdominal pain and distention, vomiting, and shock in the third trimester or immediately postpartum. Elevated transaminases, anemia, and disseminated intravascular coagulation are common, but the diagnosis can be confirmed with magnetic resonance imaging or computed tomography when time allows. Bedside ultrasound may be invaluable as a time-saving diagnostic tool. Survival requires early diagnosis and rapid treatment. Surgical intervention has included packing of the liver, resection of the involved segment or lobe (usually right), and even transplantation. Radiographically guided embolization has also been described in cases limited to a single lobe.

Acute Fatty Liver of Pregnancy (AFLP). AFLP occurs in the third trimester of pregnancy and is of variable severity but can be fatal. It occurs in about 1 in 15,000 pregnancies and is more likely to occur in preeclamptic patients. Clinical presentation reflects the severity of the disease and ranges from nausea, abdominal pain, and general malaise to progressive liver failure with jaundice, coagulopathy, encephalopathy, and uremia. Expected laboratory abnormalities include elevated transaminases, prolonged clotting times, hypoglycemia, and uremia. Liver biopsy will demonstrate centrilobular microvesicular fatty deposition with either absent or minimal inflammation and necrosis. Essential hepatic architecture is preserved and eventual regression to normal hepatic tissue is found in survivors. Treatment is delivery, the delay of which must include a thoughtful assessment of fetal viability balanced against the possibility of rapid deterioration. Liver transplantation has been described as a treatment for AFLP, but timely delivery appears to result in complete reversibility of the disease in most cases.

SYSTEMIC EFFECTS OF LIVER DISEASE

The diseased liver's pervasive impact on the function of other organ systems might be predicted by its myriad roles in health. The discussion that follows is intended to briefly outline systemic abnormalities associated with hepatic dysfunction that are of particular concern in the perioperative period.

Cardiovascular Effects of Liver Disease

The impact of chronic liver disease on the cardiovascular system is extremely complex and variable from patient to patient and under different circumstances within the same patient. The special considerations of portal hypertension are discussed with ascites in a separate section.

The cardiovascular profile of the cirrhotic patient is classically described as a hyperdynamic state with markedly increased cardiac output, low systemic vascular resistance, and modestly reduced arterial blood pressure. Despite this sustained elevation in cardiac output, functional exercise capacity of the cirrhotic is decreased. Available data show that cirrhotic patients undergoing exercise testing respond with lower than normal peak heart rates, lack of increased left ventricular ejection fraction, abnormally increased end-diastolic volumes with subnormal maximal cardiac outputs, and autonomic reflex abnormalities.[247]

Absolute intravascular volume is usually increased in cirrhotic patients, but coexisting renal disease, the impact of synthetic failure via decreased oncotic pressures, treatment of ascites with paracentesis and/or diuretics, and other factors may dramatically affect intravascular volume. Even with increased intravascular volume, the actual clinical behavior of the patient is often that of relative hypovolemia. Generalized vasodilatation,

widespread arteriovenous shunting, and depressed cardiac response are presumed to be major responsible factors. Decompensation with abrupt decreases in volume may be related to attenuated sympathetic effects on the heart and the systemic vasculature. Furthermore, while the healthy liver can displace a portion of its blood volume into the central circulation with sympathetic simulation, this compensatory mechanism is impaired or absent in the setting of cirrhosis.

Portal Hypertension and Ascites

The appreciation of esophageal variceal bleeding from cirrhotic obstruction of portal blood flow and the actual term portal hypertension are over 100 years old. The consequences of portal hypertension such as ascites, variceal hemorrhage, and encephalopathy still cause significant morbidity and mortality in advanced liver disease today.

In western societies, portal hypertension is most often associated with cirrhosis. Portal hypertension can actually be found in a variety of situations, however, and its causes have been categorized by mechanism and location. This way of considering portal hypertension incorporates both the forward and backward models of portal hypertension that have been variously favored in the past. Elevated pressure can result primarily from increased flow, increased resistance to flow, or both. If increased resistance is present, it may be prehepatic, intrahepatic (presinusoidal, sinusoidal, or postsinusoidal), or posthepatic. Box 5-2 demonstrates this categorization schema with several examples. The relative resistance of portosystemic collateral pathways, while not causal, will affect the degree of portal hypertension.

Pressure within the portal vein is usually less than 10 mm Hg, although variability is introduced by the influence of intra-abdominal pressure on the absolute venous pressure. The hepatic venous pressure gradient (HPG) can be used to control for this variability and attempt to localize the cause of increased portal venous pressure.

BOX 5–2 Categorization and Examples of Portal Hypertension Etiologies

Increased flow predominates
   (Arterial-portal fistula, splenic hemangiomatosis)
Increased resistance predominates
   Prehepatic (portal vein thrombosis, splenic vein thrombosis)
   Intrahepatic
      Presinusoidal (schistosomiasis, azathioprine)
      Sinusoidal (cirrhosis, alcoholic hepatitis, methotrexate)
      Postsinusoidal (Budd-Chiari syndrome)
   Posthepatic (caval web, cardiogenic: right-sided heart failure, tricuspid regurgitation)

HPG is the gradient between hepatic venous pressure and the wedged hepatic venous pressure. The latter, in a manner analogous to pulmonary artery occlusion pressure, estimates the intrasinusoidal pressures of the liver. Shortcomings of this measurement include variable sinusoidal communications arising from different pathologic processes causing resultant variability in pressures, as well as measurement from the efferent vessel causing occlusion artifact. When available, HPG can be used to localize etiology (e.g., HPG would be normal if the cause of portal hypertension were prehepatic) and monitor therapeutic interventions (e.g., sequential HPG can be used to verify improvement after β blockade). Portal hypertension is typically defined as an absolute pressure greater than 10 mm Hg or an HPG of greater than 5 mm Hg. The HPG at which portosystemic collaterals begin to develop appears to be 10 to 12 mm Hg in alcoholic cirrhosis.[248] These are most commonly gastroesophageal varices. Variceal bleeding is believed to be possible with an HPG of greater than 12 to 15 mm Hg, although the degree of elevation above this threshold is poorly related to bleeding risk.

Whether by the development of varices or intentional portosystemic shunt procedures, significant portal blood flow can bypass the liver to the systemic venous circulation. This circumvention of hepatocyte processing has been implicated in the prolonged and exaggerated effects of medications with high hepatic extraction, persistence of endogenous vasodilating substances usually cleared by the liver, and hepatic encephalopathy (discussed later).

Ascites is often present in the setting of severe cirrhosis and portal hypertension. As described previously, the normal sinusoid is lined with fenestrated endothelium and has no basement membrane. The normal sinusoidal pressure is low enough as to be nearly balanced by oncotic pressure. With increasing sinusoidal pressure, however, protein and fluid move into the interstitium with increased volume and increasing protein content of hepatic interstitial fluid and lymph. This flow eventually exceeds lymphatic return and accumulates in the abdomen as ascites. Interestingly, as the sinusoids develop a pseudo–basement membrane (so-called capillarization as previously described) less protein transudates through the now partially obstructed fenestrations. As a result, the protein content of the ascitic fluid can decrease with advancing disease.

The long-standing treatment of ascites includes diuretic therapy and paracentesis in conjunction with sodium restriction. Intravenous infusion of albumin with paracentesis has decreased the rapidity of ascites reaccumulation in some patients, perhaps because of the sinusoidal changes mentioned earlier. In any case, the treatment of ascites results in some decrease of intravascular volume.

Renal Effects of Liver Disease

Renal function is commonly reduced in advanced liver disease. Processes such as infection or immune-mediated disease may primarily affect both the liver and kidneys. However, in cirrhosis and sometimes in acute liver failure, renal function can deteriorate as a secondary consequence of liver dysfunction. This phenomenon is termed *hepatorenal syndrome* (HRS). Prerenal failure and acute tubular necrosis can also occur in the setting of severe liver disease. They are discussed briefly with emphasis on their sometimes difficult, but important, differentiation from hepatorenal syndrome.

HRS is the type of renal failure specifically associated with advanced liver disease. It usually occurs in patients with ascites. As previously discussed, advanced liver disease often produces a cardiovascular profile of high cardiac output with low peripheral resistance and a relative, if not absolute, hypovolemia. This can predictably result in renal dysfunction of hypoperfusion ("prerenal") etiology. However, in HRS, the decrease in renal cortical flow appears exaggerated. The reduction in total renal and especially cortical blood flow is reduced before there is any clinical evidence of renal injury. Cortical blood flow can actually be significantly decreased even with normal glomerular filtration rates. Such patients, with an increased resistive index by Doppler studies, are at high risk to proceed to renal insufficiency.[249] The proposed sites and mechanisms of renal vasoconstriction occurring paradoxically in a patient with generalized vasodilation are active topics of discussion. Suggested mediators that are abnormally produced or become imbalanced within the kidney as a result of liver disease include prostaglandins, nitric oxide, catecholamines, and endothelins.[250,251] HRS is commonly designated as type I or type II. Type I occurs acutely over days in patients with marginal hepatic function and is associated with instigating factors such as gastrointestinal bleeding, infection, or hypovolemia in about one half of cases. Type II HRS is slowly progressive and occurs in patients with better-preserved and more stable hepatic function who often have recalcitrant ascites. Diagnostic criteria[252] for HRS are (1) advanced liver disease with portal hypertension; (2) an elevated serum creatinine or decreased creatinine clearance; (3) absence of other etiology; (4) lack of response to volume expansion; and (5) absence of proteinuria, obstructive uropathy, or parenchymal renal disease. Despite specific criteria, accurate diagnosis appears to be problematic.[253] This has ramifications both for patients who may have a more reversible process that is not considered and for the interpretation of HRS series that may include (and exclude) misdiagnosed patients.

Although the kidney in HRS remains essentially unchanged histologically and function may return to normal after liver transplantation,[254] spontaneous recovery is rare and there is currently no other definitive treatment. Promising work with animal models using vasopressin analogs may be coming to fruition. The mechanism of this treatment appears to be related to vasoconstriction of the splanchnic circulation. This is theorized to improve effective blood volume and perhaps suppress rennin-angiotensin and sympathetic activity to more normal ranges. Simple volume expansion, interestingly, is not particularly effective,[255] but colloid infusion may improve the response to V1 vasopressin agonists.[256] Experience is thus far limited,[256-258] and ischemic complications were problematic in a series using ornipressin.[259]

The diagnosis of *prerenal failure* should be considered because it may well be reversible if treated promptly. The question of whether prerenal failure can progress to HRS in some patients is unanswered but must be of concern. *Acute tubular necrosis* (ATN), when it occurs, is often precipitated by a combination of sustained hypoperfusion and nephrotoxic agents such as nonsteroidal anti-inflammatory analgesics, contrast dye, and aminoglycoside antibiotics. Elevated bilirubin, which itself has been postulated to be nephrotoxic, is associated with an increased incidence of ATN.

Characteristics helpful in distinguishing prerenal failure and HRS are limited. HRS sometimes demonstrates tubular damage with proteinuria and, in fact, may progress to ATN. Urine sodium will be low in both processes, whereas urinary creatinine will be high compared with levels in the plasma. Proteinuria, high urine sodium, and low urine creatinine are typical of ATN. Volume challenge of the patient with renal dysfunction is a logical approach to diagnose and begin treatment of prerenal failure.

Pulmonary Effects of Liver Disease

The diseased liver impacts lung function in a variety of ways, sometimes with obvious mechanisms. Nearly 10% of patients with cirrhosis, for example, will develop pleural effusion. Classically termed *hepatic hydrothorax,* such effusions are initially transudative and more commonly occur on the right side. Effusion can occasionally occur in isolation but is most typically associated with ascites. In the more typical latter case, transdiaphragmatic communications between the peritoneal and pleural cavities are thought to allow movement of fluid into the chest. The impact on lung mechanics includes decreased lung volumes and pulmonary compliance, as well as elevated pleural pressures (abnormalities also caused by massive ascites). Moderate hypoxemia, thought to be an effect predominately of intrapulmonary shunt, is common, but improvement after evacuation of the effusion is unpredictable.[260] Without resolution of the hepatic process, repeated thoracenteses and perhaps portosystemic shunting may be required.

Some diseases that affect the liver will also primarily affect the lung; examples include cystic fibrosis, α_1-antitrypsin deficiency, sarcoidosis, and primary biliary cirrhosis. Several descriptions also exist of patients undergoing sclerosis of esophageal varices who develop a range of pulmonary deterioration. These problems range from worsening hypoxemia and decreased vital capacity to full-blown adult respiratory distress syndrome. The etiology of these problems may have been embolization of particular sclerosants.[261]

Two poorly understood syndromes that are sometimes confused but have very different findings and implications are *hepatopulmonary syndrome* and *portopulmonary hypertension.* Table 5-9 summarizes their contrasting definitions, signs and symptoms, and management. In hepatopulmonary syndrome, peripheral pulmonary vasculature (precapillary and capillary) has characteristic vascular dilatations. These dilatations are thought to increase the distance between enough centrally flowing red cells and the alveoli to impair oxygenation. This effect is exaggerated in the sitting position with increased basilar blood flow, accounting for the symptoms of platypnea (worsened shortness of breath in the upright position) and orthodeoxia. Supplemental oxygen will typically improve saturation, but no other medical treatments have been consistently effective. Liver transplantation is usually an effective treatment, although improvement may be seen only after several months. Portopulmonary hypertension is a distinctly different process that appears histologically similar to primary pulmonary hypertension with medial hypertrophy. Pulmonary artery pressures may respond to vasodilators such as intravenous or inhaled epoprostenol or inhaled nitric oxide. The mortality of liver transplantation in patients with portopulmonary hypertension and mean pulmonary artery pressures of greater than 40 mm Hg is considered to be prohibitively high, although there are scattered case reports of survivors.[262] At this time it appears that recent onset and aggressive preoperative therapy[263] of portopulmonary hypertension may be associated with improved outcome.

Hepatic Encephalopathy

Hepatic encephalopathy can be associated with either acute or chronic liver disease and can itself be slowly progressive or, usually with an instigating process, deteriorate rapidly. It is a neuropsychiatric disorder that should be a diagnosis of exclusion. Differential diagnoses include intracranial processes (e.g., hemorrhage, tumor, or abscess), hypoxemia, neurologic infection, sepsis, and metabolic encephalopathy. Primary neuropsychiatric disorders can have similar presentations.

Clinical observation and admittedly limited animal models have led to the generally accepted concept that hepatic encephalopathy is caused by the failure of the liver

TABLE 5–9 Distinguishing Hepatopulmonary Syndrome and Portopulmonary Hypertension

	Hepatopulmonary Syndrome	Portopulmonary Hypertension
Defining Characteristics	Liver dysfunction Intrapulmonary vascular dilatations (IPVD) Abnormal alveolar-arterial oxygen gradient (>15 mm Hg with room air) Other cardiopulmonary causes excluded	Lack of general agreement Commonly cited criteria: 　Portal hypertension 　Resting PAPm > 25 　PAOP < 15 　Other causes excluded
Common Symptoms	Platypnea Orthodeoxia Arterial desaturation	Orthopnea Dyspnea on exertion Fatigue
Common Signs and Diagnostics	Clubbing Decreased DLco CE-Echo positive	Hypoxemia with exertion Elevated PAP
Management	Oxygen supplementation Liver transplantation	Vasodilator trial

PAP, pulmonary artery pressure; PAPm, mean PAP; PAOP, pulmonary artery occlusion pressure; DLco, carbon monoxide diffusing capacity; CE-Echo positive, contrast enhanced echocardiography: positive when contrast appears in left side of heart within three to six cardiac cycles of appearance in right side of heart and in the absence of another cause.

to clear neurotoxins or their precursors arising from the gut. Box 5-3 lists several substances currently being considered in the development of hepatic encephalopathy. A brief discussion of several of these theories will provide an opportunity to also explain justifications for current treatments used in hepatic encephalopathy. *Ammonia* is generally believed to play a central role in hepatic encephalopathy. It is produced by colonic bacterial activity and small bowel deamination of glutamine, absorbed into the portal circulation and, in health, removed by the liver. Hepatic dysfunction, especially in association with portosystemic shunting, allows increased systemic ammonia concentrations. Glutamine synthetase inhibition can blunt cerebral edema and intracranial hypertension in animals with portocaval shunting and ammonia infusions.[264] This observation has supported the concept that central nervous system metabolism of ammonia with resultant increases of glutamine leads to an osmotic gradient capable of causing cerebral edema. Ammonia is also capable of altering the blood-brain barrier and influencing glutamate-associated neurotransmission.

Despite these interesting findings, blood ammonia levels have not consistently correlated with the severity of hepatic encephalopathy. Lactulose, however, is still a mainstay of treatment for hepatic encephalopathy. The therapeutic mechanisms of lactulose are purportedly both acidification of the gut and catharsis resulting in decreased ammonia absorption. Ammonia load can be further decreased with poorly absorbed antibiotics that decrease bacterial activity, decreased protein ingestion, and control of gastrointestinal bleeding. *γ-Aminobutyric acid* (GABA) has received attention because in animal models of hepatic encephalopathy both expression of GABA receptors and blood-brain GABA movement were found to be increased. With the introduction of flumazenil and other investigational benzodiazepine antagonists, interest was focused on the GABA receptor within the context of its interaction with benzodiazepines. Some patients with hepatic encephalopathy do, in fact, improve with benzodiazepine antagonists. The effect, however, is variable and of unpredictable duration. The *false neurotransmitter* or amino acid imbalance theory is based on the increased proportion of aromatic as compared with branched-chain amino acids often found in patients with hepatic encephalopathy. Increased aromatic amino acids are proposed to be the precursors for false neurotransmitters such as octopamine, tyramine, and phenethylamine. Clinically, branched-chain amino-acid supplementations have been reported to improve hepatic encephalopathy and investigation of the therapeutic mechanism is ongoing.[265]

The severity of hepatic encephalopathy is assessed on the basis of cognitive function, behavior, motor function, and level of consciousness. As shown in Table 5-10, a stage of 1 through 4 can be assigned according to these changes.

BOX 5–3 Theorized Pathogenic Substances in Hepatic Encephalopathy

Ammonia
γ-Aminobutyric acid (GABA)
True neurotransmitters
False neurotransmitters (aromatic amino acid excess)
Serotonin
Endogenous opioids
Manganese

TABLE 5-10   Stages of Hepatic Encephalopathy

Stage	1	2	3	4
Cognitive Function	Decreased attention	Obvious memory deficits	Amnesia, disorientation, incoherence	Absent
Behavior Characteristics	Irritable, anxious	Inappropriate (disinhibition)	Angry, paranoid, seizures	Absent
Motor Function	Tremor, fine motor loss	Asterixis, dysarthria, repeated blinking and yawning	Babinski reflex, nystagmus, altered deep tendon reflexes	Dilated pupils, decorticate or decerebrate posturing
Level of Consciousness	Normal, with altered sleep patterns	Lethargic, with ataxia	Confused, delirious, or stuporous	Comatose

ASSESSMENT OF PERIOPERATIVE RISK IN THE PATIENT WITH LIVER DISEASE

Estimation of perioperative risk in the patient with liver disease is problematic. Available data are often either outdated, retrospective, nonspecific to etiology, and/or of limited subject size. While acknowledging these shortcomings, generally accepted guidelines are summarized in Table 5-11, and expanded below.

Acute Hepatitis. High mortality rates from older studies are often quoted for patients undergoing elective surgery who have acute hepatitis. Patients were predominately undergoing exploratory laparotomy for the possibility of surgically correctable jaundice in an era before the availability of accurate noninvasive diagnostic techniques. These studies showed a mortality rate of approximately 10%[266,267] for viral hepatitis and nearly 55%[268,269] for alcoholic hepatitis. Acute hepatitis has thus been considered a contraindication to elective surgery, although these outcomes have not been retested in the setting of modern anesthetics and techniques.

Chronic Hepatitis. In chronic hepatitis, the patient's clinical and biochemical status should be used to assess perioperative risk. In the symptomatic patient with synthetic and/or excretory abnormalities, data from different eras indicate increased perioperative risk.[270,271] Conversely, well-compensated, asymptomatic chronic hepatitis appears to add little perioperative risk.[272]

Steatohepatitis. Fatty liver itself does not contraindicate elective surgery, whether of alcoholic or nonalcoholic etiology. It is important to verify that acute alcoholic injury is not also present and further to emphasize to the patient the importance of abstinence in avoiding direct parenchymal damage and worsening of perioperative liver abnormalities. Patients with severe steatohepatitis tend to show increased morbidity and mortality in major hepatobiliary surgery,[273] although other associated factors are surgical time and body mass index. Nonalcoholic steatohepatitis (NASH) has been presumed to be the etiology of increased cirrhosis in morbidly obese patients. Among patients undergoing gastric bariatric surgery, a voluntary

TABLE 5-11   Approach to the Patient with Liver Disease for Elective Surgery

Acute Hepatitis	Postpone surgery until normalization of biochemical profiles.
Chronic Hepatitis	Proceed with surgery if clinical course and laboratory parameters have been stable. Unspecified increased perioperative risk.
Obstructive Jaundice	Proceed with surgery, with attention to fluid resuscitation. Endoscopic or percutaneous preoperative biliary drainage controversial.
Cirrhosis: Child's A or B	Optimize and proceed with surgery. (See text for special concern in cases requiring cardiopulmonary bypass.) Coagulation: Goal of prothrombin time within 2 sec of normal. Parenteral vitamin K, if ineffective, then fresh frozen plasma and/or cryoprecipitate. Ascites: If conservative management (fluid restriction and/or diuretics) ineffective, then paracentesis. Encephalopathy: Evaluate and treat triggering processes (e.g., gastrointestinal bleeding, uremia, medications); consider lactulose.
Cirrhosis: Child's C	Postpone surgery while improving Child's classification or cancel surgery for nonsurgical management.

Adapted from: Rizvon MK, Chou CL: Surgery in the patient with liver disease. Med Clin North Am 2003;87:211-227.

multi-institutional survey[274] reported a previously undiagnosed cirrhosis incidence of nearly 6% and a mortality in this group of 4%, all deaths being postoperative. More recent data from a single institution's 48 consecutive bariatric patients found 33% to have NASH and a further 12% to have advanced fibrosis;[275] mortality figures were not reported, but NASH and fibrosis were both associated with diabetes mellitus but not body mass index in this obese population.

Cirrhosis. Cirrhosis is the liver abnormality for which most perioperative data exist and for which a generally accepted classification has been developed and verified. Specifically, the Child-Turcotte and Child-Pugh classifications of cirrhosis have been demonstrated to correlate well with perioperative mortality rates (Table 5-12). Data from the 1980s[276] and 1990s[277] show remarkably similar mortalities of approximately 10% for Child's A, 30% for Child's B, and 80% for Child's C in patients undergoing open abdominal procedures. Recent experience indicates that laparoscopic cholecystectomy[278-280] is better tolerated in Child's A and B cirrhotics, even considering higher conversion to open procedures than controls. Endoscopic intervention is often chosen for Child's C patients.

The distinction between Child's A and Child's B disease may be important in patients undergoing cardiopulmonary bypass. Two very small series indicate that Child's A patients will experience a marginal increase in complications, but reported a 50% to 80%[281,282] mortality in their Child's B patients.

ANESTHETIC MANAGEMENT

Concern for liver function may arise in a variety of clinical scenarios. A patient presenting for any elective procedure may have previously undetected laboratory abnormalities with which no symptoms have been associated. The patient with obvious jaundice or ascites, on the other hand, may present for related diagnostic or therapeutic interventions. Patients with advanced and/or life-threatening hepatic dysfunction may require interventions such as biliary decompression, partial hepatic resection, and liver transplantation; alternatively, these patients may require unrelated emergency procedures such as appendectomy, fracture repair, or cesarean delivery, with significant risk posed by their hepatic process.

The dilemmas faced by clinicians in these situations have been already implied in earlier sections. Laboratory value profiles are helpful, but not specific, in diagnosing disease processes. Perioperative data for specific diseases are limited and often reflect a variety of diagnostic criteria, anesthetic management techniques, and eras. Additionally, assessment of hepatic reserve is problematic. Although extraction tests have been used to assess hepatic function (particularly in transplant candidates)[283,284] and newer nuclear imaging techniques show promise for risk stratification in the future,[285,286] neither are well correlated with operative risk, nor are they universally available.

Anesthetic management is discussed from two perspectives. First, management issues ranging from asymptomatic laboratory abnormalities to fulminate failure are addressed. Anesthetic considerations for procedures directly involving the liver are then discussed. Supporting data, when available, are cited. Management recommendations are otherwise based on common practice, available reports, and/or the authors' opinions.

Anesthetic Management for Patients with Liver Dysfunction

Newly Discovered Asymptomatic Abnormal Laboratory Values

Previous series have reported the incidence of elevated transaminases in asymptomatic patients without prior diagnostic abnormality to range from less than 1% to greater than 10%. In the 1970s, an often-quoted study[287] found that 11 of 7620 (0.14%) patients scheduled for elective surgery had unexpected significant elevations of liver function tests. Of particular interest, 3 of these 11 patients developed jaundice even though their surgical procedures were canceled. A large series of asymptomatic patients undergoing nondirected screening indicates that the prevalence of asymptomatic elevations may be much

TABLE 5–12 Child-Pugh Classification of Cirrhosis			
Factor and Score	1	2	3
Serum Bilirubin (mg/dL)	<2.0	2.0-3.0	>3.0
Serum Albumin (g/dL)	>3.5	3.0-3.5	<3.0
Ascites	None	Easily controlled	Poorly controlled
Prothrombin Time Prolongation	0-4	4-6	>6
(INR)	(<1.7)	(1.7-2.3)	(>2.3)

The Child-Pugh score is calculated by adding the scores of the five factors (possible scores therefore range from 5-15). Child's Class is A (5 or 6), B (7, 8, or 9), or C (10 and greater).

BOX 5–4   **Differential Diagnosis of New Asymptomatic LFT Abnormalities** (See Table 5-1 for Typical Patterns)

False positive (especially likely in asymptomatic patients
  without risk factors)
Early and/or subclinical hepatitis
Nonalcoholic steatohepatitis
Drug or toxic effect
Ischemic injury
Infiltrative process
Biliary disease

higher 3 decades later. Approximately 15% of 2294 patients were found to have transaminase levels greater than normal range, and nearly 4% had levels greater than twice normal.[288] The authors considered a high prevalence of nonalcoholic steatohepatitis as a likely cause for their findings. Other likely and important diagnoses are listed in Box 5-4.

Approximately one third of asymptomatic patients without risk factors will have normal values on repeated laboratory evaluation. Conversely, acute hepatitis is still considered a contraindication to elective surgery. The cautious and often recommended path would be to postpone elective surgery until further evaluation, signs, and symptoms allow either determination of etiology or resolution of the undefined process. Other authors[289] have advocated a tiered response. In the latter approach, for example, if transaminases were elevated less than two times normal, risk factors for acute hepatitis would be reassessed. If the absence of risk factors was confirmed, this algorithm would then proceed to elective surgery. Regardless of the approach chosen, careful reassessment of the patient's history is indicated as outlined in Box 5-5. The divided opinion of experts reflects the unanswered dilemma for the clinician, which is to determine when acute hepatitis has been adequately excluded to justify the delivery of an anesthetic for elective surgery.

BOX 5–5   **Asymptomatic Laboratory Abnormalities: Critical Questions and Further Diagnostic Strategy to Discuss with Patient and/or Primary Medical Doctor**

Reassess risk factors for acute hepatitis.
  Viral hepatitis exposures
  Toxic exposures
  Alcohol history
  Medication history
Repeat liver panel laboratory studies (LFTs).
Order viral hepatitis laboratory studies, especially with even
  marginal indication from history.
Consider hepatology consultation for:
  Worsening LFTs and/or positive viral serology
  Transaminases that remain more than twice normal

Suspected or Known Acute Hepatitis

Patients with acute hepatitis should not be subjected to an anesthetic for an elective procedure. Some patients will require urgent surgery (1) without time for a definitive diagnosis or resolution of asymptomatic laboratory abnormalities or (2) with known acute hepatitis. It seems prudent to manage the former group with the same principles that would be applied for known acute hepatitis, and so these situations will be discussed together. (Acute hepatic failure is an entirely different entity that is discussed separately.) It is generally accepted (with supporting data but without absolute proof) that decreased hepatic blood flow is an important cause of perioperative hepatic dysfunction in patients with acute hepatitis and that efforts should therefore be made to maintain total blood flow to the liver. Peripheral procedures will have less impact than abdominal procedures, but procedure location is usually mandated by circumstance. In animal models and humans, it appears that halothane decreases total hepatic blood flow by decreasing both portal venous and hepatic arterial blood flow[290,291] and should be avoided. Isoflurane is the best studied alternative and appears to preserve hepatic blood flow markedly better than does halothane. Total intravenous anesthesia may prove to be another reasonable alternative in this setting. Positive-pressure ventilation and positive end-expiratory pressure of themselves would be expected to decrease liver flow,[292] but spontaneous ventilation with an elevated carbon dioxide and splanchnic sympathetic stimulation could also be detrimental. Drugs with known or suspected hepatotoxicity should be avoided, if possible. Examples are given in the prior discussion of hepatotoxins; an incomplete list is included in Box 5-6.

BOX 5–6   **Acute Hepatitis for Urgent Surgery: Intraoperative Management**

Preserve hepatic blood flow.
  Avoid halothane (isoflurane is best-studied alternative and
    better preserves flow).
  Consider regional anesthesia if procedure and coagulation
    allows.
  Maintain normocapnia.
  Avoid PEEP if possible.
  Provide generous volume maintenance.
Avoid medications with situational potential hepatotoxicity
  whenever possible. Examples:
  Halothane
  Acetaminophen, particularly in the alcoholic patient
  Sulfonamides, tetracycline, and penicillins
  Amiodarone
Perform postoperative surveillance clinically and biochemically
  for progression of hepatic dysfunction.
Suspect infectious etiology.
  Provider exposures treated as high risk for viral hepatitis

Cirrhosis

As previously described, cirrhosis is a sequela of many different types of liver injury and represents a histologic diagnosis rather than a single disease process. The key elements of disruption of normal architecture by scarring with nodules of regenerating parenchyma are common to all causes, but some causes have typical associated findings. Common causes of cirrhosis are listed in Box 5-7. These and several less common causes are detailed in previous sections, and a more complete list can be found in Box 5-1.

Ironically, the cirrhotic patient often suffers more from extrahepatic manifestations of his disease than from loss of hepatic parenchyma, per se. Such issues as coagulopathy and altered drug metabolism are important considerations, to be sure, but the anesthesiologist must be cognizant of a wide range of comorbidities and complications that occur with cirrhosis. Several important considerations are listed in Box 5-8.

Portal hypertension has already been discussed in terms of its role in the development of significant varices and ascites. The patient's history should be reviewed for portosystemic shunts such as a surgical splenorenal shunt or the now more common TIPS (transjugular intrahepatic portal systemic shunt) procedure. *Ascites* is important preoperatively for many reasons. Its presence may have led to treatment with spironolactone, paracentesis, or, in resistant cases, even the placement of a peritoneal-systemic shunt. All of these treatment modalities may result in blood volume and electrolyte abnormalities, which should be assessed preoperatively. Enthusiastic paracentesis can also cause or exacerbate hypoalbuminemia, depending on the character of the ascites.

All patients with cirrhosis and especially known portal hypertension should be considered to be at risk for having *esophageal varices.* These dilated veins communicating blood from the hypertensive portal system to lower

---

BOX 5–8 Comorbidities and Complications of Cirrhosis

Portal hypertension
Ascites
Variceal bleeding
Hypoalbuminemia
Coagulopathy
Renal dysfunction (hepatorenal syndrome as extreme presentation)
Central nervous system effects (hepatic encephalopathy as extreme presentation)
Hepatopulmonary syndrome
Pleural effusion(s)
Portopulmonary hypertension
Glucose intolerance
Circulatory changes: high cardiac output and low systemic vascular resistance

---

pressure systemic veins can be the source of massive bleeding. They may be treated with endoscopic sclerotherapy. Blind instrumentation of the esophagus should be undertaken with extreme caution if not avoided completely.

Abnormal PT and *hypoalbuminemia* reflect decreased synthetic reserve and/or increased loss or consumption. If time permits, the response to vitamin K can be determined, but otherwise fresh frozen plasma is often used to bring the PT within acceptable range. Hypofibrinogenemia or dysfibrinogenemia from altered synthesis and fibrinolysis may also be responsible for coagulopathy and may be treated with cryoprecipitate. *Thrombocytopenia,* thought to be caused by both splenic sequestration and decreased peripheral survival, should be addressed as required by the procedure in question. Qualitative abnormalities of platelet function, including abnormal activation, may also exist but are difficult to assess. Implications of the other listed comorbidities and complications of cirrhosis have been described in previous sections.

Review of the patient's history must recognize the multisystemic impact of cirrhosis. If time allows, correctable abnormalities of coagulation, metabolic status, and intravascular status, should be addressed preoperatively. Child's classification (see Table 5-12 and its earlier discussion) should be evaluated for some general sense of perioperative risk. It is important to remember that most patients with significant cirrhosis have at least some degree of cognitive dysfunction and memory lapse; verification of history and signs of early encephalopathy should be sought from objective observers. Other important considerations are listed in Box 5-9.

The course of cirrhosis can be stable for long periods, but this belies the minimal systemic reserve that is often present. Indeed, perturbations that would be minor and well tolerated in the healthy patient may precipitate decompensation in the cirrhotic patient. Dietary indiscretions,

---

BOX 5–7 Common Causes of Cirrhosis

Alcohol
Viral hepatitis
   Hepatitis B, C, and D (Delta)
Nonalcoholic steatohepatitis
Metabolic
   Wilson's disease
   Hemochromatosis
   α_1-Antitrypsin deficiency
   Diabetes mellitus
   Galactosemia
Autoimmune
Drug or toxin other than alcohol
Primary biliary cirrhosis
Cholestasis (prolonged)
Cystic fibrosis

BOX 5–9   Critical Questions to Ask Patients and/or Their Primary Medical Doctor

Etiology of cirrhosis
Complications of cirrhosis, particularly related to Child's classification
History of disease progression
History of therapeutic interventions
Current medications
Deterioration of status associated with current illness
Seek reliable confirmation: suspect patient's cognitive function and memory

infection, minor trauma, and medication interruptions, for example, may not be tolerated. In the same sense, procedures that would be considered minor in most patients may be major challenges to the cirrhotic patient, especially in the case of high Child's classification and/or significant preoperative deterioration.

Cirrhotic patients should be managed perioperatively with many of the same considerations as the patient with acute hepatitis (see previous section). Box 5-10 includes common additional cardiovascular, coagulation, and metabolic abnormalities that must also be addressed. Correction of PT to within 2 seconds of normal is generally recommended for invasive procedures. If time allows, vitamin K can be administered parenterally. Typically, however, fresh frozen plasma is used initially. Cryoprecipitate can be added if necessary. Portal hypertension and ascites may be present. Changes in pharmacokinetics and pharmacodynamics should be expected but are unpredictable. Drugs with high hepatic extraction are especially affected by portosystemic shunting of blood; highly protein-bound medications are affected by hypoalbuminemia with variable offset by increased gamma globulins, and the effects of drugs such as vasopressors (decreased) and sedatives (increased) may be altered.

Acute Liver Failure

Acute liver failure or fulminant hepatic failure can occur rarely with any number of insults to the liver that result in the loss of sufficient hepatic parenchyma to precipitate acute decompensation. Diagnosis of the syndrome requires acute hepatocellular failure (without prior significant liver disease) and encephalopathy. The time interval between onset of illness and progression to encephalopathy may be correlated with both etiology and prognosis. Ischemic hepatitis and many toxic injuries, for example, progress to encephalopathy in a matter of days; viral hepatitis and cryptogenic failure are more typically associated with a month between onset and the development of encephalopathy. Additionally, the presence of jaundice for more than a week before encephalopathy may indicate a poor prognosis. These observations have led to the use of various nomenclatures (Box 5-11) for acute hepatic failure. The discussion here uses the original definition in an attempt to avoid confusion.

Worldwide, the most common causes of acute liver failure are drugs, particularly acetaminophen, and viral hepatitis. Box 5-12 lists the more common causes in approximate order of likelihood for centers in the United Kingdom and

BOX 5–10   Anesthetic Preparation and Management in Cirrhosis

Consider same issues as in acute hepatitis (see previous discussion):
Preserve hepatic blood flow.
    Avoid halothane (Isoflurane is best studied alternative and better preserves flow).
    Consider regional anesthesia if procedure and coagulation allows.
    Maintain normocapnia.
    Avoid PEEP if possible.
    Provide generous volume maintenance.
Avoid medications with situational potential hepatotoxicity whenever possible. Examples:
    Halothane
    Acetaminophen, particularly in the alcoholic patient
    Sulfonamides, tetracycline, and penicillins
    Amiodarone
AND
Anticipate presence or development of abnormalities of:
    Coagulation
        Attempt to correct prothrombin time to within 2 seconds of normal.
        Consider cryoprecipitate if fresh frozen plasma ineffective or fibrinogen abnormality.

Correct thrombocytopenia appropriately for procedure.
Anticipate higher than normal blood loss for procedure.
Hemodynamics
Anticipate relative hypovolemia, worsened by treatment of ascites.
Assess for presence of high cardiac output, low peripheral resistance.
Suspect portal hypertension and/or variceal bleeding, even without history.
Anticipate depressed response to ionotropes and vasopressors.
Consider invasive monitoring.
Pharmacokinetics and pharmacodynamics
Altered volume of distribution may occur.
    Decreased serum albumin, increased gamma globulins.
    Intravascular volume is unpredictable, especially with ascites treatment.
Portosystemic shunted blood bypasses liver.
    Drugs highly extracted by liver especially affected.
Increased sensitivity to sedative medications may be present.

BOX 5–11 Nomenclatures of Acute Hepatic Failure

Original definition of acute hepatic failure or fulminant hepatic failure
Hepatocellular failure (jaundice or coagulopathy)
No prior diagnosis of significant liver disease
Encephalopathy within 8 weeks of onset
Nomenclature refinements based on syndrome development
Subfulminant hepatic failure
  Encephalopathy develops between 2 weeks and 3 months
    after jaundice.
Fulminant hepatic failure
  Encephalopathy develops within 2 weeks of jaundice
Hyperacute liver failure
Encephalopathy develops within 1 week of jaundice.
Acute liver failure
  Encephalopathy develops between 1 and 4 weeks of jaundice.
Subacute liver failure
  Encephalopathy develops between 5 and 12 weeks after
    jaundice.

BOX 5–13 Comorbidities and Complications Seen with Acute Liver Failure

Encephalopathy
  Cerebral edema with elevated intracranial pressure
  Other causes such as hypoxemia, electrolyte abnormality,
    hypoglycemia
Hemorrhage
  Gastrointestinal: typically gastric ulceration and not
    variceal origin
  Coagulopathy
Respiratory failure
  Adult respiratory distress syndrome
  Pneumonia and/or aspiration in encephalopathic patient
Renal failure
  Hypovolemia
  Acute tubular necrosis
  Hepatorenal syndrome
Hypoglycemia
Hypotension
  Relative hypovolemia
  Generalized vasodilatation
Sepsis

United States. The causes listed as uncommon have been reported as the cause of acute failure. The differential diagnosis of acute liver failure is very limited. Sepsis may be associated with cholestasis, disseminated intravascular coagulation, and encephalopathy without actual hepatocellular destruction. Factor VIII will often be suppressed in disseminated intravascular coagulation of sepsis but not in acute liver failure. Decompensation of chronic liver disease can also be confused with acute liver failure, particularly when a reliable patient history is not available.

Acute liver failure is a medical emergency, often of the gravest proportions. Etiology-specific therapy should be implemented when it exists. *N*-Acetylcysteine, for example, is used to treat acetaminophen toxicity, whereas emergency delivery is indicated for failure associated with fatty liver of pregnancy. A major dilemma occurs for the intensivist managing acute liver failure. Some patients, with appropriate supportive care, can survive with recovery of hepatic function. Patients with acetaminophen toxicity and hepatitis A are more likely to fall into this group. Others are

unlikely to survive without liver transplantation. There has been much interest and effort expended in devising,[293] verifying,[294-296] and refining[297] methods to separate these two groups. The patient who may be a candidate for transplantation should be transported to an experienced transplant center without delay. This allows the dual processes of constant reassessment of prognosis for recovery and transplant candidacy to be implemented.

Anesthesia should not be administered to patients with acute liver failure except for potentially life-saving emergency procedures. Management issues encompass not only the issues previously discussed for acute hepatitis but also attention to often severe neurologic, hemodynamic, and metabolic derangements. Boxes 5-13 and 5-14 outline relevant systemic effects of acute liver failure and additional information that should be sought from the critical care team, respectively.

Direct measurement of intracranial pressure (ICP) can be invaluable for advanced encephalopathy. Placement of a monitoring device does have substantial risk of bleeding

BOX 5–12 Etiology of Acute Liver Failure

Common
  Acetaminophen toxicity
  Hepatitis B
  Cryptogenic
  Hepatitis A (most common worldwide cause)
  Toxicity other than acetaminophen
Uncommon
  Wilson's disease
  Vascular disease
  Pregnancy associated
  Ischemia
  Reye's syndrome
  Infections other than hepatitis A and B

BOX 5–14 Critical Questions to Ask Patients and/or Medical Team

Any evidence of preexisting liver disease
Presumptive cause of acute liver failure
  Treatment instituted if appropriate (e.g., acetaminophen
    poisoning)
Course of neurologic deterioration
  Measures instituted to control intracranial pressure
Metabolic, cardiovascular, and coagulation support required
  thus far

and infection in this setting. Clinical indicators of damaging ICP increases under anesthesia, however, may be both delayed and insensitive. If direct monitoring is not available, patients should be presumed to have elevated ICP with poor intracranial elastance. Maintenance of adequate cerebral perfusion pressure may be problematic because of relative hypovolemia and generalized vasodilatation.

Hemorrhage should be anticipated in acute liver failure. Severe coagulopathy often requires extensive transfusion. Gastrointestinal bleeding tends to be related to stress ulcerations, rather than the variceal bleeding found in chronic liver disease. Hypoglycemia can be profound because of decreased intake and loss of hepatic release. Adult respiratory distress syndrome (ARDS) occurs frequently in acute liver failure and can present a dilemma in attempting to avoid hypercapnia for ICP concerns while avoiding ventilatory pressure and volume lung injury in ARDS. Renal failure has been attributed to prerenal mechanisms, hepatorenal syndrome, and acute tubular necrosis. Regardless of etiology, patients with acute liver failure frequently require hemofiltration or hemodialysis, and nephrotoxic medications should be avoided whenever possible.

Invasive hemodynamic monitoring, like ICP devices, must be considered to incur a higher than normal risk in the patient with acute liver failure. Considering the interplay of systemic abnormalities just outlined, however, management of these patients typically requires invasive monitoring. Finally, it is unlikely that coagulation abnormalities can be fully corrected. The possibility of large volume transfusion requirements should be anticipated with adequate venous access, fluid warming devices, personnel, and blood bank support.

Anesthetic management issues are summarized in Box 5-15.

Anesthetic Management for Procedures Involving the Hepatobiliary System

Transjugular Intrahepatic Portosystemic Shunt (TIPS or TIPSS)

The TIPS procedure, in use since 1989, is sometimes referred to as transjugular intrahepatic portosystemic *stent* shunt in earlier literature. This terminology emphasized the importance of stenting open hepatic tissue to avoid the loss of patency that had been experienced with the original technique of ballooning without stent placement. With the refinement of this procedure, patients were provided with portosystemic shunting to relieve portal hypertension without undergoing major surgery. Characteristics of patients presenting for TIPS can be found in Box 5-16. The essentials of TIPS involve placing a catheter into the hepatic vein via the right jugular approach, passage of a specialized needle and then guidewire into a major tributary of the portal vein, and then passage of an angioplasty balloon and metallic stent over this wire to create and maintain a tract through the hepatic tissue. Mortality is increased in patients undergoing emergency TIPS for variceal bleeding, renal insufficiency, marked elevations of bilirubin, and/or coagulopathy resistant to treatment. Early mortality may approach 80% in

---

BOX 5–15   Anesthetic Preparation and Management in Acute Liver Failure

Consider same issues as in acute hepatitis (see previous section):
Preserve hepatic blood flow.
　Avoid halothane (isoflurane is best studied alternative and better preserves flow).
　Consider regional anesthesia if procedure and coagulation allows.
　Maintain normocapnia.
　Avoid PEEP if possible.
　Provide generous volume maintenance.
Avoid medications with situational potential hepatotoxicity whenever possible. Examples:
　Halothane
　Acetaminophen, particularly in the alcoholic patient
　Sulfonamides, tetracycline and penicillins
　Amiodarone
Suspicion of infectious etiology
　Provider exposures treated as high risk for viral hepatitis.
AND
Anticipate elevated intracranial pressure (ICP) with compromised cerebral perfusion pressure.
　Assess with direct ICP monitoring if available.

Elevate the patient's head.
　Consider osmotic diuresis.
　Consider barbiturates.
　Consider hypertonic saline.
　Avoid systemic hypotension.
Consider electroencephalography to detect seizure activity perioperatively.
Anticipate hypoglycemia, sometimes profound, with added perioperative stress.
Prepare for adult respiratory distress syndrome.
　Consider PEEP (in conflict with ICP concerns and hepatic perfusion).
　Consider decreased tidal volumes with permissive hypercapnia (in conflict with ICP).
Anticipate hypotension.
　Relative hypovolemia.
　Hemorrhage.
　Extensive vasodilation.
Prepare for massive transfusion requirements.
　Alert blood bank.
　Secure adequate venous access.
Utilize invasive hemodynamic monitoring.

BOX 5–16   Characteristics of Patients Presenting for TIPS

Diagnoses in Patients Requiring TIPS
Portal hypertension, most commonly from cirrhosis, with:
   Bleeding varices and/or
   Ascites failing medical management

Comorbidities Common in Patients Requiring TIPS
Comorbidities of cirrhosis (see earlier discussion), especially:
   Bleeding varices
      Emergency procedure associated with increased mortality
   Ascites
      Recent paracentesis and/or diuretic therapy may cause
        hypovolemia
   Cardiovascular
      Typically high cardiac output and low peripheral
        vascular resistance
      Depressed response to inotropes and vasopressors

patients with more than one of these risk factors.[298] In one small series, patients with Child-Pugh class C disease not only failed to have resolution of ascites but also had worse mortality than patients randomized to repeated paracentesis.[299] In a larger series of 60 patients, mortality without liver transplant was similar in TIPS and paracentesis groups at 1 and 2 years, although multivariate analysis demonstrated association of TIPS with survival not requiring registration for liver transplantation.[300] Complications that can lead to significant morbidity have been reported. Puncture of the liver capsule or injury to a hepatic artery can occur with extensive bleeding. Increased central venous pressure has been observed after

shunting, and the cirrhotic with poor cardiac function may decompensate: myocardial infarction has been reported. Encephalopathy is a risk of any portosystemic shunting procedure, for reasons described in the prior discussion of hepatic encephalopathy. Hemolysis from mechanical trauma was prevalent in some early series of TIPS but has become a less common issue in recent years. Modern TIPS procedures maintain a patency rate of greater than 90% per year. When necessary, revision or repeat TIPS have become commonplace in active centers.

Anesthetic considerations for patients undergoing TIPS are, in essence, those of managing the patient with cirrhosis complicated by ascites and/or portal hypertension, except for the rare patient who presents with presinusoidal or venous causes of portal hypertension. The reader is referred to the earlier section dealing with this patient group; for convenience the summary of key points is duplicated in Box 5-17. Although some centers perform TIPS with the patient under sedation, most cases are performed using general anesthesia. Sedated patients report significant pain during intrahepatic dilation and stent deployment. The unpredictable response of patients with advanced cirrhosis to sedative and narcotic medications should also be considered in choosing between sedation and general anesthesia.

Biliary Tract Procedures

Cholecystectomy, Choledochal Cyst Excision, and Biliary Tumor Resection. General characteristics of patients undergoing procedures of the biliary tract are listed in Box 5-18.

BOX 5–17   Anesthetic Management of Patients for TIPS (See section regarding management of patients with cirrhosis)

Preserve hepatic blood flow.
   Avoid halothane (isoflurane is best studied alternative and
      better preserves flow).
   Consider regional anesthesia if procedure and coagulation
      allows.
   Maintain normocapnia.
   Avoid PEEP if possible.
   Provide generous volume maintenance.
Avoid medications with situational potential hepatotoxicity
  whenever possible. Examples:
   Halothane
   Acetaminophen, particularly in the alcoholic patient
   Sulfonamides, tetracycline, and penicillins
   Amiodarone
Suspect infectious etiology.
   Provider exposures treated as high risk for viral hepatitis.
Anticipate presence or development of abnormalities of:
  Coagulation
    Attempt to correct prothrombin time to within 2 seconds
      of normal.
    Consider cryoprecipitate if fresh frozen plasma is
      ineffective or fibrinogen abnormality.

    Correct thrombocytopenia appropriately for procedure.
    Anticipate higher than normal blood loss for procedure.
  Hemodynamics
    Anticipate relative hypovolemia, worsened by treatment
      of ascites.
    Assess for presence of high cardiac output, low peripheral
      resistance.
    Suspect portal hypertension and/or variceal bleeding,
      even without history.
    Anticipate depressed response to inotropes and
      vasopressors.
    Consider invasive monitoring.
  Pharmacokinetics and pharmacodynamics
    Altered volume of distribution
      Decreased serum albumin, increased gamma
        globulins
      Intravascular volume unpredictable, especially with
        ascites treatment
    Portosystemic shunted blood bypasses liver
      Drugs highly extracted by liver especially affected
    Increased sensitivity to sedative medications may
      be present

BOX 5–18   Characteristics of Patients Undergoing Procedures of the Biliary Tract

Diagnoses in Patients Requiring Biliary Tract Procedures
Cholecystectomy
    Cholelithiasis
    Cholecystitis
    Choledocholithiasis
Biliary duct tumor
Choledochal cyst

Comorbidities and Complications Associated with Biliary Tract Disease
Respiratory embarrassment from abdominal pain
Obstructive jaundice
Coagulopathy from vitamin K malabsorption with chronic
  biliary obstruction
Cholelithiasis increased with:
    Female gender
    Obesity
    Cystic fibrosis
Crohn's disease
    Sickle cell anemia

BOX 5–19   Anesthetic Preparation and Management for Biliary Tract Surgery

Check for elevated prothrombin time.
    Vitamin K may correct if time allows, otherwise use fresh
      frozen plasma.
Pay attention to volume status when vomiting, decreased oral
  intake, or fever is present.
Consider rapid-sequence induction or awake intubation in
  patients with nausea and vomiting.
Perioperative opioids may cause spasm of sphincter of Oddi.
Blood loss typically is minimal unless complex biliary repair
  or coagulopathy.
Open procedures
    Pain can significantly affect respiratory status and be
      difficult to manage.
    Consider epidural analgesia or intercostals nerve blocks.
Laparoscopic procedures
    Pneumoperitoneum associated with:
      Increased incidence of pneumothorax and
        pneumomediastinum
      Subcutaneous emphysema
      Decreased venous return
      Increased peak inspiratory pressures
      Hypercapnia from insufflated CO_2 and decreased
        pulmonary compliance

Although open cholecystectomy is still performed in selected patients with anticipated technical difficulties or coexisting disease such as advanced cirrhosis or bleeding diathesis, most institutions now plan laparoscopic cholecystectomy in over 90% of cases. Indications for cholecystectomy are cholelithiasis, choledocholithiasis, and cholecystitis. Patients in this group are often otherwise healthy, although cirrhotic patients often require cholecystectomy and may present the challenges of coagulopathy and portal hypertension. Patients with severe cardiopulmonary disease may poorly tolerate the pneumoperitoneum required for laparoscopic surgery; conversely, postoperative pulmonary function after laparoscopy is superior to that of open, high abdominal surgery.

The extrahepatic biliary tree may uncommonly be the site of primary tumors or cystic dilation (choledochal cysts) that may present as symptoms of cholangitis, pancreatitis, or cholecystitis. Surgical excision is required and, depending on location, may be technically challenging and result in extensive blood loss.

Endoscopic retrograde cholangiopancreatography (ERCP) has become a cornerstone in the assessment and often the management of patients with suspected biliary obstruction. It is typically implemented after suspicious ultrasound, computed tomography, and/or magnetic resonance imaging. There is a great deal of institutional variation in the management of patients undergoing ERCP, ranging from sedation to general anesthesia. Trends that appear to be emerging are the increased use of conscious sedation or general anesthesia in referral centers undertaking more complex procedures and the cooperative development by involved professional societies of national management guidelines.[301]

Anesthetic preparation (Box 5-19) should focus on any coexisting diseases and complications, with medical optimization as time allows. Even healthy patients with biliary disease will often be profoundly hypovolemic and may be actively experiencing nausea and vomiting. Narcotics should be titrated with the awareness that their stimulation of the sphincter of Oddi may precipitate worsened pain in the conscious patient preoperatively and technical failure of cholangiography intraoperatively. Atropine, glycopyrrolate, naloxone, and glucagon have all been reported to reverse this narcotic-induced spasm. Transfusion is typically not required, and the procedure itself mandates no monitoring beyond that dictated by general patient condition.

Hepatic Resection

A wide range of patients undergo hepatic resection (Box 5-20). Living-directed donors are healthy individuals whose excised lobes will be transplanted into another patient. Most other patients have either benign or malignant primary hepatic tumors or metastatic tumors to the liver. This large group may have a variety of associated disease processes such as cirrhosis and, of course, any number of unrelated diseases. More rarely, patients near extremis may require resection for problems such as trauma or pregnancy-associated rupture with uncontrolled bleeding.

Recent technologic applications such as intraoperative sonography, ultrasonic suction aspiration, harmonic scalpels, and the argon laser coagulator have become a

BOX 5-20   Characteristics of Patients Undergoing Hepatic Resection

Diagnoses of Patients Requiring Hepatic Resection
  Living directed donor
  Hepatic tumor
  Trauma
  Pregnancy-associated hepatic rupture

Comorbidities That May Be Seen in Patients Requiring Hepatic Resection
  Chronic hepatitis, particularly hepatitis C
  Cirrhosis
    Markedly decreases liver's regenerative capacity
  Primary benign or malignant hepatic tumor with biliary obstruction
  Numerous cancers with metastases to the liver

routine part of liver resections in many centers. Hepatic cryotherapy, originally as an open procedure[302] and now under radiologic guidance, has been utilized for lesions otherwise unresectable because of underlying liver disease or anatomic position. For whatever reasons, overall morbidity and mortality of tumor resection and/or destruction has improved remarkably in recent experience.

The anesthetic management of patients undergoing liver resection (Box 5-21) does have two areas of interesting controversy. The first involves fluid management. The traditional school of thought has been that the patient should be kept relatively euvolemic or even slightly hypervolemic during dissection. The logic is that, as in any procedure with the risk of sudden blood loss, the patient can be more rapidly resuscitated when hemorrhage occurs from a point of euvolemia instead of already being hypovolemic. The other approach is to minimize fluids throughout dissection so as to generate a low central venous pressure (CVP). This is augmented by intermittent occlusion of vascular inflow by some surgeons. Here, the logic is that CVP is a critical determinant in hepatic venous pressures so that the lower the CVP, the lower the

BOX 5-21   Anesthetic Preparation and Management

Define volume management strategy (low central venous pressure vs. euvolemia).
Consider risk and benefits of epidural catheter placement.
Consider invasive hemodynamic monitoring.
Secure adequate intravenous access for massive transfusion.
Alert blood bank of potential for extensive transfusion requirements.
Consider use of cell salvage and rapid infusion device.
Anticipate possibility of postoperative hepatic insufficiency.
  Hypoglycemia
  Coagulopathy
Anticipate common postoperative complications of atelectasis, effusion, and pneumonia.

bleeding from cut hepatic surfaces. This approach has been adopted at many centers and has support in recent literature.[303-307] It should be emphasized that following resection and confirmation of hemostasis, fluid resuscitation is undertaken. Proponents of this approach believe that the presumed increased risks of organ hypoperfusion, possible hemorrhage in a hypovolemic patient, and even air embolism are outweighed by the improved surgical conditions and decreased blood loss and transfusion requirements that have been reported.

Postoperative analgesia is another interesting area of discussion.[308-310] Many centers routinely place epidural catheters for pain management, whereas others do not. Although postoperative pain is significant in this upper abdominal chevron incision, many anesthesiologists fear that the postoperative fluctuations of coagulation that may be seen in any major abdominal procedure will be dangerously accentuated with the resection of large amounts of hepatic tissue. There are limited data to guide the clinician in weighing the risk of epidural catheter placement in a patient who may become coagulopathic against the presumed benefits, especially pulmonary,[311-313] of epidural analgesia.

The possibility of massive blood loss always exists in these procedures. The blood bank should be alerted, and appropriate venous access should be attained. Cell salvage may be used if cancer and infection are not present.

Liver Transplantation

Orthotopic Liver Transplantation. Liver transplantation has, in two decades, made a remarkable transition from a procedure of desperate last resort to a commonly recommended therapy (Table 5-13). In the United States, data indicate 80% to 90% one-year survival across all groups and 70% to 80% five-year survival. With improved survival, recurrences of infection (first hepatitis B, and now hepatitis C) as well as the morbidities of long-term immunosuppression have become management issues. Indeed, transplantation can be viewed as exchanging an otherwise untreatable disease (e.g., cirrhosis or acute liver failure) with the treatable disease of immunosuppression. The most common available diagnoses of current U.S. liver transplant candidates are listed for adult and pediatric patients in Box 5-22. Box 5-23 briefly lists important anesthetic considerations in liver transplant cases.

The Previously Transplanted Patient. The remarkable improvement in patients surviving liver transplantation and the number of transplantations performed means that more patients will present for surgery who have had a liver transplant. Many of these patients seek all health care at their transplant center. However, it is likely that for practical and economic reasons or medical urgency that many patients will seek care elsewhere. Faced with this

TABLE 5–13 Anesthetic Management for Orthotopic Liver Transplantation

Management Issue and Common Practices	Comments
Hemodynamic Monitoring	
Direct intra-arterial pressures: radial and/or femoral arteries	Two sites often utilized, heparin-free infusion in one for laboratory samples.
Pulmonary artery catheter	Continuous cardiac output and mixed venous saturation catheters allow rapid assessment of oxygen delivery and utilization.
Transesophageal echocardiography	Particularly useful for portopulmonary syndrome, reperfusion crisis, and suspected tamponade as well as general cardiac function and fluid status. Risk exists of variceal bleeding in coagulopathic patients with esophageal varices.
Central Nervous System Monitoring	
Intracranial pressure monitoring	Indicated in fulminant liver failure with advanced encephalopathy if coagulopathy can be adequately corrected.
Laboratory monitoring	
Standard coagulation profiles	Prothrombin and partial thromboplastin times, fibrinogen levels, fibrinogen degradation products, and platelet count.
Factor activity	Readily available in some centers, allows factor specific determinations of abnormalities and therapeutic response.
Thromboelastography (TEG)	TEG was commonly used in early transplantation series. Allows "bedside" evaluation of coagulation with patterns typical of factor and platelet deficiency and fibrinolysis. Allows in-vitro assessment of factor and antifibrinolytic therapy. Still used in many centers.
Potential for Massive Transfusion and Veno-veno Bypass	
Extensive venous access	Peripheral large bore (8.5 Fr or larger) catheters allow rapid volume infusion.
Blood bank protocol	10-20 units of packed red blood cells, fresh frozen plasma, and platelets should be available. Many cases require that several units of cells and plasma be verified and at the bedside.
Rapid infusion devices	Many centers use rapid infusion pump devices capable of infusing 1 L or more of fluid in a minute. Careful attention to overpressure alarms and catheter sites is important to avoid pressurized extravasation.
Cell salvage	Cell salvage is commonly used when cancer or infection is not suspected. Large volumes of processed cells will dilute platelets and coagulation factors. Impact on fibrinolysis is controversial.
Veno-veno bypass	Utilization ranges from routine to selected or rare in different centers. Flow from femoral and portal vein to axillary or internal jugular vein maintains venous return during caval interruption. (Piggyback transplantation requires partial or short caval occlusion, typically veno-veno bypass is not utilized.[59])

situation, the anesthesiologist should evaluate the function of the transplanted liver through history, examination, and routine liver panel studies as described for patients in general. Within a few months of transplantation serum bilirubin and transaminase levels should return toward or to normal range. AST changes, in particular, are monitored as indications of graft rejection. Alkaline phosphatase and GGT are more likely to remain elevated after transplant and must be considered in their trends rather than absolute values.

Conservative management of the patient with the transplanted liver would be to apply the principles discussed for the patient with acute hepatitis. There are, however, little data to indicate that the transplanted liver is at particularly increased risk for perioperative dysfunction. Immunosuppressive protocols should be maintained and their pharmacologic interactions with perioperative medications considered.

Special Considerations

Postoperative Liver Dysfunction

Every anesthesiologist should be prepared to provide at least initial consultation and/or care for the postoperative patient with liver dysfunction. The specter of hepatic necrosis from halothane exposure still looms large in the minds and literature of many colleagues in other specialties. As discussed previously, halothane is rarely a cause of severe hepatic injury, and newer volatile agents have

BOX 5–22 Most Common Diagnoses of U.S. Patients Registered for Liver Transplantation

Adult
- Cirrhosis from hepatitis C
- Cirrhosis from alcohol
- Cryptogenic cirrhosis
- Primary biliary cirrhosis
- Autoimmune cirrhosis
- Cirrhosis from hepatitis B
- Acute liver failure
- Primary sclerosing cholangitis

Pediatric
- Biliary atresia (extrahepatic)
- Autoimmune cirrhosis
- Acute liver failure
- Obstructive biliary disease
- Cystic fibrosis
- Cirrhosis
- Neonatal hepatitis
- Congenital hepatic fibrosis
- Inborn errors of metabolism

extremely rarely or never been convincingly implicated. With a balanced approach, the anesthesiologist can help to ensure that the more likely, although perhaps less dramatic, causes of postoperative dysfunction are considered with recognition of their relative probability.

The reported incidence of hepatic abnormalities after anesthesia depend on preexisting state of health, population, procedure, era, and the defining criteria for dysfunction. Studies report 25% to 75% of postoperative patients develop abnormal laboratory values, but a much smaller percentage progress to clinically significant disease and/or jaundice. A variety of causes of postoperative jaundice are summarized in Box 5-24. Three general categories of postoperative abnormalities are increased bilirubin production, hepatocellular injury, and cholestatic disorders.

Bilirubin overproduction can cause jaundice in the previously healthy patient when bilirubin production exceeds hepatic processing capacity. About 250 mg of bilirubin is usually conjugated daily, but the healthy liver can conjugate up to three times that amount. Several perioperative situations can exceed this production. About 10% of transfused red cells, if older than 2 weeks, are destroyed within 1 day of administration. Similarly, red cells within hematomas are rapidly hemolyzed during resorption. The placement of stents (as discussed with early TIPSS series, for example) and mechanical valves can result in fragmentation or so-called mechanical hemolysis. Laboratory values usually show a pattern of mildly elevated AST and LDH, reduced haptoglobin, unconjugated hyperbilirubinemia, and reticulocytosis. The peripheral smear may reveal schistocytes. Unrecognized preexisting diseases can result in a relative or absolute overproduction of bilirubin. The amount of

BOX 5–23 Preoperative Considerations in the Liver Transplant Patient

Coagulation is almost universally abnormal; severity and direct causes are variable.
- Decreased or abnormal factor synthesis
- Fibrinolysis
- Disseminated intravascular coagulation
- Thrombocytopenia

Metabolic abnormalities arise from variety of causes; overall picture is unpredictable.
- Hypoglycemia in acute hepatic failure, glucose intolerance in cirrhosis
- Respiratory alkalosis common with hypoxemia-driven tachypnea
- Metabolic acidosis from peripheral shunting causing tissue hypoperfusion
- Metabolic alkalosis from volume contraction of paracentesis, diuresis, vomiting

Cardiovascular
- High cardiac output with low peripheral resistance is typical.
- Peripheral arteriovenous shunting causes paradoxical tissue ischemia.
  - Increased endogenous vasodilators usually metabolized by liver.
  - Formation of true arteriovenous fistulas
- Cardiomyopathy may occur with alcoholism, Wilson's disease, etc.

- Cardiac reserve must be adequate to tolerate rigorous challenges of transplantation.
- Pericardial effusion may require preoperative or early intraoperative drainage.
- Portopulmonary hypertension confers exceptionally high perioperative risk.

Respiratory
- Hypoxemia common
  - Ascites and pleural effusions with respiratory compromise
  - Intrapulmonary shunting from endogenous vasodilators
  - Hepatopulmonary syndrome associated with intrapulmonary vascular dilatations
- ARDS may be present, particularly in acute failure

Neurologic
- Encephalopathy common, severity variable
- Encephalopathy of acute liver failure is often associated with critical intracranial pressure elevations.
  - Direct intracranial pressure measurement is invaluable for intraoperative management.

Renal
- Dysfunction common; severity ranges from mild to hepatorenal syndrome.
- Osmotic diuretics and dopamine are often used but without proven efficacy.
- Preoperative or intraoperative hemofiltration should be considered for anuric patients.

BOX 5–24 Classification and Examples of Postoperative Jaundice

Preexisting limitation of capacity for bilirubin metabolism
  Chronic liver disease
  Gilbert's disease
Unappreciated preexisting disease with natural or accelerated progression
  Viral hepatitis
  Cirrhosis
  Autoimmune hepatitis
Hepatocellular injury
  Ischemic hepatitis
  Viral hepatitis
  Drug hepatotoxicity
Increased bilirubin load
  Breakdown of hemoglobin from transfused erythrocytes
  Resorption of large hematomas
  Hemolysis
    Mechanical (e.g., stents, cell salvage processing)
    Preexisting disease (e.g., glucose-6-phosphate dehydrogenase deficiency)
    Transfusion reaction
Intrahepatic cholestasis
  Benign postoperative cholestasis
  Medication associated
Extrahepatic biliary obstruction
  Postoperative pancreatitis
  Biliary stricture
Cholecystitis, calculous or acalculous

hemoglobin that can be conjugated decreases in Gilbert's disease. Glucose-6-phosphate dehydrogenase deficiency, sickle cell disease, and the thalassemias can result in increased hemolysis with what would usually be insignificant stress. Table 5-14 compares laboratory patterns that may be seen in postoperative liver dysfunction.

Hepatocellular necrosis can account for postoperative jaundice and transaminase abnormalities. Ischemic liver injury typically manifests 1 to 10 days after the insult. Hypoperfusion from hypotension, cardiopulmonary bypass, and mechanical interruption of flow as well as hypoxemia have been associated with this type of injury. Venous congestion from right-sided heart failure may exacerbate the damage. As previously discussed, liver blood flow is decreased with most anesthetics. In the case of unrecognized chronic disease, small decreases in blood pressure and cardiac output may not allow the hepatic arterial flow to compensate for decreased portal venous flow to the liver. Aminotransferase levels are markedly elevated, as is LDH, as previously described in patterns of hepatic injury. If liver biopsy is performed, centrilobular or panlobular necrosis is found. The injury can progress to acute liver failure with its attendant derangements as previously outlined. Treatment is supportive with insurance of perfusion and oxygen delivery.

Viral hepatitis is an unusual but important cause of postoperative jaundice. Some percentage of patients will have an acute infection with a time course that conspires to manifest perioperatively or a chronic infection that results in hepatic deterioration postoperatively. Transfusion-borne disease is less likely than preoperative infection in the current era. The disease can unfold anytime in the first 2 postoperative weeks with typical laboratory findings; previously discussed serologic studies and RNA analysis are indicated.

Anesthetic-associated injury was discussed with hepatotoxins, but a few important points are repeated here. Halothane can cause either a milder intrinsic hepatotoxicity or a severe idiosyncratic hepatotoxicity. The latter appears to occur in the range of 1 in 35,000 adult anesthetics, if the previously described risk factors are absent. Transaminases are elevated, bilirubin increases in correlation with severity, and eosinophilia is found in up to 30% of cases. The newer inhalational anesthetics are rarely, if ever, associated with hepatic injury of consequence.

TABLE 5–14 Biochemical Patterns of Postoperative Liver Dysfunction

	AST and ALT	Alkaline Phosphatase	LDH	Bilirubin	Others
Overproduction of bilirubin	AST (↑) ALT NL	Other medications	↑	↑Unconj	↑Reticulocytes schistocytes
Ischemic injury	↑ 5-100×	(↑) 2×	↑↑	(↑) 2-3×	
Viral infection	↑ > 10×	(↑)	(↑)	↑	Serologies and RNA analysis
Anesthetic associated-severe	↑ to ↑↑			↑	Leukocytosis, eosinophilia
Benign postoperative cholestasis	(↑)	↑ 3×		↑ 3×	PT (↑)
Extrahepatic cholestasis	↑	↑		↑	

AST, aspartate aminotransferase; ALT, alanine aminotransferase; LDH, lactate dehydrogenase; PT, prothrombin time; unconj, unconjugated; NL, normal; (↑), mild or no increase; ↑, increased; ↑↑, marked increase; × = times normal.

This is believed to be because of decreased biotransformation and improved hepatic perfusion as compared with halothane. *Other drugs* that should be considered in postoperative liver dysfunction are tetracycline, isoniazid, phenytoin, penicillin, acetaminophen, and sulfonamides.

Benign postoperative cholestasis occurs with or without jaundice. It tends to occur in critically ill patients. Its causes are believed to be multifactorial, having significant overlap with issues such as increased bilirubin load and hypoperfusion. Treatment is supportive, and mortality is related to processes other than cholestasis. Major infection can also cause intrahepatic cholestasis. Some authors, in fact, consider this to simply be another cause of benign postoperative cholestasis, whereas others distinguish the two. Regardless of nomenclature, infection should be considered in the differential diagnosis of postoperative cholestasis.

Extrahepatic cholestasis is a rare cause of postoperative jaundice but should be considered. Causes include cholecystitis (with or without cholelithiasis), postoperative pancreatitis, and complications of surgery that disrupt the biliary tract. Aminotransferases, alkaline phosphatase, and total bilirubin are typically mildly to moderately elevated. Total parenteral nutrition has been associated with both acalculous cholecystitis and cholelithiasis, as well as steatohepatitis and even micronodular cirrhosis with long-term administration.

A general approach to the patient with postoperative liver dysfunction is to review the history for any overlooked evidence of preexisting liver disease. A biochemical liver profile, complete blood cell count, and clotting times should be assessed. Elevations of unconjugated bilirubin can arise from breakdown of transfused red cells, hemolysis from mechanical devices or preexisting disease, hematoma resorption, or Gilbert's syndrome. Haptoglobin, reticulocyte count, and LDH can be used to help confirm the etiology. In the case of conjugated hyperbilirubinemia, further discriminating laboratory testing should be pursued. Markedly increased aminotransferases and LDH without evidence of obstruction are consistent with ischemic injury, drug-associated injury, or active viral infection. Abdominal sonography can be used to evaluate obstruction. Sepsis, total parenteral nutrition, medication effects, and acalculous cholecystitis can also cause cholestasis and conjugated hyperbilirubinemia.

CONCLUSION

The vital roles of the liver, even in health, are of a complexity and number beyond our current understanding. Patients with liver disease or undergoing procedures affecting the liver can present great challenges to the anesthesiologist. With the current surge of patients deteriorating from chronic and often undiagnosed hepatitis C and the limited number of organs available for transplantation, we can expect to care for an increasing number of patients with significant hepatic dysfunction. Recent history also demonstrates the rapid development and implementation of new procedures, often in such arenas as interventional radiology and from the experience of transplant surgery. Such innovation requires the application of basic management principles and critical review of accumulating experience.

The stated goals of this chapter included discussion of relevant hepatic structure and function, responses of the liver to injury, discussion of specific disease etiologies, and principles of anesthetic management. With these considerations, it is hoped that the anesthesiologist can more comfortably and rationally approach the management of patients with hepatic disease as well as those undergoing liver-related surgery.

References

1. Cotran RS, Kumar V, Collins T (eds): Robbins Pathologic Basis of Disease, 6th ed. Philadelphia, WB Saunders, 1999.
2. Feldman M, Friedman LS, Sleisenger MH (eds): Sleisenger & Fordtran's Gastrointestinal and Liver Disease, 7th ed. Philadelphia, WB Saunders, 2002.
3. Schuchmann M, Galle PR: Apoptosis in liver disease. Eur J Gastroenterol Hepatol 2001;13:785-790.
4. Patel T, Steer CJ, Gores GJ: Apoptosis and the liver: A mechanism of disease, growth regulation, and carcinogenesis. Hepatology 1999;30:811-815.
5. Berenguer M, Wright T: Viral hepatitis. In Feldman M, Friedman L, Sleisenger M (eds): Sleisenger & Fordtran's Gastrointestinal and Liver Diseases, 7th ed. Philadelphia, WB Saunders, 2002.
6. Ryder SD, Beckingham IJ: ABC of diseases of liver, pancreas, and biliary system: Acute hepatitis. BMJ 2001;322:151-153.
7. Cuthbert JA: Hepatitis A: Old and new. Clin Microbiol Rev 2001;14: 38-58.
8. Bower WA, Nainan OV, Han X, et al: Duration of viremia in hepatitis A virus infection. J Infect Dis 2000;182:12-7.
9. Tomida S, Matsuzaki Y, Nishi M, et al: Severe acute hepatitis A associated with acute pure red cell aplasia. J Gastroenterol 1996;31:612-617.
10. Diwan AH, Stubbs JR, Carnahan GE: Transmission of hepatitis A via WBC-reduced RBCs and FFP from a single donation. Transfusion (Paris) 2003;43:536-540.
11. Mannucci PM, Gdovin S, Gringeri A, et al: Transmission of hepatitis A to patients with hemophilia by factor VIII concentrates treated with organic solvent and detergent to inactivate viruses. The Italian Collaborative Group. Ann Intern Med 1994;120:1-7.
12. Lednar WM, Lemon SM, Kirkpatrick JW, et al: Frequency of illness associated with epidemic hepatitis A virus infections in adults. Am J Epidemiol 1985;122:226-233.
13. Kemmer NM, Miskovsky EP: Hepatitis A. Infect Dis Clin North Am 2000;14:605-615.
14. Willner IR, Uhl MD, Howard SC, et al: Serious hepatitis A: An analysis of patients hospitalized during an urban epidemic in the United States. Ann Intern Med 1998;128:111-114.
15. Vento S, Garofano T, Renzini C, et al: Fulminant hepatitis associated with hepatitis A virus superinfection in patients with chronic hepatitis C. N Engl J Med 1998;338:286-290.
16. Keeffe EB: Is hepatitis A more severe in patients with chronic hepatitis B and other chronic liver diseases? Am J Gastroenterol 1995;90:201-205.
17. Glikson M, Galun E, Oren R, et al: Relapsing hepatitis A: Review of 14 cases and literature survey. Medicine (Baltimore) 1992;71: 14-23.

18. Craig AS, Schaffner W: Clinical practice: Prevention of hepatitis A with the hepatitis A vaccine. N Engl J Med 2004;350:476-481.

19. Prevention of hepatitis A infections: Guidelines for use of hepatitis A vaccine and immune globulin. American Academy of Pediatrics Committee on Infectious Diseases. Pediatrics. 1996;98:1207-1215.

20. Avgerinos A, Armonis A, Manolakopoulos S, et al: Endoscopic sclerotherapy versus variceal ligation in the long-term management of patients with cirrhosis after variceal bleeding: A prospective randomized study. J Hepatol 1997;26:1034-1041.

21. Lai CL, Ratziu V, Yuen MF, et al: Viral hepatitis B. Lancet 2003;362:2089-2094.

22. Alter MJ, Mast EE: The epidemiology of viral hepatitis in the United States. Gastroenterol Clin North Am 1994;23:437-455.

23. Huo TI, Wu JC, Wu SI, et al: Changing seroepidemiology of hepatitis B, C, and D virus infections in high-risk populations. J Med Virol 2004;72:41-45.

24. Christensen PB, Krarup HB, Niesters HG, et al: Outbreak of hepatitis B among injecting drug users in Denmark. J Clin Virol 2001;22:133-141.

25. Kidd-Ljunggren K, Broman E, Ekvall H, et al: Nosocomial transmission of hepatitis B virus infection through multiple-dose vials. J Hosp Infect 1999;43:57-62.

26. Webster GJ, Hallett R, Whalley SA, et al: Molecular epidemiology of a large outbreak of hepatitis B linked to autohaemotherapy. Lancet 2000;356:379-384.

27. Schreiber GB, Busch MP, Kleinman SH, et al: The risk of transfusion-transmitted viral infections: The Retrovirus Epidemiology Donor Study. N Engl J Med 1996;334:1685-1690.

28. Brook MG: Sexually acquired hepatitis. Sex Transm Infect 2002;78:235-240.

29. Alter MJ, Margolis HS: The emergence of hepatitis B as a sexually transmitted disease. Med Clin North Am 1990;74:1529-1541.

30. Akbar SM, Horiike N, Onji M, et al: Dendritic cells and chronic hepatitis virus carriers. Intervirology 2001;44:199-208.

31. Chin R, Locarnini S: Treatment of chronic hepatitis B: Current challenges and future directions. Rev Med Virol 2003;13:255-272.

32. Rehermann B: Immune responses in hepatitis B virus infection. Semin Liver Dis 2003;23:21-38.

33. Hyams KC: Risks of chronicity following acute hepatitis B virus infection: A review. Clin Infect Dis 1995;20:992-1000.

34. Milich DR, Jones JE, Hughes JL, et al: Is a function of the secreted hepatitis B e antigen to induce immunologic tolerance in utero? Proc Natl Acad Sci U S A 1990;87:6599-6603.

35. Harpaz R, McMahon BJ, Margolis HS, et al: Elimination of new chronic hepatitis B virus infections: Results of the Alaska immunization program. J Infect Dis 2000;181:413-418.

36. Chang MH, Chen CJ, Lai MS, et al: Universal hepatitis B vaccination in Taiwan and the incidence of hepatocellular carcinoma in children. Taiwan Childhood Hepatoma Study Group. N Engl J Med 1997;336:1855-1859.

37. Chernesky MA, Browne RA, Rondi P: Hepatitis B virus antibody prevalence in anaesthetists. Can Anaesth Soc J 1984;31:239-245.

38. Browne RA, Chernesky MA: Viral hepatitis and the anaesthetist. Can Anaesth Soc J 1984;31:279-286.

39. Browne RA, Chernesky MA: Infectious diseases and the anaesthetist. Can J Anaesth 1988;35:655-665.

40. Yuen MF, Lai CL: Treatment of chronic hepatitis B. Lancet Infect Dis 2001;1:232-241.

41. Niederau C, Heintges T, Lange S, et al: Long-term follow-up of HBeAg-positive patients treated with interferon alfa for chronic hepatitis B. N Engl J Med 1996;334:1422-1427.

42. Yuen MF, Hui CK, Cheng CC, et al: Long-term follow-up of interferon alfa treatment in Chinese patients with chronic hepatitis B infection: The effect on hepatitis B e antigen seroconversion and the development of cirrhosis-related complications. Hepatology 2001;34:139-145.

43. Dienstag JL, Schiff ER, Wright TL, et al: Lamivudine as initial treatment for chronic hepatitis B in the United States. N Engl J Med 1999;341:1256-1263.

44. Dienstag JL, Goldin RD, Heathcote EJ, et al: Histological outcome during long-term lamivudine therapy. Gastroenterology 2003;124: 105-117.

45. Allen MI, Deslauriers M, Andrews CW, et al: Identification and characterization of mutations in hepatitis B virus resistant to lamivudine. Lamivudine Clinical Investigation Group. Hepatology 1998;27:1670-1677.

46. Marcellin P, Chang TT, Lim SG, et al: Adefovir dipivoxil for the treatment of hepatitis B e antigen-positive chronic hepatitis B. N Engl J Med 2003;348:808-816.

47. Perrillo R, Schiff E, Yoshida E, et al: Adefovir dipivoxil for the treatment of lamivudine-resistant hepatitis B mutants. Hepatology 2000;32:129-134.

48. Rizzetto M, Canese MG, Arico S, et al: Immunofluorescence detection of new antigen-antibody system (delta/anti-delta) associated to hepatitis B virus in liver and in serum of HBsAg carriers. Gut 1977;18:997-1003.

49. Taylor JM: Replication of human hepatitis delta virus: Recent developments. Trends Microbiol 2003;11:185-190.

50. McCruden EA, Hillan KJ, McKay IC, et al: Hepatitis virus infection and liver disease in injecting drug users who died suddenly. J Clin Pathol 1996;49:552-555.

51. Navascues CA, Rodriguez M, Sotorrio NG, et al: Epidemiology of hepatitis D virus infection: Changes in the last 14 years. Am J Gastroenterol 1995;90:1981-1984.

52. Lettau LA, McCarthy JG, Smith MH, et al: Outbreak of severe hepatitis due to delta and hepatitis B viruses in parenteral drug abusers and their contacts. N Engl J Med 1987;317:1256-1262.

53. Wu JC, Chen CM, Sheen IJ, et al: Evidence of transmission of hepatitis D virus to spouses from sequence analysis of the viral genome. Hepatology 1995;22:1656-1660.

54. Hoofnagle JH: Type D (delta) hepatitis. JAMA 1989;261:1321-1325.

55. Rosina F, Cozzolongo R: Interferon in HDV infection. Antiviral Res 1994;24:165-174.

56. Lauer GM, Walker BD: Hepatitis C virus infection. N Engl J Med 2001;345:41-52.

57. Choo QL, Kuo G, Weiner AJ, et al: Isolation of a cDNA clone derived from a blood-borne non-A, non-B viral hepatitis genome. Science 1989;244:359-362.

58. Alter MJ, Kruszon-Moran D, Nainan OV, et al: The prevalence of hepatitis C virus infection in the United States, 1988 through 1994. N Engl J Med 1999;341:556-562.

59. Donahue JG, Munoz A, Ness PM, et al: The declining risk of post-transfusion hepatitis C virus infection. N Engl J Med 1992;327: 369-373.

60. Wasley A, Alter MJ: Epidemiology of hepatitis C: Geographic differences and temporal trends. Semin Liver Dis 2000;20:1-16.

61. Ohto H, Terazawa S, Sasaki N, et al: Transmission of hepatitis C virus from mothers to infants. The Vertical Transmission of Hepatitis C Virus Collaborative Study Group. N Engl J Med 1994;330:744-750.

62. Conte D, Fraquelli M, Prati D, et al: Prevalence and clinical course of chronic hepatitis C virus (HCV) infection and rate of HCV vertical transmission in a cohort of 15,250 pregnant women. Hepatology 2000;31:751-755.

63. Thomas DL, Villano SA, Riester KA, et al: Perinatal transmission of hepatitis C virus from human immunodeficiency virus type 1-infected mothers. Women and Infants Transmission Study. J Infect Dis 1998;177:1480-1488.

64. Granovsky MO, Minkoff HL, Tess BH, et al: Hepatitis C virus infection in the mothers and infants cohort study. Pediatrics 1998;102:355-359.

65. Paccagnini S, Principi N, Massironi E, et al: Perinatal transmission and manifestation of hepatitis C virus infection in a high risk population. Pediatr Infect Dis J 1995;14:195-199.

66. Zanetti AR, Tanzi E, Paccagnini S, et al: Mother-to-infant transmission of hepatitis C virus. Lombardy Study Group on Vertical HCV Transmission. Lancet 1995;345:289-291.

67. Lavanchy D: Hepatitis C: Public health strategies. J Hepatol 1999;31:146-151.

68. Kage M, Ogasawara S, Kosai K, et al: Hepatitis C virus RNA present in saliva but absent in breast-milk of the hepatitis C carrier mother. J Gastroenterol Hepatol 1997;12:518-521.

69. Soto B, Rodrigo L, Garcia-Bengoechea M, et al: Heterosexual transmission of hepatitis C virus and the possible role of coexistent human immunodeficiency virus infection in the index case: A multicentre study of 423 pairings. J Intern Med 1994;236:515-519.

70. Couzigou P, Richard L, Dumas F, et al: Detection of HCV-RNA in saliva of patients with chronic hepatitis C. Gut 1993;34:S59-S60.

71. Sagnelli E, Gaeta GB, Felaco FM, et al: Hepatitis C virus infection in households of anti-HCV chronic carriers in Italy: A multicentre case-control study. Infection 1997;25:346-349.

72. Bronowicki JP, Venard V, Botte C, et al: Patient-to-patient transmission of hepatitis C virus during colonoscopy. N Engl J Med 1997;337:237-240.

73. Esteban JI, Gomez J, Martell M, et al: Transmission of hepatitis C virus by a cardiac surgeon. N Engl J Med 1996;334:555-560.

74. Ross RS, Viazov S, Gross T, et al: Transmission of hepatitis C virus from a patient to an anesthesiology assistant to five patients. N Engl J Med 2000;343:1851-1854.

75. Poynard T, Yuen MF, Ratziu V, et al: Viral hepatitis C. Lancet 2003;362:2095-2100.

76. Poynard T, Marcellin P, Lee SS, et al: Randomised trial of interferon alpha2b plus ribavirin for 48 weeks or for 24 weeks versus interferon alpha-2b plus placebo for 48 weeks for treatment of chronic infection with hepatitis C virus. International Hepatitis Interventional Therapy Group (IHIT). Lancet 1998;352:1426-1432.

77. Pawlotsky JM: Use and interpretation of virological tests for hepatitis C. Hepatology 2002;36:S65-S73.

78. NIH Consensus Statement on Management of Hepatitis C: 2002. NIH Consensus & State-of-the-Science Statements 2002;19:1-46.

79. Afdhal NH: Diagnosing fibrosis in hepatitis C: Is the pendulum swinging from biopsy to blood tests? Hepatology 2003;37:972-974.

80. Gebo KA, Herlong HF, Torbenson MS, et al: Role of liver biopsy in management of chronic hepatitis C: A systematic review. Hepatology 2002;36:S161-S172.

81. Dienstag JL: The role of liver biopsy in chronic hepatitis C. Hepatology 2002;36:S152-S160.

82. Lindsay KL, Trepo C, Heintges T, et al: A randomized, double-blind trial comparing pegylated interferon alfa-2b to interferon alfa-2b as initial treatment for chronic hepatitis C. Hepatology 2001;34:395-403.

83. Fried MW, Shiffman ML, Reddy KR, et al: Peginterferon alfa-2a plus ribavirin for chronic hepatitis C virus infection. N Engl J Med 2002;347:975-982.

84. Manns MP, McHutchison JG, Gordon SC, et al: Peginterferon alfa-2b plus ribavirin compared with interferon alfa-2b plus ribavirin for initial treatment of chronic hepatitis C: A randomised trial. Lancet 2001;358:958-965.

85. Jaeckel E, Cornberg M, Wedemeyer H, et al: Treatment of acute hepatitis C with interferon alfa-2b. N Engl J Med 2001;345:1452-1457.

86. Worm HC, van der Poel WH, Brandstatter G: Hepatitis E: An overview. Microbes Infect 2002;4:657-666.

87. Naik SR, Aggarwal R, Salunke PN, et al: A large waterborne viral hepatitis E epidemic in Kanpur, India. Bull World Health Organ 1992;70:597-604.

88. Robson SC, Adams S, Brink N, et al: Hospital outbreak of hepatitis E. Lancet 1992;339:1424-1425.

89. Khuroo MS, Dar MY: Hepatitis E: Evidence for person-to-person transmission and inability of low dose immune serum globulin from an Indian source to prevent it. Indian J Gastroenterol 1992;11:113-116.

90. Linnen J, Wages J Jr, Zhang-Keck ZY, et al: Molecular cloning and disease association of hepatitis G virus: A transfusion-transmissible agent. Science 1996;271:505-508.

91. Stapleton JT: GB virus type C/hepatitis G virus. Semin Liver Dis 2003;23:137-148.

92. Alter HJ, Nakatsuji Y, Melpolder J, et al: The incidence of transfusion-associated hepatitis G virus infection and its relation to liver disease. N Engl J Med 1997;336:747-754.

93. Pessoa MG, Terrault NA, Detmer J, et al: Quantitation of hepatitis G and C viruses in the liver: Evidence that hepatitis G virus is not hepatotropic. Hepatology 1998;27:877-880.

94. Polgreen PM, Xiang J, Chang Q, et al: GB virus type C/hepatitis G virus: A non-pathogenic flavivirus associated with prolonged survival in HIV-infected individuals. Microbes Infect 2003;5:1255-1261.

95. Craig P: *Echinococcus multilocularis*. Curr Opin Infect Dis 2003;16:437-444.

96. Lewis JW Jr, Koss N, Kerstein MD: A review of echinococcal disease. Ann Surg 1975;181:390-396.

97. Ersahin Y, Mutluer S, Guzelbag E: Intracranial hydatid cysts in children. Neurosurgery 1993;33:219-224; discussion 224-225.

98. Pandey M, Chaudhari MP: Primary hydatid cyst of sacral spinal canal: Case report. Neurosurgery 1997;40:407-409.

99. Tekkok IH, Benli K: Primary spinal extradural hydatid disease: Report of a case with magnetic resonance characteristics and pathological correlation. Neurosurgery 1993;33:320-323; discussion 323.

100. Angulo JC, Sanchez-Chapado M, Diego A, et al: Renal echinococcosis: Clinical study of 34 cases. J Urol 1997;157:787-794.

101. Snodgrass D, Blome S: Cardiac hydatid disease: Report of two cases. Australas Radiol 2002;46:194-196.

102. Lygidakis NJ: Diagnosis and treatment of intrabiliary rupture of hydatid cyst of the liver. Arch Surg 1983;118:1186-1189.

103. Khoury G, Jabbour-Khoury S, Bikhazi K: Results of laparoscopic treatment of hydatid cysts of the liver. Surg Endosc 1996;10:57-59.

104. Sola JL, Vaquerizo A, Madariaga MJ, et al: Intraoperative anaphylaxis caused by a hydatid cyst. Acta Anaesthesiol Scand 1995;39:273-274.

105. Khoury G, Jabbour-Khoury S, Soueidi A, et al: Anaphylactic shock complicating laparoscopic treatment of hydatid cysts of the liver. Surg Endosc 1998;12:452-454.

106. Wellhoener P, Weitz G, Bechstein W, et al: Severe anaphylactic shock in a patient with a cystic liver lesion. Intensive Care Med 2000;26:1578.

107. Kambam JR, Dymond R, Krestow M, et al: Efficacy of histamine H1 and H2 receptor blockers in the anesthetic management during operation for hydatid cysts of liver and lungs. South Med J 1988;81:1013-1015.

108. Alagille D, Estrada A, Hadchouel M, et al: Syndromic paucity of interlobular bile ducts (Alagille syndrome or arteriohepatic dysplasia): Review of 80 cases. J Pediatr 1987;110:195-200.

109. Krantz ID, Piccoli DA, Spinner NB: Clinical and molecular genetics of Alagille syndrome. Curr Opin Pediatr 1999;11:558-564.

110. Tzakis AG, Reyes J, Tepetes K, et al: Liver transplantation for Alagille's syndrome. Arch Surg 1993;128:337-339.

111. Emerick KM, Rand EB, Goldmuntz E, et al: Features of Alagille syndrome in 92 patients: Frequency and relation to prognosis. Hepatology 1999;29:822-829.

112. Bucuvalas JC, Horn JA, Carlsson L, et al: Growth hormone insensitivity associated with elevated circulating growth hormone-binding protein in children with Alagille syndrome and short stature. J Clin Endocrinol Metab 1993;76:1477-1482.

113. Adachi T, Murakawa M, Uetsuki N, et al: Living related donor liver transplantation in a patient with severe aortic stenosis. Br J Anaesth 1999;83:488-490.

114. Choudhry DK, Rehman MA, Schwartz RE, et al: The Alagille's syndrome and its anaesthetic considerations. Paediatr Anaesth 1998;8:79-82.

115. Muller C, Jelinek T, Endres S, et al: Severe protracted cholestasis after general anesthesia in a patient with Alagille syndrome. Z Gastroenterol 1996;34:809-812.

116. Luisetti M, Seersholm N: Alpha1-antitrypsin deficiency: I. Epidemiology of alpha1-antitrypsin deficiency. Thorax 2004;59:164-169.

117. Perlmutter DH, Joslin G, Nelson P, et al: Endocytosis and degradation of alpha 1-antitrypsin-protease complexes is mediated by the serpin-enzyme complex (SEC) receptor. J Biol Chem 1990;265:16713-16716.

118. Carrell RW, Lomas DA: Alpha1-antitrypsin deficiency—a model for conformational diseases. N Engl J Med 2002;346:45-53.

119. Elliott PR, Lomas DA, Carrell RW, et al: Inhibitory conformation of the reactive loop of alpha 1-antitrypsin. Nat Struct Biol 1996;3:676-681.

120. Elliott PR, Stein PE, Bilton D, et al: Structural explanation for the deficiency of S alpha 1-antitrypsin. Nat Struct Biol 1996;3:910-911.

121. Callea F, Brisigotti M, Fabbretti G, et al: Hepatic endoplasmic reticulum storage diseases. Liver 1992;12:357-362.

122. Lomas DA, Evans DL, Finch JT, et al: The mechanism of Z alpha 1-antitrypsin accumulation in the liver. Nature 1992;357:605-607.

123. Dafforn TR, Mahadeva R, Elliott PR, et al: A kinetic mechanism for the polymerization of alpha1-antitrypsin. J Biol Chem 1999;274:9548-9555.

124. Piitulainen E, Eriksson S: Decline in FEV1 related to smoking status in individuals with severe alpha1-antitrypsin deficiency (PiZZ). Eur Respir J 1999;13:247-251.

125. Lindblad A, Glaumann H, Strandvik B: Natural history of liver disease in cystic fibrosis. Hepatology 1999;30:1151-1158.

126. Duthie A, Doherty DG, Williams C, et al: Genotype analysis for delta F508, G551D and R553X mutations in children and young adults with cystic fibrosis with and without chronic liver disease. Hepatology 1992;15:660-664.

127. Duthie A, Doherty DG, Donaldson PT, et al: The major histocompatibility complex influences the development of chronic liver disease in male children and young adults with cystic fibrosis. J Hepatol 1995;23:532-537.

128. Efrati O, Barak A, Modan-Moses D, et al: Liver cirrhosis and portal hypertension in cystic fibrosis. Eur J Gastroenterol Hepatol 2003;15:1073-1078.

129. Pozler O, Krajina A, Vanicek H, et al: Transjugular intrahepatic portosystemic shunt in five children with cystic fibrosis: Long-term results. Hepatogastroenterology 2003;50:1111-1114.

130. Bloom AI, Verstandig A: SCVIR 2002 Film Panel case 2: TIPS for bleeding varices in cystic fibrosis and liver cirrhosis. J Vasc Interv Radiol 2002;13:533-536.

131. Noble-Jamieson G, Barnes N, Jamieson N, et al: Liver transplantation for hepatic cirrhosis in cystic fibrosis. J R Soc Med 1996;89:31-37.

132. Pfister E, Strassburg A, Nashan B, et al: Liver transplantation for liver cirrhosis in cystic fibrosis. Transplant Proc 2002;34:2281-2282.

133. Knoppert DC, Spino M, Beck R, et al: Cystic fibrosis: Enhanced theophylline metabolism may be linked to the disease. Clin Pharmacol Ther 1988;44:254-264.

134. Kearns GL, Mallory GB Jr, Crom WR, et al: Enhanced hepatic drug clearance in patients with cystic fibrosis. J Pediatr 1990;117:972-979.

135. Waggoner DD, Buist NR, Donnell GN: Long-term prognosis in galactosaemia: Results of a survey of 350 cases. J Inherit Metab Dis 1990;13:802-818.

136. Widhalm K, Miranda da Cruz BD, Koch M: Diet does not ensure normal development in galactosemia. J Am Coll Nutr 1997;16: 204-208.

137. Levy HL, Sepe SJ, Shih VE, et al: Sepsis due to *Escherichia coli* in neonates with galactosemia. N Engl J Med 1977;297:823-825.

138. Vogt M, Gitzelmann R, Allemann J: Decompensated liver cirrhosis caused by galactosemia in a 52-year-old man. Schweiz Med Wochenschr 1980;110:1781-1783.

139. Bosch AM, Bakker HD, van Gennip AH, et al: Clinical features of galactokinase deficiency: A review of the literature. J Inherit Metab Dis 2002;25:629-634.

140. Bevan JC: Anaesthesia in Von Gierke's disease: Current approach to management. Anaesthesia 1980;35:699-702.

141. Ogawa M, Shimokohjin T, Seto T, et al: Anesthesia for hepatectomy in a patient with glycogen storage disease. Masui 1995;44:1703-1706.

142. Shenkman Z, Golub Y, Meretyk S, et al: Anaesthetic management of a patient with glycogen storage disease type 1b. Can J Anaesth 1996;43:467-470.

143. Kakinohana M, Tokumine J, Shimabukuro T, et al: Patient-controlled sedation using propofol for a patient with von Gierke disease. Masui 1998;47:1104-1108.

144. Mohart D, Russo P, Tobias JD: Perioperative management of a child with glycogen storage disease type III undergoing cardiopulmonary bypass and repair of an atrial septal defect. Paediatr Anaesth 2002;12:649-654.

145. Matern D, Starzl TE, Arnaout W, et al: Liver transplantation for glycogen storage disease types I, III, and IV. Eur J Pediatr 1999;158:S43-S48.

146. Rosenthal P, Podesta L, Grier R, et al: Failure of liver transplantation to diminish cardiac deposits of amylopectin and leukocyte inclusions in type IV glycogen storage disease. Liver Transpl Surg 1995;1: 373-376.

147. Stormon MO, Cutz E, Furuya K, et al: A six-month-old infant with liver steatosis. J Pediatr 2004;144:258-263.

148. Choi YK, Johlin FC Jr, Summers RW, et al: Fructose intolerance: An under-recognized problem. Am J Gastroenterol 2003;98: 1348-1353.

149. Newbrun E, Hoover C, Mettraux G, et al: Comparison of dietary habits and dental health of subjects with hereditary fructose intolerance and control subjects. J Am Dent Assoc 1980;101:619-626.

150. Edwards CQ, Cartwright GE, Skolnick MH, et al: Genetic mapping of the hemochromatosis locus on chromosome six. Hum Immunol 1980;1:19-22.

151. Simon M, Bourel M, Fauchet R, et al: Association of HLA-A3 and HLA-B14 antigens with idiopathic haemochromatosis. Gut 1976;17:332-334.

152. Feder JN, Gnirke A, Thomas W, et al: A novel MHC class I-like gene is mutated in patients with hereditary haemochromatosis. Nat Genet 1996;13:399-408.

153. Adams PC: Nonexpressing homozygotes for C282Y hemochromatosis: Minority or majority of cases? Mol Genet Metab 2000;71:81-86.

154. Harrison SA, Bacon BR: Hereditary hemochromatosis: Update for 2003. J Hepatol 2003;38:S14-S23.

155. Fletcher LM, Dixon JL, Purdie DM, et al: Excess alcohol greatly increases the prevalence of cirrhosis in hereditary hemochromatosis. Gastroenterology 2002;122:281-289.

156. Fletcher LM, Halliday JW: Haemochromatosis: Understanding the mechanism of disease and implications for diagnosis and patient management following the recent cloning of novel genes involved in iron metabolism. J Intern Med 2002;251:181-192.

157. Andrews NC: Disorders of iron metabolism. N Engl J Med 1999;341:1986-1995.

158. Feder JN, Penny DM, Irrinki A, et al: The hemochromatosis gene product complexes with the transferrin receptor and lowers its affinity for ligand binding. Proc Natl Acad Sci U S A 1998;95: 1472-1477.

159. Cardoso EM, Stal P, Hagen K, et al: HFE mutations in patients with hereditary haemochromatosis in Sweden. J Intern Med 1998;243: 203-208.

160. Powell LW, George DK, McDonnell SM, et al: Diagnosis of hemochromatosis. Ann Intern Med 1998;129:925-931.

161. Bacon BR, Powell LW, Adams PC, et al: Molecular medicine and hemochromatosis: At the crossroads. Gastroenterology 1999;116:193-207.

162. Edwards CQ, Cartwright GE, Skolnick MH, et al: Homozygosity for hemochromatosis: Clinical manifestations. Ann Intern Med 1980;93:519-525.

163. Nichols GM, Bacon BR: Hereditary hemochromatosis: Pathogenesis and clinical features of a common disease. Am J Gastroenterol 1989;84:851-862.

164. Britton RS: Metal-induced hepatotoxicity. Semin Liver Dis 1996;16: 3-12.

165. Bacon BR, Britton RS: The pathology of hepatic iron overload: A free radical—mediated process? Hepatology 1990;11:127-137.

166. Bonkovsky HL, Lambrecht RW: Iron-induced liver injury. Clin Liver Dis 2000;4:409-429, vi-vii.

167. Niederau C, Fischer R, Sonnenberg A, et al: Survival and causes of death in cirrhotic and in noncirrhotic patients with primary hemochromatosis. N Engl J Med 1985;313:1256-1262.

168. Brandhagen DJ: Liver transplantation for hereditary hemochromatosis. Liver Transpl 2001;7:663-672.

169. Prieto-Alamo MJ, Laval F: Deficient DNA-ligase activity in the metabolic disease tyrosinemia type I. Proc Natl Acad Sci U S A 1998;95:12614-12618.

170. Stoner E, Starkman H, Wellner D, et al: Biochemical studies of a patient with hereditary hepatorenal tyrosinemia: Evidence of glutathione deficiency. Pediatr Res 1984;18:1332-1336.

171. Gilbert-Barness E, Barness LA, Meisner LF: Chromosomal instability in hereditary tyrosinemia type I. Pediatr Pathol 1990;10:243-252.

172. De Braekeleer M, Larochelle J: Genetic epidemiology of hereditary tyrosinemia in Quebec and in Saguenay-Lac-St-Jean. Am J Hum Genet 1990;47:302-307.

173. Scriver CR: Human genetics: Lessons from Quebec populations. Ann Rev Genom Hum Genet 2001;2:69-101.

174. Mitchell G, Larochelle J, Lambert M, et al: Neurologic crises in hereditary tyrosinemia. N Engl J Med 1990;322:432-437.

175. Holme E, Lindstedt S: Tyrosinaemia type I and NTBC (2-(2-nitro-4-trifluoromethylbenzoyl)-1,3-cyclohexanedione). J Inherit Metab Dis 1998;21:507-517.

176. Grompe M: The pathophysiology and treatment of hereditary tyrosinemia type 1. Semin Liver Dis 2001;21:563-571.

177. Terlato NJ, Cox GF: Can mucopolysaccharidosis type I disease severity be predicted based on a patient's genotype? A comprehensive review of the literature. Genet Med 2003;5:286-294.

178. Man TT, Tsai PS, Rau RH, et al: Children with mucopolysaccharidoses— three case reports. Acta Anaesthesiol Sin 1999;37:93-96.

179. Baines D, Keneally J: Anaesthetic implications of the mucopolysaccharidoses: A fifteen-year experience in a children's hospital. Anaesth Intensive Care 1983;11:198-202.

180. Walker RW, Allen DL, Rothera MR: A fibreoptic intubation technique for children with mucopolysaccharidoses using the laryngeal mask airway. Paediatr Anaesth 1997;7:421-426.

181. Walker RW, Colovic V, Robinson DN, et al: Postobstructive pulmonary oedema during anaesthesia in children with mucopolysaccharidoses. Paediatr Anaesth 2003;13:441-447.

182. Vas L, Naregal F: Failed epidural anaesthesia in a patient with Hurler's disease. Paediatr Anaesth 2000;10:95-98.

183. Yoskovitch A, Tewfik TL, Brouillette RT, et al: Acute airway obstruction in Hunter syndrome. Int J Pediatr Otorhinolaryngol 1998;44:273-278.

184. Busoni P, Fognani G: Failure of the laryngeal mask to secure the airway in a patient with Hunter's syndrome (mucopolysaccharidosis type II). Paediatr Anaesth 1999;9:153-155.

185. Vogler C, Barker J, Sands MS, et al: Murine mucopolysaccharidosis VII: Impact of therapies on the phenotype, clinical course, and pathology in a model of a lysosomal storage disease. Pediatr Dev Pathol 2001;4:421-433.

186. Tokieda K, Morikawa Y, Natori M, et al: Intrauterine growth acceleration in the case of a severe form of mucopolysaccharidosis type VII. J Perinat Med 1998;26:235-239.

187. Gillett PM, Schreiber RA, Jevon GP, et al: Mucopolysaccharidosis type VII (Sly syndrome) presenting as neonatal cholestasis with hepatosplenomegaly. J Pediatr Gastroenterol Nutr 2001;33:216-220.

188. Toda Y, Takeuchi M, Morita K, et al: Complete heart block during anesthetic management in a patient with mucopolysaccharidosis type VII. Anesthesiology 2001;95:1035-1037.

189. Charrow J, Andersson HC, Kaplan P, et al: The Gaucher registry: Demographics and disease characteristics of 1698 patients with Gaucher disease. Arch Intern Med 2000;160:2835-2843.

190. Cox TM, Schofield JP: Gaucher's disease: Clinical features and natural history. Baillieres Clin Haematol 1997;10:657-689.

191. Hollak CE, Corssmit EP, Aerts JM, et al: Differential effects of enzyme supplementation therapy on manifestations of type 1 Gaucher disease. Am J Med 1997;103:185-191.

192. Hollak CE, Aerts JM, Goudsmit R, et al: Individualised low-dose alglucerase therapy for type 1 Gaucher's disease. Lancet 1995; 345:1474-1478.

193. Hollak CE, Levi M, Berends F, et al: Coagulation abnormalities in type 1 Gaucher disease are due to low-grade activation and can be partly restored by enzyme supplementation therapy. Br J Haematol 1997;96:470-476.

194. Kita T, Kitamura S, Takeda K, et al: Anesthetic management involving difficult intubation in a child with Gaucher disease. Masui 1998;47:69-73.

195. Tobias JD, Atwood R, Lowe S, et al: Anesthetic considerations in the child with Gaucher disease. J Clin Anesth 1993;5:150-153.

196. Garcia Collada JC, Pereda Marin RM, Martinez AI, et al: Subarachnoid anesthesia in a patient with type I Gaucher disease. Acta Anaesthesiol Scand 2003;47:106-109.

197. Dell'Oste C, Vincenti F: Anaesthetic management of children with type II and III Gaucher disease. Minerva Pediatr 1997;49:495-498.

198. Kolodny EH: Niemann-Pick disease. Curr Opin Hematol 2000;7: 48-52.

199. Liscum L, Klansek JJ: Niemann-Pick disease type C. Curr Opin Lipidol 1998;9:131-135.

200. Bujok LS, Bujok G, Knapik P: Niemann-Pick disease: A rare problem in anaesthesiological practice. Paediatr Anaesth 2002;12:806-808.

201. Daloze P, Delvin EE, Glorieux FH, et al: Replacement therapy for inherited enzyme deficiency: Liver orthotopic transplantation in Niemann-Pick disease type A. Am J Med Genet 1977;1:229-239.

202. Smanik EJ, Tavill AS, Jacobs GH, et al: Orthotopic liver transplantation in two adults with Niemann-Pick and Gaucher's diseases: Implications for the treatment of inherited metabolic disease. Hepatology 1993;17:42-49.

203. Cantz M, Ulrich-Bott B: Disorders of glycoprotein degradation. J Inherit Metab Dis 1990;13:523-537.

204. Wolman M: Wolman disease and its treatment. Clin Pediatr (Phila) 1995;34:207-212.

205. Krivit W, Peters C, Dusenbery K, et al: Wolman disease successfully treated by bone marrow transplantation. Bone Marrow Transplant 2000;26:567-570.

206. Gross U, Hoffmann GF, Doss MO: Erythropoietic and hepatic porphyrias. J Inherit Metab Dis 2000;23:641-661.

207. Crimlisk HL: The little imitator—porphyria: A neuropsychiatric disorder. J Neurol Neurosurg Psychiatry 1997;62:319-328.

208. Gonzalez-Arriaza HL, Bostwick JM: Acute porphyrias: A case report and review. Am J Psychiatry 2003;160:450-459.

209. Elder GH, Hift RJ, Meissner PN: The acute porphyrias. Lancet 1997;349:1613-1617.

210. Harrison GG, Meissner PN, Hift RJ: Anaesthesia for the porphyric patient. Anaesthesia 1993;48:417-421.

211. Jensen NF, Fiddler DS, Striepe V: Anesthetic considerations in porphyrias. Anesth Analg 1995;80:591-599.

212. Stevens JJ, Kneeshaw JD: Mitral valve replacement in a patient with acute intermittent porphyria. Anesth Analg 1996;82:416-418.

213. McNeill MJ, Bennet A: Use of regional anaesthesia in a patient with acute porphyria. Br J Anaesth 1990;64:371-373.

214. Soonawalla ZF, Orug T, Badminton MN, et al: Liver transplantation as a cure for acute intermittent porphyria. Lancet 2004;363: 705-706.

215. Nguyen L, Blust M, Bailin M, et al: Photosensitivity and perioperative polyneuropathy complicating orthotopic liver transplantation in a patient with erythropoietic protoporphyria. Anesthesiology 1999;91:1173-1175.

216. Meerman L, Haagsma EB, Gouw AS, et al: Long-term follow-up after liver transplantation for erythropoietic protoporphyria. Eur J Gastroenterol Hepatol 1999;11:431-438.

217. Bloomer JR, Rank JM, Payne WD, et al: Follow-up after liver transplantation for protoporphyric liver disease. Liver Transpl Surg 1996;2:269-275.

218. Lock G, Holstege A, Mueller AR, et al: Liver failure in erythropoietic protoporphyria associated with choledocholithiasis and severe post-transplantation polyneuropathy. Liver 1996;16:211-217.

219. de Torres I, Demetris AJ, Randhawa PS: Recurrent hepatic allograft injury in erythropoietic protoporphyria. Transplantation 1996;61:1412-1413.

220. Wilson S: Progressive lenticular degeneration: A familial nervous disease associated with cirrhosis of the liver. Brain 1912;34:295-509.
221. Riordan SM, Williams R: The Wilson's disease gene and phenotypic diversity. J Hepatol 2001;34:165-171.
222. Gitlin N: Wilson's disease: The scourge of copper. J Hepatol 1998;28:734-739.
223. El-Youssef M: Wilson disease. Mayo Clin Proc 2003;78:1126-1136.
224. Cox DW: Genes of the copper pathway. Am J Hum Genet 1995;56:828-834.
225. Valentine JS, Gralla EB: Delivering copper inside yeast and human cells. Science 1997;278:817-818.
226. Schaefer M, Roelofsen H, Wolters H, et al: Localization of the Wilson's disease protein in human liver. Gastroenterology 1999;117:1380-1385.
227. Cauza E, Maier-Dobersberger T, Polli C, et al: Screening for Wilson's disease in patients with liver diseases by serum ceruloplasmin. J Hepatol 1997;27:358-362.
228. Saito T: Presenting symptoms and natural history of Wilson disease. Eur J Pediatr 1987;146:261-265.
229. McCullough AJ, Fleming CR, Thistle JL, et al: Diagnosis of Wilson's disease presenting as fulminant hepatic failure. Gastroenterology 1983;84:161-167.
230. Tissieres P, Chevret L, Debray D, et al: Fulminant Wilson's disease in children: Appraisal of a critical diagnosis. Pediatr Crit Care Med 2003;4:338-343.
231. Wilson DC, Phillips MJ, Cox DW, et al: Severe hepatic Wilson's disease in preschool-aged children. J Pediatr 2000;137:719-722.
232. Dening TR, Berrios GE: Wilson's disease: A prospective study of psychopathology in 31 cases. Br J Psychiatry 1989;155:206-213.
233. Dening TR, Berrios GE: Wilson's disease: Psychiatric symptoms in 195 cases. Arch Gen Psychiatry 1989;46:1126-1134.
234. Klepach GL, Wray SH: Bilateral serous retinal detachment with thrombocytopenia during penicillamine therapy. Ann Ophthalmol 1989;13:201-203.
235. Umeki S, Konishi Y, Yasuda T, et al: D-Penicillamine and neutrophilic agranulocytosis. Arch Intern Med 1985;145:2271-2272.
236. Brewer GJ: Tetrathiomolybdate anticopper therapy for Wilson's disease inhibits angiogenesis, fibrosis and inflammation. J Cell Mol Med 2003;7:11-20.
237. Askari FK, Greenson J, Dick RD, et al: Treatment of Wilson's disease with zinc: XVIII. Initial treatment of the hepatic decompensation presentation with trientine and zinc. J Lab Clin Med 2003;142:385-390.
238. Geissler I, Heinemann K, Rohm S, et al: Liver transplantation for hepatic and neurological Wilson's disease. Transplant Proc 2003;35:1445-1446.
239. Sutcliffe RP, Maguire DD, Muiesan P, et al: Liver transplantation for Wilson's disease: Long-term results and quality-of-life assessment. Transplantation 2003;75:1003-1006.
240. Suzuki S, Sato Y, Ichida T, et al: Recovery of severe neurologic manifestations of Wilson's disease after living-related liver transplantation: A case report. Transplant Proc 2003;35:385-386.
241. Popper H: Aging and the liver. Prog Liver Dis 1986;8:659-683.
242. Lacaine F, LaMuraglia GM, Malt RA: Prognostic factors in survival after portasystemic shunts: Multivariate analysis. Ann Surg 1985;202:729-734.
243. Hosking SW, Bird NC, Johnson AG, et al: Management of bleeding varices in the elderly. BMJ 1989;298:152-153.
244. Poupon RE, Lindor KD, Cauch-Dudek K, et al: Combined analysis of randomized controlled trials of ursodeoxycholic acid in primary biliary cirrhosis. Gastroenterology 1997;113:884-890.
245. Combes B, Luketic VA, Peters MG, et al: Prolonged follow-up of patients in the U.S. multicenter trial of ursodeoxycholic acid for primary biliary cirrhosis. Am J Gastroenterol 2004;99:264-268.
246. Levy C, Angulo P: Ursodeoxycholic acid and long-term survival in primary biliary cirrhosis. Am J Gastroenterol 2004;99:269-270.
247. Grose RD, Nolan J, Dillon JF, et al: Exercise-induced left ventricular dysfunction in alcoholic and non-alcoholic cirrhosis. J Hepatol 1995;22:326-332.
248. Roberts LR, Kamath PS: Pathophysiology of variceal bleeding. Gastrointest Endosc Clin North Am 1999;9:167-174.
249. Platt JF, Ellis JH, Rubin JM, et al: Renal duplex Doppler ultrasonography: A noninvasive predictor of kidney dysfunction and hepatorenal failure in liver disease. Hepatology 1994;20:362-369.
250. Lang F, Tschernko E, Haussinger D: Hepatic regulation of renal function. Exp Physiol 1992;77:663-673.
251. Salo J, Fernandez-Esparrach G, Gines P, et al: Urinary endothelin-like immunoreactivity in patients with cirrhosis. J Hepatol 1997;27:810-816.
252. Arroyo V, Gines P, Gerbes AL, et al: Definition and diagnostic criteria of refractory ascites and hepatorenal syndrome in cirrhosis. International Ascites Club. Hepatology 1996;23:164-176.
253. Watt K, Uhanova J, Minuk GY: Hepatorenal syndrome: Diagnostic accuracy, clinical features, and outcome in a tertiary care center. Am J Gastroenterol 2002;97:2046-2050.
254. Gonwa TA, Klintmalm GB, Levy M, et al: Impact of pretransplant renal function on survival after liver transplantation. Transplantation 1995;59:361-365.
255. Gines P, Guevara M, De Las Heras D, et al: Review article: Albumin for circulatory support in patients with cirrhosis. Aliment Pharmacol Ther 2002;16:24-31.
256. Ortega R, Gines P, Uriz J, et al: Terlipressin therapy with and without albumin for patients with hepatorenal syndrome: Results of a prospective, nonrandomized study. Hepatology 2002;36:941-948.
257. Ganne-Carrie N, Hadengue A, Mathurin P, et al: Hepatorenal syndrome: Long-term treatment with terlipressin as a bridge to liver transplantation. Dig Dis Sci 1996;41:1054-1056.
258. Le Moine O, el Nawar A, Jagodzinski R, et al: Treatment with terlipressin as a bridge to liver transplantation in a patient with hepatorenal syndrome. Acta Gastroenterol Belg 1998;61:268-270.
259. Guevara M, Gines P, Fernandez-Esparrach G, et al: Reversibility of hepatorenal syndrome by prolonged administration of ornipressin and plasma volume expansion. Hepatology 1998;27:35-41.
260. Agusti AG, Cardus J, Roca J, et al: Ventilation-perfusion mismatch in patients with pleural effusion: Effects of thoracentesis. Am J Respir Crit Care Med 1997;156:1205-1209.
261. Bindrim SJ, Schutz SM: Respiratory function after injection sclerotherapy of oesophageal varices. Gastrointest Endosc 1995;42:191-193.
262. Tominaga M, Furutani H, Segawa H, et al: Perioperative management of living-donor liver transplantation in two patients with severe portopulmonary hypertension. Masui 2003;52:729-732.
263. Tan HP, Markowitz JS, Montgomery RA, et al: Liver transplantation in patients with severe portopulmonary hypertension treated with preoperative chronic intravenous epoprostenol. Liver Transpl 2001;7:745-749.
264. Blei AT, Olafsson S, Therrien G, et al: Ammonia-induced brain edema and intracranial hypertension in rats after portacaval anastomosis. Hepatology 1994;19:1437-1444.
265. Iwasa M, Matsumura K, Watanabe Y, et al: Improvement of regional cerebral blood flow after treatment with branched-chain amino acid solutions in patients with cirrhosis. Eur J Gastroenterol Hepatol 2003;15:733-737.
266. Harville DD, Summerskill WH: Surgery in acute hepatitis. JAMA 1963;184:257-261.
267. Powell-Jackson P, Greenway B, Williams R: Adverse effects of exploratory laparotomy in patients with unsuspected liver disease. Br J Surg 1982;69:449-451.
268. Greenwood SM, Leffler CT, Minkowitz S: The increased mortality rate of open liver biopsy in alcoholic hepatitis. Surg Gynecol Obstet 1972;134:600-604.
269. Mikkelsen WP, Kern WH: The influence of acute hyaline necrosis on survival after emergency and elective portacaval shunt. Major Probl Clin Surg 1974;14:233-242.
270. Hargrove MD Jr: Chronic active hepatitis: Possible adverse effect of exploratory laparotomy. Surgery 1970;68:771-773.
271. Higashi H, Matsumata T, Adachi E, et al: Influence of viral hepatitis status on operative morbidity and mortality in patients with primary hepatocellular carcinoma. Br J Surg 1994;81:1342-1345.

272. Runyon BA: Surgical procedures are well tolerated by patients with asymptomatic chronic hepatitis. J Clin Gastroenterol 1986;8:542-544.

273. Behrns KE, Tsiotos GG, DeSouza NF, et al: Hepatic steatosis as a potential risk factor for major hepatic resection. J Gastrointest Surg 1998;2:292-298.

274. Brolin RE, Bradley LJ, Taliwal RV: Unsuspected cirrhosis discovered during elective obesity operations. Arch Surg 1998;133:84-88.

275. Beymer C, Kowdley KV, Larson A, et al: Prevalence and predictors of asymptomatic liver disease in patients undergoing gastric bypass surgery. Arch Surg 2003;138:1240-1244.

276. Garrison RN, Cryer HM, Howard DA, et al: Clarification of risk factors for abdominal operations in patients with hepatic cirrhosis. Ann Surg 1984;199:648-655.

277. Mansour A, Watson W, Shayani V, et al: Abdominal operations in patients with cirrhosis: Still a major surgical challenge. Surgery 1997;122:730-735; discussion 735-736.

278. Puggioni A, Wong LL: A meta-analysis of laparoscopic cholecystectomy in patients with cirrhosis. J Am Coll Surg 2003;197:921-926.

279. Fernandes NF, Schwesinger WH, Hilsenbeck SG, et al: Laparoscopic cholecystectomy and cirrhosis: A case-control study of outcomes. Liver Transpl 2000;6:340-344.

280. Yeh CN, Chen MF, Jan YY: Laparoscopic cholecystectomy in 226 cirrhotic patients: Experience of a single center in Taiwan. Surg Endosc 2002;16:1583-1587.

281. Klemperer JD, Ko W, Krieger KH, et al: Cardiac operations in patients with cirrhosis. Ann Thorac Surg 1998;65:85-87.

282. Hayashida N, Shoujima T, Teshima H, et al: Clinical outcome after cardiac operations in patients with cirrhosis. Ann Thorac Surg 2004;77:500-505.

283. Oellerich M, Armstrong VW: The MEGX test: A tool for the real-time assessment of hepatic function. Ther Drug Monit 2001;23:81-92.

284. Petrolati A, Festi D, De Berardinis G, et al: ^{13}C-methacetin breath test for monitoring hepatic function in cirrhotic patients before and after liver transplantation. Aliment Pharmacol Ther 2003;18:785-790.

285. Hwang EH, Taki J, Shuke N, et al: Preoperative assessment of residual hepatic functional reserve using ^{99m}Tc-DTPA-galactosyl-human serum albumin dynamic SPECT. J Nucl Med 1999;40:1644-1651.

286. Onodera Y, Takahashi K, Togashi T, et al: Clinical assessment of hepatic functional reserve using ^{99m}Tc DTPA galactosyl human serum albumin SPECT to prognosticate chronic hepatic diseases—validation of the use of SPECT and a new indicator. Ann Nucl Med 2003;17:181-188.

287. Schemel WH: Unexpected hepatic dysfunction found by multiple laboratory screening. Anesth Analg 1976;55:810-812.

288. Patt CH, Yoo HY, Dibadj K, et al: Prevalence of transaminase abnormalities in asymptomatic, healthy subjects participating in an executive health-screening program. Dig Dis Sci 2003;48:797-801.

289. Maze M, Bass NM: Anesthesia and the hepatobiliary system. In Miller R (ed): Anesthesia. Philadelphia, Churchill Livingstone, 2000, p 1964.

290. Gelman S, Dillard E, Bradley EL Jr: Hepatic circulation during surgical stress and anesthesia with halothane, isoflurane, or fentanyl. Anesth Analg 1987;66:936-943.

291. Gatecel C, Losser MR, Payen D: The postoperative effects of halothane versus isoflurane on hepatic artery and portal vein blood flow in humans. Anesth Analg 2003;96:740-745.

292. Brienza N, Revelly JP, Ayuse T, et al: Effects of PEEP on liver arterial and venous blood flows. Am J Respir Crit Care Med 1995;152:504-510.

293. O'Grady JG, Alexander GJ, Hayllar KM, et al: Early indicators of prognosis in fulminant hepatic failure. Gastroenterology 1989;97:439-445.

294. Pauwels A, Mostefa-Kara N, Florent C, et al: Emergency liver transplantation for acute liver failure: Evaluation of London and Clichy criteria. J Hepatol 1993;17:124-127.

295. Anand AC, Nightingale P, Neuberger JM: Early indicators of prognosis in fulminant hepatic failure: An assessment of the King's criteria. J Hepatol 1997;26:62-68.

296. Shakil AO, Kramer D, Mazariegos GV, et al: Acute liver failure: Clinical features, outcome analysis, and applicability of prognostic criteria. Liver Transpl 2000;6:163-169.

297. Farmer DG, Anselmo DM, Ghobrial RM, et al: Liver transplantation for fulminant hepatic failure: Experience with more than 200 patients over a 17-year period. Ann Surg 2003;237:666-675; discussion 675-676.

298. Russo MW, Jacques PF, Mauro M, et al: Predictors of mortality and stenosis after transjugular intrahepatic portosystemic shunt. Liver Transpl 2002;8:271-277.

299. Lebrec D, Giuily N, Hadengue A, et al: Transjugular intrahepatic portosystemic shunts: Comparison with paracentesis in patients with cirrhosis and refractory ascites: A randomized trial. French Group of Clinicians and a Group of Biologists. J Hepatol 1996;25:135-144.

300. Rossle M, Ochs A, Gulberg V, et al: A comparison of paracentesis and transjugular intrahepatic portosystemic shunting in patients with ascites. N Engl J Med 2000;342:1701-1707.

301. Faigel DO, Baron TH, Goldstein JL, et al: Guidelines for the use of deep sedation and anesthesia for GI endoscopy. Gastrointest Endosc 2002;56:613-617.

302. Littlewood K: Anesthetic considerations for hepatic cryotherapy. Semin Surg Oncol 1998;14:116-121.

303. Jones RM, Moulton CE, Hardy KJ: Central venous pressure and its effect on blood loss during liver resection. Br J Surg 1998;85:1058-1060.

304. Chen H, Merchant NB, Didolkar MS: Hepatic resection using intermittent vascular inflow occlusion and low central venous pressure anesthesia improves morbidity and mortality. J Gastrointest Surg 2000;4:162-167.

305. Chen CL, Chen YS, de Villa VH, et al: Minimal blood loss living donor hepatectomy. Transplantation 2000;69:2580-2586.

306. Otsubo T, Takasaki K, Yamamoto M, et al: Bleeding during hepatectomy can be reduced by clamping the inferior vena cava below the liver. Surgery 2004;135:67-73.

307. Smyrniotis V, Kostopanagiotou G, Theodoraki K, et al: The role of central venous pressure and type of vascular control in blood loss during major liver resections. Am J Surg 2004;187:398-402.

308. Kwan AL: Epidural analgesia for patient undergoing hepatectomy. Anaesth Intensive Care 2003;31:236-237.

309. Greenland K: Epidural analgesia for patient undergoing hepatectomy. Anaesth Intensive Care 2003;31:593-594; author reply 594.

310. Takaoka F, Teruya A, Massarollo P, et al: Minimizing risks for donors undergoing right hepatectomy for living-related liver transplantation. Anesth Analg 2003;97:297; author reply 297-298.

311. Liu S, Carpenter RL, Neal JM: Epidural anesthesia and analgesia: Their role in postoperative outcome. Anesthesiology 1995;82:1474-1506.

312. Ballantyne JC, Carr DB, deFerranti S, et al: The comparative effects of postoperative analgesic therapies on pulmonary outcome: Cumulative meta-analyses of randomized, controlled trials. Anesth Analg 1998;86:598-612.

313. Jayr C, Thomas H, Rey A, et al: Postoperative pulmonary complications: Epidural analgesia using bupivacaine and opioids versus parenteral opioids. Anesthesiology 1993;78:666-676; discussion 22A.

314. Moreno-Gonzalez E, Meneu-Diaz JG, Fundora Y, et al: Advantages of the piggy back technique on intraoperative transfusion, fluid consumption, and vasoactive drugs requirements in liver transplantation: A comparative study. Transplant Proc 2003;35:1918-1919.

6 Obesity and Nutritional Disorders

LARS E. HELGESON, MD

OBESITY

Obesity is not an uncommon disease. According to statistics from the Centers for Disease Control and Prevention (CDC), in the United States the incidence of overweight/obesity in adults is rising to alarming levels and is, in fact, becoming the norm. In 1994, 56% of the population was classified as overweight and 23% was classified as obese. In 2002 the overweight figure was 65% and the obese figure was 31% (Fig. 6-1).[1] A significantly higher percentage of minorities than whites are classified as obese (Table 6-1).[2] Most alarming is the rise in childhood obesity. In 1963, 4% of children 6 to 17 years of age were overweight. In 1994, 11% were overweight; and in 2004 the figure was 15% (Table 6-2). This trend shows no sign of abating. Long-term consequences for these children are substantial. They have a significantly greater chance of developing associated medical problems, such as diabetes, hypertension, and heart disease, at a much earlier age. They are also much more likely to suffer from depression and social isolation.

The United States is not alone with this epidemic. Currently, half the populations of Russia and the United Kingdom are classified as overweight or obese. Developing countries are "catching up" in this regard; 15% of China is classified as overweight, and the number is growing.[3] In parts of Africa, overweight children outnumber underweight children by a ratio of 3:1.

According to the World Health Organization, "overweight and obesity are now so common that they are replacing the more traditional public health concerns such as under-nutrition and infectious diseases."[4] Globally, there are now as many overnourished people as undernourished people. Obesity causes greater morbidity and mortality then tobacco and alcohol combined.[5]

Pathophysiology

The degree of obesity is most commonly and easily measured by the body mass index (BMI) which is calculated as mass (in kilograms) per height (in meters) (Box 6-1).[2] Using the BMI as a diagnostic tool is very useful, with certain limitations.[6]

Simplistically, obesity is caused by caloric intake above metabolic needs. Realistically, the causes of obesity are multiple, complex, and interconnected to varying degrees. Several causes are outlined in Box 6-2.

Most cases of obesity appear to be related to a lack of a sense of satiety. How is it that one individual would be satisfied with a 2100 kcal/day diet whereas another would feel unsatisfied with twice that? Obesity is not a choice or a sign of "weakness." It should be considered both a behavioral and medical condition that needs to be dealt with like any other disease state. Clearly, there are very strong biologically driven underpinnings. Metabolically, satiety has multiple feedback loops with complex interactions involving hormones, neural peptides, and proteins that are further complicated by social, genetic, and environmental factors.

The role played by societal dietary norms is clear. In many developed and developing countries, traditional dietary norms are such that overweight/obesity is uncommon. As these norms become displaced by high-fat fast food and other refined food products, the incidence of overweight and obesity rises. It is hard to miss the saturation advertising of snack food, fast food, and soft drinks (including "super-sizing") in many societies. These factors combine with sedentary lifestyles to cause the vast majority of overweight and obesity.

Pharmacologic agents occasionally contribute to obesity. Table 6-3 outlines several implicated medications. Affected individuals represent a small minority.

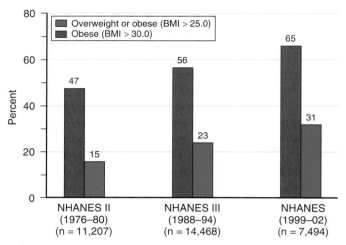

FIGURE 6–1 Age-adjusted prevalence of overweight and obesity among U.S. adults, age 20-74 years. (Age-adjusted by direct method to the year 2000 Bureau of the Census estimates using the age groups 20-39, 40-59, and 60-74 years.)

and bedridden patients. (2) Bodybuilders often have a mass of more then 100 kg and would certainly have a BMI of 30 or more kg/m², suggesting obesity. These individuals have a very low body fat percentage and could never be mistaken as being obese on appearance. (3) Lastly, the hypermuscular and obese patient would have a misleadingly high BMI.

Alternative methods of assessing body fat include abdominal girth taping, standardized height-weight tables, bioelectric impedance analysis, hydrostatic weighing, and skinfold caliper measurements (anthropometry). Each of these techniques has its own set of limitations.

Comorbidities

Even in "merely" overweight individuals (BMI of 28 kg/m²) there is undeniably an increased risk of poor health and premature death.[7-10] Obesity is closely associated with several other disease states (Box 6-3). It is true that certain disease states such as hypothyroidism, diabetes, and Cushing's syndrome can cause obesity. Most often it is the obesity that is the *cause* (not the effect) of many diseases. Table 6-5 outlines the increase in prevalence of several disease states directly attributable to obesity.

There are several pathophysiologic implications, depending on the distribution of fat. Android (truncal) distribution, more commonly seen in males, is associated with an increased incidence of cardiovascular disease and increased oxygen consumption (VO_2). Gynecoid distribution is usually seen in females; it is found predominantly on the buttocks and thighs and is less distinctly associated with cardiovascular disease. It is also less metabolically

Obesity can often be "diagnosed" simply by appearance. Obese individuals generally appear obese. However, it is important to evaluate the *degree* of obesity. Obesity is most commonly quantified by utilizing the BMI as outlined in Table 6-4. This method does have its limitations. There are three subtypes of individual in which BMI is misleading: (1) A sarcopenic individual is defined as having a relative decrease in lean body mass and a relative increase in body fat yet will have a normal BMI. This can occur in elderly

TABLE 6–1   Overweight and Obesity Prevalence by Ethnicity

Population Group	Prevalence of Overweight and Obesity in Adults BMI ≥ 25	Prevalence of Obesity in Adults BMI ≥ 30	Prevalence of Overweight in Children Ages 6-11	Prevalence of Overweight in Adolescents Ages 12-19
Total population	129,250,000	61,200,000		
Total males	64,660,000	26,370,000		
Total females	64,590,000	34,830,000		
Black				
Males	60.7%	28.1%	17.1%	20.7%
Females	77.3%	49.7%	22.2%	26.6%
Mexican American				
Males	74.7%	28.9%	27.3%	27.5%
Females	71.9%	39.7%	19.6%	19.4%
Hispanic				
Males	66.2%	21.8%		
Females	56.6%	23.3%		

BMI, body mass index.
Modified from American Heart Association: Heart Disease and Stroke Statistics—2003, American Heart Association, Dallas.

TABLE 6–2 Prevalence (%) of Overweight Among Children and Adolescents Ages 6-19 Years for Selected Years 1963-1965 Through 1999-2000

Age (Yr)*	1963-1965 1966-1970†	1971-1974	1976-1980	1988-1994	1999-2000
6-11	4%	4%	7%	11%	15%
12-19	5%	6%	5%	11%	15%

*Excludes pregnant women starting with 1971-1974. Pregnancy status not available for 1963-1965 and 1966-1970.
†Data for 1963-1965 are for children 6-11 years of age; data for 1966-1970 are for adolescents 12-17 years of age, not 12-19 years.
Adapted from Centers for Disease Control and Prevention National Center for Health Services: Prevalence of Overweight Among Children and Adolescents: United States, 1999/2000. Available at http://cdc.gov/nchs/products/pubs/pubd/hestats/overweight99.htm

active than android distribution.[11] Intra-abdominal fat is particularly associated with increased cardiovascular risk.[12]

The degree of expression of these comorbidities is highly variable, which must be taken into account whenever providing care to an obese patient.

Airway

A typical obese patient's bone structure is no different then that of a typical lean patient. Traditional parameters such as thyromental distance, narrow palate, receding chin, and overbite are equally applicable in the obese and lean patient. For most overweight/obese individuals, the excess fat has no significant impact on airway management.[13,14] There is a subset of individuals whose airways are narrowed by redundant pharyngeal tissue. Obstruction is most often seen at the retropalatal level, but other sites may be involved.[15,16] Even modestly overweight people can be affected by obstructive sleep apnea (OSA).[17] This symptom suggests that mechanical obstruction is likely, as the patient's level of consciousness diminishes. Except in

super morbidly obese patients, the degree of pharyngeal tissue redundancy is not reliably predicted by external appearance. Neck flexion/extension is more commonly impaired in patients with a BMI greater than 40, owing to prominent fat stores on the anteroposterior neck, submental area, and anteroposterior chest wall.

Respiratory/Metabolic

Basal metabolic rate is related to body surface area and is usually normal. However, obese individuals have increased production of carbon dioxide (Vco_2) and increased oxygen consumption (Vo_2).[18] It was previously thought that adipose cellular metabolism was responsible for this increase. It has now been shown that this increased metabolism is primarily due to increased effort for movement and work of breathing due to "mass loading" of the

---

BOX 6–1   Calculation of Body Mass Index

Body Mass Index (BMI) = Mass in kilograms divided by height in meters^2 (BMI = kg/m^2)

BOX 6–2   Etiology of Obesity

Sedentary lifestyle
Dietary norms
Familial/genetic tendencies
Intrinsic physiologic tendency
Emotional/behavioral
Disease states (e.g., diabetes, hypothyroidism, Cushing's syndrome, hypothalamic lesions, Prader-Willi syndrome)
Pharmacologic

TABLE 6–3   Drugs Contributing to the Etiology Of Obesity

Glucocorticoids

Hypoglycemic agents
  Insulin, sulfonylureas

Antidepressants
  Amitriptyline, imipramine, desipramine, fluvoxamine

Central nervous system agents
  Valproic acid, methysergide, metergoline

Antihypertensives
  Clonidine, prazosin, propranolol

Sex hormones
  Progestogens

Miscellaneous
  Phenothiazine, cyproheptadine, lithium

Adapted from Atkinson RL: A 33-year-old woman with morbid obesity. JAMA 2000;283:3236-3243.

Adapted from Bessesen DH, Kushner R (eds): Evaluation and Management of Obesity. Philadelphia, Hanley & Belfus, 2002, p 2.

TABLE 6–4 Classification of Obesity and Malnutrition Using Body Mass Index

Category	BMI (kg/m^2)
Severely malnourished	<15
Moderate malnutrition	15-16.9
Mild malnutrition	17-18.5
Normal	18.6-24.9
Overweight	25-29.9
Obese	30-39.9
Morbid obesity	≥40
Super morbid	>50

TABLE 6–5 Proportion of Disease Prevalence Attributable to Obesity

Type II diabetes	57%
Hypertension	17%
Coronary heart disease	17%
Gallbladder disease	30%
Osteoarthritis	14%
Breast cancer	11%
Uterine cancer	11%
Colon cancer	11%

chest wall. The work of breathing in the morbidly obese is increased by up to 70%, compared with the nonobese.[19] These increases are much more pronounced during exertion compared to lean individuals.

Pulmonary

Obtaining preoperative pulmonary function tests (PFTs) is usually not indicated for obesity per se, because the results will not alter management. There does not seem to be any correlation between the abnormalities seen in the PFT results in obese patients and pulmonary complications,[20] although there is a correlation with airway, ventilator, and pulmonary management. Obese individuals have greater amounts of chest wall adipose tissue, including breasts in men and women. This "mass loading" has the net affect of increasing the intrathoracic pressure, which will increase the amount of alveolar compression and closure. This results in significant intrapulmonary shunting as deoxygenated pulmonary artery blood passes through nonventilated alveoli to mix with oxygenated blood in the pulmonary vein.[21] Some individuals have alveolar closure during normal, upright spontaneous breathing.[22,23] This decrease in functional residual capacity is exacerbated by mass shifting from the abdomen as the patient lies supine and further worsened by the Trendelenburg position. Figures 6-2 and 6-3 illustrate this concept. The decrease in functional residual capacity can be so significant as to drop well below closing capacity. Clinically, this means that apnea for as short as 5 seconds can result in hypoxemia.[24] A conscious patient may have difficulty remaining supine for even short periods of time and in more severe cases may become hypoxic when supine for only a few moments. This may necessitate intubation, induction, and maintenance of general anesthesia in a semi-seated position. If possible, other techniques of "off-loading" can be employed (Fig. 6-4).[25]

Postoperatively, obese patients are at increased risk of hypoxia, pulmonary atelectasis, and pneumonia.[26]

Cardiovascular

Many overweight patients have no significant cardiovascular disease, but incidental eccentric left ventricular hypertrophy is frequently found.[27] Normal left ventricular function is usually present, but diminished left ventricular compliance is common.[28] In some individuals, left ventricular diastolic dysfunction can develop, which results in greater sensitivity to changes in preload and afterload. As the duration and degree of obesity increases, so can the degree of ventricular dysfunction and, ultimately, pulmonary hypertension.[29-32]

BOX 6–3 Comorbidities of Obesity

Hypertension
Coronary artery disease
Deep venous thrombosis
Atherosclerosis
Increased stroke risk
Insulin resistance
Diabetes mellitus type II
Orthopedic (knees, hips, spine)
Psychosocial (depression, anxiety, interpersonal difficulties)
Hyperlipidemia
Gastroesophageal reflux
Sleep apnea
Obesity hypoventilation syndrome (pickwickian syndrome)
Asthma
Fatty liver
Cholecystitis and cholelithiasis
Cancer (breast, uterine, prostate, renal, colon, pancreatic, gastric)
Gout
Menstrual abnormalities
Complicated labor and childbirth
Poor surgical wound healing
Increased risk for postoperative thrombophlebitis and pneumonia

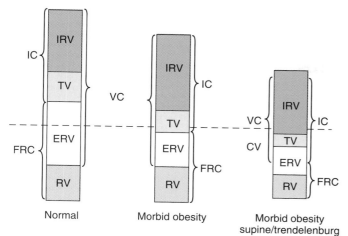

FIGURE 6–2 Comparison of lung volumes between lean and obese subjects. In some morbidly obese patients, lying supine, tidal volume (TV) can be at or below closing volume (CV). VC, vital capacity; IC, inspiratory capacity; FRC, functional residual capacity; IRV, inspiratory reserve volume; ERV, expiratory reserve volume; RV, residual volume.

Guidelines for assessing the cardiovascular risk[33] are applicable to both the obese and lean patient (Fig. 6-5). This includes the use of β blockers. Because of the diminished physical activity and increased incidence of hypertension, hyperlipidemia, and diabetes, there is an increased risk of cardiovascular disease compared with the general population. Cardiovascular disease must always be suspected, and the threshold is lower for a comprehensive cardiac evaluation.

Circulating blood volume is increased with increasing body weight. Cardiac output is increased, usually owing to increased stroke volume and an essentially unchanged heart rate.[34] This limits any increase in cardiac output that may otherwise be required.

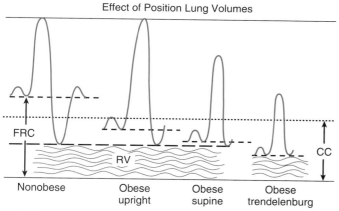

Effect of Position Lung Volumes

FIGURE 6–3 Effect of position change in various lung volumes in nonobese subject compared with markedly obese subject. FRC, functional residual capacity; RV, residual volume; CC, closing capacity. *(From Brown BR [ed]: Anesthesia and the Obese Patient. Contemporary Anesthesia Practice Series. Philadelphia, FA Davis, 1982, p 26.)*

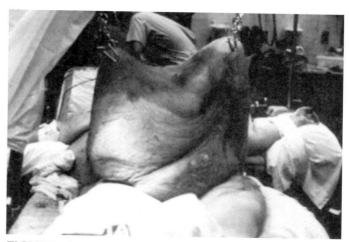

FIGURE 6–4 Patient's abdominal panniculus mechanically lifted followed by markedly improved arterial oxygenation. *(From Wyner J, Brodsky JB, Merrell RC: Massive obesity and arterial oxygenation. Anesth Analg 1981;60:691-693.)*

Perioperative Concerns

Evaluating every patient's baseline medical status is the starting point for any anesthetic. One has to know what medical conditions exist and how they can affect the patient's well being and our anesthetic management. Assuming that a patient has been properly treated for any preexisting medical conditions, maintenance of the patient's baseline medical status is the ideal preoperative situation. For example, continuing antiseizure or antihypertensive medications and tight control of diabetes through the day of surgery are well-established protocols.

If a patient's medical conditions are not properly treated, the case needs to be delayed until the medical status is stable. If the procedure cannot be delayed, then we must manage the patient as conditions present. In this context, management of the obese patient is no different than for any other patient. Obesity does present several unique issues that warrant special attention.

Emotional Issues

Obese individuals undergo a daily routine of subtle and not-so-subtle social slights, insults, and discrimination. They have had a lifetime of negative self-image, which is reinforced by almost all aspects of society. Advertising emphasizes "thin is good and fat is bad." There are embarrassing difficulties in finding clothes that fit or having difficulty fitting in a movie theater or airline seat. Consequently, an obese patient will often bring varied emotional baggage with which we must deal. There are two principles to which we must adhere when dealing with an obese patient. First, we discuss with the patient the issues that are specifically relevant to our anesthetic care which are a consequence of the patient's weight. Discussions should be "matter of fact" and should avoid glossing over issues

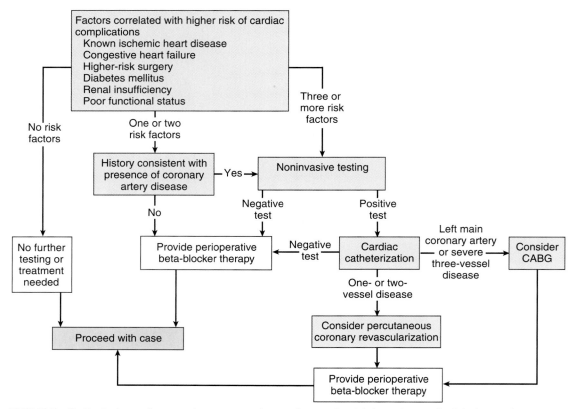

FIGURE 6–5 Pathway for assessing preoperative cardiovascular risk in patients scheduled to undergo noncardiac surgery. The decision whether to perform noninvasive testing is based on the presence of clinical risk factors, the patient's functional status, and the type of surgery scheduled. If the result of a noninvasive test is abnormal, the decision whether to perform cardiac catheterization is based on several features. The likelihood of left main coronary artery disease or severe three-vessel disease is much higher, and cardiac catheterization should be considered more strongly if ischemia is provoked at a low level of stress or persists during stress testing, if there is severe ST-segment depression, if large areas of the myocardium appear to be at risk, or if ischemia is demonstrated in a patient known to have left ventricular dysfunction at rest. Coronary artery bypass grafting (CABG) and percutaneous coronary revascularization should be performed only if justified independently of the need for noncardiac surgery.[33] *(Modified from Fleisher LA, Eagle KA: Clinical practice: Lowering cardiac risk in noncardiac surgery. N Engl J Med 2001;45:1677-1682.)*

or using euphemisms. The patient knows that he or she is obese and that there are issues related to that fact. However, we should not bring undue attention to the patient's obesity or in any way come across as judgmental or patronizing. Second, we should act compassionately and treat the obese patient with simple kindness, humanity, and respect. We should avoid any condescension, innuendo, or comments about the patient's size and avoid any "talk" with other people anywhere near the patient.

Airway

Our goal is to provide a safe anesthetic, and gaining control of the patient's airway is central to this. It is wise to optimize all factors to safely gain control of the patient's airway. Because of fat distribution on the obese patient's back and shoulders, it is necessary to build a custom ramp out of blankets to properly align the oral, laryngeal, and pharyngeal axes (Fig. 6-6). A useful reference point is an imaginary horizontal line drawn between the earlobe and sternum, as noted in Figure 6-7.

The American Society of Anesthesiologists (ASA) difficult airway algorithm, noted in Figure 6-8,[35] is a well-known and proven guideline. This algorithm is applicable to both the obese and lean patient. As noted earlier, most overweight/obese patients do not present with a difficult airway, although they do have a greater likelihood of it occurring compared with the general population.

A recent history of previous difficult or uneventful intubations should be obtained. This is the best predictor for an uneventful laryngoscopy/intubation. A thorough evaluation should be done, including the Mallampati score, atlanto-occipital mobility (neck extension), mouth opening, mandible width, neck circumference, thyromental distance, and dentition. The degree of any limitations in range of motion must be identified. One critical bit of usually missing information is the amount of fatty redundant tissue in the pharynx. This is very difficult to assess.

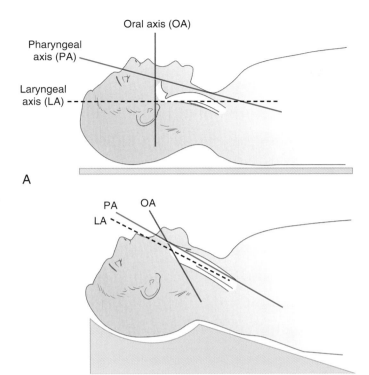

FIGURE 6–6 Schematic diagram demonstrating head position for endotracheal intubation. **A,** Successful direct laryngoscopy for exposure of the glottic opening requires alignment of the oral, pharyngeal, and laryngeal axes. **B,** Subsequent head extension at the atlanto-occipital joint serves to align the three axes, resulting in the shortest distance and most nearly straight line from the incisor teeth to glottic opening. *(Adapted from Nichol HC, Zuck D: Difficult laryngoscopy: The "anterior" larynx and the atlanto-occipital gap. Br J Anaesth 1983;55:141.)*

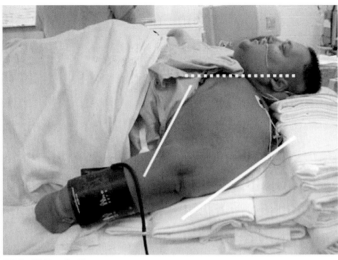

FIGURE 6–7 This figure illustrates proper positioning ("ramping") allowing optimal airway alignment in an obese patient. A useful reference point is an imaginary horizontal line drawn between the earlobe and sternum *(dashed line)*. Upper arm distortion *(solid lines)* precludes standard placement of noninvasive blood pressure cuff.

A history of significant OSA is suggestive (but not reliably predictive), as is a large-circumference neck and lateral neck radiographs, ultrasound, or computed tomographic scan.[36] A preoperative otolaryngologic evaluation may be helpful.[37] Anecdotally, another suggestive parameter is a BMI greater than 50 kg/m^2.

With excessive tissue redundancy, the only reason the airway is patent may be due to the patient's muscle tone, which will stent open the pharynx. This redundant soft tissue is likely to collapse and obstruct the pharynx after the patient loses consciousness. When induced, it may not be possible to ventilate or intubate the patient. It is these patients who have the severest form of OSA and who may later develop pickwickian syndrome.

There are many routines in the approach to management of a suspected difficult airway. Box 6-4 illustrates one approach for preparing a patient's airway for awake manipulation. One deviation from the ASA algorithm that can be very useful is performing a "direct look." A patient who is suspected of having a difficult airway is prepared as for an awake fiberoptic intubation with an antisialagogue, optimum positioning, judicious sedation, and thorough topicalization with local anesthetic. Incremental, direct laryngoscopy is performed with additional topicalization. A laryngoscopic view is obtained, not only of the vocal cord grade but with special attention paid to the amount of redundant pharyngeal tissue. If there is good visualization of the vocal cords with minimal redundancy, a standard rapid-sequence induction is indicated. If the vocal cord view is poor or there is tissue redundancy, the trachea should then be intubated with the patient awake. Induction should occur only after confirmation of proper placement. An advantage of the "direct look" is that the oropharynx is well anesthetized, should awake fiber optic intubation be necessary.

Gastrointestinal Issues

Obese patients are at significantly greater risk for aspiration (Box 6-5). As with any patient, anxiety, pain, trauma, and certain drugs all decrease gastric emptying.[38] It is well established that fasting obese preoperative patients have a gastric volume greater than 25 mL and a pH less than 2.5.[39,40] If aspirated, this volume and pH can lead to significant pulmonary parenchymal injury. Steps to minimize this risk are outlined in Box 6-6. The efficacy of cricoid pressure has been brought into question.[41,42] Whereas most sources advocate some variant of aspiration prophylaxis, aside from keeping the patient NPO, there is no real evidence to support this widespread practice. However, it is prudent to continue this standard, because it is a

Difficult Airway Algorithm

1. Assess the likelihood and clinical impact of basic management problems:
   A. Difficult ventilation
   B. Difficult intubation
   C. Difficulty with patient cooperation or consent
   D. Difficult tracheostomy

2. Actively pursue opportunities to deliver supplemental oxygen throughout the process of difficult airway management.

3. Consider the relative merits and feasibility of management choices:

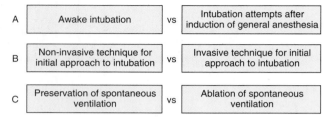

4. Develop primary and alternative strategies:

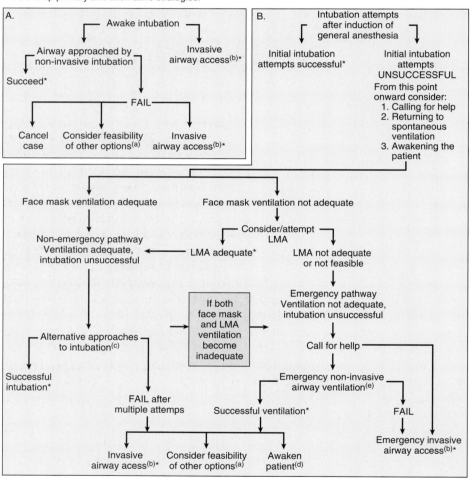

*Confirm ventilation, tracheal intubation, or LMA placement with exhaled CO_2

a. Other options include (but are not limited to): surgery utilizing face mask or LMA anesthesia, local anesthesia infiltration or regional nerve blockade. Pursuit of these options usually implies that mask ventilation will not be problematic. Therefore, these options may be of limited value if this step in the algorithm has been reached via the Emergency pathway.

b. Invasive airway access includes surgical or percutaneous tracheostomy or cricothyrotomy.

c. Alternative non-invasive approaches to difficult intubation include (but are not limited to): use of different laryngoscope blades. LMA as an intubation conduit (with or without fiberoptic guidance), fiberoptic intubation indubating stylet or tube changer, light wand, retrograde intubation, and blind oral or nasal intubation.

d. Consider re-preparation of the patient for awake intubation or canceling surgery.

e. Options for emergency non-invasive airway ventilation include (but are not limited to): rigid bronchoscope, esophageal-tracheal combitube ventilation, or transtracheal jet ventilation.

FIGURE 6–8 ASA difficult airway algorithm. *(From Practice guidelines for management of the difficult airway: A report by the American Society of Anesthesiologists task force on management of the difficult airway. Anesthesiology 1993;78: 597-602.)*

BOX 6–4 Airway Preparation for Awake Airway Manipulation

Fasting
Antisialogue
Metaclopromide
H2 blocker
(Non-particulate antacids)
Judicious sedation
Airway topical anesthesia options
  Lidocaine 4% nebulizer
  Viscous lidocaine gargle
  Direct spraying
  Transtracheal block
  Superior laryngeal nerve block
  Glossopharyngeal nerve block
Optimize airway alignment

BOX 6–6 Steps to Minimize Risk of Aspiration

NPO
H2 blocker or proton pump inhibitors the night before and morning of surgery (PO or IV)
Metoclopramide
  PO: 2 hours preinduction or
  IV: 30-45 minutes preinduction
Nonparticulate antacids, if unable to utilize H2 blockers
"Ramping," with optimal airway alignment
Awake intubation, or rapid-sequence induction using cricoid pressure

relatively benign treatment and the consequences of aspiration are severe.

Pulmonary Issues

As mentioned earlier, obese patients have a decreased functional residual capacity owing to mass loading of the chest wall, as well as transdiaphragmatic distention from the abdomen. The extent of this diminished functional residual capacity depends on the degree of obesity. Positioning of the patient for surgical needs may further diminish the functional residual capacity. Ventilator management under these conditions is challenging, to say the least. Trendelenburg positioning should be avoided, preferably using the reverse Trendelenburg position to offload the lungs, thereby improving the functional residual capacity. In select circumstances it is possible to maintain traction on the pannus, also offloading the lungs (see Fig. 6-7). Coordination with the surgeon is necessary to lessen the impact of abdominal packing and retractors. Proper prone positioning is actually less problematic then supine positioning, provided that the hanging abdomen is minimally supported.[43]

Use of positive end-expiratory pressure is often helpful because it maintains the patency of alveoli that would

BOX 6–5 Factors that Contribute to Increased Risk of Aspiration in the Obese Patient

Greater incidence of hiatal hernia
Altered geometry of gastroesophageal junction
Increased intra-abdominal pressure
Increased fasting gastric fluid volume
Decreased fasting gastric pH
Possible delayed intubation due to "difficult airway"
Possible gastric distention due to attempted mask ventilation

otherwise collapse. Careful attention must be paid to peak airway pressures to avoid barotrauma.[44] The ventilator "pressure control" setting versus "volume control" setting may be helpful in this regard. Alternatively, increasing respiratory rate and decreasing tidal volumes may be the only option. Hyperventilation resulting in hypocarbia should be avoided because of the rise in shunt fraction.[21] Ordinarily, hypoxia triggers the pulmonary hypoxic vasoconstriction response to lessen the intrapulmonary shunting. Volatile anesthetics generally blunt this response, which can result in even greater hypoxia. Initially, the obese patient's FIO_2 should begin at 1.0 and then be titrated down, using pulse oximetry as a guide.

Positioning

Even though the bone structure of obese individuals is essentially normal, the alignment is often distorted by the overlying tissue when supine. Proper "ramping" is often required for optimal airway alignment. The head must be properly supported in a neutral or slightly flexed position. One area not often considered is the lumbar spine. The buttocks can act as a fulcrum for the legs, which will extend the lumbar spine. A remedy for this is to support the knees, which will flex the hips, relieving the spine extension. Another area often ignored is the arms. With the patient lying on a ramp, the shoulders tend to extend downward (posteriorly), putting significant stress on the brachial plexus and shoulder joint. Because of the excess tissue on the upper arm, the lower arm also extends, putting excess stress on the elbow joint. It is vital to position the joints with slight flexion and to provide proper padding and support (Fig. 6-9). Abduction of the shoulder to less than 90 degrees may likewise be necessary. One solution is to simply ask the patient if there is any discomfort or if there are any stress points and to then correct this before induction of anesthesia.

Monitoring

Electrocardiography and pulse oximetry do not present any differences compared with those in the lean patient.

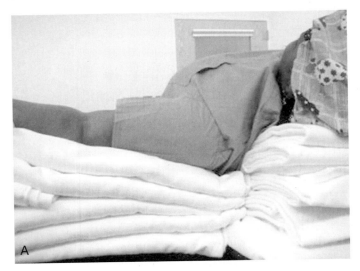

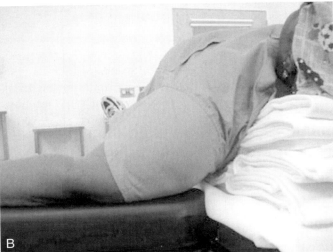

FIGURE 6–9 Illustration of proper (**A**) and improper (**B**) arm positioning. Proper positioning minimizes risk of joint, brachial plexus, and nerve compression injuries.

Central venous pressure or pulmonary artery catheter monitoring should be performed only when clinically indicated and not based on obesity alone. Frequently, the upper arms of obese patients have a pronounced cone shape (see Fig. 6-7). A noninvasive blood pressure (NIBP) cuff is designed to work on a cylindrically shaped arm. A larger NIBP cuff may reach around the arm, but the arm shape remains problematic and will often give erroneous readings, as noted in Table 6-6. There are alternatives (Fig. 6-10), which are further outlined in Table 6-7.

Pharmacokinetics/Pharmacodynamics

When providing any anesthetic, our drug dosages are calculated based on well-established protocols, as well as "titration to effect." In the obese patient, there is usually much more "titration" involved than in the lean patient.

This variability in recommendations for drugs is not clarified by the lack of consensus in the literature concerning anesthetic drugs and their pharmacokinetics and pharmacodynamics.[45-53] Table 6-8 outlines several anesthetic drugs and their suggested dosing guidelines for obese patients.

The following discussion of reference dosages is based on ideal body weight (IBW) in the obese patient. Because of the increased circulating blood volume, the volume of distribution is somewhat increased for the water-soluble drugs. Clearly, the volume of distribution for fat-soluble agents is significantly increased. However, the termination of effect and clearance is similar between the obese and lean populations. Owing to the higher levels of pseudocholinesterase in obese patients, the dosage of succinylcholine should be increased. Most nondepolarizing neuromuscular blockers should be dosed based on IBW. Mivacurium should be dosed based on IBW, but the dosage of pancuronium should be slightly increased. Interestingly, atracurium has a similar duration of action when dosed on either IBW or actual body weight.[54] Inhalation agents show no difference in minimal alveolar concentration (MAC). Because of the very low fat solubility of currently used agents, equilibrium is rapidly reached. Washout and emergence is not significantly different in the obese. Propofol dosing should be based on IBW with additional small dose titration. Recovery is similar to that in nonobese patients.[55] Thiopental induction dose should be increased somewhat.

Narcotic dosages are not well defined in obese patients, and administration should be altered judiciously, compared with a lean patient. Further clouding the situation, narcotics have significant interpatient variability. All narcotics should be titrated to effect.

Morphine is generally dosed based on IBM. Fentanyl dosage should be based on actual body mass.[51] Alfentanil has a reduced clearance and therefore a more prolonged half-life and should be dosed based on IBM, as should remifentanyl.[56]

The primary concern with narcotic use in the obese patient is postoperative respiratory depression. This concern, along with dosing uncertainty, often leads to poorly treated postoperative pain. This can lead to decreased mobility and deep breathing, which results in greater risk for deep vein thrombosis, atelectasis, and pneumonia. There must be a balance struck between the concern for respiratory depression and adequate postoperative pain control.

This degree of dosing uncertainty clearly illustrates the fact that there are multiple variable physiologic influences on anesthetic pharmacokinetics and pharmacodynamics. The suggested dosage adjustments in Table 6-8 are a reasonable starting point, but judgment and "titration" play a significant role in proper anesthetic drug administration.

TABLE 6-6   Blood Pressure Reading Discrepancies by Varied Arm Circumferences

Bladder width (cm)	12.0		15.9		18.0	
Ideal arm circumference (cm)	30.0		37.5		45.0	
Arm circumference range (cm)	26-33		33-41		>41	
Arm circumference (cm)	SBP	DBP	SBP	DBP	SBP	DBP
26	+5	+3	+7	+5	+9	+5
28	+3	+2	+5	+4	+8	+5
30	0	0	+4	+3	+7	+4
32	−2	−1	+3	+2	+6	+4
34	−4	−3	+2	+1	+5	+3
36	−6	−4	0	+1	+5	+3
40	−8	−6	−1	0	+4	+2
38	−10	−7	−2	−1	+3	+1
42	−12	−9	−4	−2	+2	+1
46	−14	−10	−5	−3	1	0
48	−16	−11	−6	−3	0	0
50	−18	−13	−7	−4	−1	−1
60	−21	−14	−9	−5	−1	−1

Modified from Graves JW, Bailey KR, Sheps SG: The changing distribution of arm circumferences in NHANES III and NHANES 2000 and its impact on the utility of the "standard adult" blood pressure cuff. Blood Press Monit 2003;8:223-227.

Pickwickian Syndrome

This term was classically described as the combination of morbid obesity, hypersomnolence, plethora, and edema[57] and originated from a prominent literary character in Charles Dickens *Oliver Twist*. This condition is commonly referred to as "obesity hypoventilation syndrome" (OHS). Owing to the mass loading of their chest walls, these individuals have difficulty adequately ventilating their lungs, resulting in poor gas exchange. They are often hypoxic and hypercapnic when awake at rest and have secondary polycythemia. They often develop pulmonary hypertension and are more prone to right-sided heart failure in advanced stages. Some reserve the term *pickwickian* for OHS patients with signs of cor pulmonale.[19] The etiology for OHS is not well understood but is related to the combination of an alteration in the brain's control of ventilation and mechanical effects on the chest wall. Patients with OHS may also have concurrent OSA, but many do not. It does not appear that OSA is the direct cause for OHS, but it may contribute in some cases.[58,59] Anesthetic implications are similar to those for the "ordinary" obese patient. These patients are more sensitive to the respiratory depression caused by narcotics and hypnotics.[60,61] The added concern of hypoxia, hypercarbia, and potential pulmonary hypertension and right-sided heart failure warrants special attention. At a minimum, baseline arterial blood gas values are appropriate as reference points for later management. These patients are more likely to have perioperative cardiopulmonary problems, so invasive monitoring should be considered, not only for intraoperative management but also for postoperative care. Management of perioperative OHS patients should reference their baseline values and not the "normal" reference parameters.

PROTEIN-ENERGY MALNUTRITION DISORDERS

This relatively recent term refers to several different under-nourished states. As the name implies, there is a dietary deficiency in protein and/or caloric intake. There is a wide range of clinical presentations, depending on patient age, acuity, severity, duration, and concurrent diseases. There is significant overlap (especially with marasmus and kwashiorkor) regarding causes, presentation, treatment, and anesthetic implications.

Protein-energy malnutrition (PEM) can be "primary," resulting from inadequate dietary intake, and is noted in developing countries and has multiple socioeconomic, political, and environmental causes. Secondary PEM is a result of decreased absorption or increased nutritional needs (as from acute or chronic illness) and is mainly seen in developed countries (Table 6-9).[62]

This discussion includes an overview of each of the various PEM syndromes. Deficiencies of specific amino acids are not discussed. For further details, the reader is referred to more in-depth sources.[62-67]

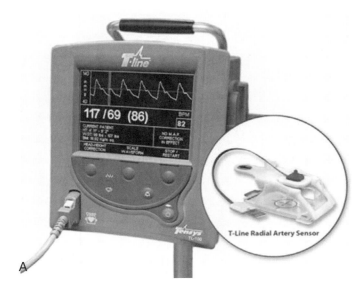

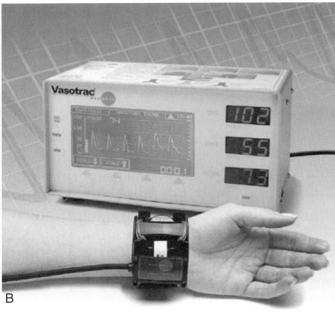

FIGURE 6–10 Alternative noninvasive blood pressure monitoring devices. **A,** T-Line by Tensys Medical. **B,** Vasotrac by Medwave.

Childhood Disorders

Kwashiorkor

The term *kwashiorkor* originated from the GA language in western Africa and refers to the child who is weaned from breast feeding when another child is born. The result is the loss of often the only source of high-quality dietary protein. It is sometimes referred to as edematous PEM. Typically, kwashiorkor occurs when weaning or shortly thereafter. It occurs most often in tropical societies where the main dietary staple is carbohydrates with low protein content (cassava, yams). This is in contrast to that in temperate countries, where the staples are grains relatively rich in proteins. Very rarely, it has occurred in developed countries in cases of child neglect or misdirected dietary restrictions. At first glance, these children appear nourished, but they have a severe protein deficiency. They are colloquially referred to as "sugar babies" (Fig. 6-11). These children's abdomens are distended not due to ascites but from edematous and distended intestine and an enlarged, fatty liver.

Marasmus

This disorder refers to a dietary deficiency of both protein and calories and is sometimes referred to as nonedematous PEM. These children's progressively starved appearance is one of emaciation with generalized muscle wasting. Later stages show virtually no subcutaneous fat and a face that appears withdrawn or "wizened," with sunken eyes and hollow cheeks. This occurs mostly in areas of famine but can occur in developed countries in cases of child abuse and neglect (Fig. 6-12). There are less severe cases of marasmus that are related to commercial formula feeding[68] and in hospitalized children undergoing treatment for other conditions.[69,70]

Marasmic Kwashiorkor

This refers to children exhibiting variable characteristics of both marasmus and kwashiorkor. The presentation is seen in children with an inconsistent diet that varies in protein and calories.

Refeeding Syndrome

This problem was first described in post–World War II victims of starvation. The logical thought was to provide a high-calorie, high-protein diet to these victims. What was not understood is "reductive adaptation," which is an energy and nutrient conserving adaptive response by severely undernourished individuals. Unfortunately, severe gastrointestinal and metabolic derangements occurred, with many patients dying as a result of the best intentions. This is an ongoing problem today. These misconceptions are common in afflicted areas, which is the reason that the mortality rate from PEM has remained virtually unchanged for the past 50 years.[71,72] The proper protocols are clearly outlined by the World Health Organization[73] and shown in simplified form in Table 6-10. These patients often have renal and electrolyte abnormalities, so intravenous hydration must be closely monitored. Gradual and progressive introduction of increasing amounts of carbohydrates, micronutrients, fats, and protein into the diet turned out to be the proper approach. The gastrointestinal mucosa is not able to process the sudden appearance of large amounts of food and must first be gradually stimulated back to normal functional levels. Additionally,

TABLE 6–7	Alternatives for Blood Pressure Monitoring
Options	**Comments**
Arterial line	Time consuming Technical problems with placement Technical problems with monitoring Some risk to patient
NIBP cuff placement on forearm	Usually reliable Simple to use Pulse pressure slightly wider than proximal placement
Vasotrac by Medwave T-Line by Tensys Medical (see Fig. 6-10)	Relatively newer technologies Near continuous NIBP monitoring at the radial artery Usually but does not always correlate with NIBP cuff or arterial line Some technical problems with use. Precise placement over radial artery required.

NIBP, Noninvasive blood pressure.

the "machinery" of cellular metabolism and physiology needs to be corrected before advancing the diet to make up for the nutritional deficiencies.[74] This concept applies both to enteral and parenteral nutrition. Cardiac dysrhythmias, heart failure, respiratory failure, liver and kidney functional derangements, coma, convulsions, and death can all occur with a too aggressive nutritional or intravenous treatment. A key concern with the refeeding syndrome is hypophosphatemia (and hypokalemia) and their sequelae.[75]

Clinical Implications

Table 6-11 outlines a comparison of kwashiorkor and marasmus to help differentiate the disorders.

Kwashiorkor is considered by some to be a subtype of marasmus, where the child has an underlying infection or other stress leading to a metabolic cascade.[76] This idea explains only some of the clinical overlap. It is important to understand the physiologic alterations and how to deal with them.

Preoperatively, these children must be nutritionally improved and it is vital that the refeeding syndrome be avoided. Problems concerning drug metabolism and distribution, myocardial, renal, and hepatic function, and electrolyte derangements are all highly unpredictable and place the child at extreme risk. Any sort of surgical procedure must be delayed, except in the direst of circumstances. Ideally, the child should be fed so as to eventually approach a "normal" height/weight ratio. Certainly, this

TABLE 6–8	Dosage of Anesthesia Drugs		
	Dosage Based on:		
Drug	**IBM**	**Adjust**	**Notes**
Propofol		✓	Increase induction dose somewhat due to increased blood volume
Thiopental		✓	Increase dose ~10% relative to IBM. Larger volume of distribution
Volatile agents	✓		No change in minimal alveolar concentration
Midazolam		✓	Increased dosage expected, relative to IBM. Titrate to effect
Narcotics	✓		Titrate to effect (see text)
Succinylcholine		✓	Increase dosage based on IBM due to ↑ plasma cholinesterase
Mivacurium		✓	Minimal data Increase somewhat relative to IBM
Rocuronium	✓		
Atracurium		✓	Based on ABM or IBM
Vecuronium	✓		
Pancuronium		✓	Increase dosage ~10% relative to IBM

ABM, actual body mass; IBM, ideal body mass, LBM, lean body mass.

TABLE 6–9   Representative Causes of Secondary Protein-Energy Malnutrition

Malabsorption
    Pancreatic insufficiency
    Pancreatitis
    Bacterial overgrowth
    Gluten-sensitive enteropathy
    Radiation enteritis
    Intestinal ischemia
    Assorted surgical alterations
    Motility diseases

Increased needs
    Sepsis
    Growth

Altered appetite
    Psychiatric/behavioral
    Chronic illness
        Cancer
        Tuberculosis
    Pharmacologic

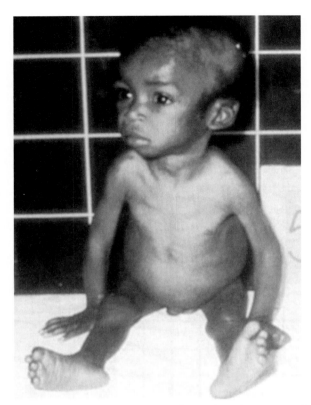

FIGURE 6–12 Marasmus. Note the profound wasting and sparse hair. *(From Zitelli BJ, Davis HW: Atlas of Pediatric Physical Diagnosis, 4th ed. Philadelphia, Mosby, 2002, p 338.)*

is usually not a realistic option. There would be an improvement in outcome if the procedure could be delayed even some days while following the guidelines of the World Health Organization of resuscitation and stabilization. This will at least begin to repair some of the cellular metabolic derangements to improve the patients' physiologic responses to the anesthetic and surgical stresses. It is difficult to give any specific anesthetic management suggestions concerning the PEM child in the acute phase of the disorder. The plan and management must be highly individualized (taking into account the physiologic changes noted in Box 6-7) and to proceed only with patience, great reluctance, and extreme care.

Adult Disorders

Refeeding Syndrome

This topic has been discussed previously in detail. This syndrome must be taken into account in all forms of adult starvation. The principles and practice are equally applicable for both adults and children and bear no further discussion here.

Anorexia Nervosa and Starvation

Anorexia nervosa is a subtype of adult starvation. It is a psychiatric/emotional disorder of primarily adolescent and young women in wealthy societies. It occurs uncommonly in males. There are societal pressures emphasizing the idea that one needs to be thin to be attractive or worthwhile. Combined with a distorted body image,[77] affected individuals diet to the point of starvation (Figure 6-13).

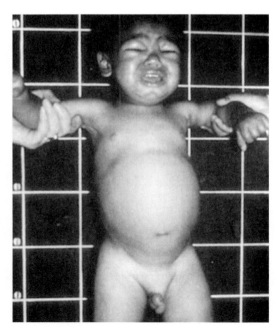

FIGURE 6–11 Kwashiorkor. This patient has a typical "sugar baby" appearance with generalized edema. Note the periorbital and limb edema. *(From Zitelli BJ, Davis HW: Atlas of Pediatric Physical Diagnosis, 4th ed. Philadelphia, Mosby, 2002, p 339.)*

TABLE 6–10 Initial Clinical Management of Severe Malnutrition

Resuscitate Acutely

- Treat fluid and electrolyte imbalance and shock: administer oxygen and glucose, reduce heat loss, give antibiotics, maintain circulation, treat vitamin A deficiency.

Stabilize

- Control energy and protein intake at maintenance: 400 kJ/kg/day (10 kcal/kg/day), 1 to 1.5 g protein/kg/day.
- Small frequent meals: eight meals every 3 hours or six meals every 4 hours throughout 24 hours.
- Correct deficiencies of specific nutrients by addition to food: potassium (4 mmol/kg/day), magnesium (0.4 mmol/kg/day), folic acid (1 mg/day), zinc (2 mg/kg/day), copper (0.3 mg/kg/day), multivitamin supplement.
- Treat bacterial infection: broad-spectrum antibiotics, cotrimoxazole or ampicillin with gentamicin.
- Treat small bowel overgrowth with metronidazole.
- Treat helminth infections with mebendazole.
- Transfuse for severe anemia.
- Topical treatment and care for skin lesions.
- Exclude tuberculosis.
- Give sensory stimulation and emotional support.

Weight Gain (Rapid Catch-Up Growth)

- Ad libitum intake to achieve at least 600 kJ/kg/day (15 kcal/kg/day), 4 g protein/kg/day.
- Continue with micronutrient supplements.
- Add supplemental iron.
- Give sensory stimulation and emotional support.

Modified from Management of the Child with Severe Malnutrition: A Manual for Physicians and Senior Health Care Workers. Geneva, World Health Organization, 1999.

Adult victims of starvation can come from different situations. They may have been prisoners or hostages, be engaged in hunger strikes, or, most often, live in an area with environmental, political, or socioeconomic upheaval. Prognosis is dependant on several variables.[78] However, there are two groups of patients with underrecognized states of malnutrition. One group is the elderly, who may be living independently in the community or in a nursing home and may be undernourished for varied reasons.[79,80] Another group is the hospitalized patients, especially the elderly, with chronic medical conditions.[81-85] These patients' nutritional status and requirements are often not adequately considered or monitored when treating their underlying medical conditions.

Clinical Implications

Starvation entails a progressive increased use of body fat for metabolic fuel. In the first 12 to 24 hours after a meal, glucose use by muscle diminishes and fatty acid production and utilization increases. Ketone body levels in the plasma gradually become elevated over the first week, which then

provides 70% of the energy to the brain. Glucose production drops significantly as fatty acid delivery to the liver increases. The net effect is to spare protein (and muscle) loss. Nevertheless, there is still a net negative nitrogen balance.[86] The body is also able to diminish energy requirements. After 7 days, the resting metabolic rate drops by 15% and, after 14 days, by 25%.[87]

In general, an adult human can withstand up to approximately a 40% decline below ideal body mass, at which point the patient will begin to systemically collapse and gradually die.[88] When the BMI falls to approximately 13 kg/m^2, death is virtually certain.[89] Virtually all organ systems are affected, with infection often being the final step to death. Often, these patients have emotional and psychiatric concerns with which we need to deal, particularly with anorexia nervosa, former prisoners and famine victims. As mentioned, whenever possible it is prudent to delay a surgical procedure until the patient's nutritional status can be improved. A severely malnourished patient undergoing an emergent surgical procedure has a significantly increased morbidity and mortality, related both to surgical and anesthetic concerns. It is vital to avoid the refeeding syndrome because such a patient is at even greater risk than in their malnourished state alone.

These surgical patients have virtually no metabolic reserve. The patient may survive the surgery but could die immediately postoperatively as a result of stress. Wound healing or a simple infection may metabolically demand more then can be delivered by the severely undernourished patient.[88,90]

There is evidence that the heart is not "spared" protein loss. There may be unsuspected myocardial atrophy with concurrent risk for arrhythmia and heart failure,[91-93] particularly when fluids are not administered cautiously.

As with children, in adults suffering severe malnutrition with an immediate surgical need it is very difficult to give specific recommendations concerning an anesthetic. It is of paramount importance to take into account the physiologic changes inherent with starvation states.

Some general suggestions include assessing the situation on a case-by-case basis. One needs to evaluate the degree and duration of undernutrition and assess the degree of organ dysfunction, particularly cardiac.[91-93] Renal and liver function should be assessed by laboratory studies of albumen, liver enzymes, blood urea nitrogen, and creatinine. We also need to investigate the degree of electrolyte abnormalities, particularly potassium and phosphorus.

Serum protein and albumin levels are decreased, but albumin levels are a more reliable and sensitive indicator of protein nutritional status. In tropical and subtropical populations with known inadequate protein intake, individuals may have normal total serum protein levels.[94] It is generally accepted that a serum albumin level below

Clinical Finding	Kwashiorkor	Marasmus
General appearance	Not cachectic May appear well fed Can have pitting edema of lower extremities Advanced cases involve edema of the arms and face	Severe generalized wasting Late in course, face has sunken or "wizened" appearance due to loss of temporal, buccal and orbital fat pads Absent edema
Appetite	Diminished	Normal until advanced, becoming minimal
Mood	Apathetic, irritable when disturbed	Irritable behavior initially Listless when advanced
Skin	Dermatosis such as dyspigmentation and hyperkeratosis due to desquamation	Dry, loose skin due to loss of subcutaneous fat. Absent turgor
Hair	Sparse Straight, dry and brittle Color changes to red or gray "Flag sign": cyclical periods of poor and good nutrition that result in alternating bands of normal and abnormal hair	Thin, sparse, brittle
Abdomen	Protuberant due to edematous intestine and hepatomegaly due to fatty infiltration No ascites	Flat with intestinal pattern easily seen
Height	Normal or stunted depending on severity and duration	Normal for age in acute cases Stunted in chronic or recurrent cases
Weight	Weight for age ~ 70% Often involves some muscle wasting, but edema can be misleading May have weight loss, but often maintain weight	Weight for age < 60% Very low weight to height ratio Significant muscle wasting
Vital signs	Not generally affected	Adaptive metabolic regulation resulting in poor thermoregulation, hypotension and bradycardia
Mortality	Higher than marasmus Treatment dependent (see text)	Lower than kwashiorkor Treatment dependent (see text)

TABLE 6–11   Comparative Diagnosis of Kwashiorkor and Marasmus

3 g/dL or a transferrin level below 200 mg/dL indicates severe protein malnutrition.

With therapeutic diets, specific serum transport proteins improve more rapidly than serum albumin. This is due to the shorter half-lives of these proteins. It is unclear if measurements of these proteins are superior to albumin for the detection of inadequate dietary protein.[95,96]

Bulimia Nervosa

This condition has a similar etiology to anorexia nervosa but presents differently. These individuals (usually in young women, with a peak incidence at age 20 years) usually appear well nourished but alternate between binge eating and vomiting. They often have primarily a psychological disorder involving self-image, obsessive-compulsive behavior, and depression. They may abuse laxatives and diuretics. There are fewer physiologic concerns than with anorexia nervosa. There may be esophageal erosions from gastric acid and diminished gastroesophageal sphincter tone, which predisposes to pulmonary aspiration. There is a greater likelihood of having metabolic and electrolyte derangements from excessive vomiting and diuretic use when compared with anorexia nervosa.

Obese Starvation

Overweight and obese patients may go on an unsupervised starvation or semi-starvation diet with unexpected complications. This sort of diet can produce rapid weight loss, but numerous vital nutrients may not be ingested. This can result in an undernourished yet obese patient. Significant deficiencies of multiple vitamins and minerals can develop, with special attention to copper, potassium, and magnesium. A deficiency of these three minerals may play an especially important roll in promoting an electrically unstable heart, particularly in patients with prolonged QT intervals on an electrocardiogram. Stress from any

BOX 6–7 Physiologic and Metabolic Effects of Protein-Energy Malnutrition with Anesthetic Implications

Hepatic:
    Altered metabolic pathways
    Depressed albumen production
    Depressed plasma cholinesterase production
Altered drug redistribution (fat soluble)
Altered neuromuscular junction activity
Altered sensitivity to narcotics
Renal function in advanced stages:
    Impaired fluid-electrolyte balance
    Impaired drug excretion

source can create an autonomic imbalance, which can then lead to arrhythmias and potentially sudden death.[93] Properly supervised and supplemented diets of this type can result in significant and safe weight loss.[97]

Micronutrient Disorders

Vitamins and minerals are highly varied in biochemical and physiologic function. They are involved in complex interactive metabolic pathways, such as carbohydrate and protein metabolism, hormone production and regulation, as well as "routine" physiologic functioning, such as neural impulse propagation or oxygen utilization in the tissues. Because of the complexity of human biochemistry and physiology, only the primary clinical implications of essential micronutrient derangements are discussed here. More in-depth information can be found in the referenced sources.

The four fat-soluble vitamins (A, D, E, and K) can be stored in significant quantities, so a dietary deficiency may not manifest clinically for up to 1 year. The water-soluble vitamins have minimal body storage (except cyanocobalamin—vitamin B_{12}) and can manifest a deficiency in a matter of weeks. The water-soluble vitamins are absorbed directly into portal blood (compared to the fat-soluble vitamins) and are excreted in the urine when plasma levels rise.

It is unusual to have isolated micronutrient abnormalities. Deficiencies often happen in concert with other micronutrient deficiencies to varying degrees, along with macronutrient deficiencies of starvation syndromes. Virtually all micronutrients are ubiquitous in foodstuffs, the result being that clinically significant deficiencies are virtually nonexistent, except in specific circumstances. Deficiencies can occur in people on unusual or highly restrictive diets but more commonly in debilitated or hospitalized patients on prolonged inappropriate total parenteral nutrition (TPN). Certain malabsorption syndromes have been implicated (Table 6-12), as well as drug-mediated deficiencies (Table 6-13).

Micronutrient excess is virtually always the result of excessive nutritional supplementation. This presents no problem with most micronutrients, because excess amounts are readily excreted. Exceptions are iron, the fat-soluble vitamins (A, D, E, K), or patients with liver or renal insufficiency/failure.

For simplicity, the minerals calcium, magnesium, and phosphorus are included in the topic of "micronutrients," even though they are often ingested in gram and multiple-gram amounts.

Fat-Soluble Vitamins

Vitamin A. Sources of this vitamin include animal (dairy, liver, fish) and plant (particularly red, orange, and yellow colored). This vitamin is involved in several functions, such as vision, epithelial differentiation, bone development and growth, immune functions, and reproduction. Vitamin A can be stored in the body for up to 1 year, but deficiencies can occur, especially in undernourished children younger than the age of 5 years. Children can develop poor visual dark adaptation, xerosis, and keratomalacia. Adults may have night blindness. Anorexia, skin erythema, and desquamation occurs, as can hepatomegaly and reproductive problems.[98-100] Toxicity can present as anorexia,

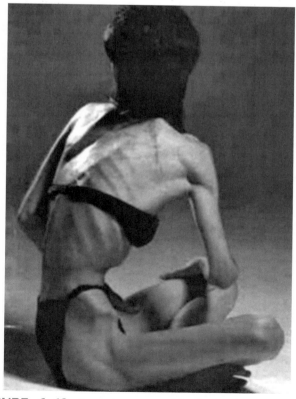

FIGURE 6–13 Anorexia nervosa. *(From "Fathers for Life,"* www.fathersforlife.org)

TABLE 6–12   Malabsorption Syndromes Associated with Micronutrient Deficiencies

Syndrome/Disorder	Deficiency
Gastrectomy	Vitamin B_{12}, vitamin D, iron, calcium
Short bowel syndrome	
Ileum resection	Iron, multiple water-soluble vitamins and minerals
Jejunum resection including duodenum	No clinically relevant deficiencies
	Vitamin B_{12} and folate
Colectomy	Impaired fluid and minerals especially electrolytes
Decreased bile production	All fat-soluble vitamins
Rapid transit/diarrhea	Often minimal sequelae
Ulcerative colitis	Severe disease results in electrolyte abnormalities
Crohn's disease	
Radiation	
Sprue/gluten intolerance	
Tropical sprue	Vitamin B_{12} and folate
Bacterial overgrowth	Vitamin B_{12} (normal folate)
	Fat-soluble vitamins

desquamation, ataxia, conjunctivitis, and alopecia. Liver problems include hepatomegaly, portal hypertension due to venous sclerosis and congestion, and cirrhosis. There is also a link between maternal oversupplementation and teratogenicity.[101-105] Deficiency or toxicity is suggested by a thorough history. The presence of Bitot spots is suggestive of a deficiency. Plasma retinol levels can be performed, along with several other tests.[106-110]

Vitamin D. This vitamin is produced with skin exposure to sunlight. People at risk for deficiency would include anyone with little exposure to sunlight (elderly, northern climates, sun sensitivities, and newborns) and in people with fat malabsorption syndromes. Vitamin D is involved in bone growth and development and is vital in the absorption of calcium and phosphorus from the intestine. A deficiency can result in hypocalcemia and in children can present as rickets. Adults can present with brittle bones and joint problems.[111-117] Toxicity due to excessive sun exposure does not occur due to cutaneous photochemical autoregulation.[118] In infants, toxicity presents with anorexia, failure to thrive, nausea and vomiting, hypertension, hypercalcemia, and renal insufficiency. Adults present additionally with soft tissue calcification of the kidney and heart, hyperphosphatemia, weakness, polyuria, polydipsia, and occasionally death. There is no readily available direct assay to assess vitamin D status.[119,120] Clinical history is central, along with an index of suspicion. Elevated plasma alkaline phosphatase released from osteoclasts is suggestive of preclinical rickets. The plasma concentration of calcidiol is possibly an indirect indicator of vitamin D body levels. Individuals with low levels of vitamin D will typically have an elevated parathyroid hormone level. These tests are of limited reliability or specificity.

Vitamin E. Sources of this vitamin include a wide variety of both plants and animals, with vegetable oils being the richest source. Deficiencies are therefore unusual. Vitamin E is an antioxidant. As such, it is centrally involved in cell membrane repair and maintenance, possibly adding mechanical stabilization. All membranes are susceptible to

TABLE 6–13   Drug-Mediated Effects on Micronutrients

Drug	Micronutrient	Effect
Omeprazole	Vitamin B_{12}	Impairs absorption
Isoniazid	Pyridoxine (B_6)	Impairs utilization, not absorption
Cholestyramine	Vitamin D, folate	Binds in gut, impairing absorption
Penicillamine	Zinc	Increases renal excretion
Sulfasalazine	Folate	Decrease absorption and blocks dependent enzymes

oxidation, particularly the mitochondria and endoplasmic reticulum. Tissues most susceptible include the erythrocytes, lung, and brain. Deficiencies are extraordinarily rare but can occur in certain fat malabsorption syndromes (e.g., cystic fibrosis), chronic cholestasis, premature infants, and the genetic disorder abetalipoproteinemia. Symptoms include ataxia, renal degeneration, hemolytic anemia, generalized weakness, retinal degeneration, ataxia, and other neurologic dysfunctions.[121] Toxicity is unusual, even with massive supplemental intake.[122,123] There are reports of muscle weakness, diplopia, and gastrointestinal distress.[123-125] Toxicity can also present by interference with the function of other fat-soluble vitamins.[124] There is no accurate method to assess vitamin E levels in the body. There are several methodologies, which have little clinical application.

Vitamin K. A significant amount of this vitamin is produced by colonic bacteria and is passively absorbed. Bacterial production was thought to be generally adequate for human needs, but this concept has been brought into doubt.[126,127] Dietary sources include vegetable oils, green leafy vegetables, and some legumes. Animal sources provide a poor to fair source. Slight intestinal absorption is facilitated by bile and pancreatic enzymes. Vitamin K is required for the proper formation of vitamin K–dependent clotting factors II (prothrombin), VII, IX and X, which are produced in the liver. Vitamin K is central for blood coagulation and clotting. A deficiency interferes with the intrinsic and extrinsic pathways of fibrinogen activation into fibrin. There are four other vitamin K–dependent clotting proteins, whose roles are less clearly understood.[128]

Human deficiencies are rare but can occur in trauma, in patients in intensive care units, and in people on chronic antibiotic therapy (decreased bacterial flora). Newborns are particularly at risk because their colonic flora is not yet developed and their diet consists of milk, which is low in vitamin K.[128,129] The primary clinical problems associated with vitamin K deficiency concerns impaired clotting and is suggested by a prolongation of prothrombin time. Coagulation and clotting times are prolonged with a risk of excessive surgical and trauma blood loss. There are unique issues with enclosed areas such as the epidural, intracranial, and pericardial spaces. There are also concerns with demineralization of bone.[130]

Toxicity from excessive supplementation of the natural form of vitamin K (phylloquinone) has not been described, owing to efficient metabolism. However, when infants have been given an excess of the synthetic form (menadione), hemolytic anemia, hyperbilirubinemia, and jaundice have been described.[123] Measurement of prothrombin time is nonspecific and merely suggestive of vitamin K status. More specific measurements are available but of limited practical use.[129,131]

Water-Soluble Vitamins

Vitamin C (Ascorbic Acid, Ascorbate). Primates, including humans, are some of the few animals not able to synthesize vitamin C. Nutritional sources include citrus and other assorted fruits and vegetables. Vitamin C is involved in the synthesis or metabolism of collagen, carnitine (fat metabolism), tyrosine (amino acid), and neurotransmitters (norepinephrine, serotonin), among other substances.[132] Additionally, it has a role as an antioxidant and is thought to be beneficial in assorted disease states, such as the common cold, cancer, cardiovascular disease, and others.[133-137] A deficiency can result in scurvy, which manifests as problems related to imperfect collagen metabolism. Common findings include bleeding gums, loose teeth, arthralgia, easy bruising, and poor wound and fracture healing. Rare in developed countries, it can occur in people with poor diets, such as alcoholics and the elderly. Toxicity can occur when dosages are well in excess of 1 g/day and can manifest as osmotic diarrhea and kidney stones.[138,139]

Vitamin B₁. Thiamine is found in many different foods, but particularly rich sources include meat, legumes, yeast, and wheat germ. Thiamine is involved in energy transformation pathways, membrane maintenance, and nerve conduction.[140,141] A deficiency can result in one of three forms of beriberi. Dry beriberi occurs in older adults with a chronic low intake and manifests with muscle weakness and wasting. Wet beriberi results in more extensive cardiovascular involvement, such as right-sided heart failure. Acute beriberi occurs primarily in infants. Thiamine deficiency is often associated with alcoholism and is due to poor diet, increased liver requirements due to liver damage, and decreased absorption. Alcoholics manifest Wernicke's encephalopathy characterized by ataxia, ophthalmoplegia, nystagmus, short-term memory loss, and confusion.[142] Massive intravenous or intramuscular doses can lead to headache, convulsions, and cardiac arrhythmias.[143-145]

Vitamin B₂. Riboflavin is widely found in different foods, particularly animal sources. It is involved in a wide variety of oxidation-reduction pathways, particularly the electron transport chain, pyruvate decarboxylation, fatty acid oxidation, monoamine oxidase synthesis, and others. There is no distinct disease associated with riboflavin deficiency. Some symptoms include photophobia, glossitis (magenta tongue), dermatitis, peripheral neuropathy, mouth edema, and perioral skin lesions. Toxicity has been described only under experimental conditions.[146]

Vitamin B₃. Niacin is found in many animal sources, as well as grains and legumes. There is a multitude of enzymes (mainly dehydrogenases) in which niacin is involved. Particularly, niacin is involved in the electron transport chain, fatty acid, cholesterol, and hormone metabolic pathways. A deficiency results in pellagra, classically described by the four Ds of dementia, dermatitis, diarrhea, and death. A deficiency can result from use of the antituberculosis drug isoniazid and from malabsorption syndromes. Toxicity is not well described. The nicotinic acid form of the vitamin is used in very large doses (over 3 g/day) to treat hypercholesterolemia. There are several side effects, including excessive histamine release, decreased bile flow, hepatic injury, dermatitis, and elevation of plasma glucose level.[138,147]

Vitamin B$_6$. Vitamin B$_6$ has several different forms. Pyridoxine is found primarily in plant foods, but the other forms are found in plant and/or animal sources. Vitamin B$_6$ is involved in a large number of enzyme systems, primarily amino acid metabolism and glycogen catabolism. A deficiency can occur in select groups: the elderly with poor nutrition, alcoholics, hemodialysis patients, and patients taking certain medications (isoniazid, penicillamine, and corticosteroids). Findings of vitamin B$_6$ deficiency include somnolence, fatigue, glossitis, stomatitis in adults, and seizures in infants.[148-150] Also seen is hypochromic, microcytic anemia due to deranged heme synthesis. Mega-dosing of vitamin B$_6$ has been suggested for the treatment of several disorders, such as atherosclerosis, autism, and depression. While there has been some success, there are some toxic risks, such as neuropathy resulting in paresthesias, unsteady gait, and numb hands and feet.[123,138,151]

Vitamin B$_{12}$. All dietary cobalamin is produced by bacteria and obtained almost exclusively from animal sources. One exception is legumes, where the cobalamin is produced by nitrogen fixing bacteria.[152] Cobalamin is involved in amino acid metabolism and the Krebs cycle.

Nitrous oxide has been shown to interfere with cobalamin function. Patients who are cobalamin deficient and undergo a nitrous oxide anesthetic may manifest an acute deterioration of nervous system function.[152-154]

Cobalamin deficiency can result from a strict vegetarian (vegan) diet, but usually only after 1 and up to 20 or more years, owing to adequate body stores and minimal excretion.[155] Most cases occur from poor absorption rather then inadequate dietary intake. Megaloblastic macrocytic anemia can result with a gradual onset. The anemia can be abated by giving large doses of folate, but the neurologic impairment is caused by gradual demyelination and will not be improved by folate administration. The neurologic deficit is probably related to diminished vitamin B$_{12}$–dependent production of methionine.[156] There is no direct clinical measure of an individual's cobalamin level.

Pantothenic Acid. This vitamin is widely found in virtually all foodstuffs. In fact, the Greek term *pantos* translates as "everywhere." Pantothenic acid is integral to the structure of coenzyme A, which is central for energy metabolism in the Krebs cycle and assorted other metabolic pathways. Deficiency occurs only in severely malnourished individuals and can present as vomiting, fatigue, weakness, and the "burning feet syndrome." Toxicity has not been described.[157]

Biotin. This vitamin was at one time known as vitamin H. Biotin is widely available in most foods and is also produced by colonic bacteria. Raw egg whites can bind to biotin and prevent its absorption. It is important in several metabolic pathways, such as the Krebs cycle, metabolism of fatty acids, and certain amino acids. Deficiency presents as several nonspecific features, such as anorexia, alopecia, dermatitis, hallucinations, and muscle pains. Toxicity has not been described.[158]

Folic Acid. Folate is found in green vegetables, legumes, and liver. Fruits and meats are poor sources. Folate is a component of amino acid metabolism and is involved in purine and pyrimidine synthesis. There is a synergism between folate and vitamin B$_{12}$ whereby the availability of vitamin B$_{12}$ frees up the "trapped" metabolite of folate. A deficiency of folate can manifest as megaloblastic anemia after several months, and megaloblastic anemia due to vitamin B$_{12}$ deficiency manifests after a much longer period. As mentioned in the discussion of vitamin B$_{12}$, this sign can be masked by large doses of folate. Toxicity is difficult to accomplish[159] but can present as insomnia, malaise, irritability, and gastrointestinal symptoms.

Minerals

The micro and macro minerals are outlined in Table 6-14. Most minerals are found in all foods to varying degrees, and most diets result in adequate intake. In undernutrition states, most individuals have adequate body reserves for most circumstances. Under these conditions, low total body levels of any mineral are relatively unimportant compared with the issue of PEM. In other words, the consequences of PEM usually manifest prior to any mineral deficiency. Toxic levels of dietary minerals do not occur, except under conditions of renal dysfunction.

Deficiencies can occur in long-term patients in intensive care units. These individuals are under immense physiologic stress, requiring large amounts of assorted minerals, particularly magnesium. Often, these hospitalized patients have poor or no enteral intake and are frequently receiving incomplete enteral or parenteral supplementation.

Of special note are the assorted nutritional supplements that are taken by increasing numbers of patients. Many of these mineral supplements have no direct impact on our care. However, other supplements are not purely "mineral supplements." Herbal supplements often claim to help a variety of patient concerns, such as preventing osteoporosis in perimenopausal women. Some of the other

TABLE 6-14   Microminerals and Macrominerals

Mineral	Sources	Primary Functions	Deficiency Findings	Toxicity
Calcium	Dairy, sardines, dark green leafy vegetables, legumes	Bone and teeth structure Muscle contraction Blood clotting Multiple regulatory enzyme pathways	Rickets Osteomalacia Osteoporosis Tetany Chronic hypertension and colon cancer	Acutely can result in hypercalcemia Seen only in renal disease
Magnesium	Legumes, nuts, grains, soybeans, seafood	Bone physiology Protein metabolism Nerve impulses Multiple enzymes	Usually only seen in alcoholism or renal disease Depression, tetany, muscle weakness, nausea, convulsions	Nausea, weakness, depression, double vision, slurred speech
Phosphorus	Meat, fish, eggs, dairy, legumes, nuts, grains	Bone physiology, especially energy cell utilization membranes	*Rare* Rickets Osteomalacia Neuromuscular abnormalities Skeletal and hematologic abnormalities	*Rare* Seen only in infants taking phosphorus-fortified formulations
Sodium	Table salt, meat, seafood, dairy, most vegetables, grains Poor source: fruit	Cellular electrical activity, especially neural Muscle contraction	*Rare* Anorexia Nausea Muscle atrophy	Seen only in renal disease
Potassium	Fresh and dried fruit, especially bananas, potatoes, beans, dairy	Cellular and electrical activity, especially neural	Does not happen from dietary deficiencies Occurs due to disturbance Muscle weakness, apathy, confusion, cardiac arrhythmias	Seen only in renal patients or iatrogenic Intractable cardiac arrhythmias
Chloride	Table salt, meat, seafood, dairy, most vegetables, grains Poor source: fruit	Primary anion: maintains electrical neutrality, pH balance	Anorexia, weakness, metabolic acidosis, lethargy	
Sulfur	Meats, dairy, legumes, nuts	Component of sulfur-containing amino acids and assorted metabolic pathways	Unknown	
Iodine	Seafood, liver eggs; iodized salt	Thyroid hormone synthesis	Cretinism (children), myxedema, goiter	None known
Iron	Organ meats, shellfish, nuts, legumes, green leafy vegetables	Critical for formation of hemoglobin and myoglobin Cytochrome function	Lethargy, fatigue, anemia, dysphagia angular stomatitis	Hemochromatosis Hemosiderosis
Zinc	Meats, whole grains, wheat germ	Enzymes in pathways involving energy metabolism, protein and collagen synthesis	Poor wound healing Diminished growth Hair, nail, and skin changes	Nausea/vomiting, abdominal cramps, bloody diarrhea
Copper	Organ meat, shellfish, whole grains, eggs, legumes	Synthesis of neurotransmitters, collagen, and lipid Facilitates iron utilization	Anemia, bone problems, hair and nail abnormalities	Nausea/vomiting Diarrhea Hematuria Oliguria/anuria
Fluorine	Fish, meat, grain legumes	Bone and teeth maintenance	Dental caries Bone fractures	Nausea/vomiting Cardiac arrhythmia

ingredients in many "natural" supplements may pose an anesthetic risk.[160-163]

The topic of "minerals" overlaps the topic of cellular physiology, electrolytes, and their homeostasis. Table 6-14 references primarily nutritional concerns. Discussions concerning electrolyte balance and physiology or causative disease states are more appropriately addressed in relevant internal medicine, biochemistry, and physiology texts.

CONCLUSION

Obesity presents a complex anesthetic challenge. The degree of obesity, comorbidities, and management issues are variable and interrelated. Associated medical and management concerns must always be considered, despite a negative history. Alternately, not all obese patients have coexisting diseases such as hypertension, diabetes, difficult airway, and so forth. Vigilance is particularly relevant in this population group.

A patient with severe PEM presents his or her own set of unique challenges. The "take-home" point is that the complexity and extraordinary degree of metabolic uncertainty are associated with profound management challenges. Due to the highly variable and unpredictable nature of these derangements, management must be highly individualized, with flexibility and vigilance being the cornerstone. Micronutrient abnormalities seldom present as isolated entities, due to the fact that most micronutrients are found in a wide variety of foods. Occasionally, isolated deficiencies occur under specific circumstances, such as with unusual and restricted diets. In developed societies, micronutrient deficiencies occur most frequently in elderly, debilitated patients with prolonged hospitalizations. In less developed societies, micronutrient deficiencies occur most commonly as a result of PEM, but they are often not recognized owing to the overriding issues of PEM. Micronutrient toxicity may present in cases of renal insufficiency or when consuming very large amounts of a particular food, but generally it occurs only with excessive supplementation.

References

1. Centers for Disease Control and Prevention: Prevalence of Overweight and Obesity Among Adults: United States 1999-2000. Atlanta, CDC, 2002.
2. American Heart Association: Heart Disease and Stroke Statistics. AHA, Dallas, 2003.
3. Kushner RF: Defining the scope of the problem of obesity. In Bessesen DN, Kushner RF (eds): Evaluation and Management of Obesity. Philadelphia, Hanley & Belfus, 2002.
4. World Health Organization: Preventing and Managing the Global Epidemic of Obesity. In Report of the WHO Consultation on Obesity. Geneva, WHO, 1997.
5. Sturm R: The effects of obesity, smoking, and drinking on medical problems and costs: Obesity outranks both smoking and drinking in its deleterious effects on health and health costs [see comment]. Health Affairs 2002;21:245-253.
6. Pories WJ: So you think we are bariatric surgeons? Think again [see comment]. Obesity Surg 2003;13:673-675.
7. Fine JT, Colditz GA, Coakley EH, et al: A prospective study of weight change and health-related quality of life in women. JAMA 1999;282:2136-2142.
8. Willett WC: Goals for nutrition in the year 2000 [see comment]. CA Cancer J Clin 1999;49:331-352.
9. Bender R, Jockel KH, Richter B, et al: Body weight, blood pressure, and mortality in a cohort of obese patients. Am J Epidemiol 2002;156:239-245.
10. Owens TM: Morbid obesity: The disease and comorbidities. Crit Care Nurs Q 2003;26:162-165.
11. Bray GA, Gray DS: Obesity: I. Pathogenesis. West J Med 1988;149:429.
12. Peiris AN, et al: Adiposity, fat distribution, and cardiovascular risk. Ann Intern Med 1989;110:867-872.
13. Brodsky JB: Positioning the morbidly obese patient for anesthesia. Obesity Surg 2002;12:751-758.
14. Brodsky JB, Lemmens HJ, Brock-Utne JG, et al: Morbid obesity and tracheal intubation [see comment]. Anesth Analg 2002;94:732-736; table of contents.
15. Nishimura T, Suzuki K: Anatomy of oral respiration: Morphology of the oral cavity and pharynx. Acta Otolaryngol Suppl (Stockh) 2003;550:25-28.
16. Hudgel DW: Variable site of airway narrowing among obstructive sleep apnea patients. J Appl Physiol 1986;1403-1409.
17. Frey WC, Pilcher J: Obstructive sleep-related breathing disorders in patients evaluated for bariatric surgery. Obesity Surg 2003;13:676-683.
18. Luce JM: Respiratory complications of obesity. Chest 1980;78:626-631.
19. Koenig SM: Pulmonary complications of obesity. Am J Med Sci 2001;249-279.
20. Crapo RO, Kelly TM, Elliott CG, Jones SB: Spirometry as a preoperative screening test in morbidly obese patients. Surgery 1986;763-768.
21. In-nami H, Kikuta Y, Nagi H, et al: The increase in pulmonary venous admixture by hypocapnia is enhanced in obese patients. Anesthesiology 1985;63:A520.
22. Unterborn J: Pulmonary function testing in obesity, pregnancy, and extremes of body habitus. Clin Chest Med 2001;22:759-767.
23. Sanders MH: The upper airway and sleep-disordered breathing: Getting the big picture. [see comment]. Am J Respir Crit Care Med 2003;509-510.
24. Jense HG, et al: Effect of obesity on safe duration of apnea in anesthetized humans. Anesth Analg 1991;72:89-93.
25. Wyner J, Brodsky JB, Merrell RC: Massive obesity and arterial oxygenation. Anesth Analg 1981; 60:691-693.
26. Eichenberger A, Proietti S, Wicky S, et al: Morbid obesity and postoperative pulmonary atelectasis: An underestimated problem. Anesth Analg 2002;95:1788-1792, table of contents.
27. Carabello BA, Gittens L: Cardiac mechanics and function in obese normotensive persons with normal coronary arteries. Am J Cardiol 1987;59:469-473.
28. Chakko S, Alpert M., Alexander JK: Obesity and ventricular function in man. In Alpert AJ (ed): The Heart and Lung in Obesity. Armonk, NY, Futura 1998, pp 57-76.
29. Thakur V, Richards R, Reisin E: Obesity, hypertension, and the heart. Am J Med Sci 2001;242-248.
30. Iacobellis G, Ribaudo MC, Leto G, et al: Influence of excess fat on cardiac morphology and function: Study in uncomplicated obesity. Obes Res 2002;767-773.
31. Stoddard MF, Tseuda K, Thomas M, et al: The influence of obesity on left ventricular filling and systolic function. Am Heart J 1992;694-699.
32. Messerli FH, Sundgaard-Riise K, Reisin E, et al: Disparate cardiovascular effects of obesity and arterial hypertension. Am J Med 1983;74:808-812.
33. Eagle KA, Berger PB, Calkins H, et al: ACC/AHA guideline update for perioperative cardiovascular evaluation for noncardiac surgery—executive summary a report of the American College of Cardiology/American Heart Association Task Force on Practice Guidelines (Committee to Update the 1996 Guidelines on Perioperative Cardiovascular Evaluation for Noncardiac Surgery). Anesth Analg 2002;94:1257-1267.

34. Alexander JK: Obesity and the heart. Curr Probl Cardiol 1980;5:1-41.

35. American Society of Anesthesiologists: Practice guidelines for management of the difficult airway: An updated report by the American Society of Anesthesiologists Task Force on Management of the Difficult Airway. Anesthesiology 2003;98:1269-1277.

36. Ezri T, Gewurtz G, Sessler DI, et al: Prediction of difficult laryngoscopy in obese patients by ultrasound quantification of anterior neck soft tissue. Anaesthesia 2003;58:1111-1114.

37. Norton ML, Brown AC: Evaluating the patient with a difficult airway for anesthesia. Otolaryngol Clin North Am 1990;23:771-785.

38. Stoelting R: NPO and aspiration: New perspectives. In ASA Annual Meeting Refresher Course Lectures. Park Ridge, IL, American Society of Anesthesiologists, 2000, pp 1-7.

39. Schreiner MS: Gastric fluid volume: Is it really a risk factor for pulmonary aspiration? [see comment]. Anesth Analg 1998;87:754-756.

40. Vaughan RW, Bauer S, Wise L: Volume and pH of gastric juice in obese patients. Anesthesiology 1975;43:686-689.

41. Brimacombe JR, Berry AM: Cricoid pressure [see comment]. Can J Anaesth 1997;44:414-425.

42. Chassard D, Tournadre JP, Berrada KR, Bouletreau P: Cricoid pressure decreases lower oesophageal sphincter tone in anaesthetized pigs. Can J Anaesth 1996;43:414-417.

43. Pelosi P, Croce M, Calappi E, et al: Prone positioning improves pulmonary function in obese patients during general anesthesia. Anesth Analg 1996;83:578-583.

44. Sprung J, Whalley DG, Falcone T, et al: The effects of tidal volume and respiratory rate on oxygenation and respiratory mechanics during laparoscopy in morbidly obese patients [see comment]. Anesth Analg 2003;97:268-274, table of contents.

45. Bouillon T, Shafer SL: Does size matter? [see comment]. Anesthesiology 1998;89:557-560.

46. Blouin RA, Warren GW: Pharmacokinetic considerations in obesity. J Pharm Sci 1999;88:1-7.

47. Blouin RA, Kolpek JH, Mann HJ: Influence of obesity on drug disposition. Clin Pharm 1987;6:706-714.

48. Hirota K, Ebina T, Sato T, et al: Is total body weight an appropriate predictor for propofol maintenance dose? Acta Anaesthesiol Scand 1999;43:842-844.

49. Greenblatt DJ, Abernathy DR, Locniskar A, et al: Effect of age, gender, and obesity on midazolam kinetics. Anesthesiology 1984;61:27-35.

50. Bentley JB, Borel JD, Vaughan RW, et al: Weight, pseudocholinesterase activity, and succinylcholine requirement. Anesthesiology 1982;57:48-49.

51. Bentley JB, Borel JD, Gillespie TJ: Fentanyl pharmacokinetics in obese and non-obese patients. Anesthesiology 1981;55:A177.

52. Oberg B, Poulsen TD: Obesity: An anaesthetic challenge. Acta Anaesthesiol Scand 1996;40:191-200.

53. Egan TD, Huizinga B, Gupta SK, et al: Remifentanil pharmacokinetics in obese versus lean patients [see comment]. Anesthesiology 1998;89:562-573.

54. Varin F, Ducharme J, Theoret Y, et al: Influence of extreme obesity on the body disposition and neuromuscular blocking effect of atracurium. Clin Pharmacol Ther 1990;48:18-25.

55. Servin F, Farinotti R, Haberer JP, Desmonts JM: Propofol infusion for maintenance of anesthesia in morbidly obese patients receiving nitrous oxide: A clinical and pharmacokinetic study. Anesthesiology 1993;78:657-665.

56. See reference 53.

57. Beckelmann AG, Burwell CS, Robin ED, Whaley RD: Extreme obesity associated with alveolar hypoventilation. Am J Med 1956;21:811-818.

58. Kessler R, Chaouat A, Schinkewitch P, et al: The obesity-hypoventilation syndrome revisited: A prospective study of 34 consecutive cases [see comment]. Chest 2001;120:369-376.

59. Weitzenblum E, Chaouat A: Hypoxic pulmonary hypertension in man: What minimum daily duration of hypoxaemia is required? [comment]. Eur Respir J 2001;18:251-253.

60. Boushra NN: Anaesthetic management of patients with sleep apnoea syndrome [erratum appears in Can J Anaesth 1996 Nov;43(11):1184]. Can J Anaesth 1996;43:599-616.

61. Dhonneur G, Combes X, Leroux B, Duvaldestin P: Postoperative obstructive apnea. Anesth Analg 1999;89:762-767.

62. Heird WC: Food insecurity, hunger, and undernutrition. In Behrman RE, Kliegman R, Jenson HB (eds): Nelson Textbook of Pediatrics, 17th ed, Philadelphia, WB Saunders, 2004.

63. Shils ME, Olson JS, Shike M, et al: Modern Nutrition in Health and Disease, 9th ed. Philadelphia, Williams & Wilkins, 1999.

64. Linder MC: Nutritional Biochemistry and Metabolism with Clinical Applications, 2nd ed. New York, Elsevier, 1991.

65. Gropper SS, Smith JL, Groff JL: Advanced Nutrition and Human Metabolism, 4th ed. Belmont, NY, Thomson Wadsworth, 2002.

66. Leleiko NS, Horowitz M: Nutritional deficiency states. In Rudolph CD, Rudolph AM, Hostetter MK, et al (eds): Rudolph's Pediatrics, 21st ed. New York, McGraw-Hill, 2003.

67. Jackson AA: Severe malnutrition. In Warrell DA, Cox TM, Firht JD, et al (eds): Oxford Textbook of Medicine, 4th ed. Oxford University Press, 2003.

68. Centers for Disease Control and Prevention: Severe malnutrition among young children—Georgia, January 1997-June 1999. JAMA 2001;285:2573-2574.

69. Hendricks KM, Duggan C, Gallagher L, et al: Malnutrition in hospitalized pediatric patients: Current prevalence. Arch Pediatr Adolesc Med 1995;149:1118-1122.

70. Reilly JJ, Weir J, McColl JH, Gibson BE: Prevalence of protein-energy malnutrition at diagnosis in children with acute lymphoblastic leukemia. J Pediatr Gastroenterol Nutr 1999;29:194-197.

71. Ashworth A: Treatment of severe malnutrition [see comment]. J Pediatr Gastroenterol Nutr 2001;32:516-518.

72. Schofield C, Ashworth A: Why have mortality rates for severe malnutrition remained so high? Bull World Health Org 1996;74:223-229.

73. World Health Organization: Management of the child with severe malnutrition: A manual for physicians and senior health workers. Geneva, WHO, 1999.

74. Solomon SM, Kirby DF: The refeeding syndrome: a review [see comment]. JPEN J Parenter Enter Nutr 1990;14:90-97.

75. Knochel JP: The clinical status of hypophosphatemia: An update. N Engl J Med 1985;313:447-449.

76. Keusch GT: The history of nutrition: malnutrition, infection and immunity. J Nutr 2003;133:336S-340S.

77. Waller G, Hodgson S: Body image distortion in anorexia and bulimia nervosa: The role of perceived and actual control [see comment]. J Nerv Ment Dis 1996;184:213-219.

78. Collins S, Myatt M: Short-term prognosis in severe adult and adolescent malnutrition during famine: Use of a simple prognostic model based on counting clinical signs. JAMA 2000;284:621-626.

79. Nourhashemi F, Andrieu S, Rauzy O, et al: Nutritional support and aging in preoperative nutrition. Curr Opin Clin Nutr Metab Care 1999;2:87-92.

80. McCormack P: Undernutrition in the elderly population living at home in the community: A review of the literature. J Adv Nurs 1997;26:856-863.

81. Ennis BW, Saffel-Shrier S, Verson H: Diagnosing malnutrition in the elderly. Nurse Pract 2001;26:52-56, 61-62, 65.

82. Hoffer LJ: Clinical nutrition: I. Protein-energy malnutrition in the inpatient [see comment]. Can Med Assoc J 2001;165:1345-1349.

83. Dudek SG: Malnutrition in hospitals: Who's assessing what patients eat? Am J Nurs 2000;100:36-42; quiz 42-43.

84. Waitzberg DL, Correia MI: Nutritional assessment in the hospitalized patient. Curr Opin Clin Nutr Metab Care 2003;6:531-538.

85. Sullivan DH, Sun S, Walls RC: Protein-energy undernutrition among elderly hospitalized patients: A prospective study. JAMA 1999;281:2013-2019.

86. Cahill GF Jr: Starvation in man. Clin Endocrinol Metab 1976;5:397-415.

87. Klein S, Jeejeebhoy KN: The malnourished patient: In Feldman M, Friedman LS, Sleisenger MH (eds): Sleisenger and Fordtran's Gastrointestinal and Liver Disease, 7th ed. Philadelphia, WB Saunders, 2002.

88. Mora RJ: Malnutrition: Organic and functional consequences. World J Surg 1999;23:530-535.

89. Henry CJ: Body mass index and the limits of human survival. Eur J Clin Nutr 1990;44:329-335.

90. Hensle TW: The impact of surgery on the starving patient. Compr Ther 1978;4:24-32.

91. Webb JG, Kiess MC, Chan-Yan CC: Malnutrition and the heart. Can Med Assoc J 1986; 135:753-758.

92. Schocken DD, Holloway JD, Powers PS: Weight loss and the heart: Effects of anorexia nervosa and starvation. Arch Intern Med 1989;149:877-881.

93. Fisler JS: Cardiac effects of starvation and semistarvation diets: Safety and mechanisms of action. Am J Clin Nutr 1992;56(1 Suppl): 230S-234S.

94. Beaton GH, McHenry EW: Nutrition: A Comprehensive Treatise. Vol. 3. New York, Academic Press, 1966.

95. Winkler MF, Gerrior SA, Pomp A, Albina JE: Use of retinol-binding protein and prealbumin as indicators of the response to nutrition therapy [see comment]. J Am Dietet Assoc 1989;89:684-687.

96. Sawicky CP, Nippo J, Winkler MF, Albina JE: Adequate energy intake and improved prealbumin concentration as indicators of the response to total parenteral nutrition. J Am Dietet Assoc 1992;92:1266-1268.

97. Ahmed W, Flynn MA, Alpert MA: Cardiovascular complications of weight reduction diets. Am J Med Sci 2001;321:280-284.

98. Tanumihardjo SA: Assessing vitamin A status: Past, present and future. J Nutr 2004;134:290S-293S.

99. Fiore P, DeMacro R, Sacco O, et al: Nightblindness, xerophthalmia, and severe loss of visual acuity due to unnecessary dietary restriction. Nutrition 2004;20:477.

100. Kapil U: Impact of single/multiple micronutrient supplementation on child health. Indian J Pediatr 2004;71:983-984.

101. Wiegand UW, Hartmann S, Hummler H: Safety of vitamin A: Recent results. Int J Vitam Nutr Res 1998;68:411-416.

102. Mulder GB, Manley N, Grant J, et al: Effects of excess vitamin A on development of cranial neural crest-derived structures: A neonatal and embryologic study. Teratology 2000;62:214-226.

103. Allen LH, Haskell M: Estimating the potential for vitamin A toxicity in women and young children. J Nutr 2002;132(9 Suppl): 2907S-2919S.

104. Fishman RA: Polar bear liver, vitamin A, aquaporins, and pseudotumor cerebri [comment]. Ann Neurol 2002;52:531-533.

105. Perrotta S, Nobili B, Rossi F, et al: Infant hypervitaminosis A causes severe anemia and thrombocytopenia: Evidence of a retinol-dependent bone marrow cell growth inhibition. Blood 2002;99:2017-2022.

106. Shrestha AK, Duncan B, Taren D, et al: A new, simple, inexpensive means of testing functional vitamin A status: The night vision threshold test (NVTT): A preliminary field-test report. J Trop Pediatr 2000;46:352-356.

107. Congdon NG, West KP Jr: Physiologic indicators of vitamin A status. J Nutr 2002;132(9 Suppl):2889S-2894S.

108. de Pee S, Dary O: Biochemical indicators of vitamin A deficiency: Serum retinol and serum retinol binding protein. J Nutr 2002; 132(9 Suppl):2895S-2901S.

109. Erhardt JG, Estes JE, Pfeiffer CM, et al: Combined measurement of ferritin, soluble transferrin receptor, retinol binding protein, and C-reactive protein by an inexpensive, sensitive, and simple sandwich enzyme-linked immunosorbent assay technique. J Nutr 2004;134:3127-3132.

110. Ferraz IS, Daneluzzi JC, Vannucchi H, et al: Detection of vitamin A deficiency in Brazilian preschool children using the serum 30-day dose-response test. Eur J Clin Nutr 2004;58:1372-1377.

111. Peng LF, Serwint JR: A comparison of breastfed children with nutritional rickets who present during and after the first year of life. Clin Pediatr 2003;42:711-717.

112. Dawodu A, Agarwal M, Hossain M, et al: Hypovitaminosis D and vitamin D deficiency in exclusively breast-feeding infants and their mothers in summer: A justification for vitamin D supplementation of breast-feeding infants. J Pediatr 2003;142:169-173.

113. Wharton B, Bishop N: Rickets. Lancet 2003;362:1389-1400.

114. Nuti R, Martini G, Valenti R, et al: Vitamin D status and bone turnover in women with acute hip fracture. Clin Orthop Rel Res 2000;422:208-213.

115. Kirubakaran C, Ranjini K, Scott JX, et al: Osteopetrorickets. J Trop Pediatr 2004;50:185-186.

116. Bloom E, Klein EJ, Shushan D, Feldman KW: Variable presentations of rickets in children in the emergency department. Pediatr Emerg Care 2004;20:126-130.

117. Reginato AJ, Coquia JA: Musculoskeletal manifestations of osteomalacia and rickets. Best Pract Res Clin Rheumatol 2003;17:1063-1080.

118. Webb AR, Holick MF: The role of sunlight in the cutaneous production of vitamin D3. Annu Rev Nutr 1988;8:375-399.

119. Peacey SR: Routine biochemistry in suspected vitamin D deficiency. J R Soc Med 2004;97:322-325.

120. Thompson K, Morley R, Grover SR, Zacharin MR: Postnatal evaluation of vitamin D and bone health in women who were vitamin D deficient in pregnancy, and in their infants. Med J Aust 2004;181:486-488.

121. Sokol RJ: Vitamin E deficiency and neurologic disease. Annu Rev Nutr 1988;8:351-373.

122. Zondlo Fiume M: Final report on the safety assessment of tocopherol, tocopheryl acetate, tocopheryl linoleate, tocopheryl linoleate/oleate, tocopheryl nicotinate, tocopheryl succinate, dioleyl tocopheryl methylsilanol, potassium ascorbyl tocopheryl phosphate, and tocophersolan. Int J Toxicol 2002;21(Suppl 3):51-116.

123. Vitamin preparations as dietary supplements and as therapeutic agents. Council on Scientific Affairs. JAMA 1987;257(14):1929-1936.

124. Bieri JG, Corash L, Hubbard VS: Medical uses of vitamin E. N Engl J Med 1983;308:1063-1071.

125. Traber MG, Packer L: Vitamin E: Beyond antioxidant function. Am J Clin Nutr 1995;62(6 Suppl):1501S-1509S.

126. Suttie JW: The importance of menaquinones in human nutrition. Annu Rev Nutr 1995;15:399-417.

127. Ferland G, Sadowski JA, O'Brien ME: Dietary induced subclinical vitamin K deficiency in normal human subjects [see comment]. J Clin Invest 1993;91:1761-1768.

128. Olson RE: The function and metabolism of vitamin K. Annu Rev Nutr 1984;4:281-337.

129. Jie K, Hamulyak K, Gijsbers B, et al: Serum osteocalcin as a marker for vitamin K status in pregnant women and their newborn babies. Thromb Haemost 1992;68:388-391.

130. Binkley N, Suttie JW: Vitamin K nutrition and osteoporosis. J Nutr 1995;125:1812-1821.

131. Sadowski J, Hood S: The applications of methods used for the evaluation of vitamin K nutritional status in human and animal studies. In Suttie JW (ed): Current Advances in Vitamin K Research. New York, Elsevier, 1988, pp 453-463.

132. Levine M: New concepts in the biology and biochemistry of ascorbic acid. N Engl J Med 1986;314:892-902.

133. Abudu N, Miller JJ, Attaelmannan M, Levinson SS: Vitamins in human arteriosclerosis with emphasis on vitamin C and vitamin E. Clin Chim Acta 2004;339:11-25.

134. Hemila H: Vitamin C and the common cold. Br J Nutr 1992; 67:3-16.

135. De Tullio MC, Arrigoni O: Hopes, disillusions and more hopes from vitamin C. Cell Mol Life Sci 2004;61:209-219.

136. Tamayo C, Richardson MA: Vitamin C as a cancer treatment: State of the science and recommendations for research. Alternative Ther Health Med 2003;9:94-101.

137. Padayatty SJ, Katz A, Wang Y, et al: Vitamin C as an antioxidant: Evaluation of its role in disease prevention. J Am Coll Nutr 2003;22:18-35.

138. Alhadeff L, Gualtieri CT, Lipton M: Toxic effects of water-soluble vitamins. Nutr Rev 1984;42:33-40.

139. Levine M, Dhariwal KR, Welch RW, et al: Determination of optimal vitamin C requirements in humans. Am J Clin Nutr 1995;62(6 Suppl): 1347S-1356S.

140. McCormick DB: The co-enzyme function of thiamin (Peters et al., 1929-1937). J Nutr 1997;127(5 Suppl):1038S-1039S.

141. Eisinger J: Thiamin and cognitive impairment [comment]. J Am Coll Nutr 1997;16:96-98.

142. Wood B, Currie J: Presentation of acute Wernicke's encephalopathy and treatment with thiamine. Metab Brain Dis 1995;10:57-72.

143. Davis RE, Icke GC, Hilton JM: High serum thiamine and the sudden infant death syndrome. Clin Chim Acta 1982;123:321-328.

144. Hori M, Nakayama Y, Noguichi Y, Kowa Y: Chronic toxicity and teratological test of thiamine monophosphate disulfide. J Vitaminol 1966;12:42-48.

145. Wrenn KD, Murphy F, Slovis CM: A toxicity study of parenteral thiamine hydrochloride. Ann Emerg Med 1989;18:867-870.

146. Minami H, Soto K, Maeda T, et al: Hypoxia potentiates ultraviolet A–induced riboflavin cytotoxicity. J Invest Dermatol 1999; 113:77-81.

147. McKenney JM, Proctor JD, Harris S, Chinchili VM, et al: A comparison of the efficacy and toxic effects of sustained- vs immediate-release niacin in hypercholesterolemic patients [see comment]. JAMA 1994;271:672-677.

148. Barthelemy H, Chouvet B, Cambazard F: Skin and mucosal manifestations in vitamin deficiency. J Am Acad Dermatol 1986;15:1263-1274.

149. Bitsch R: Vitamin B$_6$. Int J Vitam Nutr Res 1993;63:278-282.

150. Brussaard JH, Lowik MR, van den Berg H, et al: Dietary and other determinants of vitamin B$_6$ parameters. Eur J Clin Nutr 1997;51(Suppl 3):S39-S45.

151. Berger AR, Schaumburg HH, Schroeder C, et al: Dose response, coasting, and differential fiber vulnerability in human toxic neuropathy: A prospective study of pyridoxine neurotoxicity. Neurology 1992;42:1367-1370.

152. Seetharam B, Alpers DH: Absorption and transport of cobalamin (vitamin B$_{12}$). Annu Rev Nutr 1982;2:343-369.

153. Metz J: Cobalamin deficiency and the pathogenesis of nervous system disease. Annu Rev Nutr 1992;12:59-79.

154. Flippo TS, Holder WD Jr: Neurologic degeneration associated with nitrous oxide anesthesia in patients with vitamin B$_{12}$ deficiency. Arch Surg 1993;128:1391-1395.

155. Herbert V: Staging vitamin B-12 (cobalamin) status in vegetarians. Am J Clin Nutr 1994;59(5 Suppl):1213S-1222S.

156. Metz J: Pathogenesis of cobalamin neuropathy: Deficiency of nervous system S-adenosylmethionine? Nutr Rev 1993;51:12-15.

157. Fox H: Pantothenic acid. In Robert B, Rucker (ed): Handbook of Vitamins. New York, Marcel Dekker, 3rd ed. 1991, pp 429-451.

158. Rucker RB: The water soluble vitamins. In Groff SS, Gropper SS, Groff JL (eds): Advanced Nutrition and Human Metabolism. 4th ed. Belmont, NY, Thomson Wadsworth, 2002.

159. Butterworth CE Jr, Tamura T: Folic acid safety and toxicity: A brief review. Am J Clin Nutr 1989;50:353-358.

160. Ang-Lee MK, Moss J, Yuan CS: Herbal medicines and perioperative care [see comment]. JAMA 2001;286:208-216.

161. Crowe S, McKeating K: Delayed emergence and St. John's wort. Anesthesiology 2002;96:1025-1027.

162. Crowe S, Fitzpatrick G, Jamaluddin MF: Use of herbal medicines in ambulatory surgical patients. Anaesthesia 2002;57:203-204.

163. Tsen LC, Segal S, Pothier M, Bader AM: Alternative medicine use in presurgical patients [erratum appears in Anesthesiology 2000 Nov;93(5):1371]. Anesthesiology 2000;93:148-151.

7 Renal Diseases

Maurizio Cereda, MD, Jiri Horak, MD, and Patrick Neligan, MD

RENAL PHYSIOLOGY

There are three major anatomic demarcations in the kidney: the cortex, the medulla, and the renal pelvis. The cortex receives most of the blood flow and is mostly concerned with reabsorbing filtered material. The medulla is a highly metabolically active area that serves to concentrate the urine. The pelvis collects urine for excretion.

The functional unit of the kidney is the nephron. There are five parts of the nephron: (1) the glomerulus, which is the blood-kidney interface where plasma is filtered from capillaries into the Bowman's capsule; (2) the proximal convoluted tubule, which reabsorbs most of the filtered load, including nutrients and electrolytes; (3) the loop of Henle, which, depending on its length, concentrates urine by increasing the osmolality of surrounding tissue and filtrate; (4) the distal convoluted tubule, which reabsorbs water and sodium depending on needs; and (5) the collecting system, which collects urine for excretion. There are two types of nephrons, those localized to the cortex and those extending into the medulla. The latter are more metabolically active and are characterized by long loops of Henle.

Renal blood flow is 25% of cardiac output (1200 mL/min). Of this, renal plasma flow is about 660 mL/min, and 120 mL/min is filtered out of the blood and into the nephron. Ultimately, approximately 1.2 mL of this fluid is excreted as urine (1% of filtered load). The three major determinants of glomerular filtration rate (GFR) are (1) renal blood flow and renal perfusion pressure; (2) the hydrostatic pressure difference between the tubule and the capillaries; and (3) the surface area available for ultra-filtration (Fig. 7-1).

Proximal Tubule

In the proximal tubule, two thirds of filtered sodium, water, and chloride are reabsorbed along with most of the filtered glucose, amino acids, bicarbonate, and vitamins. Sodium is actively pumped out of the tubule, and water follows passively.

Loop of Henle

There are two parts to the loop, a thin descending limb and a thick ascending limb. The loop functions to generate an osmotic gradient in the medulla, so that urine can be concentrated or left dilute, depending on the body's fluid and electrolyte needs. A sodium-potassium-chloride ($Na^+/K^+/2Cl^-$) pump actively extracts these electrolytes from the tubular fluid in the thick ascending limb, which is impermeable to water (Fig. 7-2). Increased interstitial sodium and chloride leads to a dramatic increase in medullary osmolality. In addition, the loop and distal tubule are impermeable to urea but the collecting duct is not.

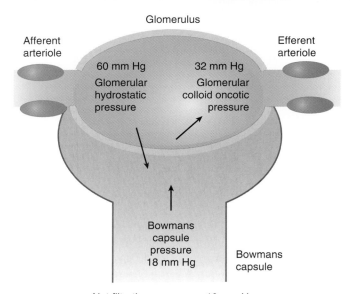

FIGURE 7–1 Filtration and filtration pressure.

Consequently, urea is concentrated in the tubules and significantly increases the osmolality of tubular fluid. When this fluid enters the collecting duct, urea diffuses along the concentration gradient into the interstitium, thereby increasing medullary tonicity further. This provides an osmotic gradient for the reabsorption of water from tubular fluid in the distal tubule and collecting duct.

Fluid delivered to the distal convoluted tubule is hypotonic. As this fluid passes down through this tubule and the collecting duct it is exposed to very high osmolar pressures in the surrounding tissues. If the patient is dehydrated, the pituitary gland produces antidiuretic hormone (ADH, vasopressin), making the collecting ducts permeable to water. Water is rapidly reabsorbed along the concentration gradient. In the absence of ADH a dilute urine is excreted.

Extracellular fluid volume depends on the amount of sodium in the body, so one of the essential roles of the kidney is sodium conservation. If the extracellular volume drops, a complex series of neurohormonal interactions lead to the release of aldosterone, which makes the collecting ducts permeable to sodium, which is reabsorbed.

Autoregulation of Blood Flow and Medullary Hypoxia

Renal blood flow is directed mostly to the cortex to optimize glomerular filtration and the reabsorption of solute. By contrast, blood flow to the renal medulla is low, to preserve osmotic gradients and enhance urinary concentration. The process of urine production and fluid and electrolyte conservation is intensely energy dependent. The anatomic distribution of medullary vasculature is designed in a hairpin manner to enhance countercurrent exchange; oxygen diffuses from arterial to venous vasa recta, which leaves the outer medulla deficient in oxygen. The medullary Po_2 is in the range of 10 to 20 mm Hg, contrasting to the Po_2 in the cortex, which is about 50 mm Hg.[1]

Intense demand for oxygen and nutrients and tenuous supply leaves the medulla and its tubules susceptible for ischemic injury. To maintain blood flow, and continuous filtration, a system of autoregulation operates in the kidney. Thus, production of tubular fluid is constant over a wide range of blood pressures.

The kidney neither autoregulates or perfuses at low blood pressures; this appears to be a protective effect because the medulla is relatively hypoxemic. Treatment for oliguria, under these circumstances, is to increase the renal perfusion pressure.

Oliguria, therefore, signals low renal perfusion, and the kidney protects itself from ischemia. The term *acute renal success* has been used to describe this phenomenon.[2] The coupling of blood flow and urinary concentration is essential for the operation of the nephron, and medullary hypoxia is the inevitable consequence. If excessive, medullary blood flow disrupts the osmolality gradients (built up by countercurrent exchange); if it is too slow, anoxia injures the tubules. Thus diminution of function, manifest as oliguria, has evolved as a protective mechanism for the medulla.[3]

A variety of differing physiologic mechanisms are involved in this regulation of blood flow and tubular transport in the renal medulla (Table 7-1). Loop diuretics increase the partial pressure of oxygen within the medulla, although it is unknown and unclear if this is a beneficial effect.[4,5]

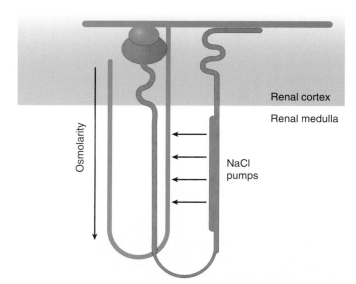

FIGURE 7–2 Sodium chloride is actively pumped from the thick ascending limb of the loop of Henle.

TABLE 7–1 Mechanisms Regulating Blood Flow and Tubular Transport in the Renal Medulla

Medullary Vasodilators

Nitric oxide
Prostaglandin E_2
Adenosine
Dopamine
Urodilatin

Medullary Vasoconstrictors

Endothelin
Angiotensin II
Vasopressin

Inhibitor of Transport in the Medullary Thick Limbs

Prostaglandin E_2
Adenosine
Dopamine
Platelet-activating factor
Cytochrome P450–dependent arachidonate metabolites
Tubuloglomerular feedback

Certain agents are known to worsen renal medullary hypoxia and these include amphotericin B, nonsteroidal anti-inflammatory drugs (NSAIDs), angiotensin II, calcium, myoglobin, and radiographic contrast agents.[3]

SPECIFIC RENAL DISEASES

Based on the structures involved, renal diseases can have glomerular or tubular origin. In the former, the glomerular structures are damaged and deposits of antigen, antibodies, and complement can be detected by microscopy. Typically, patients with glomerular diseases present with various degrees of hematuria, proteinuria, and salt and water retention. In tubular diseases, the tubular cells or the peritubular interstitium are more severely affected than the glomerulus. Abnormal handling of electrolytes characterizes these diseases.

Glomerular Diseases

Glomerulonephritis

Glomerulonephritis is an important cause of renal impairment, accounting for 10% to 15% of cases of end-stage renal failure in the United States, following only diabetes and hypertension in importance.[6] It is defined as a disease characterized by intraglomerular inflammation and cellular proliferation associated with hematuria with secondary renal impairment over days to weeks. Hematuria in patients with glomerulonephritis is characterized by the presence of dysmorphic red cells[7] or red cell casts in the urine, findings that differentiate hematuria of glomerular origin from extraglomerular bleeding.

In primary glomerulonephritis, disease is almost entirely restricted to the kidneys, as in IgA nephropathy or post-streptococcal glomerulonephritis, whereas in secondary glomerulonephritis kidney involvement occurs in association with more diffuse inflammation, as in systemic lupus erythematosus or systemic vasculitis.

Both humoral and cell-mediated immune mechanisms play a part in the pathogenesis of glomerular inflammation.[8] A unique initiating stimulus is followed by a common pathway of inflammation with activation of the coagulation and complement cascades and production of proinflammatory cytokines[9] and, subsequently, fibrotic events. Inflammatory, proliferative, and fibrotic changes may affect specific cells of the kidney differently or may result in more global changes with particular patterns resulting in a spectrum of clinical presentations. Thus, many of the underlying diseases can produce a spectrum of clinical pictures.

Patients with glomerulonephritis generally present with one of five clinical syndromes: (1) asymptomatic hematuria, (2) acute glomerulonephritis, (3) rapidly progressive glomerulonephritis, (4) the nephrotic syndrome, or (5) chronic glomerulonephritis.

Asymptomatic hematuria refers to either macroscopically or microscopically detected blood in the urine of patients who have normal GFRs and no evidence of a systemic disease known to affect the kidneys. IgA nephropathy, mesangioproliferative glomerulonephritis, is a common cause of asymptomatic hematuria that is often associated with a simultaneous respiratory or gastrointestinal tract infection. IgA nephropathy occurs in all age groups, with a peak incidence in the second and third decades.[10,10a] Despite a mild clinical presentation with benign hematuria, end-stage renal disease (ESRD) ultimately develops in 20% to 40% of patients 5 to 25 years after diagnosis.[11] There is no cure for IgA nephropathy. In patients at high risk of ESRD, glucocorticoids with or without adjunctive cytotoxic agents have been used in an attempt to retard the progression of this disease.

The renal lesion of Henoch-Schönlein purpura (HSP) is almost identical to that of the more severe variants of IgA nephropathy. However, as a small vessel vasculitis, HSP also has the systemic features of a purpuric rash largely affecting the lower limbs, arthritis or arthralgia, and abdominal pain sometimes in association with rectal bleeding. The disease is most common in subjects who are younger than 20 years of age. Renal involvement can also occur in adults where it is thought to carry a worse prognosis. Although hematuria and proteinuria are the most common renal presentations, up to 29% of patients may present with a combined nephritic and nephrotic picture.

Acute glomerulonephritis is a syndrome characterized by the abrupt onset of macroscopic hematuria, oliguria, and acute renal failure. It manifests with a sudden decrease in the GFR and with fluid retention, resulting in generalized edema and hypertension. Urinary protein excretion varies widely in this syndrome, but the rate is generally less than 3 g of protein per day. Edema probably results from renal sodium retention caused by the sudden decrease in the GFR.

Post-streptococcal glomerulonephritis is the best known example of endocapillary glomerulonephritis, the most common form of acute glomerulonephritis, and is representative of a larger group of postinfectious glomerulonephritis in which acute glomerular injury results from immune events triggered by a variety of bacterial, viral, and protozoal infections. In the United States and Europe this lesion is increasingly seen in infections such as endocarditis after intravenous drug abuse.

Deposits of IgG and C3 are regularly found within glomeruli and suggest that immune-complex formation is involved. However, it remains unclear whether the associated inflammation is mediated by circulating immune complexes, complexes formed in situ, or both.[12]

Poststreptococcal glomerulonephritis is an acute, reversible disease characterized by spontaneous recovery in the vast majority of patients. Typically, gross hematuria and edema develop 7 days to 12 weeks after the streptococcal infection. Spontaneous resolution of the clinical manifestations is generally rapid: diuresis usually ensues within 1 to 2 weeks, and the serum creatinine concentration returns to baseline within 4 weeks.

Poststreptococcal glomerulonephritis predominantly affects children between the ages of 2 and 10 years, but it also occurs in adults. Almost 10% of patients are older then 40.[13,14] Although most patients eventually have a complete recovery, hypertension, recurrent or persistent proteinuria, and chronic renal insufficiency develop in some.[15] The long-term prognosis of patients with poststreptococcal glomerulonephritis has been controversial. The reported incidence of chronic renal insufficiency can be as high as 20%.[13,15,16]

Rapidly progressive glomerulonephritis is a rare clinical syndrome characterized by signs of glomerulonephritis (hematuria, proteinuria, and red cell casts) and a rapid decline in renal function that can lead to end-stage renal failure within days to weeks. It accounts for only 2% to 4% of all cases of glomerulonephritis. Although causes are heterogeneous, the pathologic hallmark of this syndrome is the presence of extensive cellular crescents surrounding most glomeruli. Crescents result from the proliferation of parietal epithelial cells and mononuclear phagocytes within Bowman's capsule.[17] Rapidly progressive glomerulonephritis with glomerular crescent formation can be superimposed on primary glomerular diseases,[17,18] and it has been associated with infectious and multisystemic diseases as well, including vasculitides, cryoglobulinemia, and systemic lupus erythematosus. It can also occur as a primary disorder.

Rapidly progressive glomerulonephritis is classified pathologically according to the presence or absence of immune deposits and their character on immunofluorescence microscopy. Linear deposition of immunoglobulin along the glomerular basement membrane is detected in approximately 20% of patients. This type of rapidly progressive glomerulonephritis has two peaks of onset age, one in the third decade with a male preponderance and the second in the sixth and seventh decades affecting both sexes equally.[19] Associated lung involvement is more common in young men (Goodpasture's disease), whereas isolated damage to the kidneys is more common in older patients. Lung hemorrhage is the most common cause of death during early disease and should be suspected with hemoptysis or when a chest radiograph shows alveolar shadowing without restriction by anatomic fissures and with sparing of the upper zones.

Granular immune-complex deposition is detected in an additional 30% of patients.[17] In the remaining patients, no immune deposits are detectable in glomeruli ("pauci-immune" disease). Serologically, however, these diseases are linked in about 90% of cases by the finding of antineutrophil cytoplasmic antibodies. This category is represented by microscopic polyangiitis, Wegener's granulomatosis, and idiopathic crescentic glomerulonephritis. Microscopic polyangiitis is associated with cutaneous (purpura), neurologic (mononeuritis multiplex), or gastrointestinal vasculitis together with renal failure. Pulmonary symptoms, due to nongranulomatous arteriolar vasculitis and capillaritis, are present in only 50% of cases. By contrast, Wegener's granulomatosis is dominated by pulmonary manifestations with upper and lower pulmonary hemorrhage due to granulomatous vasculitis, respiratory tract involvement, and cavitating lung lesions, which are seen by radiography.

Unless complicated by systemic disease, rapidly progressive glomerulonephritis typically has an insidious onset, with nonspecific symptoms such malaise and lethargy. Urinalysis invariably demonstrates hematuria (usually dysmorphic red cells) and moderate proteinuria; nephrotic-range proteinuria occurs in less than 30% of patients.[17]

Rapidly progressive glomerulonephritis should be treated aggressively. A delay in the diagnosis and initiation of therapy increases the risk of ESRD, and the likelihood of renal recovery is poor without therapy.[20-22] Glucocorticoids and cyclophosphamide are the main therapeutic agents.[23] Plasma exchange is commonly used to remove circulating pathogenic autoantibodies in patients with glomerular basement membrane disease.[24]

Chronic glomerulonephritis is a syndrome manifested by progressive renal insufficiency in patients with glomerular inflammation, hematuria, and, often, hypertension. The kidney is the organ most commonly affected by systemic lupus erythematosus, and lupus nephritis is one of the most serious manifestations of this autoimmune disease. The clinical spectrum of lupus nephritis ranges from mild urinary abnormalities to acute and chronic renal failure. Patients, most commonly women in their 20s and 30s with a black preponderance, frequently suffer from lethargy, arthralgia or arthritis, rashes, and the symptoms of pleurisy and pericarditis in the months before presentation.[25] Clinically significant nephritis develops most commonly within 3 years after diagnosis and rarely develops after 5 years.[26] Asymptomatic hematuria or non-nephrotic proteinuria may be the only clues to renal involvement and should prompt further tests for other evidence of glomerular disease. Although tubulointerstitial nephritis can be a prominent component of lupus nephritis, immune-complex glomerulonephritis is the primary histopathologic finding.

Nephrotic syndrome presents as "heavy" proteinuria (protein excretion >3 g/day), hypoalbuminemia, edema, and varying degrees of hyperlipidemia and lipiduria.

The most common histologic lesions associated with primary nephrotic syndrome are focal segmental glomerulosclerosis, membranous glomerulopathy, minimal change disease, and membranoproliferative glomerulonephritis.[27,28] Diabetes is the most common cause of nephrosis (Table 7-2). Among the nondiabetic glomerulopathies, minimal change disease accounts for the majority of the cases of nephrosis in children whereas membranous glomerulopathy causes most of the adult cases.[29] Idiopathic membranoproliferative glomerulonephritis generally affects persons between the ages of 5 and 30 years and has a slight female predominance. The recent recognition of a causal relation between hepatitis C infection and membranoproliferative glomerulonephritis has led to the suggestion that this virus may be responsible for as many as 60% of cases previously deemed to be idiopathic.[30] Patients present 10 to 15 years after infection in middle age and have subclinical liver disease with mild biochemical abnormalities. Renal disease is often seen in the context of cryoglobulinemia. Patients suffer malaise, anemia, peripheral neuropathy, polyarthralgia, and a purpuric rash, together with lower limb ulceration and Raynaud's disease.

Approximately half of patients with membranoproliferative glomerulonephritis present with the nephrotic syndrome, whereas the remainder present with either acute glomerulonephritis or asymptomatic urinary abnormalities.

TABLE 7–2 Differential Diagnosis of Nephrotic Syndrome

Diabetes
Minimal change disease
Membranous glomerulopathy
Human immunodeficiency virus infection
Hepatitis
Cancer

Some degree of renal functional impairment is evident in half of patients at presentation. Spontaneous remissions are rare, and the disease generally has a chronic, progressive course.

The use of cytotoxic drugs and glucocorticoids has not proved to be consistently beneficial. Nephrotic syndrome also occurs as a complication of a wide variety of systemic diseases, cancer, infections, and drug therapy.

Depending on the disease that causes it, nephrotic syndrome may be reversible or eventually result in renal failure, whereas in other cases it may respond to corticosteroid and immunosuppressant therapy. Angiotensin-converting enzyme (ACE) inhibitors are often used in both hypertensive and nonhypertensive patients, because they are known to limit urinary protein loss. Fluid management can be particularly complex in patients with nephrotic syndrome, and assessment of their volume status may require invasive monitoring. Low plasma oncotic pressure causes diffuse interstitial edema owing to leakage of fluid from the intravascular space and may result in low intravascular volume,[31] particularly in patients who are undergoing aggressive diuretic treatment. These subjects may benefit from intravenous albumin administration rather than from large volume crystalloid administration. It has been suggested that plasma volume can be increased in some nephrotic patients, owing to enhanced sodium and water reabsorption at the tubular level.[32] In these cases, diuretic therapy may be necessary. Patients with nephrotic syndrome tend to respond poorly to diuretics because of the binding of these drugs with intratubular albumin. Therefore, higher and more frequent diuretic doses or the combined use of loop diuretics and thiazides may be needed.[33] The low proteinemia associated with nephrotic syndrome significantly affects the pharmacokinetics of drugs with a high protein binding, and therefore the dosing of most anesthetic drugs should be reduced accordingly.[32]

Patients with nephrotic syndrome have a particularly high frequency of cardiovascular disease and should undergo a thorough cardiac evaluation before higher risk surgeries. In fact, altered apolipoprotein metabolism causes hyperlipidemia while loss of anticoagulant plasma proteins leads to a hypercoagulable state. The risk of thromboembolic events is near 50%,[34] and these patients require diligent prophylactic anticoagulation with heparin and compressive devices (Table 7-3).

Tubulointerstitial Diseases

Nephritis

Acute interstitial nephritis is characterized by a peritubular inflammation causing renal insufficiency, sterile pyuria, and leukocyte casts (Table 7-4). Hematuria and proteinuria are also observed but are of lower degree than in

TABLE 7–3   Preparation and Intraoperative Management in Patients with Nephrotic Syndrome

- Perform cardiac risk stratification.
- Measure albumin concentration.
- Assess volume status; consider invasive monitoring.
- Reduce doses of drugs with high protein binding.
- Provide venous thromboembolism prophylaxis.

glomerular diseases. Altered sodium reabsorption and reduced urine-concentrating ability are more frequent than edema and hypertension.[29] Systemic manifestations such as rash, fever, and peripheral eosinophilia are often observed. Acute interstitial nephritis is caused by drugs, particularly antibiotics and NSAIDS, but can be caused also by infectious and autoimmune diseases. Discontinuation of the offending agent usually results in renal recovery, but corticosteroids can be necessary in some cases.

Pyelonephritis is an acute interstitial inflammation caused by a bacterial infection. Fever and signs of acute infection are usually observed, although the inflammatory response can be blunted in elderly and immunosuppressed patients. Pyelonephritis can be a cause of septic shock, particularly in hospitalized patients.

Chronic tubulointerstitial nephropathy is a slowly evolving interstitial inflammation and is a relatively common cause of chronic renal failure. Patients usually have pyuria, mild proteinuria, and minimal or no hematuria. Tubular dysfunction characterizes this disease, with hyperkalemia, non-gap metabolic acidosis, and polyuria. Chronic tubulointerstitial nephropathy can be caused by chronic ingestion of NSAIDS and acetaminophen.[35] Other drugs, such as cyclosporine and tacrolimus, toxins, autoimmune and neoplastic disorders can cause chronic tubulointerstitial nephropathy.

Disorders of Tubular Function

Bartter's syndrome is characterized by sodium, chloride, and potassium wasting. It is caused by a defect of the $Na^+/K^+/2Cl^-$ transporter in the thick ascending limb of the loop of Henle and is inherited with an autosomal recessive pattern.[36] Two forms of this syndrome exist: a neonatal one, characterized by polyhydramnios, and a classic form with onset at 2 or 3 years of life, characterized by polyuria, failure to thrive, and vomiting. Bartter's syndrome is diagnosed based on hypokalemia, hypochloremic metabolic alkalosis, and increased urinary concentrations of sodium, potassium, and chloride. Patients with Bartter's syndrome are not hypertensive, although renin, angiotensin, and aldosterone levels are elevated. Renal prostaglandin production is typically increased. Bartter's syndrome is treated acutely with saline infusion and potassium supplementation. The syndrome responds to chronic inhibition of prostaglandin synthesis, probably owing to a reduction of cortical blood flow.[29]

Gitelman's syndrome is an autosomal recessive disorder of the Na^+/Cl^- transporter in the distal convoluted tubule, it has similar features to Bartter's syndrome, but it has a later onset and is characterized by hypocalciuria and hypomagnesemia.[36]

Liddle's syndrome is an autosomal dominant disorder characterized by constant activation of the epithelial sodium channel in the collecting tubule in spite of low aldosterone levels. Patients present in their teenage years with hypertension, polyuria, failure to thrive, and hypokalemia. Treatment includes salt restriction, potassium supplementation, and lifelong administration of triamterene or amiloride.[29]

Pseudohypaldosteronism type I is an autosomal dominant resistance to the action of aldosterone, characterized by renal sodium loss and decreased sodium concentrations in sweat and saliva. The levels of aldosterone and its metabolites are typically increased. The onset is in early life, with failure to thrive, vomiting, and hyponatremia. Respiratory tract infections are common and resemble cystic fibrosis. Treatment mainly consists of sodium supplementation and is particularly important during periods of stress, such as illness or surgery.

Fanconi's syndrome is a global dysfunction of the proximal tubules, resulting in urinary loss of amino acids, glucose, bicarbonate, sodium, potassium, and phosphate. The main clinical manifestations are growth retardation, rickets, hyperchloremic acidosis, polyuria, dehydration, and symptomatic hypokalemia. Fanconi's syndrome has multiple causes that may lead to dysfunction of different tubular channels. Among the inherited causes, *cystinosis* is the most important one and is an autosomal recessive disorder that leads to generalized lysosomal cystine accumulation with renal and extrarenal manifestations. Other inherited causes of Fanconi's syndrome are Wilson's disease,

TABLE 7–4   Signs of Nephritis

Acute interstitial nephritis	Sterile pyuria, leukocyte casts, eosinophiluria, eosinophilia
Chronic tubulointerstitial nephropathy	Polyuria, acidosis, hyperkalemia
Pyelonephritis	Pyuria, bacteriuria, signs of infection, flank pain

galactosemia, and glycogenosis. Acquired causes of Fanconi's syndrome include heavy metal poisoning and exposure to multiple drugs such as tetracycline and chemotherapeutics. Treatment involves sodium and fluid replacement, correction of acidosis and hypokalemia, vitamin D and phosphate supplementation, and correction of the underlying causes when possible. Cystinosis usually evolves to ESRD within 10 years from diagnosis. The early use of cysteamine decreases lysosomal cystine and delays the evolution of renal failure, avoiding renal transplant in some cases.[37]

Renal tubular acidosis (RTA) is a group of differing renal tubular defects that have in common abnormalities of handling sodium and chloride. Normal renal function, and indeed control of acid-base balance, requires the kidney to excrete a net load of chloride over sodium, because dietary intake of these ions is roughly similar. In RTA the nephron excretes insufficient chloride, reducing the strong ion difference and resulting in metabolic acidosis.[38-40] Similarly, pseudohypoaldosteronism appears to result from high chloride reabsorption.[41] Bartter's syndrome is caused by a mutation in the gene encoding the chloride channel, *CLCNKB,* that regulates the $Na^+/K^+/2Cl^-$ cotransporter NKCC2.[42]

Proximal renal tubular acidosis (type II) is a problem of sodium and chloride handling in the proximal tubule leading to hypokalemic non-gap metabolic acidosis. It may occur alone, presumably secondary to a genetic defect, or as part of Fanconi's syndrome. Proximal RTA is defined by the inability to acidify the urine below a pH of 5.5. In some cases there is excess urinary elimination of sodium and its companion anion bicarbonate owing to mutations in the gene *SLC4A4,* encoding the Na^+/HCO_3^- cotransporter NBC-1.[43] Treatment is by administration of sodium either as sodium acetate or as sodium bicarbonate. Hypokalemia is due to activation of aldosterone secretion due to hypovolemia. This type of acidosis is most commonly caused by Fanconi's syndrome, but it can be also isolated. The diagnosis of proximal tubular acidosis can be confirmed by urine alkalinization to more than 7.5 after an intravenous sodium bicarbonate load.[29]

Hypokalemic distal tubular acidosis (type I) is due to an abnormality of chloride excretion in the distal tubule. There is a parallel reduction in the excretion of NH_4^+. In its autosomal dominant form, distal RTA is associated with mutations in the gene encoding the Cl^-/HCO_3^- exchanger AE1 or band 3 protein.[44]

Patients have severe metabolic acidosis with serum bicarbonate levels close to 10 mmol/L and are unable to acidify urine to less than a pH of 5.5. Hypovolemia and hyperaldosteronism cause hypokalemia. The patients frequently present with kidney stones due to hypercalciuria, which is caused by increased calcium mobilization from bone buffers. The most common cause of this type of acidosis is Sjögren's syndrome.

Hyperkalemic distal renal tubular acidosis (type IV) is caused by impaired excretion of both chloride and potassium ions in the distal tubule, leading to non-gap acidosis and hyperkalemia. There is an abnormality in the genes encoding the WNK1 and WNK4 kinases, which are responsible for transcellular conductance of chloride.[45] There is an association with diminished secretion of aldosterone. Urine pH is usually lower than 5.5, unlike type I acidosis. The acquired version of type IV RTA is usually mild and is often associated with chronic renal insufficiency. Its most common cause is diabetes mellitus, but exposure to NSAIDs and cyclosporine is a possible cause. Patients need treatment when the hyperkalemia is significant. Use of fludrocortisone, thiazides, and sodium bicarbonate can be considered.[29]

Renal Cystic Diseases

Renal cysts can be observed in a significant percentage of the population and are usually asymptomatic. Polycystic kidney is a severe inherited disease that can be transmitted in an autosomal recessive or dominant manner. The recessive form has an incidence of 1 in 20,000 live births and usually results in perinatal death due to extreme renal enlargement causing pulmonary compression and hypoplasia. The dominant form occurs in 1 of 800 live births and results in significant disease by adult age. The pathogenesis involves alteration in the synthesis of the tubuloepithelial membrane receptor polycistin.[46] At the age of presentation, the kidneys are massively enlarged and patients complain of flank pain, hypertension, hematuria, and recurrent pyelonephritis. This disease leads to ESRD in 50% of the cases.[29] Ten percent of cases also have cerebral arterial aneurysms. Therapy includes management of hypertension, prevention of kidney infections, and renal transplantation. Some cases may require nephrectomy due to recurrent severe pyelonephritis or to discomfort from the massive kidney enlargement.

Renal Involvement in Systemic Diseases

Hypertension and Diabetes

Long-standing, poorly controlled hypertension frequently causes renal dysfunction and causes approximately 20% of the cases of ESRD.[47] African-American ethnicity is a particular risk factor for this complication. Hypertension initially causes functional alterations in the renal circulation, with rightward displacement of the autoregulatory curve (Fig. 7-3), followed by permanent histologic changes at the arteriolar level.[48]

When autoregulation is completely lost, both systemic hypotension and hypertension may result in worsening renal function. High glomerular intravascular pressures cause increased capillary permeability and

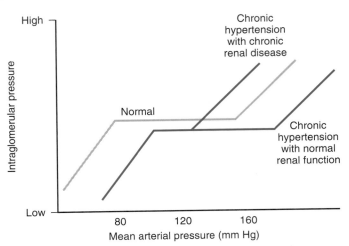

FIGURE 7–3 The relationship between intraglomerular pressure and mean arterial pressure follows a typically sigmoid curve due to autoregulation of afferent and efferent vessel tone with the effect of maintaining a constant glomerular blood flow in spite of significant changes in blood pressure. In hypertensive patients, this relationship is shifted to the right but maintained. When renal disease superimposes, the curve becomes more linear and changes in blood pressure directly affect glomerular blood pressure and flow. *(From Palmer BF: Renal dysfunction complicating the treatment of hypertension. N Engl J Med 2002;347:1256-1261.)*

proteinuria[49] whereas low blood pressure results in renal cell ischemia.

Accelerated hypertension is a particular condition in which an extremely elevated blood pressure causes a significant acute renal injury characterized by marked proteinuria. The goal in the management of patients with this condition should be to obtain an acute reduction in diastolic blood pressure to less than 120 mm Hg followed by further reductions over a time frame of weeks. In patients who present with accelerated hypertension, excessively rapid correction of blood pressure can lead to renal ischemic injury.

Diabetes mellitus is the most important cause of ESRD. Although type 1 diabetes is more frequently associated with renal involvement, the prevalence of patients with type 2 diabetes and renal disease has increased, probably owing to longer survival of these patients. Diabetic nephropathy is characterized by proteinuria, the extent of which predicts the onset and the outcome of renal insufficiency.[50] Proteinuria is not only a marker of renal disease, but it also contributes to causing further renal damage.[51] In fact, it has been shown in animal models that excessive tubular reabsorption of protein may cause interstitial inflammation, scarring, and fibrosis.[49] Poorly controlled blood pressure, hyperglycemia, and hypercholesterolemia are risk factors for the development of diabetic nephropathy,[52] and, therefore, control of these factors is important in the prevention or the limitation of diabetic kidney disease. Improved glycemic control has been shown to reduce the incidence of diabetic

nephropathy.[53] Strict blood pressure control has beneficial effects on the kidney in diabetic patients,[54] and its benefit is probably higher for those patients with significant proteinuria.[55] Although the blood pressure goal can be reached with any agent, ACE inhibitors are more effective in slowing nephropathy than other classes of antihypertensive drugs both in diabetic and in nondiabetic patients.[56] This effect of ACE inhibitors is probably related to their ability in reducing or preventing proteinuria.[57] Similar renoprotective effects have been shown also with angiotensin receptor blockers.[58] The use of ACE inhibitors in patients with compromised renal function is often associated with a moderate increase in serum creatinine and potassium levels. This effect should be seen as a normal response to decreased blood pressure and a marker of drug effectiveness rather than a sign of deterioration of renal function and an indication to discontinuation of ACE inhibitor therapy.[48] Calcium channel blockers also have beneficial effects on renal function, although the use of amlodipine was associated with adverse outcomes in African-American patients with hypertensive nephropathy. Additional measures proposed to slow the progression of chronic diabetic and nondiabetic nephropathy are dietary protein intake restriction, smoking cessation, and lipid-lowering medications.

Sickle Cell Disease

Sickle cell disease is the cause of a significant nephropathy with manifestations that can include hematuria, papillary necrosis due to occlusion of vasa recta, acute renal failure due to renal hypoperfusion or rhabdomyolysis, and chronic renal failure due to glomerulosclerosis. Proteinuria is detected in a high percentage of patients. An inability to concentrate urine is the hallmark of sickle cell nephropathy and is due to loss of the countercurrent exchange mechanism from loss of perfusion to the vasa recta. The intraoperative management of patients with sickle cell nephropathy should follow the general recommendations on sickle cell management, with additional care to avoid renal hypoperfusion.[59]

Vascular Diseases of the Kidney

Chronic atherosclerotic stenosis of the renal arteries is a relatively common condition in the population with advanced age and with extrarenal atherosclerosis, as shown by angiographic studies.[60] Renal artery stenosis can cause progressive ischemic nephropathy and, when bilateral, it results in significant renal dysfunction. However, this condition is often underdiagnosed, mainly owing to the lack of specific chemical markers of renal ischemic disease. Most often, the diagnosis is made by radiologic investigations such as duplex ultrasonography, angiography, computed tomography, or magnetic resonance imaging angiography.

Although renal artery atherosclerosis is often associated with systemic hypertension, correction of the stenosis does not always result in blood pressure normalization, because hypertension is more likely to be essential in the majority of cases.[61] Thrombosis of the renal artery may complicate preexisting stenosis or may be caused by hypercoagulability, trauma, or aortic dissection; and it can precipitate acute renal failure. Fibromuscular dysplasia of the renal artery occurs mainly in young women and still has no known causes. Unlike atherosclerotic stenosis, this condition is associated with renovascular hypertension and rarely causes renal failure.[62]

Medical management of renal artery stenosis is centered on control of hypertension, and ACE inhibitors are the drugs of choice for this purpose, although inhibition of angiotensin-mediated efferent tone may precipitate renal failure in patients with bilateral renal artery stenosis. Surgical correction of renal artery stenosis is aggravated by a significant rate of complications, particularly in patients with coexisting aortic disease, and is probably not indicated in patients with advanced nephropathy.[61] The use of percutaneous angioplasty and stenting has emerged as an attractive alternative to the surgical corrective approach.[63]

Chronic Renal Failure

Chronic renal failure (CRF) has become increasingly frequent in the western world,[64] reaching a prevalence of 0.1% in the United States. Data from the U.S. Renal Data System showed a 104% increase in the prevalence of CRF between 1990 and 2001.[65] The prevalence is higher in advanced ages and in certain ethnic groups such as the African American and Native American.[66] Recent studies have detected an impressively high rate of mild to moderate renal dysfunction in the U.S. population, particularly in the elderly (Fig. 7-4).[67] These patients are at risk for progression to renal failure if further kidney damage is superimposed.

An elevated number of patients with CRF undergo surgeries for reasons that may or may not be related to kidney disease; therefore, understanding the pathophysiology and the clinical management of these patients is highly important for the anesthesiologist. In fact, CRF significantly complicates perioperative management and has a relevant impact on surgical outcomes. In patients with CRF necessitating dialysis, mortality rates of 4% after general surgery and of 10% after cardiac surgery have been reported, with morbidity rates approaching 50%.[68] This increased rate of complications is probably due to the low renal reserve of patients with CRF and to their reduced ability to respond to the stress, fluid load, and tissue trauma caused by surgery. However, additional morbidity is created by the organ dysfunctions and the coexisting diseases frequently met in these patients.

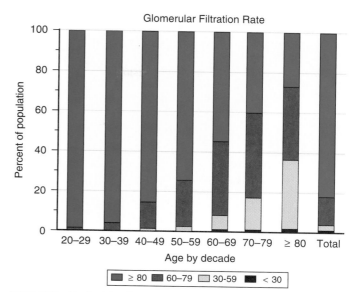

FIGURE 7–4 Distribution of glomerular filtration rate (expressed as mL/min/1.73 m² BSA) by age for nondiabetic subjects. *(From Clase CM, Garg AX: Classifying kidney problems: Can we avoid framing risks as diseases? BMJ 2004;329:912-915.)*

Pathophysiology

Many different renal and extrarenal pathologic conditions result in the loss of glomerular function as their "final common pathway." Renal dysfunction is progressive and is usually divided in stages according to the GFR (Table 7-5).[69]

Proteinuria is also used as an index of the severity of kidney disease and can be used to predict renal survival.[70] The loss of GFR can be accelerated by events such as intercurrent diseases, nephrotoxins, and surgery. Eventually, ESRD is reached when the GFR decreases below a critical point and the kidney is unable to maintain homeostasis unless renal replacement therapy is initiated.

When renal tissue is lost, surviving nephrons undergo adaptive changes, with tubular hypertrophy, afferent vessel vasodilation, and increased glomerular blood flow.[71] By increasing tubular excretion or reabsorption of water and solutes, these changes allow the remaining nephrons to compensate for lost tissue and to maintain near-normal handling of the glomerular ultrafiltrate. On the other side, these same changes seem to accelerate the progression of kidney disease. Glomerular capillary hypertension due to afferent vasodilation causes glomerulosclerosis, increased endothelial permeability, and proteinuria. The latter probably promotes further renal damage,[70,72] because excessive tubular reabsorption of urinary protein may cause peritubular inflammation, scarring, and fibrosis.[71]

A progressive inability to maintain tight control of body fluid composition follows the exhaustion of renal compensatory mechanisms. Patients with very low GFR are prone to sodium accumulation and to hypervolemia,

TABLE 7–5   Stages of Renal Dysfunction

Stage	Description	Creatinine Clearance (~GFR)(mL/min/1.73 m^2)	Metabolic Consequences
1	Normal or increased GFR; people at increased risk or with early renal damage	>90	
2	Early renal insufficiency	60-89*	Concentration of parathyroid hormone starts to rise (GFR ~60-80)
3	Moderate renal failure (chronic renal failure)	30-59	Decrease in calcium absorption (GFR < 50) Lipoprotein activity falls Malnutrition Onset of left ventricular hypertrophy Onset of anemia (erythropoietin deficiency)
4	Severe renal failure (pre–end-stage renal disease)	15-29	Triglyceride concentrations start to rise Hyperphosphatemia Metabolic acidosis Tendency to hyperkalemia
5	End-stage renal disease (uremia)	<15	Azotemia develops

GFR, glomerular filtration rate.
*May be normal for age.
Adapted from Parmar MS: Chronic renal disease. BMJ 2002;325:85-90.

because they may not be able to excrete the equivalent of their sodium intake. When the regulation of urine osmolality and of free water excretion is impaired, changes in water intake may cause sodium concentration abnormalities. Inability to excrete potassium by the distal tubule results in accumulation of this electrolyte. Patients with CRF usually tolerate significant hyperkalemia, partly due to increased intestinal excretion. However, acute processes such as acidosis, surgery, and tissue necrosis can trigger rapid increases in serum potassium and cause life-threatening arrhythmias. Decreased phosphate excretion causes accumulation of this electrolyte and its precipitation in tissues together with calcium. Hypocalcemia is also caused by deficient renal production of vitamin D and by lower intestinal absorption of calcium, and it results in secondary hyperparathyroidism, bone reabsorption, and renal osteodystrophy.

Patients with renal failure develop a metabolic acidosis that is initially associated with hyperchloremia and normal anion gap. When renal failure becomes severe, inability to excrete titratable acids causes an increased anion gap.

The uremic syndrome characterizes renal decompensation and is due to accumulation of catabolic byproducts. Although the severity of uremia is usually quantified from the serum urea nitrogen levels, this syndrome is caused by accumulation of different substances and by several hormonal and metabolic dysfunctions. Central nervous system manifestations may range from personality changes to coma and seizures, and their onset is more related to the rapidity of the onset of azotemia than to its absolute level. Peripheral and autonomic neuropathies are relatively common and cause sensory loss, gastroparesis, and sympathetic dysregulation. Uremia causes gastric mucosal irritation and gastric ulcers in a significant fraction of patients who have uncompensated renal failure. Uremic patients have a bleeding diathesis even when coagulation times are normal. This bleeding tendency is caused by a platelet dysfunction resulting from inadequate release of von Willebrand factor and factor VIII by the endothelial cells.[73] Renal failure may also cause a predisposition to thrombosis due to hyperfibrinogenemia, antiphospholipid antibodies, hyperhomocysteinemia, and anticoagulatory protein C deficiency. Patients with CRF typically have a significant anemia that is mainly due to deficient production of erythropoietin, although gastrointestinal bleeding and iron deficiency may contribute to its genesis.

Multiple cardiovascular derangements are associated with CRF. Hypertension is usually due to fluid overload but also to neuroendocrine imbalances. Patients with CRF often have significant left ventricular hypertrophy and enlargement, associated with systolic and diastolic dysfunction, and are prone to heart failure.[74] Anemia significantly contributes to the adverse effects of CRF on the cardiovascular system, by increasing cardiac output and myocardial oxygen demand and by causing left ventricular hypertrophy and enlargement.[73] Uremic pericarditis is not frequent in patients on dialysis, but it should be considered because, if present, it can be complicated by pericardial hemorrhage and tamponade.

TABLE 7–6	Signs of Uremic Emergency
Fluid overload	Hypertension, pulmonary edema, peripheral edema
Electrolyte imbalance	Hyperkalemia, hyponatremia, hypocalcemia
Acid-base abnormalities	Increased anion gap, hyperchloremia, low plasma CO_2, hyperventilation
Encephalopathy	Seizures, coma, decreased airway reflexes, obtundation
Systemic hypoperfusion	Congestive heart failure, cardiac tamponade
Bleeding diathesis	Normal platelet counts and coagulation times, increased bleeding times

TABLE 7–8 Signs of Inadequate Dialysis
Anorexia, nausea, vomiting, diarrhea
Peripheral neuropathy
Weakness, poor functional status
Decreased alertness
Ascites, pericarditis
Hypertension, fluid overload
Persistent anemia despite erythropoietin
Small urea reduction with dialysis

Clinical Presentations

Patients with CRF often present with a history of a known kidney disease that has been medically managed along its evolution and that has relatively controlled manifestations. Therefore, many patients with CRF present in a compensated state and with relatively mild symptoms. Vague malaise or nocturia may be the only complaints. However, some patients may present with the signs and the symptoms of acute renal decompensation and uremic emergency (Table 7-6), a condition that should be rapidly addressed by a nephrologist and that often requires emergent initiation of hemodyalis.[73] This is more likely to happen in patients with rapidly progressing or unrecognized renal disease. In other patients, an acute event or illness may overcome the residual renal reserve or cause further kidney damage, precipitating acute on chronic renal failure (Table 7-7).

Patients who have been receiving chronic dialysis usually present in a relatively compensated state, but they may have signs of hypovolemia if fluid removal has been

TABLE 7–7 Causes of Acute on Chronic Renal Failure
Dehydration
Infection
Uncontrolled hypertension
Renal disease exacerbation
Heart failure
Nephrotoxins
Urinary obstruction
Major surgery

overzealous. When either the dose or the timing of dialysis is inadequate (Table 7-8), some of the clinical manifestations of uremia resurface.[75] Pericardial effusions due to uremic pericarditis are slow to evolve and rarely result in tamponade, but they should be suspected in the presence of hypotension, pulsus paradoxus, and jugular vein enlargement.

Anemia accounts for many of the symptoms and signs observed in CRF patients, such as malaise, low exercise ability, decreased mental acuity, left ventricular dilatation, and hypertrophy. Most of these manifestations improve if anemia is corrected by erythropoietin administration.[73] Patients who are not receiving dialysis are typically undernourished due to anorexia and hypercatabolism associated to CRF. Additionally, some patients may be receiving a low protein diet as an attempt to delay the need for dialysis and to limit the progression of renal disease.[64] The protein weight loss is often masked by the increase in body water content. Patients who do receive dialysis should be fed an adequate amount of protein, because currently available dialysis systems afford efficient solute-clearing capabilities and protein intake limitation is unnecessary.[75] The clinical manifestations of renal osteodystrophy are usually evident only when bone and renal disease are advanced and include bone and joint pain, lytic lesions on radiographs, and, occasionally, spontaneous bone fractures.[73] Growth retardation and bone deformities are common in children. Pruritus is common in patients with severe renal failure, particularly in those on dialysis, and is probably caused by calcium precipitation in the skin.

Patients receiving hemodialysis have a surgically created access that can consist of a native arteriovenous fistula or a synthetic graft. Some patients may present with a hemodialysis catheter placed in a central or femoral vein. Dialysis access sites are at high risk of clotting and infection and should be inspected for patency and local irritation. Long-term dialysis patients have a long history of peripheral and central cannulation and may present a challenge for central access.

Differential Diagnosis

Any diseases that damage the kidney at the glomerular or tubular level may progress to CRF. Diabetes and hypertension are by large the most important causes of ESRD, accounting together for more than 60% of cases in the United States.[65] Glomerular diseases and tubulointerstitial diseases cause 18% and 7% of cases of ESRD, followed by cystic kidney disease (5%).[64]

The differential diagnosis is usually straightforward and based on history, imaging, and laboratory analysis (Table 7-9). Renal biopsy is indicated in patients with unexplained CRF who do not have atrophic kidneys on ultrasound and in patients with nondiabetic nephrotic syndrome.[73] Establishing a differential diagnosis is important, especially when the condition causing renal failure can be controlled and further renal damage can be prevented, such as with vasculitis, drug-induced nephropathy, autoimmune disease, renal ischemia, and infectious diseases.

Given the high prevalence of diabetes and hypertension in patients with CRF it is not surprising that the most important comorbidities associated with CRF involve the cardiovascular system (Table 7-10). Cardiac disease is the most important cause of death in patients with ESRD.[66,74] Congestive heart failure is present in 40% of patients receiving dialysis and is an important predictor of death. Seventy-five percent of CRF patients have left ventricular hypertrophy and diastolic dysfunction at the time of initiation of dialysis.[74] Left ventricular dysfunction improves with dialysis, correction of anemia, and renal transplant.[75] Coronary artery disease is common in patients with CRF, with a reported prevalence of 40%,[76] and it is an important cause of ventricular dysfunction and mortality. The "classic" risk factors contribute to the prevalence of coronary artery disease, but renal failure itself might be an independent risk factor for this condition. This hypothesis has been suggested by the fact that significant coronary artery

TABLE 7–9 Differential Diagnosis of Chronic Renal Failure

Diabetes
Hypertension
Glomerulonephritis
Cystic kidney disease
Ischemic renal disease
Pyelonephritis
Analgesic nephropathy
Hereditary diseases
Autoimmune diseases
Vasculitis

TABLE 7–10 Comorbidities of Chronic Renal Failure

Hypertension
Diabetes
Coronary artery disease
Congestive heart failure
Dyslipidemia
Peripheral vascular disease
Immune depression

disease is observed also in CRF patients who are neither hypertensive nor diabetic.[76]

Hypertension is almost universal in renal failure and is both an important causative factor for renal disease, as discussed earlier, and as a manifestation of fluid overload and endocrine dysregulation. Hyperlipidemia has a high prevalence in CRF patients, and it manifests with increases in triglycerides and in very low density lipoproteins, and with decreases in high-density lipoproteins.[73] Patients with nephrotic syndrome have a 90% prevalence of hypercholesterolemia. Control of hyperlipidemia is important not only to decrease the risk of coronary artery disease but also because it might reduce proteinuria and help to preserve glomerular function.

Patients with advanced renal disease are particularly prone to infections and to delayed wound healing and may not respond to certain immunizations, such as hepatitis B. This is partly due to malnutrition but also to specific deficiencies in humoral and cell-mediated immunity, such as impaired phagocytosis, defective lymphocyte function, and impaired antibody response.[73] Hemodialysis does not completely correct this immunodeficiency and causes additional risk of infection. Patients on dialysis have impaired febrile response even with severe infections and are at particularly high risk for staphylococcal infections and tuberculosis.[75]

When CRF is associated with vasculitis and autoimmune diseases, the systemic manifestations of these diseases should be remembered, particularly when they affect the cardiovascular and respiratory system as seen, for example, with Goodpasture's disease, lupus, and rheumatoid arthritis.

Preoperative Evaluation and Preparation

The preoperative evaluation of the patient with CRF should start with a thorough history and physical examination and should focus on the comorbidities associated with kidney diseases and on the signs and symptoms of uremia, fluid overload, and inadequate dialysis. Laboratory studies should be aimed at assessing electrolyte concentrations, acid-base status, urea and creatinine levels, hematocrit, platelet count, and coagulation. Electrolytes should not be measured immediately after dialysis, owing to incomplete equilibration between plasma and intracellular fluids. Platelet dysfunction is not related to a low platelet count, and it can be detected only using the bleeding time, measured as the time to cessation of hemorrhage after a standardized skin incision.[77] However, this test seems to have a limited predictive value for clinical bleeding and is uncommonly used. Patients who are receiving adequate dialysis are less likely to have significant platelet dysfunction and their risk of bleeding should not be excessive. A chest radiograph is usually ordered to rule out fluid overload, although it may probably be avoided in younger patients who are adequately dialyzed, have good exercise tolerance, and are undergoing lower risk surgeries. An electrocardiogram is obtained to screen for changes caused by myocardial ischemia and by electrolyte abnormalities.

The cardiac risk stratification of patients with CRF is not straightforward. In fact, the sensitivity and specificity of symptoms such as chest pain and reduced exercise tolerance is reduced, compared with the population without renal disease. Silent myocardial ischemia is relatively common owing to the frequency of diabetes and of autonomic neuropathy whereas dyspnea on exertion may be caused also by fluid overload. At the same time, the classic signs of congestive heart failure may be absent in patients who have ventricular dysfunction but are receiving adequate dialysis. The cardiac evaluation of CRF patients is further complicated by the fact that noninvasive evaluation has a decreased accuracy in this population. In renal transplantation candidates, myocardial scintigraphy and dobutamine stress echocardiography had less than 75% sensitivity for significant coronary artery disease as detected by angiography and had poor predictive power for myocardial events.[78] Therefore, in CRF patients undergoing higher risk surgeries the threshold for requesting a cardiac evaluation and for obtaining a coronary angiogram should be probably lower than in the nonrenal population.[76] An evaluation algorithm proposes that renal transplantation candidates who are asymptomatic for myocardial ischemia but have diabetes or are older than age 50 years should undergo noninvasive cardiac evaluation, followed by coronary arteriography and revascularization if indicated.[79] According to this same algorithm, patients who are symptomatic for ischemia or heart failure should all receive an invasive evaluation. Although no evidence is available in patients undergoing nontransplant surgeries, it is reasonable to follow a similar approach for procedures with similar and higher risk. The outcomes of revascularization in patients with CRF are worse compared with the remaining population. Percutaneous balloon angioplasty has a higher rate of restenosis in renal than in nonrenal patients, although better results have been obtained with stent placement.[80] Coronary artery bypass

graft in renal failure patients has a higher perioperative morbidity and mortality, but it may have a lower rate of restenosis and higher long-term survival compared with angioplasty.[76]

In preparation for elective surgery, patients with ESRD should receive dialysis the day before the operation. This is essential to achieve a volume status as close to normovolemic as possible, to allow the patient to tolerate fluid loads associated with surgery, and to obtain normal electrolyte concentrations. On the other hand, excessive fluid removal may cause hypovolemia and make the patient prone to intraoperative hemodynamic instability. The dialysis records, when available, can help to assess the adequacy of dialysis. Urea should decrease more than 65% during a dialysis session. Dry weight, defined as the lowest weight tolerated in absence of hypovolemic symptoms, is recorded to monitor the efficacy of fluid removal and ideally should be relatively stable over time, with 3% to 4% weight gain between sessions.[81] Dialysis should not be given immediately before the surgery because of the possibility of causing rapid fluid shifts and hypokalemia. In the case of emergent surgery, it may be possible to proceed without dialysis if a minimal weight gain between treatments is documented; however, patients with signs of fluid overload or with life-threatening hyperkalemia may need emergent dialysis before the operation if time allows. Otherwise, patients have to be managed medically and receive dialysis after the operation. Significant hyperkalemia, when present, can be temporarily controlled with pharmacologic means. Intraoperative use of ultrafiltration is relatively common during on-pump cardiac surgery,[82] and it also has been reported during noncardiac surgery.[83,84] Potassium levels above 5.5 mEq/L are usually considered a contraindication to elective surgery because tissue trauma and cell death can cause potassium to increase to life-threatening levels. Hypokalemia should not be treated unless at life-threatening levels.

Blood pressure should be optimized before elective surgery. Current recommendations for long-term CRF management set a blood pressure goal of lower than 130/80 mm Hg in patients with CRF.[76] Hypertension in CRF patients is usually volume dependent and responds to adequate dialysis, but most patients will also require pharmacologic therapy.[75] Perioperative β blockers should be considered for patients at increased cardiac risk. Hypertension management is important not only for myocardial protection but also because the use of certain antihypertensive drugs such as ACE inhibitors and angiotensin receptor blockers has been shown to limit the evolution of renal disease.

Control of anemia is important because anemia is an important cause of left ventricular hypertrophy, heart failure, and angina. Hematocrit should be optimized before surgery. For ambulatory ESRD patients, hemoglobin of 11 to 12 g/dL is considered optimal,[75] and this value is also used as a target before surgery, although this practice is not supported by clinical evidence. The target hemoglobin level can be achieved by increasing erythropoietin administration if time allows or by transfusion for urgent surgery. Correction of anemia also helps to improve the platelet dysfunction of renal failure.[85] If platelet dysfunction is suspected or documented, it can be treated by administration of desmopressin or cryoprecipitate, both of which increase the level of von Willebrand factor and improve the interaction between platelets and endothelial cells.[73] Their onset of action is rapid, which renders both drugs useful intraoperatively. However, the prolonged use of desmopressin is limited by induction of tachyphylaxis. Estradiol is also effective in the treatment of platelet dysfunction, but its peak effect is delayed for several days. Most commonly encountered chronic medications in patients with CRF are listed in Table 7-11.

Acute Renal Failure

Acute renal failure (ARF) refers to a variety of syndromes leading to abrupt reduction in GFR. ARF refers to a reduction in renal function, not necessarily renal damage, and it may occur de novo or in a patient with preexisting chronic renal disease.

Renal failure manifests as acute reduction in urinary output (oliguria) or an increase in the circulating concentration of nitrogenous waste products, which ultimately lead to the syndrome of uremia. In clinical practice, serum urea and creatinine are used as measurable markers of uremia but are not responsible for it. Oliguria is defined as a urine volume of less than 400 to 500 mL/24 hr. Oliguria is not necessary for the diagnosis of ARF, although it is often the presenting sign. Unfortunately, there is no consensus on an operational definition of ARF. Indeed, the term "failure" is problematic, because it does not separate extrarenal and renal components.[86]

The ARF syndromes have traditionally been classified into three major categories on the basis of their pathophysiology: prerenal, renal, and postrenal ARF. Prerenal ARF is associated with a reduction in renal blood flow and glomerular perfusion, secondary to hypotension or hypovolemia. In the initial stages there is no damage to the tubules; however, if it is sustained, ischemic injury results. Postrenal ARF is characterized by acute obstruction to the urinary tract. The obstruction can be at any level in the urinary tract from the renal pelvis to the urethra; however, for obstruction proximal to the urinary bladder to result in ARF it must be bilateral or occur in the setting of a single functional kidney. Abdominal compartment syndrome (see later) appears to combine prerenal and postrenal components. Intrinsic ARF is associated with renal parenchymal injury. This results from ischemic or toxic injury to renal tubular epithelial cells (acute tubular necrosis) and from glomerular, vascular, and interstitial inflammatory disease processes (Table 7-12).

Acute Tubular Necrosis

Acute tubular necrosis (ATN) results in ARF due to a number of processes. Medullary ischemia results from hypoxic injury to the thick limb of the loop of Henle. This leads to sloughing of cells (casts), which block tubular flow. The tubular pressure builds up and glomerular filtration is inhibited. Ischemic ATN is common in perioperative medicine, resulting from hypovolemia, hypotension, deliberate ischemia, such as application of suprarenal cross clamps (in cardiac and aortic surgery). ATN also results from a variety of toxic insults. These include aminoglycoside and glycopeptide (vancomycin) antibiotics, NSAIDs, radiographic contrast, pigment (rhabdomyolysis), heavy metals, and solvents.

The clinical course of ATN can be divided into three phases: initiation, maintenance, and recovery. The initiation phase refers to the period in which the kidney is injured and progression is potentially preventable. When renal failure becomes established there may be a dramatic reduction in GFR, manifest as oliguria, with accumulation of nitrogenous waste products of metabolism and the development of uremia, confusion and cognitive decline, pericarditis, platelet dysfunction, and so on. This phase lasts days to weeks. The recovery phase lasts 4 to 6 weeks and is characterized by poor renal concentrating capacity and polyuria. Cellular repair takes place, and GRF gradually returns to normal.

TABLE 7–11	List of Chronic Medications That Are Common in Chronic Renal Failure
Hypertension	β Blockers, calcium channel blockers, angiotensin-converting enzyme inhibitors, angiotensin antagonists
Fluid overload	Thiazides, furosemide
Osteodystrophy and hypocalcemia	Calcium supplements, phosphate binders, calcitriol
Diabetes	Insulin, oral hypoglycemics
Anemia	Erythropoietin, iron

TABLE 7–12 Causes of Intrinsic Acute Renal Failure
Acute Tubular Necrosis
Ischemia
Hypotension
Hypovolemic shock
Sepsis
Cardiac arrest
Cardiopulmonary bypass
Drug-Induced Nephropathy
Aminoglycosides
Radiocontrast agents
Amphotericin
Cisplatin
Pigment Nephropathy
Intravascular hemolysis
Cryoglobulinemia
Rhabdomyolysis
Acute Interstitial Nephritis **Drug-Induced**
Penicillins
Cephalosporins
Sulfonamides
Rifampin
Phenytoin
Furosemide
Nonsteroidal anti-inflammatory drugs (NSAIDs)
Infection-Related
Bacterial infection
Viral infections
Rickettsial disease
Tuberculosis
Endocarditis
Systemic Diseases
Systemic lupus erythematosus
Multiple myeloma
Diabetes mellitus
Amyloidosis
Acute glomerulonephritis
Poststreptococcal glomerulonephritis
Rapidly progressive glomerulonephritis
Vascular Syndromes
Hemolytic-uremic syndrome
Thrombotic thrombocytopenic purpura
Systemic vasculitis
Renal artery thromboembolism
Renal vein thrombosis

Renal Function Tests

A normally functioning kidney is able to conserve salt and water. A sensitive indicator of tubular function is sodium handling because the ability of an injured tubule to reabsorb sodium is impaired, whereas an intact tubule can maintain this reabsorptive capacity in the face of a hemodynamic stress. With a prerenal insult, the urine sodium concentration should be less than 20 mEq, and the calculated fractional excretion of sodium (FENa) should be less than 1% [FENa = $(U_{Na}/P_{Na}) \div (U_{Creatinine}/P_{Creatinine})$]. Urinary osmolality is high in prerenal syndrome. If the patient has tubular damage for any reason the urinary sodium concentration will be greater than expected (>80 mEq) and the urinary osmolality low.

There is very little consensus as to what exactly constitutes ARF. In clinical practice, urea, a breakdown product of protein that is partially reabsorbed, and creatinine, a metabolic byproduct of muscle metabolism that is partially secreted, are used as markers for renal failure. Serum urea underestimates GFR. Serum creatinine is a better marker, assuming that muscle turnover is constant. Hence, in a trauma victim, when there may be significant muscle injury, creatinine may underestimate renal function. Serum creatinine is very insensitive to even substantial declines in GFR. The GFR may be reduced by up to 50% before the serum creatinine level becomes elevated. Creatinine overestimates the GFR, so it is difficult to assess true renal function using the serum creatinine value. Conventional wisdom relates that a doubling of the serum creatinine level is indicative of renal failure. However, this may be misleading in patients with reduced muscle turnover (i.e., critically ill or elderly patients). The creatinine clearance has been used as a method of overcoming these problems. The most commonly used method of calculation is:

$$\text{Creatinine clearance (mL/min)} = [(140 - \text{Age}) \times (\text{Wt})]/(72 \times \text{Creatinine})^*$$

There are many reasons why this calculation may be inaccurate, including variations in creatinine production from person to person and from time to time. Furthermore, the weight as an index of muscle mass may be inaccurate in obese or edematous (particularly in critical care) patients. A more effective method would be to compare what is in the urine to what is in the serum as a measure of clearance.

The serum creatinine level is usually falsely raised by error inherent in measurement. The urinary creatinine level is falsely raised by tubular secretion. These errors tend to cancel each other out, so the following equation gives a reasonably accurate estimate of GFR:

$$\text{Creatinine clearance} = (\text{Urinary creatinine [mg/ml]} \times \text{Urinary volume}) \times 100/\text{Serum creatinine}$$

Finally, the differences in the way the kidneys handle urea and creatinine is of diagnostic value (Table 7-13). It is known that urea is reabsorbed and creatinine is not.

*Multiply by 0.85 if female.

TABLE 7-13   Evaluation of Oliguria

Parameter	Prerenal	Acute Tubular Necrosis
U:P osmolality	>1.4:1	1:1
U:P creatinine	>50:1	<20:1
Urine sodium (mEq/L)	<20	>80
Fractional excretion of sodium (%)	<1	>3
RFI %	<1%	>1%
Creatinine clearance (mL/min)	15-20	<10
Blood urea nitrogen/creatinine	>20	<10

U:P, urine:plasma; RFI, renal failure index, calculated as urinary sodium/(urinary creatinine/serum creatinine).

In dehydration (prerenal syndrome) the ratio of urea to creatinine is elevated (from a factor of 10 to a factor of 20).

In conclusion, if renal dysfunction is suspected, concentrating capacity (urinary sodium and osmolality) and GFR (creatinine clearance) should be measured. Renal failure index (RFI) is a consolidated figure that may be used as a single score. It is calculated as follows:

$$\text{Renal failure index (RFI)} = \text{Urinary sodium}/(\text{Urinary creatinine/Serum creatinine}).$$

Urinary microscopy is a useful diagnostic technique for ARF, particularly in the early stages. The presence of different cells or casts indicate the etiology of the disease process (Table 7-14).

Trauma-Associated Renal Failure

ARF is a frequent complication of major trauma, often associated with severe hypovolemia and ATN. This is prevented with early, aggressive volume resuscitation and control of the source of bleeding.

Rhabdomyolysis

Rhabdomyolysis refers to the release of large quantities of muscle cell contents as the result of traumatic or nontraumatic injury of skeletal muscle. There is a linear relationship between the degree of trauma and the likelihood of developing pigment nephropathy, as quantified by the serum creatine phosphokinase level. In addition to myoglobin, the protein primarily responsible for renal injury, there is a dramatic increase in the serum concentration of intracellular ions: phosphate, potassium, and magnesium. The serum calcium concentration subsequently falls dramatically.

Four mechanisms are believed to contribute to the development of ARF in myoglobinuria: hypovolemia,

TABLE 7-14   Urinalysis Findings in Acute Renal Failure

Type of Renal Injury	Urinalysis
Prerenal	Benign or hyaline casts
Acute tubular necrosis	Heme granular or epithelial cell casts
Acute interstitial nephropathy	WBCs, WBC casts, eosinophils, proteinuria
Acute glomerulonephritis	RBCs, dysmorphic RBCs, RBC casts, proteinuria
Postrenal	Benign ± hematuria

WBC, white blood cell; RBC, red blood cell.

renal vasoconstriction, heme-mediated proximal tubular cell toxicity, and intratubular cast formation. Renal perfusion rapidly decreases after muscle cell injury as a result of massive fluid sequestration into the injured tissue. There is a dramatic increase in the circulating concentration of renal vasoconstrictors: epinephrine, norepinephrine, endothelin and angiotensin II. Usually myoglobin is reabsorbed by the proximal tubule and metabolized by releasing free iron, which is soaked up by glutathione, but in rhabdomyolysis this mechanism is overwhelmed. Free heme proteins scavenge nitrous oxide, contributing to vasoconstriction, and generate free radicals, which are nephrotoxic. In addition, in the presence of an acidic urine, myoglobin binds with a renal excretory protein (Tamm-Horsfall) to form a cast that obstructs the tubules and causes ATN.

Although rhabdomyolysis was first described in trauma, it also occurs in other circumstances (Table 7-15). Presenting symptoms in rhabdomyolysis usually reflect the primary disease process with superimposed symptoms of muscle injury or renal failure. Occasionally the patient may present with acute limb compartment syndrome.

TABLE 7–15 Causes of Rhabdomyolysis
Traumatic Causes
Crush injury
Lightning strike/electrocution
Immobilization
Extensive burns
Heat-Related Causes
Heatstroke
Overexertion (marathon running)
Malignant hyperthermia
Neuroleptic malignant syndrome
Inflammatory Causes
Polymyositis
Dermatomyositis
Sepsis
Snake bites
Toxic Causes/Associations
Alcohol
Cocaine
Amphetamine
Ecstasy (MDMA)
LSD
HMG-CoA reductase inhibitors

This may result from a closed fracture of crush injury or inappropriate surgical closure. The patient complains of pain, swelling, tenderness, and bruising. Where there is neurovascular impairment the pain is severe. Urgent fasciotomy is required. Rhabdomyolysis is suspected by the presence of tea-colored urine and a rising creatine phosphokinase level. If the diagnosis cannot be separated from hemoglobinuria, microscopic examination of the urine is necessary. The patient may develop severe hyperkalemia, hyperphosphatemia, hyperuricemia, and lactic acidosis. Profound hypocalcemia may develop as the result of deposition of calcium salts in injured muscle.

Several strategies have been proposed to prevent the development of ARF in rhabdomyolysis. The only approach supported by evidence is aggressive volume replacement. The nature of the fluid (isotonic, hypotonic) is less important than the absolute volume. Urinary alkalization with sodium bicarbonate or sodium acetate is unproven, as is the use of mannitol to promote diuresis.[87,88]

Abdominal Compartment Syndrome

The abdominal compartment syndrome refers to an abrupt increase in intra-abdominal pressure leading to organ dysfunction. This results in hypotension, respiratory compromise, liver and mesenteric ischemia and renal failure. Abdominal compartment syndrome most commonly is seen in trauma patients who require massive volume resuscitation. Extravasation of large quantities of resuscitation fluid into the bowel wall leads to massive edema and abdominal hypertension. It may also occur in settings associated with mechanical limitations of the abdominal wall, such as tight surgical closures or scarring after burn injuries, that reduce abdominal compliance. Renal insufficiency results from decreased renal perfusion and correlates with the severity of the increased intra-abdominal pressure. Oliguria usually develops when the intra-abdominal pressure exceeds 15 mm Hg; anuria usually develops at pressures greater than 30 mm Hg. The specific cause of renal abdominal compartment syndrome is unclear. There is no correlation between intra-abdominal pressure and urinary output. Venous compression and obstruction undoubtedly plays a part, along with direct cortical compression and aortic and renal artery compression.

The diagnosis of abdominal compartment syndrome is based on clinical suspicion and measurement of bladder pressures. This is achieved by injecting 50 mL of saline into the empty bladder through the Foley catheter. The tubing of the drainage bag is cross clamped and a 16-gauge needle is inserted through the aspiration port and connected to a pressure transducer.

Treatment consists of abdominal decompression—usually surgical. The abdominal wall is opened, and the fascia is left open. This is covered by a wound device or the skin. Once edema has subsided, the abdominal wound is closed, although definitive surgery may be delayed for a year or more. If abdominal hypertension is suspected, the anesthesiologist must weigh the cost and benefit of further fluid resuscitation. There is a direct relationship between the volume of crystalloid administered and the incidence of abdominal compartment syndrome. In this situation, colloid resuscitation is probably preferable.[89-91]

Perioperative Renal Dysfunction

Renal dysfunction is relatively common in the postoperative period. Its frequency is higher in certain types of surgery such as aortic reconstruction, where a 25% rate has been reported.[92] Postoperative renal dysfunction manifests with a spectrum of severity that can range from mild defects to renal failure requiring dialysis. When acute renal failure superimposes to other underlying diseases, a significant increase in morbidity and mortality is observed[93,94] but even a moderate renal dysfunction can worsen surgical outcomes. In fact, long-term survival after cardiac surgery is decreased in patients who have moderate renal impairment postoperatively[95] and longer postoperative hospital stays have been observed in patients with mild renal dysfunction after vascular surgery.[96] Thus, the importance of perioperative renal morbidity cannot be underestimated and its prevention assumes a particular importance. Unfortunately, none of the strategies that have been so far proposed to protect from this complication is supported by strong clinical evidence. The study of risk reduction of renal complications is therefore continuing.

Pathophysiology

The kidney is subject to multiple harmful events in the perioperative period. Among these, renal hypoperfusion is one of the most important factors that contribute to renal dysfunction.[97] The most common causes of decreased renal blood flow are hypovolemia, heart failure, and vascular clamping. Renal hypoperfusion results in hypoxic damage to the outer portion of the renal medulla, an area that is exquisitely sensitive to hypoxia. In fact, this region receives a poor blood supply relative to its high oxygen consumption owing to intense solute reabsorption by the thick segment of the loop of Henle. Alterations in ionic pumps, loss of intracellular adenosine triphosphate, increased intracellular calcium, tubular epithelial cell swelling and sloughing are characteristically observed during renal hypoxic damage. Additionally, hypoxic injury might render the kidney more sensitive to subsequent ischemic events, as suggested by the loss of renovascular autoregulation observed in animals after renal ischemia.[97]

Nephrotoxic substances are also important contributors to renal injury, and it is recognized that their effect is synergistically increased by concomitant renal ischemia and hypoperfusion.[98] One of the mechanisms of contrast dye nephropathy, a common cause of perioperative renal dysfunction, is probably the ultrafiltration of a high osmotic load that, by stimulating an increased tubular solute reabsorption, may increase tubular oxygen consumption and favor cell hypoxia. Anti-inflammatory drugs acutely injure renal cells by inhibiting formation of prostaglandins and their effect is enhanced when the kidney is hypoperfused. In fact, prostaglandins are generated during renal hypoperfusion with the effect of maintaining blood flow to the peritubular vessels and to decrease tubular reabsorption. Suppression of their formation may lead to tubular cell ischemia. Finally, preexisting renal disease, diabetes, hypertension, and chronic ischemia increase the susceptibility of the kidney to superimposed ischemic or chemical insults.[99] This is related to lower renal functional reserve, to impaired renovascular autoregulation as seen in hypertensive patients, and to the fact that the effects of renal insults are often permanent and probably add to each other in a cumulative manner in the course of a life span.

Risk Factors

The risk of perioperative renal dysfunction is significantly affected by patient-related factors such as advanced age,[92] left ventricular dysfunction,[93] and preexisting renal insufficiency.[93] A significant part of the population has mild to moderate renal dysfunction, particularly in the elderly (see Fig. 7-4),[67] and is at increased risk for progression to renal failure if further renal damage is superimposed in the perioperative period. The presence of diabetes and systemic hypertension is associated with increased risk for postoperative renal dysfunction, although it is not clear whether this is an independent risk factor or it is rather a consequence of preexisting renal insufficiency. Cholestasis is associated with an increased risk of renal morbidity, probably owing to increased endotoxemia.[100] Recently, evidence of a genetic predisposition to postoperative renal impairment has been reported. In a prospective study on patients undergoing cardiac surgery, certain alleles of the apolipoprotein E genotype have been associated with higher postoperative elevation of creatinine,[101] suggesting that risk stratification might be accomplished by gene testing in the future. Table 7-16 lists the risk factors for perioperative renal dysfunction.

Among surgery-related factors, extensive surgery, high intraoperative blood loss, and transfusion requirement significantly increase the risk for renal dysfunction,[92] but vascular and cardiac surgery are associated with the highest risk of renal morbidity. In particular, the incidence of postoperative renal morbidity after aortic surgery is high and has not decreased in recent times, in spite of improvements of surgical and anesthetic management. In patients undergoing aortic thoracoabdominal aneurism repair, Rectenwald and colleagues detected a 28% incidence of renal dysfunction that was associated with worsened outcomes.[102] Patients undergoing vascular surgery have a high incidence of preoperative kidney disease[92] owing to their comorbidities, a fact that partly explains the high frequency of perioperative renal morbidity in this population. Both proximal location and prolonged duration of aortic cross-clamping[103] are associated with worsened renal function after aortic surgery. Renal injury after aortic clamping is related not only to parenchymal ischemia but also to inflammatory activation and ischemic reperfusion injury of the bowel. Avoidance of aortic cross-clamping with endovascular repair should prevent these complications. The most recent randomized controlled study comparing endovascular and open infrarenal aortic aneurism repair showed a similarly low incidence of renal complications in both study arms, a finding that was probably due to the low rate of renal complications in patients with only infrarenal aneurisms.[104] Newer devices allowing repair of more proximal aneurysms that would otherwise require suprarenal clamping have the potential of decreasing the incidence of renal complications in the future.

Patients undergoing cardiac surgery have a high risk of renal complications, and the risk is further increased with valve replacement.[105] In a prospective cohort study in patients undergoing cardiac surgery, Chertow and coworkers

TABLE 7–16   Risk Factors for Perioperative Renal Dysfunction and Anesthetic Management

Patient Factors	
Preexisting renal disease	Optimize volume status and cardiac output, intravenous fluids and/or inotropes; consider invasive hemodynamic monitoring and/or transesophageal echography.
Heart failure	Optimize blood pressure management before surgery; maintain near-basal blood pressure introperatively.
Advanced age	
Hypovolemia	
Sepsis	
Diabetes	
Hypertension	
Cholestasis	
Surgical Factors	
Vascular surgery	Optimize volume status and cardiac output.
Heart surgery	Consider mannitol for vascular clamping, although there is little supporting evidence.
Major abdominal surgery	
Trauma	
Transplant	
Pharmacologic Factors	
Antimicrobials	Avoid hypovolemia.
NSAIDS	Avoid nephrotoxic antimicrobials, or optimize schedule and formulation.
Contrast dye	Avoid NSAIDs in patients at risk.
	Avoid contrast studies or give *N*-acetylcysteine, bicarbonate; consider ultrafiltration.

identified 10 risk factors for renal morbidity and stratified patients in three groups with increasing risk (Table 7-17).[106] This model has been validated in a broader population of patients and may provide a guide for the risk stratification of patients undergoing this type of surgery.[107] Renal impairment after cardiac surgery is related to renal hypoperfusion, inflammatory activation by the cardiopulmonary bypass, and endotoxemia resulting from bowel ischemia. However, it is not clear whether the avoidance of cardiopulmonary bypass decreases the incidence of postoperative renal failure. The finding of a significant decrease in renal impairment with off-pump surgery[108,109] has not been confirmed in all studies.[110,111] The largest randomized controlled study comparing off-pump with on-pump coronary bypass did not specifically address renal morbidity but showed comparable outcomes and better cost-effectiveness with off-pump technique.[112]

Renal Replacement Therapy

Renal replacement therapy involves the use of semipermeable biocompatible membranes to remove nitrogenous waste products, ion products of metabolism and fluid from the body. Indications for renal replacement therapy are listed in Table 7-18. There are three types: intermittent hemodialysis, peritoneal dialysis, and continuous renal replacement therapy. Two processes underlie renal replacement therapy: diffusion and convection.

Diffusion is a process in which the movement of solutes along an electrochemical gradient from a compartment in which they are in high concentration to one in which they are in lower concentration (Fig. 7-5). An electrolyte solution runs countercurrent to blood flowing on the other side of a semipermeable (small-pore) filter. Small molecules such as urea move along the concentration gradient into the dialysate fluid. Larger molecules are poorly removed by

TABLE 7–17   Independent Risk Factors for Acute Renal Failure After Cardiac Surgery

Valvular surgery
Decreased creatinine clearance
Intra-aortic balloon pump
Prior heart surgery
New York Heart Association class IV
Peripheral vascular disease
Ejection fraction < 35%
Pulmonary rales
Chronic obstructive pulmonary disease
Systolic hypertension or hypotension

Modified from Chertow GM, Lazarus JM: Preoperative renal risk stratification. Circulation 1997;95:878-884.

this process. Solute removal is directly proportional to the dialysate flow rate.

Convection/ultrafiltration is a process in which solute is carried across a semipermeable membrane in response to a transmembrane pressure gradient (a process known as solvent drag). This mimics the actual situation in the normal human kidney (Fig. 7-6). The rate of ultrafiltration depends on the porosity of the membrane and on the hydrostatic pressure of the blood, which depends on blood flow. This is very effective in removal of fluid and middle-sized molecules, which are thought to cause uremia.

Intermittent hemodialysis is the most widely used and effective modality. Large amounts of fluid can be removed, and electrolyte abnormalities can be rapidly corrected. The system includes a double-lumen intravenous catheter or arteriovenous fistula, a pump that forces blood into a filter (semipermeable membrane), dialysate fluid (usually deionized water) that flows in and out, and a return line to the patient. The blood flow rate is 200 to 400 mL/min, the dialysate flow is approximately 500 mL/min, the filtration rate is between 300 and 2000 mL/hr, and urea clearance is 150 to 250 mL/min. With this high flow and clearance rate patients, depending on the extent of their catabolism, only require 3 to 4 hours of dialysis, two or three times a week. There are dramatic fluid and osmotic shifts between the intravascular and extravascular compartments, causing transient hypotension and disequilibrium. Many critically ill patients cannot tolerate this. With hemodialysis, preferential solute and water removal from blood occurs as blood courses through the dialyzer and comes in "contact" with dialysate across a closed network of semipermeable membranes. These membranes allow diffusive movement of non–protein-bound solutes according to their molecular size and chemical gradients between the dialysate and blood. Water and sodium removal depends on a hydrostatic transmembrane

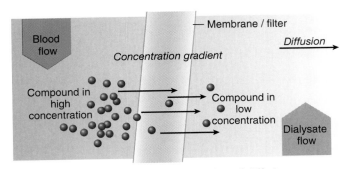

FIGURE 7–5 Schematic representation of diffusion.

pressure gradient between the dialysate and blood that is set up by the head of pressure of blood moving into the dialyzer, resistance to blood return to the patient, and negative pressure in the dialysate compartment created by rapid countercurrent flow of dialysate through it. Anticoagulation with heparin is the standard method for preventing thrombosis of the extracorporeal circuit during acute intermittent dialysis.

Dialysis disequilibrium syndrome is a self-limited condition characterized by nausea, vomiting, headache, altered consciousness, and rarely seizures or coma. It typically occurs after a first dialysis in very uremic patients. The syndrome is triggered by rapid movement of water into brain cells following the development of transient plasma hypo-osmolality as solutes are rapidly cleared from the bloodstream during dialysis. The incidence of this complication has fallen in recent years with the more gradual institution of dialysis and the precise prescription of dialysis to include such variables as membrane size, blood flow rate, and sodium profile.

Peritoneal dialysis has the advantage of being simple and cost effective. A small tube is surgically inserted into the peritoneal cavity. Dextrose is infused into the peritoneum and left in situ for 4 to 6 hours. Waste products diffuse along the concentration gradient into the fluid, which is drained over 30 to 40 minutes. The major disadvantages of peritoneal dialysis are poor solute clearance, poor uremic control, risk of peritoneal infection, and mechanical obstruction of pulmonary and cardiovascular performance.

TABLE 7–18 **Indications for Renal Replacement Therapy**
Oliguria (urine output < 200 mL/12 hr)
Anuria (urine output < 50 mL/12 hr)
Hyperkalemia (K^+ > 6.5 mEq/L)
Severe acidemia (pH < 7.1)
Azotemia (urea > 180 mg/dL)
Pulmonary edema
Uremic encephalopathy
Uremic pericarditis
Uremic neuropathy/myopathy
Severe dysnatremia (Na^+ > 160 or < 115 mEq/L)
Hyperthermia
Drug overdose with dialyzable toxin

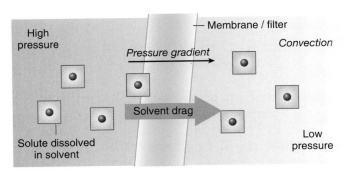

FIGURE 7–6 Schematic representation of convection.

Continuous renal replacement therapy is used in intensive care units to treat hemodynamically unstable patients. In critical illness the phenomenon of capillary leak increases the interstitial volume and makes patients edematous. This makes the clearance of solute difficult to calculate and indeed implement. Continuous techniques lead to more effective urea and water clearance. Continuous renal replacement therapy combines dialysis and ultrafiltration, and has been used to manage patients with acute renal failure, shock, sepsis, and massive fluid overload. Typical blood flow rates are 120 to 150 mL/min and dialysate rates of 1 to 4 L/hr. A more aggressive version—high-volume ultra-filtration—is in widespread use, in particular, in patients with sepsis-induced renal failure. In high-volume ultrafiltration up to 35 mL/kg/hr is ultrafiltered from the patient.[113] Cole and colleagues have suggested that this may be an effective method of reducing pressor requirements in sepsis.[114]

Renal Transplantation

Renal transplantation provides better survival and quality of life than dialysis for patients with ESRD. There is a long-term survival advantage associated with cadaveric ("deceased donor kidney" is preferred by the Association of Organ Procurement Organizations) renal transplantation over dialysis. This difference is most pronounced in patients with diabetes and glomerulonephritis as causes of ESRD.[115-117]

Ideally, renal transplantation should precede the need for dialysis. The unfavorable relationship between time spent on dialysis therapy and outcome has been shown to be progressive. Four years of dialysis therapy confers approximately 70% of additional mortality and graft loss compared with transplantation before the dialysis therapy.[118,119] Renal transplantation may lead to complete resolution of cardiovascular complications, systolic dysfunction, left ventricular hypertrophy, left ventricular dilatation, or uremia,[120] as well as other comorbidities related to ESRD.[121]

The rate of cadaveric kidney donation remains at approximately 9,000 per year despite persistent public education and legislative adjustments to facilitate the organ donation process. Thus, the wait for a cadaveric kidney can be as long as several years. Meanwhile, the mean annual mortality of dialysis patients waiting for a transplant is between 6% and 10%.[115] Fortunately, major progress has been made in increasing the numbers of living kidney donors. In 2001, for the first time in the United States, the number of living donors exceeded the number of cadaveric donors.[122]

The introduction of cyclosporine in 1983 and a series of effective new immunosuppressive agents—corticosteroids, tacrolimus, mycophenolate, azathioprine, and sirolimus—and protocols in following years led to low mortality rates

and a 1-year graft survival rate close to 90% by the mid 1990s.[123-125] Antilymphocyte antibodies are now used in addition to immunosuppressants.[126,127]

In 1987, the United Network for Organ Sharing (UNOS) began to administer the Organ Procurement and Transplantation Network under contract with the U.S. Department of Health and Human Services. An allocation algorithm was developed that ranked patients according to their waiting time and provided points for varying degrees of human leukocyte antigen matching in an effort to use organs in an equitable fashion.

The algorithm for cadaveric donor kidney allocation between 1995 and October 2002 is listed in Table 7-19, together with subsequent changes. The algorithm requires constant re-evaluation as the reality of the expanding waiting list changes with time and new information regarding the implications of previous policy decisions becomes available.

Anesthetic Considerations

Because of the presence of coexisting disease in the population with chronic renal failure, a more extensive preoperative evaluation is required. One proposed management strategy for patients with ESRD who are candidates for transplantation is shown in Figure 7-7.

Anesthesia monitoring should be selected based on specific cardiac comorbidities. A pulmonary artery pressure catheter is rarely required, but it should be considered in patients with severe coronary artery disease and left ventricle dysfunction, moderate to severe valvular abnormalities, or significant pulmonary artery hypertension.

Volume status can vary with the time since the last dialysis. Intraoperative volume expansion increases renal blood flow and is associated with improved graft function.[128-132] Only administration of mannitol combined with volume expansion has been shown to decrease the incidence of acute tubular necrosis after transplantation.[133,134] Hydroxyethyl starch solutions should be used with caution because of their potential worsening effect on renal function.[135]

Hemostasis

Multiple hemostatic abnormalities have been associated with ESRD.[136] Abnormal platelet function and decreased levels of both factor VIII and von Willebrand factor are common. Preoperative dialysis improves platelet function and is the mainstay of the prevention of uremic bleeding, although it is not always immediately effective. Desmopressin, 0.3 µg/kg, given intravenously 1 hour before surgery, and cryoprecipitate, 10 units over 30 minutes, effective in 1 hour, offer an alternative and effective treatment for the temporary reversal of uremic bleeding in patients who require urgent invasive procedures.[137,138]

TABLE 7–19   UNOS Point System for Cadaver Kidney Allocation Before October 2002 with Subsequently Implemented, Adopted, and Proposed Changes

Category	Points Assigned Before October 2002	Changes
Time of waiting	1 point assigned to the patient waiting the longest, fractions proportionately assigned to the remainder, 1 additional point for each full year waiting	No change
Estimation of wait	From time of UNOS registration after GFR < 20 mL/min Time lost during inactivity	From time of dialysis or GFR < 20 mL/min* No loss for inactivity†
Antigen mismatch	7 points for 0 B and DR mismatch 5 points for 1 B or DR mismatch 2 points for 2 B or DR mismatch	2 points for 0 DR mismatch 1 point for 1 DR mismatch‡
Panel-reactive antibody	4 points, if panel-reactive antibody > 80%	No change
Pediatric	4 points for age < 11 y; 3 points for age of 11 y but < 18 y	No change
ECD kidneys	Waiting time-based allocation‡	No category

GFR, glomerular filtration rate; B, blood; DR, donor-related; ECDs; all donors > 60 years or donors > 50 years with a history of hypertension, renal dysfunction, or nontraumatic cause of death.
*Proposed changes.
†Adopted.
‡Subsequently implemented.
From Danovitch GM, Cecka JM: Allocation of deceased donor kidneys: Past, present, and future. Am J Kidney Dis 2003;42:882-890.

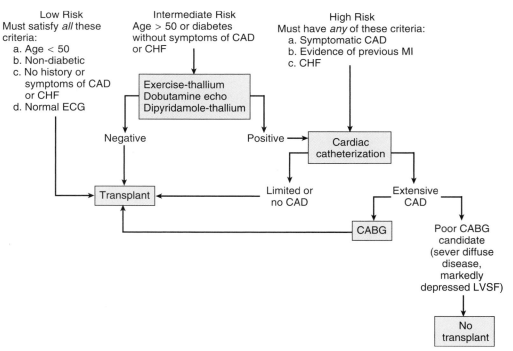

FIGURE 7–7 Management strategy for ESRD patients who are candidates for transplantation. CABG, coronary artery bypass grafting; CAD, coronary artery disease; CHF, congestive heart failure; ECG, electrocardiogram; echo, echocardiogram; LVSF, left ventricular systolic function; MI, myocardial infarction. *(From De Lemos JA, Hillis LD: Diagnosis and management of coronary artery disease in patients with end-stage renal disease on hemodialysis. J Am Soc Nephrol 1996;7:2044-2054.)*

Hyperkalemia

Mild to moderate hyperkalemia leading to direct, aldosterone-independent, renal potassium secretion is now considered to be an adaptive response.[139] Stable serum potassium levels of 5.0 to 5.5 mmol/L before surgery should be tolerated.

INTRAOPERATIVE CONSIDERATIONS FOR THE PATIENT WITH RENAL DISEASE

Hemodynamic Management

Intraoperative hemodynamic management of the renal patient is challenging. In patients who are anuric or oliguric, intravenous fluid administration should be limited to the correction of losses, given their reduced tolerance to fluid overload. In patients who have residual renal function, hypotension, hypovolemia, and renal hypoperfusion may accelerate the progression to ESRD and should be avoided. However, the frequent coexistence of systolic and diastolic left ventricular dysfunction renders these patients prone to having low cardiac output. Additionally, many patients present to surgery with poorly controlled hypertension while their kidneys cannot tolerate large swings in blood pressure due to compromised autoregulation. Therefore, patients with renal disease undergoing higher-risk procedures often need invasive hemodynamic monitoring with arterial, central venous, and pulmonary artery catheters. There are no definite recommendations guiding the choice of monitoring techniques. In fact, the accuracy of filling pressures to estimate patient volume status is questionable,[140] while no benefit of the routine intraoperative use of pulmonary artery catheters has been documented.[141] The choice of hemodynamic monitoring should be based on the history and characteristics of the individual patient and should be directed to specific hemodynamic goals such as optimization of cardiac output. The use of intraoperative transesophageal echocardiography for hemodynamic and volume status monitoring may have a role in patients with renal disease.

The available evidence guiding the choice of intravenous fluids is still scanty but the use of balanced solutions rather than normal saline offers advantages such as avoidance of hyperchloremic acidosis. Potassium-containing solutions are usually avoided in anuric patients with higher potassium levels, although the potassium intake associated with administration of moderate amounts of these fluids is minimal. It is still unclear whether the use of colloids benefits renal patients. Renal toxicity of dextran is known, but alterations in renal function have been reported also with hetastarch, and the safety of its use in patients with renal insufficiency is unclear.[142] However, in one study hetastarch given in a 15-mL/kg dose did not cause renal damage in patients with no preexisting renal disease[143]

and more recent hetastarch formulations with added balanced solutions and with lower molecular weight have improved the safety profile of this drug.[144,145] Albumin administration should probably be reserved for patients with nephrotic syndrome with very low serum albumin levels.

Intravenous access is usually difficult in patients with ESRD, and central venous access is often needed. The veins and arteries of the nondominant upper extremity should be spared from vascular cannulation, because they may be needed for dialysis access in the future. Subclavian vein cannulation should also be avoided because this procedure is frequently complicated by thrombosis, which compromises dialysis access.

Pharmacologic Choices

The anesthetic management of patients with renal failure is complicated by the fact that the pharmacokinetics of several anesthetic drugs are significantly altered. Drugs that are lipid insoluble, are ionized, and that undergo significant renal excretion are more heavily affected by kidney dysfunction. Although renal failure does not always increase the duration of a single dose of these drugs, repeat administration or infusion should be at reduced dosage and the effect should be monitored if possible. Renal failure may also affect the response to more liposoluble drugs that are not mainly excreted by the kidney. In fact, some drugs are biotransformed by the liver to active metabolites that do undergo significant renal excretion and, therefore, can be accumulated in patients with renal failure. Additionally, all drugs that are highly protein bound have an increased free fraction in the presence of hypoproteinemia, such as with nephrotic syndrome. Finally, the response to hypnotic drugs is often increased in uremic patients, an effect that has been ascribed to higher permeability of the hematoencephalic barrier. Table 7-20 lists various anesthetic choices in patients with chronic renal failure.

Induction

Doses of induction agents should be decreased significantly owing to increased free fraction of these drugs, particularly when barbiturates are used. The same consideration applies to benzodiazepines when used for induction or as premedicants. Propofol is not significantly excreted by the kidney; and, although patients with ESRD have slightly increased volume of distribution for this drug, the half-life of propofol is not significantly prolonged in these patients.[146] A higher induction dose requirement for propofol has been reported in one study comparing patients with ESRD with normal patients, a result that has been ascribed to concomitant anemia and a hyperdynamic circulatory state.[147] The choice of anesthetic

TABLE 7-20   Choices of Anesthetic Agents for Renal Patients

Agent Type	Preferred	Used with Caution	Avoided
Inhaled agents	Isoflurane Desflurane	Enflurane Sevoflurane	Methoxyflurane
Induction agents	Etomidate Ketamine	Thiopental Propofol Midazolam	Diazepam Lorazepam
Opioids	Fentanyl Remifentanil Alfentanil	Morphine Hydromorphone	Meperidine
Neuromuscular blockers	Cisatracurium Atracurium Mivacurium	Vecuronium Succinylcholine Rocuronium	Pancuronium Doxacurium

induction dose should also consider the possible presence of autonomic dysfunction, hypovolemia, pericardial tamponade, and the preoperative use of ACE inhibitors,[148] all factors that can cause hypotension after induction of anesthesia. A safe induction strategy is a slow titration of anesthetic and sedative agents, unless rapid-sequence induction is indicated.

Ketamine is hepatically metabolized, has a short redistribution half life, is well tolerated hemodynamically, and is indicated in patients at risk for hypotension. However, the active metabolites norketamine and dehydronorketamine are renally excreted and have the theoretical potential for accumulation after prolonged use.[149] Etomidate can be used in hemodynamically unstable patients, given the good hemodynamic profile of this drug. The use of prolonged infusions of etomidate is contraindicated owing to adrenal suppression and to the possible accumulation of the solvent propylene glycol in patients with renal failure.

Muscle Relaxants

Rapid-sequence induction is often indicated in patients with renal failure, owing to the high incidence of gastroparesis. Succinylcholine is not contraindicated as long as there is no preexisting hyperkalemia. In fact, this drug causes a transient increase in serum potassium levels but this effect in renal patients is similar to normal subjects.[150] The use of succinylcholine in absence of significant adverse effects has been reported also in moderately hyperkalemic patients.[151] Rocuronium is an acceptable alternative to succinylcholine for rapid-sequence induction if a longer paralysis can be accepted. Renal failure does not affect the response to a single dose of rocuronium. The elimination of rocuronium is mainly biliary, although a 26% renal excretion has been measured in humans.[152] Its duration of action is only slightly prolonged after repeat doses.[153] In fact, the plasma clearance of this

drug is not affected by renal dysfunction, although the volume of distribution is increased, resulting in a longer half-life.

Pancuronium has an increased half-life when creatinine clearance is lower than 50 mL/min,[154] and, therefore, its prolonged or repeat administration should be avoided. Owing to the presence of alternative muscle relaxants that are less affected by renal dysfunction, pancuronium is usually avoided in these patients. Vecuronium is mainly biotransformed and excreted by the liver, with only a 15% renal excretion. However, its duration of action is prolonged in patients with ESRD. This effect is due to a decreased clearance, to an increased response to blood concentrations of the drug, and to accumulation of the active metabolite 3-desacetyl-vecuronium.[155] Although the prolonged infusion of vecuronium for muscle relaxation in the intensive care unit should be avoided, the intraoperative use of this drug in patients with chronic renal failure is safe, provided that the appropriate dose adjustments and neuromuscular monitoring are implemented.

Doxacurium, another nondepolarizing muscle relaxant, is mainly excreted by the kidney, and the time to recovery from muscle relaxation is significantly increased in patients with creatinine clearance lower than 40 mL/min.[156] Atracurium and its isomer cisatracurium are the most attractive options for patients with renal failure. In particular, cisatracurium is more potent and leads to less histamine liberation than atracurium, and for these reasons it has become popular. Both drugs undergo non–organ-dependent elimination by the Hoffman reaction, with a non–dose-dependent clearance, and with production of laudanosine.[157] Although accumulation of laudanosine caused cerebral irritation in experimental models, there are no reports of seizures caused by cisatracurium in humans.[158]

Even when the elimination of muscle relaxant is prolonged owing to renal failure, the use of reversal agents is still safe, because these drugs undergo significant renal excretion (50% in the case of neostigmine) and their duration of action is prolonged by renal dysfunction.[159] Additionally, reversal of muscle relaxation with neostigmine is not delayed after a single dose of vecuronium.[160]

Maintenance and Postoperative Period

The effects of inhaled anesthetics in patients with and without renal dysfunction have been discussed previously. Although most of the intravenous agents used during anesthesia and postoperatively undergo hepatic metabolism, some of them undergo transformation to active metabolites that are renally excreted and may accumulate during renal failure. This effect is more significant after prolonged use, such as in the postoperative period. Morphine undergoes 10% conjugation to morphine-6-glucuronide, a molecule with very high potency that rapidly accumulates in the cerebrospinal fluid of patients in renal failure[161] and that may lead to significant sedation. Morphine-6-glucuronide has significant interindividual variability, probably owing to genetic polymorphism at the opioid receptor,[162] and has a delayed onset, probably from a slow transfer through the hematoencephalic barrier.[163]

Morphine-6-glucuronide can be cleared by hemodialysis. Similar to morphine, meperidine and hydromorphone are transformed to neurotoxic metabolites and should be used with care or avoided. Remifentanil, fentanyl, and alfentanil do not have active metabolites and are well tolerated in patients with renal failure.

Among the benzodiazepines, midazolam, lorazepam, and diazepam are transformed to renally excreted metabolites and should be used with care, particularly during postoperative sedation. Additionally, current lorazepam formulations contain propylene glycol, a renally excreted toxic substance that accumulates after prolonged high-dose administration in patients with renal failure.[164]

The use of total intravenous anesthesia with propofol, remifentanil, and cisatracurium has been proposed for renal patients and is probably safe.[165] However, the advantage of such complex and costly strategy is unclear given the safety of current inhalation anesthetics.

Regional anesthesia is commonly chosen in renal patients, particularly for peripheral procedures such as creation of arteriovenous fistulas, for which brachial plexus blocks are a popular choice. Central neuraxial blockade can be used safely, provided that it is remembered that renal patients are prone to hemodynamic instability and hypotension when sympathetic blockade is superimposed to preexisting autonomic dysfunction. The occurrence of epidural hematoma after neuraxial block has been reported in a patient with chronic renal failure,[166] and a high index of suspicion should be maintained. However, this is probably a very rare event in patients who are adequately dialyzed.

Effects of Perioperative Drugs on Renal Function

Anesthetics

Anesthetic agents affect kidney function mainly through their systemic effects. In fact, most anesthetics depress cardiac output and blood pressure, causing a decrease in renal perfusion that can be corrected by adequate volume and hemodynamic support. Surgical stress may alter glomerular blood flow by promoting local vasoconstriction through sympathetic activation, whereas hypovolemia may trigger inappropriate secretion of ADH, which, independently from serum osmolality, causes decreased excretion of free water and of urine. These alterations are usually transient unless hypovolemia and renal hypoperfusion are not corrected.

The evidence that some inhalational anesthetics can lead to altered renal function has raised the concern that renal morbidity may be caused by these agents. Both methoxyflurane and enflurane have been shown to cause impairment in urine concentrating ability and ADH-resistant polyuria.[167-169] This effect has been ascribed to the fact that both these gases are highly biotransformed, because the minimally metabolized isoflurane and desflurane are not associated with renal effects,[170,171] even when they are administered for an extended time.[172] Renal injury from anesthetic gases is related to liberation of inorganic fluoride.[173] In experimental studies, fluoride has been shown to cause damage of the collector duct cell and crystal deposition at the mitochondrial level, probably resulting in impairment of Na^+, K^+ ATPase and of water reabsorption.[174] Based on animal dose-response curves, a critical fluoride level of 50 μM is considered toxic to the kidney.[175] Sevoflurane has been associated with liberation of fluoride near the toxic range.[176,177] Alterations in sensitive biochemical markers of altered renal functions have been observed when sevoflurane was administered to healthy volunteers, as compared with desflurane.[178] However, no alterations in blood urea nitrogen or creatinine were observed with sevoflurane in these volunteers. Multiple clinical studies have failed to show clinically significant renal function alterations after administration of sevoflurane.[179-181] This discrepancy between sevoflurane and methoxyflurane, in spite of comparable serum fluoride levels, may be explained by the faster clearance of the former agent, which results in shorter exposure of renal cells to increased fluoride. However, the recent finding that methoxyflurane, and not sevoflurane, undergoes significant microsomal biotransformation in the kidney, with resulting higher intraparenchymal fluoride concentrations, may explain why actual renal injury does not seem related to serum fluoride concentrations.[182]

Sevoflurane is degraded to the vinyl ether named compound A when administered at low fresh gas flow

(<1 L/min) and particularly when baralyme absorbers of smaller size are used. Compound A induces dose-related nephrotoxicity in animal models,[183] and the concern that toxic blood levels of this substance are possible in humans undergoing low flow sevoflurane anesthesia has resulted in considerable concern and in a warning by the U.S. Food and Drug Administration against the use of sevoflurane at fresh gas flows less than 2 L/min. However, there is little evidence that sevoflurane leads to clinically significant renal alterations compared with other inhaled anesthetic agents, as observed by Mazze and colleagues in a retrospective analysis of 1941 patients undergoing sevoflurane anesthesia.[184] This can be explained by the fact that compound A levels in humans are well below the levels observed in animal studies and that human kidney is probably less sensitive to this substance than rat kidney, owing to different biotransformation. The concern that sevoflurane might exacerbate preexisting renal disease has been also raised. However, renal toxicity has not been detected when sevoflurane was administered in patients with renal insufficiency with a relatively high flow of 4 L/min.[185]

Antibiotics and Contrast Dyes

Several antimicrobial agents that are commonly used in the perioperative period are known to be nephrotoxic. Aminoglycosides are associated with a significant incidence of renal failure. The common practice of monitoring the blood levels of these drugs has not been shown to prevent injury, whereas once-daily administration seems to be protective, compared with the traditional three times per day schedule.[186] The common antifungal amphotericin-B is associated with a nephropathy that can be attenuated by fluid administration and by the use of the lipid-complexed forms of the drug.[187] Newer drugs, such as voriconazole, may have less nephrotoxicity with similar antifungal effectiveness, compared with amphotericin.[188]

Administration of radiographic contrast dye is relatively common in the perioperative period and is an important cause of renal dysfunction or failure in hospitalized patients. Risk factors for contrast dye nephropathy include previous renal disease, older age, hypovolemia, heart failure, and diabetes.[189] Noniodinated dyes with low osmolarity have been shown to be somewhat less harmful to the kidney. Excessive osmolar load, renovascular vasoconstriction, and oxidant damage are thought to be involved in the pathogenesis of contrast dye nephropathy. Until recently, intravenous hydration was the only strategy proven to have some effectiveness in preventing this nephropathy in high-risk patients, whereas furosemide and mannitol had no positive effect.[190] More recently, the use of N-acetylcysteine combined with intravenous

hydration and administered before and after the contrast dye has been shown to protect against worsened renal injury in patients with chronic renal failure.[191] However, these encouraging results have not been confirmed in another study.[192]

More recently, intravenous hydration using a sodium bicarbonate solution had a lower incidence of contrast medium–related nephropathy compared with normal saline, in patients with creatinine values greater than 1.1 mg/dL.[193] Finally, the use of continuous hemofiltration during percutaneous coronary intervention in patients with chronic renal failure reduced the incidence of nephropathy, compared with intravenous saline infusion alone.[194] Hemofiltration was associated also with a reduction of in-hospital and 1-year mortality, a result that underlines the clinical relevance of contrast medium–induced nephropathy and the importance of its prevention.

Nonsteroidal Anti-inflammatory Drugs

Several NSAIDs have been associated with acute and chronic nephropathy. This condition can be diagnosed by specific computed tomographic findings, and its classic presentation is papillary necrosis.[195] The pathophysiologic mechanisms are multiple and include an allergic-mediated nephritis, a direct toxicity due to chronic high dosage exposure, and medullary ischemia from inhibition of prostaglandin formation.[196] Although there is a clear association between nephropathy and the use of excessive analgesic doses, the incidence of this condition in patients taking usual doses of these drugs is unknown. The incidence of nephropathy due to NSAIDs in surgical patients with no preexisting renal disease is probably very limited, although case reports of adverse renal events exist in the literature, particularly with the use of ketorolac.[197] Renal dysfunction is more likely if NSAIDs are administered to patients who have preexisting renal disease, who are hypovolemic, and who are receiving other nephrotoxic drugs.[198] Perioperative administration of ketorolac did not cause renal dysfunction in patients receiving high-flow sevoflurane anesthesia.[199] Diclofenac did not cause a decrease in glomerular function in elderly patients who had a baseline creatinine clearance of higher than 40 mL/min/1.73 m^2.[200] It is still not clear whether the use of selective cyclooxygenase inhibitors lowers the incidence of renal side effects.[201]

Antihypertensive Agents

ACE inhibitors are commonly used by hypertensive patients and have proven benefits in patients with congestive heart failure, coronary artery disease, and renal insufficiency. In the last group ACE inhibitors decrease urinary protein excretion and seem to delay the progression of renal insufficiency. Angiotensin receptor antagonists are a new class of drugs that have been recently introduced in the therapy for patients with ACE inhibitor intolerance and seem to share the same benefits of these drugs. Although the acute preoperative administration of ACE inhibitors seems to have favorable effects on renal perfusion,[202] investigators have reported that patients who are chronically managed with these drugs have pronounced hypotension after induction of anesthesia if the drug is not stopped before the day of the surgery.[203] Similar results have been observed in patients taking angiotensin receptor antagonists.[204] These results have been ascribed to an impairment of angiotensin-mediated hemodynamic regulation, as suggested by a bigger hypotensive response to hypovolemia in animals pretreated with these drugs.[205] Additionally, Cittanova and coworkers have shown in a prospective observational study that chronic use of ACE inhibitors predicts postoperative renal dysfunction, expressed as a 20% reduction in creatinine clearance.[206] However, the results of this study are limited by its retrospective design, although confounding factors such as the presence of heart failure were accounted for. Besides, increases in creatinine concentration are commonly observed during ACE inhibition and are not due to permanent kidney damage. The clinical relevance of the renal dysfunction reported by Cittanova and coworkers is unclear; therefore, routine discontinuation of these drugs before surgery cannot be recommended.

Risk Modification and Renal Protection Strategies

A considerable amount of research has been invested in trying to identify effective strategies that could alter the course of perioperative renal dysfunction, and several agents have been shown to afford renal protection from toxic or ischemic insults in animal models. Unfortunately, none of these agents has been demonstrated to be effective in well-conducted clinical trials. Among these agents dopamine has been known for a long time to cause a selective renal vasodilation when infused with a low rate owing to a specific action on dopaminergic receptors. This effect has been shown to result in increased sodium and water excretion in animals,[207] and it has been hypothesized that the use of dopamine at low dosages may result in protection from renal injury. The use of dopamine in patients with high risk for renal damage or with established renal failure has widely spread. However, recent evidence from well-conducted studies does not support this practice. In a blinded, randomized study by Lassnigg and colleagues comparing low-dose dopamine to placebo or furosemide in cardiac surgery patients, dopamine did not improve creatinine clearance, urine output, or sodium

excretion in the postoperative period.[208] Additional evidence that dopamine does not improve renal outcomes is provided by a randomized study by Bellomo and associates on patients with systemic inflammatory response syndrome and acute renal dysfunction. In this study, dopamine decreased neither creatinine concentrations nor the number of patients requiring renal replacement therapy.[209]

Mannitol is also considered to be a renoprotective agent, owing to its ability to increase urine output, decrease tubular cell swelling, and scavenge oxygen radicals. This drug is often used during cardiac and vascular surgery, although the evidence supporting this use is very poor.[210] Loop diuretics block ion pumps and may reduce tubular cell oxygen consumption, theoretically providing protection from ischemia.[97] However, in the study by Lassnigg and coworkers on cardiac surgery patients, the group treated with furosemide had significantly worsened creatinine clearance and a higher number of patients with renal injury, compared with the dopamine and placebo groups.[208] It is worth noticing that the furosemide group had the highest urine output, compared with the other two groups. Evidence in patients with acute renal failure[211] suggests that the use of diuretics to increase urine output may be associated with worsened outcomes, although the results have not been confirmed in one study.[212] These results combined suggest that using pharmacologic agents to increase urine output may not necessarily lead to improved outcomes in patients with renal dysfunction or who are at high risk for it.

Other agents have been suggested to be renoprotective. Among these, calcium channel blockers might protect from tubular cell hypoxia by decreasing intracellular calcium and have been shown to limit tubular damage during cardiac surgery.[213] ADH analogues and other dopamine receptor agonists such as fenoldopam might also have a renoprotective action. However, evaluation in larger clinical trials is awaited before reverting to their routine use with the intent to limit or improve renal injuries in high-risk patients. In the meanwhile, the only recommendations that can be made, in the perioperative management of the patients at high-risk for renal dysfunction, are to try to limit exposure to known insults by avoiding or carefully using nephrotoxic drugs, choose noncontrast imaging studies when possible[214] or use one of the available protection techniques, and select lower risk surgical procedures. Given the importance of ischemic injury in the determination of renal dysfunction in the perioperative period, restoration and maintenance of normovolemia can be considered as the most effective renal protection strategy. This can be a challenging task, given the limitations of the available monitoring techniques and the uncertainties on the quantity and the quality of the optimal intraoperative fluid management.

References

1. Brezis M, Heyman SN, Dinour D, et al: Role of nitric oxide in renal medullary oxygenation: Studies in isolated and intact rat kidneys. J Clin Invest 1991;88:390-395.
2. Thurau K, Boylan JW: Acute renal success: The unexpected logic of oliguria in acute renal failure. Am J Med 1976;61:308-301
3. Brezis M, Rosen S: Hypoxia of the renal medulla—its implications for disease. N Engl J Med 1995;332:647-655.
4. Heyman SN, Rosen S, Epstein FH, et al: Loop diuretics reduce hypoxic damage to proximal tubules of the isolated perfused rat kidney. Kidney Int 1994;45:981-985.
5. Cantarovich F, Rangoonwala B, Lorenz H, et al: High-dose furosemide for established ARF: A prospective, randomized, double-blind, placebo-controlled, multicenter trial. Am J Kidney Dis 2004;44:402-409.
6. U.S. Renal Data Systems. USRDS 1997 annual data report. Bethesda, MD, National Institutes of Health, National Institute of Diabetes and Digestive and Kidney Diseases, April 1997.
7. Pollock C, Lui P-L, Gyory AZ, et al: Dysmorphism of urinary red blood cells—value in diagnosis. Kidney Int 1989;36:1045-1049.
8. Cibrik DM, Sedor JR: Immunopathogenesis of renal disease. In Greenberg A (ed): Primer on Kidney Diseases, 2nd ed. San Diego, CA, Academic Press, 1997, pp 141-149.
9. Hricik DE, Chung-Park M, Sedor JR: Glomerulonephritis. N Engl J Med 1998;339:888-899.
10. Emancipator SN: IgA nephropathy: Morphologic expression and pathogenesis. Am J Kidney Dis 1994;23:451-462.
10a. Julian BA, Waldo FB, Rifai A, Mestecky J: IgA nephropathy, the most common glomerulonephritis worldwide: A neglected disease in the United States? Am J Med 1988;84:129-132.
11. Davin J-C, Ten Berge IJ, Weening JJ: What is the difference between IgA nephropathy and Henoch-Schönlein purpura nephritis? Kidney Int 2001;59:823-834.
12. Holm SE: The pathogenesis of acute post-streptococcal glomerulonephritis in new lights. APMIS 1988;96:189-193.
13. Tejani A, Ingulli E: Poststreptococcal glomerulonephritis: Current clinical and pathologic concepts. Nephron 1990;55:1-5.
14. Rodríguez-Iturbe B, García R: Isolated glomerular diseases: Acute glomerulonephritis. In Holliday MA, Barratt TM, Vernier RL (eds): Pediatric Nephrology, 2nd ed. Baltimore, Williams & Wilkins, 1987, pp 407-419.
15. Schacht RG, Gluck MC, Gallo GR, Baldwin DS: Progression to uremia after remission of acute poststreptococcal glomerulonephritis. N Engl J Med 1976;295:977-981.
16. Roy S III, Pitcock JA, Etteldorf JN: Prognosis of acute poststreptococcal glomerulonephritis in childhood: Prospective study and review of the literature. Adv Pediatr 1976;23:35-69.
17. Kerr PG, Lan HY, Atkins RC: Rapidly progressive glomerulonephritis. In Schrier RW, Gottschalk CW (eds): Diseases of the Kidney, 6th ed. Boston, Little, Brown, 1997, vol 2, pp 1619-1644.
18. Bolton WK: Rapidly progressive glomerulonephritis. Semin Nephrol 1996;16:517-526.
19. Merkel F, Pullig O, Marx M, et al: Course and prognosis of anti-basement membrane antibody mediated disease: Report of 35 cases. Nephrol Dial Transplant 1994;9:372-376.
20. Hogan SL, Nachman PH, Wilkman AS, et al: Prognostic markers in patients with antineutrophil cytoplasmic autoantibody-associated microscopic polyangiitis and glomerulonephritis. J Am Soc Nephrol 1996;7:23-32.
21. Lal DPSS, O'Donoghue DJ, Haeney M: Effect of diagnostic delay on disease severity and outcome in glomerulonephritis caused by anti-neutrophil cytoplasmic antibodies. J Clin Pathol 1996;49:942-944.
22. Heilman RL, Offord KP, Holley KE, Velosa JA: Analysis of risk factors for patient and renal survival in crescentic glomerulonephritis. Am J Kidney Dis 1987;9:98-107.
23. Nachman PH, Hogan SL, Jennette JC, Falk RJ: Treatment response and relapse in antineutrophil cytoplasmic autoantibody-associated microscopic polyangiitis and glomerulonephritis. J Am Soc Nephrol 1996;7:33-39.

24. Levy JB, Pusey CD: Still a role for plasma exchange in rapidly progressive glomerulonephritis? J Nephrol 1997;10:7-13.
25. Madaio MP, Harrington JT: The diagnosis of glomerular diseases: Acute glomerulonephritis and the nephrotic syndrome. Arch Intern Med 2001;161:25-34.
26. Baldwin DS, Gluck MC, Lowenstein J, Gallo GR: Lupus nephritis: Clinical course as related to morphologic forms and their transitions. Am J Med 1977;62:12-30.
27. Hricik DE, Kassirer JP: The nephrotic syndrome. Dis Mon 1982;28:1-56.
28. Haas M, Meehan SM, Karrison TG, Spargo BH: Changing etiologies of unexplained adult nephrotic syndrome: A comparison of renal biopsy findings from 1976-1979 and 1995-1997. Am J Kidney Dis 1997;30:621-631.
29. Johnson RJ, Feehally J: Comprehensive Clinical Nephrology. St. Louis, Mosby, 2003, pp xvii, 1229.
30. Johnson RJ, Willson R, Yamabe H, et al: Renal manifestations of hepatitis C virus infection. Kidney Int 1994;46:1255-1263.
31. Schrier RW, Fassett RG: A critique of the overfill hypothesis of sodium and water retention in the nephrotic syndrome. Kidney Int 1998;53:1111-1117.
32. Orth SR, Ritz E: The nephrotic syndrome. N Engl J Med 1998;338:1202-1211.
33. Brater DC: Diuretic therapy. N Engl J Med 1998;339:387-395.
34. Bellomo R, Atkins RC: Membranous nephropathy and thromboembolism: Is prophylactic anticoagulation warranted? Nephron 1993;63:249-254.
35. DeBroe ME, Elseviers MM: Analgesic nephropathy. N Engl J Med 1998;338:446-452.
36. Scheinman SJ, Guay-Woodford LM, Thakker RV, et al: Genetic disorders of renal electrolyte transport. N Engl J Med 1999;340:1177-1187.
37. Gahl WA, Thoene JG, Schneider JA: Cystinosis. N Engl J Med 2002;347:111-121.
38. Rodriguez-Soriano J: New insights into the pathogenesis of renal tubular acidosis—from functional to molecular studies. Pediatr Nephrol 2000;14:1121-1136.
39. Fencl V, Leith DE: Stewart's quantitative acid-base chemistry: Applications in biology and medicine. Respir Physiol 1993;91:1-16.
40. Corey HE: Stewart and beyond: New models of acid-base balance. Kidney Int 2003;64:777-787.
41. Choate KA, Kahle KT, Wilson FH, et al: WNK1, a kinase mutated in inherited hypertension with hyperkalemia, localizes to diverse Cl^--transporting epithelia. Proc Natl Acad Sci U S A 2003;100:663-668.
42. Shaer AJ: Inherited primary renal tubular hypokalemic alkalosis: A review of Gitelman and Bartter syndromes. Am J Med Sci 2001;322:316-332.
43. Igarashi T, Inatomi J, Sekine T, et al: Mutations in SLC4A4 cause permanent isolated proximal renal tubular acidosis with ocular abnormalities. Nat Genet 1999;23:264-266.
44. Sabatini S, Kurtzman NA: Biochemical and genetic advances in distal renal tubular acidosis. Semin Nephrol 2001;21:94-106.
45. Wilson FH, Disse-Nicodeme S, Choate KA, et al: Human hypertension caused by mutations in WNK kinases. Science 2001;293:1107-1112.
46. Wilson PD: Polycystic kidney disease. N Engl J Med 2004;350:151-164.
47. Levey AS: Clinical practice: Nondiabetic kidney disease. N Engl J Med 2002;347:1505-1511.
48. Palmer BF: Renal dysfunction complicating the treatment of hypertension. N Engl J Med 2002;347:1256-1261.
49. Remuzzi G, Bertani T: Pathophysiology of progressive nephropathies. N Engl J Med 1998;339:1448-1456.
50. Riz E, Orth SR: Nephropathy in patients with type 2 diabetes mellitus. N Engl J Med 1999;341:1127-1133.
51. Rossing P, Hommel E, Smidt UM, Parving HH: Impact of arterial blood pressure and albuminuria on the progression of diabetic nephropathy in IDDM patients. Diabetes 1993;42:715-719.
52. Ravid M, Brosh D, Ravid-Safran D, et al: Main risk factors for nephropathy in type 2 diabetes mellitus are plasma cholesterol levels,

mean blood pressure, and hyperglycemia. Arch Intern Med 1998;158:998-1004.

53. Intensive blood-glucose control with sulphonylureas or insulin compared with conventional treatment and risk of complications in patients with type 2 diabetes (UKPDS 33). UK Prospective Diabetes Study (UKPDS) Group. Lancet 1998;352:837-853.

54. Nielsen FS, Rossing P, Gall MA, et al: Long-term effect of lisinopril and atenolol on kidney function in hypertensive NIDDM subjects with diabetic nephropathy. Diabetes 1997;46:1182-1188.

55. Peterson JC, Adler S, Burkart JM, et al: Blood pressure control, proteinuria, and the progression of renal disease. The Modification of Diet in Renal Disease Study. Ann Intern Med 1995;123:754-762.

56. Ruggenenti P, Perna A, Gherardi G, et al: Renoprotective properties of ACE-inhibition in non-diabetic nephropathies with non-nephrotic proteinuria. Lancet 1999;354:359-364.

57. Ruggenenti P, Fassi A, Ilieva AP, et al: Preventing microalbuminuria in type 2 diabetes. N Engl J Med 2004;351:1941-1951.

58. Brenner BM, Cooper ME, de Zeeuw D, et al: Effects of losartan on renal and cardiovascular outcomes in patients with type 2 diabetes and nephropathy. N Engl J Med 2001;345:861-869.

59. Firth PG, Head CA: Sickle cell disease and anesthesia. Anesthesiology 2004;101:766-785.

60. Harding MB, Smith LR, Himmelstein SI, et al: Renal artery stenosis: Prevalence and associated risk factors in patients undergoing routine cardiac catheterization. J Am Soc Nephrol 1992;2:1608-1616.

61. Safian RD, Textor SC: Renal-artery stenosis. N Engl J Med 2001;344:431-442.

62. Slovut DP, Olin JW: Fibromuscular dysplasia. N Engl J Med 2004;350:1862-1871.

63. Zeller T, Frank U, Muller C, et al: Predictors of improved renal function after percutaneous stent-supported angioplasty of severe atherosclerotic ostial renal artery stenosis. Circulation 2003;108:2244-2249.

64. Levey A: Clinical practice: Nondiabetic kidney disease. N Engl J Med 2002;347:1505-1511.

65. Centers for Disease Control and Prevention: State-specific trends in chronic kidney failure—United States, 1990-2001. MMWR Morbid Mortal Wkly Rep 2004;53:918-920.

66. Incidence and prevalence of ESRD. United States Renal Data System. Am J Kidney Dis 1998;32(2 Suppl 1):S38-S49.

67. Clase CM, Garg AX, Kibert BA: Classifying kidney problems: Can we avoid framing risks as diseases? BMJ 2004;329:912-915.

68. Kellerman PS: Perioperative care of the renal patient. Arch Intern Med 1994;154:1674-1688.

69. Parmar MS: Chronic renal disease. BMJ 2002;325:85-90.

70. Locatelli F, Marcelli D, Comelli M, et al: Proteinuria and blood pressure as causal components of progression to end-stage renal failure. Northern Italian Cooperative Study Group. Nephrol Dial Transplant 1996;11:461-467.

71. Remuzzi G, Bertani T: Pathophysiology of progressive nephropathies. N Engl J Med 1998;339:1448-1456.

72. Rossing P, Hommel E, Smidt UM, Parving HH: Impact of arterial blood pressure and albuminuria on the progression of diabetic nephropathy in IDDM patients. Diabetes 1993;42:715-719.

73. Johnson RJ, Feehally J: Comprehensive Clinical Nephrology. St. Louis, Mosby, 2003, pp xvii, 1229.

74. Foley RN, Parfrey PS, Sarnak MJ: Epidemiology of cardiovascular disease in chronic renal disease. J Am Soc Nephrol 1998;9 (12 Suppl):S16-S23.

75. Ifudu O: Care of patients undergoing hemodialysis. N Engl J Med 1998;339:1054-1062.

76. Gupta R, Birnbaum Y, et al: The renal patient with coronary artery disease: Current concepts and dilemmas. J Am Coll Cardiol 2004;44:1343-1353.

77. Steiner RW, Coggins C, Carvalho AC: Bleeding time in uremia: A useful test to assess clinical bleeding. Am J Hematol 1979;7:107-117.

78. De Lima JJ, Sabbaga E, Vieira ML, et al: Coronary angiography is the best predictor of events in renal transplant candidates compared with noninvasive testing. Hypertension 2003;42:263-268.

79. Lewis MS, Wilson RA, Walker KW, et al: Validation of an algorithm for predicting cardiac events in renal transplant candidates. Am J Cardiol 2002;89:847-850.

80. Tadros GM, Herzog CA: Percutaneous coronary intervention in chronic kidney disease patients. J Nephrol 2004;17:364-368.

81. Jaeger JQ, Mehta RL: Assessment of dry weight in hemodialysis: an overview. J Am Soc Nephrol 1999;10:392-403.

82. Journois D: Hemofiltration during cardiopulmonary bypass. Kidney Int 1998;Suppl 66:S174-S177.

83. van der Hoven B, van der Spoel JI, Scheffer GJ, et al: Intraoperative continuous hemofiltration for metabolic management in acute aortoiliac occlusion. J Clin Anesth 1998;10:599-602.

84. Blackwell MM, Chavin KD, Sistino JJ, et al: Perioperative perfusion strategies for optimal fluid management in liver transplant recipients with renal insufficiency. Perfusion 2003;18:55-60.

85. Gotti E, Mecca G, Valentino C, et al: Renal biopsy in patients with acute renal failure and prolonged bleeding time: A preliminary report. Am J Kidney Dis 1985;6:397-399.

86. Bellomo R, Kellum J, Ronco C: Acute renal failure: Time for consensus. Intensive Care Med 2001;27:1685-1688.

87. Holt SG, Moore KP: Pathogenesis and treatment of renal dysfunction in rhabdomyolysis. Intensive Care Med 2001;27:803-811.

88. Allison RC, Bedsole DL: The other medical causes of rhabdomyolysis. Am J Med Sci 2003;326:79-88.

89. Balogh Z, McKinley BA, Cox CS Jr, et al: Abdominal compartment syndrome: The cause or effect of postinjury multiple organ failure. Shock 2003;20:483-492.

90. Balogh Z, McKinley BA, Cocanour CS, et al: Patients with impending abdominal compartment syndrome do not respond to early volume loading. Am J Surg 2003;186:602-607.

91. Shafi S, Kauder DR: Fluid resuscitation and blood replacement in patients with polytrauma. Clin Orthop 2004;37-42.

92. Godet G, Fleron MH, Vicaut E, et al: Risk factors for acute postoperative renal failure in thoracic or thoracoabdominal aortic surgery: A prospective study. Anesth Analg 1997;85:1227-1232.

93. Levy EM, Viscoli CM, Horwitz RI: The effect of acute renal failure on mortality: A cohort analysis. JAMA 1996;275:1489-1494.

94. Chertow GM, Christiansen CL, Cleary PD, et al: Prognostic stratification in critically ill patients with acute renal failure requiring dialysis. Arch Intern Med 1995;155:1505-1511.

95. Chertow GM, Levy EM, Hammermeister KE, et al: Independent association between acute renal failure and mortality following cardiac surgery. Am J Med 1998;104:343-348.

96. Huynh TT, Miller CC 3rd, Estrera AL, et al: Determinants of hospital length of stay after thoracoabdominal aortic aneurysm repair. J Vasc Surg 2002;35:648-653.

97. Lameire N, Vanholder R: Pathophysiologic features and prevention of human and experimental acute tubular necrosis. J Am Soc Nephrol 2001;12(Suppl 17):S20-S32.

98. Brezis M, Rosen S: Hypoxia of the renal medulla—its implications for disease. N Engl J Med 1995;332:647-655.

99. Novis BK, Roizen MF, Aronson S, Thisted RA: Association of preoperative risk factors with postoperative acute renal failure. Anesth Analg 1994;78:143-149.

100. Wahbah AM, el-Hefny MO, Wafa EM, et al: Perioperative renal protection in patients with obstructive jaundice using drug combinations. Hepatogastroenterology 2000;47:1691-1694.

101. Chew ST, Newman MF, White WD, et al: Preliminary report on the association of apolipoprotein E polymorphisms, with postoperative peak serum creatinine concentrations in cardiac surgical patients. Anesthesiology 2000;93:325-331.

102. Rectenwald JE, Huber TS, Martin TD, et al: Functional outcome after thoracoabdominal aortic aneurysm repair. J Vasc Surg 2002;35:640-647.

103. Wahlberg E, Dimuzio PJ, Stoney RJ, et al: Aortic clamping during elective operations for infrarenal disease: The influence of clamping time on renal function. J Vasc Surg 2002;36:13-18.

104. Prinssen M, Verhoeven EL, Buth J, et al: A randomized trial comparing conventional and endovascular repair of abdominal aortic aneurysms. N Engl J Med 2004;351:1607-1618.

105. Bove T, Calabro MG, Landoni G, et al: The incidence and risk of acute renal failure after cardiac surgery. J Cardiothorac Vasc Anesth 2004;18:442-445.

106. Chertow GM, Lazarus JM, Lew NL, et al: Preoperative renal risk stratification. Circulation 1997;95:878-884.

107. Fortescue EB, Bates DW, Chertow GM: Predicting acute renal failure after coronary bypass surgery: Cross-validation of two risk-stratification algorithms. Kidney Int 2000;57:2594-2602.

108. Bucerius J, Gummert JF, Walther T, et al: On-pump versus off-pump coronary artery bypass grafting: Impact on postoperative renal failure requiring renal replacement therapy. Ann Thorac Surg 2004;77:1250-1256.

109. Stallwood MI, Grayson AD, Mills K, Scawn ND: Acute renal failure in coronary artery bypass surgery: Independent effect of cardiopulmonary bypass. Ann Thorac Surg 2004;77:968-972.

110. Gamoso MG, Phillips-Bute B, Landolfo KP, et al: Off-pump versus on-pump coronary artery bypass surgery and postoperative renal dysfunction. Anesth Analg 2000;91:1080-1084.

111. Schwann NM, Horrow JC, Strong MD 3rd, et al: Does off-pump coronary artery bypass reduce the incidence of clinically evident renal dysfunction after multivessel myocardial revascularization? Anesth Analg 2004;99:959-964.

112. Nathoe HM, van Dijk D, Jansen EW, et al: A comparison of on-pump and off-pump coronary bypass surgery in low-risk patients. N Engl J Med 2003;348:394-402.

113. Ronco C, Bellomo R, Homel P, et al: Effects of different doses in continuous veno-venous haemofiltration on outcomes of acute renal failure: A prospective randomised trial. Lancet 2000;356:26-30.

114. Cole L, Bellomo R, Journois D, et al: High-volume haemofiltration in human septic shock. Intensive Care Med 2001;27:978-986.

115. Wolfe RA, Ashby VB, Milford EL, et al: Comparison of mortality in all patients on dialysis, patients on dialysis awaiting transplantation, and recipients of a first cadaveric transplant. N Engl J Med 1999;341:1725-1730.

116. Rabbat CG, Thorpe KE, Russell JD, Churchill DN: Comparison of mortality risk for dialysis patients and cadaveric first renal transplant recipients in Ontario, Canada. J Am Soc Nephrol 2000;11:917-922.

117. Ojo AO, Hanson JA, Meier-Kriesche H, et al: Survival in recipients of marginal cadaveric donor kidneys compared with other recipients and wait-listed transplant candidates. J Am Soc Nephrol 2001;12:589-597.

118. Meier-Kriesche HU, Port FK, Ojo AO, et al: Effect of waiting time on renal transplant outcome. Kidney Int 2000;58:1311-1317.

119. Danovitch GM, Cecka JM: Allocation of deceased donor kidneys: Past, present, and future. Am J Kidney Dis 2003;42:882-890.

120. Ferreira SR, Moises VA, Tavares A, Pacheco-Silva A: Cardiovascular effects of successful renal transplantation: A 1-year sequential study of left ventricular morphology and function and 24-hour blood pressure profile. Transplantation 2002;74:1580-1587.

121. Nampoory MR, Das KC, Johny KV, et al: Hypercoagulability, a serious problem in patients with ESRD on maintenance hemodialysis, and its correction after kidney transplantation. Am J Kidney Dis 2003;42:797-805.

122. United Network for Organ Sharing National kidney data. Available at: http://www.unos.org.

123. Hariharan S, Johnson CP, Bresnahan BA, et al: Improved graft survival after renal transplantation in the United States 1988-1996. N Engl J Med 2001;342:605-611.

124. Gonwa T, Johnson C, Ahsan N: Randomized trial of tacrolimus + mycophenolate mofetil or azathioprine versus cyclosporine + mycophenolate mofetil after cadaveric kidney transplantation: Results at three years. Transplantation 2003;75:2048-2053.

125. Johnson RWG: Sirolimus (Rapamune) in renal transplantation. Curr Opin Nephrol Hypertens 2002;11:603-607.

126. Goggins WC, Pascual MA, Powelson JA: A prospective, randomized clinical trial of intraoperative versus postoperative thymoglobulin in adult cadaveric renal transplant recipients [abstract]. Transplantation 2003;76:798-802.

127. Szczech LA, Feldman HI: Effect of anti-lymphocyte antibody induction therapy on renal allograft survival. Transplant Proc 1999;31:9S-11S.

128. Luciani J, Frantz P, Thibault P, et al: Early anuria prevention in human kidney transplantation: Advantage of fluid load under pulmonary arterial pressure monitoring during surgical period. Transplantation 1979;28:308-312.

129. Carlier M, Squifflet JP, Pirson Y, et al: Maximal hydration during anesthesia increases pulmonary arterial pressures and improves early function of human renal transplants. Transplantation 1982;34:201-204.

130. Thomsen HS, Lokkegaard H, Munck O: Influence of normal central venous pressure on onset of function in renal allografts. Scand J Urol Nephrol 1987;21:143-145.

131. Dawidson IJ, Sandor ZF, Coorpender L, et al: Intraoperative albumin administration affects the outcome of cadaver renal transplantation. Transplantation 1992;53:774-782.

132. Dawidson IJ, Ar'Rajab A: Perioperative fluid and drug therapy during cadaver kidney transplantation. Clin Transpl 1992;267-284.

133. Tiggeler RG, Berden JH, Hoitsma AJ, Koene RA: Prevention of acute tubular necrosis in cadaveric kidney transplantation by the combined use of mannitol and moderate hydration. Ann Surg 1985;201:246-251.

134. Van Valenberg PL, Hoitsma AJ, Tiggeler RG, et al: Mannitol as an indispensable constituent of an intraoperative hydration protocol for the prevention of acute renal failure after renal cadaveric transplantation. Transplantation 1987;44:784-788.

135. Boldt J, Priebe HJ: Intravascular volume replacement therapy with synthetic colloids: Is there an influence on renal function? Anesth Analg 2003;96:376-382.

136. Jubelirer SJ: Hemostatic abnormalities in renal disease. Am J Kidney Dis 1985;5:219-225.

137. Chen KS, Huang CC, Leu ML, et al: Hemostatic and fibrinolytic response to desmopressin in uremic patients. Blood Purif 1997;15:84-91.

138. Davenport R: Cryoprecipitate for uremic bleeding. Clin Pharm 1991;10:429.

139. Gennari FJ, Segal AS: Hyperkalemia: An adaptive response in chronic renal insufficiency. Kidney Int 2002;62:1-9.

140. Michard F, Boussat S, Chemla D, et al: Relation between respiratory changes in arterial pulse pressure and fluid responsiveness in septic patients with acute circulatory failure. Am J Respir Crit Care Med 2000;162:134-138.

141. Sandham JD, Hull RD, Brant RF, et al: A randomized, controlled trial of the use of pulmonary-artery catheters in high-risk surgical patients. N Engl J Med 2003;348:5-14.

142. Schortgen, F, Lacherade JC, Bruneel F, et al: Effects of hydroxyethyl starch and gelatin on renal function in severe sepsis: A multicentre randomised study. Lancet 2001;357:911-916.

143. Dehne MG, Muhling J, Sablotzki A, et al: Hydroxyethyl starch (HES) does not directly affect renal function in patients with no prior renal impairment. J Clin Anesth 2001;13:103-111.

144. Boldt J: New light on intravascular volume replacement regimens: What did we learn from the past three years? Anesth Analg 2003;97:1595-1604.

145. Ragaller MJ, Theilen H, Koch T: Volume replacement in critically ill patients with acute renal failure. J Am Soc Nephrol 2001;12(Suppl 17):S33-S39.

146. Ickx B, Cockshott ID, Barvais L, et al: Propofol infusion for induction and maintenance of anesthesia in patients with end-stage renal disease. Br J Anesth 1998;81:854-860.

147. Goyal P, Puri GD, Panday CK, Srivastva S: Evaluation of induction doses of propofol: Comparison between endstage renal disease and normal renal function patients. Anesth Intensive Care 2002;30:584-587.

148. Coriat P, Richer C, Douraki T, et al: Influence of chronic angiotensin-converting enzyme inhibition on anesthetic induction. Anesthesiology 1994;81:299-307.

149. Pedraz JL, Lanao JM, Dominguez-Gil A: Kinetics of ketamine and its metabolites in rabbits with normal and impaired renal function. Eur J Drug Metab Pharmacokinet 1985;10:33-39.
150. Thapa S, Brull SJ: Succinylcholine-induced hyperkalemia in patients with renal failure: An old question revisited. Anesth Analg 2000;91:237-241.
151. Schow AJ, Lubarsky DA, Olson RP, Gan TJ: Can succinylcholine be used safely in hyperkalemic patients? Anesth Analg 2002;95:119-122.
152. Proost JH, Eriksson LI, Mirakhur RK, et al: Urinary, biliary and faecal excretion of rocuronium in humans. Br J Anaesth 2000;85:717-723.
153. Cooper RA, Mirakhur RK, Wierda JM, Maddineni VR: Pharmacokinetics of rocuronium bromide in patients with and without renal failure. Eur J Anesthesiol 1995;11:43-44.
154. Murray MJ, Coursin DB, Scuderi PE, et al: Double-blind, randomized, multicenter study of doxacurium vs. pancuronium in intensive care unit patients who require neuromuscular-blocking agents. Crit Care Med 1995;23:450-458.
155. Sakamoto H, Takita K, Kemmotsu O, et al: Increased sensitivity to vecuronium and prolonged duration of its action in patients with end-stage renal failure. J Clin Anesth 2001;13:193-197.
156. Fisher DM, Reynolds KS, Schmith VD, et al: The influence of renal function on the pharmacokinetics and pharmacodynamics and simulated time course of doxacurium. Anesth Analg 1997;89:786-795.
157. Kisor DF, Schmith VD, Wrgin WA, et al: Importance of the organ-independent elimination of cisatracurium. Anesth Analg 1996;83:1065-1071.
158. Lien CA, Schmith VD, Belmont MR, et al: Pharmacokinetics of cisatracurium in patients receiving nitrous oxide/opioid/barbiturate anesthesia. Anesthesiology 1996;84:300-308.
159. Bevan DR, Archer D, Donati F, et al: Antagonism of pancuronium in renal failure: No recurarization. Br J Anaesth 1982;54(1): 63-8.
160. Dhonneur G, Rebaine C, Slavov V, et al: Neostigmine reversal of vecuronium neuromuscular block and the influence of renal failure. Anesth Analg 1996;82:134-138.
161. D'Honneur G, Gilton A, Sandouk P, et al: Plasma and cerebrospinal fluid concentrations of morphine and morphine glucuronides after oral morphine: The influence of renal failure. Anesthesiology 1994;81:87-93.
162. Lotsch J, Zimmermann M, Darimont J, et al: Does the A118G polymorphism at the mu-opioid receptor gene protect against morphine-6-glucuronide toxicity? Anesthesiology 2002;97:814-819.
163. Angst MS, Buhrer M, Lotsch J: Insidious intoxication after morphine treatment in renal failure: Delayed onset of morphine-6-glucuronide action. Anesthesiology 2002;92:1473-1476.
164. Al-Khafaji AH, Dewhirst WE, Manning HL, et al: Propylene glycol toxicity associated with lorazepam infusion in a patient receiving continuous veno-venous hemofiltration with dialysis. Anesth Analg 2002;94:1583-1585, table of contents.
165. Dahaba AA., von Klobucar F, Rehak PH, List WF: Total intravenous anesthesia with remifentanil, propofol and cisatracurium in end-stage renal failure. Can J Anaesth 1999;46:696-700.
166. Basta M, Sloan P: Epidural hematoma following epidural catheter placement in a patient with chronic renal failure. Can J Anaesth 1999;46:271-274.
167. Mazze RI, Shue GL, Jackson SH: Renal dysfunction associated with methoxyflurane anesthesia: A randomized, prospective clinical evaluation. JAMA 1971;216:278-288.
168. Barr GA, Cousins MJ, Mazze RI, et al: A comparison of the renal effects and metabolism of enflurane and methoxyflurane in Fischer 344 rats. J Pharmacol Exp Ther 1974;188:257-264.
169. Mazze RI, Trudell JR, Cousins MJ: Methoxyflurane metabolism and renal dysfunction: Clinical correlation in man. Anesthesiology 1971;35:247-252.
170. Litz RJ, Hubler M, Lorenz W, et al: Renal responses to desflurane and isoflurane in patients with renal insufficiency. Anesthesiology 2002;97:1133-1136.
171. Spencer EM, Willatts SM, Prys-Roberts C: Plasma inorganic fluoride concentrations during and after prolonged (>24 hr) isoflurane sedation: Effect on renal function. Anesth Analg 1991;73:731-737.
172. Kong KL, Tyler JE, Willatts SM, Prys-Roberts C: Isoflurane sedation for patients undergoing mechanical ventilation: Metabolism to inorganic fluoride and renal effects. Br J Anaesth 1990;64:159-162.
173. Taves DR, Fry BW, Freeman RB, Gillies AJ: Toxicity following methoxyflurane anesthesia: II. Fluoride concentrations in nephrotoxicity. JAMA 1970;214:91-95.
174. Cittanova, ML, Lelongt B, Verpont MC, et al: Fluoride ion toxicity in human kidney collecting duct cells. Anesthesiology 1996;84:428-435.
175. Cousins MJ, Mazze RI: Methoxyflurane nephrotoxicity: A study of dose response in man. JAMA 1973;225:1611-1616.
176. Kobayashi Y, Ochiai R, Takeda J, et al: Serum and urinary inorganic fluoride concentrations after prolonged inhalation of sevoflurane in humans. Anesth Analg 1992;74:753-757.
177. Frink EJ Jr, Ghantous H, Malan TP, et al: Plasma inorganic fluoride with sevoflurane anesthesia: Correlation with indices of hepatic and renal function. Anesth Analg 1992;74:231-235.
178. Eger EI 2nd, Gong D, Koblin DD, et al: Dose-related biochemical markers of renal injury after sevoflurane versus desflurane anesthesia in volunteers. Anesth Analg 1997;85:1154-1163.
179. Frink EJ Jr, Ghantous H, Malan TP, et al: Plasma inorganic fluoride with sevoflurane anesthesia: Correlation with indices of hepatic and renal function. Anesth Analg 1992;74:231-235.
180. Smith I, Ding Y, White PF: Comparison of induction, maintenance, and recovery characteristics of sevoflurane N₂O and propofol-sevoflurane-N₂O with propofol-isoflurane-N₂O anesthesia. Anesth Analg 1992;74:253-259.
181. Hara T, Fukusaki M, Nakamura T, Sumikawa K: Renal function in patients during and after hypotensive anesthesia with sevoflurane. J Clin Anesth 1998;10:539-545.
182. Kharasch ED, Hankins DC, Thummel KE: Human kidney methoxyflurane and sevoflurane metabolism: Intrarenal fluoride production as a possible mechanism of methoxyflurane nephrotoxicity. Anesthesiology 1995;82:689-699.
183. Gonsowski CT, Laster MJ, Eger EI 2nd, et al: Toxicity of compound A in rats: Effect of increasing duration of administration. Anesthesiology 1994;80:566-573.
184. Mazze RI, Callan CM, Galvez ST, et al: The effects of sevoflurane on serum creatinine and blood urea nitrogen concentrations: A retrospective, twenty-two-center, comparative evaluation of renal function in adult surgical patients. Anesth Analg 2000;90:683-688.
185. Conzen PF, Nuscheler M, Melotte A, et al: Renal function and serum fluoride concentrations in patients with stable renal insufficiency after anesthesia with sevoflurane or enflurane. Anesth Analg 1995;81:569-575.
186. Prins JM, Buller HR, Kuijper EJ, et al: Once versus thrice daily gentamicin in patients with serious infections. Lancet 1993;341:335-339.
187. Walsh TJ, Finberg RW, Amdt C, et al: Liposomal amphotericin B for empirical therapy in patients with persistent fever and neutropenia. National Institute of Allergy and Infectious Diseases Mycoses Study Group. N Engl J Med 1999;340:764-771.
188. Walsh TJ, Pappas P, Winston DJ, et al: Voriconazole compared with liposomal amphotericin B for empirical antifungal therapy in patients with neutropenia and persistent fever. N Engl J Med 2002;346:225-234.
189. Mehran R, Aymong ED, Nikolsky E, et al: A simple risk score for prediction of contrast-induced nephropathy after percutaneous coronary intervention: Development and initial validation. J Am Coll Cardiol 2004;44:1393-1399.
190. Solomon R, Werner C, Mann D, et al: Effects of saline, mannitol, and furosemide to prevent acute decreases in renal function induced by radiocontrast agents. N Engl J Med 1994;331:1416-1420.
191. Tepel M, van der Giet M, Schwarzfeld C, et al: Prevention of radiographic-contrast-agent-induced reductions in renal function by acetylcysteine. N Engl J Med 2000;343:180-184.
192. Durham JD, Caputo C, Dokko J, et al: A randomized controlled trial of N-acetylcysteine to prevent contrast nephropathy in cardiac angiography. Kidney Int 2002;62:2202-2207.

193. Merten GJ, Burgess WP, Gray LV, et al: Prevention of contrast-induced nephropathy with sodium bicarbonate: A randomized controlled trial. JAMA 2004;291:2328-2334.

194. Marenzi G, Marana I, Lauri G, et al: The prevention of radiocontrast-agent-induced nephropathy by hemofiltration. N Engl J Med 2003;349:1333-1340.

195. DeBroe ME, Elseviers MM: Analgesic nephropathy. N Engl J Med 1998;338:446-452.

196. Ronco PM: Drug-induced end-stage renal disease. N Engl J Med 1994;331:1711-1712.

197. Sivarajan M, Wasse L: Perioperative acute renal failure associated with preoperative intake of ibuprofen. Anesthesiology 1997;86:1390-1392.

198. Jaquenod M, Ronnhedh C, Cousins MJ, et al: Factors influencing ketorolac-associated perioperative renal dysfunction. Anesth Analg 1998;86:1090-1097.

199. Laisalmi M, Teppo AM, Kovusalo AM, et al: The effect of ketorolac and sevoflurane anesthesia on renal glomerular and tubular function. Anesth Analg 2001;93:1210-1213.

200. Fredman B, Zohar E, Golan E, et al: Diclofenac does not decrease renal blood flow or glomerular filtration in elderly patients undergoing orthopedic surgery. Anesth Analg 1999;88:149-154.

201. McCrory CR, Lindahl SGE: Cyclooxygenase inhibition for perioperative analgesia. Anesth Analg 2002;95:169-176.

202. Licker M, Bednarkiewicz M, Neidhart P, et al: Preoperative inhibition of angiotensin-converting enzyme improves systemic and renal haemodynamic changes during aortic abdominal surgery. Br J Anaesth 1996;76:632-639.

203. Coriat P, Richer C, Douraki T, et al: Influence of chronic angiotensin-converting enzyme inhibition on anesthetic induction. Anesthesiology 1994;81:299-307.

204. Bertrand M, Godet G, Meersschaert K, et al: Should the angiotensin II antagonists be discontinued before surgery? Anesth Analg 2001;92:26-30.

205. Ryckwaert F, Colson P, Andre E, et al: Haemodynamic effects of an angiotensin-converting enzyme inhibitor and angiotensin receptor antagonist during hypovolaemia in the anaesthetized pig. Br J Anaesth 2002;89:599-604.

206. Cittanova ML, Zubicki A, Savu C, et al: The chronic inhibition of angiotensin-converting enzyme impairs postoperative renal function. Anesth Analg 2001;93:1111-1115.

207. Bello-Reuss E, Higashi Y, Kaneda Y: Dopamine decreases fluid reabsorption in straight portions of rabbit proximal tubule. Am J Physiol 1982;242:F634-F640.

208. Lassnigg A, Donner E, Grubhofer G, et al: Lack of renoprotective effects of dopamine and furosemide during cardiac surgery. J Am Soc Nephrol 2000;11:97-104.

209. Bellomo R, Chapman M, Finfer S, et al: Low-dose dopamine in patients with early renal dysfunction: A placebo-controlled randomised trial. Australian and New Zealand Intensive Care Society (ANZICS) Clinical Trials Group. Lancet 2000;356:2139-2143.

210. Conger JD: Interventions in clinical acute renal failure: What are the data? Am J Kidney Dis 1995;26:565-576.

211. Mehta RL, Pascual MT, Soroko S, et al: Diuretics, mortality, and nonrecovery of renal function in acute renal failure. JAMA 2002;288:2547-2553.

212. Uchino S, Doig GS, Bellomo R, et al: Diuretics and mortality in acute renal failure. Crit Care Med 2004;32:1669-1677.

213. Piper SN, Kumle B, Maleck WH, et al: Diltiazem may preserve renal tubular integrity after cardiac surgery Can J Anesth 2003;50:285-292.

214. Carpenter JP, Fairman RM, Barker CF, et al: Endovascular AAA repair in patients with renal insufficiency: Strategies for reducing adverse renal events. Cardiovasc Surg 2001;9:559-564.

8 Neurologic Diseases

DIMITRY BARANOV, MD, TOM KELTON, MD, HEATHER McCLUNG, MD,
KEITH SCARFO, DO, and JAMES G. HECKER, PhD, MD

Over the past decade there have been advances in the diagnosis and treatment of neurologic diseases, in part from information gleaned from genetics.

BASAL GANGLIA AND CEREBELLAR DISORDERS

Disorders of the basal ganglia and cerebellum are linked by motor signs and symptoms and by location of pathology in the extrapyramidal motor system. The extrapyramidal system consists of the basal ganglia, striatum (caudate, putamen), globus pallidus, subthalamic nucleus, and substantia nigra (Fig. 8-1).[1] Motor functions are coordinated through the nuclei of the basal ganglia and cerebellum via the cortical/brain stem/spinal system.[2] Damage to elements of this system, or to the extrapyramidal tracts,

can lead to movement disorders, commonly negative symptoms or signs (e.g., akinesia, bradykinesia, loss of reflexes) or positive symptoms or signs (e.g., chorea, athetosis, ballismus, dystonia), and contraction abnormalities.[2]

Extrapyramidal disorders can be divided into loss of function due to deficits and symptoms due to loss of inhibitory inputs. Impairments in patient-initiated movements are described as *hypokinesia, bradykinesia,* or *akinesia,* depending on rapidity of voluntary movements. *Muscle tone* is defined as resistance to passive movement. *Rigidity* refers to a constant resistance to passive movement, whereas *cogwheel rigidity* (Parkinson's disease) is jerky resistance. *Chorea* refers to involuntary, rapid, widespread, jerky, arrhythmic movements that are slower than myoclonic jerks. *Ataxia* is cerebellar incoordination of voluntary movements. Ataxia is usually thought of as purely loss of

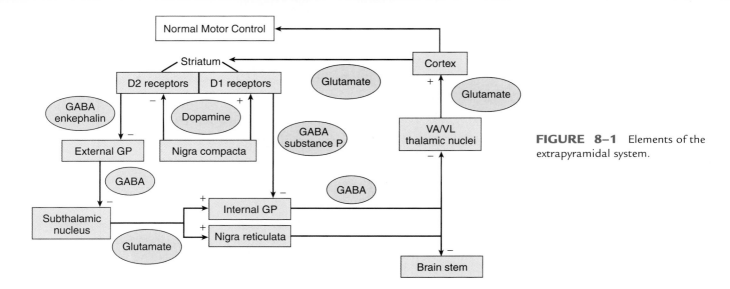

FIGURE 8–1 Elements of the extrapyramidal system.

motor coordination, but it may result from profound sensory loss as well. *Athetosis,* an inability to maintain any part of the body in a voluntary muscle position, is slower than chorea and is most often found in the hands. *Dystonia* is a persistent increase of muscle tone, most often involving the trunk rather than extremity muscle groups, which results in a fixed or shifting abnormal postures. Focal dystonias include spastic torticollis. *Hemiballismus* is used to describe violent, unilateral, proximal limb movements on one side only. *Double athetosis* is a combination of athetosis and chorea in all four limbs.

Damage to extrapyramidal tracts can occur as a result of central nervous system (CNS) trauma, chronic neurodegenerative disease, stroke, ischemic CNS disease, drug therapy, or hypoxic encephalopathies. The neurotransmitters most involved in basal ganglia function include acetylcholine, inhibitory γ-aminobutyric acid (GABA) projection neurons, and glutamate, as well as the neuromodulators substance P, enkephalins, somatostatins, and neuropeptide Y. Catecholamines probably also act as neuromodulators with modest effects, with the exception of dopamine in the substantia nigra and striatum, where it plays a critical role in Parkinson's disease. The motor strip in the cerebral cortex receives both inhibitory and excitatory modulation from the basal ganglia, with feed-forward and feed-back connections to the basal ganglia/thalamus/corticospinal system. Table 8-1 compares several of the more common bradykinesias and hyperkinetic movement disorders and contrasts them to other neurologic diseases that can also manifest as movement disorders. The most common of the movement disorders is Parkinson's disease (PD).

Parkinson's Disease (Paralysis Agitans)

Pathology and Diagnosis. Parkinson's disease is characterized by the loss of pigmented cells in the substantia nigra and pigmented nuclei, as well as by a neurotransmitter imbalance caused by a relative dopamine deficiency in the caudate nucleus and putamen. An as yet unidentified environmental agent has been postulated as causative for PD.[2] Experimentally, a Parkinson's model can be created by ablation (surgical or 1-methyl-4-phenyl-1,2,3,6-tetra-hydropyridine [MPTP]) of pigmented cells of the substantia nigra. MPTP is degraded by monoamine oxidase B (MAO-B), causing a toxic metabolite and destruction of the substantia nigra. The remaining pigmented cells in the substantia nigra contain eosinophilic inclusions called Lewy bodies, which are also seen in all cases of idiopathic PD. These inclusions are characteristic of numerous neurodegenerative diseases. The inhibitory effects of dopamine in the basal ganglia are normally opposed by the excitatory modulation by acetylcholine. The etiology can also be due to manganese poisoning, encephalitis, CNS trauma (pugilistica), carbon monoxide exposure, or chronic reserpine, phenothiazine, or butyrophenone use. In the United States the incidence is approximately 1% in those older than age 65 years. The incidence is highest in the 40- to 70-year age group, with peak onset in the sixth decade. Diagnosis is made on the basis of the characteristic stooped posture, axial instability, shuffling, unsteady gait, expressionless face (hypokinetic dysarthria), rigidity, paucity of movement (bradykinesia), and pill-rolling tremor. Up to one third of PD patients develop dementia as well. Tremors are dampened with intentional movement or with complete relaxation.

Treatment of PD is based on achieving a balance between cholinergic and striatal dopaminergic activity. Levodopa (L-dopa) crosses the blood-brain barrier and is the mainstay of treatment. It is converted in the CNS by dopa-decarboxylase to dopamine, which does not appreciably cross the blood-brain barrier. L-Dopa is co-administered with carbidopa or benserazide decarboxylase inhibitors to minimize the systemic dopamine effects. Other therapies used for treatment of PD include

TABLE 8-1   Comparison of Movement Dysfunction Disorders

Disease	Chorea/Dystonia/Dyskinesia	Dementia/Mental Retardation	Ataxia (Volitional Coordination)	Muscle Weakness/Atrophy	Sensory Loss	Hereditary?
Huntington's disease	Chorea	Memory, affect	Yes	Yes	No	Yes
Parkinson's disease	Dystonia/Dyskinesia	Affect	Yes	Disuse atrophy	Yes	Some
Guillain-Barré syndrome	None	No	Possible	Yes	Yes	Risk factors
Rheumatic chorea	Chorea	Emotional lability	Possible	Hypotonia	No	No
Amyotrophic lateral sclerosis (ALS), spinal motor atrophy (SMA)	Spasticity Limb and bulbar weakness	No	No	Yes	ALS rare SMA no	Some
Alzheimer's disease	Rare	Dementia	No	No	No	No
Friedreich's ataxia	Spasticity occasionally chorea	No	Yes	Yes	Yes	Yes
Torsion dystonia	Dystonia	No	Yes	No	No	Yes
Spastic torticollis	Dystonia	No	Yes	No	No	Yes
Diffuse Lewy body disease	Possible	Possible	Some	Rare	Rare	No
Multiple system atrophy (old: olivopontocerebellar atrophy)	Dysturia possible	Some variants	Yes	Yes	Rare	Some
Other rare diseases causing these signs/symptoms	Drug-induced chorea (phenothiazines, haloperidol, phenytoin); lupus; thyrotoxicosis; polycythemia vera; stroke; tumor; vascular; striatonigral degeneration with autonomic dysfunction (Shy-Drager); Wilson's; Hallervorden-Spatz; progressive supranuclear palsy (Steele-Richardson-Olzenski)	Diffuse cortical atrophy; Lewy body inclusions; pick (lobar sclerosis); thalamic degeneration; cortical-basal ganglionic degeneration; cerebrocerebellar degeneration (Greenfield)	Non-Friedreich's ataxia; paraneoplasm; alcohol or nutritional; Holmes familial cortical cerebellar atrophy; Marie-Foix-Alajouanine; Gerstmann-Straüssler-Scheinken; Machedo-Joseph; autosomal dominant late onset	Bulbar palsy; primary lateral sclerosis; hereditary progressive atrophy and spastic paraplegia	Hereditary sensory neuropathies; hereditary sensory-motor neuropathies (Charcot-Marie-Tooth); hypertrophic interstitial polyneuropathy (Dejerine-Sottas disease)	

Adapted from Adams RD, Victor M, Ropper AH (eds): Principles of Neurology. New York, McGraw-Hill, 1997, pp 1048, 1081.

selegiline and rasagiline (second generation), MAO-B inhibitors are used to block the degradation of dopamine, which often delays the need for L-dopa. Dopamine agonists (i.e., bromocriptine, ropinirole, pergolide, apomorphine, and pramipexole) or catechol-*o*-methyl transferase (COMT) inhibitors (i.e., tolcapone, entacapone) are used early in the disease or in combination with L-dopa to minimize the dose of L-dopa.

Common side effects of chronic dopamine delivery include nausea and vomiting, myocardial irritability, decreased intravascular volume, and orthostatic hypotension due to suppression of the renin-angiotensin axis, confusion, psychiatric symptoms and depression, and the classic "on-off" phenomenon seen with rapid shifts from mobility to immobility and involuntary movements. Dyskinesias are the limiting factor in therapy and are treated by decreasing the dose of L-dopa and adding the anticholinergics trihexyphenidyl (Artane) and benztropine mesylate (Cogentin) or by using the dopaminergics bromocriptine, lisuride, or pergolide or the antiviral amantadine, which releases presynaptic dopamine. Clozapine is sometimes effective for treatment of drug-induced psychosis. Stereotactic lesions in the globus pallidus have been tried to alleviate the tremors and rigidity. Adrenal medullary grafts and, more recently, stem cell transplants have shown progress in animal models of PD.

Preoperative Assessment and Perioperative Considerations. Preoperative assessment should focus on the effectiveness of treatment. Hypotension due to relative hypovolemia, autonomic dysfunction, and depleted norepinephrine stores is possible. Treatment of hypotension should be with volume as needed and with direct-acting agents such as phenylephrine, rather than ephedrine.

Therapeutic drugs should be continued through the morning of surgery. Medications that could cause extrapyramidal symptoms (e.g., phenothiazines, butyrophenones [Droperidol]), and metoclopramide (Reglan) should be held. One should be aware of the potential for increased catecholamine-induced tachyarrhythmias with L-dopa and Halothane (rarely used in the United States anymore). Ketamine has the potential for a hypertensive response but has been used without incident, and opioids such as fentanyl have a potential for an exacerbation of muscle rigidity. Morphine was reported to decrease dyskinesia in low doses but to increase dyskinesias at high doses.[3] Use of inhaled anesthetics has been associated with an increase in rigidity postoperatively. Propofol blocks the tremors of PD in the immediate postoperative period.[4] Although there is no contradiction to regional anesthesia, there was one report of increased potassium after succinylcholine use that was most likely related to denervation.[5] Most reports indicate that the use of succinylcholine or nondepolarizing neuromuscular blockers is acceptable.[6,7] Diphenhydramine (Benadryl), a centrally acting

anticholinergic, can be used for control of tremor in the awake patient.

The patient's routine doses should be resumed as soon as possible in the postoperative period. There is an increased incidence of laryngospasm and respiratory failure and obstructive ventilation in the postoperative period.[1]

Sydenham's Chorea (Rheumatic Chorea)

Pathology and Diagnosis. Rheumatic chorea is a movement disorder often seen in female children with a prior exposure to β-hemolytic streptococci. It persists despite improvements in medical care, even in the developed world. Females are affected more than males, and children have a higher incidence than adults.[8,9] There also appears to be a familial predisposition to the disease.[10] The choreatic movements occur more often in the upper extremities and tend to cease during sleep. The pathology of chorea is uncertain, with degeneration in the cortex, basal ganglia, substantia nigra, and cerebellum, and sometimes including arteritis.

Symptoms include emotional lability, irritability, and occasional severe mental retardation. Diagnosis is based on observation of the characteristic choreiform movements in a child. The differential diagnosis includes any of the other basal ganglia diseases that have choreiform signs (e.g., Huntington's disease, neuroleptics, phenytoin, oral contraceptives, lupus, thyrotoxicosis, polycythemia vera, hyperosmolar nonketotic hyperglycemia, and chorea gravidarum).

Perioperative Considerations. Diagnostic workup includes electrocardiographic (ECG) and cardiac evaluation, as well as antibiotic prophylaxis for β-streptococcal rheumatic heart disease. Although rarely fatal, ECG abnormalities and endocarditis are seen at increased frequency in asymptomatic siblings. Treatment is symptomatic, and the mainstays have been corticosteroids, barbiturates, and phenothiazines; levodopa is used for the Parkinson-like features. Because of an extremely limited anesthetic experience, there are few anesthetic contraindications other than potential interactions with the drugs used for symptomatic therapy. As in the treatment of PD, propofol will likely decrease choreiform movements in the postoperative period.

Huntington's Chorea

Pathology and Diagnosis. Huntington's disease (Huntington's chorea) is a monohybrid autosomal dominant disease (chromosome 4, CAG repeat) with complete penetrance. It is another example of polyglutamine expansion diseases and is related to the cerebellar ataxias.[11] It has an incidence of 4 per 1 million and is characterized by severe atrophy of the caudate nucleus and putamen bilaterally, less atrophy of the globus pallidus and basal ganglia, and diffusely enlarged ventricles. The mutant Huntington protein interacts with both transcription factors and the ubiquitin-proteasome pathway,[12,13] but pathology seems to be limited to the CNS. Increases in somatostatin and dopamine and decreases in GABA are seen in these brain regions. Onset occurs between ages 35 and 40, with earlier onset in successive generations, known as anticipation. Clinically, the disease is marked by chorea, athetosis, dysarthria, ataxia, and dementia. Mood, cognitive, and self-control changes may occur much earlier, correlating with increases in the motor components.[2] Although butyrophenones and phenothiazines help suppress movement, therapies are limited. Delivery of brain-derived neurotrophic factor (BDNF), glial cell line–derived neurotrophic factor (GDNF), or ciliary derived neurotrophic factor (CDNF) to lateral ventricles has shown promise in animals.[14,15]

Perioperative Considerations. One case of delayed recovery from thiopental has been described,[16] although other case reports document no problems with thiopental or propofol for induction or with the use of inhaled anesthetics and nondepolarizing neuromuscular blockage (NDNMB).[17-23] Decreased pseudocholinesterase activity is seen; and although only a single case of delayed recovery from succinylcholine has been reported,[24] one should be aware of the potential for a delayed recovery from succinylcholine.[20] Neither nondepolarizing nor depolarizing muscle relaxants are contraindicated,[25] although there is a potential for delayed recovery from pseudocholinesterase-dependent NDNMB. Butyrophenones and phenothiazines may alleviate choreiform movements. Because anticholinergic effects may worsen choreiform movements, glycopyrrolate should be used instead of atropine to avoid central CNS effects.

Spasmodic Torticollis and Other Focal Dystonias

Pathology and Diagnosis. Also known as craniocervical spasms, spasmodic torticollis belongs to a group of restricted dyskinesias and dystonias in which only one or a few muscle groups are primarily affected. Spasmodic torticollis consists of contractile spasms of the scalene, sternocleidomastoid (SCM), and upper trapezius muscles, and secondary dystonia of the arm, trunk, neck, and facial musculature, with rotation and partial extension of the head (torticollis).[2] No neuropathologic changes have been found, and these disorders may be related to an imbalance in the dopamine pathway in the striatum. Other restricted dyskinesias include Meige's syndrome (blepharospasm), oromandibular dystonia (lip retraction and pursing), and spasmodic dysphonia (spasm with attempted speech). Symptoms begin in early adulthood and can be easily diagnosed by abnormal electromyographic (EMG) activity

in the sternocleidomastoid, trapezius, and posterior cervical muscles. The disorder is characterized by simultaneous activation of both agonist and antagonist muscles in the same muscle group. Surgical treatments to transect the SCM or spinal accessory nerves and the first three cervical motor roots have been used to alleviate symptoms, but complications can include phrenic nerve injury and dysphagia owing to an inability to lift the chin. EMG-guided botulism toxin injections every 3 to 4 months have been shown to be effective in up to 90% of patients. Treatments may lose efficacy if antibodies to the toxin develop. There are no contraindications to anesthetics. Spasms are relieved with muscle relaxants, whereas N_2O at concentrations above 50% relieves dystonia.[26] There is one case report of spastic torticollis during general anesthesia in a patient who was receiving chlorpromazine (Thorazine) preoperatively.[27]

Torsion dystonia (Oppenheim's disease or dystonia musculorum deformans) is an autosomal dominant disease most often seen in adulthood, although forms of this disorder with variable penetrance are occasionally seen. An autosomal recessive form is seen occasionally in children of Jewish ancestry.[2]

Clinically the disease is characterized by torsion spasms, involuntary twisting, and vertebral column movements, with possible lordosis, scoliosis, or a fixed cervical spine. Treatment attempts have included L-dopa, bromocriptine, carbamazepine, diazepam, tetrabenazine, trihexyphenidyl, and clonazepam, with limited improvements in symptoms. Although there are no contraindicated anesthetic agents, awake fiberoptic techniques may be indicated for airway control. Symptoms are relieved during sleep or heavy sedation.[28] Other forms of hereditary and nonhereditary dystonias include Wilson's disease (inherited error in copper transport, with absent ceruloplasmin globulin), Creutzfeldt-Jakob disease (prion, with earlier onset variant), double athetosis (status marmoratus), and Hallervorden-Spatz (globus pallidus pigmentary degeneration).

MOTOR NEURON DEGENERATION

Motor neuron diseases are characterized by variable, progressive, degenerative loss of motor neurons in the frontal cortex, the ventral horn of the spinal cord, and lower cranial nerve medullary nuclei, leading to muscle weakness, atrophy, corticospinal tract signs, and wasting in the spinal cord, brain stem, and motor cortex, with intact intellect and sensory system.[29] Pathology shows loss of anterior horn cells in the spinal cord and lower brain stem, in which loss of large fibers precedes that of small fibers. Astrocytes and lipofuscin fill in for the deleted neurons. In addition to the depleted large motor nerve fibers, there is a loss of muscarinic, cholinergic, glycinergic, and benzodiazepine receptors, up to and including

TABLE 8–2   Degenerative Motor Neuron Diseases
Amyotrophic lateral sclerosis (ALS) 　Progressive muscular atrophy 　Primary lateral sclerosis 　Pseudobulbar palsy
Inherited motor neuron diseases 　Autosomal-recessive spinal muscular atrophy 　　Type I: Werdnig-Hoffman, acute 　　Type II: Werdnig-Hoffmann, chronic 　　Type III: Kugelberg-Welander 　　Type IV: Adult-onset disease 　Familial ALS 　Familial ALS with dementia or Parkinson's disease (Guam) 　Other 　　Arthrogryposis multiplex congenita 　　Progressive juvenile bulbar palsy (Fazio-Londe) 　　Neuroaxonal dystrophy
Associated with other degenerative disorders 　Olivopontocerebellar atrophies 　Peroneal muscle atrophy
Friedreich's ataxia
Guillain-Barré syndrome 　Baló's disease
Acute disseminated encephalomyelitis following measles, chickenpox, smallpox, and (rarely) mumps, rubella, or influenza
Acute and subacute necrotizing hemorrhagic encephalitis 　Acute encephalopathic form (Hurst's disease) 　Subacute necrotic myelopathy 　Acute brain purpura

the motor cortex. Recently, superoxide dismutase (SOD) mutations have been found in these patients, leading to the possibility that increased free radicals may contribute significantly to disease progression. We will consider several representatives of the motor neuron diseases,[29] including amyotrophic lateral sclerosis (ALS) (mixed upper and lower motor neuron disease), Friedreich's ataxia (mixed), and spinal muscle atrophy (lower motor neurons), before we consider polyneuropathies. Because the classification of these diseases is uncertain, mixed upper and lower motor neuron diseases with sensory involvement could also be considered in the general category of polyneuropathies as well (Table 8-2).

Amyotrophic Lateral Sclerosis

Pathophysiology and Diagnosis. The most common example of a motor neuron disease is ALS, a progressive degeneration of both lower motor neurons, leading to amyotrophy, and upper motor neurons, leading to hyperreflexia and spasticity (due to "laterally sclerotic" corticospinal tracts). Primary disease is limited to the motor cortex and efferent pathways.[2] If motor nuclei of the lower brain stem

are most affected, it is termed *progressive bulbar palsy.* Weakness and atrophy in the absence of corticospinal tract signs is termed *progressive spinal muscle atrophy.* The selective motor neuron death of ALS spares intellect, voluntary movement, and the sensory system. The extraocular and sacral parasympathetic neurons for bowel and bladder are also spared. It is autosomal dominant with an age-dependent penetrance, and the gene defect appears to map to chromosome 21 in some cases. This relentlessly progressive disease attacks both upper and lower motor neurons. The incidence is about 2 per 100,000. Onset is highest in the 40- to 50-year age group, and men are affected more frequently than women. Sporadic forms account for 90% of the cases, whereas familial forms account for the rest. Onset at an earlier age is seen in rare familial autosomal dominant and recessive forms. By far the highest incidence is found in the Mariana and Guam Islands, in three clusters that are associated with Parkinson's dementia.[2] ALS is also sometimes associated with malignancy.

Pathologic examination reveals that astrocytic gliosis has replaced the lost motor neurons, and neurofilament, intracellular, and ubiquinated inclusions are also common in pathologic examination. Diagnosis is made with magnetic resonance spectroscopy, EMG, and nerve conduction studies, with a decrease in the number of motor units but an increase in the size of single motor action potentials. EMG shows fasciculations, fibrillations, and denervation, but conduction is only slightly delayed. Interestingly, sensory evoked potentials are abnormal. Clinically, fine motor awkwardness and early spastic weakness is seen, with atrophy, hyperreflexia, mild spasticity, fasciculations and involvement of the limbs gradually progressing to all extremities and motor neurons. Bulbar symptoms are seen in striated muscles, thereby affecting speech, swallowing, and facial spasms with emotional responses. Fasciculations may be visible under the skin owing to contractions of muscle fiber bundles and may worsen with exercise and fatigue. Dementia is rare. Over 100 mutations in the *SOD1* gene have been reported in familial ALS.[30] Besides SOD mutations,[31] other proposed causes include excitotoxicity, mitochondrial dysfunction, apoptosis, heavy metal exposure, and GM_2 ganglioside accumulation. There are no effective therapies, although Storkebaum[32] reported improvements in an animal model of ALS after intracerebroventricular vascular endothelial growth factor (VEGF) delivery.

Perioperative Considerations. Supportive treatment includes respiratory support, aspiration precautions, feeding tubes, and walkers. Because of the involvement of respiratory function and bulbar muscles, particular care must be given to prevention of aspiration and the need for ventilatory support. Succinylcholine should be avoided owing to the potential for hyperkalemic response from denervated muscle.[33] Case reports also indicate an increased sensitivity to NDNMB.[34] Successful epidural and general anesthesia without NDNMBs has been reported.[35,36] Cyclophosphamide, interferon, minocycline, and tyrosine-releasing hormone (TRH) infusion have all been tried, with limited improvement in motor function. Gabapentin has shown some promise in animal studies, and more recently the antiglutamate drug riluzole has slowed disease progression.[37-39]

Friedreich's Ataxia

Pathophysiology and Diagnosis. Friedreich's ataxia is a prototype of a progressive ataxia involving the spinal cord, peripheral nerves, heart, and pancreas. Incidence is 1 per 50,000 in whites, and the disorder accounts for one half of all hereditary ataxia.[40] Other similar lesions include cerebellar lesions such as familial cortical cerebellar atrophy, brain stem lesions such as familial cerebellar and olivopontocerebellar degeneration, and olivopontocerebellar atrophy. These are autosomal recessive (GAA repeat, mapping to chromosome 9q13) with an autosomal dominant subset (with four distinct chromosomal loci), with onset from 10 to 30 years of age. Pathology is caused by a loss of function in the frataxin gene, which encodes for a mitochondrial protein, presumably leading to increased oxidative stress.[41,42] Gross pathology is characterized by degeneration of long descending and ascending fibers in the spinal cord, posterior columns, corticospinal and spinocerebellar tracts, with fibrosis, gliosis, and atrophy of the dorsal root ganglions. This is a mixed upper and lower motor neuron disease with predominantly cerebellar atrophy. Clinically, patients exhibit ataxia, nystagmus, absent lower limb reflexes, spasticity, weakness, dysarthria, and, finally, atrophy. Friedreich's ataxia is associated with diabetes mellitus, cardiomyopathy, pes cavus, kyphoscoliosis, restrictive respiratory function, and hypertrophic cardiomyopathy with myocardial muscle degeneration and a potential for congestive heart failure. The ECG often shows sinus tachycardia and arrhythmias and is abnormal in 95% of cases. Diagnosis is by genetic testing, magnetic resonance imaging (MRI), and electrophysiologic studies (EPS). The differential diagnosis for ataxia includes alcoholic-nutritional, drug abuse, ataxia-telangiectasia, autosomal dominant Roussy-Levy variant of hereditary neuropathy type I idiopathic atrophy, neoplasm, or cerebellar stroke. Whereas 5-hydroxytryptophan (serotonin) seems to improve cerebellar symptoms, there are no treatments.

Perioperative Considerations. Anesthetic considerations are similar to those of the motor neuron degenerative diseases: regional anesthesia is not contraindicated, and care should be taken with onset and recovery of NDNMB, with particular attention to bulbar and respiratory function.

Cardiomyopathy and bulbar dysfunction are implicated most often as the cause of death. One recent case report described general anesthesia with endotracheal intubation, a propofol/alfentanil infusion, and no use of muscle relaxants, without complication.[43]

Spinal Muscular Atrophy

Pathophysiology and Diagnosis. Spinal muscular atrophy (SMA) is characterized by peripheral motor nerves without involvement of upper motor neurons. Some types are more frequent in infancy and childhood, but all types appear to map to chromosome 5 and appear to be autosomal recessive. They are a leading cause of heritable infant deaths, trailing only cystic fibrosis in the category of autosomal recessive disease. SMA may also be seen in other diseases, such as Friedreich's ataxia.

Infantile SMA, also known as Werdnig-Hoffman disease or SMA type I, is a rapid, progressive disease of infancy, causing hypotonic weakness and usually death within the first year of age. SMA type II is a slightly slower form of SMA; it is also progressive but can be seen in adolescents or young adults. SMA type III (Kugelberg-Welander disease) is a more indolent variant with prominent spastic weakness manifested in late childhood and affecting muscles of the trunk and proximal limbs. SMA type IV is a slowly progressive adult-onset variant.

Perioperative Considerations. The etiology of the impaired neuromuscular transmission is not yet known. Decreases in choline acetyltransferase, part of the ACh synthesis pathway, are seen secondary to degeneration of the anterior horn cells, and the decreased acetylcholine leads to an increased sensitivity to NDNMB. One should avoid succinylcholine because of the increased potassium release and myotonia-like contractions. Because of the potential for aspiration and respiratory weakness, careful dosing and attention to reversal of neuromuscular blockade (NMB) are important. Likewise, high blocks with regional anesthetics may exacerbate the respiratory and/or bulbar muscle weakness but regional anesthesia is not absolutely contraindicated. Case reports describe both regional[44] and general anesthesia[45,46] for SMA II and III patients. Watts[47] used total intravenous (IV) anesthesia and a laryngeal mask airway (LMA), while Habib and colleagues[48] described the use of alfentanil and propofol, without NMB, for direct laryngoscopy and intubation for an abdominal procedure.

PERIPHERAL NERVE DISEASE AND THE POLYNEUROPATHIES

Peripheral nerve disease covers a wide variety of causation and clinical entities (Table 8-3). The peripheral nervous system (PNS), which encompasses all neural structures

TABLE 8–3   Principal Neuropathic Syndromes

I. Syndrome of Acute Motor Paralysis with Variable Disturbance of Sensory and Autonomic Function
A. Guillain-Barré syndrome (GBS; acute inflammatory polyneuropathy; acute autoimmune neuropathy)
B. Acute axonal form of GBS
C. Acute sensory neuro(no)pathy syndrome
D. Diphtheritic polyneuropathy
E. Porphyric polyneuropathy
F. Certain toxic polyneuropathies (thallium, triorthocresyl phosphate)
G. Rarely, paraneoplastic
H. Acute pandysautonomic neuropathy
I. Tick paralysis
J. Critical illness polyneuropathy

II. Syndrome of Subacute Sensorimotor Paralysis
A. Symmetrical polyneuropathies
1. Deficiency states: alcoholism (beriberi), pellagra, vitamin B_{12} deficiency, chronic gastrointestinal disease
2. Poisoning with heavy metals and solvents: arsenic, lead, mercury, thallium, methyl *n*-butyl ketone, *n*-hexane, methyl bromide, ethylene oxide, organophosphates (TOCP, etc.), acrylamide
3. Drug toxicity: isoniazid, ethionamide, hydralazine, nitrofurantoin and related nitrofurazones, disulfiram, carbon disulfide, vincristine, cisplatin, paclitaxel, chloramphenicol, phenytoin, pyridoxine, amitriptyline, dapsone, stilbamidine, trichloethylene, thalidomide, clioquinol, amiodarone, adulterated agents such as L-tryptophan, etc.
4. Uremic polyneuropathy
5. Subacute inflammatory polyneuropathy
B. Asymmetrical neuropathies (mononeuropathy multiplex)
1. Diabetes
2. Polyarteritis nodosa and other inflammatory angiopathic neuropathies (Churg-Strauss, hypereosinophilic, rheumatoid, lupus, Wegener granulomatosis, isolated peripheral nervous system vasculitis)
3. Mixed cryoglobulinemia
4. Sjögren-sicca syndrome
5. Sarcoidosis
6. Ischemic neuropathy with peripheral vascular disease
7. Lyme disease
C. Unusual sensory neuropathies
1. Wartenberg migrant sensory neuropathy
2. Sensory perineuritis
D. Meningeal-based nerve root disease (polyradiculopathy)
1. Neoplastic infiltration
2. Granulomatous and infectious infiltration: Lyme, sarcoid, etc.
3. Spinal diseases: osteoarthritic spondylitis, etc.
4. Idiopathic polyradiculopathy

III. Syndrome of Chronic Sensorimotor Polyneuropathy
A. Less chronic, acquired forms
1. Paraneoplastic: carcinoma, lymphoma, myeloma, and other malignances
2. Chronic inflammatory demyelinating polyneuropathy (CIDP)

3. Paraproteinemias
4. Uremia (occasionally subacute)
5. Beriberi (usually subacute)
6. Diabetes
7. Connective tissue diseases
8. Amyloidosis
9. Leprosy
10. Hypothyroidism
11. Benign sensory form in the elderly
B. Syndrome of more chronic polyneuropathy, genetically determined forms
1. Inherited polyneuropathies of predominantly sensory type
a. Dominant mutilating sensory neuropathy in adults
b. Recessive mutilating sensory neuropathy of childhood
c. Congenital insensitivity to pain
d. Other inherited sensory neuropathies, including those associated with spinocerebellar degenerations, Riley-Day syndrome, and the universal anesthesia syndrome
C. Inherited polyneuropathies of mixed sensorimotor types
1. Idiopathic group
a. Peroneal muscular atrophy (Charcot-Marie-Tooth; hereditary motor-sensory neuropathy [HMSN], types I and II)
b. Hypertrophic polyneuropathy of Dejerine-Sottas, adult and childhood forms
c. Roussy-Levy polyneuropathy
d. Polyneuropathy with optic atrophy, spastic paraplegia, spinocerebellar degeneration, mental retardation, and dementia
e. Hereditary liability to pressure palsy
2. Inherited polyneuropathies with a recognized metabolic disorder
a. Refsum's disease
b. Metachromatic leukodystrophy
c. Globoid-body leukodystrophy (Krabbe's disease)
d. Adrenoleukodystrophy
e. Amyloid polyneuropathy
f. Porphyric polyneuropathy
g. Anderson-Fabry disease
h. Abetalipoproteinemia and Tangier disease

IV. Neuropathy Associated with Mitochondrial Disease

V. Syndrome of Recurrent or Relapsing Polyneuropathy
A. Guillain-Barré syndrome
B. Porphyria
C. Chronic inflammatory demyelinating polyneuropathy
D. Certain forms of mononeuritis multiplex
E. Beriberi or intoxications
F. Refsum's disease, Tangier disease

VI. Syndrome of Mononeuropathy or Plexopathy
A. Brachial plexus neuropathies
B. Brachial mononeuropathies
C. Causalgia
D. Lumbosacral plexopathies
E. Crural mononeuropathies
F. Migrant sensory neuropathy
G. Entrapment neuropathies

From Adams RD, Victor M, Ropper AH (eds): Principles of neurology. New York, McGraw-Hill, 1997.

outside of the spinal cord and brain stem, includes a broad variety of cell types, nerve fibers, anatomic variability, and function. Likewise, the pathologic conditions capable of affecting the PNS at multiple points are also incredibly variable. Signs and symptoms of polyneuropathies can therefore include impaired motor function, spasm and fasciculations, reflex changes, sensory loss, pain and paresthesia, dysesthesias, ataxia, tremor, trophic changes, and autonomic dysfunction. These can all have acute or chronic onset and duration.

Guillain-Barré syndrome (GBS) is an example of a polyneuropathy with motor, sensory, and autonomic components. The anesthetic considerations of the polyneuropathies in general will be discussed using GBS as an illustrative example. In actuality, diagnosis of a specific etiology for a mixed polyneuropathy can be challenging. In large studies a sizable fraction of patients remain without a specific diagnosis of causative agent. Polyneuropathies that might be encountered frequently by anesthesia providers include those due to ischemia, diabetes, drugs, rheumatoid arthritis, lupus, sarcoid, Sjögren's disease, paraneoplasm, acquired metabolic syndrome, uremia, and alcohol. Of particular interest are the polyneuropathy of critical illness[49,50] and a report of acute quadriplegia and myopathy attributed to prolonged NMB and corticosteroid use.[51] The inherited polyneuropathies are covered later in this chapter. Individual neuropathies due to trauma, radiation, reflex sympathetic dystrophy (RSD), or inflammation of individual peripheral nerves are not covered here.

Guillain-Barré Syndrome

Pathology and Diagnosis. Guillain-Barré syndrome, also known as acute idiopathic polyneuritis or acute inflammatory polyneuropathy, is a cell-mediated immunologic response against peripheral nerves, with a number of variant forms (Table 8-4).[52-57] It is found worldwide, in both sexes and all ages, with an incidence of about 1.5 per 100,000. Pathologic examination demonstrates perivascular lymphocytic and inflammatory cell infiltration, segmental demyelination, and wallerian degeneration along entire peripheral nerves and scattered throughout the PNS. Damage is primarily axonal and is thought to be due to an immune-mediated response to myelin proteins.[58] In 60% to 70% of cases, GBS is preceded by a mild gastrointestinal or respiratory influenza-like illness by 1 to 3 weeks, with *Campylobacter jejuni,* Epstein-Barr virus (EBV), or cytomegalovirus (CMV) most frequently identified.[59] Other preceding events that have been statistically associated with GBS include surgery, other viral illness, vaccination, and lymphomatous disease. GBS is characterized by paresthesias, numbness, and progression to weakness that is mostly symmetrical. Distal extremities are affected first, followed by proximal upper extremities and cranial muscles in 50% of cases. Pain and aches accompany variable sensory loss and areflexia.

Signs and symptoms can be limited solely to lower extremities or can lead to total muscular paralysis with paresthesias and autonomic dysfunction (hypotension and hypertension, sinus tachycardia or bradycardia, diaphoresis or loss of sweating, and orthostatic hypotension). Hyponatremia, the syndrome of inappropriate antidiuretic hormone (SIADH), and diabetes insipidus can also occur. Nerve conduction studies show reduced amplitude of motor evoked potentials, slowed conduction, prolonged latency, and prolonged F waves. Diagnosis is made with an increased finding of protein in the cerebrospinal fluid (CSF) with a normal cell count. The differential diagnosis includes the muscular dystrophies, acute spinal cord injury, transverse myelitis or myelopathy,

---

TABLE 8–4   Guillain-Barré Syndrome and Its Variant Forms

Form of Guillain-Barré Syndrome	Incidence/Occurrence	Motor or Sensory	Characteristic Signs	Suspected Etiology
Acute inflammatory demyelinating polyneuropathy	Most common in developed countries of Europe and North America	Both motor and sensory	85%-90% of cases; peripheral nerve demyelination	Cell-mediated immune, and humoral, attacks myelin and Schwann cells
Acute motor axonal neuropathy	Mainly northern China;	Motor only; axonal damage	Seasonal; higher incidence of respiratory failure	Immune, motor axons; higher association with *Campylobacter jejuni*
Acute motor-sensory neuropathy	Prolonged course	Resembles pure variant but with some sensory	Axonal damage of both motor and sensory	
Miller-Fisher variant		No significant weakness, but can involve cranial nerves	Ataxia, ophthalmoplegia, areflexia	Often *Campylobacter jejuni* also, antibodies to cranial nerve myelin

Data from references 54-59.

renal failure, polyneuropathy of critical illness, prolonged corticosteroid use, chronic neuromuscular blockade, and acute hyperphosphatemia. Treatment consists of symptomatic support of respiration and hemodynamics, as well as aspiration precautions. Corticosteroids have not proven efficacious, but plasmapheresis within the first 2 weeks after onset has been useful.[60] Recovery is usually spontaneous and full.

Perioperative Considerations. The anesthetic management is the same as that for motor neuron degeneration. Succinylcholine should be avoided because of the potential for potassium release, and there should be increased awareness of the potential for increased sensitivity to NDNMB. An arterial line may be useful for patients with autonomic dysfunction, and postoperative ventilation may be necessary because of reduced respiratory function. Regional anesthesia is controversial owing to a limited number of case reports claiming an association with onset of disease, although use for obstetrics has also been reported.[61] Both general anesthesia with limited or no use of NDNMBs[62-64] and regional anesthesia have been reported for poly(dermato)myositis, which has proximal muscle weakness and myalgias similar to GBS.

ABNORMALITIES OF METABOLISM AND CIRCULATION OF THE CSF PATHWAYS

The balance between CSF formation, intracranial pressure (ICP), circulation, and absorption determines CSF hydrostatic pressure and the distribution of CSF within the CNS. There is 50 to 150 mL of CSF in the adult, and it is divided into two main compartments: an intracranial compartment, consisting of primarily lateral ventricles and the third ventricle, and the spinal subarachnoid space. CSF is generated primarily in the choroid plexus at a rate of 21 to 22 mL/hr. In the absence of pathologic or vascular changes, CSF production, flow, and uptake determine CSF pressure and ventricular volume. CSF production occurs mainly in the choroid plexus in the ventricles at a rate of 500 to 600 mL/day and is due to a combination of active transport and passive filtration from blood plasma. CSF formation is affected by numerous drugs and conditions, including temperature, CSF pressure, hypocapnia, and venous pressure. Electrolytes and glucose equilibrate with CSF in the ventricles and subarachnoid space. Ionized drugs enter the CSF slowly, except for those taken up by a facilitated diffusion membrane transport. Diffusion of water, sodium, and hypotonic or hypertonic fluids occurs rapidly, and the CSF is in dynamic equilibrium with blood and intracellular fluid in the brain.

CSF bulk flow occurs from the lateral ventricles through the foramina of Monro to the third ventricle, through the aqueduct of Silvius to the fourth ventricle. CSF exits the fourth ventricle through the two lateral foramina of Luschka and the foramen of Magendie (medially) into the perimedullary and perispinal subarachnoid spaces, then to the brain stem, basal cistern, and cerebral hemispheres. CSF bathes the intracranial and spinal subarachnoid spaces from the cisterna magna, with considerable to and fro bulk flow across the various foramina as a result of cardiac oscillations and movement. A pressure gradient with arterial pulsations is observed to fall with direction of CSF flow, from 60 mm Hg in the lateral ventricles to 50 mm Hg in the cistern to 30 mm Hg in the lumbar subarachnoid space. CSF is taken up by bulk filtration at several sites, primarily the arachnoid villa in the sagittal sinus. Each ventricle normally contains 25 to 40 mL. Obstruction of the foramina or increased production can lead to hydrocephalus.

The blood-brain barrier is made up of both blood-CSF and brain-CSF barriers of varying "barrier" effectiveness and includes capillary endothelium, plasma membrane adventitia, and pericapillary foot processes of astrocytes. Drugs that affect CSF production include digoxin, furosemide, corticosteroids, and acetazolamide. Aminophylline increases CSF production by increasing the Na^+,K^+-ATPase active transport. The effects of most opioids are modest, and the effects of anesthetic agents on the balance between production and absorption is usually small. Artru,[65-67] in a series of classic studies in dogs, showed little effect of isoflurane, halothane, or fentanyl on CSF production, although ketamine and enflurane increased CSF production. More recently, Sugioku[68] showed decreased CSF production in rabbits with sevoflurane anesthesia, confirmed an increase in production with enflurane, and showed increased CSF absorption with N_2O. Artru[69] showed no significant alterations in CSF production or absorption by sevoflurane or remifentanil.

Hydrocephalus

Pathophysiology and Diagnosis. Hydrocephalus is defined as excessive ventricular CSF, most commonly due to foraminal obstruction (noncommunicating), but it can also be due to overproduction or impaired absorption (communicating). Congenital hydrocephalus is seen in 0.3% due to Arnold-Chiari malformation, Dandy-Walker cysts, myelomeningocele, aqueductal stenosis, arachnoid cysts, neoplasms, and vascular malformations. Acquired hydrocephalus can result from meningitis, intraventricular or subarachnoid hemorrhage, trauma, or neoplasm.[2]

Hydrocephalus may be acute or chronic in onset, and diagnosis is most commonly made by computed tomography (CT) or MRI. Chronic hydrocephalus may present as headache and nausea, whereas the rapid increase in CSF pressure in acute hydrocephalus can also cause vomiting, confusion, and lethargy. Signs include irregular respiration, papilledema, decorticate or decerebrate posturing, bradycardia, hypertension, and ECG changes due to brain stem compression and transtentorial herniation. Ventricular hydrocephalus is treated with an intraventricular catheter or surgical correction of a physical obstruction, whether due to neoplasm, malformation, or clot. Ventricular catheters are most commonly shunted to peritoneal, pleural, or, less commonly, atrial, choledochal, or vesicular spaces.[70]

Perioperative Considerations. Anesthetic considerations are similar to other neurosurgical procedures, with particular attention to the potential for increased ICP and avoidance of abrupt or severe changes in CSF pressures or volumes due to the abnormal drainage. One of the rare case reports in a small series of patients described a variable response of ICP after induction of anesthesia with ketamine.[71] Oversedation, hypercarbia, hypoxia, anxiety, and hyperventilation should be avoided. Rapid decompression can cause subdural hematoma secondary to bridging veins from the dura or upward herniation of the brain stem, causing bradycardia, irregular respiration, or ECG changes.

Normal-Pressure Hydrocephalus

Pathophysiology and Diagnosis. Normal-pressure hydrocephalus is common in the elderly and is associated with hypertension and atherosclerotic heart disease.[72] The exact incidence in the United States is not known, but as many as 1 in 25,000 people worldwide may have this disorder and as many as 6% of patients with dementia appear to have it. It may be seen occasionally in pediatric patients as well. Symptoms include forgetfulness, inattention, impaired thought process, and memory difficulty. Signs include ataxia, urinary incontinence, and cognitive dysfunction.[73] CT or MRI shows ventricular enlargement with normal to low lumbar opening CSF pressures. Pathology is due to hydrocephalic compression, periventricular (especially frontal subcortical) hypoperfusion, and secondary stretching of periventricular vascular and white matter structures.[74] CSF shunting is only beneficial in less than 50% of patients.[75-77] The differential diagnosis includes all of the other causes of dementia in the elderly.[78] Anesthetic management is similar to that for hydrocephalus.

Pseudotumor Cerebri

Pathophysiology and Diagnosis. Pseudotumor cerebri or idiopathic intracranial hypertension (previously also called "benign" intracranial hypertension) is defined as an increased ICP with normal CSF composition, normal CNS imaging studies, and no known etiology. The pathology that has been proposed to account for pseudotumor cerebri is probably due to increased CSF production or increased cerebral venous pressure; increased sagittal sinus pressure, leading to low conductance CSF outflow, extracellular edema; and increased brain volume, with the resultant compression of venous sinuses and decreased CSF absorption.[79,80] The increased CSF and intracranial pressures may be a compensatory increase in an attempt to restore CSF bulk absorption.[81] Incidence is about 0.9 per 100,000. In children, both males and females are affected equally, but in adults more women are diagnosed. In adults, pseudotumor cerebri presents as a throbbing or episodic headache, nausea, vomiting, or blurred vision. Headaches are most often worst in the morning and are exacerbated by Valsalva maneuvers and movement. Visual changes are manifested as a blind spot, field cuts with inferonasal field cut, diplopia, or blindness. This diagnosis is most common in obese women and can be self-limited. Signs include papilledema, abnormal third or lateral ventricles, effaced cerebral sulci, and elevated ICP pressures (as high as 300 to 600 mm Hg). CSF composition is normal, and, remarkably, consciousness is not altered. The diagnosis is one of exclusion, and the differential diagnosis includes cerebral venous thrombosis, increased ICP due to neoplasm, infection, or inflammatory process.

Perioperative Considerations. Multiple causes are associated with pseudotumor cerebri. Treatment is initially medical therapy (Table 8-5), mainly with diuretics, but serial lumbar punctures with drainage may also be used. If medical management fails or visual changes progress, CSF shunts,

TABLE 8–5 Causes Associated with Pseudotumor Cerebri
Endocrine
Addison's disease, menarche, pregnancy, hypo/hyperthyroid, hypoparathyroidism, pseudohypoparathyroidism, empty sella syndrome
Dietary
Obesity, hypo-/hypervitaminosis A, vitamin D deficiency, malnutrition
Drugs
Corticosteroid withdrawal, estrogen, oral contraceptives, lithium, tetracycline, trimethoprim-sulfamethoxazole, nitrofurantoin, nalidixic acid, thyroid supplements, danazol
Impaired Cerebral Venous Drainage
Otitis media, mastoiditis, idiopathic cerebral venous/dural sinus thrombosis, superior vena cava syndrome, arteriovenous malformation, right-sided heart failure, jugular vein ligation, subclavian vein, thrombosis
Others
AIDS, systemic lupus erythematosus, polyarteritis nodosa, polycythemia vera, anemia (pernicious, iron deficiency), Guillain-Barré syndrome, thrombocytopenia

usually lumboperitoneal, may be attempted but have a high failure and complication rate.[82,83]

Optic nerve decompression is sometimes used to salvage visual loss[84] and can attenuate headaches.[85-87] Anesthetic management is the same for hydrocephalus, but regional anesthesia is not absolutely contraindicated.[88]

Syringomyelia and Syringobulbia

Pathophysiology and Diagnosis. Syringomyelia is an enlarged CSF-filled cavity in the spinal cord, whereas syringobulbia is a comparable cavity in the brain stem. Hydromyelia refers to a cavity in the central canal. Syringomyelia can be communicating, often in conjunction with Chiari malformations, or noncommunicating. Syringomyelia is progressive, with loss of pain and temperature sensation in the upper extremities, with preserved touch and proprioception, possible hyporeflexia, and extremity atrophy.[2] Deep tendon reflexes can be lost, and loss of paraspinous muscles can result in scoliosis.

Syringobulbia most commonly presents as a throbbing occipital headache and can lead to lower cranial nerve dysfunction, including motor and sensory changes of the tongue, vocal cords, and sensation of the face. Traumatic syrinx formation can manifest itself as pain radiating to the neck and upper extremities.[89] Diagnosis is by CT with contrast medium enhancement, or by MRI, although it may be found after a failed subarachnoid block.[90] Pathologic examination shows a syrinx cavity filled with CSF and reactive gliosis histology, but without inflammation or ischemia. Noncommunicating syringomyelia can be the result of spinal cord trauma, tumor, or arachnoiditis.

Perioperative Considerations. Surgery is intended to drain the syrinx cavity and to relieve the spinal cord compression, either by craniocervical decompression, in the case of communicating syringomyelia, or with laminectomy and shunting, in the case of noncommunicating syringomyelia. Patients should be treated as if they have an acute spinal cord injury, because they can exhibit autonomic hyperreflexia, impaired sympathetic responses, impaired temperature regulation, and respiratory difficulty. Succinylcholine is contraindicated, and the response to NDNMBs can be variable.[91] Syringobulbia involvement of the cranial nerves may lead to impaired airway protection.

SPINAL CORD INJURY

Pathophysiology and Diagnosis. Acute spinal cord injury (SCI) affects some 220,000 individuals in the United States each year. The majority are young adult males, and the injuries are commonly associated with alcohol or other substances of abuse and with motor vehicle accidents. Acute trauma resuscitation is covered in Chapter 17, and we only briefly review specific neurologic considerations after acute and chronic SCI here.

Anesthetic Management of Acute SCI. Any trauma patient should be considered to be at risk for brain or spinal cord injury and treated appropriately with cervical spine precautions and examination for head or neck injuries that might possibly have been overlooked while treating other life-threatening injuries. Rarely, vertebral artery injuries can occur in conjunction with cervical spine injuries and should be in the differential diagnosis in patients with CNS trauma and signs and symptoms consistent with cerebellar or brain stem injury (e.g., gait, balance, nausea/vomiting, hemodynamics, respiration, cranial nerve dysfunction).[92] Elderly trauma patients are at increased risk for flexion and extension injuries, which can lead to central cord syndrome, with symptoms of variable sensory loss below the level of spinal cord injury, lower extremity weakness, and urinary dysfunction. Acute SCI can lead to loss of sympathetic and autonomic reflexes, responses, and tone (spinal shock). This is manifested as cardiovascular and autonomic instability, loss of reflexes, and flaccid paralysis.[93] Symptomatic inotropic, chronotropic, and respiratory support is indicated. These patients are at risk for possible neurogenic pulmonary edema, myocardial irritability and arrhythmias, hypoactive and hyperactive sympathetics and autonomics. Risks of abdominal atony and ileus, distention, malfunction of the diaphragm, and increased risks of aspiration should all be considered. Ongoing secondary injury after trauma to the spinal cord may cause extension of the initial injury, with further loss of function and increased respiratory or cardiovascular compromise. Quadriplegia may be associated with hyperdynamic vagal responses owing to loss of sympathetic or cardioaccelerator fibers. Bronchi may be hyperresponsive from increased tone after SCI as well.

Anesthetic Management of Chronic SCI. Unfortunately, patients with a chronic SCI are not uncommon and frequently present for urologic or orthopedic procedures. Multiple organ systems can be affected by the injury, and the level of SCI determines organ system involvement. Higher lesions (those above T4 to T6) can cause significant impairment of hemodynamics and cardiovascular reflexes.[94] These changes are due to damage to the sympathetic chain, chronic loss of cardiovascular and cerebrovascular tone, increased renin-angiotensin activity, and resultant changes in intravascular volume. Respiratory function may be impaired because of diaphragmatic and chest wall mechanics and ventilation-perfusion mismatch. Patient positioning for optimal spontaneous respiration must be balanced with the potential for orthostatic hypotension. Other common coexisting diseases include renal dysfunction (i.e., infection, stones, insufficiency, failure), anemia, pressure necrosis and sores, osteoporosis, pain, and lack of temperature regulation.

Autonomic hyperreflexia is found in the majority of SCI patients with lesions above T6. It is defined as a generalized autonomic overactivity in response to stimuli, out of proportion to the intensity of the stimulus. Common stimuli include bladder or intestinal distention, but it may also include uterine contractions or surgical skin incision. Signs and symptoms include hypertension, bradycardia, headache, visual changes, sweating, piloerection below the level of the lesion with vasodilation above the level of the lesion, and cardiac arrhythmias.[94] Untreated autonomic hyperreflexia can lead to hypertensive crisis, stroke, seizures, and death. The pathology involves the unopposed sympathetic thoracolumbar tract, with impaired descending spinal inhibitory pathways. Anesthesia can be regional or general, and the key is effective anesthesia, regardless of the technique chosen. Treatment of hypertensive crisis should include calcium channel blockade (nicardipine, nifedipine), vasodilators (nitroprusside, hydralazine), or α-adrenergic antagonists (phentolamine, phenoxybenzamine). Centrally acting antihypertensives (clonidine, methyldopa) are not as effective in acute treatment, and β blockers alone are contraindicated due to the resultant unopposed α-adrenergic activity. Epidural anesthesia has been used to treat autonomic hyperreflexia in a quadriplegic patient.[95]

DEMYELINATING DISEASES

The most common demyelinating diseases are classified into two groups, multiple sclerosis and diffuse cerebral sclerosis. Multiple sclerosis has three subtypes that include chronic relapsing encephalomyopathy, neuromyelitis optica, and the acute form of multiple sclerosis. Diffuse myelinoclastic cerebral sclerosis, also known as Schilder's disease, usually has a relapsing remitting course and affects primarily children, but it can present in young adulthood and may mimic intracranial neoplasm or abscess.[15] Definitive pathologic findings include neuronal myelin sheath destruction, perivascular inflammatory infiltration, which is mainly perivenular in white matter, and a lack of fiber tract wallerian or secondary degeneration. Although similar in pathology, the leukodystrophies and Krabbe's disease primarily affect infants and involve abnormal myelin production, or dysmyelination. In addition, with recent advances in genomics, the etiology for several of these leukodystrophies has been genetically linked to transport proteins and enzymes responsible for myelin production.[96]

Multiple Sclerosis

Pathophysiology and Diagnosis. Multiple sclerosis (MS) is an autoimmune disorder mediated by inducible T cells and autoantibodies that target CNS myelin. In the United States roughly 400,000 men and women are diagnosed with MS, with a twofold to threefold higher prevalence in women.[97] There is a well-established geographic correlation in the incidence of MS, with the highest rates (30 to 80/100,000) found in Northern Europe and northern climates in North America, followed by southern regions of Europe and the United States (6 to 14/100,000). The lowest incidence (1 in 100,000) is seen in equatorial latitudes. There is a bimodal distribution of MS patients, with one third presenting between 45 and 60 years of age and the majority between 20 and 40 years of age. Despite extensive epidemiologic studies, it appears that MS is influenced by unknown environmental factors and familial genetics rather than ethnicity or comorbidities. First-degree relatives demonstrate up to 14 times the incidence of MS. In this group there has been a remarkable similarity between HLA-B7 and HLA-Dw2 antigens. Many researchers and clinicians believe that there is an underlying autoimmune component to MS in light of the fact that the diagnostic criteria include evidence of CSF antibodies of the IgG type.

The typical MS patient experiences unpredictable bouts of neurologic deficits, secondary to random CNS sclerotic lesions, followed by variable periods of latency, hence the chronic relapsing clinical course. These nonspecific sclerotic lesions can present acutely over several hours or chronically over months to years with evolving motor, neurologic and cognitive deficits depending on the location and size of the lesion(s). At the cellular level the clinical symptoms are thought to be secondary to circulating activated myelin-reactive T cells with locally associated edema. This theory is further supported by the often rapid response to immunosuppression to decrease inflammation and edema.[97]

Research is currently focused on identifying genetic loci that are linked to MS and could potentially lead to diagnostic and therapeutic advances. Genetic testing research for diagnostic and treatment purposes has not been conclusive to date, because demyelinating diseases have been linked to several enzyme cascades and antigenic expression in the HLA groups. Several genomic screens have been undertaken to locate such genes but have not provided consistent gene localization, except for the major histocompatibility complex on chromosome 6p21 and a locus on chromosome 19q13.[98] A T-cell β chemokine known as the RANTES (*r*egulated upon *a*ctivation, *n*ormal T-cell *e*xpressed and *s*ecreted) gene has been found in sclerotic lesions in the CNS of MS patients post mortem. There appears to be a significant correlation with certain polymorphisms of this gene and its relation to onset and mortality.[99] The Multiple Sclerosis Genetics Group, which is a multicenter research consortium, has multiple studies underway trying to identify inherited and inducible genetic loci for MS.

Common clinical manifestations include paresthesias, weakness, bulbar deficits affecting cranial nerve function, abnormal extremity tone, cerebellar ataxia or diplopia, and bladder or bowel dysfunction; however, the severity and multitude of symptoms depends on the gross burden of sclerotic lesions in the CNS.

Factors that have been clinically established as exacerbating MS include stressful events such as emotional and physical trauma, infections, surgery, and the peripartum period. Hormonal and temperature fluctuations appear to have a clinical correlation with exacerbations as well. Davis[99a] demonstrated that a temperature rise of 0.5°F blocks nerve conduction in previously demyelinated nerve fibers. Previously, Edmund and Fog documented clinical deterioration with temperature elevations in 75% of MS patients.[100]

Diagnostic criteria for MS are based on clinical, laboratory, and radiologic findings. The most useful appear to be MRI evidence of CNS plaques (typically periventricular) that are separate in time and space and are supported by abnormal evoked potentials of the somatosensory, visual, and auditory type. CSF may show abnormal oligoclonal antibodies. Current therapies for MS are not curative but attempt to ameliorate acute exacerbations and prevent future recurrences. Most MS flares respond to glucocorticoid therapy in the early phases, but many patients fail to respond to corticosteroids as their number of exacerbations increases. Patients with optic neuritis respond to oral and intravenous adrenocorticotropic hormone and prednisone in the acute phases and experience fewer relapses. Other immunosuppressive agents, such as cyclophosphamide, cytarabine, and azathioprine, have shown intermittent success at preventing the number and severity of relapses but are not without side effects. Patients with severe motor spasticity and bladder dysfunction are treated with antispastic medications, which provide some relief. Alternative therapies that are not clinically proven but that have been tried in severely resistant cases include plasmapheresis, hyperbaric oxygen therapy, linoleate supplementation, and interferons.

Perioperative Considerations. Although not directly correlated with anesthetic medications, the clinical course of MS may fluctuate in the perioperative period. Periods of stress, whether emotional or physical, often coincide with a deterioration of MS symptoms. There have been no randomized studies that implicate general anesthesia as an exacerbating factor for MS flares; however, there are rare case reports of disease exacerbation associated with perioperative fevers.

Anesthetic induction agents and inhaled gases have no demonstrable adverse effects on nerve conduction and have not been definitively implicated in the literature as contributing to progression of any neurodegenerative disorders. However, several agents used commonly during general anesthesia might affect nerve conduction and thus affect MS patients. Temperature fluctuations have been implicated in nerve conduction inhibition in demyelinated nerve fibers. Drugs that are commonly administered under anesthesia include the anticholinergics atropine and glycopyrrolate. At the doses used during surgery these drugs have not been shown to significantly raise temperatures enough to elicit symptoms or predict exacerbations. An earlier account of sodium thiopental being deleterious for MS patients undergoing surgery or sedation has now been discounted.[101-104] The use of depolarizing muscle relaxants also carries theoretical risks in MS patients, more specifically those with profound neurologic deficits that often cause upregulation of motor end plate acetylcholine receptors and the hyperkalemic response to depolarization. We have not found any studies that implicate nondepolarizing muscle relaxants in neurologic sequelae perioperatively; thus, their use appears to be safe.

Local and regional anesthesia remains a controversial topic in MS patients because of their pharmacodynamics on nerve conduction. In clinical practice it is common for clinicians to perform lumbar puncture for diagnosis and clinical response to therapies, and there are no significant data to suggest an exacerbation of symptoms with said procedure.[105] With the pathology of demyelination in MS one might expect that the potential for neurotoxicity with local anesthetics administered in the epidural or intrathecal space would be higher. However, several retrospective studies have not demonstrated a significant increase in MS exacerbations with either epidural or spinal local anesthetic administration.[106-111] Although unproven, many clinicians believe that repeated doses of local anesthetics for regional anesthesia carry a potentially increased risk for neurotoxicity, both locally and centrally, because the blood-brain barrier may be more permeable owing to chronic inflammatory changes. In light of this concept, many believe that lower concentrations of local anesthetics should be utilized and combined with narcotics, because there have been no reports of significant adverse events with epidural or intrathecal opioids. Regardless of the technique utilized, MS patients should be informed of the potential side effects and risks of perioperative exacerbations.

Based on the historical and clinical data available there appear to be no absolute contraindications for general or regional anesthesia in the MS population. As a standard preoperative assessment these patients should have a well-documented neurologic examination, as well as a postoperative assessment for any new findings. During surgery there should be close attention to thermoregulation, because pyrexia has been described to elicit MS exacerbations in a perioperative setting. Chronic immunosuppressive therapy should be maintained or continued; however, there is no clinical evidence to support the use of stress doses of corticosteroids perioperatively.

Mucopolysaccharidoses

Pathophysiology and Diagnosis. The mucopolysaccharidoses (MPS) are hereditary lysosomal storage disorders caused by the deficiency of various enzymes necessary for the metabolism of glycosaminoglycans (GAG), previously called mucopolysaccharides. Excess accumulation of partially degraded glycosaminoglycans within cells causes cellular dysfunction. The faulty metabolism results in serious structural and functional abnormalities in a wide variety of tissues, particularly bone and cartilage. There are now 9 MPS disorders, classified as types I through IX, based on enzyme deficiency and severity of the phenotype. With the exception of Hunter's syndrome (MPS II), which is an X-linked disorder, the MPS are inherited in an autosomal recessive pattern. The cumulative incidence is estimated at 1 in 20,000 live births. Table 8-6 outlines the classification system and summarizes the associated clinical features.

Diagnosis is made by elevated GAG concentration in urine or demonstration of enzyme deficiency in leukocytes. Treatment options include enzyme replacement, bone marrow transplantation, and cord blood transplantation. These therapies are symptomatic and may alter the natural progression of the disease but do not prevent eventual decline in function. The MPS continue to worsen as the patient grows older, and most patients will die of pulmonary or cardiac complications.

Perioperative Considerations. The anesthetic implications of this disease are extensive and relate to the end organ dysfunction and anatomic distortions experienced by this patient population. Complications with general anesthesia are common, and morbidity and mortality are primarily due to airway issues. Upper airway abnormalities such as macroglossia, hypertrophic tonsils and adenoids, patulous lips, micrognathia, friable tissues, copious secretions, and restrictive temporomandibular joint movement can hinder adequate ventilation. Many patients have obstructive breathing at baseline, with sleep apnea and need for continuous positive airway pressure. Bone marrow transplant can reverse upper airway obstruction.[112] Lower airway abnormalities from deposition of GAG in the epiglottis and tracheal wall distort the airway, and difficulties with intubation can increase with age as this process continues.[113] A short neck with a narrow, anterior larynx accompanied by possible cervical instability or history of cervical fusion offer additional airway challenges, particularly in

TABLE 8–6 Classification of Mucopolysaccharidoses*,†

Syndrome	MPS Type	Incidence	Clinical Features
Hurler	IH	1/100,000	Severe skeletal and cardiac abnormalities, coarse facies, airway obstruction, hepatosplenomegaly, hydrocephalus, mental retardation, corneal opacities, and hearing loss
Hurler-Scheie	IH/IS	1/115,000	Intermediate in severity with significant joint involvement, hepatosplenomegaly, micrognathia, and near-normal mentation.
Scheie	IS	1/500,000	Mildest MPS I with life span of several decades Aortic valve disease common Normal facies and intelligence
Hunter	II	1/100,000	Mild to severe forms Physical disease similar to MPS I with slower progression Less mental retardation but aggressive behavior
Sanfillippo A-D	III A-D	1/30,000	Primarily central nervous system involvement with progressive mental retardation and aggressive behavior Each subtype is the result of a different enzyme deficiency. III C is the mildest form.
Morquio	IV A and B	Rare	Skeletal disease and ligament laxity with high incidence of odontoid dysplasia and atlantoaxial instability Normal intelligence and survival to middle age Both types have severe and mild forms.
Maroteaux-Lamy	VI	Rare	Severe skeletal disease similar to MPS I but normal intelligence Severity variable
Sly	VII	Rare	Variable physical presentation with psychomotor retardation
Hyaluronidase deficiency‡	IX	Very rare	Short stature, acetabular erosion, periarticular masses

*MPS V and VIII no longer in use.
†Goetz C (ed): Textbook of clinical neurology, 2nd ed. Philadelphia, Saunders, 2003, pp. 611–612
‡Natowicz MR, Short MP, Wang Y, et al: Clinical and biochemical manifestations of hyaluronidase deficiency. N Eng J Med 1996; 335(14):1029–1033.

those with Hurler's syndrome (MPS I). Incidence of difficult and failed intubations is reported as 54% and 23%, respectively.[114,115] Tracheotomy is also technically difficult, owing to a large mandible, short neck, and retrosternal trachea and was impossible even post mortem in one case report.[116,117]

Cardiac abnormalities also result from MPS. Mitral and aortic valves thicken, causing insufficiency that may progress to cardiomyopathy.[118] Deposition of GAG in the walls of arterial blood vessels causes systemic hypertension and coronary artery disease. Coronary lesions are diffuse and can lead to ischemia or sudden death. Coronary angiography may not predict the severity of the diseases.[112,119] Pulmonary hypertension secondary to chronic hypoxemia of pulmonary disease and airway obstruction can lead to right-sided heart failure.

Pulmonary dysfunction is another frequent complication. Kyphoscoliosis causes a restrictive disease with recurrent pneumonia and ventilation-perfusion mismatch, resulting in chronic hypoxemia and hypercarbia. Patients with Morquio's syndrome (MPS IV) are also prone to atlantoaxial instability and odontoid dysplasia. This can lead to central apnea from cord compression.[120]

Neurologic complications of MPS vary depending on the particular classification. Developmental delay and sleep disturbance are common. Vertebral subluxation can occur at any level of the spinal column and compromise the spinal cord. Communicating hydrocephalus frequently develops and can cause increased ICP. Seizures are uncommon in most of these patients.

Patients with MPS present for surgery frequently, most commonly for ear, nose, and throat procedures and hernia repairs. Anesthetic management should begin with a preoperative evaluation that establishes which type of MPS is involved and what components of the disease are present.[115] Careful review of cardiac, pulmonary, and neurologic function are paramount, and workup may include an electrocardiogram, chest radiograph, neck films, pulmonary function tests, and echocardiogram, as indicated. Preoperative flexion-extension films to evaluate stability of the cervical spine are recommended in those with Morquio's syndrome.[121] Detailed inspection of the airway, review of old anesthesia records, and neck imaging can help predict airway difficulties.[115] However, the airway can worsen with time and disease progression. Age and level of mental retardation are also important considerations in planning an anesthetic. Premedication with benzodiazepines can be helpful in the uncooperative patient but should be avoided in those with an airway prone to obstruction. An antisialagogue should be administered to decrease secretions but used cautiously in patients with heart disease.

Because most reported anesthetic complications in this population involve airway or positioning difficulties, regional anesthesia may be a safer option.[122-124] Regional technique may prove problematic if the patient cannot lie flat because of skeletal pain or respiratory compromise or is unable to cooperate because of mental retardation.[121] If general anesthesia is required, the airway can be secured before induction with topicalization of the airway and awake fiberoptic intubation. A reverse guidewire technique is also possible after appropriate sedation.

When inducing general anesthesia before securing the airway, inhalation induction with spontaneous ventilation is recommended.[123,125] For those unable to cooperate with inhalation induction, intravenous induction with ketamine has been used successfully.[123] Intravenous access should be established before induction, and difficult airway equipment should be immediately available. Nasotracheal intubation is discouraged because of anatomically altered nasal passages and friable tissues. Recent literature has shown that the laryngeal mask airway can be used successfully in this population for maintenance of adequate ventilation during general anesthesia and for assistance with fiberoptic intubation through the laryngeal mask airway.[126] Limited use of the angulated video-intubation laryngoscope has also facilitated intubation in MPS patients with cervical spine instability.[127] Intraoperative considerations include careful positioning to avoid cervical subluxation and arterial cannulation in patients with severe pulmonary or cardiac dysfunction.[120] Narcotics should be titrated carefully to avoid respiratory depression. There are no reported abnormal responses to muscle relaxants or anesthetic agents. Extubation should be performed with caution in these patients, because they have increased incidence of atelectasis and airway obstruction secondary to traumatic tissue edema.

HEREDITARY PERIPHERAL NEUROPATHIES

Inherited disorders of peripheral nerves are a part of a much larger group of inherited or acquired polyneuropathies that often coexist with systemic, infectious, and metabolic diseases (e.g., diabetes mellitus, thyroid disease, neoplastic syndromes) or are caused by exposure to various agents (e.g., heavy metals, alcohol, certain medications). As such, the hereditary neuropathies are a common and very diverse group of genetically determined neurologic diseases. They are primarily characterized by a dysfunction of peripheral sensory neurons in the presence of additional muscle weakness or autonomic system dysfunction. However, a dysfunction of the central nervous and other organ systems is more prominent in some types of hereditary neuropathies, which is of special relevance to the anesthesiologist treating these patients. Historically, classification of these disorders was primarily based on clinical manifestations and eponyms were used to designate a specific combination of clinical symptoms (e.g., Riley-Day syndrome, Charcot-Marie-Tooth disease). However, significant phenotypic variability led to nosologic confusion. Modern classification of hereditary neuropathies is based on clinical and electrophysiologic characteristics, modes of inheritance, and underlying genetic mutations. The hereditary neuropathies are usually divided into three major groups according to their main clinical manifestation—predominantly motor involvement, predominantly sensory or autonomic involvement, or neither. These major groups are further divided into types (usually based on differences in clinical presentation, pathology, nerve conductivity studies) and subtypes (based on genetic characteristics). Table 8-7 provides information about some of the more prevalent hereditary types of polyneuropathies; a comprehensive description can be found in a recent review.[128]

In the previous edition of this textbook, traditional eponymic classification was used. This approach is still used in many, even most, recent anesthesia textbooks. However, we believe that use of the modern classification with cross-referencing to traditional eponyms is

warranted in this edition. All major medical reference databases use this classification, and patients seen in clinical anesthesia practice will be increasingly likely to have a diagnosis defined by this new terminology, which is widely accepted in the mainstream neurologic practice.

Hereditary Primary Motor Sensory Neuropathies, Including Charcot-Marie-Tooth Disease

The hereditary motor sensory neuropathies (HMSNs) represent a spectrum of disorders caused by a specific mutation in one of several myelin genes that results in defects in myelin structure, maintenance, and formation. The association of different mutations within the same gene with various clinical phenotypes is a common finding in this group of peripheral neuropathies. This variability suggests that these disorders represent a spectrum

TABLE 8–7 Hereditary Peripheral Neuropathies

Hereditary Peripheral Neuropathies	Clinical Manifestations and Underlying Pathologic Process	Inheritance Patterns	Electrophysiologic Findings
Hereditary Primary Motor Sensory Neuropathies (HMSN)			
HMSN type 1 (Charcot-Marie-Tooth disease type 1 or CMT 1)—five identified subtypes	Demyelinating disorder, distal weakness, onset in first or second decade of life, slow-progressing, onion bulbs	Autosomal dominant	Moderate to severe reduction in nerve conduction velocities
HMSN type 2 (Charcot-Marie-Tooth disease type 2 or CMT 2)—eight identified subtypes	Neuroaxonal (not demyelinating) disorder, distal weakness, slow progressing	Autosomal dominant	Normal to mildly reduced nerve conduction velocities
HMSN type 3 (Dejerine-Sottas or congenital hypomyelinating neuropathy)—three identified subtypes	Demyelinating disorder, severe hypotonia in early childhood or at birth, onion bulbs	Autosomal dominant	Very severe reduction in nerve conduction velocities
HMSN type 4—seven identified subtypes)	Large group of disorders with typically early severe presentation and rapidly progressing, demyelinating, sometimes prominent sensory deficit	Autosomal recessive	Very severe reduction or absent nerve conduction velocities
Hereditary Primary Sensory Autonomic Neuropathies (HSAN)			
HSAN type 1 (hereditary sensory radicular neuropathy)	Small axon loss, acromutilation	Autosomal dominant	—
HSAN type 2 (congenital sensory neuropathy)	Large and small axon loss	Autosomal recessive	—
HSAN type 3 (Riley-Day syndrome or familial dysautonomia)	Large and small axon loss, with dysautonomic crises, lack of lacrimation	Autosomal recessive	—
HSAN type 4 (congenital insensitivity to pain with anhidrosis)	Congenital sensory neuropathy with anhidrosis, C-axon loss	Autosomal recessive	—
Other Hereditary Neuropathies			
Hereditary neuropathy with pressure palsy			
Hereditary brachial plexopathy			
Giant axonal neuropathy			

of related phenotypes caused by an underlying defect in peripheral nervous system myelination. The HMSNs, otherwise known as Charcot-Marie-Tooth disease (CMTD), have been classified as types 1 through 7, which are further subdivided, thus consisting of close to 30 clinical syndromes. The vast majority of these syndromes are very rare and have never been reported in the anesthesia literature. The space limitations of this text, in addition to the paucity of relevant anesthesia references, do not allow a detailed description of all currently identified phenotypes. Therefore, only types 1 and 2 (CMT1 and CMT2), and 3, which together are the most common hereditary peripheral neuropathies,[129] will be discussed. Combined prevalence in the population is close to 40 per 100,000.

Pathophysiology and Diagnosis. HMSN type 1, or CMT1, is a demyelinating disorder of peripheral nerves, which most often presents in the first or early second decade of life, although infants can also be affected.[130] Significant family history is typical. Diffuse slowing of nerve conduction velocity and gradually progressing distal muscle weakness and early loss of coordination characterize CMT1. It is associated with loss of reflexes, pes cavus foot deformity, and hammertoes. Later, distal calf atrophy develops (classic "stork leg deformity"), in combination with gradual loss of proprioception and sense of vibration. Abnormal concentric myelin formations are called onion bulbs and are found around the peripheral axons. These are a characteristic feature of CMT1, usually revealed by the sural nerve biopsy. The CMT1A subgroup of patients may present with proximal muscle wasting and weakness. Dematteis and colleagues also observed obstructive sleep apnea in this subtype of patients, with a high degree of correlation between the severity of neuropathy and degree of obstruction.[131] Even later changes include atrophy of the intrinsic hand and foot muscles, footdrop, palpable hypertrophy of the peripheral nerves, and possible development of scoliosis and kyphosis. Disease exacerbation may occur in pregnancy.[132] Life expectancy is unaffected.

HMSN type 2, or CMT2, also called axonal CMT, is a heterogeneous disorder with normal or borderline nerve conduction velocity. It is primarily an axonal, and not a demyelinating, disorder, with neuropathy being a result of neuronal death and wallerian degeneration (no onion bulbs on biopsy). The clinical course is similar to that of CMT1, but sensory symptoms predominate over motor symptoms and peripheral nerves are not palpable. Patients with CMT2C subtype display significant degree of vocal cord and diaphragm weakness, resulting in obstructive sleep apnea, which is of interest to the anesthesiologist.[133]

Onset is usually in the second or third decades of life but can be in early childhood with rapid clinical progression.

TABLE 8-8   Differential Diagnosis of Hereditary Motor Sensory Neuropathies

Genetic Neuropathies

Refsum's disease
Metachromatic leukodystrophy
Familial brachial plexus neuropathy
Adrenomyeloneuropathy
Pelizaeus-Merzbacher disease
Amyloid neuropathies

Acquired Neuropathies

Metabolic Disease
   Diabetes mellitus
   Thyroid disease
   Vitamin B_{12} deficiency
Infectious
   Neurosyphilis
   Leprosy
   Human immunodeficiency virus
Others
   Chronic alcoholism
   Heavy metal intoxications
   Vasculitis
   Neoplastic syndromes
   Chronic inflammatory demyelinating polyneuropathy

HMSN type 3 includes two syndromes: Dejerine-Sottas syndrome and congenital hypomyelinating neuropathy (CHM). Both of these syndromes are characterized by profound hypotonia, presenting in early infancy or at birth, in the case of CHM. Dejerine-Sottas syndrome is clinically similar to CMT1, although its manifestations are more severe and appear in early childhood.

The preoperative preparation of HMSNs may be complicated owing to similarity in clinical presentation with other genetic or acquired polyneuropathies (Table 8-8).

No specific treatments for HMSNs are available. Symptomatic supportive care consists of orthopedic corrective joint procedures for pes cavus and scoliosis deformities and physical and occupational therapy. Orthopedic procedures are usually staged, ranging from soft tissue procedures and osteotomies to triple arthrodesis. Multiple administrations of general or regional anesthesia might be required.

Preoperative preparation of patients with HMSNs is dictated by the extent of clinical involvement and coexisting morbidities.

The degree of motor neurologic involvement should be evaluated, and affected muscle groups should be noted. Atrophic denervated muscles usually display significant resistance to nondepolarizing muscle relaxants and are unreliable for monitoring of neuromuscular blockade.

The CMT1 and CMT2C patients should be evaluated for restrictive pulmonary disease related to scoliosis and diaphragmatic weakness and potential obstructive sleep apnea. Respiratory insufficiency has been described in patients with CMT.[134-136] Careful planning for extubation and a possible need for postoperative respiratory support may be necessary in these patients.

Patients with HMSNs may have undetected cardiac conduction abnormalities.[137,138] Although this association is not strong, all patients with an HMSN should have a preoperative ECG.

Pregnancy often leads to exacerbation of the symptoms of CMTD and, in combination with diaphragmatic splitting, can lead to respiratory compromise.[136]

Intraoperative Considerations.

The anesthetic experience for HMSN types 1, 2, and 3 is limited to a number of case reports[136,137,139-145] and retrospective reviews.[146,147] Despite the absence of strong evidence advocating for or against the use of specific anesthetic agents or particular anesthetic techniques, a number of important concerns have been raised in the literature regarding anesthetic management of these patients.

Malignant Hyperthermia. Although drugs triggering malignant hyperthermia (MH) have been used in patients with CMTD without complication,[146,147] there are two reports of MH during general anesthesia in patients with CMTD.[142] In these reports the authors advocate against the use of succinylcholine and volatile agents. Furthermore, an approach postulating that any patient with a neuromuscular disease should be considered to be at increased risk for MH adds to this controversy. The review of the available literature describing anesthesia management in patients with HMSNs indicates that the majority of authors prefer to avoid administering MH-triggering agents in patients with HMSN types 1, 2, and 3, in part owing to medicolegal considerations.

Succinylcholine use in these patients is associated with increased risk of malignant arrhythmias secondary to exaggerated hyperkalemic response.[148] Although succinylcholine has been used in CMTD without untoward effects,[146,147] it seems appropriate to avoid its use in any patient with suspected muscular denervation.

Nondepolarizing muscle relaxants have been used successfully in patients with HMSNs without indications of prolonged duration of action.[146,147,149,150] However, some authors express reasonable concern that adequate monitoring of neuromuscular blockade could be complicated due to altered responses on the affected muscles, which are not always obvious during clinical assessment.[151] Additionally, there is at least one case report of prolonged neuromuscular block with vecuronium.[152] Inadequate reversal of neuromuscular blockade in patients with preexisting respiratory compromise can lead to serious complications. It is advocated by some authors to avoid the use of nondepolarizing muscle relaxants in such patients whenever possible.[139,141,145]

Neuroaxial anesthetic techniques have been successfully used in patients with HMSNs without untoward effects, including for vaginal delivery and cesarean section.[136,144,145,153,154] However, some authors correctly point out that medicolegal concerns have to be taken into considerations when designing anesthesia plans for these patients.[136,145] Despite lack of evidence that anesthesia affects the course of preexisting neuromuscular disease, regional anesthesia may be erroneously blamed for any subsequent deterioration in sensory or motor deficits. This is especially true in pregnancy, which, as pointed out earlier, is associated with exacerbation of neurologic symptoms in women with CMTD. Additionally, the choice between general or regional/neuraxial anesthesia in patients with CMTD complicated by respiratory compromise is guided by the preservation of respiratory function in the perioperative period. In patients with phrenic nerve involvement, whose respiration depends on accessory muscles, regional block involving intercostal muscles can lead to acute respiratory failure.[136] On the other hand, there are case reports of patients with CMTD who required prolonged respiratory support after general anesthesia.[155,156]

Hypnotic Anesthetic Agents. Patients with CMT1 have been reported to demonstrate increased sensitivity to thiopental, correlating with the degree of motor and sensory deficit.[157] However, propofol and total intravenous anesthesia have been successfully used in these patients without untoward effects.[140,143]

In summary, anesthetic management in the vast majority of patients with HMSNs appears to be uncomplicated and should be directed to accommodate any coexisting systemic conditions.

Hereditary Sensory and Autonomic Neuropathies

The hereditary sensory and autonomic neuropathies (HSANs) are a diverse and constantly expanding group of disorders affecting the development of autonomic and sensory neurons. Until recently, seven such disorders have been described, with familial dysautonomia (HSAN type III), also known as Riley-Day syndrome, and HSAN type IV, also known as congenital insensitivity to pain with anhidrosis (CIPA), being by far the most recognized and well understood. All HSANs are manifested by both sensory and autonomic dysfunction present at variable degree, with a unique feature for all types being absence of a normal axon flare response after intradermal injection of histamine phosphate. The reported anesthetic experience for HSANs is limited to anesthesia management of patients with familial dysautonomia (HSAN III) and CIPA (HSAN IV). The clinical presentation, diagnosis, and management of other HSANs have been reviewed.[158]

Familial Dysautonomia (HSAN Type III, or Riley-Day Syndrome)

Pathophysiology and Diagnosis. Familial dysautonomia (FD) is a rare genetic disorder that affects, almost exclusively, persons of Ashkenazi Jewish extraction. It is the most prevalent and well studied of all HSANs. Development of autonomic and sensory neurons is impaired, resulting in reduced population of nonmyelinated and small-diameter myelinated axons. The sympathetic neurons are primarily affected, and sympathetic ganglia are small. The parasympathetic neurons and large axons are generally spared. FD presents at birth and progresses with age. In the past, more than 50% of patients died before 5 years of age. Today, due to improvements in diagnosis and treatment, newborns diagnosed with FD have more than a 50% chance to live past 30 years of age.

Although FD has close to 100% penetrance, the presentation of the disease at different life stages is highly variable. Autonomic dysfunction is the most prominent feature of this disease, presenting the most impediment to normal functioning, and usually overshadows the sensory deficits. The clinical diagnosis is usually established soon after birth by demonstrating the presence of the following main criteria: absence of tears with emotional crying, absence of lingual fungiform papillae, hypotonic or absent patellar reflexes, and absence of axon flare to intradermal injection of histamine in children of Ashkenazi Jewish descent. Many other systems are affected at various stages in life, and the myriad of clinical manifestations of FD can be divided into two main groups: sensory dysfunction and autonomic dysfunction (Table 8-9).

Differential diagnosis typically does not present a problem, considering availability of genetic testing and the fact that this disease is restricted to Ashkenazi Jews. However, many other conditions have some similar symptoms of autonomic and sensory dysfunction. All HSANs, cranial nerve and/or nuclear dysplasias, cri du chat syndrome, and Möbius syndrome can have some of the features found in FD. Many eye conditions share similar ocular manifestations with those of FD.

Treatment in FD is symptomatic. Diazepam is the most effective treatment for dysautonomic crisis with

---

TABLE 8–9 Familial Dysautonomias: Sensory and Autonomic Dysfunction

Sensory System	Syncopal episodes produced by various stimuli (e.g., full bladder, large bowel movement)
Decreased pain sensation, often with hypersensitivity of palms, sole, neck, and genital areas; decreased temperature sensation	Postural hypotension (can develop in older patients)
Visceral sensation intact	*Dysautonomic Crisis*
Sense of vibration and proprioception affected in older individuals; ataxia	Episodes of severe nausea and vomiting associated with agitation, hypertension, tachycardia, excessive sweating and salivation; easily triggered by emotional or physical stress, arousal from sleep
Hypotonia in younger children, often disappears with age; decreased tendon reflexes	**Other Manifestations**
Prone to self-injury; unrecognized fractures; scoliosis and joint deformities	**Renal System**
Autonomic System	Dehydration azotemia
Gastrointestinal System	Progressive loss of renal function with age
Impaired oropharyngeal coordination; impaired swallowing, resulting in dysphagia and frequent aspirations in newborns and infants	**Central Nervous System and Developmental**
Abnormal esophageal motility; decreased lower esophageal sphincter pressure; esophageal reflux	Emotional lability, probably related to catecholamine imbalance
Gastrointestinal dysmotility, complicated by cyclical vomiting (part of dysautonomic crisis)	Prolonged breath holding with crying, decerebrate posturing, syncope, cyanosis; may be misinterpreted as seizures
Respiratory System	Normal intelligence
Recurrent pneumonias due to aspirations	Delayed development
Insensitivity to hypoxia and hypercapnia (no ventilatory response)	**Ocular Manifestations**
Low tolerance for hypoxia; profound hypotension and bradycardia in response to hypoxia	Absence of overflow tears with emotional crying in all patients
Cardiovascular System	Corneal insensitivity; abrasions and spontaneous injuries; ulcers
Rapid severe orthostatic hypotension without compensatory tachycardia	Optic neuropathy increasing with age
Episodes of severe hypertension and tachycardia as part of dysautonomic crisis	**Laboratory Findings**
	Elevated blood urea nitrogen
	Hyponatremia associated with excessive sweating
	Catecholamine imbalance—elevated DOPA:DHPG ratio

vomiting. It also normalizes blood pressure and heart rate in these patients. Increased salt and fluid intake is used to treat dehydration and hyponatremia and associated postural hypotension. Fludrocortisone and midodrine are also used for this purpose. Surgical procedures performed on these patients include gastrostomies in majority of patients before 5 years of age to provide fluids and alimentations in patients with dysphagia; fundoplication for treatment of gastroesophageal reflux and associated pneumonia; and spinal fusions for severe scoliosis.

Preoperative Preparation. Anesthesia for surgical procedures had been associated with great risks in patients with FD.[159-161] Recent progress in the understanding of existing risks and improved preoperative preparation resulted in significantly improved perioperative outcomes.[162-165] Good working knowledge of FD manifestations and a systematic approach to preoperative assessment is essential for successful anesthetic management of these patients.

The respiratory system should be evaluated for signs of chronic or acute infections due to repeated aspirations. Chest radiography is warranted in all patients. In patients with restrictive pulmonary disease due to chronic pneumonias and scoliosis arterial blood gas analysis is included.

Severe intraoperative hypotonia is a well-recognized risk of general anesthesia.[159-161] Cardiac output is dependent on preload due to lack of compensatory sympathetic response to hypotonia. Correction of existing dehydration and hyponatremia is essential for intraoperative hemodynamic stability in these patients. Intravenous prehydration with crystalloids is often recommended to achieve euvolemic status preoperatively.[165,166]

Patients are evaluated for the presence and severity of gastroesophageal reflux. Antacids need to be administered preoperatively to affected patients.

Renal function is assessed to rule out significant renal failure, which can affect the choice of muscle relaxants.

Patients with FD are prone to anticipation anxiety that can trigger dysautonomic crisis. Preoperative medication with benzodiazepines is recommended. Preoperative medication with opioids is contraindicated owing to the concern of increased sensitivity to the agents.

Intraoperative Considerations. Intraoperative management of FD patients is directed toward better cardiovascular stability, prevention of pulmonary aspiration, prevention of postoperative respiratory compromise, and adequate postoperative pain control. Invasive hemodynamic monitoring (intra-arterial line and central venous catheters) has been advocated in the past but was not used in one reported series without untoward effects.[162,165] It appears reasonable to use it in patients with postural hypotension and for extensive surgery with large fluid shifts. Immediate preinduction administration of fluid bolus

can reduce blood pressure variation. Blood pressure instability intraoperatively is treated by additional fluid boluses and direct-acting vasopressors, if the patient is unresponsive to administration of fluids. Any episodes of desaturation are promptly addressed by increased oxygen concentration to avoid profound hypotension and bradycardia owing to lack of hypoxic compensatory responses.

Rapid-sequence induction with cricoid pressure should be considered in patients with gastroesophageal reflux and a history of repeated aspirations.

Careful planning for extubation, postoperative ventilatory support, and weaning from the respirator in the ICU should be part of the routine postoperative management for these patients. In the past, FD patients frequently required prolonged ventilation in the ICU setting after general anesthesia. Reports indicate that with alternative techniques, such as epidural[162] or local anesthesia, or deep propofol sedation with spontaneous ventilation,[165] these patients can recover from anesthesia very quickly without need for postoperative respiratory support.

Although patients with FD have decreased perception of pain and temperature, their visceral perception is intact and they need sufficient levels of anesthesia and postoperative pain control. Postoperative pain should be promptly treated to avoid dysautonomic crisis. Nonsteroidal anti-inflammatory drugs (NSAIDs) or paracetamol will suffice in the many cases. Opioids should be used cautiously to avoid respiratory depression. Regional techniques can be useful.[162]

There have been no reports of adverse or prolonged responses to any specific anesthetic agents or muscle relaxants. For appropriate surgical procedures, regional anesthesia is well tolerated.[162] Use of deep propofol sedation for endoscopic outpatient procedures has been reported, with excellent results.[165]

Body temperature needs to be carefully monitored owing to impaired temperature control in these patients. The eyes should be lubricated and protected at all times.

In conclusion, FD is a serious anesthetic challenge that can be hazardous in these patients without proper preoperative preparations and intraoperative management. However, current approaches have resulted in significantly reduced mortality and morbidity in these patients.

Congenital Insensitivity to Pain with Anhidrosis (CIPA, or HSAN type IV)

Pathophysiology and Diagnosis. CIPA is a rare autosomal recessive neuropathy characterized by recurrent episodic fever, anhidrosis (absence of sweating), pain insensitivity, self-mutilating behavior, and mental retardation.[158] Death from hyperthermia has been reported in infants with CIPA. Besides anhidrosis, it differs from FD by complete insensitivity to superficial and deep painful stimuli and normal lacrimation, much milder autonomic dysfunction, with absent postural hypotension or dysphagia. Self-inflicted multiple injuries are typical for these patients. This is often accompanied by accidental trauma, burns, wound infections, skin ulcers, joint deformities, and osteomyelitis.

There is only limited anesthetic experience in patients with CIPA.[167-169] Okuda and associates[167] suggest three important considerations in the anesthesia management of patients with CIPA: anxiety alleviation, temperature control, and adequate pain control. Despite congenital insensitivity to pain, general anesthesia was found to be necessary. Overall requirements of general anesthetics necessary for maintaining stable hemodynamics have been found to be only slightly reduced. General anesthesia was used in all patients in these reports without any adverse reactions to the intravenous or inhalational anesthetic agents, opioids, and succinylcholine. In one report, a patient died following intraoperative cardiac arrest without clear cause, although the authors suspected that the high concentration of halothane used (2%) could be responsible.[168] Previous recommendations against the use of atropine (or other anticholinergic drugs) to avoid hyperpyrexia in these patients was not supported by the results reported in this series. Many patients received atropine without any untoward effects.

NEURODEGENERATIVE DISORDERS WITH AUTONOMIC FAILURE

Autonomic failure (or dysautonomia), with its protean range of manifestations and symptoms, is a common part of an immensely diverse group of disorders in which some or all elements of the autonomic nervous system are affected. Autonomic failure to a various degree is a part of the presentation of many systemic diseases (e.g., diabetes mellitus, amyloidosis), infectious diseases (e.g., leprosy, human immunodeficiency virus, rabies), immune disorders (e.g., acute dysautonomia, Guillain-Barré syndrome), paraneoplastic disorders, hereditary autonomic disorders (e.g., all HSANs, dopamine β-hydroxylase deficiency), and neurodegenerative disorders, to name just a few. A comprehensive discussion on various aspects of autonomic dysfunction in these conditions can be found in most neurology and medical textbooks. In this chapter we discuss only the most prevalent neurodegenerative disorders in which autonomic failure plays a prominent role, presenting a significant anesthetic challenge.

Parkinson's disease (PD), dementia with Lewy-body disorder (DLB), multiple system atrophy (MSA), and pure autonomic failure disorder (PAF) are all neurodegenerative disorders of unclear etiology, presenting with variable degrees of autonomic dysfunction. Based on the differences in the neuropathology, these disorders can be divided into two subgroups: Lewy-body syndromes (PD, DLB, and PAF) and multiple system atrophy (MSA).

All these disorders are characterized by the presence of α-synuclein (hence, these disorders are often called synucleinopathies) in the neuronal (Lewy bodies, as in Lewy body syndromes) or glial (GCIs, as in MSA) cytoplasmic inclusions. In PD, neurodegeneration is predominant in the substantia nigra and other brain stem nuclei and in peripheral autonomic neurons. Motor dysfunction is more prominent than autonomic failure in PD patients. Neuronal degeneration in PAF is restricted to peripheral autonomic neurons, hence the symptoms of pure autonomic failure without other manifestations. Extensive cortical involvement, in addition to degeneration of brain stem nuclei and peripheral autonomic neurons, is characteristic for DLB, which presents as severe dementia associated with parkinsonism and autonomic failure.

In MSA, cytoplasmic inclusions are found in the glial cells (GCIs) and not neurons (Lewy body). These are associated with degenerative changes in the central neurons in basal ganglia, cortex, and spinal cord but not in peripheral autonomic neurons. Two phenotypes of MSA are currently identified based on the predominant clinical picture of parkinsonism (MSA-P) or cerebellar dysfunction (MSA-C). In the past, the patients with a predominant picture of autonomic failure were diagnosed with Shy-Drager syndrome. Today this term is rarely used, because all patients with MSA have a significant degree of autonomic dysfunction.[170]

Autonomic failure in patients with Lewy body syndromes and MSA is typically manifested by orthostatic and postprandial hypotension, bladder dysfunction, gastrointestinal motility disorders, and erectile sexual dysfunction. Orthostatic and postprandial hypotension is often the most disabling and early aspect of dysautonomia in many of these patients. Many other symptoms of autonomic dysfunction described in the section on familial dysautonomia can be present. The differential diagnosis can be very difficult owing to frequent overlapping of the clinical picture between these conditions, especially in the initial stages of the disease process. Definitive diagnosis in some disorders could be established only on postmortem histopathologic examination. However, thorough clinical examination helps to distinguish between PD, LBD, MSA, and PAF (Table 8-10). The subject of neurodegenerative disorders with autonomic failure has been reviewed.[170,171]

Anesthetic management of PD is described elsewhere in this chapter. Although DLB is the second most common cause of dementia after Alzheimer's disease, there are no reports of anesthetic management in the literature. It appears reasonable to assume that the principles of anesthetic management of patients with DLB are common to those in patients with other forms of dementia. In DLB patients with advanced dysautonomia the same precautions should be taken as in patients with MSA.

TABLE 8–10 Differential Diagnosis of Multiple System Atrophy, Parkinson's Disease, Pure Autonomic Failure, and Dementia with Lewy Bodies

Characteristic	Multiple System Atrophy	Parkinson's Disease	Pure Autonomic Failure	Dementia with Lewy Bodies
Central nervous system involvement	Multiple involvements	Multiple involvements	Unaffected	Multiple involvements
Site of lesions	Mainly preganglionic, central; degeneration of interomediolateral cell columns	Peripheral autonomic postganglionic neurons	Mainly peripheral autonomic postganglionic neurons; loss of ganglionic neurons	Cortex, brain stem, peripheral autonomic postganglionic neurons
Progression	Fast, median survival 6-8 years after first symptoms	Slow	Slow, up to 15 years and longer	Slow
Prognosis	Poor	Good	Good	Moderate to poor
Autonomic dysfunction	Early onset, severe	Late onset, usually mild to moderate	Severe, usually the only manifestation	Unclear, but can be severe
Extrapyramidal involvement	Common	Common	Absent	Common
Cerebellar involvement	Common	Common	Absent	Common
Lewy bodies	Mostly absent	Primarily in substantia nigra	Present in autonomic neurons	Cortex, brain stem, hippocampus
Glial cytoplasmic inclusions (postmortem staining)	Present	Absent	Absent	Absent
Response to chronic levodopa therapy	Poor	Good		Moderate
Dementia	Uncommon	Usually not severe, in 25%-30% of patients	Uncommon	Early, severe, rapidly progressing dementia

Adapted from Marti MJ, Tolosa E, Campdelacreu J: Clinical overview of the synucleinopathies. Mov Disord 2003;18(Suppl 6):S21-S27; and Kaufmann H, Biaggioni I: Autonomic failure in neurodegenerative disorders. Semin Neurol 2003;23:351-363.

Multiple System Atrophy

In 1998, Consensus Committees representing the American Autonomic Society and the American Academy of Neurology defined MSA as a sporadic, progressive, neurodegenerative disorder of undetermined etiology, characterized by features in the three clinical domains of parkinsonism, autonomic failure, and cerebellar or pyramidal dysfunction. In the past, the terms' "striatonigral degeneration," "olivopontocerebellar atrophy," and "Shy-Drager syndrome" were used, depending on the predominance of clinical symptoms in any of these three domains.

MSA is a fatal disease that typically presents in the fourth to sixth decade of life with a mean disease duration of 6 years from the onset of symptoms. Because of the significant similarity of clinical presentation to other neurodegenerative disorders, it is often not diagnosed until later stages. Parkinsonism is a predominant symptom in 80%, and cerebellar dysfunction is seen in 20% of all patients. Parkinsonism is usually not responsive to antiparkinsonian medications, which helps to differentiate it from PD. The most common and early presentation of autonomic dysfunction is urinary incontinence and erectile dysfunction (in male patients). Orthostatic hypotension is found in half of these patients and is usually mild. Reduced heart rate variability and absence of compensatory tachycardia during hypotension is characteristic. Paradoxically, supine hypertension is present in more than half of patients with MSA and complicates their management. Recurrent syncopes are signs of severe orthostatic hypotension. Severe constipation, fecal incontinence, and decreased sweating are other signs of autonomic dysfunction in MSA.

Obstructive sleep apnea or central sleep apnea and sleep-related inspiratory stridor associated with bilateral vocal cord paresis or dysfunction have been reported in MSA patients.[172]

There are no currently available treatments that can modify the clinical course or address the underlying pathologic process. All the treatments are symptomatic, intended for improving the quality of life in these patients. Orthostatic hypotension is treated with administration of fludrocortisone or milrinone (oral adrenergic vasoconstrictor). The presence of significant supine hypertension limits the use of vasopressors. Erythropoietin has been reported to be useful in the treatment of patients with associated anemia and severe hypotension. Tracheostomy and respiratory support is reserved for the patients with stridor and central sleep apnea.

Intraoperative Considerations. Perioperative management of patients with MSA is a formidable challenge, owing to potential hemodynamic instability and possible respiratory compromise in the postoperative period. A few case reports in the literature indicate no adverse effects to most commonly used anesthetic agents.[173-183] The management is directed at ensuring hemodynamic stability by the use of invasive hemodynamic monitoring, adequate preoperative hydration, and maintenance of normovolemia with fluid replacement intraoperatively. Preoperative optimization of fludrocortisone therapy is recommended. There is some controversy in the literature regarding the potentially unpredictable response to vasopressor amines due to sympathetic hypersensitivity caused by autonomic denervation.[175,184] Therefore, it is recommended to administer vasoactive medications very cautiously in much smaller doses than usual. However, vasopressors have been used without any adverse effects for treatment of hypotension intraoperatively, when titrated judiciously.[176,177,183]

Significant intraoperative supine hypertension has been reported with minimal response to labetalol but a profound hypotension after hydralazine administration.[185] The hypotension responded only to vasopressin infusion. It appears that short-acting vasodilators such as sodium nitroprusside may be a better choice for the treatment of intraoperative supine hypertension. The hypertensive episodes in autonomic failure are particularly responsive to transdermal nitroglycerin.[186]

Neuraxial anesthesia techniques have been successfully employed in patients with MSA, including for labor and delivery, with a greater degree of hemodynamic stability, also avoiding possible difficulties with extubation in these patients.[174,179,180,182,187] It is speculated that patients with autonomic failure are less likely to respond with hypotension to sympathectomy caused by neuraxial block because they are already sympathectomized. The data in the literature support this hypothesis.

When general anesthesia is opted for, careful planning for extubation and postoperative monitoring of the respiration in the ICU setting is warranted, especially in patients with a history of stridor or central or obstructive sleep apnea.

Pure Autonomic Failure

Pure autonomic failure (PAF) is a sporadic, slow-progressing neurodegenerative disorder of the autonomic nervous system that typically affects individuals in their sixth decade of life. It is characterized by an isolated impairment of the peripheral and central autonomic nervous system. No symptoms of parkinsonism, cerebellar dysfunction, or dementia are typically present. The orthostatic hypotension in this syndrome is typically very severe and more disabling than in other neurodegenerative disorders with autonomic failure. Other symptoms of autonomic failure are similar to those seen in MSA. The prognosis, however, is much better.

There is only one case report in the literature of general anesthesia without complications in a patient with PAF.[188] It is not very clear from the abstract provided whether the patient also had epidural anesthesia performed. However, the authors advocate the use of epidural anesthesia and invasive hemodynamic monitoring for greater hemodynamic stability.

It seems that the same principles of anesthetic management that are used for patients with MSA should be applied when managing PAF patients.

NEUROECTODERMAL DISORDERS

Neuroectodermal disorders belong to a group of congenital malformations affecting structures of ectodermal origin and are characterized by coexistent skin and nervous system lesions. Neurofibromatosis types I (von Recklinghausen's disease) and II, von Hippel-Lindau disease (VHL), tuberous sclerosis, and Sturge-Weber syndrome are of particular interest to anesthesiologists, owing to the multiple anesthetic challenges that patients with these disorders may present. Patterns of inheritance, genetic characteristics, and encoded proteins associated with identified genetic mutations are provided in Table 8-11. Neurofibromatoses, von Hippel-Lindau disease, and tuberous sclerosis are also often called phakomatoses on the basis of the patchy ophthalmologic manifestations observed in these disorders. There has been significant progress in the understanding of the pathogenesis of phakomatoses, which is characterized by loss of function of various tumor suppressor genes, which, in turn, leads to the development of benign or malignant tumors in many tissues.[189] Although the inheritance patterns and pathogenesis of Sturge-Weber are unknown, it is usually discussed together with phakomatoses, owing to the similarity of the clinical manifestations and to the distribution of lesions observed in

TABLE 8–11 Patterns of Inheritance, Genetic Characteristics and Encoded Proteins Associated with Identified Genetic Mutations in Neuroectodermal Disorders

Disorder	Pattern of Inheritance	Genetic Mapping and Protein Product
Neurofibromatosis I (von Recklinghausen's disease)	Autosomal dominant trait, familial transmission in 50%; the rest are spontaneous mutations Complete penetrance, variable expression	*NF1* gene on chromosome 17, truncated (nonfunctional) neurofibromin
Neurofibromatosis II		*NF2* tumor suppressor gene on chromosome 22, truncated merlin Other genes may be involved.
Von Hippel-Lindau disease	Autosomal dominant trait with variable high penetrance	*VHL* gene on chromosome 3, VHL protein Other genes may be involved.
Tuberous sclerosis	Autosomal dominant trait; 1 in 3 familial transmission, the rest spontaneous mutations or mosaicism Complete penetrance, variable expression	*TSC1* gene on chromosome 9 and *TSC2* on chromosome 16, encoding for hamatrin and tuberin, respectively
Sturge-Weber syndrome	Not inherited	Unknown

these disorders.[190] All these disorders are chronic conditions, in which there is increasing pathology over the patient's lifetime.

Neurofibromatoses

Pathophysiology and Diagnosis. Neurofibromatoses are genetic disorders of the nervous system primarily affecting the development and growth of neural tissues and causing subsequent growth of neural tumors. They are divided into type I, or NF1, also known by its eponym as von Recklinghausen's disease, and type II, or NF2. The former is much more common and accounts for 90% of all neurofibromatoses. These two types have different causes, and their clinical manifestations and diagnostic criteria differ significantly (Table 8-12). Other rare forms of neurofibromatosis have been defined and reviewed.[191]

Preoperative Preparation. While evaluating a patient diagnosed with neurofibromatosis for surgery and anesthesia, it is important to make a distinction between NF1 and NF2. Unlike patients with NF1, in which associated pathology may involve all systems in the body, relevant clinical manifestations of NF2 are largely limited to intracranial pathology.[192] It is worth mentioning that although NF2 is much less prevalent in the general population (1:210 000) than NF1 (1:5000), most of the patients with NF2 will require surgical removal of cranial nerve schwannomas, an NF2 primary manifestation. As a result, anesthesiologists in neurosurgical practice frequently see these patients whereas in general practice the likelihood of seeing patients with NF2 is very low. To date, most anesthetic and medical literature concerned with management of neurofibromatosis is limited to NF1. Here, we cover mainly the issues related to the perioperative

management of NF1 patients. The specifics of NF2 anesthetic management are addressed when relevant.

The severity of clinical manifestations of NF1 varies greatly between patients and usually increases over the patient's lifetime. NF1 might involve multiple organ systems, thus presenting a formidable challenge to an anesthesiologist. Familiarity with the clinical manifestations of NF1 and a systematic approach to preoperative assessment of these patients are essential to successful anesthetic management.[192]

Airway Assessment. Thorough assessment of the airway is important in NF1 patients. Neurofibromas associated with NF1 can affect any segment of the airway. Intraoral lesions have been reported in up to 5% of patients with NF1, involving the tongue and the laryngeal and pharyngeal structures, leading to obstruction and dyspnea.[192] Plexiform and major subcutaneous neurofibromas are commonly found in the cervical region and parapharyngeal spaces. Large lesions can cause significant airway distortion and/or obstruction. Unanticipated sudden airway obstruction following induction of general anesthesia has been reported requiring emergency tracheostomy.[193,194] Large neurofibromas originating in the posterior mediastinum, retroperitoneal space, or cervical paraspinal areas can lead to progressive compression of the distal airway.[195,196] Additionally, involvement of the recurrent laryngeal nerve can result in unilateral vocal cord paralysis.[197] Cranial nerve involvement due to the large intracranial tumors found in neurofibromatosis can lead to impairment and loss of effective gag reflex and swallowing mechanisms,[192] which can leave the airway unprotected after extubation in these patients.

Additionally, some NF1 patients can have macrocephaly, mandibular abnormalities, and undiagnosed cervical spine instability, further complicating airway

TABLE 8–12   Pathologic Findings, Clinical Manifestations, and Diagnosis of Neurofibromatosis Types 1 and 2

	Type 1	Type 2
Neural Tissue Tumors	Neurofibromas (major feature) of the skin, peripheral nerves, and along nerve roots; plexiform neurofibromas (can become malignant), astrocytomas (not malignant), optic nerve gliomas	Vestibular (often called acoustic neuromas) or other cranial nerve schwannomas (main feature), spinal schwannomas, astrocytomas, meningiomas, ependymomas
Cutaneous Manifestations	Café-au-lait spots (usually the first symptom), cutaneous neurofibromas	Rare
Ocular Manifestations	Pigmented iris hamartomas or Lisch nodules	None
Central Nervous System (Besides Tumors)	Epilepsy, hydrocephalus, mild mental retardation more frequent than in general population	Intracerebral calcifications
Cardiovascular Involvement	Essential hypertension, renovascular (renal artery stenosis) hypertension, pheochromocytoma-related hypertension, vascular neurofibromatosis, aortic and cerebral aneurysms, obstruction of major thoracic vessels by neurofibromas	None
Pulmonary Involvement	Fibrosing alveolitis	None
Osseous Involvement	Many bone abnormalities, including chest deformities, kyphoscoliosis, sphenoid and occipital bone dysplasia, long-bone deformities, etc.	None
Other Systems	Neurofibromas of gastrointestinal system, intestinal carcinoid tumors, association with multiple endocrine neoplasia type III, which includes pheochromocytoma, NF1, and medullary thyroid carcinoma	None
Diagnostic Criteria	Cutaneous (95% of adult patients), nodular (peripheral nerves) and plexiform (30%) neurofibromas, café-au-lait spots, Lisch nodules (95%), optic nerve glioma	Bilateral acoustic neuromas or first-degree relative with NF2 in combination with unilateral acoustic neuroma, meningioma, glioma, or schwannoma
Symptoms	Symptomatic picture of NF1 is immensely diverse and determined by degree of involvement of various systems in the body. Severity of symptoms varies widely between patients	Tinnitus, poor balance caused by eighth nerve tumors. Headache, facial pain, facial numbness and other symptoms related to pressure effect of growing neural lesions

management. Patients with neurofibromas involving the cervical spine should be evaluated for cervical instability, including radiography, neck CT, or MRI as needed.

Cardiovascular Assessment. All NF1 patients should be screened for hypertension, which is common, and is caused by renal artery stenosis, catecholamine-secreting nodular plexiform neurofibroma, or pheochromocytoma (found in up to 1% of patients).[198] In patients with hypertension that is paroxysmal or resistant to routine treatment, it is essential to exclude pheochromocytoma, which is associated with high intraoperative morbidity and may lead to death if not detected preoperatively.[192] All patients with NF1 should be questioned for the presence of brief headaches, anxiety attacks, palpitations, and night sweats, which are common for pheochromocytoma. Coarctation of the abdominal or thoracic aorta is another rare cause of hypertension in NF1.

Other cardiovascular pathologic processes associated with NF1 include vena caval obstruction by mediastinal tumors, generalized vasculopathy caused by vascular nodular proliferation, and potential association with hypertrophic cardiomyopathy.[192]

Pulmonary Assessment. Pulmonary function should be evaluated for the presence of restrictive lung disease, which can be caused by kyphoscoliosis, intrapulmonary neurofibromas, and progressive pulmonary fibrosis associated with NF1.[192] Patients are questioned for the presence of cough or dyspnea. Chest radiography and arterial blood gas analysis are ordered if pulmonary involvement is suspected. It will help evaluate the need for postoperative ventilation and admission to an intensive care unit.

CNS Assessment. CNS tumors are major manifestations of both NF1 and NF2. Therefore, all patients must be evaluated for undiagnosed CNS tumors and increased ICP. Absence of intracranial or intraspinal tumors on earlier examinations cannot be relied on, because new asymptomatic tumors in different locations can appear over time. Also, new neurologic symptoms should not be ascribed to the preexisting CNS lesions and the possibility of new pathology should be explored.

Additionally, these patients should be assessed for the presence of epilepsy and questioned for the nature of their seizures and type of anticonvulsant therapy. The possibility of cerebral aneurysms or intracranial internal carotid artery stenosis should be investigated if the patient is symptomatic.[199] The brain stem structures can also be affected by neurofibroma or gliomas, which can lead to central hypoventilation, requiring ventilation support with prolonged weaning after surgery.[200] Mild mental retardation may be present in these patients, and the degree of the patient's cooperation should be evaluated.

Other Systems. Patients with NF1 may have carcinoid tumors, especially in the duodenum,[192] and present with carcinoid syndrome and significant risk of perioperative morbidity and mortality. Symptoms of carcinoid syndrome include flushing, bronchoconstriction, diarrhea, and right-sided heart lesions. Perioperative management of patients with carcinoid syndrome has been reviewed.[201] The association of NF1, carcinoid tumor, and pheochromocytoma would make the correct diagnosis especially difficult.[202]

NF1 in pregnancy presents an increased risk of severe hypertension, potentially rapid growth of CNS lesions, and intracranial hypertension. Patients should be assessed for the presence of an intraspinal tumor before the decision to employ neuraxial anesthesia is made. The association of pregnancy, NF1 and pheochromocytoma carries very high risks.[192]

Intraoperative Considerations. Anesthetic experience in patients with neurofibromatosis is limited to few case reports. The anesthetic challenges in these patients are many, and anesthetic management should be designed, based on the existing pathology and its severity.

Awake fiberoptic intubation is the preferred approach in patients with airway lesions, although even elective awake fiberoptic intubation can fail when gross anatomic distortion is present.[203] In pediatric or mentally impaired patients, an asleep fiberoptic intubation in a spontaneously breathing patient should be considered. Sevoflurane induction followed by fiberoptic intubation in spontaneously breathing patients has been successfully employed.[204] In all NF1

patients with complicated airway, advanced planning as outlined in the American Society of Anesthesiologists' guidelines for the difficult airway management[205] is advised. A difficult airway cart and possibly equipment for emergency tracheostomy should be immediately available, depending on the severity of airway distortion.

The severity of the cardiovascular or cerebrovascular pathology will dictate the extent of hemodynamic monitoring. An intra-arterial catheter is advised in all patients with severe hypertension and associated cerebrovascular pathology to ensure appropriate cerebral perfusion pressure. Use of central venous and/or pulmonary artery catheter should be reserved for patients with active pheochromocytoma, carcinoid syndrome, and cardiac lesions with advanced cardiac disease.

Neuraxial anesthesia should not be performed in patients with increased intracranial pressure or intraspinal lesions. The presence of significant kyphoscoliosis might also complicate conduction of neuraxial anesthesia. If it is perceived that neuraxial anesthesia is preferable because of the high risk of general anesthesia, spinal cord neurofibromas and intracranial hypertension need to be ruled out using CT or MRI.[206]

Although there have been many reports of altered response to nondepolarizing muscular blockers and succinylcholine, the results of a large retrospective study indicate that the response to various muscular blockers is unchanged in patients with neurofibromatoses.[192,207] However, neuromuscular blockade should be monitored, especially in NF1 patients with renal impairment or those receiving anticonvulsant therapy. Succinylcholine should be avoided in the presence of neurologic deficit.

There are no contraindications to any specific anesthetic agents. Potent inhalational agents and nitrous oxide should be used with caution in patients with large intracranial tumors and increased ICP.

Positioning of NF1 patients may be complicated by gross deformities of the chest, spine, or the neck. Potential cervical instability should be considered when positioning these patients. The combination of chest deformities and intrathoracic neurofibromas can lead to severe hemodynamic compromise caused by the sternal compression of the heart in the prone position.[208]

Careful planning for extubation is warranted in patients with difficult airway. Postoperative respiratory support and slow weaning may be necessary in patients with restrictive lung disease of hypoventilation syndromes due to the brain stem involvement.

Von Hippel-Lindau Disease

Pathophysiology and Diagnosis. Von Hippel-Lindau disease (VHLD) is an autosomal dominant neoplastic syndrome of variable expression. It is characterized by the development of various benign or malignant tumors and cystic

TABLE 8–13   Von Hippel-Lindau Disease: Distribution of Lesions by Organs, Frequency, Age at Onset and Clinical Symptomatology

	Frequency in Patients	Mean Age at Onset (yr)	Clinical Symptoms
CNS			
Retinal hemangioblastoma	25%-60%	25	Glaucoma, vision loss, blindness
CNS hemangioblastomas			
Cerebellum	44%-72%	33	Headache, nausea, ataxia, motor and sensory
Brainstem	10%-25%	32	deficits, hearing loss; pain syndromes
Spinal cord	13%-50%	33	
Lumbosacral nerve roots	<1%	Unknown	
Supratentorial	<1%	Unknown	
Endolymphatic sac tumors (petrous bone papillary adenoma)	11%	22	Hearing loss, tinnitus, vertigo, facial paresis
Syringomyelia	80% (in patients with CNS lesions)		
Visceral			
Renal cell carcinoma or cysts	25%-60%	39	Hematuria, flank pain
Pheochromocytoma	10%-20%	30	Often asymptomatic, with sudden hypertensive crisis
Pancreatic tumor or cysts	35%-70%	36	Abdominal pain, jaundice
Epididymal cystadenoma	25%-60%	Unknown	
Broad ligament cystadenoma	Unknown	Unknown	

lesions in many organ systems.[209] Whereas hemangioblastomas of the retina and the CNS are the most typical lesions found in VHLD patients, lesions of many other visceral organs are frequently found. Organ distribution of the lesions associated with VHLD, their frequency, mean age at onset, and relevant clinical symptoms can be found in Table 8-13. It is important to understand that the clinical presentation of VHLD is highly variable and progressive. Various tumors can affect multiple organs at the same time. Penetrance of VHLD increases with age, reaching 90% by the age of 60.[210] In the past, the majority of patients with VHDL died of complications of the renal cell carcinoma and CNS hemangioblastomas. With improvements in the treatment and diagnosis of VHDL, including serial screening and a multidisciplinary approach to management of these patients, their life expectancy has significantly improved.[209] Over their lifetime, the majority of patients with VHLD require surgical treatment under general anesthesia for the CNS hemangioblastomas, sometimes preceded by embolization, pheochromocytomas, and renal cell carcinoma.

Preoperative Preparation. There are a number of serious anesthetic concerns in patients with VHLD that need to be considered during preoperative evaluation. These patients need to be evaluated for the presence of pheochromocytomas, CNS lesions, and renal function impairment due to renal cell carcinoma.

Pheochromocytomas in VHLD can be multiple, bilateral, and, in some patients, the only manifestation of the disease, with 5% of the tumors being malignant. Although pheochromocytomas are found only in 10% to 20% of VHLD patients, the recent preoperative screening for hidden pheochromocytomas is essential because of the high potential for perioperative hypertensive crisis, and potential mortality associated with undiagnosed pheochromocytoma, especially in pregnancy.[211] The subject of anesthesia for a patient with pheochromocytoma has been reviewed and covered in Chapter 13.[212] Definitive diagnosis is based on demonstrating excessive production of catecholamines, by measuring urine and blood levels of catecholamines and urinary metanephrines, and supported by imaging tests (CT and MRI).[210]

CNS Hemangioblastomas. Patients with VHLD should be evaluated for the presence, distribution, and size of the CNS lesions. Symptoms of increased ICP or local mass effect can be present in these patients, as described in Table 8-13. The postoperative central hypoventilation syndrome and bulbar palsy with impairment of swallowing mechanisms have been reported after removal of brain stem hemangioblastomas.[213] Postoperative respiratory support and careful planning for extubation is warranted.

Intraoperative Considerations. The experience of anesthetic management of patients with VHLD is limited to a few case reports in the literature.[214-222] The choice of anesthesia and monitoring in these patients is dictated by the type of surgery performed and the extent of the existing pathology. For example, the anesthetic management for a patient undergoing posterior fossa decompression in the sitting position for the excision of intramedullary hemangioblastoma is very different from what it would be for nephrectomy for renal cell carcinoma. There is no contraindication to use of any specific anesthetic agents.

The use of an intra-arterial catheter is indicated for craniotomy and pheochromocytoma removal. Use of a central venous and/or pulmonary artery catheter is warranted for the removal of pheochromocytoma.

Neuraxial anesthesia has been successfully used for cesarean section or delivery in patients with VHLD.[214,216,220,222] However, risks related to use of neuraxial anesthesia in patients with an asymptomatic spinal cord and/or cerebellar hemangioblastomas should be carefully considered.[223]

Tuberous Sclerosis

Pathophysiology and Diagnosis. Tuberous sclerosis (TS) complex is inherited as an autosomal dominant trait with a prevalence in the general population of 1 in 50,000 to 300,000 people. It is a multisystem disorder primarily characterized by cutaneous and neurologic involvement. However, cardiac, pulmonary, and renal involvement have also been reported.[189] The clinical picture of TS is determined by what organs are involved and the extent of that involvement. However, the most frequent clinical presentation of TS is generalized or partial seizures, which typically start in early childhood. The severity and onset of the seizure disorder correlate with degree of developmental problems.[189]

The characteristic skin lesions are usually the first evidence of TS, with the most common being hypopigmented macula in different shapes (90%), adenoma sebaceum (50%), "shagreen" patches, café-au-lait spots, fibromas, and angiomas. The CNS pathology consists of subependymal nodules or giant cell astrocytomas (90%) and hamartomatous regions in the cortex called tubers, which give the name to the disorder and are believed to be the cause of seizures (80% to 100%) and mental retardation (50%). Developmental delays, mental retardation, and behavioral problems are found in 45% to 70% of patients with TS. Cardiac rhabdomyomas are present in up to 50% of infants with TS and often regress with age.[224] A high incidence of congenital heart disease in patients with TS has been reported.[224] Cardiac abnormalities secondary to TS can lead to obstruction of flow, congestive heart failure, arrhythmias, conduction delays, and preexcitation. Renal lesions composed of primary renal cysts and angiomyolipomas are found in half of all patients with TS. Renal angiomyolipomas are associated with early-onset severe hypertension and may result in renal hemorrhage.

Pulmonary cysts and lymphangiomyomatosis have been reported. Pleural thickening can lead to recurrent spontaneous pneumothorax. Upper airway fibromas and papillomas, involving the tongue, the palate, and, sometimes the larynx or the pharynx, have been reported in TS patients.

There is no specific treatment for the majority of TS manifestation, except for the standard medical anticonvulsant therapy. Based on the clinical series,[224] many of the patients with TS require general anesthesia for diagnostic or operative procedures in their childhood. The majority of them will do so for the surgical treatment of intractable seizures due to tuberous lesions.

Preoperative Preparation. Preoperative evaluation of patients with TS should be directed toward determination of the extent of neurologic, cardiovascular, pulmonary/airway, and renal involvement.

Data on the nature of seizure disorder, anticonvulsant medications and their effectiveness, degree of mental retardation, and behavioral problems should be collected. Patient cooperation is also assessed. Increased ICP due to intracranial lesions should be excluded.

Cardiovascular assessment includes an ECG and is performed in all patients to exclude arrhythmias, conduction defects, or preexcitation, which are often found in patients with rhabdomyomas. If heart involvement is suspected, an echocardiography and chest radiograph are performed to rule out congenital heart disease and congestive heart failure due to rhabdomyomas or TS pulmonary involvement.

The upper airway should be evaluated for the presence of TS nodular tumors. A history of spontaneous pneumothorax is noted, because it can recur and is associated with high mortality. Chest radiography and arterial blood gas analysis are ordered if pulmonary involvement is suspected. It will help evaluate the need for postoperative ventilation and admission to an intensive care unit.

Renal function should be assessed and associated hypertension ruled out.

Intraoperative Considerations. The experience of anesthetic management of patients with TS is limited to a number of case reports and retrospective series reported in the literature.[224-229] No specific anesthetic agents are contraindicated in TS, and the choice of anesthetic is determined by the magnitude of the surgical procedure and the severity of TS.

Airway management might be complicated in patients with airway lesions, and alternatives to direct laryngoscopy should be considered. Careful planning for extubation in these patients is warranted and is based on the size of the airway masses and extent of pulmonary involvement.

Anticonvulsant therapy should be optimized before surgery and continued throughout the perioperative period.

Anesthetic management is tailored to prevent exacerbation of seizures.

Neuromuscular blockade should be monitored with a nerve stimulator. The patients on chronic anticonvulsive therapy may have higher requirements for nondepolarizing muscle relaxants.[230]

Regional anesthesia is not contraindicated in TS patients and has been safely employed.[226]

Sturge-Weber Syndrome

Pathophysiology and Diagnosis. Sturge-Weber syndrome (SWS) is a rare congenital (not heritable) vascular disorder of unknown etiology.[190] Its hallmark manifestations are a facial angioma (port-wine stain) and a leptomeningeal angioma. The facial angioma, besides presenting a serious aesthetic problem for the patient, can also involve the eye structures, leading to glaucoma. In cases of increased intraocular pressure refractory to medication, surgical intervention is recommended. The leptomeningeal angioma is associated with progressive neurologic symptoms, such as seizures (80%), hemiparesis, mental retardation (50% to 66%), behavioral problems, visual field defects, and hydrocephalus. Seizures are treated with anticonvulsant therapy but may be refractory in more than 50% of cases. In refractory cases, hemispherectomy or limited surgical excision of epileptogenic tissue has been performed successfully. Differential diagnosis of SWS is not problematic, because clinical features do not overlap with other disorders. Prognosis for SWS patients is determined largely by the severity of seizures and by the size of leptomeningeal angioma. However, the disease is typically not fatal. There is no specific treatment for SWS, although the cutaneous, ocular, and neurologic manifestations of SWS are managed medically or surgically with mixed success.

Preoperative Preparation. Most of the patients with SWS requiring a surgical procedure will need it for the surgical treatment of facial or ocular angioma or removal of intracranial leptomeningeal angioma causing seizures that are refractory to medical therapy. Preoperative evaluation of patients with SWS should be directed toward determination of the extent of neurologic pathology and associated symptoms. Patients should be evaluated for signs of increased ICP and hydrocephalus. If the surgical procedure is not for the treatment of seizures, optimization of anticonvulsant therapy should be considered.

Intraoperative Consideration. There is little evidence in the literature to support any particular anesthetic approach to these patients. Two case reports in the literature describing anesthetic management of patients with SWS[231,232] do not provide information regarding adverse reactions to particular anesthetic regimens. Adverse outcomes related to use of general anesthesia are also not reported in the surgical literature concerned with the management of patients with SWS.

POSTERIOR FOSSA ANOMALIES AND ARNOLD-CHIARI MALFORMATIONS

The Arnold-Chiari malformation is a somewhat archaic eponym that is often used in the anesthesia literature to denote a group of congenital posterior fossa anomalies. This group of disorders includes many other disorders besides Chiari type I (CM I) and type II (CM II) malformations, and the list grows every year (Table 8-14). A great deal of semantic confusion, which exists in the literature regarding precise definition and classification of this group of disorders, can be explained by rapid progress being made in the neuroimaging characterization of existing pathology and in the understanding of brain stem and cerebellar development. However, the current lack of understanding of etiology and pathogenesis in most of these conditions precludes a complete classification that would be accepted in all the different fields of medicine involved with the management of these disorders. This topic has been reviewed.[233] It is out of the scope of this text to provide discussion about all of the posterior fossa anomalies. Therefore, we will limit ourselves to discussion of the CM I and CM II, which constitute the vast majority of all posterior fossa anomalies in the general population. The rest of these disorders, or at least some of them, and their characteristic features are presented in Table 8-14. It is worth mentioning that in the past the term *Arnold-Chiari malformation* was often used as a combined term for different types of posterior fossa abnormalities or used interchangeably with Chiari type I and II. To avoid this semantic confusion we use the Chiari I and II malformation definition, which is most commonly used in the modern literature.

Chiari I Malformation

Pathophysiology and Diagnosis. CM I is anatomically defined as an extension of the cerebellar tonsils below the foramen magnum. It is not associated with caudal displacement of the medulla or supratentorial abnormalities. The etiology of CM I is not well established. The small size of the posterior fossa causing the cerebellar displacement is the most likely explanation. Downward tonsillar displacement is not associated with any actual malformations of the cerebellum or midbrain structures found in most other posterior fossa anomalies.

The CM I is associated with the various skeletal and CNS abnormalities listed in Table 8-15. The diagnosis of the CM I in otherwise asymptomatic patients is made progressively more often during the investigation of these abnormalities with neuroimaging techniques.[234]

TABLE 8–14   Pathophysiology, Clinical Features and Associated Pathology in the Posterior Fossa Anomalies

Malformation Type	Pathophysiology	Clinical Features	Associated Pathology
Chiari type I malformation	Cerebellar tonsils displaced into cervical spinal canal, small posterior fossa	Usually presents in late teens or adult years; wide variety of neurologic symptoms caused by the upper cervical canal compression	Syringomyelia, syringobulbia, scoliosis, skeletal anomalies
Chiari type II malformation	Cerebellar vermis and brain stem displaced into cervical spinal canal	Presents at birth or early infancy; lower brain stem and cranial nerves dysfunction; could be medical emergency	Myelomeningocele and other lumbosacral neural tube closure defects, hydrocephalus, syringomyelia
Chiari type III malformation (very rare)	Cerebellum displaced into large occipital encephalocele	Respiratory and swallowing disorders, cranial nerves deficits, dystonias; often fatal	Corpus callosum agenesis, tentorium dysplasia, midbrain deformities
Dandy-Walker malformation	Cyst-like dilation of the fourth ventricle, enlarged posterior fossa, hypoplasia and anterior rotation of cerebellar vermis	Very heterogeneous in presentation, depending on associated pathology; ataxia, brain stem dysfunction, mental retardation (varies), hydrocephalus	Corpus callosum agenesis, brain stem anomalies, hydrocephalus
Jourbet's syndrome (extremely rare)	Cerebellar vermis aplasia	Motor hypotonia, ataxia, behavioral delay	Occipital meningocele, scoliosis, hydrocephalus, hepatic fibrosis
Cerebellar disruptions (very rare)	Cerebellar tissue loss	Motor deficits, mental retardation, often early death	
Pontocerebellar hypoplasia (very rare)	Pontine hypoplasia, cerebellar hypoplasia	Severe developmental disorders, seizures, often early death	-
Rhombencephalosy-napsis (extremely rare)	Cerebellar hemispheres fusion, vermis agenesis, fusion of dentate nuclei and superior cerebellar peduncles	Variable presentation; mental retardation, epilepsy, spasticity common	Hydrocephalus, ventriculomegaly

The signs and symptoms of the CM I can be divided into those caused by the compression of dural or neural structure by the displaced cerebellar tonsils and those related to the progressive development of syringomyelia (Table 8-16). The patients with CM I usually become symptomatic in the late teens. However, some may first display symptoms at a more advanced age, even in the presence of the syringomyelia.[235]

The differential diagnosis in CM I with syringomyelia is complex owing to a wide range of neurologic symptoms and signs observed in this condition. Many neurologic diseases of the spinal cord and cerebellum, including MS, SMA, ALS, spinocerebellar ataxias, mononeuropathy multiplex, cervical disc degenerative disease, and others have similar clinical picture. However, use of the CNS and skeletal imaging studies resolves most of these difficulties. A paucity of imaging findings in the presence of a florid clinical neurologic picture might make it difficult to differentiate CM I from hematomyelia, astrocytoma, or ependymoma of the spinal cord, Leigh disease, or necrotizing myelopathy.

Preoperative Preparation. The majority of situations in which patients with CM I will require anesthesia for a surgery fall under two categories:

1. Suboccipital craniectomy with or without cervical laminectomies for the decompression of neural structures trapped in the foramen magnum. Occasionally, decompression or shunting of the coexisting syrinx is required.

TABLE 8–15   Abnormalities Associated with Chiari Malformation Type 1

Associated Abnormality	Important Features
Skeletal	
Basilar impression	Decreased overall cervical spine mobility combined with cervical spine instability, increased risk of neurologic injury from minor trauma
Atlanto-occipital fusion	
Klippel-Feil syndrome	
Atlantoaxial assimilation	
Scoliosis	Common finding in patients with syringomyelia
Central Nervous System	
Syringomyelia	Usually maximal in the cervical cord

TABLE 8–16 Signs and Symptoms in Chiari Type 1 Malformation

Signs and Symptoms	Important Features
Caused by Compression at the Craniocervical Junction	
Occipital/posterior cervical pain	Associated with Valsalva maneuver
Weakness	Typically caused by the distortion of the medulla
Sensory deficits	
Hyperreflexia	
Babinski response	
Vocal cord paralysis, hoarseness, dysarthria	Typically caused by the involvement of the lower cranial nerves
Dysphagia, recurrent aspirations	
Sleep apnea	
Sinus bradycardia, syncope	
Ataxia	Symptoms of the rare cerebellar syndrome
Nystagmus	
Caused by Syringomyelia	
Upper limb weakness with atrophy	Usually starts distally at the hand and spreads proximally
Suspended sensory loss	Pain and temperature loss; touch and position preserved
Progressive scoliosis	
Lower motor neuron paralysis	

2. Anesthesia for labor and delivery and cesarean section in parturients with CM I.

Generally, both categories pose similar anesthetic risk, although their preoperative neurologic status typically differs. The patients scheduled for craniectomy already present with some degree of neurologic involvement, which indicates significant compression of the neural elements in the craniocervical junction. Most pregnant patients diagnosed with CM I are either asymptomatic or have already undergone surgical correction.[236]

Neurologic assessment is directed toward evaluation of signs of brain stem compression or cranial nerve involvement: vocal cord dysfunction, ventilation disorders, swallowing control. It is important to determine whether any neurologic symptoms are exacerbated with laughing, coughing, or exertion or during flexion-extension of the neck. Symptoms of increased intracranial pressure are sought. Appropriate imaging studies should be performed in all patients with suspected CM I. The presence of syringomyelia is determined even in patients without a clinical picture of myelopathy, especially in parturients, in whom neuraxial anesthesia is considered. The presence and location of motor deficit is noted to avoid overdosing nondepolarizing muscle relaxants by monitoring neuromuscular blockade on denervated muscles.

Autonomic function should be evaluated in patients with significant brain stem involvement. Subclinical autonomic dysfunction, a well-recognized condition in CM I, can result in unstable hemodynamics, lack of compensatory responses to hypotension, hypoxia, and hypocarbia intraoperatively.[237,238] The absence of heart rate beat-to-beat variability and lack of cardiac responses to postural maneuvers are good predictors of autonomic dysfunction.

Cervical spine assessment is directed toward evaluation of possible associated cervical spine abnormalities listed in Table 8-15. Limited range of motion could be due to cervical spine fusion combined with hypermobility between fused segments. Therefore, lateral and anteroposterior flexion-extension cervical spine radiographs are recommended.

Intraoperative Considerations.
General Anesthesia for Neurosurgical Procedures. There are a number of case reports in the literature regarding anesthetic management of these patients for suboccipital decompression.[238-242] There is no evidence that any

TABLE 8–17 Chiari Malformation Type II Clinical Presentation in Early and Late Childhood

	Signs and Symptoms	Implications
Children ≤ 2 Yr		
Increasing hydrocephalus Brain stem dysfunction Ninth and 10th cranial nerve dysfunction	Inspiratory stridor due to vocal cords abduction paralysis/paresis, apneic episodes (including cyanotic expiratory apnea of central origin), swallowing difficulties, chronic aspirations, weak gag reflex, dysphagia, malnutrition	Often emergency presentation; life threatening; shunt placement is lifesaving (although not in all infants)
Older Children		
Cervical myelopathy Syringomyelia	Weakness and spasticity of upper extremities, occipital headache, craniocervical pain, ataxia, sensory loss, scoliosis	Slowly progressing, rarely life threatening; decompressive surgery is often performed after normal cerebrospinal fluid shunt function confirmed

particular anesthetic agents are contraindicated for these patients. Although in one case the patient developed asystole after dural incision and draining of CSF, the patient promptly responded to atropine and ephedrine administration without sequelae.[242]

During induction of anesthesia and positioning, flexion-extension of the neck should be limited to prevent further compression of the neural structures. Fiberoptic bronchoscopic intubation, awake or asleep, is recommended in patients with skeletal cervical spine abnormalities and unstable cervical spine.[243] Careful planning for extubation, and possibly postoperative respiratory support with slow weaning, is indicated in patients with pronounced brain stem compression and cranial nerve involvement, owing to increased risk of postoperative ventilatory failure[238] or compromised upper airway reflexes.[244-246] Use of invasive monitoring is usually limited to the arterial line for measuring blood pressure and blood gases analysis in the postoperative period, if needed. Although, in the past, suboccipital decompression was often performed in the sitting position and was associated with high risk of venous air embolism, it is routinely performed in the prone position today. For this reason there is no need for right atrial catheter placement.

Anesthesia for Labor and Delivery. There are a number of case reports[247-253] and retrospective series[236] on anesthetic management in this group of patients. In patients without an elevated ICP or significant neurologic symptomatology at the time of delivery, it seems to be safe to employ epidural, spinal, or general anesthesia with inhalational agents, whether for vaginal delivery or cesarean section. In those patients with increased intracranial pressure and neurologic deficits associated with syringomyelia the risks and benefits for any form of anesthesia should be carefully weighed, bearing in mind that dural puncture may result in the sudden neurologic deterioration caused by further cerebellar herniation.[252,253] For labor, a combination of cervical and pudendal blocks, supplemented by parenteral opioids, could be the safest approach.[236] For a cesarean delivery, general endotracheal anesthesia directed toward preventing ICP elevations should be considered. Other considerations mentioned in the section for decompressive suboccipital craniotomy are also valid in these patients.

Chiari II Malformation, Myelomeningocele, and Hydrocephalus

Pathophysiology and Diagnosis. CM II is very distinct in its presentation, anatomy, prognosis, and outcomes from CM I. One of the most striking features of CM II is that it is present in practically every child born with meningomyelocele (MMC). Conversely, CM II is diagnosed only in children with MMC.[254] Additionally, hydrocephalus is found

or will develop in more than 80% of children born with MMC and CM II and often presents as a medical emergency requiring urgent shunt placement. Therefore, we are going to discuss these conditions and their implications for anesthesia care together.

Although the etiology of the CM II is not well understood, one of the possible and most likely explanations has been proposed by McLone and Knepper.[255] According to their theory, both open neural tube defect and incomplete spinal occlusion lead to CSF leakage out of the fetal spinal canal and ventricular system. The lack of ventricular CSF distention precludes the full development of the normal size posterior fossa, which, in turn, leads to the caudal displacement of the rapidly developing cerebellum into the spinal canal along with the brain stem. Anatomically, CM II is characterized by the caudal displacement of the cerebellar vermis (not the cerebellar tonsils, as in CM I) below the foramen magnum. The vermis could reach as far down as the upper thoracic spinal canal as the child ages. Other neuroanatomic anomalies typically found in CM II include small upward rotated cerebellum, caudal displacement of the medulla (and sometimes the pons) into the spinal canal, small posterior fossa, multiple ventricular anomalies, and small fourth ventricle and the aqueduct. The foramen magnum is often enlarged. Additionally, hypoplasia or aplasia of cranial nerve nuclei is often present (20%). Other associated abnormalities of MMC and CM II include neurogenic bladder, neurogenic bowel, multiple orthopedic deformities, and lower extremity fractures. These latter conditions often require repeated corrective surgical procedures under general anesthesia.

It is important to understand that the first indication of possible CM II in the newborn is the presence of MMC, which will require urgent repair. However, these neonates must be evaluated for the signs and symptoms of CM II. Asymptomatic CM II is the most common cause of death in children with MMC younger than 2 years of age. Close to one third of patients with MMC will develop symptoms of brain stem compression, and one third of them will die[254] before the age of 5 years. Therefore, all symptomatic CM II patients should be aggressively evaluated for hydrocephalus and considered for CSF shunt placement. Symptomatic CM II in children younger than 2 years typically has a different presentation than in older children (Table 8-17).

Preoperative Preparation. Most children with CM II undergo MMC repair procedure in the first hours of their life. The principles of anesthetic management for MMC repair can be found in most pediatric anesthesia texts. All other procedures typically required by these patients during their lifetime can be divided into three categories: emergency decompressive surgery or CSF shunt placement in stridorous infants, elective decompressive procedure (e.g., cervical laminectomies), or corrective surgical procedures for associated pathology (e.g., bladder surgery, orthopedic procedures) in patients without obvious symptoms of CM II.

Emergency Procedures. These patients should be evaluated for the signs of vocal cord dysfunction and breathing disorders. Patients with these symptoms may develop respiratory depression, such as apneic spells and vocal cord paralysis, even if the ICP is well controlled.[244,256] They should be monitored postoperatively in the ICU for the signs of apnea and the compromised airway. Careful planning for extubation is recommended. Volemic status should be evaluated in patients with unrepaired MMC, with potentially significant loss of CSF.

Elective Procedures. The most important step in the surgical and anesthetic preoperative evaluation of these patients is to rule out nonfunctioning shunt or latent hydrocephalus. Otherwise, the considerations are similar to those described in patients with CM I.

Intraoperative Considerations. Anesthetic management in the literature on CM II is limited to two case reports and a series. There are no clear contraindications to any particular anesthetic agents. Positioning of the patient may be a challenge, especially in those cases when shunt placement is performed simultaneously with MMC repair. Extremes of the neck flexion or extension should be avoided to prevent further compression of neural structures in the upper cervical canal.

Inhalational mask induction, even in the asymptomatic child, can be complicated by apneic spells and laryngospasm.[257]

In the past, when suboccipital decompressive craniectomy and duraplasty was performed, an increased risk of inadvertent hemorrhage from the occipital or transverse sinuses had to be considered in these patients. This life-threatening complication was associated with venous air embolism and carried very high mortality. This surgery is rarely recommended today. However, invasive hemodynamic monitoring is indicated for decompressive cervical laminectomies.

Succinylcholine should be avoided in patients with motor deficits, which are typically present in these patients after MMC repairs or as a result of cervical myelopathies. Neuromuscular blockade should be monitored on the limbs not affected by motor deficits to avoid overdosing.

Intraoperative considerations for orthopedic, urologic, and other corrective procedures in asymptomatic patients are similar to those in patients with CM I.

KLIPPEL-FEIL SYNDROME AND OTHER CERVICAL SPINE DISORDERS OF CHILDHOOD

Anesthetic care of patients with cervical spine disorders resulting from congenital or developmental alterations in childhood represent a unique and complex challenge. Increased susceptibility to cervical spine injury and subsequent neurologic deficit, often combined with anatomically difficult airway, are common for this diverse group of disorders of different etiology. Understanding of the anatomic and pathophysiologic features of these disorders, thorough preoperative evaluation, and appropriate early management are essential in prevention of neurologic injury and other anesthetic complications in these patients.[258,259] Klippel-Feil syndrome is a member of this group and is often mentioned in the anesthetic literature. It also presents one of the most formidable anesthetic challenges. For simplicity of presentation, other disorders in this section are discussed in conjunction with the discussion of the preoperative evaluation and anesthetic management of this syndrome.

Pathophysiology and Diagnosis. Klippel-Feil syndrome is a rare (1 in 42,000 births) congenital anomaly of the cervical spine typically characterized by fusion of two

---

TABLE 8–18 Cervical Spine Disorders		
Disorder	**Cervical Spine Abnormalities**	**Symptoms**
Down syndrome	Occipitocervical or atlantoaxial instability	Muscle weakness, gait abnormality, neck pain
Achondroplasia	Foramen magnum stenosis, lumbar spine stenosis, cervical instability is uncommon	Severe sleep apnea and sudden death in early childhood
Spondyloepiphyseal dysplasia	Odontoid hypoplasia and/or os odontoideum with atlantoaxial instability	Persistent hypotonia, motor developmental delay
Mucopolysaccharidoses, Morquio syndrome	Odontoid hypoplasia with atlantoaxial instability and progressive myelopathy, extradural soft tissue hypertrophy	Severe neurologic compromise secondary to upper cervical spinal cord compression, sudden death
Isolated odontoid anomalies: aplasia, hypoplasia, os odontoideum	Progressive atlantoaxial instability	Symptoms of upper cervical spinal cord injury, sudden death

or more cervical vertebrae. It is unclear whether Klippel-Feil syndrome is a discrete entity with common genetic etiology or a phenotypic presentation of a heterogeneous group of congenital spinal deformities.[260] The classic triad of short neck, low posterior hairline, and limitations of cervical motion are found in less than half of patients with this condition. Other common associated findings include congenital scoliosis (50% of patients), renal abnormalities (one third of patients), the Sprengel deformity (congenital elevation of scapula), hearing impairment, posterior fossa dermoid cysts, and congenital heart disease (the most frequent being ventricular septal defect). Overall decreased neck mobility is the most common physical finding. This finding is often combined with hypermobility between fused vertebral segments, which puts these patients at high risk for either spontaneous neurologic injury, or neurologic injury as a result of minor trauma.[261] Many neurologic symptoms caused by cranial nerve abnormalities, cervical radiculopathy, or myelopathy are typically found in the second or third decade of life. Most neurologic manifestations are secondary to chronic compression of the cervical spinal cord, pons, medulla, and stretching of the cranial nerves. Sudden neck movement or minor falls can cause basilar artery insufficiency and syncope. Tetraplegia has been reported as a result of minor trauma in these patients.[261] This syndrome is often classified into three different types, depending on the location of the fused cervical vertebrae. The presentation of clinical and anatomic features of this syndrome varies widely, ranging from mild deformity to severe disability.

Alternative Conditions. Cervical spine abnormalities similar to those observed in Klippel-Feil syndrome are frequently seen in other uncommon disorders listed in Table 8-18.[258] Cervical instability, increased risk of severe neurologic injury from minor trauma, and difficult airway is common for all of these conditions. A full description of these disorders and relevant anesthetic issues can be found either in the subsequent sections of this chapter or other chapters of this book.

Preoperative Preparation. Preoperative assessment in patients with cervical spine disorders should primarily be directed at the evaluation of degree of cervical instability present, preexistent neurologic impairment, and the evaluation of airway. A previous uneventful anesthetic history is a poor predictor of difficult airway or neurologic complications in patients with Klippel-Feil syndrome, because cervical fusion becomes progressively worse with time.[262] Therefore, lateral and anteroposterior flexion-extension cervical spine radiographs are recommended. Cervical MRI is indicated to assess the degree of neurologic involvement, such as cord compression and myelopathy. Other perioperative considerations should

include the following:

1. Congenital heart defects and cardiac conduction abnormalities. Preoperative ECG and echocardiography are indicated.
2. Assessment of pulmonary function, which could be severely compromised in patients with chest deformities and advanced scoliosis. Consider chest radiography and pulmonary function tests.
3. Renal function. Patients with Klippel-Feil syndrome should be evaluated for kidney anomalies and renal failure.

Intraoperative Considerations. Anesthetic experience in Klippel-Feil syndrome patients is limited to a number of case reports.[243,259,263-267] The main anesthetic challenge in these patients is airway management and positioning.

Airway Management. Awake fiberoptic intubation is the preferred approach whenever possible.[243,263,267] However, most pediatric and mentally impaired (Down syndrome) patients are not suitable candidates, and asleep fiberoptic intubation in a spontaneously breathing patient should be considered. Direct laryngoscopy is likely to be difficult owing to multiple facial, neck, and chest deformities. However, when direct laryngoscopy is chosen, a neutral neck axis needs to be maintained to avoid neurologic sequelae. The laryngeal mask airway can be used to ventilate these patients, although intubation via laryngeal mask may be technically difficult.[264]

Positioning. Positioning of patients with Klippel-Feil syndrome may be difficult owing to multiple head, neck, and thoracic deformities. Great care must be taken to avoid any cervical tension or sudden neck movements while positioning these patients. It is important to understand that the risk of neurologic injury in these patients is not limited to laryngoscopy and intubation and may develop thereafter.[259,263,268]

Regional anesthesia has been successfully performed in these patients[265,266] and might be preferable if indicated, to avoid potential neurologic and respiratory complications related to airway management. It can be difficult to perform considering various spine deformities associated with this condition.

Neuromuscular Blockade. Succinylcholine should be avoided in the presence of neurologic deficit. In patients with associated renal anomalies accompanied by renal failure, the use of nondepolarizing muscle relaxants for which excretion is dependent on renal function is contraindicated.

Other Issues. Careful planning for extubation is warranted in patients with significantly compromised pulmonary function and after very difficult intubation. There are no contraindications to any specific anesthetic drugs in these patients.

Acknowledgment

This chapter is based on the chapter on Neurologic Diseases in the third and fourth editions of Anesthesia and Uncommon Diseases, authored by Drs. Martz, Schreibman, and Matjasko, who provided a comprehensive approach. We have reorganized this chapter by sections, keeping some of the disease categories but changing others to reflect current neurology nomenclature.

References

1. Nicholson G, Pereira AC, Hall GM: Parkinson's disease and anaesthesia. Br J Anaesth 2002;89:904-916.
2. Adams RD, Victor M, Ropper AH (eds): Principles of Neurology. New York, McGraw-Hill, 1997.
3. Berg D, Becker G, Reiners K: Reduction of dyskinesia and induction of akinesia induced by morphine in two parkinsonian patients with severe sciatica. J Neural Transm 1999;106:725-728.
4. Anderson BJ, Marks PV, Futter ME: Propofol: Contrasting effects in movement disorders. Br J Neurosurg 1994;8:387-388.
5. Gravlee GP: Succinylcholine-induced hyperkalemia in a patient with Parkinson's disease. Anesth Analg 1980;59:444-446.
6. Cooperman LH: Succinylcholine-induced hyperkalemia in neuromuscular disease. JAMA 1970;213:1867-1871.
7. Muzzi DA, Black S, Cucchiara RF: The lack of effect of succinylcholine on serum potassium in patients with Parkinson's disease. Anesthesiology 1989;71:322.
8. Veasy LG, Tani LY, Hill HR: Persistence of acute rheumatic fever in the intermountain area of the United States. J Pediatr 1994;124:9-16.
9. Carapetis JR, Currie BJ: Rheumatic chorea in northern Australia: A clinical and epidemiological study. Arch Dis Child 1999;80:353-358.
10. Aron, AM, Freeman, JM, Cavalcanti, F: The natural history of Sydenham's chorea: Review of the literature and long-term evaluation with emphasis on cardiac sequelae. Am J Med 1965;38:83.
11. Trottier Y, Lutz Y, Stevanin G, et al: Polyglutamine expansion as a pathological epitope in Huntington's disease and four dominant cerebellar ataxias. Nature 1995;378:403-406.
12. Schaffar G, Breuer P, Boteva R, et al: Cellular toxicity of polyglutamine expansion proteins: Mechanism of transcription factor deactivation. Mol Cell 2004;15:95-105.
13. Bence NF, Sampat RM, Kopito RR: Impairment of the ubiquitin-proteasome system by protein aggregation. Science 2001;292:1552-1555.
14. Kells AP, Fong DM, Dragunow M, et al: AAV-mediated gene delivery of BDNF or GDNF is neuroprotective in a model of Huntington disease. Mol Ther 2004;9:682-628.
15. Bloch J, Bachoud-Levi AC, Deglon N, et al: Neuroprotective gene therapy for Huntington's disease, using polymer-encapsulated cells engineered to secrete human ciliary neurotrophic factor: results of a phase I study. Hum Gene Ther 2004;15:968-975.
16. Davies DD: Abnormal response to anaesthesia in a case of Huntington's chorea. Br J Anaesth 1966;38:490-491.
17. Soar J, Matheson KH: A safe anaesthetic in Huntington's disease? Anaesthesia 1993;48:743-744.
18. Farina J, Rauscher L: Anaesthesia and Huntington's chorea: A report of two cases. Br J Anaesth 1977;49:1149-1167.
19. Browne M: Anaesthesia in Huntington's chorea. Anaesthesia 1982;38:65.
20. Gupta K, Leng CP: Anaesthesia and juvenile Huntington's disease. Paediatr Anaesth 2000;10:107-109.
21. Gaubatz CL, Wehner RJ: Anesthetic considerations for the patient with Huntington's disease. AANA J 1992;60:41-44.
22. Cangemi CF Jr, Miller RJ: Huntington's disease: Review and anesthetic case management. Anesth Progress 1998;45:150-153.
23. Nagele P, Hammerle AF: Sevoflurane and mivacurium in a patient with Huntington's chorea. Br J Anaesth 2000;85:320-321.
24. Gualandi W, Bonfanti G: [A case of prolonged apnea in Huntington's chorea]. Acta Anaesth 1968;19(Suppl 6):235-238.
25. Mitra S, Sharma K, Arora S, et al: Repeat anesthetic management of a patient with Huntington's chorea. Can J Anaesth 2001;48:933-934.
26. Gillman MA, Sandyk R: Nitrous oxide ameliorates spasmodic torticollis. Eur Neurol 1985;24:292-293.
27. Stemp LI, Taswell C: Spastic torticollis during general anesthesia: Case report and review of receptor mechanisms. Anesthesiology 1991;75:365-366.
28. Steen SN: Anesthetic management for basal ganglia surgery in patients with movement disorders. Anesth Analg 1965;44:66-69.
29. Worms PM: The epidemiology of motor neuron diseases: A review of recent studies. J Neurol Sci 2001;191:3-9.
30. Andersen PM, Sims KB, Xin WW, et al: Sixteen novel mutations in the Cu/Zn superoxide dismutase gene in amyotrophic lateral sclerosis: A decade of discoveries, defects and disputes. Amyotroph Lateral Scler Other Motor Neuron Disord 2003;4:62-73.
31. Turner JB, Atkin DJ, Farg AM, et al: Impaired extracellular secretion of mutant superoxide dismutase 1 associates with neurotoxicity in familial amyotrophic lateral sclerosis. J Neurosci 2005;1:108-117.
32. Storkebaum E: Treatment of motoneuron degeneration by intracerebroventricular delivery of VEGF in a rat model of ALS. Neuroscience 2005;8:85-92.
33. Gronert GA, Lambert EH, Theye RA: The response of denervated skeletal muscle to succinylcholine. Anesthesiology 1973;39:13-22.
34. Rosenbaum KJ, Neigh JL, Strobel GE: Sensitivity to nondepolarizing muscle relaxants in amyotrophic lateral sclerosis: Report of two cases. Anesthesiology 1971;35:638-641.
35. Otsuka N, Igarashi M, Shimodate Y, et al: [Anesthetic management of two patients with amyotrophic lateral sclerosis (ALS)]. [Japanese]. Masui 2004;53:1279-1281.
36. Hara K, Sakura S, Saito Y, et al: Epidural anesthesia and pulmonary function in a patient with amyotrophic lateral sclerosis. Anesth Analg 1996;83:878-879.
37. Lacomblez L, Bensimon G, Leigh PN, et al: Dose-ranging study of riluzole in amyotrophic lateral sclerosis. Amyotrophic Lateral Sclerosis/Riluzole Study Group II. Lancet 1996;347:1425-1431.
38. Mitsumoto H: Riluzole—what is its impact in our treatment and understanding of amyotrophic lateral sclerosis? Ann Pharmacother 1997;31:779-781.
39. Miller RG, Mitchell JD, Lyon M, Moore DH: Riluzole for amyotrophic lateral sclerosis (ALS)/motor neuron disease (MND). Cochrane Database Syst Rev 2002;(2):CD001447.
40. Labuda M, Labuda D, Miranda C: Unique origin and specific ethnic distribution of the Friedreich ataxia GAA expansion. Neurology 2000;54:2322.
41. Durr A, Cossee M, Agid Y, et al: Clinical and genetic abnormalities in patients with Friedreich's ataxia. N Engl J Med 1996;335:1169-1175.
42. Campuzano V, Montermini L, Molto MD, et al: Friedreich's ataxia: Autosomal recessive disease caused by an intronic GAA triplet repeat expansion. Science 1996;271:1423-1427.
43. Levent K, Yavuz G, Kamil T: Anaesthesia for Friedreich's ataxia: Case report. Min Anestesiol 2000;66:657-660.
44. Buettner AU: Anaesthesia for caesarean section in a patient with spinal muscular atrophy. Anaesth Intensive Care 2003;31:92-94.
45. Kitson R, Williams V, Howell C: Caesarean section in a parturient with type III spinal muscular atrophy and pre-eclampsia. Anaesthesia 2004;59:94-95.
46. McLoughlin L, Bhagvat P: Anaesthesia for caesarean section in spinal muscular atrophy type III. Int J Obstet Anesth 2004;13:192-195.
47. Watts JC: Total intravenous anaesthesia without muscle relaxant for eye surgery in a patient with Kugelberg-Welander syndrome. Anaesthesia 2003;58:96.

48. Habib AS, Helsley SE, Millar S, et al: Anesthesia for cesarean section in a patient with spinal muscular atrophy. J Clin Anesth 2004;16:217-219.

49. De Jonghe B, Sharshar T, Lefaucheur JP, et al: Groupe de Reflexion et d'Etude des Neuromyopathies en Reanimation: Paresis acquired in the intensive care unit: A prospective multicenter study. JAMA 2002;288:2859-2867.

50. Deem S, Lee CM, Curtis JR: Acquired neuromuscular disorders in the intensive care unit. Am J Respir Crit Care Med 2003;168:735.

51. Larsson L, Li X, Edstrom L, et al: Acute quadriplegia and loss of muscle myosin in patients treated with nondepolarizing neuromuscular blocking agents and corticosteroids: Mechanisms at the cellular and molecular levels. Crit Care Med 2000;28:34-45.

52. Feasby TE, Gilbert JJ, Brown WF, et al: An acute axonal form of Guillain-Barré polyneuropathy. Brain 1986;109:1115-1126.

53. Yuki N, Yoshino H, Sato S, Miyatake T: Acute axonal polyneuropathy associated with anti-GM1 antibodies following *Campylobacter* enteritis. Neurology 1990;40:1900-1902.

54. McKhann GM, Cornblath DR, Griffin JW, et al: Acute motor axonal neuropathy: A frequent cause of acute flaccid paralysis in China. Ann Neurol 1993;33:333-342.

55. Visser LH, Van der Meche FG, Van Doorn PA, et al: Guillain-Barré syndrome without sensory loss (acute motor neuropathy): A subgroup with specific clinical, electrodiagnostic and laboratory features. Dutch Guillain-Barré Study Group. Brain 1995;118:841-847.

56. Ho TW, Mishu B, Li CY, et al: Guillain-Barré syndrome in northern China: Relationship to *Campylobacter jejuni* infection and anti-glycolipid antibodies. Brain 1995;118:597-605.

57. Fisher M: An unusual variant of acute idiopathic polyneuritis (syndrome of ophthalmoplegia, ataxia and areflexia). N Engl J Med 1956;255:56-57.

58. Hahn AF: Guillain-Barré syndrome. Lancet 1998;352:635-641.

59. Jacobs BC, Rothbarth PH, Van der Meche FG, et al: The spectrum of antecedent infections in Guillain-Barré syndrome: A case-control study. Neurology 1998;51:1110-1115.

60. Osterman PO, Fagius J, Lundemo G, et al: Beneficial effects of plasma exchange in acute inflammatory polyradiculoneuropathy. Lancet 1984;2:1296-1299.

61. Brooks H, Christian AS, May AE: Pregnancy, anaesthesia and Guillain-Barré syndrome. Anaesthesia 2000;55:894-898.

62. Ohta M, Nishikawa N, Kida H, Miyao S: [Anesthetic management of two patients with polymyositis]. Masui 2000;49:1371-1373, 2000. Japanese.

63. Fujita A, Okutani R, Fu K: [Anesthetic management for colon resection in a patient with polymyositis]. Masui 1996;45:334-336. Japanese.

64. Rockelein S, Gebert M, Baar H, Endsberger G: [Neuromuscular blockade with atracurium in dermatomyositis]. Anaesthesist 1995;44:442-444. German.

65. Artru AA: Relationship between cerebral blood volume and CSF pressure during anesthesia with isoflurane or fentanyl in dogs. Anesthesiology 1984;60:575-579.

66. Artru AA: Effects of halothane and fentanyl on the rate of CSF production in dogs. Anesth Analg 1983;62:581-585.

67. Artru AA: Isoflurane does not increase the rate of CSF production in the dog. Anesthesiology 1984;60:193-197.

68. Sugioka S: [Effects of sevoflurane on intracranial pressure and formation and absorption of cerebrospinal fluid in cats]. Masui 1992;41:1434-1442. Japanese.

69. Artru AA, Momota T: Rate of CSF formation and resistance to reabsorption of CSF during sevoflurane or remifentanil in rabbits. J Neurosurg Anesth 2000;12:37-43.

70. Walchenbach R, Geiger E, Thomeer RT, Vanneste JA: The value of temporary external lumbar CSF drainage in predicting the outcome of shunting on normal pressure hydrocephalus. J Neurol Neurosurg Psychiatry 2002;72:503-506.

71. Kaul HL, Jayalaxmi T, Gode GR, Mitra DK: Effect of ketamine on intracranial pressure in hydrocephalic children. Anaesthesia 1976;31:698-701.

72. Krauss JK, Regel JP, Vach W, et al: Vascular risk factors and arteriosclerotic disease in idiopathic normal-pressure hydrocephalus of the elderly. Stroke 1996;27:24-29.

73. Tsai TC, He CC, Wu SZ, et al: Normal pressure hydrocephalus found after anesthesia—a case report. Acta Anaesth Sin 2003;41:197-200.

74. Kristensen B, Malm J, Fagerland M, et al: Regional cerebral blood flow, white matter abnormalities, and cerebrospinal fluid hydrodynamics in patients with idiopathic adult hydrocephalus syndrome. J Neurol Neurosurg Psychiatry 1996;60:282-288.

75. Vanneste JA: Three decades of normal pressure hydrocephalus: Are we wiser now? J Neurol Neurosurg Psychiatry 1994;57:1021-1025.

76. Black PM: Idiopathic normal-pressure hydrocephalus: Results of shunting in 62 patients. J Neurosurg 1980;52:371-377.

77. Wikkelso C, Andersson H, Blomstrand C, et al: Normal pressure hydrocephalus: Predictive value of the cerebrospinal fluid tap-test. Acta Neurol Scand 1986;73:566-573.

78. Knopman DS: An overview of common non-Alzheimer dementias. Clin Geriatr G Med 2001; 17(2):281-301.

79. Malm J, Kristensen B, Markgren P, Ekstedt J: CSF hydrodynamics in idiopathic intracranial hypertension: A long-term study. Neurology 1992;42:851-858.

80. Owler BK, Parker G, Halmagyi GM, et al: Pseudotumor cerebri syndrome: Venous sinus obstruction and its treatment with stent placement. J Neurosurg 2003;98:1045-1055.

81. Karahalios DG, Rekate HL, Khayata MH, Apostolides PJ: Elevated intracranial venous pressure as a universal mechanism in pseudotumor cerebri of varying etiologies. Neurology 1996;46:198-202.

82. Jain N, Rosner F: Idiopathic intracranial hypertension: Report of seven cases. Am J Med 1992;93:391-395.

83. Rosenberg ML, Corbett JJ, Smith C, et al: Cerebrospinal fluid diversion procedures in pseudotumor cerebri. Neurology 1993;43:1071-1072.

84. Spoor TC, McHenry JG: Long-term effectiveness of optic nerve sheath decompression for pseudotumor cerebri. Arch Ophthalmol 1993;111:632-635.

85. Kelman SE, Heaps R, Wolf A, Elman MJ: Optic nerve decompression surgery improves visual function in patients with pseudotumor cerebri. Neurosurgery 1992;30:391-395.

86. Corbett JJ, Thompson HS: The rational management of idiopathic intracranial hypertension. Arch Neurol 1989;46:1049-1051.

87. Kelman SE, Sergott RC, Cioffi GA, et al: Modified optic nerve decompression in patients with functioning lumboperitoneal shunts and progressive visual loss. Ophthalmology 1991;98:1449-1453.

88. Abouleish E, Ali V, Tang RA: Benign intracranial hypertension and anesthesia for cesarean section. Anesthesiology 1985;63:705-707.

89. Biyani A, el Masry WS: Post-traumatic syringomyelia: A review of the literature. Paraplegia 1994;32(11):723-731.

90. Adler R, Lenz G: Neurological complaints after unsuccessful spinal anaesthesia as a manifestation of incipient syringomyelia. Eur J Anaesthesiol 1998;15:103-105.

91. Agusti M, Adalia R, Fernandez C, Gomar C: Anaesthesia for caesarean section in a patient with syringomyelia and Arnold-Chiari type I malformation. Int J Obstet Anesth 2004;13:114-116.

92. Deen HG Jr, McGirr SJ: Vertebral artery injury associated with cervical spine fracture: Report of two cases. Spine 1992;17:230-234.

93. Atkinson PP, Atkinson JL: Spinal shock. Mayo Clin Proc 1996;71: 384-389.

94. Hambly PR, Martin B: Anaesthesia for chronic spinal cord lesions. Anaesthesia 1998;53:273-289.

95. Murphy DB, McGuire G, Peng P: Treatment of autonomic hyperreflexia in a quadriplegic patient by epidural anesthesia in the postoperative period. Anesth Analg 1999;89:148-149.

96. Noetzel MJ: Diagnosing "undiagnosed" leukodystrophies: The role of molecular genetics. Neurology 2004;62:847-848.

97. Kenealy SJ, Pericak-Vance MA, Haines JL: The genetic epidemiology of multiple sclerosis. J Neuroimmunol 2003;143:7-12.

98. Haines JL, Bradford Y, Garcia ME, et al: Multiple Sclerosis Genetics Group: Multiple susceptibility loci for multiple sclerosis. Hum Mol Genet 2002;11:2251-2256.

99. Gade-Andavolu R, Comings DE, MacMurray J, et al: RANTES: A genetic risk marker for multiple sclerosis. Multiple Sclerosis 2004;10:536-539.

99A. Davis FA, Michael FA, Neer D: Serial hyperthermia testing in multiple sclerosis related to circadian temperature variations. Acta Neurol Scand 1973;49(1):63-74

100. Edmund J, Fog T: Visual and motor instability in multiple sclerosis. Arch Neurol Psychiatry 1955;73:316-320.

101. Siemkowicz E: Multiple sclerosis and surgery. Anaesthesia 1976;31:1211-1216.

102. Baskett PJ, Armstrong R: Anaesthetic problems in multiple sclerosis: Are certain agents contraindicated? Anaesthesia 1970;25:397-401.

103. Bamford C, Sibley W, Laguna J: Anesthesia in multiple sclerosis. Can J Neurol Sci 1978;5:41-44.

104. Kytta J, Rosenberg PH: Anaesthesia for patients with multiple sclerosis. Ann Chir Gynaecol 1984;73:299-303.

105. Schapira K, Poskanzer DC, Miller H: Familial and conjugal multiple sclerosis. Acta Neurol Scand 1966;42(Suppl 19):83-84.

106. Warren TM, Datta S, Ostheimer GW: Lumbar epidural anesthesia in a patient with multiple sclerosis. Anesth Analg 1982;61:1022-1023.

107. Berger JM, Ontell R: Intrathecal morphine in conjunction with a combined spinal and general anesthetic in a patient with multiple sclerosis. Anesthesiology 1987;66:400-402.

108. Bader AM, Hunt CO, Datta S, et al: Anesthesia for the obstetric patient with multiple sclerosis. J Clin Anesth 1988;1:21-24.

109. Leigh J, Fearnley SJ, Lupprian KG: Intrathecal diamorphine during laparotomy in a patient with advanced multiple sclerosis. Anaesthesia 1990;45:640-642.

110. Crawford JS: Regional analgesia for patients with chronic neurological disease and similar conditions. Anesthesia 1981;36:821-822.

111. Abouleish E: Neurological diseases. In James FM, Wheeler AS (eds): Obstetric Anesthesia: The Complicated Patient. Philadelphia, FA Davis, 1988, pp 110-111.

112. Belani KG, Krivit W, Carpenter BL, et al: Children with mucopolysaccharidosis: Perioperative care, morbidity, mortality, and new findings. J Pediatr Surg 1993;28:403-408.

113. Baines D, Keneally J: Anaesthetic implications of the mucopolysaccharidoses: A fifteen-year experience in a children's hospital. Anaesth Intensive Care 1983;11:198-202.

114. Walker RW, Darowski M, Morris P, Wraith JE: Anaesthesia and mucopolysaccharidoses: A review of airway problems in children. Anaesthesia 1994;49:1078-1084.

115. Herrick IA, Rhine EJ: The mucopolysaccharidoses and anaesthesia: A report of clinical experience. Can J Anaesth 1988;35:67-73.

116. Shinhar SY, Zablocki H, Madgy DN: Airway management in mucopolysaccharide storage disorders. Arch Otolaryngol Head Neck Surg 2004;130:233-237.

117. Hopkins R, Watson JA, Jones JH, Walker M: Two cases of Hunter's syndrome—the anaesthetic and operative difficulties in oral surgery. Br J Oral Surg 1973;10:286-299.

118. Wippermann CF, Beck M, Schranz D, et al: Mitral and aortic regurgitation in 84 patients with mucopolysaccharidoses. Eur J Pediatr 1995;154:98-101.

119. Braunlin EA, Hunter DW, Krivit W, et al: Evaluation of coronary artery disease in the Hurler syndrome by angiography. Am J Cardiol 1992;69:1487-1489.

120. Morgan KA, Rehman MA, Schwartz RE: Morquio's syndrome and its anaesthetic considerations. Paediatr Anaesth 2002;12:641-644.

121. Tobias JD: Anesthetic care for the child with Morquio syndrome: General versus regional anesthesia. J Clin Anesth 1999;11:242-246.

122. Kempthorne PM, Brown TC: Anaesthesia and the mucopolysaccharidoses: A survey of techniques and problems. Anaesth Intensive Care 1983;11:203-207.

123. Sjogren P, Pedersen T, Steinmetz H: Mucopolysaccharidoses and anaesthetic risks. Acta Anaesthesiol Scand 1987;31:214-218.

124. King DH, Jones RM, Barnett MB: Anaesthetic considerations in the mucopolysaccharidoses. Anaesthesia 1984;39:126-131.

125. Diaz JH, Belani KG: Perioperative management of children with mucopolysaccharidoses. Anesth Analg 1993;77:1261-1270.

126. Walker RW: The laryngeal mask airway in the difficult paediatric airway: An assessment of positioning and use in fibreoptic intubation. Paediatr Anaesth 2000;10:53-58.

127. Dullenkopf A, Holzmann D, Feurer R, et al: Tracheal intubation in children with Morquio syndrome using the angulated video-intubation laryngoscope. Can J Anaesth 2002;49:198-202.

128. Klein CJ: Pathology and molecular genetics of inherited neuropathy. J Neurol Sci 2004;220:141-143.

129. Mersiyanova IV, Ismailov SM, Polyakov AV, et al: Screening for mutations in the peripheral myelin genes PMP22, MPZ and Cx32 (GJB1) in Russian Charcot-Marie-Tooth neuropathy patients. Hum Mutat 2000;15:340-347.

130. Roy EP III, Gutmann L, Riggs JE: Longitudinal conduction studies in hereditary motor and sensory neuropathy type 1. Muscle Nerve 1989;12:52-55.

131. Dematteis M, Pepin JL, Jeanmart M, et al: Charcot-Marie-Tooth disease and sleep apnoea syndrome: A family study. Lancet 2001;357:267-272.

132. Rudnik-Schoneborn S, Rohrig D, Nicholson G, Zerres K: Pregnancy and delivery in Charcot-Marie-Tooth disease type 1. Neurology 1993;43:2011-2016.

133. Yoshioka R, Dyck PJ, Chance PF: Genetic heterogeneity in Charcot-Marie-Tooth neuropathy type 2. Neurology 1996;46:569-571.

134. Eichacker PQ, Spiro A, Sherman M, et al: Respiratory muscle dysfunction in hereditary motor sensory neuropathy, type I. Arch Intern Med 1988;148:1739-1740.

135. Nathanson BN, Yu DG, Chan CK: Respiratory muscle weakness in Charcot-Marie-Tooth disease: A field study. Arch Intern Med 1989;149:1389-1391.

136. Reah G, Lyons GR, Wilson RC: Anaesthesia for caesarean section in a patient with Charcot-Marie-Tooth disease. Anaesthesia 1998;53:586-588.

137. Tetzlaff JE, Schwendt I: Arrhythmia and Charcot-Marie-Tooth disease during anesthesia. Can J Anaesth 2000;47:829.

138. Yim SY, Lee IY, Moon HW, et al: Hypertrophic neuropathy with complete conduction block—hereditary motor and sensory neuropathy type III. Yonsei Med J 1995;36:466-472.

139. Ginz HF, Ummenhofer WC, Erb T, Urwyler A: [The hereditary motor-sensory neuropathy Charcot-Marie-Tooth disease: Anesthesiologic management—case report with literature review]. Anaesthesist 2001;50:767-771. German.

140. Gratarola A, Mameli MC, Pelosi G: Total intravenous anaesthesia in Charcot-Marie-Tooth disease: Case report. Min Anestesiol 1998;64:357-360.

141. Niiyama Y, Kanaya N, Namiki A: [Anesthetic management for laparoscopic surgery in a patient with Charcot-Marie-Tooth disease]. Masui 2003;52:524-526. Japanese.

142. Roelofse JA, Shipton EA: Anaesthesia for abdominal hysterectomy in Charcot-Marie-Tooth disease: A case report. S Afr Med J 1985;67:605-606.

143. Sugino S, Yamazaki Y, Nawa Y, et al: [Anesthetic management for a patient with Charcot-Marie-Tooth disease using propofol and nitrous oxide]. Masui 2002;51:1016-1019. Japanese.

144. Tanaka S, Tsuchida H, Namiki A: [Epidural anesthesia for a patient with Charcot-Marie-Tooth disease, mitral valve prolapse syndrome and IInd degree AV block]. Masui 1994;43:931-933. Japanese.

145. Huang J, Soliman I: Anaesthetic management for a patient with Dejerine-Sottas disease and asthma. Paediatr Anaesth 2001;11:225-227.

146. Antognini JF: Anaesthesia for Charcot-Marie-Tooth disease: A review of 86 cases. Can J Anaesth 1992;39:398-400.

147. Greenberg RS, Parker SD: Anesthetic management for the child with Charcot-Marie-Tooth disease. Anesth Analg 1992;74:305-307.

148. Cooperman LH: Succinylcholine-induced hyperkalemia in neuromuscular disease. JAMA 1970;213:1867-1871.

149. Baraka AS: Vecuronium neuromuscular block in a patient with Charcot-Marie-Tooth syndrome. Anesth Analg 1997;84:927-928.

150. Naguib M, Samarkandi AH: Response to atracurium and mivacurium in a patient with Charcot-Marie-Tooth disease. Can J Anaesth 1998;45:56-59.

151. Fiacchino F, Grandi L, Ciano C, Sghirlanzoni A: Unrecognized Charcot-Marie-Tooth disease: Diagnostic difficulties in the assessment of recovery from paralysis. Anesth Analg 1995;81:199-201.

152. Pogson D, Telfer J, Wimbush S: Prolonged vecuronium neuromuscular blockade associated with Charcot-Marie-Tooth neuropathy. Br J Anaesth 2000;85:914-917.

153. Scull T, Weeks S: Epidural analgesia for labour in a patient with Charcot-Marie-Tooth disease. Can J Anaesth 1996;43:1150-1152.

154. Sugai K, Sugai Y: [Epidural anesthesia for a patient with Charcot-Marie-Tooth disease, bronchial asthma and hypothyroidism]. Masui 1989;38:688-691. Japanese.

155. Brian JE Jr, Boyles GD, Quirk JG Jr, Clark RB: Anesthetic management for cesarean section of a patient with Charcot-Marie-Tooth disease. Anesthesiology 1987;66:410-412.

156. Byrne DL, Chappatte OA, Spencer GT, Raju KS: Pregnancy complicated by Charcot-Marie-Tooth disease, requiring intermittent ventilation. Br J Obstet Gynaecol 1992;99:79-80.

157. Kotani N, Hirota K, Anzawa N, et al: Motor and sensory disability has a strong relationship to induction dose of thiopental in patients with the hypertropic variety of Charcot-Marie-Tooth syndrome. Anesth Analg 1996;82:182-186.

158. Axelrod FB, Hilz MJ: Inherited autonomic neuropathies. Semin Neurol 2003;23:381-390.

159. Kritchman MM, Schwartz H, Paper EM: Experiences with general anesthesia in patients with familial dysautonomia. JAMA 1959;170:529-533.

160. McCaughey TJ: Familial dysautonomia as an anaesthetic hazard. Can Anaesth Soc J 1965;12:558-568.

161. Axelrod FB, Donenfeld RF, Danziger F, Turndorf H: Anesthesia in familial dysautonomia. Anesthesiology 1988;68:631-635.

162. Challands JF, Facer EK: Epidural anaesthesia and familial dysautonomia (the Riley Day syndrome): Three case reports. Paediatr Anaesth 1998;8:83-88.

163. Szold A, Udassin R, Maayan C, et al: Laparoscopic-modified Nissen fundoplication in children with familial dysautonomia. J Pediatr Surg 1996;31:1560-1562.

164. Udassin R, Seror D, Vinograd I, et al: Nissen fundoplication in the treatment of children with familial dysautonomia. Am J Surg 1992;164:332-336.

165. Wengrower D, Gozal D, Gozal Y, et al: Complicated endoscopic pediatric procedures using deep sedation and general anesthesia are safe in the endoscopy suite. Scand J Gastroenterol 2004;39:283-286.

166. Beilin B, Maayan C, Vatashsky E, et al: Fentanyl anesthesia in familial dysautonomia. Anesth Analg 1985;64:72-76.

167. Okuda K, Arai T, Miwa T, Hiroki K: Anaesthetic management of children with congenital insensitivity to pain with anhidrosis. Paediatr Anaesth 2000;10:545-548.

168. Rozentsveig V, Katz A, Weksler N, et al: The anaesthetic management of patients with congenital insensitivity to pain with anhidrosis. Paediatr Anaesth 2004;14:344-348.

169. Tomioka T, Awaya Y, Nihei K, et al: Anesthesia for patients with congenital insensitivity to pain and anhidrosis: A questionnaire study in Japan. Anesth Analg 2002;94:271-274.

170. Marti MJ, Tolosa E, Campdelacreu J: Clinical overview of the synucleinopathies. Mov Disord 2003;18(Suppl 6):S21-S27.

171. Kaufmann H, Biaggioni I: Autonomic failure in neurodegenerative disorders. Semin Neurol 2003;23:351-363.

172. Isono S, Shiba K, Yamaguchi M, et al: Pathogenesis of laryngeal narrowing in patients with multiple system atrophy. J Physiol 2001;536:237-249.

173. Dewhurst A, Sidebottom P: Anaesthetic management of a patient with multiple system atrophy (Shy-Drager syndrome) for urgent hip surgery. Hosp Med 1999;60:611.

174. Gomesz FA, Montell M: Caudal anaesthesia in the Shy-Drager syndrome. Anaesthesia 1992;47:1100.

175. Hack G, Engels K, Greve I, Rapp S: [Anesthesiologic implications in the Shy-Drager syndrome—a case report]. Anasth Intensivther Notfallmed 1990;25:362-366. German.

176. Harioka T, Miyake C, Toda H, et al: [Anesthesia for Shy-Drager syndrome; effects of elastic bandage, phenylephrine, and IPPV]. Masui 1989;38:801-804. Japanese.

177. Hashimoto H, Nishiyama T, Nagase Y, et al: [Anesthesia for emergency surgery in a patient with Shy-Drager syndrome]. Masui 2001;50:40-41. Japanese.

178. Hutchinson RC, Sugden JC: Anaesthesia for Shy-Drager syndrome. Anaesthesia 1984;39:1229-1231.

179. Malinovsky JM, Cozian A, Rivault O: Spinal anesthesia for transurethral prostatectomy in a patient with multiple system atrophy. Can J Anaesth 2003;50:962-963.

180. Niquille M, Van Gessel E, Gamulin Z: Continuous spinal anesthesia for hip surgery in a patient with Shy-Drager syndrome. Anesth Analg 1998;87:396-399.

181. Saarnivaara L, Kautto UM, Teravainen H: Ketamine anaesthesia for a patient with the Shy-Drager syndrome. Acta Anaesthesiol Scand 1983;27:123-125.

182. Tsen LC, Smith TJ, Camann WR: Anesthetic management of a parturient with olivopontocerebellar degeneration. Anesth Analg 1997;85:1071-1073.

183. Yazawa R, Kondo T, Miyashita T, et al: [Anesthetic management of a patient with olivopontocerebellar atrophy using heart rate variability (HRV)]. Masui 2004;53:55-58. Japanese.

184. Bevan DR: Shy-Drager syndrome: A review and a description of the anaesthetic management. Anaesthesia 1979;34:866-873.

185. Vallejo R, DeSouza G, Lee J: Shy-Drager syndrome and severe unexplained intraoperative hypotension responsive to vasopressin. Anesth Analg 2002;95:50-52.

186. Shannon J, Jordan J, Costa F, et al: The hypertension of autonomic failure and its treatment. Hypertension 1997;30:1062-1067.

187. McBeth C, Murrin K: Subarachnoid block for a case of multiple system atrophy. Anaesthesia 1997;52:889-892.

188. Kida K, Mori M, Yoshitake S, et al: [Anesthetic management for a patient with pure autonomic failure]. Masui 1997;46:813-817. Japanese.

189. Korf BR: The phakomatoses. Clin Dermatol 2005;23:78-84.

190. Baselga E: Sturge-Weber syndrome. Semin Cutan Med Surg 2004;23:87-98.

191. Ruggieri M: The different forms of neurofibromatosis. Childs Nerv Syst 1999;15:295-308.

192. Hirsch NP, Murphy A, Radcliffe JJ: Neurofibromatosis: Clinical presentations and anaesthetic implications. Br J Anaesth 2001;86:555-564.

193. Crozier WC: Upper airway obstruction in neurofibromatosis. Anaesthesia 1987;42:1209-1211.

194. Reddy AR: Unusual case of respiratory obstruction during induction of anaesthesia. Can Anaesth Soc J 1972;19:192-197.

195. Dodge TL, Mahaffey JE, Thomas JD: The anesthetic management of a patient with an obstructing intratracheal mass: A case report. Anesth Analg 1977;56:295-298.

196. el Oakley R, Grotte GJ: Progressive tracheal and superior vena caval compression caused by benign neurofibromatosis. Thorax 1994;49:380-381.

197. Rees G: Neurofibroma of the recurrent laryngeal nerve. Chest 1971;60:414-418.

198. Delgado JM, de la Matta MM: Anaesthetic implications of von Recklinghausen's neurofibromatosis. Paediatr Anaesth 2002;12:374.

199. Zhao JZ, Han XD: Cerebral aneurysm associated with von Recklinghausen's neurofibromatosis: A case report. Surg Neurol 1998;50:592-596.

200. Sforza E, Colamaria V, Lugaresi E: Neurofibromatosis associated with central alveolar hypoventilation syndrome during sleep. Acta Paediatr 1994;83:794-796.

201. Vaughan DJ, Brunner MD: Anesthesia for patients with carcinoid syndrome. Int Anesthesiol Clin 1997;35:129-142.

202. Wheeler MH, Curley IR, Williams ED: The association of neurofibromatosis, pheochromocytoma, and somatostatin-rich duodenal carcinoid tumor. Surgery 1986;100:163-169.

203. Wulf H, Brinkmann G, Rautenberg M: Management of the difficult airway: A case of failed fiberoptic intubation. Acta Anaesthesiol Scand 1997;41:1080-1082.

204. Wang CY, Chiu CL, Delilkan AE: Sevoflurane for difficult intubation in children. Br J Anaesth 1998;80:408.

205. Practice guidelines for management of the difficult airway: An updated report by the American Society of Anesthesiologists Task Force on Management of the Difficult Airway. Anesthesiology 2003;98:1269-1277.

206. Dounas M, Mercier FJ, Lhuissier C, Benhamou D: Epidural analgesia for labour in a parturient with neurofibromatosis. Can J Anaesth 1995;42:420-422.

207. Richardson MG, Setty GK, Rawoof SA: Responses to nondepolarizing neuromuscular blockers and succinylcholine in von Recklinghausen neurofibromatosis. Anesth Analg 1996;82:382-385.

208. Alexianu D, Skolnick ET, Pinto AC, et al: Severe hypotension in the prone position in a child with neurofibromatosis, scoliosis and pectus excavatum presenting for posterior spinal fusion. Anesth Analg 2004;98:334-335.

209. Lonser RR, Glenn GM, Walther M, et al: von Hippel-Lindau disease. Lancet 2003;361:2059-2067.

210. Hes FJ, van der Luijt RB, Lips CJ: Clinical management of Von Hippel-Lindau (VHL) disease. Neth J Med 2001;59:225-234.

211. Harrington JL, Farley DR, van Heerden JA, Ramin KD: Adrenal tumors and pregnancy. World J Surg 1999;23:182-186.

212. O'Riordan JA: Pheochromocytomas and anesthesia. Int Anesthesiol Clin 1997;35:99-127.

213. Wang C, Zhang J, Liu A, Sun B: Surgical management of medullary hemangioblastoma: Report of 47 cases. Surg Neurol 2001;56:218-226.

214. Berl M, Dubois L, Belkacem H, et al: [Von Hippel-Lindau disease and obstetric anaesthesia: 3 cases report]. Ann Fr Anesth Reanim 2003;22:359-362. French.

215. Boker A, Ong BY: Anesthesia for Cesarean section and posterior fossa craniotomy in a patient with von Hippel-Lindau disease. Can J Anaesth 2001;48:387-390.

216. Demiraran Y, Ozgon M, Utku T, Bozkurt P: Epidural anaesthesia for Caesarean section in a patient with von Hippel-Lindau disease. Eur J Anaesthesiol 2001;18:330-332.

217. Ercan M, Kahraman S, Basgul E, Aypar U: Anaesthetic management of a patient with von Hippel-Lindau disease: A combination of bilateral phaeochromocytoma and spinal cord haemangioblastoma. Eur J Anaesthesiol 1996;13:81-83.

218. Gurunathan U, Korula G: Unsuspected pheochromocytoma: von Hippel-Lindau disease. J Neurosurg Anesthesiol 2004;16:26-28.

219. Joffe D, Robbins R, Benjamin A: Caesarean section and phaeochromocytoma resection in a patient with Von Hippel Lindau disease. Can J Anaesth 1993;40:870-874.

220. Matthews AJ, Halshaw J: Epidural anaesthesia in von Hippel-Lindau disease: Management of childbirth and anaesthesia for caesarean section. Anaesthesia 1986;41:853-855.

221. Mugawar M, Rajender Y, Purohit AK, et al: Anesthetic management of von Hippel-Lindau syndrome for excision of cerebellar hemangioblastoma and pheochromocytoma surgery. Anesth Analg 1998;86:673-674.

222. Wang A, Sinatra RS: Epidural anesthesia for cesarean section in a patient with von Hippel-Lindau disease and multiple sclerosis. Anesth Analg 1999;88:1083-1084.

223. Monge E, Botella M, Rueda ML, Navia J: [Anesthesia for cesarean section in a patient with von Hippel-Lindau disease]. Rev Esp Anestesiol Reanim 2002;49:377-380. Spanish.

224. Shenkman Z, Rockoff MA, Eldredge EA, et al: Anaesthetic management of children with tuberous sclerosis. Paediatr Anaesth 2002;12:700-704.

225. Papaioannou EG, Staikou CV, Lambadarioui A, et al: Anesthetic management of a patient with tuberous sclerosis presenting for renal transplantation. J Anesth 2003;17:193-195.

226. Tsukui A, Noguchi R, Honda T, et al: Aortic aneurysm in a four-year-old child with tuberous sclerosis. Paediatr Anaesth 1995;5:67-70.

227. Ong EL, Koay CK: Tuberous sclerosis presenting for laparotomy. Anaesth Intensive Care 2000;28:94-96.

228. Nott MR, Halfacre J: Anaesthesia for dental conservation in a patient with tuberous sclerosis. Eur J Anaesthesiol 1996;13:413-415.

229. Lee JJ, Imrie M, Taylor V: Anaesthesia and tuberous sclerosis. Br J Anaesth 1994;73:421-425.

230. Soriano SG, Kaus SJ, Sullivan LJ, Martyn JA: Onset and duration of action of rocuronium in children receiving chronic anticonvulsant therapy. Paediatr Anaesth 2000;10:133-136.

231. Ceyhan A, Cakan T, Basar H, et al: Anaesthesia for Sturge-Weber syndrome. Eur J Anaesthesiol 1999;16:339-341.

232. Batra RK, Gulaya V, Madan R, Trikha A: Anaesthesia and the Sturge-Weber syndrome. Can J Anaesth 1994;41:133-136.

233. Boltshauser E: Cerebellum-small brain but large confusion: A review of selected cerebellar malformations and disruptions. Am J Med Genet A 2004;126:376-385.

234. Steinbok P: Clinical features of Chiari I malformations. Childs Nerv Syst 2004;20:329-331.

235. Takigami I, Miyamoto K, Kodama H, et al: Foramen magnum decompression for the treatment of Arnold Chiari malformation type I with associated syringomyelia in an elderly patient. Spinal Cord 2005;43:249-251.

236. Chantigian RC, Koehn MA, Ramin KD, Warner MA: Chiari I malformation in parturients. J Clin Anesth 2002;14:201-205.

237. Nogues MA, Newman PK, Male VJ, Foster JB: Cardiovascular reflexes in syringomyelia. Brain 1982;105:835-849.

238. Williams DL, Umedaly H, Martin IL, Boulton A: Chiari type I malformation and postoperative respiratory failure. Can J Anaesth 2000;47:1220-1223.

239. Kakinuma H, Saito Y, Sato H, Kobayashi T: [Blind orotracheal intubation using Trachilight in a pediatric patient with Arnold-Chiari malformation]. Masui 1999;48:1253-1254. Japanese.

240. Keyaki A, Makita Y, Nabeshima S, et al: [Surgical management of syringomyelia associated with Arnold-Chiari malformation, primary IgA deficiency and chromosomal abnormality—a case report]. Nippon Geka Hokan 1990;59:161-167. Japanese.

241. Nakayama Y, Sonoda H, Namiki A: [Propofol anesthesia for a patient with Arnold-Chiari deformity]. Masui 1998;47:726-729. Japanese.

242. Sellery GR: Intraoperative problem during surgery for Chiari malformation. Can J Anaesth 2001;48:718.

243. Daum RE, Jones DJ: Fibreoptic intubation in Klippel-Feil syndrome. Anaesthesia 1988;43:18-21.

244. Choi SS, Tran LP, Zalzal GH: Airway abnormalities in patients with Arnold-Chiari malformation. Otolaryngol Head Neck Surg 1999;121:720-724.

245. Ruff ME, Oakes WJ, Fisher SR, Spock A: Sleep apnea and vocal cord paralysis secondary to type I Chiari malformation. Pediatrics 1987;80:231-234.

246. Wynn R, Goldsmith AJ: Chiari type I malformation and upper airway obstruction in adolescents. Int J Pediatr Otorhinolaryngol 2004;68:607-611.

247. Agusti M, Adalia R, Fernandez C, Gomar C: Anaesthesia for caesarean section in a patient with syringomyelia and Arnold-Chiari type I malformation. Int J Obstet Anesth 2004;13:114-116.

248. Landau R, Giraud R, Delrue V, Kern C: Spinal anesthesia for cesarean delivery in a woman with a surgically corrected type I Arnold Chiari malformation. Anesth Analg 2003;97:253-255.

249. Nel MR, Robson V, Robinson PN: Extradural anaesthesia for caesarean section in a patient with syringomyelia and Chiari type I anomaly. Br J Anaesth 1998;80:512-515.

250. Semple DA, McClure JH: Arnold-Chiari malformation in pregnancy. Anaesthesia 1996;51:580-582.

251. Sicuranza GB, Steinberg P, Figueroa R: Arnold-Chiari malformation in a pregnant woman. Obstet Gynecol 2003;102:1191-1194.

252. Barton JJ, Sharpe JA: Oscillopsia and horizontal nystagmus with accelerating slow phases following lumbar puncture in the Arnold-Chiari malformation. Ann Neurol 1993;33: 418-421.

253. Hullander RM, Bogard TD, Leivers D, et al: Chiari I malformation presenting as recurrent spinal headache. Anesth Analg 1992;75: 1025-1026.

254. Stevenson KL: Chiari type II malformation: Past, present, and future. Neurosurg Focus 2004;16:E5.

255. McLone DG, Knepper PA: The cause of Chiari II malformation: A unified theory. Pediatr Neurosci 1989;15:1-12.

256. Nishino H, Kinouchi K, Fukumitsu K, et al: [Anesthesia and perioperative management in infants with Chiari type II malformation]. Masui 1998;47:982-986. Japanese.

257. Shiraishi M, Minami K, Horishita T, Shigematsu A: [Difficult ventilation during induction of anesthesia in a patient with Arnold-Chiari malformation type II]. Masui 2001;50:776-778. Japanese.

258. Herman MJ, Pizzutillo PD: Cervical spine disorders in children. Orthop Clin North Am 1999;30:457-466, ix.

259. Naguib M, Farag H, Ibrahim A: Anaesthetic considerations in Klippel-Feil syndrome. Can Anaesth Soc J 1986;33:66-70.

260. Tracy MR, Dormans JP, Kusumi K: Klippel-Feil syndrome: Clinical features and current understanding of etiology. Clin Orthop 2004;183-190.

261. Nagib MG, Maxwell RE, Chou SN: Identification and management of high-risk patients with Klippel-Feil syndrome. J Neurosurg 1984;61:523-530.

262. Thompson E, Haan E, Sheffield L: Autosomal dominant Klippel-Feil anomaly with cleft palate. Clin Dysmorphol 1998;7:11-15.

263. Farid IS, Omar OA, Insler SR: Multiple anesthetic challenges in a patient with Klippel-Feil syndrome undergoing cardiac surgery. J Cardiothorac Vasc Anesth 2003;17:502-505.

264. Sakai H, Takizawa K, Miura N, Suzuki M: [Anesthetic management of a child with Klippel-Feil syndrome associated with severe scoliosis]. Masui 2001;50:645-647. Japanese.

265. O'Connor PJ, Moysa GL, Finucane BT: Thoracic epidural anesthesia for bilateral reduction mammoplasty in a patient with Klippel-Feil syndrome. Anesth Analg 2001;92:514-516.

266. Dresner MR, Maclean AR: Anaesthesia for caesarean section in a patient with Klippel-Feil syndrome: The use of a microspinal catheter. Anaesthesia 1995;50:807-809.

267. Burns AM, Dorje P, Lawes EG, Nielsen MS: Anaesthetic management of caesarean section for a mother with pre-eclampsia, the Klippel-Feil syndrome and congenital hydrocephalus. Br J Anaesth 1988;61:350-354.

268. Hall JE, Simmons ED, Danylchuk K, Barnes PD: Instability of the cervical spine and neurological involvement in Klippel-Feil syndrome: A case report. J Bone Joint Surg Am 1990;72:460-462.

9 Muscle Diseases

MICHAEL K. URBAN, MD, PHD, and SALIM LAHLOU, MD

Since the writing of this chapter by J. D. Miller and H. Rosenbaum, the genetic defects and molecular mechanisms involved in many of the muscle diseases have been elucidated. In some cases this makes the management of patients with these diseases easier. However, it still requires an astute clinician to make the diagnosis of a muscle disease and assess the magnitude of the compromise in normal physiologic functions. Complaints of fatigue, weakness, and polymyalgias are commonly reported symptoms. These are nonspecific symptoms whose etiology may extend from neuromuscular disorders through rheumatologic problems to psychiatric conditions. A detailed neuromuscular physical examination and routine diagnostic testing, including electromyography (EMG), serum electrolytes, thyroid function tests, and serum creatine kinase evaluation may not provide a definitive diagnosis. In fact, many of these patients may have a final nonspecific diagnosis of "fibromyalgia" or chronic fatigue syndrome, but some will have life-threatening muscle disorders that must be recognized if they are to have any chance of effective treatment.

Perioperative respiratory complications are a major concern for patients with muscular diseases. General anesthesia and surgery, particularly abdominal and thoracic, result in postoperative pulmonary changes, specifically a loss of lung volumes and an increase in the alveolar-arterial gradient. This is the reason for a postoperative pulmonary complication rate of 25% to 48%. Patients with chronic respiratory muscle weakness have a higher incidence of postoperative respiratory complications because of the loss of respiratory reserve. In addition, their inability to take deep inspirations and cough makes them more susceptible to atelectasis and pneumonia. However, a preoperative diagnosis of respiratory compromise may be difficult in patients with skeletal muscle weakness, because their respiratory reserve is rarely challenged. Preoperative pulmonary function testing of these patients provides an assessment of the severity of the pulmonary disease and potential pulmonary risk of undergoing the planned procedure. Patients with deteriorating skeletal muscle strength can also develop kyphoscoliosis with concomitant restrictive lung disease.

If possible, the administration of muscle relaxants should be avoided and, when required, a long-acting agent should be avoided. Hypomotility of the gastrointestinal tract may lead to delayed gastric emptying and increase the risk of pulmonary aspiration. This would favor securing the airway via rapid-sequence induction with succinylcholine; however, in some muscle diseases this has been associated with ventricular fibrillation, rhabdomyolysis, and malignant hyperthermia.

Because some of these patients will also have a cardiomyopathy, the depressant effects of volatile anesthetics may provoke congestive heart failure. The respiratory depressant effects of a narcotic anesthetic may, however, require prolonged postoperative respiratory support. In all cases, after general anesthesia one must anticipate the possibility of postoperative ventilation and, once extubated, the need for intensive respiratory therapy. Regional anesthesia avoids some of the complications of general anesthesia and may provide a vehicle for postoperative analgesia without employing narcotics. However, even if regional techniques are employed to reduce anesthetic requirements and provide postoperative pain management, it may still be necessary to protect the airway and ensure adequate oxygenation during the procedure through the use of general endotracheal anesthesia.

These points are all common considerations when anesthetizing patients with muscle diseases. In this chapter our goal is to delineate the characteristics of specific muscle diseases and how these diseases will impact on our perioperative plans.

MUSCULAR DYSTROPHIES

Muscular dystrophies are a group of hereditary myopathic diseases characterized by progressive weakness. Clinical presentation is heterogeneous, from severe fatal childhood forms to relatively benign adult forms. They are all best characterized by painless degeneration and atrophy of skeletal muscles without evidence of muscle denervation.[1] Originally these diseases were characterized on the basis of their clinical presentation, for example, limb-girdle myopathy. The discovery of dystrophin and related molecules has given "muscular dystrophy" a molecular biologic basis for diagnosis, genetic mapping, and treatment.[2] Dystrophin is a large (427-kb) rod-shaped protein, which comprises about 5% of the membrane-associated cytoskeletal protein[3,4]; its gene is located on the short arm of the X chromosome. Dystrophin, with several other sarcolemmal proteins, stabilizes the muscle surface membrane during contraction and relaxation (Fig. 9-1). The dystrophin-associated complex binds intracellular actin to the extracellular basal lamina, which mechanically stabilizes the sarcolemma during muscle contraction.

Pathophysiology

Muscular dystrophies are characterized by degeneration of the skeletal muscle fibers and replacement with fibrous and fatty connective tissue, without accumulation of metabolic intermediate substrates. There is no evidence for direct neurologic involvement. The breakdown of the muscle fiber sarcolemma occurs early in the disease, with an influx of calcium and the activation of proteases, and the eventual destruction of tissue by inflammatory elements.

Duchenne's dystrophy (DMD, also called pseudo-hypertrophic dystrophy) is the most common form, seen in 1 per 3500 births. The myopathy is associated with

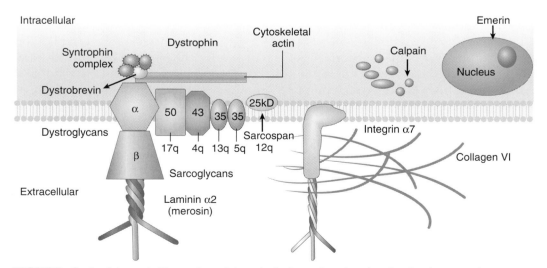

FIGURE 9–1 Schematic illustration of the principal extrajunctional molecules that are relevant to muscular dystrophy. *(Reprinted from Molnar MJ, Karpati MJ: Muscular dystrophies related to deficiency of sarcolemmal proteins. In Schapira AH, Griggs RC [eds]: Muscle Diseases. Boston, Butterworth-Heinemann, 1999, p 84.)*

mutations of the dystrophin gene located in the Xp21 stripe, inherited as a sex-linked recessive trait, with most of the reported cases being male. However, there are well-documented cases in females with a severity ranging from full Duchenne's to mild weakness. Transmission of this disease in female offspring of normal fathers can occur when there is early inactivation of the normal X chromosome (Lyon hypothesis). Only one X chromosome is active in any cell, with inactivation of the other X-chromosome occurring early in embryogenesis. Some heterozygotic females with Duchenne's dystrophy would then be expected to carry the abnormal X chromosome as the only active dystrophin gene in most cells. Female children with Turner's syndrome (XO) would also present with the disease. It is unclear whether heterozygotic females pose the same anesthetic risks as males with DMD.[5]

Diagnosis and Differential Diagnosis

Progressive and symmetrical skeletal muscle weakness and wasting are the prominent features of DMD.[6] The initial clinical presentation involves a waddling gait, frequent falling, and difficulty climbing stairs owing to proximal muscle weakness in the pelvic girdle. There is also weakness in the shoulder girdle and trunk erectors, leading to thoracolumbar scoliosis. Certain muscles, particularly the calves, demonstrate early hypertrophy. The pelvic girdle and proximal leg muscle weakness is responsible for Gowers' sign, the child climbing up his or her legs to stand up. However, usually until age 3 to 5 the child's condition goes undiagnosed. This is rapidly followed by atrophy of the other proximal muscles. All muscles are ultimately involved except for the cranial muscles and the external anal sphincter. Because of lack of denervation, there is intact sensation, but the proximal deep tendon reflexes disappear in half of the cases by age 10. The earlier the onset, the more rapid the downhill course. Usually the child is unable to walk by age 9 to 11 years. Joint contractures appear during this period, due to the uneven loss of agonist and antagonist muscle groups. Degeneration of cardiac muscle leads to a dilated cardiomyopathy. Scarring of the posterobasal portion of the left ventricle produces tall right precordial R waves and deep left precordial Q waves in the electrocardiogram. Mitral regurgitation may also be present due to papillary muscle dysfunction. Respiratory muscle weakness is detectable by age 10, but the diaphragm is usually spared. Inability to cough and clear secretions predisposes these patients to pneumonia, which is often fatal by about the third decade. These patients also have lower than average intelligence and mild cerebral atrophy, presumably due to the lack of normal brain dystrophin. About 15% of patients have a much slower disease course, which stabilizes about the time of puberty. Some clinicians believe that exercise enhances muscle destruction; however, physical therapy that involves passive movement to prevent contractures and resistive exercises for the lungs to increase endurance may be helpful. Because contractures represent a major disability for DMD patients, they often have elective operative procedures to relieve these contractures. Hence, perioperative complications that prolong their inactivity may actually exacerbate their condition by preventing the important postoperative physical therapy.

The plasma muscle enzymes aldolase and creatine kinase (CK) levels are elevated severalfold early in the progression of the disease. The MB fraction of CK, normally present only in heart muscle, cannot be used as a guide to cardiac injury because it is also elevated, owing to the destruction of regenerating skeletal muscle in DMD.[7,8] CK levels are highest (50 to 100 times normal) up to age 3 years and then decrease by about 20% per year as muscle atrophies. Increased plasma levels of liver enzymes have also been noted (aminotransferases, lactate dehydrogenase); however, liver damage has not been described in DMD, suggesting a skeletal origin. Skeletal muscle biopsy early in the disease process may demonstrate necrosis and phagocytosis of muscle fibers, as well as areas of vigorous muscle regeneration. Immunostaining reveals the complete lack of dystrophin at the surface of the muscle fibers. Although DNA testing can detect multiple deletions, duplications, and point mutations in the dystrophin gene, proximal limb muscle biopsy remains the standard for diagnosis.

In Table 9-1 we have listed the other less common forms of muscular dystrophy and their clinical course. Becker muscular dystrophy (BMD) is an allelic variant of DMD in which the mutated dystrophin gene produces a reduced amount of a truncated dystrophin protein. The pace of muscle destruction in BMD is much slower, so that affected males are able to procreate, increasing the number of individuals with the disease. However, it is usually fatal from respiratory or cardiac complications between ages 30 to 60. Facioscapulohumeral dystrophy (FSHD) is the third most common muscular dystrophy, with a pattern of progressive muscular weakness involving the face, scapular stabilizers, proximal arm, and fibula. Patients with FSHD usually present with shoulder weakness and scapular winging. FSHD is also associated with retinal abnormalities and hearing loss, but the cardiac muscle is usually spared. The limb-girdle muscular dystrophies (LGMD) are a heterogeneous grouping of *sarcoglycanopathies,* a class of transmembrane proteins that associate with dystrophin in a glycoprotein complex.[9] Common clinical features include early involvement of the proximal muscles of the legs followed by shoulder muscles with scapular winging. Affected individuals have a characteristic stance of lordosis, abducted hips, and hyperextended knees. The facial and ocular musculature is usually spared. There are usually no associated cognitive or cardiac abnormalities. Onset is in late childhood with slow progression. In contrast to most muscular dystrophies that affect the proximal musculature, the distal myopathies affect the forearms, hands, and lower legs.

TABLE 9–1   Comparison Between Duchenne's and Other Forms of Muscular Dystrophies

	Inheritance	Clinical Course	Comorbidities and Anesthetic Concerns
Becker's Dystrophy	X-linked, same locus as Duchenne's Reduced amount and abnormal dystrophin	Later onset (age 12 years) More benign course Death in early 40s, most commonly due to pneumonia	Cardiac involvement less frequent and less severe but heart failure common cause of death Pseudohypertrophy common Reports of cardiac arrests intraoperatively and postoperatively (patients at risk for rhabdomyolysis)
Emery-Dreifuss Dystrophy	X-linked	Slow progression Early contractures in elbow, ankles, and neck Significant cardiac risk with common sudden death between ages 30 and 60 years	Early atrial arrhythmias progressing to asystole: prophylactic ventricular pacemaker suggested Possible cardiomyopathy, ventricular fibrosis and cardiomegaly Possible difficult intubation secondary to limitation of neck motion (although flexion is more limited than extension)
Rigid Spine Syndrome	X-linked?	Slow progression Painless limitation of neck and trunk motions	Severe restrictive lung disease Weakness of respiratory muscles Cardiomyopathy Scoliosis Difficult intubation
Facioscapulohumeral (Landouzy-Dejerine) Dystrophy	Autosomal dominant inheritance	Onset in adolescence Weakness of pectoral, orbicularis shoulder and pelvic muscles (less than Duchenne's) Life span minimally affected	Rare cardiac involvement Abnormal vital capacity Normal CO_2 response curve Frequent upper respiratory tract infections Postoperative respiratory complications
Limb Girdle Dystrophy	Five subtypes predominantly autosomal recessive Severe childhood autosomal recessive dystrophy gene located on 17q12-21	Two most common subtypes: Erb's type (early onset, shoulder girdle primarily involved) Leyden-Möbius (late onset, pelvic girdle involvement) Severity between Duchenne's and fascioscapulohumeral dystrophy[5]	Variable cardiac involvement Sinus tachycardia and right bundle branch block most common ECG abnormalities Early severe diaphragmatic weakness (hypoventilation, hypercarbia) Heart transplant in severe childhood autosomal recessive dystrophy[6]
Distal Myopathies	Autosomal dominant	Welander's myopathy: onset after age 30 years, seen mostly in Sweden, affects hands most frequently Markesberry's dystrophy: onset in fifth decade, feet involvement Early adult-onset myopathy: involvement of anterior or posterior compartment of legs	Possible cardiomyopathy secondary to interstitial fibrosis of the heart muscle in Markesberry's dystrophy[6]

Continued

TABLE 9-1   Comparison Between Duchenne's and Other Forms of Muscular Dystrophies—cont'd

	Inheritance	Clinical Course	Comorbidities and Anesthetic Concerns
Oculopharyngeal Muscular Dystrophy		Onset after age 30 years, slow progression Weakness of pharyngeal muscles, ptosis, limbs, extraocular muscles (rare diplopia) Similar symptoms to ocular myasthenia gravis[13,14] No dysarthria, dyspnea	Common dysphagia, dyscoordination of posterior pharynx and involvement of esophagus causing aspiration and inanition[6] Sensitivity to muscle relaxants[13,14]; anticipate mechanical ventilation postoperatively Anticholinesterase agents do not reverse weakness Normal sensitivity to vecuronium in a case report[15]
Congenital Muscular Dystrophy	Fukuyama form, autosomal recessive	Onset at birth Proximal more than distal muscles involved Slow progression Creatine kinase slightly elevated Death by age 10 years in Fukuyama form (seen frequently in Japan)	Seizures and mental retardation in Fukuyama form

Anesthetic Considerations

Patients with muscular dystrophies often require surgery for muscle biopsy, the correction of scoliosis, the release of contractures, and exploratory laparotomy for ileus (Table 9-2). The operative risk is the lowest early in the course of the disease, before the patient has significant comorbidities. Hence, it is imperative to determine the severity of the disease and the associated comorbidities. Fifty to 70 percent of the patients with muscular dystrophy demonstrate some cardiac abnormality, although these are clinically significant in only 10% of patients and often in the terminal phase of the disease. No correlation has been established between the severity of the cardiac disease and the severity of the skeletal disease. Necrosis and fibrosis of the myocardium in DMD is typically limited to the posterobasal and lateral free walls of the left ventricle, whereas in the other muscular dystrophies the fibrosis may be more diffusely dispersed. Dysrhythmias occur frequently, even after minor emotional trauma. Complex ventricular premature beats correlate with both abnormal left ventricular function and an increased incidence of sudden death.[10]

Patients for operative procedures should have a recent echocardiogram. Echocardiography will demonstrate mitral valve prolapse in 10% to 25% of the patients. It may also show posterobasilar hypokinesis in a thin-walled ventricle and a slow relaxation phase with normal contraction characterizing the cardiomyopathy seen in DMD. However, preoperative echocardiography may not always reflect the ability of the diseased myocardium to respond to perioperative stress.[11] Heart failure can occur during anesthesia for major surgery even with normal preoperative echocardiography and electrocardiography, and sudden death can occur even in patients with fully compensated cardiac status. Angermann and associates[12] have advocated the use of stress echocardiography using angiotensin to detect latent heart failure and identify inducible contraction abnormalities.

Atrial and atrioventricular conduction defects with bradycardia are common in Emery-Dreifuss muscular dystrophy (EDMD), and again the severity of heart disease does not correlate with the degree of skeletal muscle involvement. Several anesthesiologists have recommended preoperative prophylactic cardiac pacing in EDMD patients undergoing general anesthesia and to have emergency pacing available when any form of anesthesia is used. Regional anesthesia has been used successfully in EDMD patients for lengthening of both Achilles tendons; in one case a temporary transvenous pacemaker was inserted before administration of the anesthetic.[13,14] In addition, EDMD patients may prove difficult to intubate and careful assessment with cervical radiography should be undertaken preoperatively. A total intravenous anesthetic or a nitrous/narcotic technique that omits volatile anesthetics and depolarizing agents (to avoid malignant hyperthermia [MH] triggering agents) would seem appropriate if a general anesthesia technique cannot be avoided.[13] To date, however, MH has not been described in EDMD.

Perioperative respiratory complications are a major concern when anesthetizing patients with muscular dystrophy. As previously discussed, at the end of the first decade

TABLE 9–2   Anesthetic Issues in Muscular Dystrophy

Potent Inhalational Anesthetics	Use is not recommended because they may trigger a malignant hyperthermia–like syndrome in patients with Duchenne's muscular dystrophy and depress myocardial contractility.
Hypnotics	Pentothal when used should be given in small increments. Propofol has been recommended as the preferred hypnotic, but higher than expected doses may be required for induction. Consideration should also be given to the myocardial status of the patient,[21] because some of these patients have significant cardiomyopathy, and the reduction in heart rate and decreased contractility with an induction dose of propofol may lead to profound hypotension and reduced end organ perfusion.
Opioids	The use of narcotics eliminates the use of myocardial depressants or inhalational agents; however, consideration should be given to the use of short-acting opioids and/or the need for postoperative ventilation.
Muscle Relaxants	The administration of nondepolarizing muscle relaxants is usually followed by an increased response, both in maximal effect and duration of action.[20] The recovery from neuromuscular blockade in muscular dystrophy patients has been reported to be three to six times longer than in healthy adults. In addition, postoperative pulmonary complications have been associated with the use of long-acting neuromuscular blocking agents. The combined effects of primary smooth muscle abnormalities, inactivity, and general anesthesia induces gastric dilatation, delayed gastric emptying, and the risk of pulmonary aspiration. Regional anesthesia may be a good alternative to general anesthesia to avoid the risk of triggering agents, respiratory depression, and the ability to use local anesthetics for postoperative analgesia.

of life; reductions in inspiration, expiration, vital capacity, and total lung capacity become prominent and reflect the weakness of respiratory muscles.

Decreased ability to cough and the accumulation of oral secretions predispose muscular dystrophy patients to postoperative respiratory tract infections. Respiratory insufficiency, however, may not be apparent because impaired skeletal muscle function prevents these patients from exercising enough to exceed their limited breathing capacity. Preoperative pulmonary function studies are valuable in determining the postoperative course of these patients.

Patients with a vital capacity of greater than 30% of the predicted value can usually be extubated immediately after surgery. With progression of the disease (vital capacity less than 30% of predicted) and the added morbidity of kyphoscoliosis, which can contribute to a restrictive respiratory pattern, postoperative ventilatory support will be required. Delayed pulmonary insufficiency may occur up to 36 hours postoperatively, even if the patient's skeletal muscle strength may appear to have returned to its preoperative level.

Sleep apnea may also compound the respiratory problems and may contribute to development of pulmonary hypertension. Preoperative introduction to chest physiotherapy and nasal continuous positive airway pressure (CPAP), and their use early in the postoperative period, has been shown to be effective in decreasing the incidence of respiratory complications.

Sometimes the first indication that a child has muscular dystrophy is an unexplained cardiac arrest or myoglobinuria with MH-like findings during general anesthesia.[15] Breucking and colleagues[16] investigated 200 families with muscular dystrophy of the Duchenne and Becker types who had received a total of 444 anesthetics. Sudden cardiac arrests occurred in 6 patients with undiagnosed disease at the time they received a general anesthetic of an inhalational agent and/or succinylcholine. There were also nine less severe incidents consisting of fever, rhabdomyolysis, and masseter spasm. The authors recommended the avoidance of the triggering agents succinylcholine and volatile anesthetics to decrease the risk of severe anesthetic complications. In earlier reports, Cobham,[17] in 1964, and Richards,[18] in 1972, did not note any temperature rise or cardiac arrest after using virtually all anesthetic agents available at that time in DMD patients. Richards reported the use of halothane 37 times and that of succinylcholine 12 times, all without subsequent problems. Nevertheless, since those publications there have been several case reports describing life-threatening complications (dysrhythmias, cardiac arrest, rhabdomyolysis) after anesthesia with muscle relaxants and inhalational agents. The anesthetic complications often seemed to parallel the severity of the muscle disease. Succinylcholine has been involved in the majority of lethal complications in patients with unsuspected DMD,[16] leading the U.S. Food and Drug Administration in 1992 to issue a warning with regard to the administration of succinylcholine in young children and adolescents. Larach and coworkers[19] reported that 48% of pediatric patients with cardiac arrest during anesthesia had an unrecognized myopathy, and 67% of them were associated with succinylcholine-induced hyperkalemia. It is speculated that an inherent membrane defect in DMD renders the muscle more susceptible to injury induced by anesthetics and depolarization with succinylcholine. Recent case reports[20,21] have documented the use of propofol, narcotics, and nondepolarizing muscle relaxants in

DMD patients without complications, but, as with the earlier series of uneventful anesthetics with triggering agents, large series are required to document their safety.

MYOTONIAS

Myotonias are a group of muscle diseases in which the pathognomonic finding is *muscle stiffness*. The process consists of slowed muscle relaxation after vigorous contraction. In some patients the stiffness may resolve with repeated muscle contractions, whereas in others it may be exacerbated. It is usually worse if a period of rest is followed by a period of exercise, and it can be provoked by cold. Myotonia results from an abnormality in the electrical properties of the sarcolemma, predisposing the muscle membrane to becoming easily depolarized. This results in a characteristic EMG pattern of repetitive discharges (myotonic runs). A diagnostic clinical sign of myotonia is *percussion myotonia:* after being struck by a percussion hammer, the muscle continues to contract for a period of time and becomes transiently indented.

Myotonic Dystrophy

Myotonic dystrophy (DM, Steinert's disease) is extremely variable in presentation, from asymptomatic cases to congenital DM with respiratory insufficiency and mental retardation (Table 9-3).[22] It is an autosomal dominant worldwide disease with an estimated frequency of 1 in 8000. The genetic defect is a result of the abnormal expansion of the nucleotide CTG on chromosome 19, which codes for a serine-threonine protein kinase. The relationship between the genetic defect and the clinical findings is still unknown. However, knockout mice that completely lack this enzyme develop normally. Expressivity of the genetic defect must also be variable, since within a family one can detect both minimally affected and severely affected individuals.

TABLE 9–3 Clinical Features of Myotonic Dystrophy

Neuromuscular	Myotonia, weakness Reduced deep tendon reflexes
Eye	Cataract, ptosis Ophthalmoparesis, retinal pigmentation
Endocrine	Testicular atrophy, diabetes, pituitary dysfunction, hyperparathyroidism
Skin	Frontal balding, pilomatrixoma
Cardiovascular	Hypotension, syncope, palpitations, mitral valve prolapse, sudden death
Gastrointestinal	Dysphagia, pseudo-obstruction
Central Nervous System	Mental retardation
Immune System	Reduced immunoglobulins

The characteristic sign of DM is myotonia; however, myotonia is absent in congenital myotonia and gradually appears during childhood. In the congenital variant hypotonia, respiratory distress and cranial muscle weakness occur at birth. In these infants motor development is delayed and is often accompanied by mental retardation. In the adult form of DM symptoms appear during the second and fourth decades of life, with progressive muscular weakness. This muscle weakness and wasting are the most disabling features of DM. Wasting is usually most prominent in the cranial musculature and distal limb muscles. Temporalis and masseter muscle atrophy leads to the classic appearance of the *hatchet face*. Deep tendon reflexes are usually reduced or absent. Weakness of the muscles of the vocal cord apparatus results in a nasal speech and the propensity to aspiration pneumonia. The limb muscles first affected lead to footdrop and weak handshake.

DM is a multisystem disease and can affect the heart (conduction system), smooth muscle (impaired intestinal motility), eye (cataracts), brain (mental retardation), and endocrine system (e.g., testicular atrophy, insulin resistance, hypometabolism). The cardiac conduction abnormalities are common and may cause sudden death. In one report 57% of the DM patients had conduction defects, with one third with first-degree atrioventricular block unresponsive to atropine. Many of these patients also have an associated cardiomyopathy, and congestive heart failure can also be a cause of death. Because anesthetics can increase vagal tone or induce arrhythmias, transthoracic pacing should be readily available.

The pulmonary complications of DM are the result of hypotonia, chronic aspiration, and central hypoventilation. Weakness of the respiratory muscles will result in alveolar hypoventilation, hypercapnia, and hypoxemia and increasing somnolence. In some cases an increased respiratory effort is required in one group of respiratory muscles (diaphragm) to overcome the myotonia in other respiratory muscles (intercostals). Smooth muscle atrophy leading to poor gastric motility, coupled with a diminished protective cough reflex, promotes aspiration. Recurrent aspiration pneumonia in some cases leads to chronic pulmonary damage such as bronchiectasis. The hypersomnolence seen with DM is often associated with CO_2 retention and appears to be primarily a central nervous system (CNS) manifestation of the disease.

Because DM is a systemic disease, anesthetic management must include consideration of the multiple manifestations of the disease. All of these patients must be treated as though they have both a cardiomyopathy and cardiac conduction defects. Medications that increase vagal tone or anesthetic plans that result in hypoxia may result in high cardiac conduction blocks. Hence, transthoracic pacing and antiarrhythmic medications should be readily available. If possible, inhalational agents should be avoided, owing to their myocardial depressant and conduction system effects.[23] Because these patients are at risk for aspiration, they should be kept at NPO status and relatively rapid protection of the airway should be achieved with an endotracheal tube. However, succinylcholine will produce contractures lasting for several minutes, rather than relaxation, and these contractures can be severe enough to prevent intubation and ventilation. These contractures are *not* inhibited by nondepolarizing agents. Other agents may also induce myotonic contractures, including methohexital and etomidate, as well as a case report with propofol. The reversal of neuromuscular blockage by neostigmine could precipitate a myotonic response; thus it is advisable to use shorter-acting nondepolarizing muscle relaxants or avoid relaxation. Myotonic contractions can occur, however, in the presence of neuromuscular blocking agents and neuraxial anesthesia, because direct stimulation of the muscle (surgical stimulation) may result in contraction. The combination of central respiratory depression and weak respiratory musculature makes these patients vulnerable to the respiratory depressants effects of most sedatives, hypnotics, and narcotics. Therefore, when possible, regional anesthesia would be the preferred anesthetic and when general anesthesia is required the patients must be monitored postoperatively. The myotonic responses to DM can be treated with phenytoin (4–6 mg/kg/day) or quinine (0.3 to 1.5 g/day).

A recently recognized variant of DM is proximal myotonic myopathy (PROMM). This disorder has features in common with DM such as the facial muscle weakness and frontal balding, but the muscle weakness and stiffness is predominantly confined to proximal rather than distal muscles.

Myotonia Congenita

This is a distinct entity from the congenital onset of DM, which usually presents with severe systemic involvement. There are two forms of this disease, one described by Thomsen in 1876 as a autosomal dominant trait and one described by Becker in the 1950s whose inheritance is recessive. Both forms are the result of mutations in the gene that codes for the major chloride channel.[24] The Thomsen variant is a mild disease with generalized myotonia, usually recognized in early childhood due to frequent falling. Cranial and upper limb musculature is the most severely affected, sometimes resulting in difficulty chewing. The myotonic responses occur after a rest interval and may result in the patient falling to the ground in a rigid state. Some patients have an athletic appearance owing to muscle hypertrophy. Many patients have lid lag and blepharospasm, which is myotonia of the lid musculature. The Becker recessive variant is similar to the dominant form, except that the myotonia is usually more severe and presents later in life (after 10 years) and does not progress in severity beyond the third decade. These patients are usually handicapped in their daily activities because of leg muscle stiffness and generalized weakness. The stiffness of myotonia is treated with medications that reduce the increased excitability of the cell membrane by acting at the sodium channel (local anesthetics, antiarrhythmics).

Myotonia Fluctuans

Becker also described individuals with the dominant form of nondystrophic myotonia in which muscle stiffness fluctuated from day to day. These individuals do not experience muscle weakness, are not sensitive to cold, and do have stiffness (myotonia) that is provoked by exercise after an interval of rest. The stiffness that occurs after heavy exercise may last 30 minutes to 2 hours with periods of days or weeks between incidents.[25] There have been several reports of adverse anesthetic events with the use of succinylcholine in these patients.[26] A variant of this disorder has been described in which the myotonia occurs *during* exercise and is not relieved by warming a cold limb. In another variant with persistent and sometimes severe myotonia, increased serum potassium will aggravate the myotonia. Children with this disorder may experience acute hypoventilation and coma after eating a meal rich in potassium, owing to myotonia of the thoracic muscles. Often these children are misdiagnosed as having a seizure disorder. Clearly, mutations of the sodium-chloride channels of muscle can result in several different clinical syndromes, including the systemic form found in DM.

METABOLIC MYOPATHIES

For muscles to contract they require energy (adenosine triphosphate [ATP]), which is provided from the metabolism of glycogen, glucose, and fatty acids. The metabolic pathways of all three converge into acetyl coenzyme A (acetyl-CoA), which within the mitochondrion is oxidized through the Krebs cycle and respiratory chain to ATP (Fig. 9-2). With regard to myopathies, defects in this process are substrate use defects (involving glycogenoses) or disorders of lipid metabolism. Tsujino and colleagues contend that patients with muscle substrate use diseases present with two major clinical presentations: (1) acute, recurrent, reversible muscle dysfunction that manifests as exercise intolerance or myalgia and (2) fixed, often progressive weakness.[27] Those disorders presenting as acute reversible muscle weakness can usually be differentiated into defects in glycogen or lipid metabolism based on their presentation. Because glycogen metabolism is important for intense aerobic exercise, patients with defects in glycogen metabolism experience muscle cramping and weakness after strenuous exercise, whereas patients with lipid metabolic defects often complain of muscle

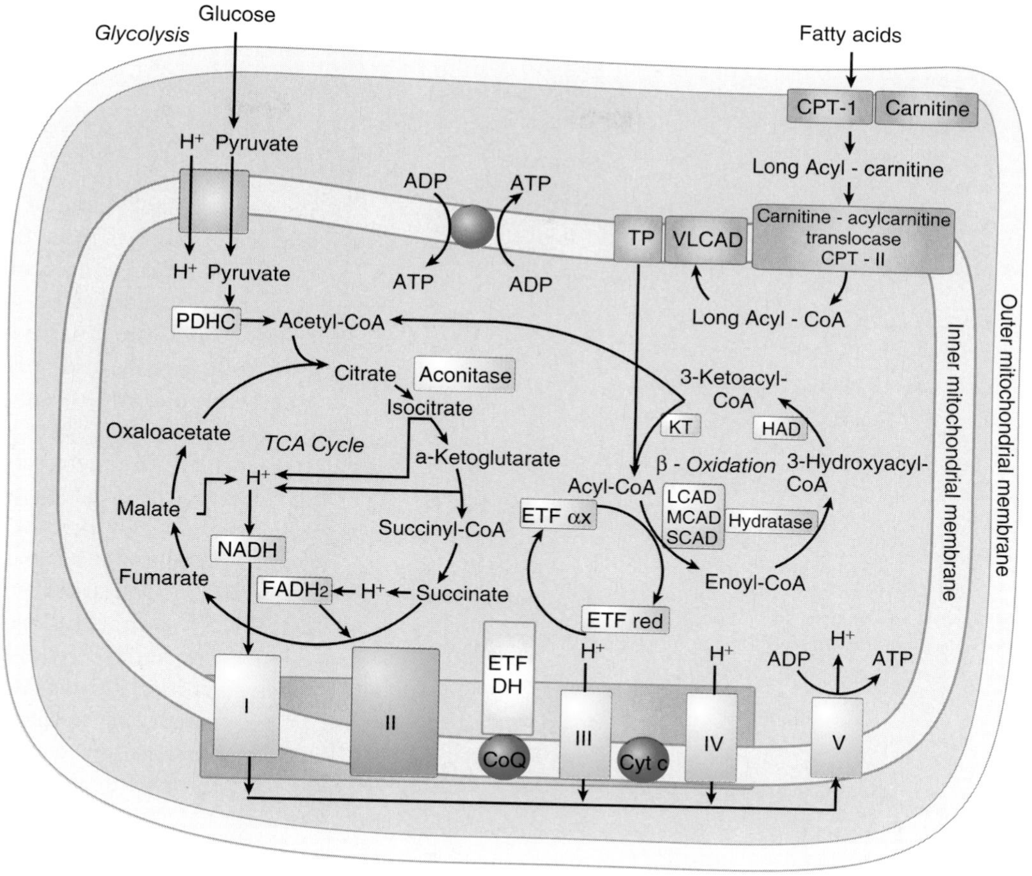

FIGURE 9–2 Schematic representation of substrate metabolism. Respiratory chain complexes encoded exclusively by nuclear DNA are solid; complexes encoded by both nuclear and mitochondrial DNA are cross-hatched. *(Reprinted from Rosenberg RN, Prusiner SB, DiMauro S, Barchi RL [eds]: The Molecular and Genetic Basis of Neurological Disease. Boston, Butterworth-Heinemann, 1997, p 201.)*

cramping or weakness after prolonged moderate exercise. Prolonged fasting can exacerbate these conditions and lead to respiratory muscle fatigue and myoglobinuria.

Metabolic myopathies of infancy or early childhood, however, usually present as multisystem disorders. The *floppy infant syndrome* is the simplified clinical description for children with different metabolic myopathies. These children are at risk for respiratory complications because they have diminished cough reflex and regularly aspirate. The metabolic defects are likely to result in developmental defects in the CNS, cardiomyopathy, and cardiac conduction defects. In addition, the progressive atrophy of skeletal musculature will lead to contractures and scoliosis.[28]

Glycogen Storage Myopathies

These disorders are the result of muscle enzymatic defects in glycogenolytic or glycolytic pathways leading to the accumulation of glycogen. The myopathy is not, however, caused by the accumulation of glycogen but by the block in energy production, *substrate use disease*. The glycogen storage diseases were assigned roman numerals in the order of their discovery and classified as muscle diseases of glycogenosis by Cori (Fig. 9-3). We will discuss these

myopathic nonlysosomal glycogenoses in their enzymatic sequential order.[28,29]

Debranching Enzyme Deficiency (Type III, Cori-Forbes Disease)

This is a disease of childhood with hepatomegaly and liver dysfunction, growth retardation, and fasting hypoglycemia that often resolves spontaneously around puberty. The enzyme has two catalytic functions, a transferase that transfers a glucosyl unit to the acceptor chain of the phosphorylase-limit dextrin (PLD) and then the glucosyl unit is hydrolyzed. Infusion of fructose, as well as a high-protein diet, will increase blood glucose levels, since gluconeogenesis is not affected. Those cases that do not resolve at puberty have early evidence of muscle involvement, both skeletal and cardiac. However, clinical myopathy is not common and usually manifests later (third and fourth decade), after the liver symptoms have remitted. Serum CK is increased in patients with myopathy. The myopathy presents as weakness rather than exercise intolerance, cramps, or myoglobinuria. There can be wasting of the distal leg and intrinsic hand muscles, which can lead to a diagnosis of motor neuron disease.

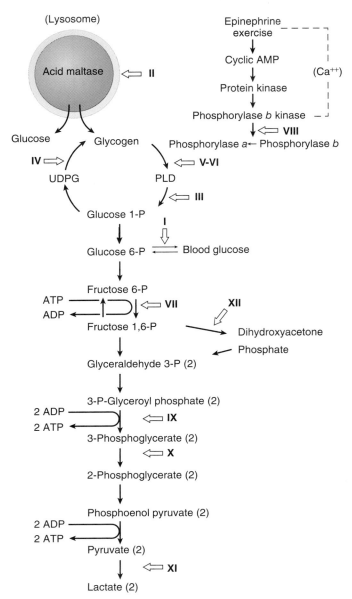

FIGURE 9–3 Scheme of glycogen metabolism and glycolysis. Roman numerals refer to glycogenosis enzymatic defects. *(From Tsujinao S, Nonaka I, DiMauro S: Glycogen storage myopathies. Neurol Clin 2000;18:127.)*

The course is slowly progressive and usually not incapacitating.

Branching Enzyme Deficiency (Type IV, Anderson's Disease)

The branching enzyme catalyzes the last step in glycogen biosynthesis by attaching short glucosyl chains to a peripheral chain of the nascent glycogen. In the enzyme-deficient state the abnormal unbranched glycogens precipitate and are no longer available for glucose production. The clinical manifestations include hepatosplenomegaly, cirrhosis, hypotonia, muscle wasting, and cardiomegaly. Most individuals affected with the disease die early. Patients who survive to maturity may also exhibit central and peripheral nervous system dysfunction.

Myophosphorylase Deficiency (Type V, McArdle's Disease)

Patients typically exhibit exercise intolerance with myalgia, cramping, stiffness, and weakness of the muscles exercised. The exercise intolerance usually develops during the teenage years, but weakness is usually not manifested until later decades. Most patients learn to adapt to their limited exercise tolerance and only later in life does the fixed proximal weakness impose significant limitations in lifestyle. If exercise continues with cramping, myoglobinuria may occur with subsequent renal failure. In this disease, as well as some of the other muscle glycolygenoses, the three to five times normal increase in venous lactate levels observed when an isolated muscle is made ischemic does <u>not</u> occur.

A distinct variant exists that exhibits severe generalized weakness, respiratory insufficiency, and death in infancy. Type V deficiency may also be associated with some cases of sudden infant death syndrome (SIDS).

Phosphorylase initiates glycogen degradation by removing 1,4-glucosyl residues from the outer branches of the glycogen molecule, leaving a phosphorylase-limit-dextran (PLD) molecule with four glucosyl units, which are then degraded by the debranching enzyme leading to glucose-1-phosphate. There are three isoenzymes expressed in muscle, brain, and liver. The brain contains both muscle and brain isoenzymes, which is why specific brain defects have not been characterized. The disease is transmitted as an autosomal recessive trait with localization on chromosome 11.

Because prolonged muscle ischemia can lead to permanent muscle weakness with atrophy and myoglobinuria with renal failure, tourniquets should be avoided. Since experimentally limited muscle exercise tolerance has been extended with glucose infusions, glucose-containing solutions should be infused intraoperatively. Adequate hydration and mannitol infusions when urine output decreases should be employed to prevent myoglobinuria. Succinylcholine should be avoided to prevent muscle fasciculations and breakdown. For the same reason, postoperative shivering should be avoided by using a warmer for intravenous fluids and warming blankets.

Muscle Phosphofructokinase Deficiency (Type VII, Tauri's Disease)

Phosphofructokinase (PFK) deficiency is similar to myophosphorylase deficiency in its clinical presentation and diagnosis. This enzyme converts fructose-6 and fructose-1-phosphate to fructose-1,6-diphosphate, with the defect thus blocking the metabolism of glycogen, glucose, and fructose. As with myophosphorylase deficiency, prolonged ischemic exercise in PFK may result in muscle necrosis and myoglobinuria. However, renal failure is not as common in PFK as it is in myophosphorylase. Because the enzyme defect also effects erythrocytes, some patients also exhibit increased hemolysis with jaundice. PFK is a tetrameric enzyme that is under the control of three structural genes (M, L, P), but only the M gene subunit is expressed in mature muscle, whereas erythrocytes express both the M and L subunits. The absence of anemia in PFK patients is related to the fact that erythrocytes can synthesize a functional enzyme with the L subunit. The defect in the M gene is transmitted as an autosomal trait on chromosome 1.

Phosphorylase B Kinase Deficiency (Type VIII)

Phosphorylase B kinase has a pivotal role in both the degradation and synthesis of glycogen. The enzyme phosphorylates glycogen phosphorylase to an active form while at the same time phosphorylating glycogen synthase to an inactive form; thus, when glycogen degradation is turned on, synthesis is turned off. Phosphorylase B kinase deficiency can be classified into different groups dependent on clinical presentation: liver disease of childhood exhibiting hepatomegaly, growth retardation, delayed motor development, hyperlipidemia, and fasting hypoglycemia, inherited as either a X-linked recessive or an autosomal recessive trait; liver and muscle disease characterized by hepatomegaly and nonprogressive myopathy of childhood, inherited as an autosomal recessive trait; muscle disease in which the patients exhibit weakness of exercising muscles with myalgias, cramps, and myoglobinuria, inherited as a X-linked recessive trait; and fatal infantile cardiomyopathy, inherited as an autosomal recessive trait. The anesthetic considerations would be similar for the previously mentioned deficits, except where the degree of liver disease required modifications.

Phosphoglycerate Kinase Deficiency (Type IX)

Phosphoglycerate kinase (PGK) catalyzes the formation of 3-phosphoglycerate and ATP. Because the enzyme is transcribed from a single gene that is expressed in all tissues except sperm, there is considerable clinical variability. The major clinical presentations include hemolytic anemia, CNS dysfunction (mental retardation, behavioral abnormalities, seizures, stroke), and exercise myopathies. These major clinical features occur with equal frequency in enzyme-deficient patients, but rarely do all appear in the same patient. It is inherited as a X-linked trait.

Phosphoglycerate Mutase Deficiency (Type X)

Phosphoglycerate mutase (PGAM) catalyzes the interconversion of 2-phosphoglycerate and 3-phosphoglycerate. Clinical features include myopathy with exercise intolerance, cramps, and myoglobinuria. It is inherited as an autosomal trait, manifesting variable heterozygotic symptoms.

Muscle Lactate Dehydrogenase Deficiency (Type XI)

Lactate dehydrogenase (LDH) is a tetramer that is composed of two distinct subunits, M and H, which can be arranged into five isoenzymes. The M subunit is the predominant form in skeletal muscle. Hence, patients with the M-type deficit exhibit exercise weakness and recurrent myoglobinuria but not other tissue pathology.

Aldolase Deficiency (Type XII)

Aldolase is present as three isoenzymes in skeletal muscle and erythrocytes; liver, kidney, and small intestine; and neural tissue. Patients with myopathy consisting of exercise intolerance also exhibit hemolytic anemia.

Myoglobinuria

Myoglobinuria is a common metabolic abnormality among the substrate use muscle diseases. Due to an enzymatic blockage in glycogen metabolism and glycolysis, the muscle becomes starved for energy, leading to ischemia, necrosis, and the release of myoglobin into the circulation. However, the most common cause of recurrent myoglobinuria is a lipid metabolism disorder, carnitine palmitoyltransferase II (CPT II). Myoglobin is a 17,000-dalton protein with a heme prosthetic group present in muscle at a concentration of about 1 g/kg and is released during ischemia and cell death. The normal serum myoglobin concentration is about 20 ng/mL, and a serum concentration of 300 ng/mL is required for renal excretion. Visible brown discoloration of the urine with myoglobin suggests massive muscle destruction (rhabdomyolysis). Hemolysis is distinguished from myoglobinuria by a positive urine benzidine test (greater than 500 ng/mL of myoglobin) without microscopic red blood cells. Furthermore, if hemolysis is not a factor, a serum sample should be free of hemolysis. Hypovolemia and acidosis in combination with myoglobinuria increase the probability of acute renal failure. The exaggerated response of muscle fasciculations to succinylcholine, seen in children and adults with myopathies, places them at risk for myoglobinuria and renal failure. Arrhythmias may develop due to the effects of hyperkalemia, acidosis, and hypocalcemia (owing to the uptake of calcium by injured muscle). The hypocalcemia will also be exacerbated by the intravenous administration of sodium bicarbonate and the hyperventilation in patients on respirators. In these instances calcium should then be administered.

Treatment is aimed at reversing muscle destruction (rest, in many cases) and the maintenance of adequate urine output. Early vigorous fluid resuscitation reduces the incidence of renal failure during myoglobinuria. Mannitol should be administered to promote an osmotic diuresis and to scavenge the free oxygen radicals produced after reperfusion of the ischemic kidney. Alkalinization of the urine with sodium bicarbonate may prevent the precipitation of myoglobin acid hematin in the renal tubules and also reduce the risk of renal failure.

Glycogenosis Type I (von Gierke's Disease)

Patients with this disease lack glucose-6-phosphatase, which acts primarily in the liver to convert glucose-6-phosphate to glucose, where it can be utilized by the brain and other tissues that require glucose.[27] Hence, this is not primarily a muscle disease but involves a lack of energy supply for muscles and other tissues. Because glycogen synthesis continues without glycogen degradation and glucose utilization, there is excess liver glycogen deposition with hepatomegaly. Because fasting hypoglycemia can be severe and is associated with acidosis, frequent small carbohydrate feedings are required. The disease is usually accompanied by seizures, mental retardation, and growth retardation; children rarely survive beyond 2 years. However, some patients have survived into their teenage years through portocaval shunts where intestinal uptake of glucose will bypass the liver, with the administration of thyroxine and glucagons to limit glycogen synthesis. Patients for surgery should be permitted to take oral glucose solutions up to 4 hours before surgery, followed by a glucose infusion. Frequent monitoring of both blood glucose and pH is required throughout the perioperative period. Lactate-containing solutions should be avoided, because these patients lack the ability to convert lactic acid to glycogen.

Glycogenosis Type II (Pompe's Disease)

This is a lysosomal acid maltase deficiency that results in the deposition of glycogen in smooth, skeletal, and cardiac muscle. The clinical presentation takes three forms. The first is an infantile form that primarily involves cardiomegaly with congestive heart failure and death, usually before age 2. The next is a juvenile form resulting in severe proximal, truncal, and respiratory muscle weakness. An echocardiogram may reveal cardiac hypertrophy with subaortic stenosis. Muscle glycogen deposition may lead to an enlarged protruding tongue, making the patient prone to upper airway obstruction. Respiratory muscle weakness may predispose the patient to prolonged postoperative ventilatory support. Once extubated, aggressive pulmonary toilet is required to prevent pneumonia. These patients often die during the second and third decade. Finally, there is a milder adult-onset variant simulating limb-girdle dystrophy. Muscle weakness in

these patients is unclear but may involve the rupture of hypertrophied lysosomes, causing muscle destruction.

MITOCHONDRIAL MYOPATHIES

The mitochondrion is an intracellular organelle that is responsible for the majority of the energy-producing pathways. The genetics of mitochondria are complex in that the enzymes and proteins of the organelle are coded for by either mitochondrial genes or cellular genes. In addition, the mitochondrial DNA is exclusively maternally inherited and heterogeneous, such that multiple different copies of mitochondrial DNA may exist within the cell. Genetic defects in these mitochondrial enzymes are devastating to normal muscle action because the enzymes are responsible for ATP production from the mitochondrial respiratory chain and oxidative phosphorylation (Fig. 9-4).[30] Luft reported the first case of a mitochondrial disorder in 1962 in a Swedish woman with evidence of hypermetabolism, but with normal thyroid function.[31] The woman was subsequently found to have a loose coupling of oxidation and physophorylation with abnormal mitochondrial structure. The following year the morphologic criteria for mitochondrial myopathy were described (RRF, ragged-red appearance with a modification of the Gomori trichrome stain).[32] It has since been discovered that not all RRF mitochondrial diseases involve myopathy, and RRF is not always present in mitochondrial myopathies. Mitochondrial myopathies can be divided into (1) "pure" mitochondrial myopathies; (2) mitochondrial encephalomyopathies; (3) oxidative phosphorylation disorders; (4) disorders of fatty acid metabolism; and (5) disorders of pyruvate metabolism.[33-37]

For an in-depth discussion of mitochondrial myopathies, please see Chapter 14, Mitochondrial Diseases.

OXIDATIVE PHOSPHORYLATION DISORDERS

The list of neuromuscular disorders associated with mitochondrial abnormalities and specifically with defects in oxidative phosphorylation (OxPhos) continually increases.[38] In addition, defects in OxPhos have the potential to affect every tissue in the body. The major cardiac manifestation of an OxPhos deficit is hypertrophic cardiomyopathy. One of the specific metabolic defects in this process has been identified, a translocase that exchanges mitochondrial ATP for cytosolic adenosine diphosphate (ADP). Hematologic manifestations have also been associated with OxPhos lesions, specifically sideroblastic anemia in the Pearson marrow pancreas syndrome. Proximal tubular defects can also be a common kidney manifestation of pediatric OxPhos diseases. Diabetes mellitus is fairly common in pediatric OxPhos disorders and has been described in the mitochondrial disorders Kearns-Sayre,

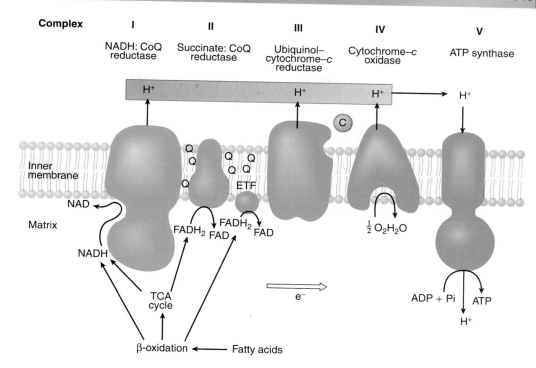

Complex	I	II	III	IV	V
	NADH: CoQ reductase	Succinate: CoQ reductase	Ubiquinol–cytochrome–c reductase	Cytochrome–c oxidase	ATP synthase

FIGURE 9–4 The mitochondrial respiratory chain and oxidative phosphorylation system. *(From Cooper JM, Clark J: The structural organization of the mitochondrial respiratory chain. In Shapira AH, Di-Mauro S [eds]: Mitochondrial Disorders in Neurology. Oxford, UK, Butterworth-Heineman. International Medical Reviews, Neurology 1994, vol 14, pp 1-30.)*

Pearson, Wolfram, and MELAS. Preoperative evaluation of these patients must include their tendency to develop lactic acidosis, feeding habits, and the utility of a glucose infusion in maintaining normal metabolism. Patients with cardiac involvement should have an echocardiogram, and patients with a history of respiratory problems (e.g., recurrent pneumonias, asthma, dyspnea) should have pulmonary function studies. Barbiturates that inhibit the respiratory chain should be avoided. Succinylcholine should also be avoided, owing to the small risk of inducing MH and lactic acidosis in myopathic patients.

OxPhos disorders can be classified according to the specific site of the biochemical defect.[39] However, patients may have an isolated defect in one complex or the genetic defect may affect several complexes. In addition, the clinical pictures of these defects often overlap. Furthermore, because the genes for OxPhos subunits may originate in either mtDNA or nuclear DNA, the specific biochemical defect does not point to the mode of inheritance. A discussion of a few of the more important syndromes associated with mitochondrial OxPhos defects follows.

Luft's Disease

As discussed earlier, in 1962 Luft described a 35-year-old woman with symptoms of hyperthyroidism (hyperhidrosis, polydipsia, polyphagia, weight loss) with normal thyroid function.[31] She was nonetheless treated for

hyperthyroidism, including thyroidectomy, without the expected results. She was subsequently found to have mitochondria of variable size with increased numbers of cristae. The biochemical defect was a loose coupling of oxidative phosphorylation; for every oxidation of hydrogen an ATP was *not* produced from ADP. Hence, more oxygen expenditure was required to achieve a normal amount of energy production. Perioperatively these patients would be at risk for hyperthermia, increased oxygen utilization, metabolic acidosis, and hypovolemia.

Complex I Deficiency

Complex I deficiency (Fig. 9-4) is one of the most common OxPhos deficits. The presentation may include isolated myopathy with exercise intolerance and lactic acidosis or a multisystemic disease.[40] The multisystemic disease includes a fatal infantile lactic acidosis with cardiomyopathy and CNS impairment.

Complex IV Deficiency

This defect usually presents before age 3 as severe infantile myopathy with failure to thrive, weakness, hypotonia, severe lactic acidosis, and associated hepatic, cardiac and renal involvement.[41] There have been reports of the myopathy improving spontaneously after age 3. This "benign" reversible infantile myopathy may be caused by a developmentally regulated OxPhos subunit.

Coenzyme Q Deficiency

Coenzyme Q is responsible for shuttling electrons between complexes I, II, and III.[41] The clinical presentation has included progressive muscle weakness starting in childhood, with associated CNS disorders. The patients improved clinically when administered 150 mg of coenzyme Q daily.

DISORDERS OF FATTY ACID METABOLISM

Muscles use long-chain fatty acids as a source of energy (Figs. 9-1 and 9-5). The fatty acids are esterified with coenzyme A (CoA) and then transported across the inner mitochondrial membrane through three steps: (1) esterification to carnitine with carnitine palmityl transferase (CPT I); (2) translocation across the membrane with carnitine acylcarnitine translocase; and (3) release as CoA by CPT II. Inherited defects have been described for each of these enzymes as well as the enzymes involved in β oxidation.[42,43] Presentation is usually in infancy as hypoketotic hypoglycemia triggered by fasting or a hypermetabolic state (infection), which may be associated with encephalopathy, hepatocellular dysfunction, and cardiomegaly.

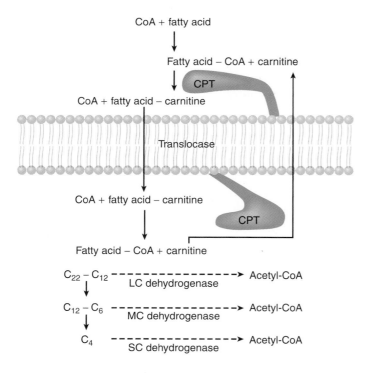

FIGURE 9–5 The transport of fatty acids into muscle mitochondria.

Carnitine Deficiency

Carnitine is synthesized in the liver and then transported to skeletal muscle, where it facilitates the transport of long-chain fatty acids into the mitochondrion. Medium-chain fatty acids do not require carnitine for transport. Because skeletal and cardiac muscle derives most of its resting, fasting, and endurance energy from fatty acid metabolism, carnitine deficiency results in weak muscles and the deposition of lipid granules. Childhood carnitine deficiency myopathy includes progressive dilated cardiomyopathy. In addition, Reye's syndrome has been associated with the deficiency, which includes vomiting, stupor, and coma. Because carnitine and medium-chain fatty acids will ameliorate the muscle weakness, they should be administered perioperatively. Corticosteroids should also be administered, because they provide an alternative transport mechanism for long-chain fatty acids. Prolonged fasting must be avoided, and glucose-containing infusions should be used.

Acyl-Coenzyme A Dehydrogenase Deficiency

The dehydrogenases break down the mitochondrial fatty acid CoA to acyl-CoA; hence, defects in these enzymes lead to the accumulation of fatty acyl-CoA and fatty carnitine acyl-CoA. The most common form is the medium-chain acyl-CoA dehydrogenase deficiency, with an incidence of 1 in 10,000. It usually presents as hypoketotic hypoglycemia during the first or second year, after fasting or a metabolic stress. The deficiency has been linked to a number of deaths from sudden infant death syndrome (SIDS). In addition, patients who survive the childhood crisis often acquire a myopathy and cardiomyopathy.

CPT Deficiency

CPT II is more common than CPT I deficiency, usually presenting in late adolescence as exercise-induced muscle cramping and myoglobinuria. Prolonged metabolic stress can result in respiratory insufficiency and renal failure from rhabdomyolysis. Serum levels of muscle CK are elevated during attacks but are usually normal between episodes. These patients exhibit normal work and oxidative capacity as long as a carbohydrate substrate is available; it is only during fasting or when glycogen stores (glucose) have been depleted that these patients have a metabolic crisis. Hence, as with several other substrate deficiency disorders, glucose should be administered perioperatively. Severe shivering and muscle contractions (succinylcholine) should also be avoided.

DISORDERS OF PYRUVATE METABOLISM

These include pyruvate dehydrogenase (PDHC) and pyruvate carboxylase (PCD) deficiency. PDHC is one of the most common presentations of congenital lactic acidosis.[44]

Clinical presentation can occur in the newborn as severe persistent lactic acidosis, usually resulting in death; can occur as a form that manifests later in infancy, associated with developmental delay, hypotonia, seizures, dysmorphic features, and intermittent episodes of lactic acidosis; and can occur in older childhood in males with ataxia, precipitated by carbohydrate meals and treated with high-fat, low carbohydrate diets.

MUSCLE CHANNELOPATHIES

This is a group of disorders that have a common molecular basis in the impairment of voltage gated skeletal muscle.[45]

Malignant Hyperthermia

Still a cause of a fatal event under anesthesia, MH was first described in 1960 by Denborough and Lovell.[46] The incidence is reported to be from 1 in 15,000 anesthetics in children to 1 in 50,000 to 100,000 anesthetics in adults. The MH syndrome is characterized by generalized muscle rigidity, unexplained increased CO_2 production, metabolic acidosis, rhabdomyolysis, elevated CK levels, hyperkalemia, and hyperthermia.[47] An increase in core temperature of 1°C every 5 minutes with elevation up to 46°C has been reported. Although the degree and duration of core temperature elevation has an effect on outcome, hyperthermia may be a late sign in the development of MH.

Pathogenesis. The syndrome is triggered by the administration of volatile anesthetics and the depolarizing muscle relaxant succinylcholine.[48] The initial presentation may be masseter spasm after the administration of succinylcholine. If succinylcholine is not administered to facilitate endotracheal intubation, the syndrome may not be recognized until later into an uncomplicated inhalational anesthetic.[49] At that point in the anesthetic, the tachycardia, hypertension, and rigid muscles might be attributed to "light" anesthesia, leading the anesthesiologist to increase the concentration of the delivered anesthetic. Only after the patient becomes red and hot, and the $ETCO_2$ has risen significantly, is the problem recognized. Muscle rigidity may make ventilation difficult, which in association with increased CO_2 production leads to both respiratory and metabolic acidosis. Furthermore, the CO_2 absorbance of the breathing circuit will become hot and exhausted, exacerbating the hyperthermia and acidosis. Cardiac arrhythmias, including ventricular tachycardia and fibrillation, the result of acidosis, hyperthermia, and catecholamine surges, are common. Bleeding may occur from the surgical site owing to the development of coagulopathies (e.g., DIC, thrombocytopenia). Acute renal failure ensues from hypotension and rhabdomyolysis. Coma will follow as a result of extreme hyperthermia and cerebral edema. The syndrome is almost always fatal if not appropriately treated. MH has also been reported in humans in response to stress or exercise.[50]

MH is a defect in the regulation of myoplasmic calcium concentration. The triggering event leads to a release of calcium from the sarcoplasmic reticulum via a voltage-dependent muscle ryanodine (RYR1) channel.[51] The RYR1 channel is regulated by calcium, ATP, calmodulin, and magnesium. Micromolar concentrations of calcium activate the RYR1 channel, whereas calcium concentrations tenfold higher (>10 µM) inhibit the channel. Mutations in the *RYR1* gene on human chromosome 19q13.1 have been linked to MH-susceptible individuals.[52] The mutant RYR1 channel is activated by lower than normal concentrations of calcium and is inhibited by higher than normal concentrations of calcium. In addition, modulation of the RYR1 receptor via calmodulin was altered such that its activating properties were dramatically increased. This ultimately leads to excess sarcoplasmic calcium with persistent contracture of myofibrils, depletion of ATP, uncoupling of oxidative phosphorylation, metabolic acidosis, and muscle necrosis. Genetic linkage studies have demonstrated that about 50% of the cases of MH can be linked to mutations in the *RYR1* gene. The *RYR1* mutation has also been linked to central core disease (a rare congenital myopathy) and to the King-Denborough syndrome. In one report it was demonstrated that in 124 MH-susceptible individuals, 23% had mutations in the *RYR1* gene.[53] In other analysis MH susceptibility was linked to the dihydropyridine (DHP) receptor gene on chromosome 7q, which also regulates skeletal muscle calcium flux.[54]

Thus, although the inheritance of MH is autosomal dominant, the molecular genetics of MH susceptibility may involve more than one genetic locus.

Diagnosis. The diagnosis of MH is based on the presentation of the clinical syndrome or the in-vitro contracture test (IVCT). The IVCT is specific for MH, but its lower sensitivity eliminates it as a practical screening test for the general surgical population. Furthermore, because many clinical scenarios can produce a hypermetabolic state and mimic MH, the diagnosis is usually made in individuals with both appropriate clinical criteria and a positive IVCT. Larach and colleagues[55] developed a clinical grading scale to assess the probability of MH susceptibility (Table 9-4). This MH scale incorporates six clinical criteria, such that the probability of MH susceptibility increases the more criteria manifested by the patient. When an individual manifests enough criteria consistent with MH, it is important that the individual undergo an IVCT, because many will be found to be non–MH susceptible. This information is important for family counseling.

TABLE 9–4 Criteria for the Clinical Grading Scale for Malignant Hyperthermia

Process	Clinical Criteria
Muscle rigidity	Generalized rigidity; masseter muscle spasm
Muscle breakdown	Creatine kinase > 20,000 U/L; myoglobinuria; plasma K > 6 mEq/L
Respiratory acidosis	End-tidal CO_2 > 55 mm Hg; $Paco_2$ > 60 mm Hg
Temperature increase	Rapidly increasing; T > 38.8°C
Cardiac involvement	Unexplained sinus tachycardia, V-tach, V-fib
Family history	Familial history of malignant hyperthermia

The IVCT is performed at only two centers in Canada and six in the United States (see *www.mhaus.org* for the addresses of MH diagnostic centers). The patient should have the muscle biopsy performed at the IVCT diagnostic center, because the test must be performed within 4 hours of excision of the muscle. The caffeine-halothane contracture test (CHCT) requires 2 g of muscle, usually harvested from the vastus lateralis or vastus medialis muscle. Regional anesthesia with sedation is preferable for the procedure, but direct infiltration of the muscle with local anesthetic is contraindicated. In the North American protocol, six longitudinal strips of muscle are hooked to force transducers and three are exposed to 3% halothane and three to caffeine. The development of a contracture of greater than or equal to 0.7g for halothane and greater than or equal to 0.3g for caffeine is considered positive for MH.[56] The specificity of this test is about 98% for tested individuals who have had an unequivocal MH episode, but the sensitivity is only 85% to 90%. Hence, with a low prevalence of the MH syndrome and 10% to 15% of normal patients testing positive, the IVCT cannot be used for routine screening. An ideal testing solution for MH would utilize a simple DNA-based test to screen surgical patients. However, as noted earlier, more than one genetic locus has been identified as being associated with MH susceptibility, and at this time our detection rate for gene mutations in known MH susceptible patients is only 23%.[53]

What about patients with masseter muscle spasm (MMS) during the induction of anesthesia? Sudden cardiac arrest after the administration of succinylcholine has been reported in normal patients with MMS but is considerably more frequent in patients with myopathies.[57] Children with muscle diseases may have a myotonic response to succinylcholine (MMS), which also includes elevated CK levels, metabolic acidosis, hyperkalemia, and dysrhythmias. This does not, however, necessarily imply that these individuals are MH susceptible. Can MMS occur in "normal" individuals after induction with succinylcholine and inhalational agents? In a study of 5000 anesthetized children, not a single child induced with pentothal developed MMS whereas the incidence of MMS was 0.5% with succinylcholine and halothane.[58] None of these patients developed MH. However, others have reported that 60% of patients with MMS tested IVCT positive for MH.[59] Because the development of the MH syndrome is potentially fatal, a non-triggering anesthetic should be used for the operation after the observation of MMS alone during anesthetic induction. The development of generalized myotonic contractions and other sequelae after succinylcholine and/or inhalational agents is abnormal, and in these cases, if possible, the anesthetic should be terminated, the patient hospitalized for observation, and the possibility of MH susceptibility investigated. Even if the patient is not MH susceptible, significant rhabdomyolysis that may occur in some muscle diseases could progress to severe metabolic acidosis, renal failure, and sudden death.

Treatment. The mortality from an MH syndrome has fallen from almost 100% to low levels due to vigilance, supportive care, withdrawal of triggering agents, and administration of dantrolene. When an MH response is suspected, dantrolene should be administered at 1 to 2 mg/kg intravenously with additional doses every 15 to 30 minutes until evidence of the acute episode has subsided. After the initial episode, the dantrolene should be continued at 1 mg/kg intravenously every 6 hours or 0.25 to 0.5 mg/kg/hr intravenously until the treatment has produced stable, normal vital signs (possibly for 24 hours, depending on the severity of the episode). Evidence of an MH relapse has been reported in about 25% of patients within 24 hours of the initial episode.[60] Each 20-mg vial of dantrolene contains 3 g of mannitol, and the vials are reconstituted in water. The most common complication of dantrolene administration is muscle weakness.

Additional responses to an MH episode should include correction of the metabolic acidosis with bicarbonate (1/2 to 2 mEq/kg), hyperventilation with 100% oxygen, and an initial fluid bolus of 10 to 20 mL/kg of cooled or room temperature normal saline. Continued fluid management will depend on the patient's urine output, electrolytes, and hemodynamic stability. Aggressive alkaline diuresis to maintain a urine output of 1 to 2 cc/kg may be required to prevent renal failure from myoglobinuria. The administration of glucose and insulin will drive potassium intracellularly and provide a substrate for maintenance of cerebral functions. Arterial blood samples and blood samples for electrolytes and CK levels should be sent regularly. It may be necessary to lavage body cavities (stomach and bladder) with cooled saline to prevent dangerous levels of hyperthermia. Muscle compartments must be evaluated to allow early treatment of compartment syndrome.

Management of the MH-Susceptible Patient. MH-susceptible patients can safely be administered general anesthesia with nitrous oxide, intravenous anesthetics, and nondepolarizing muscle relaxants. Regional anesthesia with any local anesthetic is also considered safe for MH-susceptible patients. The anesthetic circuit should not have been exposed to inhalational agents, a new CO_2 absorbent, and flushing of the anesthesia machine with a continuous flow of oxygen at 10 L/min for 20 minutes. Prophylactic loading with dantrolene appears unnecessary, because MH may still develop and effective serum dantrolene levels can be achieved after acute intravenous loading.[61] Because stress can theoretically trigger an MH response, patients should be appropriately treated with anxiolytics before their arrival in the operating room, and patients receiving a regional anesthetic should also be sedated. An MH kit with enough dantrolene to administer 10 mg/kg to a large adult, several ampules of bicarbonate, equipment for lavaging body cavities, intravenous fluids, and ice for topical cooling should be readily available.

Hyperkalemic Periodic Paralysis

Hyperkalemic periodic paralysis is inherited as an autosomal dominant trait with complete penetrance. The paralytic attacks usually begin infrequently during the first decade of life and then increase in frequency with age until they may recur daily. They often occur in the morning or after a period of rest after strenuous exercise. The attacks never occur during exercise and may be aborted if the individual begins mild exercise. The muscle weakness is accompanied by hyperkalemia, with levels up to 6 mM and a concomitant decrease in serum sodium levels. With resolution of the weakness the serum potassium level returns to normal and the patient may experience a water diuresis, creatinuria, and myalgias. The attacks can be precipitated by potassium intake, the cold, stress, glucocorticoids, and pregnancy. There are three clinical variants of the disease: with myotonia, without myotonia, and with paramyotonia. Lowering the patient's body temperature will induce weakness but not myotonia in any of the clinical variants. The myotonia that does occur in some patients is mild and rarely interferes with movement. In the paramyotonia variant the attacks include generalized weakness and paradoxical myotonia. In *paramyotonia congenita* the myotonia is induced by cold and includes hyperkalemia, but differs in that the myotonia appears during exercise and worsens with continued exercise. These individuals have the characteristic lid-lag phenomenon.[45]

The diagnosis of hyperkalemic periodic paralysis can be made via an exercise stress test. Individuals are exercised for 30 minutes to a heart rate greater than 120 beats per minute, followed by absolute rest. In normal individuals the serum potassium value will rise during the exercise phase and then decline to baseline during the rest phase. In the periodic paralysis patients, the serum potassium value will start to decline at rest but then rise again in 10 to 20 minutes with accompanying weakness.[62]

The pathogenesis of the disease involves abnormal activation of sarcolemmal sodium channels.[63] The mutation has been linked to the skeletal muscle sodium channel gene on chromosome 17q23. The mutant sodium channel responds to elevated potassium levels by increased influx of sodium and prolonged depolarization. This renders the muscle inexcitable (paralyzed) and results in a compensatory release of potassium from the cells, which may then activate more sodium channels.

Individuals with the disease may be able to attenuate attacks by ingestion of carbohydrates, continuation of mild exercise, and administration of a potassium-wasting diuretic. Preventive therapy also includes the use of potassium-wasting diuretics (hydrochlorothiazide).

Preoperative carbohydrate depletion should be avoided, if possible, by carbohydrate loading the night before surgery or starting an infusion of a glucose-containing solution. Intravenous solutions free of potassium should be administered. The electrocardiogram may show evidence of peaked T waves before a paretic attack. At that time glucose, insulin, and inhaled β agonists should be administered in an attempt to abort the paralysis. Of course the patient must be kept warm and relaxed, because both the cold and stress can trigger paralysis.

A rare variant of hyperkalemic periodic paralysis is *normokalemic periodic paralysis,* in which the serum potassium value does not increase during severe attacks. This condition includes urinary potassium retention, beneficial effects of sodium loading, and lack of beneficial effects in glucose loading. In one family the mutation was linked to the sodium channel gene on chromosome 17q.

Hypokalemic Periodic Paralysis

As with the hyperkalemic variant, the attacks in hypokalemic periodic paralysis usually begin before age 16 with infrequent attacks, which then increase in frequency to a point where they may recur daily. The attacks usually occur in the second half of the night or early in the morning. The patient may awaken in the morning paralyzed except for the cranial muscles, which are usually spared. However, respiratory function is compromised during severe attacks and fatal respiratory failure has been reported. Attacks are triggered by preceding strenuous physical activity, high carbohydrate and sodium meals, stress, and the cold. During severe attacks the serum potassium level falls to abnormal levels. Attacks can be accompanied by oliguria, constipation, diaphoresis, and sinus bradycardia. In addition, many patients may develop a permanent myopathy.[64]

The diagnosis of hypokalemic periodic paralysis is made by establishing hypokalemia during attacks and normokalemia between attacks. If an abnormally low serum potassium level is sustained, then one should consider secondary reasons for paretic attacks, including renal or gastrointestinal potassium wasting and thyrotoxic conditions. The administration of glucose and insulin may provoke an attack by driving potassium intracellularly.

Hypokalemic periodic paralysis is inherited as an autosomal dominant trait, with higher penetrance in males. The disease is linked to the L-type calcium channel DHP receptor on chromosome 1q31-32, but the pathogenesis has not been well elucidated.

Attacks can be prevented or attenuated by ingesting 2 to 10 g of potassium chloride. Patients planning to undergo surgery should not ingest a meal high in carbohydrates the night before. Electrolytes should be measured preoperatively on the day of surgery, and appropriate corrections to serum potassium should be instituted. Some patients are treated with acetazolamide to induce a mild metabolic acidosis, preventing potassium from shifting into the cell. Hypothermia should be avoided. Because an episode may precipitate respiratory failure, these patients should be monitored postoperatively.

MYASTHENIAS

These are disorders that affect the neuromuscular junction (NMJ) and are characterized by fluctuating muscle weakness and abnormal fatigability. The NMJ consists of the presynaptic and postsynaptic regions separated by the synaptic space. The nerve terminal contains acetylcholine (ACh) membrane-enclosed synaptic vesicles, which are released in response to a generated motor nerve action potential. The ACh molecules then bind to a postsynaptic receptor and induce a muscle action potential (Fig. 9-6). In addition to acquired myasthenia gravis (MG) and the Eaton-Lambert syndrome, several toxins and medications can produce myasthenic-like syndromes that affect the NMJ, including botulism, tetanus, venom poisoning, aminoglycosides, hypermagnesemia, quinidine, and organophosphate poisoning.

Acquired Myasthenia Gravis

The classic syndrome involves fluctuating weakness and fatigability involving the ocular and other muscles innervated by cranial nerves, with worsening symptoms during the day (Table 9-5). There is considerable variation in the world prevalence, from 1.2 per 1 million in Japan to 14.2 per 100,000 in West Virginia; with a female-to-male ratio of 3 to 2. MG may occur at any age, but females are more commonly affected under 40 and males more commonly affected over 60.[65]

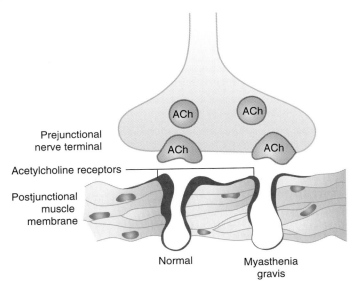

FIGURE 9–6 Schematic diagram of the neuromuscular junction, depicting the density of ACh receptors on the folds of postjunctional muscle membranes. Compared with normal folds, the density of ACh receptors is greatly reduced in the presence of myasthenia gravis. *(From Stoelting RK, Dierdorf SF: Anesthesia and Co-Existing Disease. New York, Churchill Livingstone, 1993, p 440.)*

The defect is the result of a decrease in the number of available receptors for ACh at the postsynaptic NMJ. The ACh receptors are inactivated by circulating antibodies, which block access of the receptor to ACh. Ultimately, the ACh receptor IgG complex institutes a complement-mediated lysis of the receptors in the junctional folds. Antibodies to ACh receptors are detectable in the serum in 74% to 94% of MG patients. About two thirds of

TABLE 9–5 Differential Diagnosis of Acquired Myasthenia Gravis
Symptoms
Fluctuating weakness
Fatigability of ocular and other muscles innervated by cranial nerves

Gender ratio
  Female to male 3:2
  Females ± age 40, males ± age 60

~2/3 thymic hyperplasia; 10% thymomas

In 50% of patients initial symptoms involve extraocular muscles
  Eyelid ptosis
  Sustained upward gaze
  Diplopia

Face appears expressionless
Speech is hoarse and slowed
Chewing and swallowing difficult; risk of aspiration
Dyspnea with mild to moderate exertion

the patients have thymic hyperplasia and 10% have thymomas. In about 10% of the cases MG is associated with another autoimmune disease, including hyperthyroidism, polymyositis, systemic lupus erythematosus, Sjögren's syndrome, rheumatoid arthritis, ulcerative colitis, sarcoidosis, and pernicious anemia. In addition, MG has developed in patients receiving D-penicillamine and interferon therapy and after bone marrow transplantation (Table 9-6).

In about 50% of the patients the initial symptoms involve extraocular muscles, but bulbar and limb muscles may also be included in the initial presentation. Levator palpebrae weakness leads to eyelid ptosis, which is often exacerbated by sustained upward gaze. Individuals often complain of diplopia. The face often appears expressionless with a snarling smile. Speech is usually hoarse and slowed. Chewing and swallowing of food is difficult, with a risk of aspiration. Dyspnea will occur with mild to moderate exercise. The proximal limb muscles are often more affected than the distal limb muscles. Muscle weakness is worse with repeated exercise and as the day progresses. However, the symptoms may vary daily or from week to week with periods of remission (see Table 9-5).

Although the initial symptoms are usually ocular, in about 90% of the patients the disease becomes generalized within the first year of diagnosis, with progression the most rapid during the first 3 years (Table 9-7). Prior to the 1990s the disease progressed to a complete systemic deterioration and death in one fourth of the affected patients. With the introduction of more effective therapy, the mortality from the disease has decreased dramatically. In a series of 100 patients reported by Beckman and colleagues,[65] there were no fatalities directly related to the disease. However, patients do experience episodes of respiratory failure due to bulbar involvement. A myasthenic crisis is defined as an acute exacerbation of symptoms

with respiratory compromise. In a series of 53 patients with a myasthenic crisis, 75% of the patients were extubated within 1 month of being placed on a respirator, with three deaths during the crisis and four deaths post extubation.[66] Independent risk factors associated with poor prognosis were identified, such that patients with no risk factors were all extubated within 2 weeks while patients with increasing risk factors required longer periods of respiratory support (Table 9-8).

To define the severity of the disease and the clinical prognosis, a classification for MG was devised by Osserman in 1958 and then modified in 1971 (see Table 9-7).[67]

Patients in group I are medication responsive and are not at risk for a crisis. Patients in group IIB are moderately severe, poorly responsive to medications, and are at risk for a crisis. Patients in group III have a disease that rapidly progresses over 6 months with a high risk for a crisis and often have thymomas. Patients with group IV disease have had a milder form of the disease for more than 2 years and then develop a severe, progressive form of the disease.

Neonatal myasthenia develops in about 12% of infants born to mothers with MG due to the passive transfer of ACh receptor antibodies. The symptoms of poor feeding, generalized weakness, respiratory distress, and weak cry appear a few hours after birth and usually last only 18 days.

About 30% of women with MG experience a worsening of symptoms during pregnancy. If possible, pregnancy should be planned for periods of remission when the patient is no longer receiving immunosuppressants. If the symptoms during pregnancy become debilitating,

TABLE 9–7 Classification of Myasthenia Gravis

I. Ocular Myasthenia
II. Chronic Generalized A. Mild B. Moderate
III. Acute, Fulminating
IV. Late, Severe

TABLE 9–6 Secondary Causes of Myasthenia Gravis

Hyperthyroidism
Polymyositis
Systemic lupus erythematosus
Sjögren's syndrome
Rheumatoid arthritis
Ulcerative colitis
Sarcoidosis
Pernicious anemia
Has developed in patients: Receiving D-penicillamine Receiving interferon therapy After bone marrow transplantation

TABLE 9–8 Risk Factors Associated with Prolonged Intubation After Myasthenia Gravis Crisis

Preintubation serum HCO_3^- > 30 mg/dL
Peak vital capacity < 25 mL/kg
Age > 50 years
Comorbidities: atelectasis, anemia, congestive heart failure, *Clostridium difficile* infection

these women can receive plasmapheresis and increased cholinesterase therapy.

The diagnosis of MG is usually based on the symptoms of easy fatigability and fluctuating weakness. An edrophonium chloride (Tensilon) test, however, is sometimes used to confirm the diagnosis. An initial 2 mg intravenous dose of edrophonium is administered to ascertain tolerance and then 6 to 8 mg is injected. The patient is then observed for an improvement in symptoms or the ability to complete repetitive functions. The improvement in MG symptoms is suggestive of a diagnosis of MG, and they usually last about 10 minutes. Side effects of edrophonium injection include fasciculations, sweating, nausea, abdominal cramps, and bradycardia. In addition, electrophysiologic studies can be performed, where in MG there is a decremental response of the compound action potential to repetitive electrical stimulation.

There are several therapeutic options for patients with MG, including cholinesterase inhibitors, immunosuppressants, plasma exchange, specific immunoglobulins, and thymectomy. Pyridostigmine (Mestinon), a cholinesterase inhibitor that prolongs the action of ACh at the NMJ receptor, is the first line of treatment for the symptomatic relief of MG. Pyridostigmine is dosed initially at 15 to 60 mg four times a day with resolution of symptoms within 15 to 30 minutes and a duration of 3 to 4 hours. Neostigmine bromide, a shorter-acting cholinesterase inhibitor, may be administered parenterally for acute episodes. Progressive weakness with increasing dosing of anticholinesterases may indicate the onset of a myasthenic or a cholinergic crisis. A cholinergic crisis is associated with muscarinic effects of abdominal cramps, nausea, vomiting, diarrhea, miosis, lacrimation, increased bronchial secretions, and diaphoresis. It is also possible to see significant bradycardia. These muscarinic symptoms should not be prominent during a myasthenic crisis and should be discriminated by a 2-mg edrophonium test. However, it is often difficult to distinguish these two crises and it is best to hold the anticholinesterase and support the patient with intubation and ventilation.

Thymectomy will improve the remission rate and ameliorate the progression of the disease. The best responders to thymectomy are females with hyperplastic thymus glands and high ACh receptor antibody titers. Alternate-day prednisone therapy induces remission and improves the clinical course of the disease in more than half of the patients. Azathioprine in doses of 150 to 200 mg/day in many cases also provides improvement in symptoms.

Patients for surgery and anesthesia should be warned that they may require postoperative ventilatory support. MG criteria that correlate with postoperative controlled ventilation include duration of disease greater than 6 years, presence of pulmonary disease, pyridostigmine dose greater than 750 mg/day, and preoperative vital capacity less than 2.9 L.[68] If possible, neuromuscular blocking drugs should be avoided, because the response to these medications is variable, owing to the nature of the disease and the treatment with anticholinesterases. However, patients with MG are usually resistant to succinylcholine and sensitive to nondepolarizing muscle relaxants. Hence, if rapid intubation is required, a larger dose (1.5 to 2 mg/kg) of succinylcholine should be administered.[69,70] Chronic use of anticholinesterases will also impair the effect of plasma cholinesterase. This may result in prolonged neuromuscular blockade by succinylcholine and mivacuronium. It may also reduce the metabolism of ester local anesthetics. The use of any nondepolarizing muscle relaxant should be titrated with the use of a peripheral nerve stimulator. For maintenance of anesthesia, inhalational agents might be preferred because they can be eliminated by ventilation and would not have the depressant effects that narcotics would postoperatively. One approach is to hold the patient's anticholinesterase medication 4 hours before surgery and then begin neostigmine intravenously 1 hour before emergence from anesthesia, at $1/30$ to $1/60$ the daily pyridostigmine dose infused over 24 hours. Before extubation the patient should be fully awake, have a full return to a train of four if muscle relaxants were used, and a negative inspiratory force greater than 30 cm H_2O.

Eaton-Lambert Myasthenic Syndrome

Eaton-Lambert myasthenic syndrome (ELMS) was first described in 1956 in patients with fatigable weakness and pulmonary malignancies. The weakness usually affects the proximal limb muscles, predominantly the lower limbs, with sparing of the extraocular and bulbar muscles. Symptoms are usually worse in the morning on awakening and improve during the day. Unlike MG, deep tendon reflexes are usually reduced or absent. The patients also have autonomic symptoms of dry mouth, orthostatic hypotension, hyperhidrosis, and reduced papillary light reflex. ELMS is probably due to impaired release of ACh at the nerve terminal, produced by autoantibodies directed against the voltage-gated calcium channels. It is the calcium influx into the nerve terminal that stimulates the release of ACh vesicles.[71] Because malignancy is present in about 60% of the cases of ELMS, a diagnosis of the myasthenic syndrome should elicit a search for a neoplasm.

Therapy with cholinesterases alone is usually not very effective. Muscle strength and autonomic functions can be improved with 3,4-diaminopyridine (DAP) therapy. DAP causes peripheral paresthesias, palpitations, sleeplessness, cough, diarrhea, and rare seizures. Guanidine hydrochloride, which increases the release of ACh, has also proven effective, but the severe side effects of bone marrow depression, renal tubular necrosis, cardiac arrhythmias, liver failure, and ataxia have limited its use.

These patients are sensitive to both depolarizing and nondepolarizing muscle relaxants. In addition, because ELMS patients may be treated with both DAP and pyridostigmine, antagonism of the neuromuscular blockade at the end of the surgical procedure may prove ineffective. These patients often undergo diagnostic procedures in search of occult malignancies; and because they have reduced respiratory reserve, they are at risk for respiratory failure with only a minimum of anesthetics and sedatives.[72]

INFLAMMATORY MYOPATHIES

Dermatomyositis

DM can present at any age, but usually the childhood cases present between 5 and 14 years and the adult form at 40 to 60 years. Women are usually affected more often than men. The neck flexors, shoulder girdle, and pelvic girdle muscles are the most severely affected, such that lifting their arms over the head, climbing stairs, or rising from a chair is difficult. Children usually also present with fatigue, low-grade fevers, and a rash that precedes the muscle weakness and myalgia. The classic rash includes a purplish discoloration of the eyelids with periorbital edema; papular erythematous scaly lesions over the knuckles; and a flat erythematous sun-sensitive rash over the neck, face, and anterior chest. Children also develop subcutaneous calcifications. Cardiac conduction abnormalities are common, as are congestive heart failure and myocarditis. About 10% of DM individuals also develop interstitial lung disease, with restrictive lung disease and reduced diffusing capacity. There may also be evidence of chronic pulmonary aspiration from oropharyngeal and esophageal weakness. Vasculitis of the gastrointestinal tract may result in ulcerations and perforations. In addition, necrotizing vasculitis may affect the eyes, kidneys, and lungs. Arthralgias involving all joints are a common complaint. Adult DM also is strongly associated with (up to 45%) underlying malignancies. Corticosteroids are the major therapy for DM, with the addition of more powerful immunosuppressants.[73]

Polymyositis

PM usually presents in individuals older than 20 years, with women affected more often than men. The patient usually presents as neck flexor and proximal arm and leg weakness that develops over weeks and months, but without a characteristic rash as in DM. Dysphagia is also a common symptom of PM. These patients also have similar cardiac and pulmonary complications as in DM, but there is a much lower incidence of associated malignancies. Most patients with PM improve with immunosuppressive therapy.

Inclusion Body Myositis

IBM presents with slowly progressive, distal and proximal muscle weakness, often with years from onset of symptoms to diagnosis. It is the most common inflammatory myopathy in men older than 50 years of age. Early signs of the disease include asymmetrical quadriceps and wrist/finger flexor weakness. At least 40% of the patients complain of dysphagia. IBM is not associated with cardiac abnormalities or an increased risk of cancer. The muscle biopsy demonstrates inflammation with atrophic fibers and eosinophilic cytoplasmic inclusions. Patients with IBM do not significantly improve with immunosuppressive therapy.

Overlap Syndromes

These are a group of disorders in which an inflammatory myopathy occurs in association with a connective tissue disease. These diseases include scleroderma, Sjögren's syndrome, systemic lupus erythematosus, rheumatoid arthritis, and mixed connective tissue disease. Antinuclear antibodies are seen in many of these patients.

INFECTIVE AND TOXIC MYOPATHIES

Infections, endocrine abnormalities, environmental toxins, and medications can all potentially produce myalgias and muscle weakness. In developing countries infections from parasitic infestations produce myositis and myopathies. Exogenous chemicals and the abnormal production of internal endocrine chemicals can have profound effects of skeletal muscle function. It is beyond the scope of this chapter to discuss in any detail the action of these agents on the skeletal muscle apparatus. Instead we have chosen three more common agents from each class that result in a myopathy.

Human Immunodeficiency Virus

The spectrum of findings with HIV spans asymptomatic CK elevation to generalized fatigue to severe proximal limb-girdle weakness. In one report, 18% of HIV-infected patients had muscle involvement, which included a PM-like myopathy and muscle atrophy.[74] These patients are also subject to bacterial and protozoal myopathies as a result of immunosuppressive therapy. The PM-like myopathy is progressive, is symmetrical, and usually affects the lower extremities. Dysphagia, respiratory weakness, and rashes are not part of the syndrome. HIV-infected patients also are subject to a poorly defined muscle wasting syndrome characterized by severe muscle wasting with normal or only mildly reduced muscle strength. This may be the result of generalized systemic infections, poor nutrition, and the toxins from antiviral medications.

Necrotizing Myopathy

Cholesterol-lowering medications have a propensity to produce myopathy and necrotizing myopathy. Lovastatin in combination with other medications (cyclosporine) or in patients with hepatobiliary or renal dysfunction may risk severe myopathy with rhabdomyolysis. ε-Aminocaproic acid, which is used during surgery to inhibit fibrinolysis and reduce bleeding, has been implicated in a necrotizing myopathy that affects the axial musculature. The symptoms can begin 4 or more weeks after administration of the medication and may be the result of an ischemic insult to the muscle.[75]

Thyrotoxic Myopathy

The incidence of myopathy among thyrotoxic patients has been reported to be as high as 82%. Common symptoms include myalgias, fatigue, and exercise intolerance. The weakness is predominantly proximal, and it may be associated with dysphagia and respiratory insufficiency. The sudden onset of generalized weakness with bulbar palsy has been described for thyrotoxic patients alone, but it should raise the suspicion of associated myasthenia gravis. CK levels are usually normal, except during thyroid storm, when rhabdomyolysis could lead to renal failure. The treatment of thyrotoxic myopathy is to reinstate a euthyroid condition.

References

1. Le Corre F, Plaud B: Neuromuscular disorders. Curr Opin Anesthesiol 1998;11;333-337.
2. Wagner KR: Genetic diseases of muscle. Neurol Clin 2002;20:1-27.
3. Sadoulet-Puccio HM, Kunkel LM: Dystrophin and its isoforms. Brain Pathol 1996;6:25-35.
4. Worton R: Muscular dystrophies: Diseases of the dystrophin-glycoprotein complex. Science 1995;270:755-756.
5. Bushby KM, Goodship JA, Nicholson LV, et al: Variability in clinical, genetic and protein abnormalities in manifesting carriers of Duchenne and Becker muscular dystrophy. Neuromuscul Disord 1993;3:57.
6. Emery AEH: Duchenne Muscular Dystrophy. Oxford Monographs on Medical Genetics, 2nd ed. Oxford, Oxford University Press, 1993.
7. Goedde E, Ritter H, Collsen S: Creatine kinase isoenzyme patterns in Duchenne muscular dystrophy. Clin Genet 1978;14:257.
8. Chenard E, Becone HM, Tertrain F: Arrhythmia in Duchenne muscular dystrophy: Prevalence, significance and prognosis. Neuromuscular Disord 1993;3:201.
9. Bushby KM, Beckman JS: The limb-girdle muscular dystrophies: Proposal for a new musculature. Neuromuscul Disord 1995;5:337-343.
10. Chenard E, Becone HM, Tertrain F: Arrhythmia in Duchenne muscular dystrophy: Prevalence, significance and prognosis. Neuromuscular Disord 1993;3:201.
11. Schmidt GN, Burmeister MA, Lilje C, et al: Acute heart failure during spinal surgery in a boy with Duchenne muscular dystrophy. Br J Anaesth 2003;Jun;90:800-804.
12. Angermann C, Bullinger M, Spes CH, et al: [Cardiac manifestations of progressive muscular dystrophy of the Duchenne type]. Z Kardiol 1986;75:542-551. In German.
13. Morrison P, Jago RH: Emery-Dreifuss muscular dystrophy. Anaesthesia 1991;46:33-35.
14. Shende D, Agarwal R: Anaesthetic management of a patient with Emery-Dreifuss muscular dystrophy. Anaesth Intensive Care 2002;30:372-375.
15. Farell PT: Anesthesia-induced rhabdomyolysis causing cardiac arrest: Case report and review of anesthesia and the dystrophinopathies. Anesth Intensive Care 1994;22:597-601.
16. Breucking E, Reimnitz P, Schara U, Mortier W: [Anesthetic complications: The incidence of severe anesthetic complications in patients and families with progressive muscular dystrophy of the Duchenne and Becker types]. Anaesthesist 2000;49:187-195. In German.
17. Cobham IG, Davis HS: Anesthesia for muscular dystrophy patients. Anesth Analg 1964;43:22.
18. Richards WC, Anaesthesia and serum creatine phosphokinase levels in patients with Duchenne's pseudohypertrophic muscular dystrophy. Anaesth Intensive Care 1972;1:150.
19. Larach MG, Rosenberg H, Gronert GA, Allen GC: Hyperkalemic cardiac arrest during anesthesia in infants and children with occult myopathies. Clin Pediatr 1997;36:9-16.
20. Ririe D, Shapiro F, Sethna NF: The response of patients with Duchenne's muscular dystrophy to neuromuscular blockade with vecuronium. Anesthesiology 1998;88:351-354.
21. Fairfield MC: Increased propofol requirements in a child with Duchenne muscular dystrophy [letter]. Anaesthesia 1993;48:1013.
22. Lane RJ, Shelbourne P, Johnson KJ: Myotonic dystrophy. In Lane RJ (ed): Handbook of Muscle Disease. New York, Marcel Dekker, 1966, pp 311-328.
23. Aldridge LM: Anesthetic management in myotonic dystrophy. Br J Anesth 1985;57:1119-1123.
24. Koch MC, Steinmeyer K, Lorenz C et al: The skeletal muscle chloride channel in dominant and recessive human myotonia. Science 1992;257:797-800.
25. Ricker K, Lehmann-Horn F, Moxley RT: Myotonia fluctuans. Arch Neurol 1990;47:268-272.
26. Vita GM, Olckers A, Jedlicka AE et al: Masseter spasm rigidity associated with glycine to alanine mutation in adult muscle sodium channel-subunit gene. Anesthesiology 1995;82:1097-1103.
27. Tsujino S, Nonaka I, DiMauro S: Glycogen storage myopathies. Neurol Clin 2000;18:125-150.
28. Ramchandra DS, Anisya V, Gourie-Deve M: Ketamine monoanesthesia for diagnostic muscle biopsy in neuromuscular disorders in infancy and childhood: Floppy infant syndrome. Can J Anaesth 1990;37:474-476.
29. DiMauro S, Haller RG: Metabolic myopathies: Substrate use defects. In Schapira AH, Griggs RC (eds): Muscle Diseases. Boston, Butterworth-Heinemann, 1999, pp 225-249.
30. Anderson S, Bankier AT, Barrell BG, et al: Sequence and organization of the human mitochondrial genome. Nature 1981;290:457-423.
31. Luft R, Ikkos D, Palmieri G et al: A case of severe hypermetabolism of nonthyroid origin with a defect in the maintenance of mitochondrial respiratory chain: A correlated clinical, biochemical, and morphological study. J Clin Invest 1962;41:1776-1804.
32. Engel WK, Cunningham GC: Rapid examination of muscle tissue: An improved trichrome stain method for fresh-frozen biopsy sections. Neurology 1963;13:919-923.
33. Roberts NK, Perloff JK, Kark RA: Cardiac conduction in the Kearns-Sayre syndrome: Report of 2 cases and review of 17 published cases. Am J Cardiol 1979;44:1396-1400.
34. Harvey JN, Barnett D: Endocrine dysfunction in Kearns-Sayre syndrome. Clin Endocrinol 1992;37:97-103.
35. Ciafaloni E, Ricci E, Shanske S et al: MELAS: Clinical features, biochemistry, and molecular genetics. Ann Neurol 1992;31:391-398.
36. Silvestri G, Ciafaloni E, Santorelli FM et al: Clinical features associated with the A-G transition at nucleotide 8344 of mtDNA (MERF) mutation. Neurology 1993;43:1200-1206.
37. Rahman S, Blok RB, Dahl HH et al: Leigh syndrome: Clinical features and biochemical and DNA abnormalities. Ann Neurol 1996;39: 343-351.
38. Munnich A, Rotig A, Chretien D, et al: Clinical presentations and laboratory investigations in respiratory chain deficiency. Eur J Pediatr 1996;155:262-274.

39. Turner LF, Kaddoura S, Harrington D, et al: Mitochondrial DNA in idiopathic cardiomyopathy. Eur Heart J 1998;191:725-729.

40. Robinson BH: Human complex I deficiency: Clinical spectrum and involvement of oxygen free radicals in the pathogenicity of the defect. Biochem Biophys Acta 1998;1364:271-286.

41. DiMauro S, Hirano M, Bonilla E, et al: Cytochrome oxidase deficiency: Progress and problems. In Shapiro AHV, DiMauro S (eds): Mitochondrial Disorders in Neurology. Oxford, Butterworth-Heinemann, 1994, pp 91-115.

42. Nyhan WL: Abnormalities of fatty acid oxidation. N Engl J Med 1988;319:1344-1346.

43. Stanley CA: Dissecting the spectrum of fatty acid oxidation disorders. J Pediatr 1998;132:384-386.

44. Brown GK, Otereo LJ, LeGris M, et al: Pyruvate dehydrogenase deficiency. J Med Genet 1994;31:875-879.

45. Ackerman MJ, Clapham DE: Ion channels—basic science and clinical disease. N Engl J Med 1997;336:1575-1586.

46. Denborough MA, Lovell RRH: Anesthetic deaths in a family. Lancet 1960;2:45.

47. Strazis KP, Fox AW: Malignant hyperthermia: A review of published cases. Anesth Analg 1993;77:297-304.

48. Ellis FR, Heffron JJA: Clinical and biochemical aspects of malignant hyperthermia. In Arkinson RS, Adams AP (eds): Recent Advances in Anesthesia and Analgesia. New York, Churchill-Livingstone, 1985, pp 173-207.

49. Hoenemann CW, Halene-Holtgraeve TB, Brooke M, et al: Delayed onset of malignant hyperthermia in desflurane anesthesia. Anesth Analg 2003;96:165-167.

50. Davis M, Brown R, Dickson A, et al: Malignant hyperthermia associated with exercise-induced rhabdomyolysis or congenital abnormalities and a novel RYR1 mutation in New Zealand and Australian pedigrees. Br J Anesth 2002;88:508-515.

51. Nelson TE: Malignant hyperthermia: A pharmacogenetic disease of Ca regulating proteins. Curr Mol Med 2002;2:347-369.

52. McCarthy TV, Healy JMS, Heffron JJA, et al: Localization of the malignant hyperthermia susceptibility locus to chromosome 19q12-13.2. Nature 1990;343:562-564.

53. Sei Y, Sambuughin NN, Davis EJ, et al: Malignant hyperthermia in North America. Anesthesiology 2004;101:824-830.

54. Iles D, Lehmann-Horn F, Deufel T, et al: Localization of the gene encoding the α_2-subunits of the L-type voltage-dependent calcium channel to chromosome 7q and segregation of flanking markers in malignant hyperthermia susceptible families. Hum Mol Genet 1994;3:969-975.

55. Larach MG, Localio AR, Allen GC, et al: A clinical grading scale to predict malignant hyperthermia susceptibility. Anesthesiology 1994;80:771-779.

56. Rosenberg H, Antoginni JF, Muldoon S: Testing for malignant hyperthermia. Anesthesiology 2002;96:232-237.

57. Larach MG: Hyperkalemic cardiac arrest during anesthesia in infants and children with occult myopathies. Clin Pediatr 1997;36:9-16.

58. Lazzell VA, Carr AS, Lermann J, et al: The incidence of masseter muscle rigidity after succinylcholine in infants and children. Can J Anesth 1994;41:475-479.

59. O'Flynn RP, Shutack JG, Rosenberg H, et al: Masseter muscle rigidity and malignant hyperthermia susceptibility in pediatric patients. Anesthesiology 1994;80;1228-1231.

60. Short JA, Cooper CM: Suspected recurrence of malignant hyperthermia after post-extubation shivering in the intensive care unit, 18h after tonsillectomy. Br J Anesth 1999;82:945-947.

61. Flewellen EH: Dantrolene dose response in awake man: Implications for management of malignant hyperthermia. Anesthesiology 1983;59:275-280.

62. Subramony SH, Wee AS: Exercise and rest in hyperkalemic periodic paralysis. Neurology 1986:36;173-177.

63. Ptacek IJ, George AL, Griggs RC, et al: Identification of a mutation in the gene causing hyperkalemic periodic paralysis. Cell 1991;67:1021-1027.

64. Riggs JE: Periodic paralysis: A review. Clin Neuropharmacol 1989;12:249-257.

65. Beckman R, Kuks JB, Oosterhuis HJ: Myasthenia gravis: Diagnosis and follow-up of 100 consecutive patients. J Neurol 1997;224:112-118.

66. Thomas CE, Mayer SA, Gunger Y, et al: Myasthenic crisis: Clinical features, mortality, complications, and risk factors for prolonged intubation. Neurology 1997;48:1253-1260.

67. Osserman KE, Genkins G: Studies in myasthenia gravis: Review of twenty-year experience in over 1200 patients. Mt. Sinai J Med 1971;38:497-537.

68. Eisenkraft JB, Papatestas AD, Kahn CH, et al: Predicting the need for postoperative mechanical ventilation in myasthenia gravis. Anesthesiology 1986;65:79-82.

69. Eisenkraft JB, Book WJ, Mann SM, et al: Resistance to succinylcholine in myasthenia gravis: A dose-response study. Anesthesiology 1988;69:760-763.

70. Nilsson E, Meretoja OA: Vecuronium dose-response and requirements in patients with myasthenia gravis. Anesthesiology 1990;73:28-31.

71. O-Neil JH, Murray NM, Newson-Davis J: The Lambert-Eaton myasthenic syndrome: A review of 50 cases. Brain 1988;111:577-596.

72. Small S, Ali HH, Lennon VA, et al: Anesthesia for unsuspected Lambert-Eaton myasthenic syndrome with autoantibodies and occult small cell lung carcinoma. Anesthesiology 1992;76:142-145.

73. Amanto AA, Barohm RJ: Idiopathic inflammatory myopathies. Neurol Clin 1997;15:615-648.

74. Berman A, Espinoza LR, Diaz JD, et al: Rheumatic manifestations of human immunodeficiency virus infection. Am J Med 1988;85:59-64.

75. George KK, Pourmand R: Toxic myopathies. Neurol Clin 1997;15:711-730.

10 Skin and Bone Disorders

JOHN E. TETZLAFF, MD

In this chapter a discussion is presented of the diseases and syndromes that involve the skin and bones in the context of the perioperative period. The goal is to define the anesthetic issues, including preoperative preparation, intraoperative management, and postoperative care.

Skin and bone disorders have in common alteration of the surface of the body. As a consequence, anesthetic care can be challenging. Airway management can be difficult if the anatomy is abnormal. Regional anesthesia can also be difficult or impossible for the same reason. Alterations in surface anatomy present difficult issues for positioning, and routine movement of the patient can cause significant skin lesions or bone fracture. Some of these diseases are associated with comorbidity that must be investigated preoperatively and taken into account in the perioperative care. Some of these diseases are chronic and controlled with a variety of medications that can cause organ toxicity. This knowledge will alter preoperative preparation of these patients. When these diseases create the indication for surgery, particularly urgent surgery, knowledge of the pathophysiology can guide management and decrease the risk of morbidity.

ACHONDROPLASIA AND DWARFISM

Pathophysiology. The chondrodysplasias are a group of related syndromes associated with abnormality of the size of the trunk, limbs, and skull, resulting in a disproportionate shortness of stature. Achondroplasia is the most common form of dwarfism.[1] The pathophysiology is abnormal cartilage formation, particularly at the epiphyseal growth plates.[2] Cellular structure of individual cartilage cells is abnormal.[3] Classification is based on the site of the dysplasia (e.g., epiphyseal, metaphyseal, and diaphyseal).[4] Other terms to name these diseases include "spondylo" for those that affect the spine, and "cranio" for those that involve the base of the skull. Further classification is based on age at onset (infantile) and genetic inheritance (X-linked, recessive, or autosomal dominant). The etiology is unknown but has been associated with numerous causative factors.[2]

Differential Diagnosis. Another name for achondroplasia is short-limbed dwarfism. The achondroplastic appearance is an adult less than 4 feet tall, with a large head, bulging forehead, depressed nasal bridge, prominent mandible, and short arms and legs with normal trunk size. In those that survive infancy, life expectancy is normal. Infants with this condition have shortening of the proximal part of the limbs, protuberance of the frontal skull, and depressed nasal bridge, related to shortness of the base of the skull. Lordosis, thoracolumbar kyphosis, and pelvic narrowing are present, and severe spinal stenosis is common.[1] Spinal stenosis can manifest as nerve root compression, cauda equina syndrome, thoracolumbar spinal cord compression, or high cervical cord compression due to stenosis of the foramen magnum. Quadriplegia has been reported in an achondroplastic infant due to stenosis of the foramen

TABLE 10–1 Chondroplasia: Genetics

Name	Clinical Issues	Genetics
Achondroplasia	Limbs, skull, spine	Autosomal dominant
Dystrophic dysplasia	Limbs, spine, cleft palate	Recessive
Hypochondroplasia	Limbs	Autosomal dominant
Metaphyseal dysplasia	Limbs	Recessive
Spondyloepiphyseal dysplasia	Spine, cleft palate	X-linked recessive

TABLE 10–3 Preoperative Issues for Achondroplasia Patients

Anticipated difficult airway
Laryngomalacia
Cervical spine instability
Kyphoscoliosis
Obstructive sleep apnea
Abnormal chest mechanisms

magnum caused by normal range of motion.[5] Atlantoaxial dislocation also caused high cord compromise in another infant.[6] Quadriplegia occurred after anesthesia and surgery in a diastrophic dwarf with severe kyphosis.[7]

Achondroplasia is an autosomal dominant syndrome, although family history is less obvious because fertility is low.[8] Other genetic information is contained in Table 10-1. The differential diagnosis of short stature (dwarfism) is based on a combination of clinical and radiographic features. Numerous comorbidities are associated with these syndromes and are listed in Table 10-2.

Preoperative Preparation (Table 10-3)

Because of the associated congenital defects, abnormalities of the cardiovascular and respiratory systems should

TABLE 10–2 Comorbidities Associated with Achondroplasia and the Chondrodysplasias

Malformation of the skull
Hydrocephalus
Dental abnormalities
Mental retardation
Seizure disorder
Tracheomalacia
Atlantoaxial instability (hypoplastic odontoid)
Scoliosis, kyphosis
Spinal stenosis
Difficult airway criteria
Congenital heart disease
Obstructive sleep apnea
Pulmonary hypertension
Cleft palate
Clubfoot

be actively evaluated in all patients with chondrodysplasia. Chest radiography, electrocardiography, and transthoracic echocardiogram are minimum requirements. A difficult airway will be present in a majority, complicated further by anatomic abnormality of the skull, neck, and chest. Cleft lip, cleft palate, and micrognathia may also contribute to difficult airway management. Stridor can occur spontaneously, secondary to laryngomalacia.[9] Symptomatic subglottic stenosis, requiring urgent tracheostomy for emergency surgery, has been reported.[10] The potential for atlantoaxial instability from abnormal odontoid development[1] or congenital absence of the odontoid[11] should be investigated with flexion-extension lateral cervical spine radiographs and open mouth view of the odontoid. If inconclusive, magnetic resonance imaging (MRI) of the skull and cervical spine is required. When there are cervical radicular signs or if mental retardation makes recognition impossible, high cervical stenosis should be assumed and delineated with computed tomography (CT) or MRI. When spinal cord compression is identified, decompressive laminectomy or decompression of the foramen magnum is indicated. Kyphoscoliosis can be severe, and evaluation of pulmonary reserves with chest radiography, arterial blood gas analysis, and pulmonary function tests may be required. Thoracic dystrophy can be associated with some rare dwarfism syndromes and can greatly exaggerate the ventilatory compromise with kyphoscoliosis owing to mechanical restriction of thoracic excursion. Tracheomalacia is one additional source of airway compromise and should be actively sought by identification of symptoms, CT, or flow-volume loops. Because of the shape of the head and neck, obstructive sleep apnea will be present in as many as 40% of achondroplastic patients, even in childhood.[12,13] Central sleep apnea has been reported in patients with high cervical spinal stenosis or stenosis of the foramen magnum.[13] Because there is no specific treatment for achondroplasia, there are no recurring medications. Any medication list would be related to comorbidities, such as seizure disorder or lung disease.

Intraoperative Considerations. The primary concern in achondroplasia relates to airway management. The high probability of encountering a difficult airway makes preparation for awake intubation options necessary. Reduced endotracheal tube size has been recommended.[14] Urgent airway management should be avoided because atlantoaxial instability or spinal canal stenosis puts the cervical spinal cord at risk with traditional airway maneuvers. Laryngeal mask airway (LMA) has been reported as a means to achieve oxygenation and to facilitate endotracheal intubation when it is otherwise impossible in these infants.[15] High spinal cord injury and death have been reported after routine airway management (neck flexion, extension of the occiput) in patients with atlantoaxial instability. Ventilatory difficulty should be assumed; and because of restrictive pulmonary disease, general anesthesia may be impossible without tracheal intubation. Mechanical ventilation may require a high respiratory rate and a reduced tidal volume. Volume ventilation may need to be abandoned for pressure-control ventilation.

All forms of general and regional anesthesia have been performed in patients with achondroplasia (Table 10-4). Spinal surgery, especially of the cervical spine, may require evoked potential motoring (somatosensory, motor), which modifies anesthetic options. Regional anesthesia has been reported for achondroplastic patients. Spinal and epidural anesthesia for surgery[16-18] and obstetrics[19-23] have been reported as successful, although technically difficult. Successful combined spinal/epidural anesthesia has also been reported.[24] Emergency cesarean section has been accomplished with spinal anesthesia when the issues of a difficult airway were obvious.[25] Extensive spread of small volumes of local anesthetic in the epidural space has been reported and could lead to dangerously high block if reduced volumes are not administered.[26] Peripheral nerve block and plexus block have been accomplished without incident; however, there is concern for the uncontrolled airway management issues that occur with local anesthetic induced seizure activity. The use of ketamine, succinylcholine, and nitrous oxide for cesarean section

has been reported for a full-term achondroplastic parturient who requires general anesthesia.[27] Because of the anatomic and functional abnormality of the thoracic spine, ribs, and chest, postoperative ventilatory insufficiency may occur, and extended mechanical ventilation may be necessary. The high probability of obstructive sleep apnea[12] will make postoperative pain management challenging.

Summary. Achondroplasia and other dwarfism syndromes are genetic congenital defects in the development of bones. They present as short stature and a variety of skeletal anomalies. Other associated congenital defects include congenital heart disease, cleft lip/palate, scoliosis, and clubfoot. Anesthetic management is complicated by difficult airway issues, spine abnormalities, including atlantoaxial instability, and cardiopulmonary compromise. Prolonged mechanical ventilation may be necessary.

BEHÇET'S DISEASE

Behçet's disease is an autoimmune disease manifesting as iritis[28] and ulceration of the oropharynx, perineum, and genitalia.[29] Sporadic cases involve the central nervous system (CNS), cardiovascular system, lungs, and synovial surfaces.[30,31] Less common lesions can occur in the urogenital and gastrointestinal tract. In some, fibrinolysis is impaired and recurrent thrombophlebitis and hypercoagulability can occur.

Differential Diagnosis and Clinical Manifestations (Table 10-5)

Prior to diagnosis, Behçet's disease is often confused with its numerous manifestations, defined by the major involved organ system. Skin lesions are easily confused with

---

TABLE 10–4 Anesthetic Management Issues for Achondroplasia Patients

Airway management issues
Difficult ventilation
Cervical spinal cord compression
Cervical spine instability
Technical difficulty with neuraxial block
Extensive spread of neuraxial local anesthetic
Prolonged postoperative respiratory insufficiency
Difficult acute pain control due to obstructive sleep apnea

TABLE 10–5 Clinical Manifestations of Behçet's Disease

Mucosal lesions
Spinal cord lesions
Cauda equina syndrome
Aseptic meningitis
Seizures
Intracranial thrombosis
Vasculitis
Pericardial effusion
Large vessel aneurysm or dissection
Hemoptysis, bronchiectasis
Pulmonary hypertension
Chronic renal failure

numerous other dermatologic diseases. Mucosal lesions are more specific, especially when the triad of iritis and oropharyngeal, and genital mucosal lesions is present.[32] When the CNS is involved,[33-34] serious manifestations include lesions of the spinal cord, cauda equina syndrome, aseptic meningitis, seizures, dementia, coma, and intracranial thrombosis. Dural sinus thrombosis has been reported in a patient with Behçet's disease.[35] Cardiovascular manifestations include myocarditis vasculitis,[36] pericardial effusion, valve lesions,[37] arterial occlusion, aneurysm,[38] or dissection of major blood vessels.[39] Obstruction of the superior vena cava has been reported,[40] as well as other lesions of major venous structures.[41] Pulmonary manifestations[42,43] include chronic obstructive pulmonary disease (COPD),[44] hemoptysis, bronchiectasis, pulmonary artery thrombosis, and pulmonary hypertension.[45] Glomerular lesions can precipitate chronic renal failure.[46] In patients with Behçet's involvement of the gastrointestinal tract, return of gastrointestinal function may be delayed after surgery.[47] This should also be considered in regard to drug absorbance, which can be delayed postoperatively.[48]

Preoperative Preparation (Table 10-6)

When Behçet's disease presents as major organ system involvement, these systems should be completely investigated before elective surgery. Severe neurologic manifestations[49] have usually been defined at diagnosis with MRI or CT and should be reviewed for anesthetic issues (cord compression, increased intracranial pressure [ICP], or risk of herniation). If symptoms have increased since the last study, the studies may need to be repeated. Electrocardiography and echocardiography are often needed because of the cardiovascular involvement.[50] If there are significant respiratory symptoms, arterial blood gas analysis, spirometry, and a chest radiograph should be considered. Oropharyngeal ulceration can occur and become symptomatic with onset of hemorrhage.[51] If symptoms such as stridor with exertion suggest airway compromise,

indirect laryngoscopy should be considered before elective anesthesia. Blood urea nitrogen/creatinine should be measured to identify or quantitate chronic renal disease and to reveal nephrotoxicity of treatment.[52-54] Because Behçet's disease is an inflammatory process, chronic use of anti-inflammatory and antineoplastic drugs is common. With chronic corticosteroid use, supplemental corticosteroids are necessary the day of surgery.

Intraoperative Considerations. Puncture of skin or mucous membranes is very likely to result in inflammation and nodular formation and should be kept to a minimum. This would mean that regional anesthesia would be less ideal but not contraindicated. With anesthesia of the airway, topical application of local anesthetics would be preferred to airway blocks because of potential compromise of the airway from the inflammatory response to local injection.

General anesthesia can be challenging if oropharyngeal lesions are present.[55] In extreme cases, lesions can severely reduce the lumen of the oropharynx and tracheostomy might be necessary for urgent surgery. For elective procedures, awake fiberoptic intubation would be required. Use of an LMA could aggravate lesions in the airway. If spinal cord lesions are symptomatic, use of succinylcholine can result in hyperkalemia. With cervical cord lesions, intraoperative manifestations of autonomic hyperreflexia may occur.

Summary. The anesthetic implications of Behçet's disease are related to comorbidity, mainly in the CNS, cardiovascular, and pulmonary systems (Table 10-7). In patients with severe oropharyngeal lesions, airway management can be difficult or impossible. Regional anesthesia can be utilized, but needle puncture may cause inflammation and lesion formation. General anesthesia is complicated by difficult airway management. There is risk of autonomic hyperreflexia if spinal cord lesions are present. If there is spinal cord involvement, the hyperkalemic response to succinylcholine can be exaggerated.

TABLE 10–6 Preoperative Preparation for Patients with Behçet's Disease

MRI/CT for compromised central nervous system
Electrocardiogram
Echocardiogram
Pulmonary function tests
Elective evaluation of airway
Blood urea nitrogen/creatinine
Stress-dose corticosteroids

TABLE 10–7 Anesthetic Management Issues for Patients with Behçet's Disease

Minimize skin puncture
Difficult airway management
Difficult ventilation
Lesions from needle used for regional anesthesia
Hyperkalemia with succinylcholine
Autonomic hyperreflexia

EPIDERMOLYSIS BULLOSA

Epidermolysis bullosa (EB) is a hereditary disorder of the skin and mucous membranes that causes the development of blistering of body surfaces in response to minimal trauma. The most visible abnormalities are vesicles and bullae within skin and/or mucous membranes. Abnormal healing of these lesions is a common feature, as is contracted scarring and erosion. Although skin surfaces are the primary sites of involvement, the mucous membranes of the upper gastrointestinal tract can also be extensively involved. There are several genetic variants of epidermolysis bullosa (Table 10-8).

Epidermolysis bullosa results from defects in the structural integrity of the dermal-epidermal basement membrane. In epidermolysis bullosa simplex (EBS) there is a true split through the cytoplasm of basal cells. In junctional epidermolysis bullosa (JEB) and dystrophic epidermolysis bullosa (DEB), the defect is a lack of adherence between cellular layers. Regardless, the result is a surface structure with minimal ability to withstand any shear forces. The genetic basis is probably related to abnormal gene function for keratins.

In EBS, the presentation is obvious early in life, usually when the infant begins to crawl. Sites of maximum friction are the most symptomatic (e.g., knees, elbows). JEB and DEB present later in life, because more trauma is required to elicit the abnormal response. In some of the variants, lesions can include the anus, genitourinary tract, and, ominously from the anesthesiology perspective, the larynx and vocal apparatus. Laryngeal scarring with vocal cord dysfunction or airway obstruction has been reported.[56] In EB patients, lesions of the airway can result from vigorous laryngoscopy. Esophageal obstruction and webbing has been reported.[57] Abnormality in coagulation has also been reported.[58]

Diagnosis. Epidermolysis bullosa is not subtle, and elective surgery in severe cases is uncommon. Although all surface areas are at risk, each EB patient will have areas of the body more affected than others. These sites should be identified preoperatively so that they can be protected in the perioperative period. It is particularly important to

TABLE 10–8   Genetics of Epidermolysis Bullosa Variants

Syndrome	Genetic Transmission
Epidermolysis bullosa simplex (EBS)	Autosomal dominant
Junctional epidermolysis bullosa (JEB)	Autosomal recessive
Dystrophic epidermolysis bullosa (DEB)	Variable

TABLE 10–9   Preoperative Preparation for Patients with Epidermolysis Bullosa

Stress-dose corticosteroids
Wound care
Aspiration prophylaxis
Liver function tests
Blood urea nitrogen/creatinine

identify lesions in the oropharynx or esophagus, because these may predict laryngeal involvement and risk of acute postoperative airway compromise from lesions. Fortunately, other congenital issues are not regularly associated with EB.

Preoperative Preparation (Table 10-9)

Most EB patients take chronic corticosteroids and need "stress-dose" corticosteroids on the day of surgery. Wound care and infection management/prevention are key elements for survival in EB patients and must be continued carefully in the perioperative period. EB patients with involvement of the esophagus may have severe dysphasia that can compromise airway reflexes and increase the risk of aspiration during induction or emergence from anesthesia.[59] Significant laryngeal stenosis has been reported with EB.[56] If history or symptomatology suggests an abnormal airway, a preoperative assessment with indirect laryngoscopy by an otolaryngologist may be necessary to identify existing lesions that could influence subsequent plans for airway management. Nephrotoxic and hepatotoxic agents such as cyclosporine and colchicine[60,61] have been used for treatment of EB, and preoperative preparation should address these risks when they apply.

Intraoperative Care. The key to safe anesthetic care in these patients is caution with skin and mucous membranes. The blood pressure cuff should be applied over padding and only inflated when needed. Excessive pressure or sustained inflation can cause injury and should be avoided. Placement of monitors must be done with caution.[62,63] Electrocardiographic (ECG) electrode pads can cause lesions. All positioning and patient transfers must be performed with the absolute minimum shear force applied to the body surface, and whenever possible patients should be encouraged to move themselves to decrease the risk of skin injury.[64] Spinal anesthesia for surgery has been reported.[62] Regional anesthesia for surgery or obstetrics[65] can be an excellent choice, as long as the skin at the block site is normal.[66-69] Successful brachial plexus anesthesia has also been reported in EB patients.[70] Aggressive volume or injecting pressure for infiltration should be avoided, because this can cause skin lesions. With general anesthesia, airway management can be problematic.[71] Prolonged mask ventilation could subject the face to enough friction to cause disfiguring facial lesions.[72] The physical maneuvers necessary to properly place an LMA would be likely to create lesions in the airway and should probably be avoided. Endotracheal intubation is the best approach to securing the airway but has been associated with lesions, edema, and hemorrhage.[73] This is particularly true with emergency obstetric care.[74] Atraumatic technique, the smallest possible endotracheal tube, and generous lubrication of the tube are necessary. There are no particular advantages among general anesthetic agents. Intramuscular and intravenous ketamine have been used as sole anesthesia for minor procedures.[75] The eyes should not be taped closed, but lubricated. The risk to skin surfaces from stormy emergence make rapid emergence techniques valuable. Suctioning during emergence should be gentle and limited to direct vision to avoid creating oropharyngeal lesions.[76] With intravenous drugs, the patency of intravenous access must be continuously verified, because extravasation can be associated with serious skin injury.

Summary (Table 10-10). Epidermolysis bullosa is a genetic defect in the skin and mucous membranes that decreases the tensile strength of body surfaces and results in extensive lesions from minimal trauma. Involvement of the esophagus and oropharynx can make airway management difficult, and even minimal trauma from laryngoscopy, stylettes, forceful intubation, or blind suctioning can create lesions that compromise the airway. Regional anesthesia can be selected, as long as the block site is clear of lesions. Excessive volume and/or pressure with infiltration of local anesthetic for intravenous placement or nerve block can cause skin injury. Intravenous extravasation is also associated with potential skin slough.

ERYTHEMA MULTIFORME

Erythema multiforme (EM) is a spectrum of diseases that have in common an immunologic basis for inflammatory lesions of the skin.[77-79] When involving mainly mucous membranes, it is called the Stevens-Johnson syndrome (SJS).[80] When precipitated by a bacterial skin infection it is called the staphylococcal scalded skin syndrome (SSSS). When there is a sudden onset and a large area of skin and mucous membranes is involved, the syndrome is referred to as toxic epidermal necrolysis (TEN).[81]

Pathophysiology and Clinical Manifestations (Table 10-11). The majority of the immune reactions causative for EM are triggered by systemic virus exposure, with drugs[82,83] and bacteria[84,85] causing a minority of cases.[86] Some cases have been triggered by human immunodeficiency virus (HIV)[87] or herpes. Rarely, a response that resembles EM[88] can follow radiation therapy.[89] Both the bacterially triggered (SSSS, TEN) and drug triggered (SJS) types have a more abrupt onset and fulminant course.[80] Mucocutaneous lesions of the skin adjacent to the airway and mucous membranes within the airway can cause life-threatening airway compromise. In the less-fulminant EM cases, extensive skin lesions can present in a manner indistinguishable from epidermolysis bullosa. Conjunctivitis, corneal lesions, and uveitis are common. Acute myocarditis has been associated with EM triggered by viremia. Mucosal lesions of the trachea or gastrointestinal tract can cause perforation,[90] resulting in esophageal rupture, mediastinitis, pneumothorax, bronchopleural fistula, or

TABLE 10–11 Spectrum of Erythema Multiforme
Stevens-Johnson Syndrome (SJS)
Mucous membranes
Drug Reaction
Sudden Onset, Fulminant Course
Staphylococcal Scalded Skin Syndrome (SSSS)
Skin lesions
Bacterial trigger
Sudden onset, fulminant course
Toxic Epidermal Necrolysis (TEN)
Large lesions of skin and mucous membranes
Bacterial trigger
Sudden onset, fulminant course
Erythema Multiforme (EM)
Skin, mucous membrane
Conjunctivitis, uveitis
Corneal lesions
Renal failure
Gradual onset
Variable severity

TABLE 10–10 Anesthetic Management Issues with Epidermolysis Bullosa
Padding pressure points
Careful patient transfer to avoid skin injury
Avoid high subcutaneous injection pressure
Injury from prolonged mask ventilation
Airway injury from instrumentation, stormy emergence

TABLE 10–12   Perioperative Issues with Erythema Multiforme
Skin care
Stress-dose corticosteroids
Echocardiogram to detect pericardial effusion
Detection of airway lesions
Emergency airway care (Stevens-Johnson syndrome)
Hypovolemia, electrolyte abnormality (toxic epidermal necrolysis)
Eye care

massive gastrointestinal hemorrhage. Fulminant cases may cause acute renal failure.[91]

Preoperative Preparation (Table 10-12). Mild cases of EM present no unique issues for anesthesiology or surgery. In contrast, SJS, TEN, and SSSS are phenomena that can create the need for anesthetic intervention.[92] Numerous drugs, including antimicrobials,[93] antiepileptics,[94] and antihypertensives have been reported as triggers for life-threatening airway compromise from SJS. When time permits, identifying comorbidity may allow optimization, appropriate assessment, or planning, especially if myocarditis or renal failure is known.

With EM patients, chronic skin care techniques to prevent skin injury and infection are important. Continuing this skin care into the perioperative period reduces the risks of infection and sepsis. Chronic corticosteroid therapy is common, and stress-dose corticosteroids are often required in the perioperative period. When myocarditis is known or suspected, echocardiography is required to define ventricular function and quantify pericardial effusion. If airway lesions are suspected, careful indirect laryngoscopy can identify critical lesions. In fulminant cases, this is specifically avoided to prevent acute airway compromise. With extensive acute lesions, loss of fluid and electrolytes can cause hypovolemia or electrolyte disturbances that should be identified and corrected. Severe chronic cases can be associated with cachexia and malnutrition.

Anesthetic Management

There are no unique anesthetic agents or techniques indicated in these patients. Barbiturates may precipitate SJS. Skin care is a primary issue. Skin injury from minimal trauma is a risk, and all elements of patient handling must reflect concern for this issue. Because cutaneous barriers are incompetent, surfaces must be protected from contamination, because bacteremia and sepsis could be fatal.

In fulminant cases, the anesthesia care required is often airway management. With SJS especially, anesthesia care for airway management is often urgent. All elements of management of the difficult airway may be required, including tracheostomy. When EM patients present for elective surgery, regional anesthesia is appropriate, as long as the skin at the site of the block is normal. With general anesthesia, nitrous oxide should be used with caution in light of the risk of occult barotrauma. For similar reasons, maximum peak ventilatory pressures should be kept as low as possible. In fulminant cases, dehydration and electrolyte loss intraoperatively should be considered likely. Monitoring devices can injure skin, as with epidermolysis bullosa. Unexplained arrhythmia could be a sign of acute myocarditis. Ocular care should reflect the possibility of EM involvement of the eyes.

Summary. Erythema multiforme is a syndrome with a variety of presentations. Minor cases have virtually no anesthetic implications. Severe cases can present for emergency airway management. The majority of the anesthetic management issues are related to comorbidities such as dehydration, electrolyte disturbance, renal failure, myocarditis, and ocular involvement. Most anesthetic techniques are appropriate.

ERYTHEMA NODOSUM

Pathophysiology and Clinical Manifestations. Erythema nodosum (EN) is an acute inflammatory reaction within skin and subcutaneous tissue.[95] The nodules are deep, painful, and red and most commonly represent a hypersensitivity reaction to prior inflammation or infection.[96] Some cases can be precipitated by acute streptococcal pharyngitis. Regional enteritis and ulcerative colitis have also been associated with erythema nodosum.[97] Numerous other associated features are listed in Table 10-13. Less common causes include leptospirosis,[98] toxoplasmosis,[99] Q fever,[100] and sarcoid.[101] A syndrome that resembles EN has been reported as a sequela of malignancy.[102]

TABLE 10–13 Diseases Associated with Erythema Nodosum	
Streptococcal pharyngitis	Fungal infections
Sarcoidosis	Histoplasmosis
Inflammatory bowel disease	Coccidioidomycosis
Drugs	Tuberculosis
Pregnancy	Syphilis
Yersinia enterocolitica	Gonorrhea
Measles	Rubella

In the majority of cases there is associated joint involvement, most commonly of the knees, ankles, and wrists. Permanent joint deformity is uncommon, but septic arthritis can be an indication for surgery.

Differential Diagnosis. The lesions of EN can be confused with traumatic bruising, fat necrosis, and superficial thrombophlebitis. In contrast to other dermatologic syndromes, EN is usually associated with a short interval to full resolution (3 to 6 weeks). Secondary morbidity from EN is uncommon, unless related to complications of the lesions.

Preoperative Preparation. Because the etiology of EN can be infectious, presurgical preparation should focus on identification and treatment of the infectious etiology. In cases that present for emergent surgery (e.g., infectious arthritis), the possibility of other infections should be considered, even while not delaying the surgical procedure. When the precipitating factor is sarcoid, chest radiography and spirometry should be obtained to identify limited pulmonary reserves. Arterial blood gas analysis may be indicated for severe cases. Because viremia can be etiologic for EN, other serious sequelae of viremia, such as encephalitis and myocarditis, should be considered during preparation for emergency surgery.

Intraoperative Considerations (Table 10-14). If respiratory or systemic infections are etiologic, contamination of anesthesia equipment should be prevented with either filters or a disposable circuit/carbon dioxide absorber. Both regional and general anesthesia are possible, and there are no specific recommendations regarding agents. During acute infection, there can be coincident infection of the airway that can create issues such as laryngospasm, bronchospasm, or atelectatic lobar collapse from inspissated secretion.

Summary. Erythema nodosum is a cutaneous hypersensitivity response to a variety of infectious and inflammatory disorders. Because joint involvement can occur, septic arthritis can present as an urgent indication for surgery. When sarcoidosis or pulmonary tuberculosis is causative, pulmonary compromise should be suspected. Because of the possibly infectious etiology, anesthesia equipment should be protected. There are no specific anesthetic agents or techniques either indicated or contraindicated.

FABRY'S DISEASE

Pathophysiology. Fabry's disease results from a congenital defect of glycosphingolipid caused by abnormal function of the enzyme alpha galactosidase A. The defect is transmitted as an X-linked autosomal recessive syndrome. The result is widespread deposition of neutral glycosphingolipids within most visceral structures and body fluids. The organs most affected are the vascular endothelium, smooth muscle of the cardiovascular and renal systems, cornea, kidney, reticuloendothelial system, and the ganglion and perineural cells of the nervous system.

Clinical Manifestations (Table 10-15). The consequences of lipid accumulation include excruciating pain, blue-black vascular lesions of the superficial layers of skin and mucous membranes, as well as organ dysfunction. The lesions of the mucous membranes commonly occur in the mouth and oropharynx. Some cases can occur without surface lesions.[103]

The affected organ systems present with symptoms of organ dysfunction. Cardiac disease presents early in life,[104,105] including coronary artery disease,[106] myocarditis, left ventricular hypertrophy, conduction

---

TABLE 10–14   Perioperative Issues with Erythema Nodosum

Identify infectious etiology
Quantify diminished pulmonary reserve
Detect myocarditis, encephalitis
Prevent contamination of anesthesia gear
Laryngospasm
Bronchospasm
Atelectasis

TABLE 10–15   Clinical Manifestations of Fabry's Disease

Skin lesions
Mucous membrane lesions
Coronary artery disease
Myocarditis
Cardiac conduction lesions
Valvular heart disease
Congestive heart failure
Hypertrophic cardiomyopathy
Pulmonary hypertension
Chronic renal failure
Delayed gastric emptying
Central hyperthermia
Ocular lesions
Retinal detachment/thrombosis

abnormalities,[107] valvular insufficiency,[108-110] and congestive heart failure (CHF). The progress and severity of these diseases are accelerated by the universal presence of severe hypertension. Hypertrophic cardiomyopathy has been associated with some cases of Fabry's disease.[111-113] Pulmonary hypertension from lipid accumulation in the pulmonary vasculature can occur.[114,115]

Accumulation of lipid in the kidney causes progressive loss of renal tubular units.[116] Tubules lose squamous tissue as well as the ability to exchange electrolytes. Renal blood vessels are also involved with progressive luminal narrowing. The result is progressive, chronic renal failure, and a renovascular component for hypertension. Intestinal dysfunction can occur with obstruction and delayed gastric emptying.[107,117]

Vascular lesions occur within the CNS and peripheral nervous system. Pain, hyperhidrosis, and gastrointestinal symptoms can result. Episodic fever is reported. Abnormality in the brain stem and cerebellum cause disequilibrium and abnormal temperature regulation.[118] Dementia, seizure disorder, and intracranial hemorrhage can occur. Ocular involvement[119,120] includes corneal opacity, lens involvement, and arterial lesions that can result in retinal artery thrombosis[121,122] and retinal detachment.

Diagnosis. In affected males, the diagnosis is made in childhood from skin lesions and fever of unknown origin. It can be mistakenly attributed to collagen vascular disease, rheumatic fever, or vasculitis. Fabry's disease can be diagnosed in the workup of early onset of cardiovascular, renal, or neurologic disease. Biochemical investigation is confirmatory.

Preoperative Considerations (Table 10-16). Because there is no specific treatment for Fabry's disease, preoperative preparation should focus on detection of end-organ disease. Quantification of ocular involvement should be considered to avoid the association of postoperative visual defects with surgical positioning and hemodynamic fluctuation. Measurement of blood urea nitrogen/creatinine will determine the degree of chronic renal failure. An electrocardiogram[123,124] and an echocardiogram[125] are required to detect myocardial ischemia, valve lesions, CHF, and ventricular outflow tract obstruction. Silent myocardial ischemia is likely due to lesions of the autonomic nervous system. A pharmacologic stress test may be required to determine if significant coronary artery disease is present, especially if the patient is sedentary. With an abnormal stress test or echocardiographic evidence of pulmonary hypertension, cardiac catheterization may be necessary. Careful neurologic examination is important to document peripheral lesions,[126,127] especially if regional anesthesia is planned.

Intraoperative Considerations (Table 10-17). Preoperative sedation should be considered to prevent excessive activation of the abnormal autonomic nervous system. Increased levels of monitoring may be required because of major organ system comorbidity. Abnormal temperature regulation should be assumed, and active warming and cooling devices should be present. Autonomic neuropathy is likely, and vasoactive drugs to treat sudden hypotension and hypertension should be prepared in advance.

With general anesthesia, the airway should be evaluated in advance because of oropharyngeal lesions. Agent selection is determined by comorbidity. Excellent pain control should be planned, particularly in patients with chronic pain from peripheral nerve lesions. Pain control may require carbamazine or phenytoin.[128] If morphine has been successful in treating prior pain episodes, it may be useful postoperatively.[129] If chronic pain is treated with carbamizine,[130] increased metabolism of nondepolarizing muscle relaxants should be assumed and dosing of muscle relaxants should be guided by neuromuscular blockade monitoring. Regional anesthesia is a consideration; however, autonomic instability could exaggerate the hemodynamic instability normally associated with sympathectomy from central neuraxial blocks.[131] If CNS lesions are progressive, central neuraxial block is relatively contraindicated because of the possible presence of central demyelination.

TABLE 10–16 Preoperative Preparation for Patients with Fabry's Disease
Quantify ocular involvement
Measure blood urea nitrogen/creatinine
Electrocardiogram and echocardiogram
Functional cardiac study
May need cardiac catheterization
MRI/CT if neurologic exam abnormal

TABLE 10–17 Anesthetic Management Issues with Fabry's Disease
Sedation to avoid sympathetic activations
Invasive monitoring
Temperature monitoring/control
Hemodynamic control
Airway management issues
Need for excellent analgesia
Centrally mediated chronic pain
Autonomic instability with neuraxial block

Summary. Fabry's disease is a congenital defect of glycosphingolipid metabolism that results in massive deposition of the lipoproteins in visceral structures, causing organ dysfunction. Cardiovascular, pulmonary, neurologic, renal, and ocular dysfunction are common. Anesthetic preparation and care are determined by the presence and extent of major organ system disease.

HERPES SIMPLEX

Herpes infections of the skin and mucous membranes are caused by infection with human herpes simplex virus (HSV-1 and HSV-2). Once systemic infection occurs, a primary outbreak is followed by a dormant state.[132] Recurring outbreaks result from activation. Oral and genital sites for primary infection are the most common. During the dormant state, the virus remains in the cells of the neuraxial ganglia. During the primary outbreak, the lesions are contagious by contact. After transfer to other surfaces, the viruses are only briefly contagious. Genital herpes in an active outbreak can be transferred to the neonate during transit through the birth canal. Not only is skin involved for the neonate, but devastating infection of visceral organs is a risk. Whereas genital herpes is almost always directly related to sexual contact, facial-oral infection has many causes and involves the majority of adults worldwide.[133] Reactivation is triggered by stress, fever, contact sports,[134] or surgical manipulation. The viruses move down the nerve by axonal flow and produce lesions. Numerous common lesions are listed in Table 10-18.

Diagnosis. Small, raised, confluent lesions are suggestive of the presence of the disease. The facial lesions are often confused with many other skin lesions, such as erythema multiforme, impetigo, and vaccinia. Genital herpes can be confused with fungal infections, urinary tract infection, syphilis, lymphogranuloma venereum, and genital papilloma. Mucopurulent herpes cervicitis is easily confused with infectious vaginitis. Recurrent infections are usually easily identified because of prior experience.[135]

Preoperative Considerations (Table 10-19). During primary outbreak, generalized viremia is present. Elective surgical procedures are unwise, because body fluids are contagious. Patients with herpetic whitlow can present for surgical drainage of infected finger tissue.[136] Topical and oral antiviral drugs are both therapeutic in acute episodes and part of suppression therapy to prevent outbreaks. Parenteral antiviral drugs can be lifesaving in generalized herpes and herpes encephalitis.[137-139] Detection of systemic infection is a priority. During viremia, transmission from primary lesions or systemic viremia is possible by instrumentation. This would make elective airway management during acute oral outbreak or neuraxial block during primary genital herpes unwise.

Intraoperative Care. When emergency surgery is required during acute herpetic outbreaks, all body fluids from the patient should be considered contaminated. The anesthesia machine should be protected with filters and equipment cleaned as if contaminated. Nurses and equipment aides should be warned of the risk of transmission. Simple contact cleaning is effective, and contaminated surfaces remain contagious for only a brief interval.

No particular anesthetic agents or techniques offer any advantage. Central neuraxial block during acute or systemic episodes should be avoided. Other than avoiding viral transmission to other people, recurrent lesions have no specific issues.

Summary. Acute herpetic infections are associated with systemic viremia. Elective surgery and anesthesia should be avoided to prevent dissemination of the viruses. In particular, dural puncture could induce herpes meningitis and/or encephalitis. When emergency surgery is required, the lesions should be considered contagious. Anesthesia machine protection, appropriate cleaning, and warning health care providers of risk for exposure are essential. No particular anesthetic agents are indicated or contraindicated.

TABLE 10–18   Manifestations of Herpes
Primary gingivostomatitis
Primary genital herpes
Recurrent facial-oral herpes
Herpesvirus cervicitis
Recurrent genital herpes
Herpes associated with HIV
Herpes in immunocompromised patients
Herpetic whitlow
Generalized herpes
Herpetic keratoconjunctivitis
Herpes encephalitis

TABLE 10–19   Perioperative Issues in Patients with Herpes Infection
Generalized viremia during primary outbreak
Viral transfer with airway management
Central nervous system infection with neuraxial instrumentation
Protection of anesthetic equipment
Universal precautions

MASTOCYTOSIS

Mastocytosis is caused by mast cell hyperplasia in the liver, spleen, bone marrow, lymph nodes, skin, and gastrointestinal tract.[140] Mast cells easily degranulate and symptoms related to release of mediators are common, including urticaria, flushing, abdominal pain, bone pain, diarrhea, nausea, and vomiting. This familial syndrome is based on abnormal expression of the gene that regulates mast cell production. There are a variety of manifestations of mastocytosis, and a classification system is presented in Table 10-20.

The clinical features for any given patient are determined by which mast cell mediators are produced in excess. Most patients have cutaneous lesions referred to as urticaria pigmentosa, which are small, reddish-brown, itchy lesions of the trunk and limbs. In aggressive forms, these lesions can become confluent and involve nasal and oral mucosa. Local heparin release creates a lesion with easy bruising by trivial contact. The noncutaneous manifestations of mastocytosis are related to mast cell infiltration of various organ systems. Gastritis and peptic ulcer disease result from hypersecretion secondary to increased plasma histamine levels. Abdominal pain, diarrhea, and malabsorption[141] are other manifestations directly related to mast cell invasion of gastrointestinal mucosa.[142] Liver and spleen involvement occur in some cases. The most common liver manifestation is elevation of liver enzymes, but severe cases can present as ascites and portal hypertension[143] associated with liver fibrosis.[144] Marked enlargement of the spleen occurs in a majority of cases. Bone lesions are caused by focal deposits of mast cells. Bone pain is the most common result, but pathologic fracture can occur.[145] Numerous hematologic abnormalities are associated with mastocytosis.[146] Systemic response to mediators is as varied as are the mediators chemically (Table 10-21).

Systemic mediator release can cause neuropsychiatric abnormalities, including irritability, decreased attention span, memory impairment, and secondary depression.[147,148] There is an association between mastocytosis and eosinophilic granuloma.[149]

Diagnosis. Most cases of mastocytosis are diagnosed by the characteristic skin lesions. Biopsy confirms the role of mast cells in various lesions (skin, mucous membranes, bone). Urine studies may reveal increased levels of metabolites of mast cell mediators. Without the presence of skin lesions, CT, bone scan, or endoscopy may be diagnostic. Because the systemic effects mimic other diseases with vasoactive release, workup should rule out carcinoid and pheochromocytoma by measuring urine 5-hydroxyindoleacetic acid and metanephrines.

Preoperative Considerations (Table 10-22). Gastric hypersecretion should be suspected in all mastocytosis patients. Gastric acid blockade and increased gastric emptying with metoclopramide should be considered. If liver disease is suspected, assessment of synthetic and coagulation function is required.[150] Anxiolysis may decrease mast cell activation. If chronic corticosteroids are used for treatment, stress-dose corticosteroids should be ordered for the perioperative period.

Intraoperative Consideration. Vasodilation makes hypothermia more likely, and active temperature support should be planned.[151] Release of mediators is increased by manipulation of lesions, which should be kept to the absolute minimum.[152] Bone pain indicates a risk of fracture, which should be considered during positioning. Hemodynamic instability may occur from mast cell mediator release.[153] Sudden, profound, intraoperative hypotension has been reported,[154] and epinephrine may be the intervention of choice.[155] As a result, invasive monitoring and immediate

TABLE 10–20	Manifestations of Mastocytosis
Indolent	
Syncope	
Cutaneous	
Ulcer	
Malabsorption	
Bone marrow aggregate	
Skeletal	
Liver-spleen	
Lymph gland	
Hematologic	
Myeloproliferative	
Myelodysplastic	
Aggressive	
Mastocytic leukemia	

TABLE 10–21	Mast Cell Mediators
Mediator	**Consequence**
Histamine	Pruritus, bronchoconstriction, gastric hypersecretion
Heparin	Local anticoagulation, osteoporosis
Proteases	Bone lesions
Leukotrienes	Vasopermeability, bronchoconstriction, vasoconstriction
Prostaglandin D_2	Vasodilation, bronchoconstriction
Platelet-activating factor	Vasopermeability, vasodilation, bronchoconstriction
Cytokines	Cellular activation

TABLE 10–22   Perioperative Issues with Mastocytosis

Gastric acid blockade
Delayed gastric emptying
Liver function testing
Coagulation testing
Stress-dose corticosteroids
Temperature support
Hemodynamic instability from histamine release
Invasive monitoring
Avoidance of histamine-releasing anesthetic agents
Histamine release with blood transfusion

TABLE 10–23   Mucopolysaccharidoses

Syndrome	Enzyme	Skeletal Defect
Hunter's	Sulfoiduron Sulfatase	Spine
Hurler's	α-L-Iduronidase	Face, spine
Morquio's	N-acetyl-galactose-6 sulfate sulfatose	Face, spine, femur
Scheie's	α-L-Iduronidase	Hands, face
Sanfilippo's	Heparan sulfatase	Chest, clavicle

availability of vasoactive drugs is often required. Histamine release with transfusion can be massive; pretreatment with diphenhydramine should be routine.

Regional anesthesia is acceptable, but vasodilation may accentuate the consequences of neuraxial sympathetic block. Specific agents for general anesthesia should be selected to avoid further histamine release.[156] Light anesthesia may trigger histamine release.

Summary. Mastocytosis presents numerous anesthetic implications related to release of mast cell mediators. Cutaneous, gastrointestinal, and systemic issues are most prominent. Many of the mediators have potent vasoactive properties that can alter the course of any anesthetic procedure.

MUCOPOLYSACCHARIDOSES

Mucopolysaccharidoses occur because of genetic defects in enzymes that degrade intracellular complex molecules. The action of the abnormal enzymes leads to accumulation of these partially degraded compounds and secondary cellular and organ system pathology.[157] The specific enzyme defect determines the different syndromes (Table 10-23). Accumulation of mucopolysaccharides (heparin sulfate, dermatan sulfate, and/or keratin sulfate) is the direct cause of the systemic manifestations. Accumulation occurs in CNS, peripheral nerves, ganglia, cardiac valves, coronary arteries,[158] liver, spleen, lymph nodes, retina, pituitary, and testicles. Skeletal and bony defects result from abnormal osteocytes and chondrocytes, which are enlarged and have multiple large vacuoles. In the area of the growth plates the chondrocytes are disorganized, leading to decreased growth and early closure.

Differential Diagnosis and Clinical Manifestations. Although similar, each syndrome has unique features. Hurler's syndrome results from accumulation of dermatan, and

lesser amounts of heparin.[159] The head is enlarged with abnormal faces and poor dentition. Upper airway defects are common and severe sleep apnea may be associated.[160] Airway obstruction can be progressive and symptomatic.[160] Hypoplasia of the odontoid can occur, often presenting as quadriparesis requiring fusion.[161] Short neck, flaring of the thorax and kyphoscoliosis characterize the trunk. Flexion contractures are common. Chronic dislocation and dysplasia of the hip can be present.

Cardiac defects occur because of infiltration of cardiac cells,[162] and progressive accumulation around the valves, especially the mitral valve can be observed.[163] Retardation is common, and MRI reveals multiple small cystic lesions of white matter. Acute hydrocephalus has been reported with deposition of mucopolysaccharides in the lower brain.[164] Glaucoma from mucopolysaccharide deposition has been reported.[165]

Hunter's syndrome results from accumulation of heparan sulfate. Skeletal defects include absent thoracolumbar kyphosis, pediatric carpal tunnel syndrome,[166-168] abnormal facies, structural upper airway obstruction, and mild to moderate distortion of the chest. Progressive mucopolysaccharide deposition in the upper airway leads to airway obstruction and can present as stridor and airway compromise.[169] Sleep apnea is common.[160] In one case, difficulty with endotracheal intubation during airway surgery was related to bulging false cords and glottic stenosis from deposition of mucopolysaccharides (Table 10-24).[170]

Morquio's syndrome results from accumulation of keratan sulfate and chondroitin-6-sulfate. These children are normal at birth but demonstrate spine dysplasia within 12 to 18 months. Severe thoracolumbar kyphoscoliosis occurs early in life.[171] Abnormality at the craniocervical junction is almost universal with hypoplastic odontoid,[171] atlantoaxial instability,[172,173] and, in some, severe cervical cord compression[174,175] or quadriparesis.[176] Spinal cord compression and myelopathy is a common chronic disability.[177] Dwarfism results from limited development of the trunk. Joint laxity, abnormal faces, and valgus/varus deformity of the knees are common. The CNS is usually not involved; mental retardation is uncommon.

TABLE 10–24 Comorbidities Associated with Mucopolysaccharidoses

Progressive airway obstruction
Obstructive sleep apnea
Cervical spine instability
Kyphoscoliosis
Chronic dislocation of hip
Cardiac conduction defects
Retardation
Chronic hydrocephalus
Glaucoma

Life expectancy is shortened by progressive kyphoscoliosis. Fusion of C2 to the occiput is frequently required.[178]

Preoperative Preparation (Table 10-25). Obstructive sleep apnea can be associated with pulmonary hypertension and right ventricular dysfunction. Respiratory mechanics can be compromised from airway obstruction, pectus deformities, or mechanical distortion of the thorax[179] and deposition in the tracheobronchial tree.[180] If suspected, transthoracic echocardiogram with attention to the right ventricle and right-sided valves is indicated. If a murmur is detected, echocardiography is also indicated because of the potential involvement of the aortic and mitral valves from mucopolysaccharide deposition[163,181] and the resultant cardiomyopathy.[182] Even in young children, an electrocardiogram is important because of cardiac defects from accumulation of mucopolysaccharides and early-onset coronary artery disease.[158,183] Radiographic evidence of severe thoracic deformity suggests increased risk of postoperative ventilatory insufficiency. Radiographic investigation of the cervical spine may be required if limited range of motion or abnormal surface anatomy is observed. Because odontoid development may be abnormal, atlantoaxial instability may be present. Flexion-extension cervical spine films are indicated, and if cooperation is impossible, instability must be presumed. With Hurler's

TABLE 10–25 Preoperative Issues in Patients with Mucopolysaccharidoses

Pulmonary function testing
Echocardiogram
Electrocardiogram
Chest radiograph
Cervical spine radiographs in flexion and extension
C-spine fusion

syndrome, C2-occiput fusion may be required for atlantoaxial instability owing to odontoid hypoplasia or the onset of spontaneous quadriplegia.[184]

Intraoperative Management. A large tongue, thickening of airway structures, and friable tissue make airway management more difficult. Plans for difficult airway management should be made for any patient with one of these syndromes.[185] Bronchospasm may be more common.[186] In one series, airway issues occurred in 53% of patients.[187] Death from inability to ventilate or intubate has been reported in patients with Hurler's syndrome.[188,189] Emergency tracheostomy was lifesaving in others.[183,190] Use of the LMA has been helpful in some of these children with difficult airway management, to control the airway and to assist with fiberoptic intubation.[191] LMA use has also been a failure.[192] Airway management can be challenging when cervical cord compression is symptomatic and the patient is uncooperative.[174] Transoral decompression of the brainstem and proximal cervical spine may be the chosen surgical procedure.[177] With Hurler's syndrome, progressive airway obstruction may require tracheostomy if laser decompression is not possible.[169]

Contractures may make positioning very difficult, and pressure injuries should be actively prevented. Because of tissue deposits, contractures, and bony defects, intravenous access may be very difficult. Deformities of the skeleton make regional anesthesia difficult and potentially dangerous. Even with successful catheterization of the epidural space, epidural anesthesia can be incomplete secondary to deposition of mucopolysaccharides in the epidural space.[193] Continuous spinal anesthesia has been used successfully in a child with Morquio's syndrome[194] and a child with Hurler's syndrome[195] in whom intubation could not be accomplished. During general anesthesia, recognition of acute cord compression would be difficult, and, if unrecognized, devastating neurologic injury could be the outcome[196] Massive intraoperative stroke has also been reported in a child.[197] There are no specific issues with anesthetic agents unless comorbidity is present, such as cardiac dysfunction. Complete heart block during anesthetic management has been reported.[198] Delayed awakening has been associated with Hunter's syndrome in one case.[199] Progressive respiratory failure leading to death has been reported after surgery, related to the mechanical limits of respiratory mechanics.[200] Increased sensitivity to opioids should be assumed; and because of the high probability of abnormal upper airway, airway obstruction will be even more likely during acute pain management (Table 10-26).

Summary. Patients with congenital defects in mucopolysaccharide metabolism present with anesthetic issues mainly because of skeletal structural issues. Airway management, positioning, and intravenous access problems are likely.

TABLE 10–26   Anesthetic Issues with Mucopolysaccharidoses

Difficult airway management
Difficulty with ventilation
Acute airway obstruction
Difficult positioning/injuries
Incomplete epidural block
Complete heart block
Delayed emergence
Challenging acute pain control due to obstructive sleep apnea

Asymptomatic compression of the spinal cord can be present, and spinal cord lesions from positioning during general anesthesia have been reported. Abnormality of the thorax creates diminished respiratory function and increases the probability of postoperative respiratory failure.

NEUROFIBROMATOSIS

Neurofibromatosis is a syndrome caused by the abnormal deposition of neural tissue within the nervous system, endocrine system, visceral structures, and skin.[201] The origin is congenital, with an autosomal dominant mode of transmission. Two variants are known[202]: central neurofibromatosis (10%) and von Recklinghausen's neurofibromatosis (85%).[203,204] Both have characteristic skin lesions. The central variant is associated with multiple slow-growing CNS lesions, including bilateral acoustic neuroma in most cases.[205] With the von Recklinghausen variant, osseous lesions, renal artery involvement, optic nerve compression,[206] and hydrocephalus can occur.[207] Involvement of the mid brain can cause a variety of endocrine disorders. Spinal cord lesions can create paraplegia.[208]

Clinical Manifestations (Table 10-27). Deposition of proliferating neural tissue causes organ-specific dysfunction. Proliferation in osseous tissue causes cyst formation, osteoporosis, and fracture. Long-bone fracture, osteoarthritis of weight-bearing joints, and kyphoscoliosis are potential pathophysiologic consequences. Deposition of neural tissue in the oropharynx and larynx can cause dysphagia or airway incompetence.[209,210] Interstitial lung disease can result from deposition of neural tissue.[211] Other respiratory involvement can result from chronic hypoxemia, causing pulmonary hypertension, right-sided heart strain, and respiratory failure from cor pulmonale. Obstruction of the urinary tract and/or renal artery involvement can cause renal failure. Pelvic obstruction can complicate obstetric care.[212,213] Neuroendocrine proliferation can lead to pheochromocytoma and other less common endocrinopathies.

TABLE 10–27   Clinical Manifestations of Neurofibromatosis

Bone cyst, osteoporosis, fracture
Dysphagia
Airway incompetence
Interstitial lung disease
Hydrocephalus
Retinal artery lesions
Optic nerve compress
Spinal cord compromise
Renal failure
Neuroendocrine disorders
Pelvic outlet obstruction: difficult obstetric care

Diagnosis. The diagnosis of neurofibromatosis can be delayed by the manifestations in a major organ system. The most common diagnostic evidence comes from observation of the classic skin lesions called café-au-lait spots.[214,215] The café-au-lait spots can be confused with pigmented nevus. Skin biopsy is definitive.

Preoperative Considerations (Table 10-28). The multiple sites of involvement of advanced neurofibromatosis determine the priorities for presurgical preparation. The primary site of involvement is the nervous system, which must be investigated completely. CT or MRI of the head[216] will identify masses, midline shift, or increased intracranial pressure and will demonstrate any potential risk of herniation. Occult spinal cord tumors have been reported.[217] If spinal cord involvement is suggested by weakness, pain, or other long tract signs, radiographic investigation is required. Meningocele and bony anomalies have been reported.[218,219] In particular, quantification of risk for airway management may require MRI examination of the

TABLE 10–28   Perioperative Issues for Patients with Neurofibromatosis

CT/MRI of head
Cervical spine radiographs in flexion/extension
Pulmonary function tests
Echocardiogram
Blood urea nitogen/creatinine measurement
Detection of abnormal electrolytes
Difficult airway management
Respiratory compromise with high neuraxial block
Temperature control
Abnormal response to muscle relaxants

cervical spinal cord.[220] Discovery of spinal osseous lesions would further protect the patient from spinal cord injury from fracture. The probability of pulmonary involvement can be suggested by history. If the history or physical examination (kyphoscoliosis) is positive,[221] spirometry and arterial blood gas analysis may be necessary. If there are signs of cor pulmonale, echocardiogram and even angiography may be required. If the upper airway is involved, indirect laryngoscopy should be performed by an experienced endoscopist.

Other issues that should be considered include renal failure, endocrine hyperplasia (pheochromocytoma), and optic nerve involvement. If regional anesthesia is a consideration, the site for the block must be free of lesions and anatomically normal enough to perform the block. Abnormal pituitary function is possible and occult electrolyte abnormalities should be investigated.

Intraoperative Considerations. When the airway or cervical spine is compromised, careful awake fiberoptic intubation is required. The degree of invasive monitoring is determined by the extent of major organ system compromise. When advanced pulmonary compromise is present, the possibility of prolonged postoperative mechanical ventilation must be considered.[222] In this subset of patients, central neuraxial block should be undertaken with the understanding that high levels of truncal somatic block could precipitate respiratory failure. Epidural analgesia for labor has been reported with success.[223] With advanced kyphoscoliosis, access for neuraxial block may be difficult or impossible. Even with successful epidural catheterization, the block can be incomplete because the epidural space may be partially obliterated. Abnormal temperature regulation should be assumed and active heating provided. No unique drug indications or contraindications are present, although abnormal response to muscle relaxants has been reported.[224-226]

Summary. Neurofibromatosis is a syndrome with consequences related to deposition and proliferation of abnormal neural tissue. Consequences are manifest in the central autonomic and peripheral nervous system, spine and long bones, airway, kidneys, and eyes. Anesthetic management is modified by CNS pathology, respiratory compromise, difficult airway management, endocrine and electrolyte abnormalities, and abnormal skin surface.

OSTEOGENESIS IMPERFECTA

The majority of patients with osteogenesis imperfecta (OI) have a genetic defect in the genes that creates structural collagen.[227] The subclassification of collagen found in the skeletal system, including ligament, tendon, and bone, is type I collagen. In OI there is either a quantitative defect or a structural deficiency of type I collagen.[228] Of the four or more genetic variants there is a range between extreme bone fragility that leads to death during or shortly after delivery to skeletal changes subtle enough to be confused with child abuse. The consequence of defective structural collagen is disturbance in the formation of enchondral and intramembranous bone. Ligament and tendon structure is variably defective and/or incomplete. The bone trabeculae most responsible for tensile strength are thin, and the interlinkage is diminished.

Clinical Manifestations. (Table 10-29). In the most extreme cases, multiple fractures occur during delivery. These cases are usually associated with neonatal demise. In the nonlethal forms of the disease, the most significant feature is brittle bone structure. Fractures occur from minimal force. More fractures occur in the lower extremities, perhaps because they are exposed to more trauma. The femur is fractured more often than the tibia for the same reason. Deformity of the pelvis can be extreme, and bowel obstruction from protrusion fracture of the acetabulum has been reported.[229] Spinal deformity develops because of decreased ligamentous stability, compression fractures, osteoporosis, and spondylolisthesis.[230] Kyphoscoliosis is the most common lesion, but others, including cervical spine instability/fracture[231] and upward migration of the odontoid, causing brain stem compression and altered cerebrospinal fluid flow, have been reported.[232,233] The teeth are malformed and fracture easily.[234] Blue sclera, thin sclera and cornea, and exophthalmos are common ocular abnormalities, and there has been a report of central retinal artery occlusion in the prone position in an OI patient.[235] An association with malignant hyperthermia has been reported,[236-238] although muscle biopsy from a clinical case did not test positive for malignant hyperthermia susceptibility.[239] Platelet dysfunction has been

TABLE 10–29 Clinical Manifestations of Osteogenesis Imperfecta

Multiple fractures with delivery
Fracture with minimal stress
Spinal deformity
Compression fractures
Spondylolisthesis
Abnormal dentition
Ocular lesions
Patient ductus arteriosus
Atrial septal defect
Valvular lesions

associated with OI.[240] Associated cardiac anomalies include patent ductus arteriosus, atrial septal defects, ventricular septal defects, and valvular defects.[241] Acquired cardiac defects associated with OI include aortic regurgitation,[242] mitral regurgitation from chordal rupture,[243,244] and cystic degeneration of the proximal aorta.[245]

Diagnosis. In infancy, OI can be confused with achondroplasia or other forms of dwarfism because of skeletal or skull anomalies with a common appearance. In childhood, idiopathic juvenile osteoporosis will also present in a similar manner. A confounding variable is child abuse, where fracture is also a feature of diagnosis.[246-250] In less severe forms of osteogenesis imperfecta, investigation of possible child abuse can be a cause for serious delay in diagnosis.

Preoperative Preparation (Table 10-30). The anatomic defects of osteogenesis imperfecta determine the preanesthetic preparation. Because of the nature of OI, most indications for surgery will be urgent, that is, treatment of fractures. This does not eliminate the issues of preparation. Creatine phosphokinase (CPK) levels should be measured because they can be elevated if there is risk of malignant hyperthermia. Because platelet function may be abnormal,[251] complete measurement of coagulation is indicated if there are any signs of coagulopathy, such as excessive bleeding, easy bruising, or blood with oral hygiene or bowel or bladder function.[252] Unexpected massive bleeding without an obvious surgical etiology has been reported in a patient with OI.[253] Because cor pulmonale can result from thoracic deformity, and because of associated congenital heart disease, a preoperative echocardiogram is required if a normal study is not previously known. Severe kyphosis will predict mechanical dysfunction of the lungs and should be evaluated preoperatively with spirometry.[254] Multiple issues with the skull

TABLE 10–30   Perioperative Issues with Osteogenesis Imperfecta

Creatine phosphokinase measurement: high levels suggest risk of malignant hyperthermia

Evaluation of coagulation

Electrocardiogram, echocardiogram

Central nervous system and cervical spine evaluation

Pulmonary function testing

Visual acuity

Positioning issues

Airway management issues

Bony injury during neuraxial block

Risk of malignant hyperthermia

Fracture risk with stormy emergence

and spinal column must be investigated radiographically, including brain stem compression, atlantoaxial instability, and cervical spinal cord compression. Hypoplasia or fracture of the odontoid is a significant risk[255] and must influence approaches to airway management. Basilar impression may occur, requiring decompression of the foramen magnum.[232,256-258] If undetected, normal range of motion with basilar impression[233,259] or soft odontoid[260] could cause neurologic catastrophe.[261] Minor trauma has been reported to be associated with death from brain stem compression by this same mechanism.[232] Congenital or progressive kyphoscoliosis can interfere with pulmonary function, and spirometry and arterial blood gas analysis may be indicated for major surgery, especially procedures to stabilize progressive scoliosis. Reports of retinal artery anomalies associated with OI make assessment of preoperative visual activity valuable.

Intraoperative Management. Positioning must be performed with extra care because long-bone fractures can result from minor trauma. Fragility of connective tissues makes padding important, to avoid ligament or tendon disruption. Achilles and patellar tendons are particularly at risk. Any bone is susceptible to fracture, and potential serious consequences can occur. A fatal intraoperative hemorrhage resulted from occult fracture of a rib during instrumented spine fusion, resulting in massive transfusion and coagulopathy.[262] A fracture of the femur from minor trauma caused a compartment syndrome.[263] Airway management must be gentle because fractures of the mandible, maxillary surface, and cervical spine are all possible if excessive force is applied.[264] Awake fiberoptic intubation may be the best option, although successful use of an intubating LMA has been reported.[265] Regional anesthesia is possible, but needle placement near bony structures may be problematic. Puncture of bone could cause fracture in the postoperative period. Intraosseous injection is also possible, is difficult to recognize, and could be associated with local anesthetic toxicity. However, successful use of an epidural catheter for anesthesia and postoperative analgesia for cesarean section has been reported.[266,267] Intramuscular ketamine has been used in the past as a sole anesthetic for fracture reduction,[241,268] although adequate muscle relaxation was problematic in some instances. Because there is risk of malignant hyperthermia, a nontriggering anesthetic should be planned for general anesthesia, and total intravenous anesthesia (TIVA) may be an excellent option.[269] Succinylcholine should be avoided. Metabolic acidosis without other signs of malignant hyperthermia has also been reported.[233,270,271] The risk of hyperthermia[240] requires that there be access to active cooling. Smooth emergence should be the goal, because coughing, bucking, or excitement could cause multiple fractures. When the surgical procedure is spine fusion, this is particularly important because the fusion instrumentation can be disrupted and threaten the integrity of the spinal cord.[272] Extensive cervico-occipital decompression with fusion would almost certainly require prolonged intubation and sedation before extubation.[232] Any positioning other than supine must take into account the risk of retinal artery occlusion, and external pressure on the eyes should be carefully avoided.

Summary. Anesthesia for patients with osteogenesis imperfecta is unfortunately a common experience because of the frequency of long-bone fracture, requiring fixation. Anesthetic issues arise from abnormalities of bone, including cervical spine instability, brain stem herniation, and kyphoscoliosis. Positioning must be careful, because fracture from minimal stress can occur. Similar care with airway management is necessary to avoid fracture of the mandible, maxilla, or cervical spine. Susceptibility to malignant hyperthermia must be an element of any plan for general anesthesia. Regional anesthesia should be performed with care if close to cortical bone to avoid fracture or unrecognized intraosseous injection.

OSTEOPOROSIS, OSTEOMALACIA, AND OSTEOPETROSIS

Osteoporosis is a generalized atrophy of bone that results in decreased bone mass without change in the nonmineralized elements. There is no alteration in the structural appearance of osteoporotic bone, although the tensile strength is reduced as bone density decreases. Disproportionate loss of trabecular bone is a distinguishing feature of osteoporosis.[273] When the trabecular (structural) bone volume reaches 10% or below, osteoporosis is confirmed and the risk of stress fracture becomes significant. The most common association is loss of estrogen in postmenopausal women[274] or as a product of either aging or disuse. Exercise may prevent disuse osteoporosis.[275,276] Osteoporosis has also been reported as associated with rheumatoid arthritis and osteoarthritis.[277] Reduced intestinal absorption of calcium can create osteoporosis with normal aging, in association with primary biliary cirrhosis[278,279] or chronic cholestatic liver disease.[280] Bone remodeling favors absorption more and more as a function of age. Although the tensile strength of all bone is reduced, some bones are more at risk for fracture. These include the thoracic and lumbar spine, the proximal femur, the proximal humerus, and the wrist. Compression fractures of the thoracic and lumbar spine are also common.[281] Midforearm fractures result from minimal trauma if Colles' fracture of the wrist does not occur.[274] When bone density is reduced more than 50%, spontaneous fractures of vertebral bodies may occur in response to minor compression loading, such as coughing or sneezing. Acute pain and muscle spasm are the presenting symptoms and can be the indication for surgical procedures to stabilize the spine (percutaneous

vertebroplasty). There is a clear genetic predisposition to osteoporosis, with women of Northern European descent being at highest risk.

Osteomalacia is a generalized softening of bone resulting in reduced tensile strength of bone. It results from a wide variety of causes, having in common deficient vitamin D. This can be extrinsic, as in nutritional deficiency,[282,283] or intrinsic related to malabsorption.[284,285] The result is defective or incomplete mineralization of bone. In contrast to osteoporosis, osteomalacia can occur at any age, including childhood. Bone tenderness, back pain, and abnormal gait are the most common clinical symptoms. Long-bone fractures are more likely and occur with less trauma.[286] Rarely, this can occur with symptoms of hypocalcemia when inadequate skeletal calcium is available for acute mobilization. Severe deformities of the spine (kyphoscoliosis) or pelvis (acetabular protrusio) can be the initial presentation and the indication for surgery. Radiating sciatic pain can also be both diagnostic and an indication for surgery. Skeletal muscle can have abnormal function in advanced osteomalacia, and muscle weakness can be significant. Respiratory muscle groups are not spared, and respiratory muscle failure can be accelerated. Using conservative definitions, up to 4% of geriatric hospital patients have the clinical criteria for osteomalacia. Chronic corticosteroid use can cause osteopenia,[287,288] especially associated with rheumatoid arthritis.[289,290] Comorbidities can cause osteomalacia. Hepatic osteodystrophy can occur in end-stage liver disease,[291] either based on malnutrition (alcoholism) or steatorrhea and malabsorption of vitamin D. Chronic ingestion of alcohol can impair calcium uptake by the intestine,[292,293] and osteomalacia can be the result.[294] In cholestasis, impaired absorption of vitamin D and impaired metabolism can be expected. Long-term anticonvulsant therapy can result in osteomalacia from malabsorption of calcium.[288,295] End-stage renal disease or nephrotic syndrome[296] can cause renal osteodystrophy from malabsorption of calcium and failure of mineralization of bone, secondary to abnormal vitamin D metabolism.[297] Softened bone may result in fractures proximate to large blood vessels.[298] Osteomalacia is associated with metastatic prostatic cancer.[299-301]

Osteopetrosis (marble bone disease) is a rare disorder associated with increased bone density (osteosclerosis), associated with clinical issues related to skeletal abnormality.[302] The range of severity is wide, from children with genetically based generalized skeletal defects[303] to asymptomatic adults, identified because of easy fracture and workup for metabolic bone disease.[304] Radiographic manifestations include sclerosis of bone, abnormal growth, and symmetrically increased bone mass, most obvious near the end of the long bones and pelvis. In some cases, alternating density and lucent areas can be visible radiographically, suggesting risk for pathologic or traumatic fracture.[305] Cranial nerve compression can be associated with blindness, deafness, and facial nerve paralysis.[302] Rare presentations include diffuse idiopathic skeletal hyperostosis (DISH),[306] which manifests with increased bone mass and density at ligament and tendon insertions of the spine.[307] Ankylosis can create deformity and decreased mobility. Hypertrophic osteoarthropathy is an osteopetrosis variant that occurs secondary to other disease processes, including chronic obstructive pulmonary disease, lung cancer,[308] bronchiectasis, pulmonary fibrosis, congenital heart disease, liver cirrhosis, cystic fibrosis,[309] chronic gastrointestinal disease, renal tubular acidosis,[310] cystic fibrosis, multiple myeloma,[311] and other chronic diseases. Long-bone abnormality is more likely altered compared with the trunk and vertebral column, although spondylolysis has been reported.[312] Intracranial calcification has been reported in children with osteopetrosis, associated with carbonic anhydrase II deficiency.[313] Although fracture is less common, nonunion of fracture in children is more likely.[314] Hyperostosis associated with excessive ingestion of vitamin D has been reported.[315,316]

Differential Diagnosis. The differential diagnosis of these diseases is based on radiographic examination and bone density studies. The patient with repeated fractures or a postmenopausal female with bone pain may undergo a skeletal radiographic survey. The abnormalities can include decreased bone density (osteoporosis), decreased mineralization (osteomalacia), or excessive mineralization (osteopetrosis). All have in common structural weakness of bone and increased risk of fracture.

Preoperative Preparation (Table 10-31). In patients with structural defects of bone, anatomic deformity of the airway and thorax is possible. The airway can be abnormal secondary to decreased range of motion of the neck. Despite diminished mobility, instability is also possible, secondary to fragility of the structural elements, such as the odontoid. Even if mobility is normal,

decreased tensile strength may be present. Structural abnormality of the thorax may diminish pulmonary reserves. If kyphosis, scoliosis, and/or rib cage deformity is present, chest radiography and spirometry may be indicated. Because bone pain may be an indicator of structural deficiency, an inventory of bone pain sites may be a guide to positioning issues in the operating room.

If osteoporosis is secondary to chronic corticosteroid use, stress-dose corticosteroids are indicated. Osteomalacia is often a secondary condition; and when caused by end organ failure, investigation may be required. If secondary to severe liver disease, the synthetic functions of the liver should be measured, including proteins and coagulation testing (prothrombin time, activated partial thromboplastin time). If related to chronic renal disease, blood urea nitrogen and creatinine measurements are needed to guide anesthetic care. Osteopetrosis can also be a secondary condition, and primary causes in the lungs and heart would need to be investigated and evaluated to guide anesthetic care.

Intraoperative Management. Positioning should be careful to avoid fracture. The skin is also fragile in some patients.[317] The management of the airway could be either difficult or dangerous with advanced osteoporosis. Awake fiberoptic intubation may be necessary. Positioning of the patient can be difficult, and the risk of fracture with minimal stress must be considered in all these conditions. Instrumentation of osteopetrotic bone can be difficult due to density[318] and associated with increased levels of bleeding and prolonged surgical times.[302,319] There is no interaction between anesthetic agents and structural bone disorders, unless they are secondary to other diseases (e.g., end-stage liver disease, chronic renal failure) that have independent interaction issues. Regional anesthesia can be used, but the potential for trauma to abnormal bone must be considered. Chronic compression fractures of the lumbar and thoracic spine may make access to neuraxial block sites technically difficult or impossible. Besides injury to bone, the possibility of intraosseous injection with rapid plasma uptake of local anesthetic must be considered. In patients with osteopetrosis, ankylosis of the dorsal spinal column may be present,[320,321] making neuraxial block difficult or impossible. There are no unique recovery issues.

Summary. Osteoporosis, osteomalacia, and osteopetrosis are disorders associated with reduction in the tensile strength of bone, which create indications for surgery and present anesthetic issues. These issues are focused on the skeletal anomalies that result and the comorbidities that are the primary causes of the disorders. Anesthetic care is modified by airway issues, risk of positioning injuries, and potential technical issues with regional anesthesia.

TABLE 10–31 Perioperative Issues with Structural Defects of Bone

Airway issues
Fragile cervical spine
Diminished pulmonary reserves
Stress-dose corticosteroids
Assessment of causative organ-system
Positioning issues
Risk with routine airway maneuvers
Cervical spine ankylosis
Increased risk of bleeding
Injury to bone with regional anesthesia

PAGET'S DISEASE OF BONE

Paget's disease of the bone is a process of unknown etiology that causes excessive resorption and subsequent abnormal remodeling that results in abnormally thickened bone with paradoxically reduced tensile strength. It may be related to excess parathyroid hormone or decreased calcitonin levels.[322] Paget's disease clearly has a genetic basis and is found most frequently in residents of Anglo-Saxon countries and their descendents.[323-325]

Paget's disease occurs in phases. The first phase involves active resorption of bone, and pain may occur.[326] Rapidly, new bone is deposited in an asymmetrical pattern. Pain will continue if it is present at the start of this phase, or it may occur as a new sign. The final phase is not usually associated with pain but is characterized by the proliferation of irregularly shaped trabeculae, which create a mosaic appearance in affected bone. In this final phase, the cellular content of bone is reduced, as is the tensile strength. Fracture through affected bone heals with a disorganized pattern. Collagen is prominent in the fracture callus for prolonged intervals. Vascular hypertrophy occurs during fracture repair and during the first two phases of the onset of Paget's disease. During instrumentation of this bone, bleeding will be significantly greater than normal. The abnormal remodeling of bone has been suggested as etiologic in familial cases of osteosarcoma that develop in pagetoid bone.[327-329]

Pain is the most common symptom that leads to the diagnosis of Paget's disease. Pain may be related to bone resorption, inflammation, or microfracture. Weight-bearing increases the pain in affected long bones. Pain may be caused by hyperemia after microfracture or stretching of periosteum. Weight bearing also leads to deformity, such as acetabular protrusion.[330] Osteoporosis of the skull, followed by exuberant deposition of bone and increased size and weight of the skull, can occur. Changes in the skull are commonly associated with hearing loss.[331] Excessive ossification of the foramen magnum can lead to neurologic symptoms from compression of the cerebellum in the posterior fossa or from cerebral tonsillar herniation.[332] Hydrocephalus or compression of the cervical spinal cord are possible. Hydrocephalus associated with dementia has also been reported from pathologic changes of the base of the skull related to Paget's disease.[333,334] Anatomic abnormality of the temporal bones may result in abnormal balance and hearing loss and in optic neuropathy from bony compression.[335] Paget's disease can involve the mandible, maxilla, and teeth, further increasing the abnormal configuration of the head.[336] Dental extraction is commonly more difficult and associated with increased bleeding during and after the procedure.[337] Paget's disease of the upper cervical spine can cause spinal cord compression or atlantoaxial instability.[338] Proliferation of bone can result in compression of the spinal cord or nerve roots, most particularly in the lumbar and thoracic regions,[339] or spondylitis.[340] Lumbar spinal stenosis is a common manifestation of Paget's disease, requiring surgical intervention.[341] Coincident ankylosing spondylitis has been reported.[326] Knee and hip pain associated with sclerosis and deformity are common in advanced Paget's disease.

Fractures are the most common pathologic manifestation of Paget's disease after bone pain. The incidence of nonunion of these fractures is high. Microfracture through an area of active resorption of bone during early onset of Paget's disease may lead to spread of the lesions to surrounding bone. Rarely, malignancy (osteosarcoma) may occur in bone affected by Paget's disease. Renal calculi and gout are manifestations of abnormal calcium metabolism. Excessive blood flow to bone affected by Paget's disease can cause congestive heart failure. Calcification of cardiac structures (especially valves) is common. When calcification involves the cardiac structures, arrhythmia and heart block can result. There is a correlation between Paget's disease and calcific disease of the aortic valve. Peripheral vascular disease based on arterial calcification has been reported (Table 10-32).

Diagnosis and Treatment. Paget's disease can be confused with a variety of bone disorders, including osteomalacia, osteoporosis, and osteopetrosis. The unique radiographic presentation of Paget's disease is usually the element that establishes the diagnosis.

Drug treatment is usually reserved for either symptomatic or advanced cases. Antimitotic drugs, such as colchicine, have been used for symptomatic relief, with

TABLE 10–32   Comorbidity Associated with Paget's Disease
Bone pain
Acetabular protrusion
Hypertrophy of skull
Compression at foramen magnum
Compression of cerebellum
Hydrocephalus
Hearing loss, optic neuropathy
Abnormal mandible maxilla
Cervical spine instability
Lumbar spine stenosis
High incidence of fracture
Nonunion of fracture
Osteosarcoma
Calcific cardiac conduction, valved disease
Peripheral vascular disease

the concomitant issues with bone marrow suppression.[342] Bone pain can be modified with either calcitonin[343] or biphosphonates.[344] High cardiac output can be treated with either option but may be more effective with biphosphonates.[345] The risk of osteomalacia,[346] stress,[347] and pathologic fractures[348] is higher with biphosphonates.[349-351] A limitation of calcitonin therapy is the development of resistance. Mithramycin has been used in the treatment of hypercalcemia secondary to Paget's disease.[352] It has also been used for severe bone pain refractory to other pharmacologic options. Administration is challenging since mitramycin must be administered intravenously and carefully because it is highly cytotoxic. Nausea and vomiting are commonly associated with its administration. Abnormal platelet function, hepatotoxicity, and nephrotoxicity are associated with mithramycin therapy and treatment with mithramycin should trigger evaluation of these systems.[353]

Preoperative Preparation (Table 10-33). Because of the abnormal bone metabolism, the potential for electrolyte abnormalities should be considered. If there is enlargement of the skull, CNS pathology is possible, including increased intracranial pressure and compression of the brain stem, cerebellum, and/or spinal cord. Although plain radiography of the skull will yield some information, especially if there is involvement of the maxilla or mandible, CT or MRI is needed to identify increased intracranial pressure, mass effect, or impending herniation at the foramen magnum. If there is bony abnormality of the spine, radiographic examination is required to look for spinal cord compression or anomalies that would risk injury to the spinal column during airway management. Flexion-extension films of the neck to look for atlantoaxial instability are indicated.

Because of calcific changes in the cardiovascular system, comorbidities should be sought. Basic electrocardiography may reveal lesions in the conduction system. Calcific valvular disease would be detected by cardiac auscultation, and murmurs may require evaluation by

echocardiography. Carotid bruit may trigger a carotid ultrasound. As described earlier, specific therapies for Paget's disease may necessitate detection of renal, hepatic, or platelet function abnormalities. If significant deformity of the thorax is noted, spirometry may be required to measure pulmonary reserves.

Intraoperative Issues. Airway management can be difficult related to bone changes in Paget's disease. Both pain and deformity will make positioning difficult. Excessive force should be avoided, secondary to the risk of fracture through weakened bone. Regional anesthesia can be used, but radiographic examination may be required before central neuraxial block to avoid needle instrumentation through pathologic bone. If range of motion of the spine is severely restricted, review of spine radiographs may reveal ankylosis, which presents severe technical issues for central neuraxial block.[326] Excessive bleeding occurs routinely with bone affected by Paget's disease, and increased blood loss can be expected compared with comparable procedures on nonpagetoid bone.[354] Preparation for possible massive transfusion with lower extremity joint reconstruction is indicated.[355] Sclerotic bone is more difficult to instrument, which may prolong the surgical time and further increase blood loss. There are no specific interactions between Paget's disease and anesthetic agents, except where consequences of treatment cause organ damage or dysfunction.

Summary. The anesthetic management of Paget's disease is complicated by the structural consequence of the disease, including fracture deformity and CNS dysfunction. The symptoms of Paget's disease, including pain and weak bones, present issues in patient handling in the perioperative period. When Paget's disease is symptomatic, treatment may be necessary and some of the options have anesthetic implications.

PANNICULITIS

Panniculitis is a term for a group of diseases caused by inflammation of subcutaneous tissue. The eruption of clusters of edematous masses in the subcutaneous tissue occurs most often on the trunk and thighs but can involve the neck and face. The massive inflammatory response has systemic manifestations, including malaise, myalgia,[356] fatigue, and fever.[357] In rare cases, the fat of visceral organs can be involved. Inflammation of fat around the spleen, liver, adrenals, or myocardium can cause serious organ damage. Diffuse adenopathy is common. Bone marrow suppression can cause pancytopenia and bleeding events. Rare causes include chemical panniculitis, usually from subcutaneous infection, cold panniculitis,[358] where fat necrosis is triggered by exposure to cold, infection,[359-361] and factitial panniculitis from

TABLE 10–33   Perioperative Issues with Paget's Disease
Abnormal electrolytes
Central nervous system at risk
Unstable cervical spine
Electrocardiogram, echocardiogram
Carotid ultrasound
Difficult airway management
Risk of injury with routine airway maneuvers
Excessive blood loss

self-injection. In neonates, massive subcutaneous fat necrosis can occur, but fortunately this is short lived and reasonably well tolerated.[362,363] Some forms of panniculitis are caused by serious systemic diseases, such as pancreatitis, lupus,[364,365] sarcoidosis,[366] renal failure, leukemia,[367] and lymphoma. One variant of panniculitis is associated with vasculitis in the same parts of the body in which needle trauma has induced panniculitis.[368] The consequence of the vasculitis is increased severity of tissue injury and delayed healing. Erythema nodosum is a form of panniculitis. Articular lesions have been reported.[369]

Differential Diagnosis. The lesions of panniculitis are initially confused with many other skin conditions. Lesions that are confined to subcutaneous tissue and fat are diagnostic. Although rare, panniculitis can be diagnosed during the workup of organ failure found to be associated with fat necrosis. There is an association between α-*antitrypsin deficiency and panniculitis.*

Preoperative Considerations (Table 10-34). The primary issue for presurgical preparation of patients with panniculitis focuses on care of the lesions and identification of any comorbidity caused by fat necrosis. Pressure on the lesion could cause extension. Ulcerated lesions should be protected from infection. Assessment of liver function and blood urea nitrogen/creatinine should be obtained to rule out organ dysfunction. An abnormal electrocardiogram and poor exercise tolerance could suggest cardiac involvement. When the lesions create the need for surgery (abscess, vascular compromise), evaluation should focus on functional status if fuller evaluation would delay urgent surgery. Treatment with corticosteroids mandates stress-dose corticosteroids in the perioperative period. When immunosuppressants or antimetabolites are used, organ toxicity should be investigated.

Intraoperative Considerations. Positioning can be an issue when numerous lesions are present. Anesthetic technique is dictated by other organ system involvement and urgency of surgery. If there are clusters of lesions involving either the face or neck, airway compromise should be considered. Regional anesthesia is a reasonable technique,

TABLE 10–34 Perioperative Issues in Patients with Panniculitis

Identify cause of fat necrosis
Positioning pressure causing lesions
Abscess
Vascular compromise
Stress-dose corticosteroids
Inflammation of visceral organs

as long as the needle insertion site is free of lesions. Traumatic placement of regional anesthesia or invasive monitors can create lesions.

Summary. Panniculitis is an inflammatory process that creates deep, tender lesions of fat that tend to expand and ulcerate. Although most common on the trunk and limbs, they can occur on the neck and face with potential airway issues. If generalized inflammation of fat involves fat insulating visceral organs, organ-system dysfunction can result. Perioperative care requires that positioning, regional anesthesia, or invasive monitoring not compromise lesions or increase the risk of infection.

PEMPHIGUS AND PEMPHIGOID

Pemphigus and pemphigoid are related syndromes characterized by autoimmune blistering of skin and mucous membranes. The bullae are large, soft, and superficial and range in size from 1 to 10 cm at formation. Because they are fragile, they tear easily and leave areas of inflamed, unprotected body surface area. The skin surrounding the lesions is fragile and pressure causes extension of the lesions. Mucous membranes are common sites for lesions, and the oral mucosa is involved in a majority of patients with pemphigoid and in nearly every patient with pemphigus.

The physical cause of the lesions is acantholysis, which is a breakdown of the adherence of the layers of skin and mucous membranes. With pemphigus the superficial layer is not structurally attached and lesions form from minimal trauma. With pemphigoid, the lesions are subepidermal. The lesions of pemphigoid do not extend as easily at their margins as is the case with pemphigus.

Although the most common etiology for pemphigus is idiopathic and autoimmune, there are a variety of other causes, including neonatal transmission, sun exposure, and a variety of drug reactions. The most common drug reactions are to captopril and penicillamine. In contrast to other causes, most drug-induced pemphigus resolves rapidly with elimination of the offending drug. Myasthenia gravis and thymoma have been reported to be associated with pemphigus. Rheumatoid arthritis, lupus, and cirrhosis of the liver have also been associated with pemphigus. Pemphigus may be part of a paraneoplastic syndrome.[370,371] The oral mucosal lesions of paraneoplastic pemphigus are unusually severe. The triggering neoplasms are most often lymphoma, leukemic, or thymoma.[372,373] The reverse (pemphigus as a cause of malignancy) is less likely.[374,375]

Preoperative Considerations (Table 10-35). Preoperative preparation of patients with pemphigus/pemphigoid focuses on care of the lesions, assessment of the airway,

TABLE 10–35   Perioperative Issues for Anesthetic Management for Patients with Pemphigoid

Stress-dose corticosteroids
Peripheral neuropathy with treatment (dapsone)
Patient taking immunosuppressants
Nephrotoxicity
Laryngeal/airway obstruction
Physical trauma with intubation
Airway obstruction during emergence

and consequences of treatment. First-line treatment usually begins with high-dose corticosteroid therapy[376] or bolus corticosteroid administration,[377] which should be continued through the perioperative period parenterally to deal with adrenal suppression, as well as avoiding acute exacerbation of the lesions. Dapsone has been used in some patients, but the failure rate, peripheral neuropathy,[378] and hematologic complications (anemia, hemolysis, neutropenia) have made this less common.[374,379] Rarer complications of dapsone include anaphylaxis, thrombocytopenia, and toxic epidermal necrolyis.[380] Perioperative methemoglobinemia secondary to dapsone has been reported.[381] Some patients may be receiving immunosuppressants,[382] which increase the risk of infection.[380] Because of the nephrotoxicity of some immunosuppressants (cyclosporine), renal function (blood urea nitrogen, creatinine) should be measured. Gold therapy[383] has been used and can cause liver failure,[380] and these patients should have measurement of liver function tests. A combination therapy with tetracycline and nicotinamide has been used[384] and rarely causes renal toxicity and possible acute tubular necrosis.[385] Severe dehydration and electrolyte abnormalities[386] are common in pemphigus patients with lesions covering a large surface area, and assessment of volume status and resuscitation are important preanesthetic issues. In patients with oral lesions, indirect laryngoscopy to evaluate the airway preoperatively would be valuable, recognizing the trauma that could exaggerate oropharyngeal lesions. Coexisting illnesses should be fully explored.[387]

Intraoperative Course. Elective surgery should be rare in these patients.[388] Laryngeal and airway obstruction can be the presentation of pemphigoid requiring anesthetic intervention, and tracheostomy may be required.[389] When emergency surgery is required, management of the airway is potentially life threatening.[390] Intubation could be difficult, and the physical process of placing the endotracheal tube might create lesions that could compromise the airway after extubation. Bleeding within the oropharynx could also result, even from gentle airway instrumentation.[391] Regional anesthesia is possible if the site of the block is free of lesions.[392,393]

Summary. Pemphigus and pemphigoid are autoimmune diseases of the skin that can present issues when surgery/anesthesia is required. Oral lesions are common, and airway compromise is a serious issue. Many of the treatments have issues with major organ systems that must be investigated before surgery. Because these syndromes can be induced into remission or eliminated, elective surgery should be uncommon.

PSORIASIS

Pathophysiology. Psoriasis is an inflammatory skin disease that results from epidermal proliferation and accumulation. It is the most common chronic disease of the skin. It can be triggered by bacterial or viral infection, bone marrow transplantation,[394] malignancy[395,396] or emotional stress.

Diagnosis. The lesions of psoriasis can be confused with fungal skin lesions and seborrheic dermatitis. There are no significant major organ system issues associated with psoriasis.

Preoperative Preparation. Chronic corticosteroid therapy is a common management strategy. Stress-dose corticosteroids should be provided for the perioperative period. The surface skin should be inspected to detect any areas of acute infection, which should be treated before elective surgery or regional anesthesia. Uveitis has been reported and could cause visual delay.[397] If immune suppressants are used,[398-401] renal function should be investigated. If methotrexate is used, liver toxicity should be suspected.[402,403]

Intraoperative Considerations. Trauma to psoriatic skin should be avoided. Regional blocks or invasive monitors should not be inserted through psoriatic skin. No specific agents are indicated or contraindicated. Unusual sepsis events have been associated with psoriasis[404-406] and could present in the operating room or early postoperative period.

Summary. Psoriasis is a chronic skin disease that results in large surface areas of inflamed skin. There are no anesthetic issues other than protection of the skin and avoidance of instrumentation of psoriatic skin.

PYODERMA GANGRENOSUM

Pathophysiology. Pyoderma gangrenosum (PG) is a destructive inflammatory disease of the skin.[407] The lesion begins as painful nodules that break down and erode into an ulcer.[408] These ulcers naturally expand to large sizes. Some cases are related to other systemic illness, malignancy,[409] or other autoimmune diseases.[410] Neutrophil infiltration of the dermis is causative.[411] Although mucous membranes are usually spared, lesions of the oral cavity, pharynx, and larynx have been reported in a minority of cases.[412] Intradermal injections, intravenous catheters, and surgical incision can cause new lesions. Massive edema from circumferential lesions can be the indication for surgery if distal ischemia or compartment syndrome are present. The lesions can trigger fat necrosis, also causing vascular embarrassment of limbs or panniculitis, which can trigger peritonitis. Polyarthritis can occur, and septic arthritis is an occasional presentation for urgent surgery.[411] An association with vasculitis can also present urgent need for surgery.[413,414]

Diagnosis (Table 10-36). The lesions occur as an idiopathic disease confined to the skin in a majority of cases. In the others, a systemic illness proceeds PG and is causative. Myeloma,[415] leukemia,[416-418] chronic[419] hepatitis, primary[420] biliary cirrhosis, diabetes, carcinoid, lupus,[421,422] vasculitis, and inflammatory small[423] or large[424] bowel disease are examples of precipitating causes. PG has been associated with allogenic bone marrow transplantation.[425]

Preoperative Considerations. Significant lesions around the mouth[426] can occur and should prompt further evaluation to determine if the airway is involved.[427-431] Because these lesions are associated with other diseases, presurgical preparation should focus on identifying other comorbidities. Inflammatory lesions of the lung can occur and should be investigated if symptomatic.[432,433] Chronic corticosteroid therapy requires stress-dose corticosteroids in the perioperative period. Some patients are treated with immunosuppressive drugs with organ toxicity, most notably nephrotoxicity and hepatotoxicity with methotrexate.[434] Antimetabolites can induce pancytopenia and/or coagulopathies.

Intraoperative Considerations. Pressure on existing lesions should be avoided to prevent expansion. Lesions of the oropharynx and airway should be suspected. If abnormality of voice or swallowing is detected, awake fiberoptic intubation is indicated. Regional anesthesia can be used, but the possibility of a lesion occurring at the site of the block must be considered. There is no particular anesthetic agent either indicated or contraindicated. Causative comorbidities may alter the anesthetic course.

Summary. Pyoderma gangrenosum is an inflammatory disease of the skin that causes lesions that extend and ulcerate easily. Many systemic illnesses with an inflammatory component can be associated/causative. Lesions of the oropharynx and airway have potentially serious anesthetic implications. Needle puncture and intradermal injections can cause lesions and limit the enthusiasm for regional anesthesia. When general anesthesia is selected, the possibility of lesions of the airway may make awake fiberoptic intubation the best choice.

TABLE 10–36 Causes of Pyoderma Gangrenosum

Myeloma
Leukemia
Hepatitis
Biliary cirrhosis
Diabetes
Carcinoid
Lupus
Vasculitis
Inflammatory bowel disease

References

1. Kopits SE: Orthopedic complications of dwarfism. Clin Orthop 1976;114:153-179.
2. Rimoin DL, Silberger R, Hllister DW: Chondro-osseous pathology in the chondrodystrophies. Clin Orthop 1976;114:137-152.
3. Hwang WS, Tock EPC, Tan KL, Tan LKA: The pathology of cartilage in chrondrodysplasias. J Pathol 1979;127:11-18.
4. Stanescu V, Stanescu R, Maroteaux P: Pathogenic mechanisms in osteochondrodysplasias. J Bone Joint Surg 1984;66:817-836.
5. Cohen ME, Rosenthal AD, Matson DD: Neurological abnormalities in achondroplastic children. J Pediatr 1967;71:367-376.
6. Gulati Dr, Ront D: Atlantoaxial dislocation with quadriparesis in achondroplasia. J Neurosurg 1974;40:394-395.
7. Poussa M, Merikanto J, Ryoppy S, et al: The spine in diastrophic dysplasia. Spine 1991;16:881-887.
8. Sillence DO, Rimoin DL, Lachman R: Neonatal dwarfism. Pediatr Clin North Am 1978;25:453-483.
9. Lin HJ, Sue GY, Berkowitz ID, et al: Microdontia with severe microcephaly and short stature in two brothers: Osteoplastic primordial dwarfism with dental findings. Am J Med Genet 1995;58:136-142.
10. Shiraishi N, Takakuwa K, Yamamoto N, et al: Anesthetic management of Seckel syndrome: A case report. Masui 1995;44:735-738.
11. Roberts W, Henson LC: Anesthesia for scoliosis: Dwarfism and congenitally absent odontoid process. AANA J 1995;63:332-337.
12. Sisk EA, Heatley DG, Borowski BJ, et al: Obstructive sleep apnea in children with achondroplasia: Surgical and anesthetic implications. Otolaryngol Head Neck Surg 1999;120:248-254.
13. Berkowitz ID, Raja SN, Bender KS, et al: Dwarfs: Pathophysiology and anesthetic implications. Anesthesiology 1990;73:739-759.
14. Mayhew JF, Katz J, Miner M, et al: Anesthesia for the achondroplastic dwarf. Can Anaesth Soc J 1986;33:216-221.
15. Theroux MC, Kettrick RG, Khine HH: Laryngeal mask airway and fiberoptic endoscopy in an infant with Schwartz-Jampel syndrome. Anesthesiology 1995;82:605.
16. Waltz LF, Finerman G, Wyatt GM: Anesthesia for dwarfs and other patients of pathological small stature. Can Anaesth Soc J 1975;22:703-705.
17. Nguyen TT, Papadakos PJ, Sabnis LU: Epidural anesthesia for extracorporeal shock wave lithotripsy in an achondroplastic dwarf. Reg Anesth 1997;22:102-104.
18. Kallman GN, Fening E, Obiaya MD: Anesthetic management of achondroplasia. Br J Anaesth 1986;58:117-119.

19. Cohen SE: Anesthesia for cesarean section in achondroplastic dwarfs. Anesthesiology 1980;52:264-266.

20. Morrow MJ, Black IH: Epidural anesthesia for cesarean section in an achondroplastic dwarf. Br J Anaesth 1998;81:619-621.

21. Crawford M, Dutton DA: Spinal anaesthesia for caesarean section in an achondroplastic dwarf. Anaesthesia 1992;47:1007.

22. Carstoniu J, Yee I, Halpern S: Epidural anaesthesia for caesarean section in an achondroplastic dwarf. Can J Anaesth 1992;39:708-711.

23. Ratner EF, Hamilton CL: Anesthesia for cesarean section in a pituitary dwarf. Anesthesiology 1998;89:253-254.

24. Trikha A, Goyal K, Sadera GS, Singh M: Combined spinal epidural anesthesia for vesico-vaginal fistula repair in an achondroplastic dwarf. Anaesth Intens Care 2002;30:96-98.

25. Ravenscroft A, Govender T, Rout C: Spinal anaesthesia for emergency caesarean section in an achondroplastic dwarf. Anaesthesia 1998;53:1236-1237.

26. Wardall GJ, Frame WT: Extradural anaesthesia for caesarean section in achondroplasia. Br J Anaesth 1990;64:367-370.

27. Bancroft GH, Lauria JI: Ketamine induction for cesarean section in a patient with acute intermittent porphyria and achondroplastic dwarfism. Anesthesiology 1983;59:143-144.

28. Bhisitkuk RB, Goster CS: Diagnosis and ophthalmological features of Behçet's disease. Int Ophthalmol Clin 1996;36:127-134.

29. Mangelsdorf HC, White WL, Jorizzo JL: Behçet's disease: Report of twenty-five patients from the United State with prominent mucocutaneous involvement. J Am Acad Dermatol 1996;34:745-748.

30. Mason RM, Barnes CG: Behçet's syndrome with arthritis. Ann Rheum Dis 1969;28:95-99.

31. Yurdakul S, Yazici H, Tuzuny Y: The arthritis of Behçet's disease: A prospective study. Ann Rheum Dis 1983;42:505-514.

32. Inove C, Itoh R, Kawa Y, Mizoguchi M: Pathogenesis of mucocutaneous lesions in Behçet's disease. J Dermatol 1994;21:474-481.

33. Kozin F, Haughton V, Bernhard GC: Neuro-Behçet's disease: Two cases and neuroradiologic findings. Neurology 1977;27:1148-1153.

34. O'Duffy JD, Goldstein NP: Neurologic involvement in seven patients with Behçet's disease. Am J Med 1976;61:170-179.

35. Fujikado T, Imagawa K: Dural sinus thrombosis in Behçet's disease—a case report. Jpn J Ophthalmol 1995;38:411-413.

36. McNeely MC, Jorizzo JL, Solomon AR Jr, et al: Primary idiopathic cutaneous pustular vasculitis. J Am Acad Dermatol 1986;14:939-944.

37. Nakata Y, Awazu M, Kojima Y, et al: Behçet's disease presenting with a right atrial vegetation. Pediatr Cardiol 1995;16:150-154.

38. Puckette TC, Jolles H, Proto AV: Magnetic resonance imaging confirmation of pulmonary artery aneurysm in Behçet's disease. J Thorac Imaging 1994;9:172-175.

39. Hanza M: Large artery involvement in Behçet's disease. J Rheumatol 1987;14:554-559.

40. Roguin N, Haim S, Reshef R, et al: Cardiac involvement and superior vena caval obstruction in Behçet's disease. Thorax 1978;33:375-379.

41. Sagdic K, Ozer ZG, Saba D, et al: Venous lesions in Behçet's disease. Eur J Vasc Endovasc Surg 1996;11:437-443.

42. Cadman EC, Lundberg UB, Mitchell MS: Pulmonary manifestations in Behçet's syndrome. Arch Intern Med 1976;136:944-948.

43. Efthimiou J, et al: Pulmonary disease in Behçet's syndrome. Q J Med 1986;48:259-264.

44. Ahonen AV, Stenius-Aarniala BSM, Vijanen BC, et al: Obstructive lung disease in Behçet's syndrome. Scand J Respir Dis 1978;59:44-47.

45. Tunaci A, Berkmen YM, Gokmen E: Thoracic involvement in Behçet's disease: Pathologic, clinical, and imaging features. AJR Am J Roentgenol 1995;164:51-58.

46. Herreman G, et al: Behçet's syndrome and renal involvement: A histological and immunofluorescence study of eleven renal biopsies. Am J Med Sci 1982;284:10-15.

47. Lida M, Kobayashi H, Matsumoto T, et al: Postoperative recurrence in patients with intestinal Behçet's disease. Dis Colon Rectum 1994;37:16-24.

48. Chaleby K, El-Yazigi A, Atiyeh M: Decreased drug absorption in a patient with Behçet's syndrome. Clin Chem 1987;33:1679-1685.

49. Jorizzo JL: Behçet's disease. Neurol Clin 1987;5:427-435.

50. James DG, Thomson A: Recognition of the diverse cardiovascular manifestations of Behçet's disease. Am Heart J 1982;30:457-462.

51. Powderly WG, Lombard MG, Murray FE, et al: Oesophageal ulceration in Behçet's disease presenting with haemorrhage. Ir J Med Sci 1987;156:193-195.

52. Sharquie K: Suppression of Behçet's disease with dapsone. Br J Dermatol 1984;110:493-497.

53. Yazici H, Pazarli H, Barnes CG, Tuzan Y: A controlled trial of azathioprine in Behçet's syndrome. N Engl Med 1990;322:281-288.

54. Yasui K, Ohta K, Kobayashi M, et al: Successful treatment of Behçet disease with pentoxifylline. Ann Intern Med 1996;124:891-895.

55. Turner ME: Anesthetic difficulties associated with Behçet's syndrome. Br J Anaesth 1972;44:100-103.

56. Cohen SR, Landing BH, Isaacs H: Epidermolysis bullosa associated with laryngeal stenosis. Ann Otol Rhinol Laryngol 1978;87:25-28.

57. Stewart MI, Woodley DT: Acquired epidermolysis bullosa and associated symptomatic esophageal webs. Arch Dermatol 1991;127:373-377.

58. Jio TH, Waardenberg PJ, Vermeullen HJ: Blood coagulation in epidermolysis bullosa hereditaria. Arch Dermatol 1963;88:76-83.

59. Ramadas T, Thangavelu TA: Epidermolysis bullosa and its ENT manifestations. J Laryngol Otol 1978;92:441-448.

60. Megahed M, Scharfetter-Kochnek K: Epidermolysis bullosa acquisitia—successful treatment with colchicine. Arch Dermatol Res 1994;286:35-40.

61. Cunningham BB, Kirchmann TT, Woodley D: Colchicine for epidermolysis bullosa (EBA). J Am Acad Dermatol 1996;34:781-785.

62. Farber NE, Todd RJ, Turco G: Spinal anesthesia in a patient with epidermolysis bullosa. Anesthesiology 1995;83:1364-1367.

63. Yasui Y, Yamamoto Y, Sodeyama O, et al: Anesthesia in a patient with epidermolysis bullosa. Masui 1995;44:260-263.

64. Petty WC, Gunther RC: Anesthesia for nonfacial surgery in polydysplastic epidermolysis bullosa (dystrophic). Anesth Analg 1970;49:246-245.

65. Broster T, Placek R, Eggers GWN Jr: Epidermolysis bullosa: Anesthetic management for cesarean section. Anesth Analg 1987;66:341-343.

66. Marshall BE: A comment on epidermolysis bullosa and its anesthetic management for dental operations. Br J Anesth 1963;35:724-727.

67. Kaplan R, Strauch B: Regional anesthesia in a child with epidermolysis bullosa. Anesthesiology 1987;67:262-264.

68. Dorne R, Tassaux D, Ravat F, et al: Surgery for epidermolysis bullosa in children: Value of the association of inhalation anesthesia and locoregional anesthesia. Ann Fr Anesth Reanim 1994;113:425-428.

69. Rowlingson JC, Rosenblum SM: Successful regional anesthesia in a patient with epidermolysis. Regional Anesth 1983;8:81-83.

70. Kelly RE, Koff HD, Rothaus KO, et al: Brachial plexus anesthesia in eight patients with recessive dystrophic epidermolysis bullosa. Anesth Analg 1987;66:1318-1320.

71. Smith GB, Schribman AJ: Anesthesia and severe skin disease. Anaesthesia 1984;39:443-447.

72. Reddy ARR, Wong WHW: Epidermolysis bullosa, a review of anaesthetic problems and case reports. Can Anaesth Soc J 1972;19:536-541.

73. James J, Wark H: Airway management during anesthesia in patients with epidermolysis bullosa dystrophica. Anesthesiology 1982;56:323-326.

74. Berrynill RE, Benumof JL, Saidman LJ, et al: Anesthetic management of emergency cesarean section in a patient with epidermolysis bullosa dystrophica polydysplastica. Anesth Analg 1977;57:281-286.

75. LoVerne SR, Oropollo AT: Ketamine anesthesia in dermolytic bullous disease (epidermolysis bullosa). Anesth Analg 1977;56:398-401.

76. Fisk GC, Kern IB: Anesthesia for esophagoscopy in a child with epidermolysis bullosa—a case report. Anaesth Intensive Care 1973;1:297-300.

77. Bastuji-Garin S, Rzany B, Stern RS, et al: Clinical classification of cases of toxic epidermal necrolysis, Stevens-Johnson syndrome and erythema multiforme. Arch Dermatol 1993;129:92-97.

78. Chan HL, Stern RS, Arndt KA, et al: The incidence of erythema multiforme, Stevens-Johnson syndrome and toxic epidermal necrolysis. Arch Dermatol 1990;126:43-48.

79. Huff JC, Weston WL, Tonnesen MG: Erythema multiforme: A critical review of characteristics, diagnostic criteria, and causes. J Am Acad Dermatol 1983;8:763-769.

80. Roujeau JC: The spectrum of Stevens-Johnson syndrome and toxic epidermal necrolysis. J Invest Dermatol 1994;102:28S.

81. Paquet P, Pierard GE: Erythema multiforme and toxic epidermal necrolysis: A comparative study. Am J Dermatopathol 1997;19:127-133.

82. Roujeau JC, Kelly JP, Naldi L, et al: Medication use and the risk of Stevens-Johnson syndrome or toxic epidermal necrolysis. N Engl J Med 1995;333:1600-1604.

83. Baird BJ, DeVillez RL: Widespread bullous fixed drug eruption mimicking toxic epidermal necrolysis. Int J Dermatol 1988;27:170-178.

84. Plaut MED, Mirani M: Toxic epidermal necrolysis due to E. coli. JAMA 1972;219:1629-1636.

85. Tay YK, Huff JD, Weston WL: *Mycoplasma pneumoniae* infection is associated with Stevens-Johnson syndrome, not erythema multiforme (vonHebra). J Am Acad Dermatol 1996;35:757-760.

86. Assier H, Bastuji-Garin S, Revuz J, et al: Erythema multiforme with mucous membrane involvement and Stevens-Johnson syndrome are different disorders with distinct causes. Arch Dermatol 1995;131:539-546.

87. Porteous DM, Berger TG: Severe cutaneous drug reactions (Stevens-Johnson syndrome and toxic epidermal necrolysis) in human immunodeficiency virus infection. Arch Dermatol 1991;127:740-748.

88. Kazmierowski JA, Peizner DS, Wuepper KD: Herpes simplex antigen in immune complexes of patients with erythema multiforme: Presence following recurrent herpes simplex infection. JAMA 1982;247:2547-2550.

89. Fleischer AB Jr, Rosenthal DI, Bernard SA, et al: Skin reactions to radiotherapy—a spectrum resembling erythema multiforme: Case report and review of the literature. Cutis 1992;49:35-39.

90. Carter FM, Mitchell CK: Toxic epidermal necrolysis—an unusual cause of colonic perforation. Dis Colon Rectum 1993;36:773-779.

91. Blum L, Chosidow O, Rostoker G, et al: Renal involvement in toxic epidermal necrolysis. J Am Acad Dermatol 1996;34:1088-1096.

92. Prendiville JS, Herbert AA, Greenwald MJ, et al: Management of Stevens-Johnson syndrome and toxic epidermal necrolysis in chidlren. J Pediatr 1989;115:881-885.

93. Phillips-Howard PA, Behrens RH, Dunlop J: Stevens-Johnson syndrome due to pyrimethamine/sulfadoxine during presumptive self-therapy of malaria. Lancet 1989;2:803-808.

94. Delattre JY, Satai B, Posner JB: Erythema multiforme and Stevens-Johnson syndrome in patients receiving cranial irradiation and phenytoin. Neurology 1988;38:194-197.

95. deMoragas JM: Panniculitis (erythema nodosum). In Fitzpatrick TB (ed): Dermatology in General Medicine, 2nd ed. New York, McGraw-Hill, 1979.

96. Puavilai S, Sakuntabhai A, Sriprachaya-Anunt S, et al: Etiology of erythema nodosum. J Med Assoc Thai 1995;78:72.

97. Tami LF: Erythema nodosum associated with shigella colitis. Arch Dermatol 1985;5:590.

98. Buckler JMH: Leptospirosis presenting with erythema nodosum. Arch Dis Child 1977;52:418.

99. Longmore HJA: Toxoplasmosis and erythema nodosum. BMJ 1977;1:490.

100. Conget I, Mallolas J, Mensa J, et al: Erythema nodosum and Q fever. Arch Dermatol 1987;123:867.

101. Andonopoulos AP, Asimakopoulos G, Mallioris C, et al: The diagnostic value of gastrocnemius muscle biopsy in sarcoidosis presenting with erythema nodosum and hilar adenopathy. Clin Rheumatol 1987;6:192-196.

102. Matsuoka LY: Neoplastic erythema nodosum. J Am Acad Dermatol 1995;32:361.

103. Urbain G, Peremans J, Philippart M: Fabry's disease without skin lesions. Lancet 1967;1:1-8.

104. Von Scheidt W, Eng CM, Fitzmaurice TF, et al: An atypical variant of Fabry's disease with manifestations confined to the myocardium. N Engl J Med 1991;324:395-402.

105. Ferrans VJ, Hibbs RG, Burda CD: The heart in Fabry's disease. Am J Cardiol 1969;24:95-109.

106. Fisher EA, Desnick RJ, Gordon RE, et al: Fabry disease: An unusual cause of severe coronary artery disease in a young man. Ann Intern Med 1992;117:221-224.

107. Rowe JW, Gilliam JI, Warthin TA: Intestinal manifestations of Fabry's disease. Ann Intern Med 1974;81:628-637.

108. Becker AE, Schoorl R, Balk AG, van der Heide RM: Cardiac manifestations of Fabry's disease: Report of a case with mitral insufficiency and electrocardiographic evidence of myocardial infarction. Am J Cardiol 1975;36:829-835.

109. Resnick RJ, Blieden LC, Sharp HL, et al: Cardiac valvular anomalies in Fabry disease. Circulation 1976;54:818-827.

110. Desnick RJ, Blieden LC, Sharp HL, et al: Cardiac valvular anomalies in Fabry's disease: Clinical, morphologic and biochemical studies. Circulation 1976;54:818-825.

111. Colucci WS, Lorell BH, Schoen FJ, et al: Hypertrophic obstructive cardiomyopathy due to Fabry's disease. N Engl J Med 1982;2:926-928.

112. Nagao Y, Nakashima H, Fukuhara Y, et al: Hypertrophic cardiomyopathy in late-onset variant of Fabry disease with high residual activity of α-galactosidase A. Clin Genet 1991;39:233-237.

113. Broadbent JC, Edwards WD, Gordon H, Hartzler GO: Fabry cardiomyopathy in the female confirmed by endomyocardial biopsy. Mayo Clin Proc 1981;56:623-628.

114. Barinimon EE, Guisan M, Moser KM: Pulmonary involvement in Fabry's disease: A reappraisal: Follow up of a San Diego kindred and review of the literature. Am J Med 1972;53:755-759.

115. Brown LK, Miller A, Bhuptani A, et al: Pulmonary involvement in Fabry disease. Am J Respir Crit Care Med 1997;155:1004-1010.

116. Hiraizumi Y, Kanoh M, Shigematsu H, et al: A case of Fabry's disease with granulomatous interstitial nephritis. Nippon Jinzo Gakkai Shi 1995;37:655-661.

117. Sheth KJ, Werlin SL, Freeman ME, Hodach AE: Gastrointestinal structure and function in Fabry's disease. Am J Gastroenterol 1981;76:246-251.

118. Grunnet ML, Spilsbury PR: The central nervous system in Fabry's disease. Arch Neurol 1973;28:231-236.

119. Sher NA, Letson RD, Desnick RJ: The ocular manifestations in Fabry's disease. Arch Ophthalmol 1979;97:671-676.

120. Spaeth GL, Frost P: Fabry's disease: Its ocular manifestations. Arch Ophthalmol 1965;74:760-768.

121. Zadnik K: Fabry's disease. J Am Optomet Assoc 1987;58:87-88.

122. Andersen MW, Dahl H, Fledelium H, Nielsen NV: Central retinal artery occlusion in a patient with Fabry's disease documented by scanning laser ophthalmoscopy. Acta Ophthalmol (Copenh) 1994;72:635-641.

123. Tamura T, Murayama K, Hayashi R, et al: Two cases of women with Fabry's disease detected by electrocardiographic abnormalities. Nippon-Naika-Gakkai-Zasshi 1987;75:1123-1128.

124. Yokoyama A, Yamazoe M, Shibata A: A case of heterozygous Fabry's disease with a short PR interval and giant negative T waves. Br Heart J 1987;57:296-301.

125. Goldman ME, Cantor R, Schwartz MF, et al: Echocardiographic abnormalities and disease severity in Fabry disease. Am J Coll Cardiol 1986;7:1157-1161.

126. Kocen RS, Thomas PK: Peripheral nerve involvement in Fabry's disease. Arch Neurol 1970;22:81-88.

127. Sheth KJ, Swick HM: Peripheral nerve conduction in Fabry disease. Ann Neurol 1980;7:319-323.

128. Lockman LA, Hunninghake DB, Krivit W, et al: Relief of pain of Fabry's disease by diphenylhydantoin. Neurology 1973;23:871-876.

129. Gordon KE, Ludman MD, Finley GA: Successful treatment of painful crises of Fabry's disease with low dose morphine. Pediatr Neurol 1995;12:250-251.

130. Filling-Katz M, Merrick HF, Fink JK, et al: Carbamazepine in Fabry's disease: Effective analgesia with dose-dependent exacerbation of autonomic dysfunction. Neurology 19898;39:598-600.

131. Whyte MP: Electrocardiographic PR interval in Fabry's disease. N Engl J Med 1976;294:342.

132. Corey L, Holmes KK: Genital herpes simplex virus infections: Clinical manifestations, course and complications. Ann Intern Med 1983;98:958-967.

133. Bader C, Crumpacker CS, Schnipper LE, et al: The natural history of recurrent facial-oral infection with herpes simplex virus. J Infect Dis 1978;138:897-905.

134. Becker TM, Kods R, Bailey P, et al: Grappling with herpes: Herpes gladiatorum. Am J Sports Med 1988;16:665-669.

135. Gill MJ, Arlette J, Buchan K, Tyrrell DL: Therapy for recurrent herpetic whitlow. Ann Intern Med 1986;105:631.

136. Glogau R, Hanna L, Jawetz E: Herpetic whitlow as part of genital virus infection. J Infect Dis 1977;136:689-692.

137. Whitley RJ, Cobbs CG, Alford CA, et al: Diseases that mimic herpes simplex encephalitis. JAMA 1989;262:234-239.

138. Fiddian AP, Yeo JM, Stubbings R, Dean D: Successful treatment of facial-oral herpes with topical acyclovir. BMJ 1983;286:1699-1701.

139. VanLandingham KE, Marsteller HB, Ross GW, Hayden FG: Relapse of herpes simplex encephalitis after conventional acyclovir therapy. JAMA 1988;259:1051-1053.

140. Kovenblat PE, Wedner HJ, White MP, et al: Systemic mastocytosis. Arch Intern Med 1984;144:2249-2254.

141. Reisberg IR, Oyakawa S: Mastocytosis and malabsorption, myelofibrosis and massive ascites. Am J Gastroenterol 1987;82:54-59.

142. Cherner JA, Jensen RT, Dubois A, et al: Gastrointestinal dysfunction in systemic mastocytosis: A prospective study. Gastroenterology 1988;95:657-667.

143. Bonnet P, Smadja C, Szekely AM, et al: Intractable ascites in systemic mastocytosis treated by portal diversion. Dig Dis Sci 1987;32:209-213.

144. Fonga-Djimi HS, Gottrand F, Bonnevalle M, Farriaux JP: A fatal case of portal hypertension complicating systemic mastocytosis in an adolescent. Eur J Pediatr 1995;154:819-823.

145. Johnstone PA, Mican JM, Metcalfe DD, et al: Radiotherapy of refractory bone pain due to systemic mast cell disease. Am J Clin Oncol 1994;17:328-333.

146. Lawrence JB, Friedman BS, Travis WD, et al: Hematologic manifestations of systemic mast cell disease: A retrospective study of laboratory and morphologic features and their relation to prognosis. Am J Med 1991;91:612-624.

147. Rogers MP, Bloomingdale K, Murawski BJ, et al: Mixed organic brain syndrome as a manifestation of systemic mastocytosis. Psychosom Med 1986;48:437-447.

148. McFarlin KE, Kruesi MJ, Metcalfe DD, et al: A preliminary assessment of behavioral problems in children with mastocytosis. J Psych Med 1991;21:281-288.

149. Wyre HW, Henrichs WD: Systemic mastocytosis and pulmonary eosinophilic granuloma. JAMA 1978;239:856-859.

150. Mican JM, DiBisceglie AM, Fong TL, et al: Hepatic involvement in mastocytosis: Clinicopathologic correlations in 41 cases. Hepatology 1995;22:1163-1170.

151. Scott HW, Parris WCV, Sandidge PC, et al: Hazards in operative management of patients with systemic mastocytosis. Ann Surg 1983;197:507-512.

152. Koitabashi T, Takino Y: Anesthetic management of a patient with urticaria pigmentosa. Masui 1995;44:279-286.

153. Rosenbaum KJ, Strobel GE: Anesthetic considerations in mastocytosis. Anesthesiology 1973;38:398-404.

154. Hosking MP, Warner MA: Sudden intraoperative hypotension in a patient with asymptomatic urticaria pigmentosa. Anesth Analg 1987;66:344-346.

155. Turk J, Oates JA, Roberts LJ, et al: Intervention with epinephrine in hypotension associated with mastocytosis. J Allergy Clin Immunol 1983;71:189-192.

156. Parris WCV, Scott HW, Smith BE: Anesthetic management of systemic mastocytosis: Experience with 42 cases. Anesth Analg 1986;65:511-517.

157. Kelly TE: The mucopolysaccharidoses and mucolipidoses. Clin Orthop 1976;114:116-136.

158. Brosius FC III, Roberts WC: Coronary artery disease in the Hurler syndrome: Qualitative and quantitative analysis of the extent of coronary narrowing a necropsy in six children. Am J Cardiol 1981;47:649-653.

159. Cleary MA, Wraith JE: The presenting features of mucopolysaccharidosis type IH (Hurler syndrome). Acta Paediatr 1995;84:337-339.

160. Shapiro J, Strome M, Crocker AC: Airway obstruction and sleep apnea in Hurler and Hunter syndromes. Ann Otol Rhinol Laryngol 1985;94:458-464.

161. Thomas SL, Childress MH, Quinton B: Hypoplasia of the odontoid with atlanto-axial subluxation in Hurler's syndrome. Pediatr Radiol 1985;15:353-358.

162. Renteria VG, Ferrans VJ, Roberts WC: The heart in the Hurler syndrome: Gross, histologic and ultrastructural observations in five necropsy cases. Am J Cardiol 1976;38:487-501.

163. Dangel JH: Cardiovascular changes in children with mucopolysaccharide storage diseases and related disorders clinical and echocardiographic findings in 64 patients. Eur J Pediatr 1998;157:534-538.

164. Shinnar S, Singer HS, Valle D: Acute hydrocephalus in Hurler's syndrome. Am J Dis Child 1982;136:556-557.

165. Nowaczyk MJ, Clarke JT, Morin JD: Glaucoma as an early complication of Hurler's disease. Arch Dis Child 1988;63:1091.

166. Bona I, Vial C, Brunet P, et al: Carpal tunnel syndrome in mucopolysaccharidoses: A report of four cases in child. Electromyogr Clin Neurophysiol 1994;34:471-475.

167. Haddad FS, Jones DH, Vellodi A, et al: Carpal tunnel syndrome in the mucopolysaccharidoses and mucolipidoses. J Bone Joint Surg Br 1997;79:576-582.

168. Norman-Taylor F, Fixsen JA, Sharrad WJ: Hunter's syndrome as a cause of childhood carpal tunnel syndrome: A report of three cases J Pediatr Orthop B 1995;4:106-109.

169. Adachi K, Chole RA: Management of tracheal lesions in Hurler syndrome. Arch Otolaryngol Head Neck Surg 1990;116:1205-1207.

170. Lin CM, Hsu JC, Liu HP, et al: Anesthesia for CO_2 laser surgery in patient with Hunter syndrome: Case report. Changgen Yi Xue Za Zhi 2000;23:614-618.

171. Mikles M, Stanton RP: A review of Morquio syndrome. Am J Orthop 1997;26:533-537.

172. Roach JW, Duncan D, Wenger DR, et al: Atlanto-axial instability and spinal cord compression in children: Diagnosis by computerized tomography. J Bone Joint Surg Am 1984;66:708-714.

173. Takeda E, Hashimoto T, Tayama M, et al: Diagnosis of atlantoaxial subluxation in Morquio's syndrome and spondyloepiphyseal dysplasia congenita. Acta Paediatr Jpn 1991;33:633-638.

174. Stevens JM, Kendall BE, Crockard HA, et al: The odontoid process in Morquio-Brailsford's disease: The effects of occipitocervical fusion J Bone Joint Surg Br 1991;73:851-857.

175. Piccirilli CB, Chadduck WM: Cervical kyphotic myelopathy in a child with Morquio syndrome. Childs Nerv Syst 1996;12:114-116.

176. Lipson SJ: Dysplasia of the odontoid process in Morquio's syndrome causing quadriparesis. J Bone Joint Surg Am 1997;59:340-344.

177. Ashraf J, Crockard HA, Ransford AO, et al: Transoral decompression and posterior stabilization in Morquio's disease. Arch Dis Child 1991;66:1318-1321.

178. Ransord AO, Crockard HA, Stevens JM, et al: Occipito-atlanto-axial fusion in Morquio-Brailsford syndrome: A ten-year experience. J Bone Joint Surg Br 1996;78:307-312.

179. Hope EOS, Farebrother MJB, Bainbridge D: Some aspects of respiratory function in three siblings with Morquio-Brailsford disease. Thorax 1969;28:335-341.

180. Semenza GL, Pyeritz RE: Respiratory complications of mucopolysaccharide storage disorders. Medicine 1988;67:209-219.

181. John RM, Hunter D, Swanton RH: Echocardiographic abnormalities in type IV mucopolysaccharidosis. Arch Dis Child 1990;65:746-749.

182. Hayflick S, Rowe S, Kavanaugh-McHugh A, et al: Acute infantile cardiomyopathy as a presenting feature of mucopolysaccharidosis VI. J Pediatr 1992;120:269-272.

183. Moore C, Rogers JG, McKenzie IM, Brown TC: Anesthesia for children with mucopolysaccharidoses. Anaesth Intens Care 1997;25:197-198.

184. Brill CB, Rose JS, Godmilow L, et al: Spastic quadriparesis due to C1-C2 subluxation in Hurler's syndrome. J Pediatr 1978;92: 441-443.

185. Birkinshaw KJ: Anaesthesia in a patient with an unstable neck. Anaesthesia 1975;30:46-49.

186. Man TT, Tsai PS, Rau RH, et al: Children with mucopolysaccharidosis—three case reports. Acta Anaesthesiol Sinica 1999;37:93-96.

187. Herrick IA, Rhine EJ: The mucopolysaccharidoses and anaesthesia: A report of clinical experience. Can J Anaesth 1988;35:67-73.

188. Gaitini L, Fradis M, Vaida S, et al: Failure to control the airway in a patient with Hunter's syndrome. J Laryngol Otol 1998;112:380-383.

189. Kempthorne PM, Brown TC: Anaesthesia and the mucopolysaccharidoses: A survey of techniques and problems. Anaesth Intensive Care 1983;11:203-207.

190. Ballenger CE, Swift TR, Leshner RT, et al: Myelopathy in mucopolysaccharidosis type II (Hunter syndrome). Ann Neurol 1980;7:382-385.

191. Walker RW: The laryngeal mask airway in the difficult paediatric airway: An assessment of positioning and use in fiberoptic intubation. Paediatr Anaesth 2000;10:53-58.

192. Busoni P, Fognani G: Failure of laryngeal mask airway to secure the airway in a patient with Hunter's syndrome. Paediatr Anaesth 1999;9:153-155.

193. Vas L, Naregal F: Failed epidural anesthesia in a patient with Hurler's disease. Paediatr Anaesth 2000;10:95-98.

194. Tobias JD: Anesthetic care for the child with Morquio syndrome: General versus regional anesthesia. J Clin Anesth 1999;11:242-246.

195. Sethna NF, Berde CB: Continuous subarachnoid analgesia in two adolescents with severe scoliosis and impaired pulmonary function. Reg Anesth 1991;16:333-336.

196. Linstedt U, Maier C, Joehnk H, et al: Threatening spinal cord compression during anesthesia in a child with mucopolysaccharidosis VI. Anesthesiology 1994;80:227-229.

197. Belani KG, Krivit W, Carpenter BL, et al: Children with mucopolysaccharidosis: Perioperative care, morbidity, mortality, and new findings. J Pediatr Surg 1993;28:403-408.

198. Toda Y, Takeuchi M, Morita K, et al: Complete heart block during anesthesia management in a patient with mucopolysaccharidosis type VII. Anesthesiology 2001;95:1035-1037.

199. Kreidstein A, Boorin MR, Crespi P, et al: Delayed awakening from general anesthesia in a patient with Hunter syndrome. Can J Anaesth 1994;41:423-426.

200. Jones AEP, Croley TF: Morquio syndrome and anesthesia. Anesthesiology 1979;51:261-262.

201. Wander JV, Das Gupta TK: Neurofibromatosis. Curr Probl Surg 1977;14:11-18.

202. Mulvihill JJ, Parry DM, Sherman JL, et al: Neurofibromatosis 1 (Recklinghausen disease) and neurofibromatosis 2 (bilateral acoustic neurofibromatosis). Ann Intern Med 1990; 113:39-52.

203. Riccardi VM: Von Recklinghausen neurofibromatosis. N Engl J Med 1981;305:1617-1627.

204. Roos KL, Muckway M: Neurofibromatosis. Dermatol Clin 1995;13:105-111.

205. Eldridge R: Central neurofibromatosis with bilateral acoustic neuroma. Adv Neurol 1981;29:57-65.

206. Krohel GB, Rosenberg PN, Wright JE, Smith RS: Localized orbital neurofibromas. Am J Ophthalmol 1985;100:458-464.

207. Huson SM, Thrush DC: Central neurofibromatosis. Q J Med 1985;55:231-235.

208. Rettele GA, Brodsky MC, Merin LM, et al: Blindness, deafness, quadriparesis, and a retinal malformation: The ravages of neurofibromatosis. 2. Surv Opthalmol 1996;41:135-141.

209. Chang-lo M: Laryngeal involvement in von Recklinghausen's disease: A case report and review of the literature. Laryngoscope 1977;87: 435-442.

210. Cohen SR, Landing BH, Isaacs H: Neurofibroma of the larynx in a child. Ann Otol Rhinol Laryngol 1978;87:29-34.

211. Sagel SS, Forrest JV, Askin FB: Interstitial lung disease in neurofibromatosis. South Med J 1975;68:647-652.

212. Griffits ML, Theron EJ: Obstructed labor from pelvic neurofibroma. South Afr Med J 1978;53:781.

213. Jarivs GJ, Crompton AC: Neurofibromatosis and pregnancy. Br J Obstet Gynacol 1978;85:844-846.

214. Shishiba T, Niimura M, Ohtsuka F, Tsuru N: Multiple cutaneous neurilemmomas as a skin manifestation of neurilemmomas. J Am Acad Dermatol 1984;10:744-754.

215. Crowe FW, Schull WJ: Diagnostic importance of the café-au-lait spot in neurofibromatosis. Arch Intern Med 1963;91;758-766.

216. Wishart JH: Case of tumours in the skull, dura mater, and brain. Edinburgh Med Surg J 1982;18:393-397.

217. Elster AD: Occult spinal tumors in neurofibromatosis: Implications for screening. AJR Am J Roentgenol 1995;165:956-957.

218. Leech RW, Olafson RA, Gilbertson RL, Shho DR: Intrathoracic meningocele and vertebral anomalies in a case of neurofibromatosis. Surg Neurol 1978;9:55-57.

219. Drevelengas A, Kalaitzoglou I: Giant lumbar meningocele in a patient with neurofibromatosis. Neuroradiology 1995;37:195-197.

220. Haddad FS, Williams RL, Bentley G: The cervical spine in neurofibromatosis. Br J Hosp Med 1995;53:318.

221. Chaglassian JH, Riseborogh EJ, Hall JE: Neurofibromatous scoliosis. J Bone Joint Surg Am 1976;58:695-702.

222. Fisher MM: Anesthetic difficulties in neurofibromatosis. Anaesthesia 1975;30:648-650.

223. Dounas M, Mercier FJ, Lhuissier C, Benhamou D: Epidural analgesia for labour in a parturient with neurofibromatosis. Can J Anaesth 1995;42:420-424.

224. Magbagbeola JAO: Abnormal responses to muscle relaxants in patients with von Recklinghausen's disease. Br J Anaesth 1970;42:710.

225. Yamasha M: Anaesthetic considerations in von Recklinghausen's disease (multiple neurofibromatosis). Abnormal response to muscle relaxants. Anaesthetist 1977;26:317-321.

226. Cooperman LH: Succinylcholine-induced hyperkalemia in neuromuscular disease. JAMA 1970;213:1967-1971.

227. Bullough PG, Davidson DD, Lorenzo JC: The morbid anatomy of the skeleton in osteogenesis imperfecta. Clin Orthop 1981;159: 42-57.

228. Gertner JM, Root L: Osteogenesis imperfecta. Orthop Clin North Am 1990;21:151-161.

229. Wenger DR, Abrams RA, Uaru N, et al: Obstruction of the colon due to protrusio acetabuli in osteogenesis imperfecta: Treatment by pelvic osteotomy. Report of a case. J Bone Joint Surg Am 1988;70: 1103-1107.

230. Rask MR: Spondylolisthesis resulting from osteogenesis imperfecta: Report of a case. Clin Orthop 1979;139:164-166.

231. Ziv I, Rang M, Hoffman HJ: Paraplegia in osteogenesis imperfecta: A case report. J Bone Joint Surg Br 1983;65:184-186.

232. Pozo JL, Crockard HA, Ransford AO: Basilar impression in osteogenesis imperfecta: A report of three cases in one family. J Bone Joint Surg Br 1984;66:233-238.

233. Frank E, Berger T, Tew JM Jr: Basilar impression and platybasia in osteogenesis imperfecta tarda. Surg Neurol 1982;17:116-119.

234. Levin LS: The dentition in the osteogenesis imperfecta syndromes. Clin Orthop 1981;159:64-73.

235. Bradish CF, Flowers M: Central retinal artery occlusion in association with osteogenesis imperfecta. Spine 1987;12:193-194.

236. Rampton AJ, Kelly DA, Shanahan EC, et al: Occurrence of malignant hyperpyrexia in a patient with osteogenesis imperfecta. Br J Anaesth 1984;56:1443-1445.

237. Ryan CA, Al-Ghamdi AS, Gayle M, et al: Osteogenesis imperfecta and hyperthermia. Anesth Analg 1989;68:811-814.
238. Peluso A, Cerullo M: Malignant hyperthermia susceptibility in patients with osteogenesis imperfecta. Paediatr Anaesth 1995;5:398-399.
239. Porsborg P, Astrup G, Bendixen D, et al: Osteogenesis imperfecta and malignant hyperthermia: Is there a relationship? Anaesthesia 1996;51:863-865.
240. Solomons CC, Myers DN: Hyperthermia of osteogenesis imperfecta and its relationship to malignant hyperthermia. In Gordon RA, Britt BA, Kalow W (eds): Malignant Hyperthermia. Springfield, IL, Charles C Thomas, 1971, pp 319-330.
241. Oliverio RN: Anesthetic management of intramedullary nailing in osteogenesis imperfecta: Report of a case. Anesth Analg 1973;52:232-236.
242. White NJ, Winearls CG, Smith R: Cardiovascular abnormalities in osteogenesis imperfecta. Am Heart J 1983;106:1416-1420.
243. Stein D, Kloster FE: Valvular heart disease in osteogenesis imperfecta. Am Heart J 1977;94:637-641.
244. Hammer D, Leier CV, Baba N, et al: Altered collagen composition in a prolapsing mitral valve with ruptured chordae tendineae. Am J Med 1979;67:863-866.
245. Cohen IM, Vieweg WVR, Alpert JS, et al: Osteogenesis imperfecta tarda: Cardiovascular pathology. West J Med 1977;126:228-231.
246. Taitz LS: Child abuse and osteogenesis imperfecta. BMJ 1987;295:1082-1083.
247. Paterson CR, Mcallion SJ: Osteogenesis imperfecta in the differential diagnosis of child abuse. BMJ 1996;312:351-354.
248. Ablin DS: Osteogenesis imperfecta: A review. Can Assoc Radiol J 1998;49:110-123.
249. Dent JA, Paterson CR: Fractures in early childhood: Osteogenesis imperfecta or child abuse? J Pediatr Orthop 1991;11:184-186.
250. Augarten A, Laufer J, Szeinberg A, et al: Child abuse, osteogenesis imperfecta and the grey zone between them. J Med 1993;24:171-175.
251. Solomons CC, Millar EA: Osteogenesis imperfecta—new perspectives. Clin Orthop 1973;96:299-303.
252. Estes JW: Platelet size and function in the heritable disorders of connective tissue. Ann Intern Med 1968;68:1237-1249.
253. Edge G, Okafor B, Fennelly ME, Ransford AO: An unusual manifestation of bleeding diathesis in a patient with osteogenesis imperfecta. Eur J Anaesth 1997;14:215-219.
254. Falvo KA, Klain DB, Krauss AN, et al: Pulmonary function studies in osteogenesis imperfecta. Am Rev Respir Dis 1973;108:1258-1260.
255. Meyer S, Villarreal M, Ziv I: A three-level fracture of the axis in a patient with osteogenesis imperfecta: A case report. Spine 1986;11:505-506.
256. Rush PJ, Berbrayer D, Reilly BJ: Basilar impression and osteogenesis imperfecta in a three-year-old girl: CT and MRI. Pediatr Radiol 1989;19:142-143.
257. Kurimoto M, O'Hara S, Takaku A: Basilar impression in osteogenesis imperfecta tarda: Case report. J Neurosurg 1991;74:136-138.
258. Hurwitz LJ, McSwiney RR: Basilar impression and osteogenesis imperfecta in a family. Brain 1960;83:138-149.
258. Harkey HL, Corckard HA, Stevens JM, et al: The operative management of basilar impression in osteogenesis imperfecta. Neurosurgery 1990;27:782-786.
259. Pauli RM, Gilbert EF: Upper cervical cord compression as a cause of death in osteogenesis imperfecta type II. J Pediatr 1986;108:579-581.
260. Rush GA, Burke SW: Hangman's fracture in a patient with osteogenesis imperfecta: Case report. J Bone Joint Surg Am 1984;66:778-779.
261. Ferrera PC, Hayes ST, Triner WR: Spinal cord concussion in previously undiagnosed osteogenesis imperfecta. Am J Emerg Med 1995;13:424-426.
262. Sperry K: Fatal intraoperative hemorrhage during spinal fusion surgery for osteogenesis imperfecta. Am J Forensic Med Pathol 1989;10:54-59.
263. Massey T, Garst J: Compartment syndrome of the thigh with osteogenesis imperfecta: A case report. Clin Orthop 1991;267:202-205.
264. Bergstrom L: Osteogenesis imperfecta: Otologic and maxillofacial aspects. Laryngoscope 1977;87(suppl 6):1-8.
265. Karabiyik L, Parpacu M, Kurtipek O: Total intravenous anesthesia and the use of an intubating laryngeal mask in a patient with osteogenesis imperfecta. Acta Anaesthesiol Scand 2002;46:618-619.
266. Vogel TM, Ratner EF, Thomas RC, Chitkara U: Pregnancy complicated by severe osteogenesis imperfecta: A report of two cases. Anesth Analg 2002;94:1315-1317.
267. Cunningham AJ, Donnelly M, Comerford J: Osteogenesis imperfecta: Anesthetic management of a patient for cesarean section: A case report. Anesthesiology 1984;61:91-93.
268. Libman RH: Anesthetic considerations for the patient with osteogenesis imperfecta. Clin Orthop 1981;159:123-124.
269. Baines D: Total intravenous anesthesia for patients with osteogenesis imperfecta. Paediatr Anaesth 1995;5:144.
270. Sadat-Ali M, Sankaran-Kutty M, Adu-gyamfi Y: Metabolic acidosis in osteogenesis imperfecta. Eur J Pediatr 1986;145:582-583.
271. Sadat-Ali M, Sankaran-Kutty M, Adu-gyamfi Y: Metabolic acidosis in osteogenesis imperfecta. Eur J Pediatr 1986;145:324-325.
272. Livesley PJ, Webb PJ: Spinal fusion in situ in osteogenesis imperfecta. Int Orthop 1996;20:43-46.
273. Riggs BL, Wahner HW, Dunn WL, et al: Differential changes in bone mineral density of the appendicular and axial skeleton with aging. J Clin Invest 1981;67:328-335.
274. Crilly R, Horsman A, Marshall DH, Nordin BEC: Prevalence, pathogenesis and treatment of postmenopausal osteoporosis. Aust NZ J Med 1979;9:24-30.
275. Aloia JF, Cohn SH, Babu T, et al: Skeletal mass and body composition in marathon runners. Metabolism 1978;27:1793-1796.
276. Aloia JF, Stanton HC, Ostumi JA, et al: Prevention of involutional bone loss by exercise. Ann Intern Med 1978;89:356-358.
277. Ng KC, Ravell PA, Beer M, et al: The incidence of metabolic bone disease, rheumatoid arthritis and osteoarthritis. Ann Rheum Dis 1984;43:370-377.
278. Lips P, Courpron P, Meunier PJ: Mean wall thickness of trabecular bone pockets in the human iliac crest: Changes with age. Calcif Tissue Res 1978;26:13-17.
279. Matloff DS, Kaplan MM, Neer RM, et al: Osteoporosis in primary biliary cirrhosis: Effects of 25-hydroxyvitamin D_3 treatment. Gastroenterology 1982;83:97-102.
280. Stellon AJ, Davies A, Compston J, Williams R. Osteoporosis in chronic cholestatic liver disease. Q J Med 1985;223:783-790.
281. Gallagher JC, Aaron J, Horsman A, et al: The crush fracture syndrome in post-menopausal women. Clin Endocrinol Metab 1973;2:293-315.
282. Einson P, Neustadter LM, Moncman MG: Nutritional osteomalacia. Am J Dis Child 1980;134:427-435.
283. Barzel US: Vitamin D deficiency: A risk factor for osteomalacia in the aged. J Am Geriatr Soc 1983;81:598-601.
284. Meredith SC, Rosenberg IH: Gastrointestinal-hepatic disorders and osteomalacia. Clin Endocrinol Metab 1980;9:131-150.
285. Parfitt AM, Miller MJ, Frame B, et al: Metabolic bone disease after intestinal bypass for treatment of obesity. Ann Intern Med 1978;89:193-199.
286. Chalmers J: Subtrochanteric fractures in osteomalacia. J Bone Joint Surg Br 1970;52:509-513.
287. Klein RG, Arnaud SB, Gallagher JC, et al: Intestinal calcium absorption in exogenous hypercorticolism: Role of 25-hydroxyvitamin D and corticosteroid dose. J Clin Invest 1977;60:253-259.
288. Hahn TJ: Drug-induced disorders of vitamin D and mineral metabolism. Clin Endocrinol Metab 1980;9:107-129.
289. Maddison PJ, Bacon PA: Vitamin D deficiency, spontaneous fractures and osteopenia in rheumatoid arthritis. BMJ 1974;4:433-435.
290. O'Driscoll S, O'Driscoll M: Osteomalacia in rheumatoid arthritis. Ann Rheum Dis 1980;39:1-6.

291. Compston JE: Hepatic osteodystrophy: Vitamin D metabolism in patients with liver disease. Gut 1986;27:1073-1090.

292. Krawitt EL: Ethanol inhibits intestinal calcium transport in rats. Nature 1973;243:88-89.

293. Feitelberg S, Epstein S, Ismail F, D'Amanda C: Deranged bone mineral metabolism in chronic alcoholism. Metabolism 1987;36:322-326.

294. Nilsson BE, Westlin NE: Changes in bone mass in alcoholics. Clin Orthop 1973;90:229-232.

295. Wahl TO, Gobuty AH, Lukert BP: Long-term anticonvulsant therapy and intestinal calcium absorption. Clin Pharmacol Ther 1981;30:506-512.

296. Malluche HH, Goldstein DA, Massry SG: Osteomalacia and hyperparathyroid bone disease in patients with nephrotic syndrome. J Clin Invest 1979;63:494-500.

297. Goldstein DA, Haldimann B, Sherman D, et al: Vitamin D metabolites and calcium metabolism in patients with nephrotic syndrome and normal renal function. J Clin Endocrinol Metab 1981;52:116-121.

298. Steinbach HL, Kolb FO, Gilfillan R: A mechanism of the production of pseudofractures in osteomalacia (milkman's syndrome). Radiology 1964;62:388-394.

299. Charhon SA, Chapuy MC, Delvin EE, et al: Histomorphometric analysis of sclerotic bone metastases from prostatic carcinoma with special reference to osteomalacia. Cancer 1983;51:918-924.

300. Kabadi UM: Osteomalacia associated with prostatic cancer and osteoblastic metastases. Urology 1983;21:65-67.

301. Lyles KW, Berry WR, Haussler M, et al: Hypophosphatemic osteomalacia: Association with prostatic carcinoma. Ann Intern Med 1980;93:275-278.

302. Shapiro F: Osteopetrosis: Current clinical considerations. Clin Orthop 1993;294:34-38.

303. Bollerslev J: Autosomal dominant osteopetrosis: Bone metabolism and epidemiologic, clinical, and hormonal aspects. Endocr Rev 1989;10:45-67.

304. Shapiro R, Glimcher MJ, Holtrop ME, et al: Human osteopetrosis. J Bone Joint Surg Am 1980;62:384-399.

305. Cameron HU, Dewar FP: Degenerative osteoarthritis associated with osteopetrosis. Clin Orthop 1977;127:148-153.

306. Resnick D, Niwayama G: Radiographic and pathologic features of spinal involvement in diffuse idiopathic skeletal hyperostosis (DISH). Radiology 1976;119:559-568.

307. Gall EA, Bennett GA, Bauer W: Generalized hypertrophic osteoarthropathy; a pathologic study of seven cases. Am J Pathol 1951;27:349-381.

308. Ray ES, Fisher HP: Hypertrophic osteoarthropathy in pulmonary malignancies. Ann Intern Med 1932;38:239-246.

309. Braude S, Kennedy H, Hodson M, Batten J: Hypertrophic osteoarthropathy in cystic fibrosis. BMJ 1984;288:822-823.

310. Bourke E, Delaney VP, Mosawi M, et al: Renal tubular acidosis and osteopetrosis in siblings. Nephron 1981;28:268-272.

311. Shin MS, Mowry RW, Bodie FL: Osteosclerosis (punctuate form) in multiple myeloma. South Med J 1979;72:226-228.

312. Martin RP, Deane RH, Collett V: Spondylolysis in children who have osteopetrosis. J Bone Joint Surg Am 1997;79:1685-1693.

313. Cumming WA, Ohlsson A: Intracranial calcification in children with osteopetrosis caused by carbonic anhydrase II deficiency. Radiology 1985;157:325-327.

314. Steinwender G, Hosny GA, Koch S, et al: Bilateral nonunited femoral neck fracture in a child with osteopetrosis. J Pediatr Orthop B 1995;4:213-217.

315. Davies M, Mawer EB, Freemont AJ: The osteodystrophy of hypervitaminosis D: A metabolic study. Q J Med 1986;234:911-919.

316. Stanbury SW: Vitamin D and hyperparathyroidism. J R Coll Physicians Lond 1981;15:205-2017.

317. McConkey B, Fraser GB, Bligh AS, Whiteley H: Transparent skin and osteoporosis. Lancet 1963;1:693-695.

318. Casden AM, Jaffe FF, Kastenbaum DM, et al: Osteoarthritis associated with osteopetrosis treated by total knee arthroplasty: Report of a case. Clin Orthop 1989;247:202-210.

319. Matsuno T, Katayama N: Osteopetrosis and total hip arthroplasty: Report of two cases. Int Orthop 1997;21:409-414.

320. Forestier J, Lagier R: Ankylosing hyperostosis of the spine. Clin Orthop 1971;74:65-83.

321. Vernon-Roberts B, Pirie CJ, Trenwith V: Pathology of the dorsal spine in ankylosing hyperostosis. Ann Rheum Dis 1974;33:281-288.

322. Meunier PJ, Coindre JM, Edouard CM, Arlot ME: Bone histomorphometry in Paget's disease: Quantitative and dynamic analysis of pagetic and nonpagetic bone tissue. Arthritis Rheum 1980;23:1095-1103.

323. Reasbeck JC, Goulding A, Campbell DR, et al: Radiological prevalence of Paget's disease in Dunedin, New Zealand. BMJ 1983;286:1937-1941.

324. Roper B: Paget's disease involving the hip joint. Clin Orthop Rel Res 1971;80:33-38.

325. Gardner MJ, Guyer PB, Barker DJB: Radiological prevalence of Paget's disease of bone in British migrants to Australia. BMJ 1978;1:1655-1657.

326. Franck WA, Bress NM, Singer FR, Krane SM: Rheumatic manifestations of Paget's disease of bone. Am J Med 1974;56:592-603.

327. Nassar VH, Gravanis MB: Familial osteogenic sarcoma occurring in pagetoid bone. Am J Clin Pathol 1981;76:235-239.

328. McKenna RJ, Schwinn CP, Soong KY, Higinbotham NL: Osteogenic sarcoma arising in Paget's disease. Cancer 1964;17:42-66.

329. Schajowicz F, Araujo ES, Berenstein M: Sarcoma complicating Paget's disease. J Bone Joint Surg Br 1983;65:299-307.

330. Machtey I, Rodnan GP, Benedek T: Paget's disease of the hip joint. Am J Med Sci 1966;251:524-531.

331. Sparrow NL, Duvall AJ: Hearing loss and Paget's disease. J Laryngol Otol 1967;81:601-611.

332. Epstein BS, Epstein JA: The association of cerebellar tonsillar herniation with basilar impression incident to Paget's disease. AJR Am J Roentgenol 1969;107:535-542.

333. Dohrmann PJ, Elrick WL: Dementia and hydrocephalus in Paget's disease: A case report. J Neurol Neurosurg Psychiatry 1982;45:835-837.

334. Goldhammer Y, Braham J, Kosary IZ: Hydrocephalic dementia in Paget's disease of the skull: Treatment by ventriculoatrial shunt. Neurology 1979;29:513-518.

335. Eretto P, Krohel GB, Shihab ZM, et al: Optic neuropathy in Paget's disease. Am J Ophthalmol 1984;97:505-510.

336. Smith BJ, Eveson JW: Paget's disease of bone with particular reference to dentistry. J Oral Pathol 1981;10:233-247.

337. Sofaer JA: Dental extractions in Paget's disease of bone. Int J Oral Surg 1984;13:79-84.

338. Brown HP, LaRocca H, Wickstrom JK: Paget's disease of the atlas and axis. J Bone Joint Surg 1971;53:1441-1449.

339. Siegelman SS, Levine SA, Walpin L: Paget's disease with spinal cord compression. Clin Radiol 1968;19:421-425.

340. Altman RD, Collins B: Musculoskeletal manifestations of Paget's disease of bone. Arthritis Rheum 1980;23:1121-1127.

341. Weisz GM: Lumbar canal stenosis in Paget's disease. Clin Orthop Rel Res 1986;206:223-227.

342. Theodors A, Askari AD, Wieland RG: Colchicine in the treatment of Paget's disease of bone: A new therapeutic approach. Clin Ther 1983;3:365-373.

343. Woodhouse NJY, Crosbie WA, Mohamedally SM: Cardiac output in Paget's disease: Response to long-term salmon calcitonin therapy. BMJ 1975;4:686-691.

344. Ibbertson HK, Henley JW, Fraser TR, et al: Paget's disease of bone—clinical evaluation and treatment with diphosphonate. Aust NZ J Med 1979;9:31-35.

345. Henley JW, Croxson RS, Ibbertson HK: The cardiovascular system in Paget's disease of bone and the response to therapy with calcitonin and diphosphonate. Aust NZ J Med 1979;9:390-397.

346. Fromm GA, Schajowicz F, Casco C, et al: The treatment of Paget's disease of bone with sodium etidronate. Am J Med Sci 1979;277:29-37.

347. Evans RA, Macdonald D: Diphosphonates and painful feet. Aust NZ J Med 1983;13:175-176.

348. Johnston CC Jr, Altman RD, Canfield RE, et al: Review of fracture experience during treatment of Paget's disease of bone with etidronate disodium. Clin Orthop Rel Res 1983;172:186-194.

349. Evans RA, Hills E, Dunstan CR, Wong SYP: Pathologic fracture due to severe osteomalacia following low-dose diphosphonate treatment of Paget's disease of bone. Aust NZ J Med 1983; 13:277-279.

350. Boyce BF, Smith L, Gogelman I, et al: Focal osteomalacia due to low-dose disphosphonate therapy in Paget's disease. Lancet 1984;1: 821-824.

351. Stein I, Shapiro B, Ostrum B, Beller ML: Evaluation of sodium etidronate in the treatment of Paget's disease of bone. Clin Orthop Rel Res 1977;122:347-358.

352. Elias EG, Evans JT: Mithramycin in the treatment of Paget's disease of bone. J Bone Joint Surg Am 1972;54:1730-1736.

353. Ryan WG: Treatment of Paget's disease of bone with mithramycin. Clin Orthop Rel Res 1977;127:106-110.

354. McDonald DJ, Sim FH: Total hip arthroplasty in Paget's disease. J Bone Joint Surg Am 1987;69:766-772.

355. Merkow RL, Pellicci PM, Hely DP, Salvati EA: Total hip replacement for Paget's disease of the hip. J Bone Joint Surg Am 1984;66:752-758.

356. O'Hara S, Koh C, Yanagisawa N: Myalgia as the major system in systemic panniculitis (Weber-Christian disease). Eur Neurol 1996;32:321-323.

357. Ciclitira PJ, Wight DGD, Dick AP: Systemic Weber-Christian disease. Br J Dermatol 1980;103:685-692.

358. Duncan WC, Freeman RG, Heaton CL: Cold panniculitis. Arch Dermatol 1966;94:722-725.

359. Patterson JW, Brown PC, Broecker AH: Infection-induced panniculitis. J Cutan Pathol 1989;16:183-191.

360. DeGranciansky P: Weber-Christian syndrome of pancreatic origin. Br J Dermatol 1967;79:278-283.

361. Potts DE, Mass MF, Iseman MD: Syndrome of pancreatic disease, subcutaneous fat necrosis and polyserositis. Am J Med 1975;58: 417-423.

362. Hendricks WM, Ahmad M, Gratz E: Weber-Christian disease in infancy. Br J Dermatol 1978;98:175-186.

363. Chuang SD, Chiu HC, Chang CC: Subcutaneous fat necrosis of newborn complicating hypothermic cardiac surgery. Br J Dermatol 1995;132:805-810.

364. Tuffanelli DL: Lupus erythematosus panniculitis (profundus). Arch Dermatol 1971;103:231-241.

365. Peters MS, Su WP: Lupus erythematosus panniculitis. Med Clin North Am 1989;73:1113-1118.

366. Kroll JJ, Shapiro L, Koplon BS, et al: Subcutaneous sarcoidosis with calcification. Arch Dermatol 1972;106:894-899.

367. Sumaya CV, Babu S, Reed RJ: Erythema nodosum–like lesion of leukemia. Arch Dermatol 1974;110:415-419.

368. Lee JS, Ahn SK, Lee SH: Factitial panniculitis induced by cupping and acupuncture. Cutis 1995;55:217-218.

369. Truelove LH: Articular manifestations of erythema nodosum. Ann Rheum Dis 1960;19:174-177.

370. Morioka S, Sakuma M, Ogawa H: The incidence of internal malignancies in autoimmune blistering diseases: Pemphigus and bullous pemphigoid in Japan. Dermatology 1989;82(suppl 1): 1994-1996.

371. Krain LS, Bierman SM: Pemphigus vulgaris and internal malignancy. Cancer 1974;33:1091-1095.

372. Naysmith A, Hancock BW: Hodgkin's disease and pemphigus. Br J Dermatol 1976;94:696-699.

373. Stone SP, Schroeter AL: Bullous pemphigoid and associated malignant neoplasms. Arch Dermatol 1975;111:991-994.

374. Venning VA, Millard PA, Wojnarowska F: Dapsone as first line therapy for bullous pemphigoid. Br J Dermatol 1989;120:83-92.

375. Lindelof B, Islam N, Eklund G, et al: Pemphigoid and cancer. Arch Dermatol 1990;126:66-68.

376. Siegel J, Eaglstein WH: High-dose methylprednisolone in the treatment of bullous pemphigoid. Arch Dermatol 1984;120: 1157-1165.

377. Chryssomallis F, Dimitriades A, Chaidemenos GC, et al: Steroid-pulse therapy in pemphigus vulgaris long term follow-up. Int J Dermatol 1995;34:438-442.

378. Epstein FW, Bohn M: Dapsone-induced peripheral neuropathy. Arch Dermatol 1976;112:1761-1764.

379. Bouscarat F, Chosidow O, Picard-Dahan C, et al: Treatment of bullous pemphigoid with dapsone: Retrospective study of thirty-six cases. J Am Acad Dermatol 1996;34:683-685.

380. Fine JD: Management of acquired bullous skin diseases. N Engl J Med 1995;333:1475-1479.

381. Szeremeta W, Dohar JE: Dapsone-induced methemoglobinemia: An anesthetic risk. Int J Pediatr Otorhinolaryngol 1995;33:75-80.

382. Guillaume JC, Vaillant L, Bernard P, et al: Controlled trial of azathioprine and plasma exchange in addition to prednisolone in the treatment of bullous pemphigoid. Arch Dermatol 1993;29:49-53.

383. Lever WF, Schaumburg-Lever G: Immunosuppressants and prednisone in pemphigus vulgaris. Arch Dermatol 1977;113: 1236-1241.

384. Oranje AP, Van Joost T: Pemphigoid in children. Pediatr Dermatol 1989;6:267-274.

385. Fivenson DP, Breneman DL, Rosen GB, et al: Nicotinamide and tetracycline therapy of bullous pemphigoid. Arch Dermatol 1994;130:753-758.

387. Lavie CJ, Thomas MA, Fondak AA: The perioperative management of the patient with pemphigus vulgaris and villous adenoma. Cutis 1984;34:180-183.

386. Savin JA: The events leading to the death of patients with pemphigus and pemphigoid. Br J Dermatol 1979;101:521-533.

388. Jeyaram C, Torda TA: Anesthetic management of cholecystectomy in a patient with buccal pemphigus. Anesthesiology 1975;40:600-603.

389. Drenger B, Zidebaum M, Reifen E, Leitersdorf E: Severe upper airway obstruction and difficult intubation in cicatricial pemphigoid. Anaesthesia 1986;41:1029-1031.

390. Vatashky E, Aronson JB: Pemphigus vulgaris: Anaesthesia in the traumatized patient. Anaesthesia 1982;37:1195-1198.

391. Mahalingam TG, Kathirvel S, Sodhi P: Anesthetic management of a patient with pemphigus vulgaris for emergency laparotomy. Anaesthesia 2000;55:160-162.

392. Gilsanz F, Meilan ML, Roses R, Olivera G: Regional anaesthesia and pemphigus vulgaris. Anaesthesia 1992;47:74.

393. Abouleish EI, Elias MA, Lopez M, Hebert AA: Spinal anesthesia for cesarean section in a case of pemphigus foliaceous. Anesth Analg 1997;84:449-450.

394. Gardembas-Pain M, Ifrah N, Foussard C, et al: Psoriasis after allogeneic bone marrow transplantation. Arch Dermatol 1991;126:1523-1527.

395. Stern R, Zierler S, Parrish JA: Psoriasis and the risk of cancer. J Invest Dermatol 1982;78:147-153.

396. Halprin KM, Comerford M, Taylor JR: Cancer patients with psoriasis. J Am Acad Dermatol 1982;7:633-638.

397. Yamamoto T, Yokozeki H, Katayama I, Nushioka K: Uveitis in patients with generalized pustular psoriasis. Br J Dermatol 1995;132:1023-1031.

398. Christophers E, Mrowietz U, Henneicke HH, et al: Cyclosporine in psoriasis: A multicenter dose-finding study in severe plaque psoriasis. J Am Acad Dermatol 1992;26:86-90.

399. Jegasothy BV, Ackerman CD, Todo S, et al: Tacrolimus (FK 506): A new therapeutic agent for severe recalcitrant psoriasis. Arch Dermatol 1992;128:781-785.

400. Rappersberger K, Meingassner JG, Fialla R, et al: Clearing of psoriasis by a novel immunosuppressive macrolide. J Invest Dermatol 1996;106:701-710.

401. Ellis CN, Fradin MS, Messana JM, et al: Cyclosporine for plaque-type psoriasis. N Engl J Med 1991;324:277-284.

402. Hassan W: Methotrexate and liver toxicity: Role of surveillance liver biopsy. Ann Rheum Dis 1996;55:273.

403. Roenigk HH, Auerbach R, Malibach HI, Weinstein GD: Methotrexate in psoriasis: Revised guidelines. J Am Acad Dermatol 1988;19:145-152.

404. Raza A, Maiback HI, Mandel A: Bacterial flora in psoriasis. Br J Dermatol 1976;95:603-611.

405. Marples RR, Heaton CL, Kligman AM: *Staphylococcus aureus* in psoriasis. Arch Dermatol 1973;107:568-570.

406. Payne RW: Severe outbreak of surgical sepsis due to *Staphylococcus aureus* of unusual type and origin. BMJ 1967;4:17-22.

407. Kark EC, Davis BR, Pomeranz JR: Pyoderma gangrenosum treated with clofazimine. J Am Acad Dermatol 1981;4:152-159.

408. Prystowsky JH, Kahn SN, Lazarus GS: Present status of pyoderma gangrenosum. Arch Dermatol 1989;125:57-64.

409. Gibson LE, Daoud MS, Muller SA, Perry HO: Malignant pyodermas revisited. Mayo Clin Proc 1997;72:734-739.

410. Callen JP: Pyoderma gangrenosum and related disorders. Adv Dermatol 1989;4:51-69.

411. Lazarus GS, Goldsmith LA, Rocklin RE, et al: Pyoderma gangrenosum, altered delayed hypersensitivity, and polyarthritis. Arch Dermatol 1972;105:46-51.

412. Powell FC, Schroeter AL, Perry HO: Pyoderma gangrenosum: A review of 86 patients. Am J Med 1985;55:173-186.

413. Wong E, Greaves MW: Pyoderma gangrenosum and leukocytoclastic vasculitis. Clin Exp Dermatol 1985;10:68-72.

414. Kobayashi K, Takashima I, Nagao H, Kawasaki M: A case of pyoderma gangrenosum with Takayasu's arteritis. J Transpl Med 1988;42:181-185.

415. Hoston JJ, et al: Bullous pyoderma gangrenosum and multiple myeloma. Br J Dermatol 1984;110:227-231.

416. Shore RN: Pyoderma gangrenosum, defective neutrophil chemotaxis, and leukemia. Arch Dermatol 1976;112:792-793.

417. Perry HO, Winkelmann RK: Bullous pyoderma gangrenosum and leukemia. Arch Dermatol 1972;196:901.

418. Lewis SJ, Poh-Fitzpatrick MB, Walther RR: Atypical pyoderma gangrenosum with leukemia. JAMA 1980;239:935-938.

419. Banerjee AK: Chronic active hepatitis, pyoderma gangrenosum and febrile panniculitis. Br J Clin Pract 1990;44:32-39.

420. Maturi MF, Fine JD, Schaffer EH, et al: Pyoderma gangrenosum associated with primary biliary cirrhosis. Arch Intern Med 1983;143:1261-1263.

421. Olson K: Pyoderma gangrenosum with systemic lupus erythematosus. Acta Derm Venereol (Stockh) 1971;51:233-234.

422. Selva A, Ordi J, Roca M, et al: Pyoderma gangrenosum–like ulcers associated with lupus anticoagulant. Dermatology 1994;189:182-188.

423. Basler RSW: Ulcerative colitis and the skin. Med Clin North Am 1980;65:941.

424. O'Loughlin S, Perry HO: A diffuse pustular eruption associated with ulcerative colitis. Arch Dermatol 1978;114:1061-1065.

425. Blanc D, Schreiber M, Racadot E, et al: Pyoderma gangrenosum in an allogeneic bone marrow transplant recipient. Clin Exp Dermatol 1989;14:376-379.

426. Kennedy KS, Prendergast ML, Sooy CD: Pyoderma gangrenosum of the oral cavity, nose and larynx. Otolaryngol Head Neck Surg 1987;97:487-492.

427. Curley RK, Macfarlane AW, Vickers CFH: Pyoderma gangrenosum treated with cyclosporine A. Br J Dermatol 1985;113:601-604.

428. Peter RU, Ruzicka T: Cyclosporin A in the therapy of inflammatory dermatoses. Hautarzt 1992;43:687-692.

429. Fedi MC, Quercetani R, Lotti T: Recalcitrant pyoderma gangrenosum responsive to cyclosporine. Int J Dermatol 1993;32:119-123.

430. Resnik BI, Rendon M, Kerdel FA: Successful treatment of aggressive pyoderma gangrenosum with pulse steroids and chlorambucil. J Am Acad Dermatol 1992;27:635-646.

431. Kark EC, Davis BR, Pomeranz JR: Pyoderma gangrenosum treated with clofazimine. J Am Acad Dermatol 1981;4:152-157.

432. Vignon-Pennamen MD, Zelinsky-Gurung A, Janssen F, et al: Pyoderma gangrenosum with pulmonary involvement. Arch Dermatol 1989;125:1239-1242.

433. McCulloch AJ, McEvoy A, Jackson JD, Jarvis EH: Severe steroid-responsive pneumonitis associated with pyoderma gangrenosum and ulcerative colitis. Thorax 1985;40:314-319.

434. Teitel AD: Treatment of pyoderma gangrenosum with methotrexate. Cutis 1996;57:326-328.

11 Hematologic Diseases

GREGORY FISCHER, MD, and LINDA SHORE-LESSERSON, MD

The hematologic system plays a central role in maintaining homeostasis, although its importance is often overlooked by many clinicians. It is important to understand and appreciate its many different functions, ranging from oxygen transport and hemostasis to immunity and thermoregulation.

It is beyond the scope of this chapter to give an in-depth description of all hematologic diseases. The material presented here includes the pertinent aspects of hematologic diseases that can be recognized perioperatively and may be amenable to diagnosis and selective treatment by the anesthesiologist.

ANEMIAS

Anemia is a common finding among patients presenting for surgery. It is defined as a hemoglobin concentration less than normal for age and gender. Anemia can have many different causes, making it imperative that the clinician not be content with the diagnosis of anemia alone but to initiate a search for the underlying cause. Therapeutic interventions are then tailored to treat the cause of the diagnosed anemia.

Except for severe anemia, which can be diagnosed clinically by pallor and lethargy, the diagnosis of anemia is a laboratory diagnosis. In adults, hemoglobin concentrations less than 11.5 g/dL in females and 12.5 g/dL in males are considered to be anemia. To aid in the differential diagnosis, erythrocyte indices are used to help categorize anemias and pinpoint probable causes of anemia (Table 11-1). Erythrocyte indices are defined as follows:

MCH: mean corpuscular hemoglobin (Hb × 10/RBC)
MCV: mean corpuscular volume (Hct × 10/RBC)
MCHC: mean corpuscular hemoglobin concentration (Hb/Hct)

Anemia complicates the management of patients by reducing the oxygen content in circulating blood, which in turn can reduce oxygen delivery to peripheral tissues. To avoid hypoxia the cardiovascular system must compensate by increasing cardiac output.

When interpreting the formula in Box 11-1, one sees that physically dissolved oxygen (PaO_2 × 0.003) results in only a fraction of the total oxygen content (CaO_2) found in blood. The vast majority of oxygen is bound chemically to hemoglobin. This makes it easy to understand why in states of hypoxemia one should treat the anemic patient, providing a normal PaO_2 exists, with the administration of erythrocytes, most commonly given in form of packed RBCs. Increasing FIO_2 and thus increasing PaO_2 only leads to slight increases in CaO_2.[1]

One of the controversial topics in recent years has been determining the threshold at which anesthesiologists should transfuse patients in the perioperative setting.[2-4] The best hematocrit at which the oxygen-carrying capacity is ideally matched with the rheologic properties of blood is approximately 27%. However, the "10/30 rule"

TABLE 11–1 Anemia by Erythrocyte Indices

Anemia	RBC Size	Chromatic	MCH/MCV	Reticulocytes	Serum Iron
Thalassemia	Microcytic	Hypo-	↓	↓	↑
Myelodysplastic syndrome	Microcytic	Hypo-	↓	↓	↑
Iron deficiency	Microcytic	Hypo-	↓	↓	↓
Inflammation-infection	Micro/normocytic	Hypo/normo-	↓ / ↑	↓	↓
Tumor	Micro/normocytic	Hypo/normo-	↓ / ↑	↓	↓
Hemolytic anemia	Normocytic	Normo-	Normal	↑	Normal
Hemorrhage	Normocytic	Normo-	Normal	↑	Normal
Aplastic anemia	Normocytic	Normo-	Normal	↓	Normal
Renal failure	Normocytic	Normo-	Normal	↓	Normal
Megaloblastic	Macrocytic	Hyper-	↑	Normal	Normal

Hypochromatic Microcytic Anemia	Normochromatic Normocytic Anemia	Hyperchromatic Macrocytic Anemia
MCH + MCV reduced	MCH + MCV normal	MCH + MCV increased
Serum iron increased: thalassemia, myelodysplastic syndrome	Reticulocytes increased: hemolytic anemia, hemorrhage	Normal reticulocytes: megaloblastic anemia
Serum iron decreased: iron deficiency anemia	Reticulocytes decreased: aplastic anemia, renal anemia	

Iron decrease and ferritin increase: inflammatory, infection, and tumor anemia.
MCH, mean corpuscular hemoglobin; MCV, mean corpuscular volume.

(10 g/dL hemoglobin or 30% hematocrit), once thought to be the gold standard by many clinicians, has been challenged by recent studies. There is no evidence in the literature suggesting that patients presenting to the operating room with mild anemia have increased adverse advents such as poorer wound healing, increased stroke, or myocardial infarction rates.[5] In fact, patients who receive transfusion are at high risk for perioperative infection due to the immunomodulating effects of transfusion. Thus, transfusing red cells solely on the basis of hemoglobin concentration or hematocrit is no longer considered proper care. Indications for transfusion of red cells should be based on the oxygen supply/demand ratio in the individual patient. Decreased mixed venous oxygen saturations ($S\overline{V}O_2$), serial measurements of lactate showing progressively increasing concentrations, and electrocardiographic changes suggestive of myocardial ischemia are all appropriate indications for transfusion of RBCs.[6-10] For example, Nelson and colleagues found that a hematocrit less than 27% was associated with an increased incidence of myocardial ischemia and infarction in patients undergoing infrainguinal bypass surgery.[11]

Despite great advancements in transfusion medicine, life-threatening complications still do occur. Transfusion reactions can be divided into three major pathophysiologic groups. The most common complication is the transfusion of immunologic incorrectly matched blood resulting in hemolysis. The ABO and Rhesus antigens are responsible for this reaction. Patients under general anesthesia will present with hypotension, tachycardia, and hemoglobinuria, possibly progressing to acute renal failure. Second, febrile nonhemolytic reactions are seen in 0.5% to 5% after transfusion of blood products.[12] These reactions are caused by leukocyte and thrombocyte antigens.[12,13] Third, transmission of infectious diseases (hepatitis B and C viruses and human immunodeficiency virus [HIV]) is a rare phenomenon but has serious and long-lasting consequences for the patient.[14-18]

The complications of blood product transfusion should always make the clinician weigh benefits against potential risks. Strict indications for the transfusion of blood products should be employed. Transfusion solely to achieve volume expansion or to raise the hematocrit to a certain value cannot be recommended. Finally, in a society becoming more and more conscious of the financial burden brought on by its health care system, avoiding unnecessary transfusions poses a major source of potential savings.

BOX 11–1 Formula for Calculation of Oxygen Delivery

$$DO_2 = CO \times (Hb \times SaO_2 \times 1.34 + PaO_2 \times 0.003)$$

where DO_2 = oxygen delivery; CO = cardiac output; Hb = hemoglobin concentration; SaO_2 = percent of oxygenated hemoglobin; 1.34 = Hüfner number (constant 1.34-1.36); and 0.003 = dissolved oxygen (mL/mm Hg/dL).

TABLE 11–2   Anemia and Iron Metabolism

	Serum Iron	Transferrin	Serum Ferritin
Iron deficiency	↓	↑	↓
Myelodysplastic syndrome	↑	↓	↑
β-Thalassemia	Normal-↑	Normal-↓	Normal-↑
Inflammatory or tumor associated	↓	↓	↑

Iron Deficiency Anemia

Iron deficiency anemia is the most commonly diagnosed anemia in the industrialized world. Its cause is usually due to chronic blood loss (e.g., menstruation, chronic gastrointestinal bleeding) or to increased requirements seen in pregnancy or infancy. An adult male has 50 mg/kg of iron stored in his body and requires a daily intake of 12 mg to absorb 1 mg to compensate for losses. An adult female has 35 mg/kg of iron stored and requires 15 mg to absorb 2 mg. During pregnancy the iron intake must be doubled to compensated for approximately 3 mg of daily iron losses.

Iron deficiency anemia is a microcytic/hypochromatic anemia with increased serum transferrin, low serum ferritin, and low serum iron concentrations. Microscopic examination of bone marrow reveals low to missing iron depots. The differential diagnoses to iron deficiency anemia are shown in Table 11-2. Clinically, these patients suffer from general anemia symptoms as well as from skin and mucous membrane problems. Koilonychia, hair loss, Plummer-Vinson syndrome and perlèche are all symptoms associated with iron deficiency.

The treatment of iron deficiency consists of replacing the losses either orally or parenterally and in locating the source of chronic blood loss.[19,20]

Thalassemia

Thalassemia consists of a group of inherited disorders resulting in the inability to produce structurally normal globin chains. This results in an abnormal hemoglobin molecule with subsequent hemolysis. The disorder can affect both the α and β globin chain synthesis, and depending on whether the bearer is homozygous or heterozygous the disease is called major or minor. β-Thalassemia major (Cooley's anemia) is rare and carries a poor prognosis. Patients of Mediterranean descent present with this illness in early stages of life. Patients have prehepatic jaundice, hepatosplenomegaly, and an increased susceptibility to infection. Owing to multiple blood transfusions the patients also develop secondary hemochromatosis and die of complications related to cardiac hemochromatosis (e.g., arrhythmias, congestive heart failure). α-Thalassemia is not compatible with life.

Minor thalassemias show mild anemic states with microcytic/hypochromatic erythrocyte indexes. Iron stores are normal or increased. The diagnosis is confirmed by hemoglobin electrophoresis.

Megaloblastic Anemias

Megaloblastic anemias are anemias with macrocytic/hyperchromatic erythrocyte indexes. The two most common forms are vitamin B_{12} deficiency and folic acid deficiency.

Both vitamin B_{12} and folic acid are important cofactors in the synthesis of DNA. A deficiency of either vitamin leads to an insufficient amount of DNA, resulting in the inability of bone marrow to produce an adequate amount of blood cells. This, in turn, results in very large blood cells, each packed with an abnormally high amount of hemoglobin.[21,22]

Vitamin B_{12} deficiency is most commonly caused by an autoimmune disease and results in pernicious anemia.[23] An autoantibody targeted toward the intrinsic factor leads to the inability to absorb vitamin B_{12}. Intrinsic factor is produced by gastric parietal cells and is required to absorb vitamin B_{12} (extrinsic factor) in the terminal ileum. Other causes are rare and include strict vegetarian diet, malabsorption syndromes, blind loop syndromes, and tapeworm (Diphyllobothrium latum) infection (Table 11-3).

Vitamin B_{12} deficiency can also lead to neurologic and gastroenterologic symptoms. An atrophic tongue, known as Hunter's glossitis, is a typical sequela of vitamin B_{12} deficiency. Neurologic symptoms resulting from degeneration of the lateral and posterior spinal cord columns lead

TABLE 11–3   Differential Causes of Vitamin B_{12} Deficiency

Vegetarian diet
Reduction in intrinsic factor
Pernicious anemia
Subtotal or partial gastric resection
Malabsorption syndrome
Tapeworm (Diphyllobothrium latum) infection
Blind loop syndrome

to peripheral neuropathy and gait ataxia. Depression and psychotic symptoms are also seen. Clinically, the loss of sensation to vibration is an early warning sign. The diagnosis is obtained by measuring vitamin B_{12} concentrations in plasma. At present, parenteral administration of vitamin B_{12} is the only therapeutic option available to patients.

Folic acid deficiency is the third most common cause of anemia seen in pregnancy due to increased requirements. Other risk factors for folic acid deficiency are alcoholism, abnormal dietary habits, and certain medications (methotrexate, phenytoin). Folic acid deficiency does not present with neurologic sequelae in the adult. It has, however, been linked to neural tube defects in early stages of pregnancy. The diagnosis is confirmed, as in vitamin B_{12} deficiency, by measuring plasma concentrations. Folic acid can, however, be supplemented orally.

Nitrous oxide has the ability to irreversibly oxidize the cobalt ion found in vitamin B_{12}. It would therefore seem prudent to avoid the use of nitrous oxide in patients already suffering from megaloblastic anemia to avoid a synergistic effect. Otherwise the same principles apply as in treating any other form of anemia.

Hemolytic Anemias

Hemolytic anemias can be caused by corpuscular defects of the erythrocyte or by extracorpuscular pathologic processes. Typical corpuscular hemolytic anemias are ones seen with cell membrane defects (e.g., spherocytosis), hemoglobinopathies (e.g., thalassemia, sickle cell disease) or enzyme defects within the erythrocyte (e.g., glucose-6-phosphate dehydrogenase deficiency or pyruvate kinase deficiency).

Extracorpuscular hemolytic anemias are immunologically mediated (Rh incompatibility, ABO transfusion reactions, autoimmune hemolytic anemias), the result of consumption of certain medications, caused by infectious diseases, metabolic derangements (Zieve syndrome), or the result of microangiopathic pathologic processes (hemolytic-uremic syndrome, thrombotic thrombocytopenic purpura).

Spherocytosis

Spherocytosis is one of the most common inherited hemolytic anemias. It is caused by a defect in the erythrocyte membrane, which leads to an increased permeability for sodium and water, giving the erythrocyte its typical spherical form. This renders the erythrocytes susceptible to phagocytosis in the spleen at an early age. Patients are prone to hemolytic crisis and gallstones formed primarily out of bilirubin. Normocytic anemia accompanied by signs of hemolysis (increased indirect bilirubin, increased lactate dehydrogenase, increased reticulocytes) are the typical laboratory findings. The diagnosis is confirmed by osmotic testing of the erythrocytes.

Patients with recurrent hemolytic crisis may have undergone a splenectomy. The anesthesiologist must be aware that these patients, if not properly vaccinated, are at increased risk for sepsis (overwhelming postsplenectomy sepsis).

Hemoglobinopathies

There are approximately 300 known abnormal hemoglobin molecules. Most of these pathologic globin molecules differ from the physiologic α and β chains through exchange of only one amino acid with another. It is beyond the scope of this chapter to list all hemoglobinopathies. We will concentrate on the illnesses seen most likely in daily practice.

Sickle Cell Anemia. Sickle cell anemia is the most common form of inherited hemoglobinopathy found in humans. Five to 10 percent of the African-American population are heterozygotic carriers. The mutation is in the sixth amino acid in the β chain of the hemoglobin molecule. Glutamic acid is replaced by valine.[24]

In its deoxygenated form hemoglobin S (HbS) has the tendency to precipitate, causing the erythrocytes to lose their normal biconcaval form and to take on a sickle-like structure. This leads to sludging and eventually to occlusion of the microvasculature, resulting in end organ infarction.

Heterozygotic carriers are generally asymptomatic, expressing only a sickle cell trait found in laboratory testing (HbS < 50%). However, homozygotic carriers can display sickle cell crisis as early as infancy, with signs of hemolysis and painful vaso-occlusive infarctions (spleen, kidney, bones). Due to an atrophic spleen caused by recurrent microinfarctions, patients are prone to *Streptococcus pneumoniae* and *Hemophilus influenzae* infections of the respiratory tract and osteomyelitis. The diagnosis of sickle cell anemia is made either through a microscopic sickle cell test or by hemoglobin electrophoresis.

Conventional anesthetic management is geared toward avoiding a sickle cell crisis during the perioperative period.[25] Patients should be kept well hydrated, warm, and well oxygenated. Acidosis should be avoided at all costs.[26] Sickle cell patients presenting for cardiac surgery can be appropriately managed by maintaining temperature and hemoglobin concentration. Fast-track or early extubation protocols have been utilized with success.[27] Many of the practices geared toward avoiding a sickle cell crisis are still followed in modern-day management, but some of the classic "dogmas" have been challenged during the past decade. For example, the use of tourniquets for orthopedic procedures is no longer considered an absolute contraindication.[28-30] Exchange transfusion solely with the intent to improve a laboratory value (HbS fraction < 30%) can no longer be considered proper standard of care.[31] Griffin and colleagues suggest that transfusion before elective surgery in children may not be necessary at all. The authors successfully provided anesthesia for 54 children with sickle cell disease without a transfusion. They found that smaller surgical procedures could be easily performed without complication but that pulmonary complications arose after laparotomy, thoracotomy, and tonsillectomy.[32,33] Although there are benefits for pain management and rheology that accompany the use of neuraxial anesthesia, it is still believed by many investigators that the patient with more complex sickle cell anemia is better managed using general anesthesia.[25]

The anesthesiologist is sometimes asked to assist as a pain consultant in managing an acute sickle cell crisis.[32] Adequate oxygenation, normothermia, and euvolemia are the cornerstones of management. Analgesia is achieved with opiates. Caution must be used when utilizing analgesics (e.g., nonsteroidal anti-inflammatory agents), which can potentially impair renal function, because these patients frequently suffer from renal microinfarctions with reduced baseline renal function. Vaso-occlusive crisis of the lower extremities can be managed with continuous neuraxial blocks. Occasionally a partial exchange transfusion with packed red blood cells is performed to increase the fraction of HbA greater than 50%. For rheologic reasons, the hematocrit should not exceed 35%.

In parturients with sickle cell disease, transfusion therapy is recommended to treat the complications of the disease, especially those associated with chest pain syndromes, preeclampsia, and multiple gestations.[34,35] Antibiotic prophylaxis for both mother and newborn should be actively practiced. The avoidance of adverse events during labor does not seem to be associated with the type of analgesia provided (regional vs. systemic) but appears more related to careful monitoring for the known consequences of the disease.[36]

Newer therapies are being investigated for the anesthetic management of patients with sickle cell disease. Cytotoxic agents such as hydroxyurea stimulate the production of fetal hemoglobin and are being studied in the prevention of vaso-occlusive crises. Inhaled nitric oxide and other new investigational drugs have shown promise in being able to reduce the sickling process and even to unsickle cells.

Enzyme Deficiency Anemias

Enzyme defects within erythrocytes can lead to hemolysis. The two most commonly seen defects are glucose-6-phosphate dehydrogenase deficiency and pyruvate kinase deficiency.

Glucose-6-Phosphate Dehydrogenase Deficiency. This disease is most commonly seen in individuals of African, Asian, or Mediterranean descent. The illness is inherited recessively on the X chromosome. Patients with this defect have erythrocytes containing a reduced amount of glutathione, leading to oxygenation injury of the cell membrane. A hemolytic crisis can be induced through infections or ingestion of beans and certain medications (e.g., sulfonamides, aspirin, quinidine). No specific therapy exists. Avoiding trigger substances is the only recommendation available at the present time.

Pyruvate Kinase Deficiency. This deficiency is the most common defect of the glycolysis pathway. It has an autosomal recessive pattern of inheritance. The normal erythrocyte does not have mitochondria and relies on glycolysis to produce adenosine triphosphate to maintain cellular integrity. Homozygous carriers present with hemolytic anemia, splenomegaly, and acanthocytes.

Antibody-Induced Hemolysis

Antibodies can result in two major reactions: hemolysis and agglutination. Antibodies directed against erythrocytes are either IgM or IgG in structure. IgM antibodies are larger (molecular weight 900,000 daltons) and can act like a bridge between two erythrocytes. The term *complete antibodies* is sometimes used. Examples of IgM antibodies are ABO isoagglutinins and cold agglutinins. IgG antibodies are smaller in size (150,000 daltons) and cannot form a bridge between two erythrocytes (incomplete antibodies). Examples of IgG antibodies are Rhesus (Rh) agglutinins and warm antibodies. The Coombs test is used to diagnose the presence of incomplete antibodies either already attached to the surface of erythrocytes (direct Coombs test) or in the patient's serum (indirect Coombs test).

Autoimmune Hemolytic Anemia. Autoimmune hemolytic anemias can be caused by either warm (IgG) or cold (IgM) antibodies. Seventy percent of all autoimmune hemolytic anemias are caused by warm antibodies. Warm autoimmune hemolytic anemias are seen in patients with non-Hodgkin's lymphoma, systemic lupus erythematosus, viral infection, and after ingestion of certain drugs (penicillin, α-methyldopa). These antibodies bind to the surface of erythrocytes at body temperature without causing hemolysis. The erythrocytes undergo phagocytosis in the spleen. The erythrocyte survival time can be diminished to only a few days, with erythropoiesis increased by tenfold. Fifteen percent of all patients with autoimmune hemolytic anemia present with cold antibodies. These antibodies are seen in patients after *Mycoplasma* pneumonias or mononucleosis. These antibodies lead to acrocyanosis and hemolysis as soon as intravascular temperature decreases below 25° to 30°C.

Traumatic Hemolysis

Traumatic injury to erythrocytes leading to hemolysis can be seen in patients with mechanical heart valves, intra-aortic balloon pumps, or after severe physical exertion (e.g., extreme hiking, runner's anemia).

Renal Anemia

Patients presenting for surgery with chronic renal failure (glomerular filtration rate < 30 mL/min) frequently have a normochromic, normocytic anemia owing to inadequate production of erythropoietin.[37,38] Hemoglobin concentration is generally found to be around 9 g/dL. Transfusion of packed red blood cells is necessary should signs of ischemia develop. These patients are frequently treated with recombinant human erythropoietin to raise baseline hemoglobin values.[39]

ACUTE BLOOD LOSS/HEMORRHAGIC SHOCK

One of the most challenging situations an anesthesiologist can be confronted with is having to induce a patient in hemorrhagic/hypovolemic shock. Complicating matters is the fact that acute hemorrhage is often difficult to diagnose. Laboratory values for hemoglobin are normal in the immediate period after an acute blood loss. If one loses half of his or her circulating blood volume, there will be no change in the concentration of hemoglobin unless fluid with a different hemoglobin concentration is added. In clinical practice, fluids are administered parenterally after obtaining access to the circulatory system. Advanced Trauma Life Support protocols advise administering 2 L of crystalloid solution to patients in suspected hypovolemic shock. This will lead to dilution of the original hemoglobin concentration. Providing intravenous fluids are not administered, anemia will result within hours through movement of interstitial fluid into the intravascular space. Because of this time delay the hemoglobin and hematocrit are not ideal parameters for detecting acute blood loss.

In addition to the problems encountered in the laboratory diagnosis of acute blood loss, the volume state of a patient is also extremely difficult to assess clinically. Especially in young patients, the sympathetic nervous system is capable of masking even extreme states of hypovolemia, giving the clinician a false sense of security. Subtle signs such as orthostatic hypotension, tachycardia, narrowing pulse pressure, alterations of cerebral function, and low urine output must be sought before induction of anesthesia is indicative of hypovolemia.

In an attempt to maintain adequate perfusion to the brain and myocardium the vegetative nervous system compromises perfusion to the kidneys, skeletal muscular system, and gut. This redirection in blood flow is achieved by increasing the sympathetic adrenergic tone of the vegetative nervous system, resulting in increased heart rate, systemic peripheral resistance (SVR), and narrowing pulse pressure. As a consequence of impaired tissue perfusion, lactate concentrations increase while urine output and mixed venous saturation decrease.

The treatment of acute blood loss is primarily aimed at replacing lost volume. This can be achieved by administering either crystalloid or colloid solutions. There is much debate on this subject regarding whether primarily crystalloid or colloid solutions should be employed to replace lost blood volume. The literature, however, does not clearly support the use of one over the other. Blood products need to be administered, owing to the rapid dilution of red cells and coagulation factors. The goal of therapy is aimed at restoring adequate perfusion and oxygen delivery to all organ systems. A successful course of treatment can be seen by normalization of vital signs, urine output, lactate concentrations, and $S\bar{v}O_2$. Vasopressors should be used only as a temporary resort in maintaining perfusion pressure to the myocardium and cerebrum until adequate volume replacement can be achieved.

Inducing a hypovolemic patient is one of the most challenging situations confronting anesthesiologists. All induction agents can potentially reduce the adrenergic tone needed by the organism to maintain adequate perfusion pressure to the brain and myocardium. If not corrected quickly, a vicious cycle is started that will lead to further hemodynamic deterioration. Invasive monitoring and the use of induction agents with the least suppressive effect on hemodynamics such as ketamine and etomidate are good choices. If perfusion pressure declines, the use of a vasopressor might be indicated until adequate access is obtained and volume loading begins.

DISEASES OF LEUKOCYTES

Leukocyte abnormalities rarely alter an anesthetic plan. There are, however, a few exceptions, which every anesthesiologist must know. It is the intent of this chapter to offer a brief overview of diseases associated with the leukocyte system, providing an in-depth view of the illnesses that can alter an anesthetic plan.

Lymphomas

Lymphomas are neoplasms of the lymphatic system. Clinically, they are divided into two groups: Hodgkin's disease and non-Hodgkin's lymphoma (NHL). The primary localization of these tumors is in the lymph nodes. As the disease progresses, metastatic lesions can be found in every organ. A major concern to the anesthesiologist are lesions that may obstruct the airway. Large tumor bulks can be found in the mediastinum, growing undetected until vital organs (blood vessels, heart, airway) are compressed. Mediastinal mass syndrome is the acute obstruction of the trachea or large vessels (superior vena cava, right atrium, right ventricle) by tumor mass after induction of general anesthesia. Patients frequently complain of dyspnea while in the supine position. The supine position in combination with muscle relaxation can lead to positional changes of the tumor mass and result in airway obstruction. Careful preoperative evaluation and review of the patient's computed tomographic scan can alert the anesthesiologist to this potential complication. Discussion with the patient and surgeon regarding these concerns can provoke a search for alternative means of analgesia (e.g., local anesthesia in monitored anesthesia care).

Should a general anesthetic be deemed necessary, then an inhalational induction with sevoflurane, keeping the patient breathing spontaneously and avoiding muscle relaxation, is a prudent plan. If airway compromise still occurs, then the anesthetic should be aborted and the patient awakened immediately. Awake fiberoptic intubation is another alternative, providing the bronchoscope can be passed distal to the lesion. A distal lesion, however, poses the same problems seen in conventional intubation because the end of the endotracheal tube will lie proximal to the lesion. In an urgent situation, a rigid ventilating bronchoscope must be passed immediately.

Hodgkin's Disease

Hodgkin' disease has an incidence of 3/100,000, showing a double peaked distribution in western countries during the third and sixth decades of life. Males are more frequently affected by the illness than females (3:2). Whether the Ebstein-Barr virus plays a similar role in the etiology as in the development of Burkitt's lymphoma remains unclear. Hodgkin's disease leads to immunosuppression, with increased susceptibility for tuberculosis and fungal and viral infections. Oncologists use the Ann Arbor Classification to describe the progression of disease (Table 11-4).

This classification can also be used to assess patient prognosis. The higher the grading, the worse the prognosis.

Stages I and II are primarily treated with radiation therapy. Stages III and IV are additionally treated with chemotherapy. As a result of improved medical management, the long-term survival rates have increased dramatically over the past decade. Unfortunately, the cure of Hodgkin's lymphoma comes with a price. An increasing number or "survivors" are presenting with long-term complications of the medical treatment (e.g., second neoplasms, cardiotoxicity induced by chemotherapy [doxorubicin], pulmonary toxicity through bleomycin). For patients with a history of doxorubicin therapy, assessment of cardiac function should be made, including cardiovascular testing if appropriate. Surgical patients who have been exposed to bleomycin therapy should have a complete set of PFTs if they exhibit pulmonary symptoms. This is especially helpful in patients presenting for pulmonary resection. The PFT profile of bleomycin toxicity will demonstrate a severe restrictive lung disease pattern with small lung volumes and a reduced carbon monoxide diffusion ratio.

Non-Hodgkin's Lymphomas

In contrast to Hodgkin's disease, NHL cannot be regarded as a single malignant entity but as a heterogeneous collective of neoplasia originating from T lymphocytes in lymphatic tissue. Thirty percent of cases of NHL present with a leukemic element. The incidence is reported between 5 and 10/100,000, increasing with age. As in Hodgkin's disease the male gender is more prone to acquiring the disease (1.5:1). HIV-positive patients are 1,000 times more susceptible to developing NHL than a control population.

Multiple Myeloma and Macroglobulinemia

Multiple myeloma, also known as plasmacytoma or Kahler's disease, is a malignant disorder of plasmacytes. It is classified into the group of non-Hodgkin's lymphomas. The neoplastic plasmacytes produce either a monoclonal immunoglobulin (IgG, IgA, IgD) or isolated light chains (Bence Jones plasmacytoma). During this process bone marrow is displaced by infiltration of the tumor, resulting in a loss of functioning peripheral blood cells. The tumor

TABLE 11-4 Ann Arbor Staging System for Hodgkin's Disease

Stage	Description
I	Involvement in single lymph node region or single extralymphatic site
II	Involvement in two or more lymph node regions on the same side of diaphragm
III	Involvement of lymph node regions on both sides of diaphragm; may include spleen
IV	Disseminated involvement of one or more extralymphatic organs with or without lymph node involvement

A Symptoms: without general symptoms of disease.
B Symptoms: fever, loss of weight, night sweats, pruritus.

also leads to osteolysis with a loss of normal bone architecture, resulting in an increased risk of pathologic fractures.

Patients present with high erythrocyte sedimentation rates, Bence Jones proteinuria, or a change in their protein or immunoglobulin electrophoresis. Patients will typically be anemic and have signs of coagulopathy due to thrombocytopenia, thrombocytopathy, and decreased functional plasmatic coagulation factors. Renal failure due to toxic deposition of immunoglobulin in the renal tubuli is the most common cause of mortality. Hypercalcemia resulting from increased osteoclastic activity supports the development of renal failure and can lead to hypercalcemic crisis. Ten percent of patients will develop amyloidosis. Treatment includes radiation therapy and/or chemotherapy. Prognosis is poor at present.

Macroglobulinemia or Waldenström's disease is generally seen in the aging population and caused by malignant plasmocytes producing IgM immunoglobulins. This illness is four times as seldom as multiple myeloma and is not as aggressive. Osteolysis and hypercalcemia are not seen; however, hemorrhagic diathesis caused by disorders of thrombocyte aggregation and binding of coagulation factors is observed. Hyperviscosity syndrome leading to Raynaud-like acral perfusion deficits and visual disturbances is also seen. Prognosis is better than for multiple myeloma.

Leukemias

Leukemia means "white blood" and refers to an increased amount of leukocytes seen in peripheral blood. Leukemias are divided into acute or chronic forms and myeloplastic or lymphatic forms, depending on the cell row from which the neoplasm originated.

All leukemias lead to impaired immune reactions, making patients more prone to infection. Because of the possibility of infiltration of leukemic cells into virtually all organs, a reduction in organ function can be associated with this illness.

Leukemia is treated classically with chemotherapy. The anesthesiologist should be aware of the agents employed during chemotherapy cycles. Doxorubicin is known to cause systolic dysfunction that can affect the anesthetic technique. Emerging techniques utilized to treat leukemia are allogenic bone marrow transplantation and stem cell transplantation. Treatment is generally more successful in children, with 5-year survival rate reaching 80%.

Acute Leukemia

The cornerstone for the diagnosis of an acute leukemia is the presence of immature hematopoietic cells in peripheral blood. The incidence is 4/100,000 per year. Eighty percent of acute leukemias in childhood originate from lymphatic cells; in adulthood, 80% are myelocytic. The etiology is multifactorial. Retroviruses, bone marrow damage caused by radiotherapy or chemical substances, and genetic composition of the patient (e.g., Down's syndrome, Klinefelter's syndrome) have all been linked to an increased risk for developing acute leukemia.

Chronic Myeloproliferative Disease

Chronic myeloproliferative disease incorporates four illnesses (chronic myelocytic leukemia, polycythemia vera, essential thrombocythemia, and osteomyelosclerosis). All of these diseases show a monoclonal proliferation from a myelocytic stem cell. Initially, all three cell rows are increased in number (leuko-, erythro- and thrombocytosis). Splenomegaly is common. Eventually, sclerosis of the patient's bone marrow occurs, leading to loss of its function. Extramedullary hematopoiesis is seen (liver, spleen). In the terminal phase a blast crisis is frequently seen.

Chronic leukemias develop over a prolonged period of time, sometimes taking a decade to manifest clinically. Chronic myelocytic leukemia presents as the highest concentration of leukocytes (>500,000/μL), resulting in organ infarction. Chronic lymphatic leukemia is the most common form of leukemia and increases in incidence with increasing age. Chronic myelocytic leukemia has a low degree of malignancy, allowing patients to survive for many years without impairing quality of life. Lymphadenopathy and splenomegaly are common manifestations in chronic leukemia.

Myelodysplastic Syndrome

This disease represents a heterogenic clonal stem cell pathology with qualitative and quantitative changes of hematopoiesis, peripheral cytopenia, and a high proportional amount of blast in bone marrow. It is primarily seen in the elderly (20 to 50/100,000/year in those older than age 70 years).

DISEASES OF THROMBOCYTES (PLATELETS)

Circulating platelets are anucleate discoid cells that are formed from megakaryocytes. The normal platelet count is 140,000 to 450,000/μL. Platelets have many different roles in maintaining circulation and hemostasis. Platelets form the primary phase of hemostasis, the platelet plug. This initial adhesion of platelets to the injured endothelium is responsible for the physical "healing" of the wound and for the biochemical signaling that occurs when other cells and coagulation factors are summoned to the site of injury. The platelet surface phospholipid is a critical surface on which the coagulation cascade proteases become activated and form a fibrin clot. On physical examination, the absence of normal platelet number or function can be detected by the presence of petechiae. Conversely, an excessive number of platelets or excessively activated platelets will predispose to arterial occlusive disease. Patient and family history are the most important factors in assessing platelet-related disorders.

Routine screening for platelet abnormalities is not recommended in the absence of any of the signs or symptoms. In the presence of signs of symptoms of a bleeding diathesis, a platelet count is obtained. A minimal platelet count of 50,000 to 100,000/μL is recommended before elective surgery. Spontaneous bleeding can occur with platelet counts less than 30,000/μL. Further testing such as the bleeding time and other aggregation studies will be described as they relate to individual disease states.

Thrombocytopenia

Thrombocytopenia is due to either decreased production of platelets, excessive destruction of platelets, or splenic or other sequestration. A common cause of decreased production is the result of bone marrow hypoplasia or marrow toxic drugs. Increased destruction may be drug induced or autoimmune. Thrombocytopenia also occurs in the parturient and may represent risks to maternal or fetal well-being if not recognized early.[40] A list of common causes of thrombocytopenia is found in Table 11-5.

Immune (Idiopathic) Thrombocytopenic Purpura

Immune or idiopathic thrombocytopenic purpura (ITP) is a common abnormality causing a low platelet count. It affects 0.01% of the population and is the result of autoantibodies that bind to the platelet surfaces, thus decreasing their life span.[41] It frequently affects young women and is thus encountered in the parturient.[42] Cutaneous signs such as petechiae are often the presenting feature. Treatment is not usually recommended until the platelet count is less than 30,000/μL unless the patient is having uncontrolled bleeding or major surgery. Therapy begins with corticosteroid therapy at the lowest possible dose that will lead to a response. In the presence of catastrophic bleeding, platelet transfusion can be given in conjunction with corticosteroid therapy or immune globulin therapy to decrease the immunologically mediated destruction. Plasmapheresis has also been used in conjunction with other therapies with some success. Emergent splenectomy is reserved for the patient who fails the therapies and who has life-threatening bleeding.[43]

Thrombotic Thrombocytopenic Purpura

The signs and symptoms of thrombotic thrombocytopenic purpura (TTP) consist of fever, hemolytic anemia, thrombocytopenia, renal disease, and central nervous system disease. The management of this disease consists of corticosteroids, plasmapheresis, and plasma transfusion. When TTP presents during pregnancy it can appear identical to toxemia of pregnancy. During the last trimester of pregnancy, treatment of this constellation of symptoms is delivery of the infant.

Platelet Sequestration

Platelet count will be reduced due to sequestration of platelets in the spleen. This clinical condition is almost akin to a pseudo-thrombocytopenia because the platelets are present in the body but they are not circulating in the bloodstream. Platelets adhere to extracorporeal surfaces such as a cardiopulmonary bypass circuit. This plus hemodilution accounts for most of the thrombocytopenia seen after cardiac surgery.[44]

Thrombasthenic Syndromes

In contrast to thrombocytopenia, clinical conditions in which the platelet count often falls to levels less than 30,000/μL before treatment is initiated, patients with thrombasthenic syndromes (Table 11-6) require treatment with platelet transfusion at much higher levels of platelet count because platelet function is so compromised.

TABLE 11–5 Disease States Associated with Thrombocytopenia

Impaired Production	Increased Destruction	Sequestration
Megakaryocyte dysfunction	Autoimmune (immune thrombocytopenic purpura)	Hypersplenism
Aplastic anemia	Immune (post-transfusion)	Splenomegaly
Drug (ticlopidine)	Drug (chemotherapy)	Adhesion to synthetic surfaces
Vitamin B$_{12}$/folate deficiency	Disseminated intravascular coagulation	Platelet-platelet adhesion
Myelodysplastic disorders	Thrombotic thrombocytopenic purpura Hemolytic-uremic syndrome Hemodilution Heparin-induced thrombocytopenia type 2	Heparin-induced thrombocytopenia type 1

TABLE 11–6   Platelet Disorders and Available Testing Modalities

Disorder	Pathophysiology	Testing
Bernard-Soulier syndrome	Absent GPIb	Flow cytometry, bleeding time, PFA-100
Glanzmann's thrombasthenia	Absent GPIIbIIIa	Flow cytometry, aggregation, Ultegra, TEG
Von Willebrand's disease	vWF	Bleeding time, PFA-100
Gray platelet syndrome	Alpha granule depletion	Flow cytometry, aggregation
Drug Therapy		
Aspirin ingestion	Cyclooxygenase inhibition	Aggregation, bleeding time, PFA-100, modified TEG
Clopidogrel ingestion	ADP P2Y12 inhibition	Aggregation, bleeding time, modified TEG
Abciximab	GPIIbIIIa blockade	Aggregation, flow cytometry, Ultegra
Nitroglycerin	Increased nitric oxide	Aggregation, flow cytometry

GP, glycoprotein; vWF, von Willebrand factor; TEG, thromboelastography.

von Willebrand's Disease

von Willebrand factor (vWF) is synthesized in the endothelium and in the platelet and acts as a ligand for platelet adhesion via the GPIb receptor. von Willebrand's disease is a common disorder of the vWF that frequently manifests as a bleeding disorder. It is inherited via an autosomal dominant genetic trait. Laboratory analysis of von Willebrand's disease consists of the measurement of vWF activity, vWF antigen, factor VIII activity, vWF multimeric analysis, and the bleeding time. The vWF multimeric analysis is important for the classification of the subtype of von Willebrand's disease (Table 11-7). If only factor VIII level is reduced, von Willebrand's disease can be confused with hemophilia A.[45] If only the bleeding time is prolonged, it can be confused with a primary platelet disorder. There are different subtypes of the disease that respond differently to therapy; thus, it is important to know which subtype of the disease exists in a patient.

Patients with von Willebrand's disease have a prolonged bleeding time. Clinically, they can have a range of abnormalities from mild bleeding to hemorrhagic symptoms. They often have increased mucocutaneous bleeding (during dental procedures), and women frequently present with menorrhagia.[46]

Type I disease is marked by a reduced quantity of normal vWF. The large multimers of vWF that are so critical for platelet adhesion are normal in size but reduced in quantity. Treatment of type I includes desmopressin (D-arginine vasopressin [DDAVP]), which increases the release of vWF from the endothelium and the platelet.[47,48] Desmopressin is available in intranasal or intravenous forms, and the intravenous form is often given intranasally. In patients with type I disease, a doubling of vWF activity (and factor VIII) and shortening of the bleeding time occur within 15 to 30 minutes of administration of desmopressin. The dose is 0.3 µg/kg intravenously over 30 minutes. It must be infused slowly or it will cause hypotension.

In type IIA von Willebrand's disease there is a qualitative abnormality of vWF in which there are defective platelet-vWF interactions. This is due to the absence of high- and middle-molecular-weight vWF multimers. Patients may

TABLE 11–7   von Willebrand's Disease: Laboratory Analysis and Therapy

Disease Type	vWF Activity	Antigen	Bleeding Time	Factor VIII	Treatment
Type 1	↓	↓	↑	↓	Desmopressin
Type 2A	↓	↓	↑	↓	Factor VIII concentrates
Type 2B	↓	↓	↑	↓	Factor VIII concentrates
Type 2N	Normal	Normal	↑	↓	Factor VIII concentrates
Type 3	↓↓	↓↓	↑	↓↓	Factor VIII concentrates plus desmopressin
Platelet (pseudo–von Willebrand's disease)	↓	↓	↑	↓	Platelets
Hemophilia A	Normal	Normal	Normal	↓	Factor VIII concentrates

have normal levels of vWF protein, but the protein is dysfunctional. These variants account for 15% to 30% of cases.[49-51] Type IIB von Willebrand's disease is caused by a qualitative abnormality of vWF in which there is increased platelet-vWF interaction due to an increased affinity of vWF for its platelet receptor, GPIb. The hallmark of type IIB von Willebrand's disease is an enhanced aggregation of the patient's platelets in the presence of reduced concentrations of ristocetin. In type IIB disease, a low concentration of ristocetin stimulates a full aggregation response. This form of the disease can be marked by thrombocytopenia, but there may also be increased adhesiveness and thrombosis. Thus, the administration of desmopressin as therapy is not recommended. In type IIN, there may be qualitative variants with markedly decreased affinity for factor VIII. The measured vWF activity and antigen may be normal. Type III is a severe form, with nearly complete deficiency of vWF. Usually, vWF activity and antigen are undetectable and factor VIII levels are markedly reduced. The bleeding time is prolonged, usually to more than 20 minutes. Patients with type III disease have essentially no vWF multimers. This severe form of von Willebrand's disease may be the result of a homozygous defect or a complex heterozygous defect. Desmopressin is not of benefit in patients with type III disease because they have almost no endogenous production of vWF. Platelet-type or pseudo-von Willebrand's disease is a primary platelet disorder involving the platelet receptor for vWF, GPIb. Although this is primarily a platelet disorder, patients with platelet-type, pseudo-von Willebrand's disease have absent high-molecular-weight multimers, reduced factor VIII, reduced vWF activity, and a prolonged bleeding time. The laboratory analysis is similar to patients with type IIB disease. Aggregation is enhanced in response to low concentrations of ristocetin (0.3 to 0.5 mg/mL), and mild thrombocytopenia is commonly present. Von Willebrand's disease can also be acquired. This is thought to occur by antibodies to vWF that neutralize vWF activity.

In preparation of the patient with von Willebrand's disease for surgery, baseline factor VIII and bleeding time should be obtained within 1 week of surgery. One to 2 hours before surgery, treatment with desmopressin at a dose 0.3 µg/kg should be infused. If baseline factor VIII and bleeding time were abnormal, these measures should be confirmed normal after desmopressin treatment and before surgery is begun. After surgery, these measures should be repeated once a day until wound healing is complete. Desmopressin may need to be given once daily after surgery. For more extensive surgery, factor VIII concentrates may be necessary so that desmopressin can enhance vWF activity of the administered product. Patients with type II or III disease should receive factor VIII concentrates along the same timeline as described for the treatment of type I disease. Desmopressin may cause thrombocytopenia or increased aggregation[52] in these patients, but some still suggest that it may be effective therapy in addition to replacement therapy for patients with type II and III disease. After surgery, treatment is continued every 12 hours until wound healing is complete.

Other Thrombasthenic Syndromes

Bernard-Soulier syndrome is marked by deficiency of the GPIb receptor, the major receptor responsible for platelet adhesion to collagen, vWF, and other ligands.[53] Patients with this disorder have hemorrhagic tendencies.

Glanzmann's thrombasthenia is inherited as an autosomal recessive disorder. Patients with this disorder have severe impairments in platelet aggregation, a prolonged bleeding time, and a normal platelet count. The disease is marked by the absence of the GPIIbIIIa receptor ($\alpha_{2b}\beta_3$ integrin).[53] Either component of this receptor, the α or the β component, may be absent or abnormal for the disease to be expressed. Fibrinogen binding to GPIIbIIIa induces a conformational change in the receptor, making it more likely to bind fibrinogen and further enhancing the aggregation process. GPIIbIIIa is the major receptor whereby fibrinogen bridges adjacent platelets. Thus, patients with Glanzmann's thrombasthenia have lifelong bleeding histories and require platelet transfusions to achieve normal platelet aggregation. In certain clinical scenarios such as percutaneous cardiologic intervention, pharmacologic agents are prescribed that competitively or permanently block the GPIIbIIIa receptor. The effect achieved is one of extreme platelet "paresis." If large enough doses are administered, nearly 100% of GPIIbIIIa receptors can be blocked and platelet aggregation to raw atherogenic surfaces (coronary arteries) will not occur. During drug infusion, patients are very susceptible to bleeding, but careful monitoring and drug dosing has minimized this risk. Examples of these drugs include abciximab, tirofiban, and eptifibatide. Anesthetic management of the patient with absent GPIIbIIIa function includes the transfusion of allogeneic platelets. In patients who have received GPIIbIIIa antagonist drugs, additional fibrinogen in the form of cryoprecipitate may be transfused to compete with the drug for the platelet receptor. However, this is often not done because the drugs have a higher affinity for the receptor than does the fibrinogen ligand. In emergency surgery, antifibrinolytic drugs have been used to minimize the amount of bleeding seen in these patients, but the data supporting this practice come from animal and in-vitro studies. The degree of platelet inhibition can be measured using laboratory and point-of-care tests so that an approximation of the patient's transfusion needs can be made. Laboratory testing of platelet function is discussed in a different section of this chapter.

Concomitant Drugs

In patients with thrombocytopenia and/or platelet dysfunction it is often suggested that other drugs that impair platelet function be avoided. However, many drugs and drug classes have been shown to impair platelet function in vitro.[54] The most common class of drugs would be the nitric oxide donors.[55,56] This class of drugs includes nitrates (sodium nitroprusside, nitroglycerin),[57] phosphodiesterase inhibitors (milrinone),[58] and nitric oxide itself. Nitric oxide has such a short half-life that its effects on platelet function would be short lived.[59,60] However, nitric oxide donors such as nitroprusside may clinically impair platelet function to a measurable degree in a patient whose platelet activity is already compromised.[61] Despite the fact that nitric oxide donors impair platelet function in the laboratory, this does not translate into a clinical problem.[56,62,63] In fact, when nitric oxide was compared with control inhalation after cardiopulmonary bypass, nitric oxide patients had preserved platelet counts and lower expression of GPIb. Aggregation was not different between nitric oxide and control groups.[64] The acute effects of milrinone on platelet function in vivo was also not measurable by standard laboratory or clinical tests.[65]

Antithrombotic Drug Therapy

The glycoprotein IIbIIIa (GPIIbIIIa) receptor is responsible for mediating platelet-platelet aggregation via fibrinogen bridging. Drugs that inhibit this receptor in a reversible or an irreversible fashion are potent inhibitors of platelet aggregation and include abciximab (Reopro), eptifibatide (Integrilin), and tirofiban (Aggrastat). They are frequently infused to prevent thrombus formation in patients who have undergone a high-risk coronary interventional procedure. Large-scale multicenter studies have shown that re-thrombosis and infarction rates after percutaneous angioplasty and after stent procedures have been reduced with the use of these drugs.[66] Reductions in mortality and re-infarction rates have been shown in such patient groups as diabetics and patients with prior cardiac surgery.[67]

Of the three intravenous GPIIbIIIa inhibitors, abciximab is a large monoclonal antibody that binds and causes permanent dysfunction of the GPIIbIIIa receptor, while also blocking other receptors owing to its large size. Comparative studies and head-to-head comparisons have shown that abciximab is superior to the other agents in preventing ischemic complications, which explains its prevalence of use.[68] However, its potent platelet-inhibiting properties also render it likely to cause increased episodes of major bleeding. Patients who present for surgery after having received abciximab often require a prolonged operative time to achieve hemostasis and an increased incidence of platelet transfusions.[69] By contrast, the small molecule agents eptifibatide and tirofiban are competitive blockers whose small size and half-life of approximately 2 hours make it possible to conduct cardiac surgery without an increased risk of bleeding. Studies have documented lower myocardial infarction rates[70] and similar bleeding rates in emergency coronary bypass patients who received eptifibatide compared with those that received placebo before surgery.[71]

Antiplatelet therapy has been rapidly advancing owing to the introduction of the thienopyridine derivatives ticlopidine and clopidogrel (Plavix, Sanofi). Clopidogrel has almost completely replaced ticlopidine for this use because it has a wider therapeutic index and a lesser side effect profile and is more efficacious at doses used clinically. Clopidogrel is a prodrug and requires metabolism by cytochrome P450 subtype 3A4 to form the active drug.[72-74] These drugs act by noncompetitive antagonism at one of the platelet adenosine diphosphate (ADP) receptors, the P2Y12 receptor.[75] There are three known ADP receptor subtypes: the P2X receptor is a calcium ion channel; the P2Y1 receptor is the major receptor responsible for regulating calcium influx and subsequent aggregation[76-78]; and the P2Y12 receptor inhibits cyclic adenosine monophosphate production and potentiates platelet aggregation (Fig. 11-1).

The duration of antiplatelet activity is the life span of the platelet because the P2Y12 receptor is permanently altered. The effects of clopidogrel plus aspirin are additive and sometimes synergistic, depending on the model of platelet function studied. This may explain why cardiac surgical patients having received this combination of drugs seem to have excessive postoperative bleeding.[79] Patients taking these medications at the time of cardiac surgery are at increased risk for bleeding complications and have a documented increase in transfusions and reoperations for bleeding.[73,80-85] This increase in transfusion is seen despite the careful implementation of a transfusion algorithm[82] or strict guidelines for transfusion therapy.[10,86]

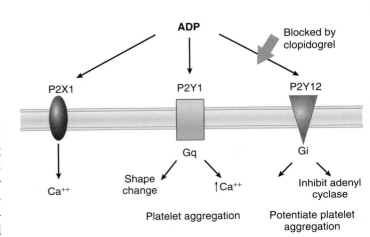

FIGURE 11–1 Role of clopidogrel in antiplatelet therapy.

The logical solution to an increased occurrence of bleeding would seem to be cessation of antithrombotic therapy in preparation for an elective surgical procedure. However, antithrombotic therapy is critical for at least 6 weeks when a bare metal stent is in situ.[87] After this period, it is believed that the stent surface has sufficient surface of neo-endothelium and is not thrombogenic.[88] The minimum period of time during which antithrombotic therapy is suggested in patients with drug-eluting stents is less well defined. The antiproliferative drugs embedded in these stents prolong the development of new endothelium and thus require longer periods (perhaps years) of antiplatelet medication.[89] It has been suggested by retrospective and case reporting that cessation of antiplatelet therapy in patients whose stent has not developed endothelium leads to thrombosis and acute myocardial infarction.

Specific monitoring of the platelet defect induced by these antithrombotic drugs would be advantageous for a number of reasons. For therapeutic efficacy, the degree to which patients are protected from thrombotic events is related to the degree of platelet inhibition. Thus, platelet function monitoring can be used for titrating drug effect. Alternatively, patients taking these medications who present for surgery can be assayed for their degree of platelet dysfunction and their risk of bleeding and need for transfusion.

Diseases or Disorders of Impaired Coagulation

Hemophilia A is inherited as an X-linked disorder. Patients with hemophilia A have insufficient production of factor VIII and thus they have severe impairments in intrinsic coagulation. This can be detected by laboratory analysis by a prolonged partial thromboplastin time. Clinically, the disease manifests as hematuria, hemarthroses, and spontaneous hemorrhage when factor VIII levels are less than 3% of normal. It is important to measure the factor VIII level so that replacement therapy can be initiated before surgery.[90] The goal of replacement therapy is to achieve 100% activity by transfusion of factor VIII concentrates. Assuming a plasma volume of 40 mL/kg, and the need for 100% functional factor VIII before surgery, the number of units of factor VIII needed can be calculated. Plasma contains 1 unit of procoagulant factor per milliliter; cryoprecipitate contains 5 to 10 units/mL, and factor VIII concentrates contain up to 40 units/mL. Factor VIII levels of greater than 30% are considered adequate for hemostasis after major surgery. Replacement therapy will have to be given twice daily in the perioperative period because the elimination half-life of factor VIII is 10 to 12 hours. Some forms of hemophilia are not easily treated with replacement factors because patients can have circulating inhibitors.

Hemophilia B is a disorder of the production of factor IX. The inheritance pattern for hemophilia B is similar to that for hemophilia A. The laboratory abnormalities are also similar in that activated partial thromboplastin time is prolonged. Replacement of factor IX is with specific procoagulant concentrates or complexes that contain high concentrations of factor IX.

Other isolated factor deficiencies are rare. Specific perioperative treatment for these disorders includes preoperative measurement of the deficient factor quantity. Replacement of that factor either in the form of factor concentrates or in a pooled plasma product should aim at bringing factor levels to 100% before surgery. Even the heat-treated factor concentrates that are manufactured carry a small risk of viral transmission because they are derived from human blood products that have been heat treated.

Thrombotic Disorders

Antithrombin III Deficiency

Antithrombin III deficiency can be inherited or acquired. The inherited form of the disease is usually marked by extremely low levels of this endogenous anticoagulant. AT3 inhibits thrombin, hence its name, but it also very effectively inhibits factors XI, X, and IX. Heparin works as an anticoagulant by enhancing the activity of AT3 by 1000-fold. Patients with congenital AT3 deficiency present with venous thromboses throughout life. They develop many complications owing to their hypercoagulable state and are unresponsive to heparin. Patients who "acquire" AT3 deficiency do so as a result of recent previous heparin administration. The continued dosing of heparin usually in intravenous form causes consumption of AT3. Thus, AT3 levels can be low and AT3 activity can also be impaired. When these patients present for cardiac surgery, they often have reduced dose-responsiveness to heparin.[91] Treatment for AT3 deficiency is replacement of AT3.[92] Specific AT3 concentrates are often available. If they are not, transfusion of plasma will replace AT3.[93] Each unit of plasma contains one unit of AT3. Measurement of preoperative levels and attempted replacement to 100% before cardiac surgery is recommended in congenital AT3 deficiency. In the acquired form of the disease it is not clear that replacement therapy is actually indicated.[94]

Protein C and S Deficiency

Proteins C and S are anticoagulant proteases that form a feedback mechanism to the coagulation cascade so that clotting does not occur unchecked. These two proteases are activated by the presence of thrombin and fibrin. It was once thought that protein C and S deficiencies were common in patients with hypercoagulable disorders.

Now it is accepted that many of the patients previously classified as protein C deficient actually had the factor V Leiden mutation.

Factor V Leiden Mutation

Factor V Leiden mutation is now known to be a common familiar disorder in European and Western cultures. Once thought to be an abnormality of activated protein C, the factor V Leiden mutation confers activated protein C resistance by virtue of the factor V molecule, which is resistant. Factor V Leiden mutations, which occur in 3% to 5% of the population, yield a resistance to activated protein C, which impairs the signaling for anticoagulation and fibrinolysis. Using a clot-based assay, in-vitro analyses evaluating the response to activated protein C in cardiac surgical patients indicate that aprotinin induces a factor V Leiden–like defect in normal plasma. In-vitro analyses from factor V Leiden patients suggest that aprotinin further exacerbates this defect in the plasma. Corroborating clinical data demonstrate that patients with factor V Leiden mutation have lesser amounts of mediastinal tube drainage and allogeneic transfusions.[95] One case report describes a patient with factor V Leiden mutation who experienced thrombosis of coronary artery revascularization grafts within a month of surgery, and other case series have described aortic thromboses after aortic replacement.[96]

Heparin-Induced Thrombocytopenia

The syndrome known as heparin-induced thrombocytopenia (HIT) develops in 5% to 28% of patients receiving heparin. HIT is commonly categorized into two subtypes. Type I is characterized by a mild decrease in platelet count and is the result of the proaggregatory effects of heparin on platelets. Type II is considerably more severe, most often occurs after more than 5 days of heparin administration (average onset time, 9 days), and is mediated by antibody binding to the complex formed between heparin and platelet factor 4 (PF4).[97,98] Associated immune-mediated endothelial injury and complement activation cause platelets to adhere, aggregate, and form platelet clots, or "white clots." Among patients developing HIT type II, the incidence of thrombotic complications approximates 20%, which in turn may carry a mortality rate as high as 40%. Demonstration of heparin-induced proaggregation of platelets confirms the diagnosis of HIT type II. This can be accomplished with a heparin-induced serotonin release assay or a specific heparin-induced platelet activation assay. A highly specific enzyme-linked immunosorbent assay for the heparin/PF4 complex has been developed and has been used to delineate the course of IgG and IgM antibody responses in patients exposed to unfractionated heparin during cardiac surgery.[99] The options for treating these patients are few.[100] If one has the luxury of being able to discontinue the heparin for 90 days, often the antibody will disappear and allow a brief period of heparinization for cardiopulmonary bypass without complication.[101] Some types of low-molecular-weight heparin have been given in HIT, but reactivity of the particular low-molecular-weight heparin with the patient's platelets should be confirmed in vitro. Supplementing heparin administration with pharmacologic platelet inhibition using prostacyclin, iloprost, aspirin, or aspirin and dipyridamole have been reported, all with favorable outcomes. Recently, the use of tirofiban with unfractionated heparin has been used in this clinical circumstance. Plasmapheresis may be used to reduce antibody levels. The use of heparin could be avoided altogether by anticoagulating with direct thrombin inhibitors such as argatroban, hirudin, or bivalirudin. These thrombin inhibitors have become the standard of care in the management of the patient with HIT type II.[102-104]

Monitoring Platelet Function

Platelet Function Tests: Point of Care

Point-of-care platelet function testing is critical to have an impact on acute medical management. The need for small sample size, rapid turnaround, ease of use, and clinical applicability make point-of-care monitoring the gold standard in the perioperative setting. Platelet function monitors can be divided into three basic and non–mutually exclusive categories: static tests, dynamic tests (nonactivated), and tests of the platelet response to an activating stimulus.

Static Tests of Platelet Function

Static tests such as the measure of β-thromboglobulin, ADP release, or the number of platelet receptors present on the surface capture only a single point in time and do not accurately reflect the dynamic environment encountered after cardiopulmonary bypass. Neither do they reflect the platelet ability to respond to an agonist.

Dynamic Tests of Platelet Function

Dynamic tests such as the bleeding time or the viscoelastic measures of clot formation better reflect the contribution of platelet function to overall clot formation because they take into account the time-dependent nature of platelet-mediated hemostasis. They are, however, nonspecific in nature owing to the absence of a platelet-specific agonist, but the tests can generally be modified to overcome this limitation.

TEG (Haemoscope, Skokie, IL) is a whole blood test of viscoelastic blood clot formation that has been used in many different clinical scenarios to diagnose coagulation abnormalities. Within 10 to 20 minutes information is obtained regarding the integrity of the coagulation cascade, platelet function, platelet-fibrin interactions, and fibrinolysis. Whole blood (360 µL) is placed into an oscillating cuvette. A piston connected to a transducer and oscillograph is immersed into the blood sample. The movement of the piston becomes coupled to the oscillating cuvette as the blood clots. This generates a signature tracing with the following parameters: reaction time (R value), coagulation time (K value), α angle, maximum amplitude (MA), amplitude 60 minutes after the maximal amplitude (A60). Respectively, these parameters measure fibrin formation, fibrinogen turnover, speed of clot formation, platelet-fibrin interactions, and fibrinolysis.

Recent modifications to the TEG have allowed for improved monitoring capabilities. Use of recombinant human tissue factor as an activator accelerates the rate of thrombin formation and shortens the time required for development of MA. Because MA is primarily reflective of clot strength and platelet function, this information can be obtained more quickly with tissue factor enhancement (5 to 10 minutes). An application of thromboelastography in the clinical arena is its use in monitoring fibrinolysis and antiplatelet therapy using either the GPIIbIIIa receptor blockers, aspirin, or clopidogrel. This has predominantly been done using modifications to the point-of-care system and is being further developed. In-vitro addition of a large dose of abciximab to the test cuvette enhances the diagnostic ability of the test to discriminate between hypofibrinogenemia and platelet dysfunction as a cause of decreased MA.[105,106]

Tests of Platelet Response to an Agonist Stimulus

The newest group of platelet function tests includes point-of-care monitors specifically designed to measure agonist-induced platelet-mediated hemostasis.

The platelet-activated clotting time, Hemostatus (Medtronic Inc., Parker, CO), measures the activated clotting time without platelet activator and compares this value to the activated clotting time obtained when increasing concentrations of a platelet-activating factor (PAF) are added. The percent reduction of the activated clotting time due to the addition of PAF is related to the ability of platelets to be activated and to shorten clotting time.[107] The assay is performed using a specific cartridge in a Heparin Management System (HMS) (Medtronic Inc., Parker, CO) device, and the Hemostatus cartridge has been found useful for monitoring platelet function during cardiac surgery.[108]

Ultegra (Accumetrics, San Diego, CA), or "rapid platelet function assay," is a point-of-care monitor designed specifically to measure the platelet response to a thrombin receptor agonist peptide (TRAP). In whole blood, it measures

TRAP activation-induced platelet agglutination of fibrinogen-coated beads using an optical detection system. Because of the importance of the GPIIbIIIa receptor in mediating fibrinogen-platelet interactions, the Ultegra has been especially useful in accurately measuring receptor inhibition in invasive cardiology patients receiving GPIIbIIIa-inhibiting drugs.[109-111]

The Platelet Function Analyzer, PFA-100 (Dade Behring, Miami, FL), is a monitor of platelet adhesive capacity that is valuable in its diagnostic abilities to identify drug-induced platelet abnormalities, Bernard-Soulier syndrome, von Willebrand's disease, and other acquired and congenital platelet defects.[112,113] The test is conducted as a modified in-vitro bleeding time. Whole blood is drawn through a chamber by vacuum and is perfused across an aperture in a collagen membrane coated with an agonist (epinephrine or ADP). Platelet adhesion and formation of aggregates will seal the aperture, thus indicating the "closure time" measured by the PFA-100. This test may be useful in detecting pharmacologic platelet dysfunction before cardiac surgery or may be able to accurately detect hypercoagulability after CPB.

"Plateletworks" (Helena Laboratories, Beaumont, TX) utilizes the principle of the platelet count ratio to assess platelet reactivity. The instrument is a Coulter counter that measures the platelet count in a standard EDTA-containing tube. Platelet count is also measured in tubes containing the platelet agonists (e.g., ADP, collagen). Addition of blood to these agonist tubes causes platelets to activate, adhere to the tube, and to be effectively eliminated from the platelet count. The ratio of the activated platelet count to the nonactivated platelet count is a function of the reactivity of the platelets. Early investigation in cardiac surgical patients indicates that this assay is useful in providing a platelet count and that it is capable of measuring the platelet dysfunction that accompanies cardiopulmonary bypass.[114] Plateletworks has also been used to study the pharmacokinetics and pharmacodynamics of clopidogrel in conjunction with other drug therapy.[72]

Platelet Aggregometry

Platelet aggregometry utilizes a photo-optical instrument to measure light transmittance through a sample of platelet-rich plasma. When exposed to a platelet agonist, the initial reversible aggregation phase results in increased light transmittance due to the platelet aggregates that decrease the turbidity of the sample. Aggregometry is considered a "gold standard" of platelet function measure.[115] It is rather labor and time intensive and is not practical for the immediate perioperative period. This is the reason for the surge in the number of point-of-care platelet function monitors being developed.

Referenes

1. Points to consider on efficacy evaluation of hemoglobin- and perfluorocarbon-based oxygen carriers. Center for Biologics Evaluation and Research. Transfusion 1994;34:712-713.
2. Wallace EL, Churchill WH, Surgenor DM, et al: Collection and transfusion of blood and blood components in the United States, 1992. Transfusion 1995;35:802-812.
3. Wallace EL, Churchill WH, Surgenor DM, et al: Collection and transfusion of blood and blood components in the United States, 1994. Transfusion 1998;38:625-636.
4. Wallace EL, Surgenor DM, Hao HS, et al: Collection and transfusion of blood and blood components in the United States, 1989. Transfusion 1993;33:139-144.
5. Shander A: Anemia in the critically ill. Crit Care Clin 2004;20:159-178.
6. Platelet transfusion therapy. National Institutes of Health Consensus Conference. Transfus Med Rev 1987;1:195-200.
7. Consensus conference: Perioperative red blood cell transfusion. JAMA 1988;260:2700-2703.
8. Consensus conference: Platelet transfusion therapy. JAMA 1987;257:1777-1780.
9. Consensus conference: Fresh-frozen plasma: Indications and risks. JAMA 1985;253:551-553.
10. Practice Guidelines for blood component therapy: A report by the American Society of Anesthesiologists Task Force on Blood Component Therapy. Anesthesiology 1996;84:732-747.
11. Nelson AH, Fleisher LA, Rosenbaum SH: Relationship between postoperative anemia and cardiac morbidity in high-risk vascular patients in the intensive care unit. Crit Care Med 1993;21:860-866.
12. Humphries JE: Transfusion therapy in acquired coagulopathies. Hematol Oncol Clin North Am 1994;8:1181-1201.
13. Mayer JE Jr, Kersten TE, Humphrey EW: Effects of transfusion of emboli and aged plasma on pulmonary capillary permeability. J Thorac Cardiovasc Surg 1981;82:358-364.
14. Curran JW, Lawrence DN, Jaffe H, et al: Acquired immunodeficiency syndrome (AIDS) associated with transfusions. N Engl J Med 1984;310:69-75.
15. Donahue JG, Munoz A, Ness PM, et al: The declining risk of post-transfusion hepatitis C virus infection. N Engl J Med 1992;327:369-373.
16. Ward JW, Bush TJ, Perkins HA, et al: The natural history of transfusion-associated infection with human immunodeficiency virus: Factors influencing the rate of progression to disease. N Engl J Med 1989;321:947-952.
17. Lackritz EM, Satten GA, Aberle-Grasse J, et al: Estimated risk of transmission of the human immunodeficiency virus by screened blood in the United States. N Engl J Med 1995;333:1721-1725.
18. Sloand EM, Pitt E, Klein HG: Safety of the blood supply. JAMA 1995;274:1368-1373.
19. Brown KE, Tisdale J, Barrett AJ, et al: Hepatitis-associated aplastic anemia. N Engl J Med 1997;336:1059-1064.
20. Young NS, Maciejewski J: The pathophysiology of acquired aplastic anemia. N Engl J Med 1997; 336:1365-1372.
21. Erbe RW: Genetic aspects of folate metabolism. Adv Hum Genet 1979;9:293-354, 367-369.
22. Erbe RW, Salis RJ: Severe methylenetetrahydrofolate reductase deficiency, methionine synthase, and nitrous oxide—a cautionary tale. N Engl J Med 2003;349:5-6.
23. Toh BH, van Driel IR, Gleeson PA: Pernicious anemia. N Engl J Med 1997;337:1441-1448.
24. Sickle-cell anemia and anaesthesia. BMJ 1965;5473:1263-1264.
25. Frietsch T, Ewen I, Waschke KF: Anaesthetic care for sickle cell disease. Eur J Anaesthesiol 2001;18:137-150.
26. Bunn HF: Pathogenesis and treatment of sickle cell disease. N Engl J Med 1997;337:762-769.
27. Djaiani GN, Cheng DC, Carroll JA, et al: Fast-track cardiac anesthesia in patients with sickle cell abnormalities. Anesth Analg 1999;89:598-603.
28. Abdulla Al-Ghamdi A: Bilateral total knee replacement with tourniquets in a homozygous sickle cell patient. Anesth Analg 2004;98:543-544, table of contents.

29. Stein RE, Urbaniak J: Use of the tourniquet during surgery in patients with sickle cell hemoglobinopathies. Clin Orthop Rel Res 1980;(151):231-233.
30. Adu-Gyamfi Y, Sankarankutty M, Marwa S: Use of a tourniquet in patients with sickle-cell disease. Can J Anaesth 1993;40:24-27.
31. Vichinsky EP, Haberkern CM, Neumayr L, et al: A comparison of conservative and aggressive transfusion regimens in the perioperative management of sickle cell disease. The Preoperative Transfusion in Sickle Cell Disease Study Group. N Engl J Med 1995;333:206-213.
32. Dix HM: New advances in the treatment of sickle cell disease: Focus on perioperative significance. AANA J 2001;69:281-286.
33. Griffin TC, Buchanan GR: Elective surgery in children with sickle cell disease without preoperative blood transfusion. J Pediatr Surg 1993;28:681-685.
34. Koshy M, Chisum D, Burd L, et al: Management of sickle cell anemia and pregnancy. J Clin Apheresis 1991;6:230-233.
35. Desforges JF, Warth J: The management of sickle cell disease in pregnancy. Clin Perinatol 1974;1:385-394.
36. Rajab KE, Skerman JH: Sickle cell disease in pregnancy: Obstetric and anesthetic management perspectives. Saudi Med J 2004;25:265-276.
37. Deutsch S: Anesthetic management in acute and chronic renal failure. Vet Clin North Am 1973;3:57-64.
38. Deutsch S: Anesthetic management of patients with chronic renal disease. South Med J 1975;68:65-69.
39. Eschbach JW, Kelly MR, Haley NR, et al: Treatment of the anemia of progressive renal failure with recombinant human erythropoietin. N Engl J Med 1989;321:158-163.
40. Kam PC, Thompson SA, Liew AC: Thrombocytopenia in the parturient. Anaesthesia 2004;59:255-264.
41. Lee LH: Idiopathic thrombocytopenia in pregnancy. Ann Acad Med Singapore 2002;31:335-339.
42. Anglin BV, Rutherford C, Ramus R, et al: Immune thrombocytopenic purpura during pregnancy: Laparoscopic treatment. JSLS 2001;5:63-67.
43. Zeller B, Helgestad J, Hellebostad M, et al: Immune thrombocytopenic purpura in childhood in Norway: A prospective, population-based registration. Pediatr Hematol Oncol 2000;17:551-558.
44. Leichtman DA, Friedman BA: The hemorrhagic complications of open-heart surgery. CRC Crit Rev Clin Lab Sci 1977;7:239-254.
45. Lee JW: Von Willebrand disease, hemophilia A and B, and other factor deficiencies. Int Anesthesiol Clin 2004;42:59-76.
46. Bowes JB: Anaesthetic management of haemothorax and haemoptysis due to von Willebrand's disease: A case report. Br J Anaesth 1969;41:894-897.
47. Plumley MH: DDAVP and anaesthesia. Anaesthesia 1988;43:898.
48. Stedeford JC, Pittman JA: Von Willebrand's disease and neuroaxial anaesthesia. Anaesthesia 2000;55:1228-1229.
49. Cohen S, Daitch JS, Amar D, Goldiner PL: Epidural analgesia for labor and delivery in a patient with von Willebrand's disease. Reg Anesth 1989;14:95-97.
50. Hepner DL, Tsen LC: Severe thrombocytopenia, type 2B von Willebrand disease and pregnancy. Anesthesiology 2004;101:1465-1467.
51. Kadir RA, Lee CA, Sabin CA, et al: Pregnancy in women with von Willebrand's disease or factor XI deficiency. Br J Obstet Gynaecol 1998;105:314-321.
52. Nichols TC, Bellinger DA, Tate DA, et al: von Willebrand factor and occlusive arterial thrombosis: A study in normal and von Willebrand's disease pigs with diet-induced hypercholesterolemia and atherosclerosis. Arteriosclerosis 1990;10:449-461.
53. Michelson AD: Flow cytometric analysis of platelet surface glycoproteins: Phenotypically distinct subpopulations of platelets in children with chronic myeloid leukemia. J Lab Clin Med 1987;110:346-354.
54. Furman MI, Liu L, Benoit SE, et al: The cleaved peptide of the thrombin receptor is a strong platelet agonist. Proc Natl Acad Sci USA 1998;95:3082-3087.
55. Bodzenta-Lukaszyk A, Gabryelewicz A, Lukaszyk A, et al: Nitric oxide synthase inhibition and platelet function. Thromb Res 1994;75:667-672.

56. Chen LY, Mehta JL: Inhibitory effect of high-density lipoprotein on platelet function is mediated by increase in nitric oxide synthase activity in platelets. Life Sci 1994;55:1815-1821.

57. Aoki H, Inoue M, Mizobe T, et al: Platelet function is inhibited by nitric oxide liberation during nitroglycerin-induced hypotension anaesthesia. Br J Anaesth 1997;79:476-481.

58. Laight DW, Anggard EE, Carrier MJ: Modulation of nitric oxide–dependent vascular and platelet function in vitro by the novel phosphodiesterase type-V inhibitor ONO-1505. J Pharm Pharmacol 1999;51:1429-1433.

59. Albert J, Norman M, Wallen NH, et al: Inhaled nitric oxide does not influence bleeding time or platelet function in healthy volunteers. Eur J Clin Invest 1999;29:953-959.

60. Albert J, Wallen NH, Broijersen A, et al: Effects of inhaled nitric oxide compared with aspirin on platelet function in vivo in healthy subjects. Clin Sci (Lond) 1996;91:225-231.

61. Cheung PY, Salas E, Schulz R, Radomski MW: Nitric oxide and platelet function: Implications for neonatology. Semin Perinatol 1997;21:409-417.

62. Bath PM, Pathansali R, Iddenden R, Bath FJ: The effect of transdermal glyceryl trinitrate, a nitric oxide donor, on blood pressure and platelet function in acute stroke. Cerebrovasc Dis 2001;11:265-272.

63. Bereczki C, Tur S, Nemeth I, et al: The roles of platelet function, thromboxane, blood lipids and nitric oxide in hypertension of children and adolescents. Prostaglandins Leukot Essent Fatty Acids 2000;62:293-297.

64. Mellgren K, Mellgren G, Lundin S, et al: Effect of nitric oxide gas on platelets during open heart operations. Ann Thorac Surg 1998;65:1335-1341.

65. Kikura M, Lee MK, Safon RA, et al: The effects of milrinone on platelets in patients undergoing cardiac surgery. Anesth Analg 1995;81:44-48.

66. Azar RR, McKay RG, Thompson PD, et al: Abciximab in primary coronary angioplasty for acute myocardial infarction improves short- and medium-term outcomes. J Am Coll Cardiol 1998;32:1996-2002.

67. Bhatt DL, Marso SP, Lincoff AM, et al: Abciximab reduces mortality in diabetics following percutaneous coronary intervention. J Am Coll Cardiol 2000;35:922-928.

68. Brown DL, Fann CS, Chang CJ: Meta-analysis of effectiveness and safety of abciximab versus eptifibatide or tirofiban in percutaneous coronary intervention. Am J Cardiol 2001;87:537-541.

69. Lemmer JH Jr: Clinical experience in coronary bypass surgery for abciximab-treated patients. Ann Thorac Surg 2000;70(2 Suppl):S33-S37.

70. Dyke CM, Bhatia D, Lorenz TJ, et al: Discussion: Immediate coronary artery bypass surgery after platelet inhibition with eptifibatide: Results from PURSUIT. Platelet Glycoprotein IIb/IIIa in Unstable Angina: Receptor Suppression Using Integrelin Therapy. Ann Thorac Surg 2000;70:866-871; discussion 871-872.

71. Bizzarri F, Scolletta S, Tucci E, et al: Perioperative use of tirofiban hydrochloride (Aggrastat) does not increase surgical bleeding after emergency or urgent coronary artery bypass grafting. J Thorac Cardiovasc Surg 2001;122:1181-1185.

72. Lau WC, Waskell LA, Watkins PB, et al: Atorvastatin reduces the ability of clopidogrel to inhibit platelet aggregation: A new drug-drug interaction. Circulation 2003;107:32-37.

73. Ng FH, Wong SY, Chang CM, et al: High incidence of clopidogrel-associated gastrointestinal bleeding in patients with previous peptic ulcer disease. Aliment Pharmacol Ther 2003;18:443-449.

74. Savi P, Combalbert J, Gaich C, et al: The antiaggregating activity of clopidogrel is due to a metabolic activation by the hepatic cytochrome P450-1A. Thromb Haemost 1994;72:313-317.

75. Defreyn G, Gachet C, Savi P, et al: Ticlopidine and clopidogrel (SR 25990C) selectively neutralize ADP inhibition of PGE1-activated platelet adenylate cyclase in rats and rabbits. Thromb Haemost 1991;65:186-190.

76. Savi P, Beauverger P, Labouret C, et al: Role of P2Y1 purinoceptor in ADP-induced platelet activation. FEBS Lett 1998;422:291-295.

77. Savi P, Bornia J, Salel V, et al: Characterization of P2x1 purinoreceptors on rat platelets: Effect of clopidogrel. Br J Haematol 1997;98:880-886.

78. Savi P, Pereillo JM, Uzabiaga MF, et al: Identification and biological activity of the active metabolite of clopidogrel [In Process Citation]. Thromb Haemost 2000;84:891-896.

79. Herbert JM, Dol F, Bernat A, et al: The antiaggregating and antithrombotic activity of clopidogrel is potentiated by aspirin in several experimental models in the rabbit. Thromb Haemost 1998;80:512-518.

80. Cavusoglu E, Cheng J, Bhatt R, et al: Clopidogrel in the management of ischemic heart disease. Heart Dis 2003;5:144-152.

81. Chen KK, Ginges I, Manolios N: Clopidogrel-associated acute arthritis. Intern Med J 2003;33:618-619.

82. Chen L, Bracey AW, Radovancevic R, et al: Clopidogrel and bleeding in patients undergoing elective coronary artery bypass grafting. J Thorac Cardiovasc Surg 2004;128:425-431.

83. Chen WH, Lee PY, Ng W, et al: Aspirin resistance is associated with a high incidence of myonecrosis after non-urgent percutaneous coronary intervention despite clopidogrel pretreatment. J Am Coll Cardiol 2004;43:1122-1126.

84. Kuchulakanti P, Kapetanakis EI, Lew R, et al: Impact of continued hospitalization in patients pre-treated with clopidogrel prior to coronary angiography and undergoing coronary artery bypass grafting. J Invasive Cardiol 2005;17:5-7.

85. Waksman R, Ajani AE, Pinnow E, et al: Twelve versus six months of clopidogrel to reduce major cardiac events in patients undergoing gamma-radiation therapy for in-stent restenosis: Washington Radiation for In-Stent restenosis Trial (WRIST) 12 versus WRIST PLUS. Circulation 2002;106:776-778.

86. Practice parameter for the use of fresh-frozen plasma, cryoprecipitate, and platelets. Fresh-Frozen Plasma, Cryoprecipitate, and Platelets Administration Practice Guidelines Development Task Force of the College of American Pathologists. JAMA 1994;271:777-781.

87. Kaluza GL, Joseph J, Lee JR, et al: Catastrophic outcomes of noncardiac surgery soon after coronary stenting. J Am Coll Cardiol 2000;35:1288-1294.

88. Wilson SH, Fasseas P, Orford JL, et al: Clinical outcome of patients undergoing non-cardiac surgery in the two months following coronary stenting. J Am Coll Cardiol 2003;42:234-240.

89. McFadden EP, Stabile E, Regar E, et al: Late thrombosis in drug-eluting coronary stents after discontinuation of antiplatelet therapy. Lancet 2004;364:1519-1521.

90. Vinckier F, Vermylen J: Dental extractions in hemophilia: Reflections on 10 years' experience. Oral Surg Oral Med Oral Pathol 1985;59:6-9.

91. Nicholson SC, Keeling DM, Sinclair ME, Evans RD: Heparin pretreatment does not alter heparin requirements during cardiopulmonary bypass. Br J Anaesth 2001;87:844-847.

92. Kanbak M: The treatment of heparin resistance with antithrombin III in cardiac surgery. Can J Anaesth 1999;46:581-585.

93. Heller EL, Paul L: Anticoagulation management in a patient with an acquired antithrombin III deficiency. J Extra Corpor Technol 2001;33:245-248.

94. Shore-Lesserson L, Manspeizer HE, Bolastig M, et al: Anticoagulation for cardiac surgery in patients receiving preoperative heparin: Use of the high-dose thrombin time. Anesth Analg 2000;90:813-818.

95. Donahue BS, Gailani D, Higgins MS, et al: Factor V Leiden protects against blood loss and transfusion after cardiac surgery. Circulation 2003;107:1003-1008.

96. Fanashawe MP, Shore-Lesserson L, Reich DL: Two cases of fatal thrombosis after aminocaproic acid therapy and deep hypothermic circulatory arrest. Anesthesiology 2001;95:1525-1527.

97. Warkentin TE, Greinacher A: Heparin-induced thrombocytopenia and cardiac surgery. Ann Thorac Surg 2003;76:638-648.

98. Warkentin TE, Kelton JG: Heparin-induced thrombocytopenia. Prog Hemost Thromb 1991;10:1-34.

99. Warkentin TE: Laboratory testing for heparin-induced thrombocytopenia. J Thromb Thrombolysis 2000;10(Suppl 1):35-45.

100. Visentin GP, Malik M, Cyganiak KA, Aster RH: Patients treated with unfractionated heparin during open heart surgery are at high risk to form antibodies reactive with heparin:platelet factor 4 complexes. J Lab Clin Med 1996;128:376-383.

101. Warkentin TE, Kelton JG: Temporal aspects of heparin-induced thrombocytopenia. N Engl J Med 2001;344:1286-1292.

102. Koster A, Crystal GJ, Kuppe H, Mertzlufft F: Acute heparin-induced thrombocytopenia type II during cardiopulmonary bypass. J Cardiothorac Vasc Anesth 2000;14:300-303.

103. Koster A, Hansen R, Grauhan O, et al: Hirudin monitoring using the TAS ecarin clotting time in patients with heparin-induced thrombocytopenia type II. J Cardiothorac Vasc Anesth 2000;14:249-252.

104. Koster A, Hansen R, Kuppe H, et al: Recombinant hirudin as an alternative for anticoagulation during cardiopulmonary bypass in patients with heparin-induced thrombocytopenia type II: A 1-year experience in 57 patients. J Cardiothorac Vasc Anesth 2000;14: 243-248.

105. Kettner SC, Panzer OP, Kozek SA, et al: Use of abciximab-modified thrombelastography in patients undergoing cardiac surgery. Anesth Analg 1999;89:580-584.

106. Mousa SA, Khurana S, Forsythe MS: Comparative in vitro efficacy of different platelet glycoprotein IIb/IIIa antagonists on platelet-mediated clot strength induced by tissue factor with use of thromboelastography: Differentiation among glycoprotein IIb/IIIa antagonists. Arterioscler Thromb Vasc Biol 2000;20:1162-1167.

107. Bode AP, Lust RM: Masking of heparin activity in the activated coagulation time (ACT) by platelet procoagulant activity. Thromb Res 1994;73:285-300.

108. Despotis GJ, Levine V, Filos KS, et al: Evaluation of a new point-of-care test that measures PAF-mediated acceleration of coagulation in cardiac surgical patients. Anesthesiology 1996;85:1311-1323.

109. Coller BS, Lang D, Scudder LE: Rapid and simple platelet function assay to assess glycoprotein IIb/IIIa receptor blockade. Circulation 1997;95:860-867.

110. Smith JW, Steinhubl SR, Lincoff AM, et al: Rapid platelet-function assay: An automated and quantitative cartridge-based method. Circulation 1999;99:620-625.

111. Steinhubl SR, Talley JD, Braden GA, et al: Point-of-care measured platelet inhibition correlates with a reduced risk of an adverse cardiac event after percutaneous coronary intervention: Results of the GOLD (AU-Assessing Ultegra) multicenter study. Circulation 2001;103:2572-2578.

112. Bock M, De Haan J, Beck KH, et al: Standardization of the PFA-100(R) platelet function test in 105 mmol/L buffered citrate: Effect of gender, smoking, and oral contraceptives. Br J Haematol 1999;106:898-904.

113. Escolar G, Cases A, Vinas M, et al: Evaluation of acquired platelet dysfunctions in uremic and cirrhotic patients using the platelet function analyzer (PFA-100): Influence of hematocrit elevation. Haematologica 1999;84:614-619.

114. Carville DG, Schleckser PA, Guyer KE, et al: Whole blood platelet function assay on the ICHOR point-of-care hematology analyzer. J Extra Corpor Technol 1998;30:171-177.

115. Ray MJ, Hawson GA, Just SJ, et al: Relationship of platelet aggregation to bleeding after cardiopulmonary bypass. Ann Thorac Surg 1994;57:981-986.

12 Infectious Diseases and Bioterrorism

PATRICK J. NELIGAN, MD

Infection has killed more soldiers in war than gunfire. Although the age of infectious diseases has all but passed in the western world, infection, and the means by which the body deals with it, remains a major problem in critical care and perioperative medicine.

A clear distinction must be made between infections, sepsis, infectiousness, and carrier states. *Infection* refers to the host response to the presence of microorganisms or tissue invasion by microorganisms. The microorganisms may be bacteria, viruses, fungi, parasites, or prions. *Sepsis* is a syndrome—the systemic inflammatory response to the microorganism and associated toxins. *Infectiousness* or contagiousness refers to the transmissibility of pathogens from one host to another. A *carrier state* refers to the persistence of a contagious organism within a host who may not demonstrate signs of infection. Each of these situations is of importance to anesthesiologists. For example, patients with fulminant surgical sepsis (e.g., necrotizing pancreatitis or gas gangrene) may come to the operating room for débridement and source control. Anesthesia management is significantly influenced by the immunologic and hemodynamic impact of sepsis.

Likewise, patients with transmissible diseases (e.g., tuberculosis, hepatitis C, or HIV) represent a significant risk to health care personnel, who may contract the diseases.[1] Finally, the dramatic events of September 2001, the subsequent anthrax scare, and the war in Iraq have refocused attention of previously eradicated infectious organisms as potential weapons of terrorism.[2]

SEPSIS, SYSTEMIC INFLAMMATORY RESPONSE SYNDROME, AND MULTIORGAN DYSFUNCTION SYNDROME

Definitions

For many years doctors attending intensive care units (ICUs) used a variety of terms to describe illnesses associated with infection or with illness that looked like infection. These terms included sepsis, septicemia, bacteremia, infection, septic shock, toxic shock, and so on. Unfortunately, there were two problems with these terms: (1) there were no strict definitions for the terms used, and often these words or phrases were used incorrectly; and

(2) an emerging body of evidence arose that led us to believe that systemic inflammation, rather than infection, was responsible for multiorgan failure. In the early 1990s a consensus conference between the American College of Chest Physicians (ACCP) and the Society for Critical Care Medicine (SCCM) laid out a new series of definitions for what is inflammation and what is sepsis (Table 12-1).[3] The reason for this is that the host response to both infectious and noninfectious injuries is similar[4]; the clinical signs are essentially the same. This inflammatory response is determined, qualitatively and quantitatively, by genetic and environmental factors.[5] Hence the term *sepsis* had come to be used, incorrectly, to describe the host response to a variety of infectious and noninfectious injuries (Fig. 12-1). A new term *SIRS* (systemic inflammatory response syndrome) was introduced to describe the process of inflammation without infection.[3] This terminology has come into common usage, albeit with some reservations.[6,7]

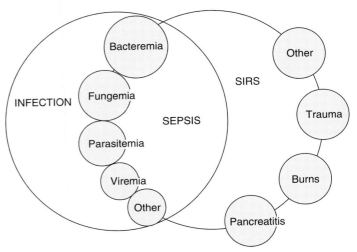

FIGURE 12–1 Infection, sepsis and SIRS. *(From Definitions for sepsis and organ failure and guidelines for the use of innovative therapies in sepsis. Consensus document ACCP/SCCM. Crit Care Med 1992;20:864-874.)*

TABLE 12–1   Definitions for Sepsis and Organ Failure and Guidelines for the Use of Innovative Therapies in Sepsis

Infection

A host response to the presence of microorganisms or tissue invasion by microorganisms.

Bacteremia

The presence of viable bacteria in circulating blood

Systemic Inflammatory Response Syndrome (SIRS)

The systemic inflammatory response to a wide variety of severe clinical insults, manifested by two or more of the following conditions:
   Temperature > 38°C or < 36°C
   Heart rate > 90 beats per minute
   Respiratory rate > 20 breaths per minute or $Paco_2$ < 32 mm Hg
   WBC count > 12,000/mm³, < 4,000/mm³, or > 10% immature (band) forms

Sepsis

The systemic inflammatory response to infection. In association with infection, manifestations of sepsis are the same as those previously defined for SIRS. It should be determined whether they are a direct systemic response to the presence of an infectious process and represent an acute alteration from baseline in the absence of other known causes for such abnormalities. The clinical manifestations would include two or more of the following conditions as a result of a documented infection:
   Temperature > 38°C or < 36°C
   Heart rate > 90 beats per minute
   Respiratory rate > 20 breaths per minute or $Paco_2$ < 32 mm Hg
   WBC count > 12,000/mm³, < 4,000/mm³, or > 10% immature (band) forms

Severe Sepsis/SIRS

Sepsis (SIRS) associated with organ dysfunction, hypoperfusion, or hypotension. Hypoperfusion and perfusion abnormalities may include, but are not limited to, lactic acidosis, oliguria, or an acute alteration in mental status.

Refractory (Septic) Shock/SIRS Shock

A subset of severe sepsis (SIRS) and defined as sepsis (SIRS)-induced hypotension despite adequate fluid resuscitation along with the presence of perfusion abnormalities that may include, but are not limited to, lactic acidosis, oliguria, or an acute alteration in mental status. Patients receiving inotropic or vasopressor agents may no longer be hypotensive by the time they manifest hypoperfusion abnormalities or organ dysfunction, yet they would still be considered to have septic (SIRS) shock.

Multiple Organ Dysfunction Syndrome (MODS)

Presence of altered organ function in an acutely ill patient such that homeostasis cannot be maintained without intervention.

From Definitions for sepsis and organ failure and guidelines for the use of innovative therapies in sepsis. Consensus document ACCP/SCCM. Crit Care Med 1992;20:864-874.

Infection, according to the 1992 definitions,[3] is a microbial phenomenon characterized by an inflammatory response to the presence of microorganisms or the invasion of normally sterile host tissue by those organisms. *Sepsis* is the presence of a systemic inflammatory response to infection. A second consensus conference was held in 2001[5] to deal with the ongoing problem with the vagueness of the definition of SIRS.[8] The strengths and weaknesses of the current sepsis definitions were reviewed. The definitions were left unchanged with the exception of an expansion in the list of signs and symptoms of sepsis to reflect the spectrum of manifestations at the bedside. These definitions have significant epidemiologic value: there is a clear increase in mortality as patients pass from SIRS, with progressive organ failure, to sepsis, to septic shock (Table 12-2).[9,10]

TABLE 12–2 Diagnostic Criteria for Sepsis

Infection,* documented or suspected, and some of the following:†

General variables
  Fever (core temperature > 38.3°C)
  Hypothermia (core temperature < 36°C)
  Heart rate > 90 beats per minute or > 2 SD above the normal value for age
  Tachypnea
  Altered mental status
  Significant edema or positive fluid balance (> 20 mL/kg over 24 hr)
  Hyperglycemia (plasma glucose > 120 mg/dL or 7.7 mmol/L) in the absence of diabetes

Inflammatory variables
  Leukocytosis (WBC count > 12,000/μL)
  Leukopenia (WBC count , 4,000/μL)
  Normal WBC count with > 10% immature forms
  Plasma C-reactive protein > 2 SD above the normal value
  Plasma procalcitonin > 2 SD above the normal value

Hemodynamic variables
  Arterial hypotension† (SBP < 90 mm Hg, MAP < 70, or an
    SBP decrease > 40 mm Hg in adults or < 2 SD below normal for age)
  $S\bar{v}o_2$ > 70%†
  Cardiac index > 3.5 L/min/m²

Organ dysfunction variables
  Arterial hypoxemia (Pao_2/Fio_2 < 300)
  Acute oliguria (urine output , 0.5 mL/kg/hr for at least 2 hr)
  Creatinine increase > 0.5 mg/dL
  Coagulation abnormalities (INR > 1.5 or aPTT > 60 seconds)
  Ileus (absent bowel sounds)
  Thrombocytopenia (platelet count < 100,000/μL)
  Hyperbilirubinemia (plasma total bilirubin > 4 mg/dL or 70 mmol/L)

Tissue perfusion variables
  Hyperlactatemia (> 1 mmol/L)
  Decreased capillary refill or mottling

WBC, white blood cell; SBP, systolic blood pressure; MAP, mean arterial pressure; $S\bar{v}o_2$, mixed venous oxygen saturation; INR, international normalized ratio; aPTT, activated partial thromboplastin time.

*Infection defined as a pathologic process induced by a microorganism.

†$S\bar{v}o_2$ sat > 70% is normal in children (normally, 75%-80%), and CI 3.5-5.5 is normal in children; therefore, NEITHER should be used as signs of sepsis in newborns or children.

Note: Diagnostic criteria for sepsis in the pediatric population are signs and symptoms of inflammation plus infection with hyperthermia or hypothermia (rectal temperature > 38.5° or < 35°C), tachycardia (may be absent in hypothermic patients), and at least one of the following indications of altered organ function: altered mental status, hypoxemia, increased serum lactate level, or bounding pulses.

From 2001 SCCM/ESICM/ACCP/ATS/SIS International Sepsis Definitions Conference. Crit Care Med. 2003;31:1250-1256.

Pathophysiology of Sepsis

The presence of pathogens in the bloodstream or tissues elicits an inflammatory response. There are five stages[4]: (1) establishment of infection, (2) preliminary systemic inflammatory response, (3) overwhelming systemic inflammatory response, (4) compensatory anti-inflammatory response, and (5) immunomodulatory failure.

Microbes possess specific virulence factors to overcome host defenses. The cell wall of gram-negative bacteria consists of an inner phospholipid bilayer and an outer layer that contains lipopolysaccharide (LPS). This consists of polysaccharide O, which protrudes from the exterior cell surface, a core polysaccharide, and a lipid component (lipid A) that faces the cell interior. Lipid A, or endotoxin, is responsible for the toxicity of this molecule. It is released with cell lysis. In meningococcemia, plasma levels of endotoxin correlate well with the development of multiorgan dysfunction syndrome (MODS).

Gram-positive organisms, such as *Staphylococcus, Streptococcus,* and *Enterococcus* actively secrete an exotoxin, which consists of two polypeptide components: the first binds the protein to the host cell, and the second has toxic effects. *Staphylococcus aureus* produces four cytolytic exotoxins, the most important of which—α toxin—punctures holes in the membranes of cells leading to osmotic lysis. In addition, *S. aureus* produces a number of superantigens that have an affinity for T-cell receptor major histocompatibility complex (MHC) class II antigen complexes. They activate a large number of T cells, leading to massive release of cytokines and toxic shock. *Clostridium difficile* produces two exotoxins: toxin A and toxin B.

In addition to toxins, bacteria possess a variety of virulence factors that contribute to the establishment of infection. For example, group A streptococci produce hyaluronidase and various proteases and collagenases, which facilitate the spread of the bacteria along tissue plains. *Staphylococcus epidermidis* produces a biofilm that coats intravascular devices and endotracheal tubes, making elimination by antibiotics almost impossible. Coliforms and *Pseudomonas* species have pili that allow the organism to bind and anchor to the epithelium, potentially a mechanism of bacterial translocation.

Fungal infections are common in the hospitalized population. Commensal organisms, such as *Candida* species, become pathogenic as a result of host factors (e.g., immunosuppression, concomitant infection, diabetes) and iatrogenic factors (e.g., multiple antibiotics, critical illness, parenteral nutrition, abdominal surgery). The gastrointestinal tract appears to be an important source of *Candida;* the mechanism of candidemia is unclear (Fig. 12-2).

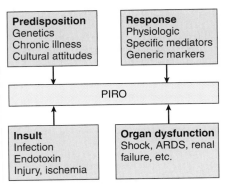

FIGURE 12–2 The PIRO model of sepsis and SIRS. *(Adapted from SCCM/ESICM/ACCP/ATS/SIS International Sepsis Definitions Conference. Crit Care Med 2003;31:1250-1256.)*

The Inflammatory Cascades

Tissue injury or pathogens (bacteria, viruses, fungi, or parasites) cause monocyte activation, which produces interleukin (IL-1, IL-6), tumor necrosis factor-alpha (TNF-α), plasminogen inactivator inhibitor-1 (PAI-1), and interferon gamma.[11,12] These cytokines subsequently modulate the release and activation of a medley of different agents: IL-8, complement, histamine, kinins, serotonin, selectins, eicosanoids, and neutrophils. This leads to local vasodilatation, release of various cytotoxic chemicals, and destruction of the invading pathogen. The release of cytotoxic material and proinflammatory cytokines results in the systemic inflammatory response: fever or hypothermia, tachypnea, tachycardia, and leukocytosis or neutropenia.

In a subgroup of patients there is an abnormal ("malignant") inflammatory response: tissue destruction by neutrophils, endothelial cell destruction, and massive systemic release of mediators. The result is vasoplegia, capillary leak, and activation of clotting cascades.

Damage to the endothelium exposes a procoagulant factor known as *tissue factor.* This exists in the subendothelial space and has a role in reparation after tissue damage. In sepsis, there is massive exposure. Tissue factor binds to activated factor VII. The resulting complex activates, in turn, factors IX and X. Factor X converts prothrombin into thrombin, which cleaves fibrinogen into fibrin—a blood clot. At the same time, the fibrinolytic system is inhibited. Cytokines and thrombin stimulate the release of PAI-1 from platelets and the endothelium. In the human body, when a clot forms, it is ultimately broken down by plasmin, which is activated by tissue plasminogen activator (TPA) from plasminogen. PAI-1 inhibits TPA.

Thrombin itself is an activator of inflammation and inhibitor of fibrinolysis. The latter is achieved by the activation of thrombin-activatable fibrinolysis inhibitor (TAFI). Thrombomodulin, another modulator of fibrinolysis, is impaired by inflammation and endothelial injury. The function of this compound is to activate protein C. Activated protein C modifies the inflammatory and coagulant response at several different levels; a deficiency occurs owing to inhibition of thrombomodulin in sepsis.

Hemodynamic Derangement in Sepsis

There are three major cardiovascular upsets in sepsis:

1. *Vasoplegia:* pathologic vasodilatation is due to loss of normal sympathetic tone, caused by the combination of local vasodilator metabolites. There is activation of adenosine triphosphate–sensitive potassium channels, leading to hyperpolarization of smooth muscle cells.[13,14] There is increased production of inducible nitric oxide synthetase (iNOS), which manufactures massive amounts of nitric oxide. In addition there is acute depletion of vasopressin.[15] Vasoplegia leads to relative hypovolemia. Vascular tone is characteristically resistant to catecholamine therapy but very sensitive to vasopressin.

2. *Reduced stroke volume* (SV): this results from the presence of a circulating myocardial depressant factor, probably TNF-α. There is reversible biventricular failure, a decreased ejection fraction, myocardial edema, and ischemia. Cardiac output is maintained by a dramatic increase in heart rate.[16]

3. *Microcirculatory failure*[17]: the small blood vessels vasodilate, and there is widespread capillary leak, maldistribution of flow, arteriovenous shunting, and oxygen utilization defects.[18] These abnormalities are incompletely understood. In addition, there is initial activation of the coagulation system and deposition of intravascular clot, causing ischemia.

The relative hypovolemia of early sepsis is virtually indistinguishable from hypovolemic or hemorrhagic shock. In response to intravascular volume depletion (distributive or hypovolemic shock), the precapillary arterioles and postcapillary venules vasoconstrict, increasing blood flow velocity, which draws fluid in from the interstitium (a net influx of fluid into the circulation). This is known as *transcapillary refill.* Fluid effectively shifts from the extravascular to the intravascular space. An oxygen debt is incurred, and there may be lactic acidosis. At this stage, patients are highly sensitive to volume resuscitation.

Eventually, persistent release of cytokines leads to depletion of reserve: there is hyperpolarization of vascular smooth muscles, massive release of iNOS, vasopressin depletion, and widespread increase in vascular permeability. The result is vasoplegia and sequestration of intravascular fluid into extracellular space. There is interstitial edema, hemoconcentration, and increased blood viscosity. There is parallel activation of clotting cascades,

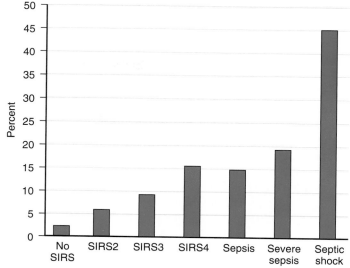

FIGURE 12–3 Mortality in SIRS/sepsis/septic shock. *(From Rangel-Frausto M, Pittet D, Costigan M, et al: The natural history of the systemic inflammatory response syndrome [SIRS]: A prospective study. JAMA 1995; 273:117-125.)*

intravascular thrombosis, and bleeding. Finally, the capacity of mitochondria to extract oxygen is impaired and multiorgan dysfunction results (Fig. 12-3).

Multiorgan Dysfunction Syndrome

The brain and kidneys are normally protected from swings in blood pressure by autoregulation. In early sepsis the autoregulation curve shifts rightward (owing to an increase in sympathetic tone). In late sepsis vasoplegia occurs and autoregulation fails, making these organs susceptible to the swings that occur in systemic blood pressure. In addition, "steal" phenomena may occur (areas of ischemia may have their blood "stolen" by areas with good perfusion). This is known as vasomotor neuropathy. Acute tubular necrosis results from cellular apoptosis, toxic injury (mechanism unclear—possibly cellular lysosomes and debris), hypotension, and hypovolemia.[19]

Patients become confused, delirious, and ultimately stuporous and comatose owing to a variety of insults: hypoperfusion injury, septic encephalopathy, metabolic encephalopathy, and, of course, drugs used for sedation.

Myocardial oxygen supply is dependent on diastolic blood pressure, which falls following vasoplegia, and on intravascular volume depletion. This may lead to ischemia. There is reversible biventricular dilatation, decreased ejection fraction, and decreased response to fluid resuscitation and catecholamine stimulation. A circulating myocardial depressant substance is responsible for this phenomenon. This substance has been shown to represent low concentrations of TNF-α and IL-1β acting in synergy on the myocardium through mechanisms that include nitric oxide and cyclic guanosine monophosphate generation.

In the lungs ventilation-perfusion mismatches occur, initially owing to increased dead space (due to hypotension and fluid shifts) and subsequently due to shunt.[20] There is increased extravascular lung water and widespread disruption of the alveolar-capillary basement membrane, leading to acute lung injury. Up to 70% of patients develop nosocomial pneumonia. It has been suggested that cytokines released as a consequence of ventilator-induced lung injury may have adverse effects at distant organs.[21] This hypothesis was confirmed from data in the Acute Respiratory Distress Syndrome (ARDS) Network trial supported by the National Institutes of Health.[22] Blood samples were obtained from 204 of the first 234 patients for measurement of plasma IL-6 concentration. Levels of this cytokine were significantly higher in the high stretch (tidal volume, 10 to 12 mL/kg) compared with the low stretch (tidal volume, 5 to 6 mL/kg) group. In addition to lower mortality, this group had a significantly lower incidence of nonpulmonary organ injury (the lung origin theory of sepsis).

There is significant hepatic dysfunction in sepsis. Uncontrolled production of inflammatory cytokines by the Kupffer cells (of the liver), primed by ischemia and stimulated by endotoxin (derived from the gut), leads to cholestasis and hyperbilirubinemia. There is decreased synthesis of albumin, clotting factors, cytochrome P450, and biliary transporters. There is impaired ketogenesis, ureagenesis, and gluconeogenesis: this is due to decreased expression of genes encoding gluconeogenic, β-oxidative, and ureagenic enzymes.[23]

Gut mucosa is usually protected from injury by autoregulation. Hypotension and hypovolemia lead to superficial mucosal injury. This results in atrophy and possible translocation of bacteria into the portal circulation and stimulates liver macrophages, causing cytokine release and amplification of SIRS (the gut origin theory of sepsis).[24,25]

Metabolic abnormalities in sepsis include hyperglycemia due to glycogenolysis, insulin resistance, and massive release of catecholamines and lactic acidosis. There is a generalized catabolic state that leads to muscle breakdown, not unlike marasmus. There is relative hypothyroidism, hypopituitarism, and adrenal insufficiency.[26,27]

Activated Protein C

Protein C is an important anticoagulant and anti-inflammatory protein. The main effect of protein C is to reduce the production of thrombin, by inactivating factors Va and VIII. Thrombin is proinflammatory, procoagulant, and antifibrinolytic.[28] In addition, protein C inhibits the influence of tissue factor on the clotting system, reduces the production of IL-1, IL-6, and TNF-α by monocytes, and has profibrinolytic properties through the inactivation of PAI-1 (it inactivates the inhibitor of the activator of the agent that converts plasminogen into plasmin).[24]

The Prowess trial has suggested that the exogenous administration of activated protein C to patients, in severe sepsis, may improve outcome.[29] However, the results of the single trial have been controversial, and there is no survival benefit in patients with severe sepsis and Apache II scores less than 25. The major clinical drawback of treatment with activated protein C is bleeding, particularly in perioperative patients.

Treating the Patient with Septic Shock

Patients with acute severe sepsis (e.g., necrotizing fasciitis or gas gangrene) are infrequently brought to the operating room for emergent source control. In this circumstance, the anesthesiologist will be required to both administer anesthesia, ensuring amnesia, analgesia, and hypnosis, and resuscitate the patient. A familiarity with modern resuscitation practices is thus important.

There are four main pillars to the management of the patient with severe sepsis: (1) immediate resuscitation, (2) empirical therapy, (3) source control, and (4) preventing further complications (Fig. 12-4).

Stage 1: Immediate Resuscitation

Immediate Stabilization (Airway and Breathing). The initial treatment priority in patients with severe sepsis is to reverse life-threatening physiologic abnormalities. The airway must be controlled and the patient oxygenated and ventilated. This usually requires endotracheal intubation and commencement of mechanical ventilation. Care must be taken when administering anesthetic agents for gaining airway control. Propofol usually causes dramatic hypotension, owing to peripheral vasodilatation and vagotonia, and should be avoided. Etomidate and ketamine are reasonable choices. Although opioids are frequently used in cardiac anesthesia for hemodynamic stability, they have significant antiadrenergic effects in sepsis and may cause dramatic hypotension. Therapies directed at slowing heart rate should be avoided, as tachycardia is the main compensatory mechanism in maintenance of cardiac output.

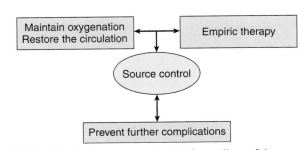

FIGURE 12-4   Treating sepsis—the four pillars of therapy.

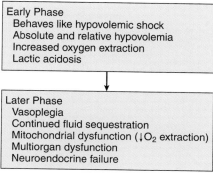

FIGURE 12–5 Two phases of sepsis resuscitation.

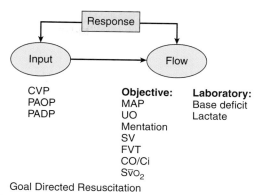

Goal Directed Resuscitation

FIGURE 12–6 Goal-directed resuscitation. CVP, central venous pressure; PAOP, pulmonary artery opening "wedge" pressure; PADP, pulmonary artery diastolic pressure; MAP, mean arterial pressure; UO, urinary output; SV, stroke volume; FVT, flow velocity time; CO, cardiac output, Ci, cardiac index, $S\bar{v}O_2$, mixed venous oxygen saturation.

After intubation, extreme care must be taken with institution of positive-pressure ventilation. The increase in intrathoracic pressure will reduce venous return: aggressive "bagging" invariably leads to severe hypotension.

Reestablishing the Circulation.

Volume Resuscitation (Fig. 12-5). In early sepsis hypotension is caused by relative hypovolemia, secondary to peripheral vasodilation. Later, hypotension is caused by myocardial depression, vasoplegia, and absolute hypovolemia secondary to capillary leak. Regardless, the initial resuscitative effort is to attempt to correct the absolute and relative hypovolemia by refilling the vascular tree. Volume resuscitation should be early (in the operating room or emergency department), aggressive, and goal directed.[30]

The choice of fluids early in resuscitation remains controversial. Initial resuscitation should include isotonic crystalloid, to replete interstitial fluid debt. Subsequent efforts are directed at maintenance of intravascular volume. If crystalloid resuscitation is continued there is significant extravasation of fluid and the patient becomes edematous.[31,32] The use of high-molecular-weight ("colloid") compounds is favored by many as a means of minimizing resuscitation volume and for potential positive oncotic effects.[31] Although the use of colloid is controversial[33,34] there is emerging evidence in support of its use in perioperative medicine and critical illness as part of a goal-directed paradigm.[35-39] The main limiting factors for colloids are availability (gelatins and pentastarches are not available in the United States) and cost. Available colloids include blood products, hydroxyethyl starches, and albumin. Previous concerns regarding albumin safety are unfounded.[40]

The goal-directed approach to resuscitation involves the use of specific monitors to measure input (fluid loading), tissue blood flow, and response (Fig. 12-6). Arterial and central lines are placed, and goals for resuscitation are set: these include a central venous pressure (CVP) of 8 to 12 cm H_2O, a mean arterial pressure (MAP) of more than 65 mm Hg, and, if the appropriate device is placed, a mixed venous oxygen saturation ($S\bar{v}O_2$) of more than 70% and an SV of between 0.7 and 1.0 mL/kg.

The Surviving Sepsis Campaign[41] promotes the use of oximetric CVP catheters to monitor input and flow (Fig. 12-7) based on the work of Rivers and colleagues.[42] Fluid is administered until the CVP reaches and stays in the target range: 8 to 12 cm H_2O for the majority of patients (Fig. 12-8). Once fluid loading has been achieved, hypotension is managed with vasopressors (norepinephrine or dopamine—see later) to a target MAP of 65 mm Hg.

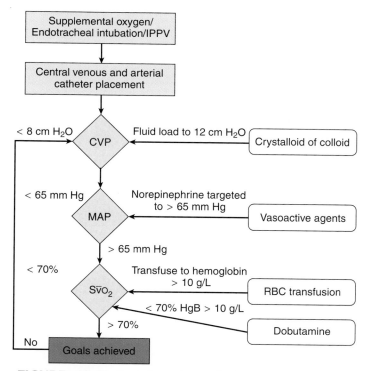

FIGURE 12–7 Goal-directed resuscitation using Oximetric CVP catheter based on the Surviving Sepsis Campaign. IPPV, intermittent positive-pressure ventilation; CVP, central venous pressure; MAP, mean arterial pressure; $S\bar{v}O_2$, mixed venous oxygen saturation; RBC, red blood cell.

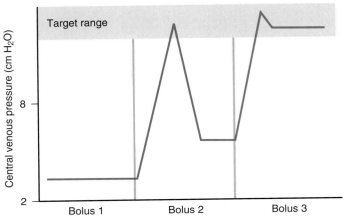

FIGURE 12–8 Goal-directed approach using central venous pressure.

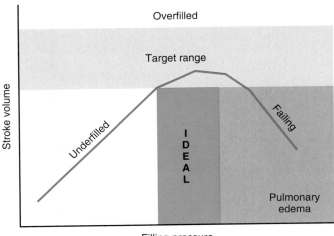

FIGURE 12–9 Using stroke volume to construct Starling curves. CVP, central venous pressure; PCWP, pulmonary capillary wedge pressure; LVEDP, left ventricular end-diastolic pressure; PADP, pulmonary artery diastolic pressure.

If the $S\bar{v}O_2$ is less than 70%, with CVP and MAP in the target range, blood is transfused until the hematocrit exceeds 30% (hemoglobin 10 g/L). If this fails to restore the $S\bar{v}O_2$, an inotrope is added, such as dobutamine or a phosphodiesterase inhibitor.

A more elegant approach involves insertion of an oximetric pulmonary artery catheter rather than a CVP line. In this paradigm, SV is used as the main end point of

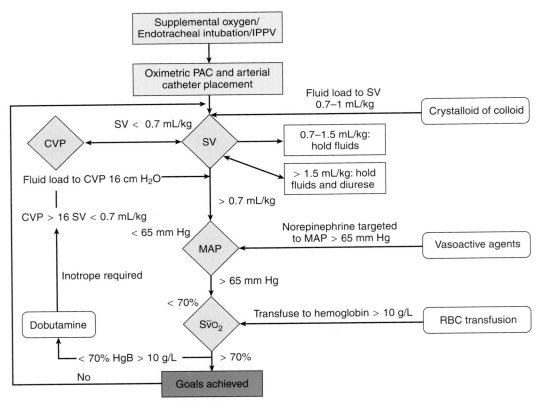

FIGURE 12–10 Algorithm for goal-directed resuscitation, using stroke volume as a measure of flow. IPPV, intermittent positive-pressure ventilation; PAC, pulmonary artery catheter; CVP, central venous pressure; SV, stroke volume; MAP, mean arterial pressure; $S\bar{v}O_2$, mixed venous oxygen saturation; RBC, red blood cell.

CVP	SvO$_2$	Stroke Volume	Clinical Impression
8 cm H$_2$O	55%	45 mL	Underfilled Underesuscitated
12 cm H$_2$O	70%	79 mL	Filled Resuscitated
18 cm H$_2$O	80%	110 mL	Overfilled Overresuscitated

FIGURE 12–11 Using the goal-directed approach to determine the effectiveness of fluid resuscitation. In this situation, the goal for stroke volume was 65 to 80 mL and for SvO$_2$ it was 70%. CVP, central venous pressure; SvO$_2$, mixed venous oxygen saturation.

resuscitation and CVP or pulmonary arterial pressure is used to determine the presence of heart failure (Fig. 12-9): a Starling curve is constructed (Fig. 12-10). Fluid is administered to the patient until the SV is in the range of 0.7 to 1 mL/kg for a sustained period (Fig. 12-11).

An SV in excess of 1.0 mL/kg is indicative of overresuscitation, and fluids are withheld until the SV drifts back into normal range. If the SV exceeds 1.5 mL/kg, serious consideration should be given to the administration of diuretics.

Vasopressor Therapy. Hypotension, unresponsive to fluid therapy, in sepsis is an indication for vasopressor use (Table 12-3). The ideal pressor agent would restore blood pressure while maintaining cardiac output and preferentially perfuse the midline structures of the body (brain, heart, splanchnic organs, and kidneys). Currently, norepinephrine is the agent of choice in the fluid-resuscitated patient.

Norepinephrine. Norepinephrine has pharmacologic effects on both α_1 and β_1 adrenoceptors. In low dosage ranges, the beta effect is noticeable and there is a mild increase in cardiac output. In most dosage ranges, vasoconstriction and increased mean arterial pressure are evident. Norepinephrine does not increase heart rate. The main beneficial effect of norepinephrine is to increase organ perfusion by increasing vascular tone. Studies that have compared norepinephrine to dopamine head to head have favored the former in terms of overall improvements in oxygen delivery, organ perfusion, and oxygen consumption. Norepinephrine is more effective at fulfilling targeted end points than dopamine,[43] is less metabolically active than epinephrine, and reduces serum lactate levels. Norepinephrine significantly improves renal perfusion and splanchnic blood flow in sepsis,[44,45] particularly when combined with dobutamine.[45]

Dopamine. Dopamine has predominantly β-adrenergic effects in low to moderate dose ranges (up to 10 MIC/kg/min), although there is much interpatient variability. This effect may be due to its conversion to norepinephrine in the myocardium and its activation of adrenergic receptors. In higher dose ranges, α-adrenoceptor activation increases and causes vasoconstriction. The agent is thus a mixed inotrope and vasoconstrictor. At all dose ranges it is a potent chronotrope. There has been much controversy about the other metabolic functions of this agent. Dopamine is a potent diuretic (it neither saves nor damages the kidneys).[46] Dopamine has complex neuroendocrine effects: it may interfere with thyroid[47] and pituitary[47] function and have an immunosuppressive effect.[48] Overall, there is no benefit to dopamine administration over norepinephrine.

Dobutamine. Dobutamine is a potent $\beta1$ agonist, with predominant effects in the heart where it increases myocardial contractility and thus SV and cardiac output. Dobutamine is associated with much less increase in heart rate than dopamine. In sepsis, dobutamine, although a vasodilator, increases oxygen delivery and consumption. Dobutamine appears particularly effective at splanchnic resuscitation, increasing pHi (gastric mucosal pH) and improving mucosal perfusion in comparison with dopamine.[49]

Epinephrine. Epinephrine has potent β_1, β_2, and α_1-adrenergic activity, although the increase in MAP in sepsis is mainly from an increase in cardiac output (SV). There are three major drawbacks from using this drug: (1) epinephrine increases myocardial oxygen demand; (2) it increases serum glucose lactate, which may be due to either worsening of perfusion to certain tissues or to a calorigenic effect

TABLE 12–3	Pharmacologic Support of the Circulation in Sepsis				
Agent	α_1	β_1	β_2	**Heart Rate**	**Organs Perfused**
Epinephrine	++++	++++	++++	↑↑↑↑	Skin, muscle
Norepinephrine	++++	++++	++	↑↑	Central organs
Dopamine	++	++	++++	↑↑↑↑	Skin, muscle
Phenylephrine	++	–	–	–	No real change

(increased release and anaerobic breakdown of glucose); and (3) epinephrine appears to have adverse effects on splanchnic blood flow,[50] redirecting blood peripherally as part of the fight or flight response.

The metabolic and hemodynamic effects makes epinephrine an unsuitable first-line agent in sepsis.

Phenylephrine. Phenylephrine is an almost pure α_1 agonist with moderate potency. Although widely used in anesthesia to treat iatrogenic hypotension, it is an ineffective agent in sepsis. Phenylephrine is a less effective vasoconstrictor than norepinephrine or epinephrine. Compared with norepinephrine, phenylephrine reduces splanchnic blood flow, oxygen delivery, and lactate uptake.[51]

Vasopressin. Vasopressin has emerged as an additive vasoconstrictor in septic patients who have become resistant to catecholamines.[52] There appears to be a quantitative deficiency of this hormone in sepsis,[15,53-55] and administration in addition to norepinephrine surprisingly increases splanchnic blood flow and urinary output. The most efficacious dose appears to be 0.04 unit/min,[56] and this is not titrated. This relatively low dose has little or no effect on normotensive patients.

Stage 2: Empirical Therapy—Antibiotics

The selection of specific antibiotics depends on:

- The presumed site of infection (see Table 12-1).
- Gram's stain results
- Suspected or known organisms
- Resistance patterns of the common hospital microbial flora
- Patient's immune status (especially neutropenia and immunosuppressive drugs), allergies, renal dysfunction, and hepatic dysfunction.
- Antibiotic availability, hospital resistance patterns, and clinical variables of the patient to be treated

Suggested Antimicrobial Regimens.

Sepsis Source Unknown. Combining either antipseudomonal cephalosporin (ceftazidine) or antipseudomonal penicillin (piperacillin + azobactam) (particularly if anaerobes are suspected) with either an aminoglycoside (gentamycin or amikacin) or a fluoroquinolone (ciprofloxacin) can be done. If an antipseudomonal cephalosporin is used and anaerobes are a possible cause, the addition of metronidazole or clindamycin should be considered.

- Piperacillin + tazobactam/imipenem + gentamycin/ciprofloxacin

Catheter-Related Bloodstream Infection. There is a strong possibility of infection with staphylococci, coagulase positive or negative.

- Vancomycin should be added to, for example, piperacillin + tazobactam. Once the infecting organisms have been isolated, the spectrum of antimicrobials should be narrowed (if methicillin-resistant *S. aureus* (MRSA) is isolated, the piperacillin + tazobactam should be discontinued).
- Vancomycin + piperacillin + tazobactam or ciprofloxacin

Community-Acquired Pneumonia. The most likely organisms are pneumococci, *Mycoplasma,* and *Legionella.* The patient requires coverage for both gram-positive and atypical organisms.

- Cephalosporin IV + macrolide PO or fluoroquinolone
- Cefuroxime/ceftriaxone IV + azithromycin PO or levofloxacin

Intra-abdominal Sepsis. The most likely infecting organisms are Enterobacteriaceae, enterococci, *S. pneumoniae,* and anaerobes. Broad-spectrum treatment is required, without cover for *Pseudomonas.*

- Penicillin + β-lactam inhibitor or ampicillin + aminoglycoside + antianaerobic agent
- Ampicillin + sulbactam or piperacillin + tazobactam or ampicillin + gentamicin/aztreonam + metronidazole or imipenem

Urosepsis. The most common organisms causing urinary tract infections are Enterobacteriaceae and enterococci, and the treatment is ciprofloxacin or ampicillin and gentamicin. In this case, however, the patient has been admitted from a nursing home and *Pseudomonas* is a strong possibility. Twin therapy is often required, not mixing β-lactam antibiotics:

- Antipseudomonal quinolone or aminoglycoside plus antipseudomonal penicillin or cephalosporin.
- Ciprofloxacin/gentamicin/amikacin plus piperacillin or ceftazidine

Cellulitis. The most likely organisms are streptococci and staphylococci. If the infection is community acquired, then cloxacillin is adequate. Again, this patient was institutionalized and the infection must be treated as hospital acquired:

- Vancomycin + gentamycin

Necrotizing Fasciitis. Type 1 (see later) is due to group A streptococci, and type 2 is polymicrobial and due to streptococci, staphylococci, *Bacteroides,* and *Clostridium.*[57]

- Penicillin (high dose) or ciprofloxacin (if penicillin allergic) + clindamycin
- Add ampicillin + sulbactam or piperacillin + tazobactam

Meningococcemia. Bacterial meningitis is meningococcal septicemia until otherwise proven. The most likely alternative organisms are pneumococci, *Hemophilus influenzae,* and, rarely, Enterobacteriaceae and Listeria.

- Third-generation cephalosporin + vancomycin (if penicillin-resistant *S. pneumoniae* suspected) + ampicillin (if *Listeria* suspected)
- Cefotaxime + vancomycin

Stage 3: Source Control

Source control is the essential curative measure in the management of sepsis and the associated inflammatory response. Although there is a myriad of potential causes of sepsis, beyond medical causes, such as pneumonia or meningitis, source control can be neatly summarized by applying the four Ds rule (Fig. 12-12)[41]: abscesses should be *d*rained, necrotic tissue should be *d*ébrided, infected *d*evices removed and recurrent sources of infection/inflammation (e.g., cholecystitis or diverticulitis) *d*efinitively controlled. This represents the major involvement of anesthesiologists within the sepsis paradigm: patients travel to the operating room for source control under anesthesia.

Stage 4: Prevention of Further Complications

A significant aspect of the critical care management of septic patients is prevention of complications. This applies also to their perioperative care. Many patients with acute severe sepsis have a concomitant hypoxic lung injury (e.g., ARDS) requiring intensive mechanical ventilatory support. This usually involves the application of high mean airway pressures to prevent de-recruitment of involved lung tissue. It is imperative that lung volume be maintained perioperatively. If the patient is requiring more than 10 cm H$_2$O of positive end-expiratory pressure

(PEEP) or is on inverse-ratio pressure-controlled or airway pressure-release ventilation then the following guidelines should be followed:

1. The operating room mechanical ventilator must be of sufficient capacity to maintain high mean airway pressure. Although some modern ventilators have this capacity, the majority of "bag in bottle" bellows are insufficient. When there is doubt, the patient should be transferred to the operating room with their ICU ventilator.
2. Extreme care must be taken to avoid disconnection from the ventilator: even short periods of disconnection (i.e., for changing from ventilator to anesthesia machine) may result is significant de-recruitment of the lung and life-threatening hypoxemia.
3. The endotracheal tube should be clamped before disconnections to maintain lung recruitment.
4. If accidental disconnection should occur, sustained inflation maneuvers should be performed to re-recruit the lung.
5. Critically ill patients are usually nursed in the semi-recumbent position. Patients lie supine in the operating room. This often results in an increase in chest wall elastance, requiring higher levels of PEEP to maintain lung volumes.
6. The standard of care in the management of patients with ARDS is to limit end inspiratory lung volumes to a plateau pressure of 30 cm H$_2$O or less and a tidal volume of 6 mL/kg or less.[31] This is to avoid "volutrama," a ventilator-associated lung injury.[58]

Care must be taken to maintain circulating volume and blood flow to tissues. During surgical débridement of, for example, necrotizing pancreatitis or fasciitis, handling of inflamed or infected tissues usually leads to significant systemic release of cytokines, worsening vasoplegia and increasing myocardial depression. The anesthesiologist must be careful to titrate vasopressors and bolus fluids in response to rapidly changing hemodynamics.

Patients with severe sepsis are at significant risk of secondary organ injuries, particularly to the liver and kidneys. Medications that are renally metabolized or excreted (e.g., pancuronium, morphine) should be used with caution. Aminoglycosides and glycopeptides (e.g., vancomycin) must be administered with reference to pharmacokinetics. Nonsteroidal anti-inflammatory agents should be avoided, because they may precipitate acute renal failure, worsen coagulopathy, and induce upper gastrointestinal bleeding in a vulnerable population. Although hepatic metabolism is well preserved in patients with liver dysfunction in sepsis, consideration should be given to the use of agents metabolized independently of the liver (e.g., cisatracurium rather than vecuronium or pancuronium; remifentanil rather than fentanyl or morphine).

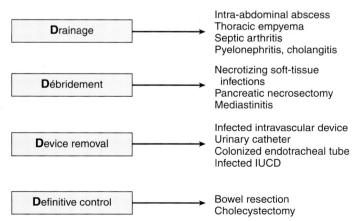

FIGURE 12–12 The 4 Ds of source control. IUCD, intrauterine contraceptive device.

The choice of anesthesia agents is dependent on a number of factors. Many patients are transported to the operating room in an induced coma (e.g., lorazepam or midazolam plus morphine or hydromorphone infusions), and little additional anesthesia is required. In the awake patient, in whom anesthesia is being induced, care should be taken as described previously. For maintenance of anesthesia, sufficient agents must be administered to maintain hypnosis and amnesia. Frequently this is not possible with volatile agents, owing to peripheral vasodilatation and hypotension. Ketamine is a good alternative, particularly if accompanied by an infusion of fentanyl or remifentanil or hydromorphone.

Patients with acute severe sepsis are at high risk for perioperative bleeding, owing to sepsis-induced coagulopathy and thrombocytopenia. Aggressive volume repletion with red cells, thawed plasma, and platelets is recommended. Activated protein C (drotrecogin alfa activated) significantly increases the risk of bleeding and must be discontinued at least 2 hours before surgical procedures and not restarted until at least 2 hours after surgery (Table 12-4).

TRANSMISSIBLE INFECTIONS AND ANESTHESIA

Hepatitis B and C

Hepatitis B

Hepatitis B is a small, double-stranded DNA hepadnavirus. It is spread by sexual intercourse, with a high degree of infectivity, via secretions and blood products. Health care workers are at particularly high risk of exposure through handling of blood/tissue or needle-stick injuries.

The outer core of the virus contains a surface antigen (HBsAg) that elicits production of a neutralizing antibody (anti-HBs). In addition, the body generates a separate antibody (anti-HBc) against the viral core antigen (HBcAg). A third viral antigen—the hepatitis B e antigen (HBeAg)—is also released from the core. The presence of this antigen in the serum is indicative of active viral replication. The presence of the antibody to this particle (anti-HBe) is indicative of the end of active viral replication.

Clinical and Pathologic Features. One to 6 weeks after exposure, HBsAg appears in the serum; its disappearance after 6 months indicates recovery (Fig. 12-13). The presence of HBsAg for greater than 6 months indicates chronic disease/carrier status (5% to 10% of infections). Past exposure of immunization can be detected by anti-HBs. In the majority of patients, anti-HBs does not rise to detectable levels until several weeks after the disappearance of the surface antigen and remains detectable for life. There may be a window in which neither antibody nor antigen are detectable. Consequently, another test is required to ensure diagnosis. This is to detect the presence of IgM antibody directed against the core antigen (IgM-anti-HBc), which is the earliest discernible anti–hepatitis B antibody. The presence of HBeAg implies high infectivity—it is usually present from 1.5 to 3 months after acute infection. The presence of anti-HBc indicates past exposure (see Fig. 12-13).

TABLE 12–4 Perioperative Care of the Patient with Established Severe Sepsis

Monitoring	Continuation of all monitoring procedures in the ICU
Fluid Administration	Fluid administration should be goal directed based on predetermined end points.
Anesthesia Agents	Determined by hemodynamic stability, whether the patient will tolerate volatile agents, preexisting infusions (e.g., lorazepam and morphine), pharmacokinetics, etc.
Mechanical Ventilation	Transport with ICU ventilator if PEEP >10 cm H_2O, inverse ratio pressure controlled or airway pressure release ventilation in use. Avoid ventilator disconnection (use clamp). Accidental disconnection should be followed by recruitment maneuvers. Inhaled nitric oxide or prostacyclin should be continued.
Vasopressors	Vasopressors should be continued; additional bags of medication should be available to avoid catastrophic cessation. Corticosteroids (for adrenal insufficiency) should be continued.
Nutrition	Gastric feeds should be discontinued 6 hours before surgery; postpyloric feeds may be continued (at the discretion of the anesthesiologist). Total parenteral nutrition should be continued.
Coagulation	All anticoagulants should be stopped before surgery. Activated protein C should be stopped 2 hours before surgery.
Renal Replacement Therapy	Continuous renal replacement therapy should be stopped 6 hours before surgery to allow autoreversal of heparin.
Antimicrobials	Dosage based on predicted microbes, resistance patterns of patient and hospital, renal function, and pharmacokinetics.

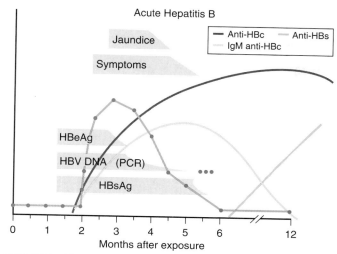

Acute Hepatitis B

FIGURE 12–13 The serologic course of acute hepatitis B. *(From Goldman L, Bennett JC [eds]: Cecil Textbook of Medicine, 21st ed. Philadelphia, WB Saunders, 2002.)*

After exposure, the incubation period is approximately 12 weeks, with resolution of symptoms after 30 to 60 days. Symptoms include a prodrome of pyrexia, anorexia, myalgia, urticaria, and nausea, followed by jaundice, hepatosplenomegaly, and lymphadenopathy. There is an increase in serum bilirubin and hepatic transaminases. Five to 10 percent of patients go on to develop chronic active hepatitis.

Anesthesia Implications. Patients who are acutely infected with hepatitis B who present for surgery represent a unique risk for health care personnel, particularly anesthesiologists. Universal precautions should be taken when dealing with tissues or body fluids (Table 12-5). Following needle-stick injury, the risk of developing clinical hepatitis B or serologic conversion, in a worker who is not immune, if the blood is positive for both HBsAg and HBeAg is approximately 25% and 50%, respectively. If the blood is HBsAg positive and HBeAg negative, however, the respective risks are only 3% and 30%.

Health care workers who have antibodies to hepatitis B virus either from pre-exposure vaccination or prior infection are not at risk. In addition, if a susceptible worker is exposed to hepatitis B virus, postexposure prophylaxis with hepatitis B immune globulin and initiation of hepatitis B vaccine is more than 90% effective in preventing hepatitis B infection (see Table 12-6 for recommendations).

Hepatitis C

Hepatitis C is the most common chronic bloodborne viral infection in the United States. It affects 300 million people worldwide, including 4 million Americans. The virus involved, a single strand of RNA, was first identified

TABLE 12–5 Universal Precautions

1. **Barrier protection** should be used at all times to prevent skin and mucous membrane contamination with blood, body fluids containing visible blood, or other body fluids (cerebrospinal, synovial, pleural, peritoneal, pericardial, and amniotic fluids, semen and vaginal secretions). Barrier protection should be used with ALL tissues. The type of barrier protection used should be appropriate for the type of procedures being performed and the type of exposure anticipated. Examples of barrier protection include disposable laboratory coats, gloves, and eye and face protection.

2. **Gloves** are to be worn when there is potential for hand or skin contact with blood, other potentially infectious material, or items and surfaces contaminated with these materials.

3. Wear **face protection** (face shield) during procedures that are likely to generate droplets of blood or body fluid to prevent exposure to mucous membranes of the mouth, nose, and eyes.

4. Wear **protective body clothing** (disposable laboratory coats) when there is a potential for splashing of blood or body fluids.

5. **Wash hands** or other skin surfaces thoroughly and immediately if contaminated with blood, body fluids containing visible blood, or other body fluids to which universal precautions apply.

6. **Wash hands immediately** after gloves are removed.

7. **Avoid accidental injuries** that can be caused by needles, scalpel blades, laboratory instruments, etc., when performing procedures, cleaning instruments, handling sharp instruments, and disposing of used needles, pipettes, etc.

8. Used needles, disposable syringes, scalpel blades, pipettes, and other sharp items are to be placed in **puncture-resistant containers** marked with a biohazard symbol for disposal.

in 1989. The infection is primarily spread by parenteral administration of blood, blood products, and needle sharing among intravenous drug abusers.

Clinical and Pathologic Features. The incubation period is 6 to 10 weeks. The majority of patients remain asymptomatic. Fifty to 70 percent of infected patients develop chronic hepatitis C, of which 50% will develop cirrhosis over a period of 20 to 30 years. Hepatitis C is a leading cause of hepatic failure in the United States. Forty percent of patients who undergo hepatic transplantation have this disease.

The nosocomial risk of hepatitis C seroconversion after a single incident of a needle stick in the health care setting is estimated to be in the 2% to 8% range. Needle-stick injury with hollow needles is associated with a 6- to 10-fold greater likelihood of transmission than when it

TABLE 12–6   Recommended Postexposure Prophylaxis for Exposure to Hepatitis B Virus

Vaccination and Antibody Response Status of Exposed Workers*	Treatment		
	Source HBsAg[†] Positive	Source HBsAg Negative	Source Unknown or Not Available for Testing
Unvaccinated	HBIG[‡] × 1 and initiate HB vaccine series[§]	Initiate HB vaccine series	Initiate HB vaccine series
Previously vaccinated known responder[‖]	No treatment	No treatment	No treatment
Known nonresponder[¶]	HBIG × 1 and initiate revaccination or HBIG × 2**	No treatment	If known high risk source, treat as if source were HBsAg positive
Antibody response unknown	Test exposed person for anti-HBs[††] 1. If adequate,[‖] no treatment is necessary. 2. If inadequate,[¶] administer HBIG × 1 and vaccine booster.	No treatment	Test exposed person for anti-HBs 1. If adequate,[‖] no treatment is necessary. 2. If inadequate,[¶] administer vaccine booster and recheck titer in 1-2 months.

*Persons who have previously been infected with HBV are immune to reinfection and do not require postexposure prophylaxis.
[†]Hepatitis B surface antigen.
[‡]Hepatitis B immune globulin; dose is 0.06 mL/kg intramuscularly.
[§]Hepatitis B vaccine.
[‖]A responder is a person with adequate levels of serum antibody to HBsAg (i.e., anti-HBs ≥ 10 mIU/mL).
[¶]A nonresponder is a person with inadequate response to vaccination (i.e., serum anti-HBs < 10 mIU/mL).
**The option of giving one dose of HBIG and reinitiating the vaccine series is preferred for nonresponders who have not completed a second three-dose vaccine series. For persons who previously completed a second vaccine series but failed to respond, two doses of HBIG are preferred.
[††]Antibody to HBsAg.
From Updated U.S. Public Health Service Guidelines for the Management of Occupational Exposures to HBV, HCV, and HIV and Recommendations for Postexposure Prophylaxis. MMWR Morbid Mortal Weekly Rep 2001;50(RR-11):22.

occurs from contaminated solid-bore needles. There is no vaccine or effective immunoglobulin for these patients. Seroconversion is confirmed by the detection of hepatitis C virus RNA in the serum. Treatment is targeted at a sustained virologic response using interferon alfa and ribavirin. This results in normalization of serum transaminase levels in 50% of patients.

Anesthesia Implications. The anesthesiologist and operating room staff are particularly vulnerable to acquiring hepatitis C by way of needle-stick injury or from contaminated blood or tissues. Patients with a known history of hepatitis B or C or high-risk patients (e.g., intravenous drug abusers) should be managed with strict barrier precautions (see Table 12-5). High-quality gloves (or two pairs of gloves) should be worn. Hands must be rigorously washed after gloves are removed, and contaminated gloves should be disposed of rapidly. Barrier protection of the eyes and mouth is imperative. Contaminated needles should not be recapped, manipulated with both hands, or manually removed from a syringe. They should be disposed of, alongside contaminated sutures and other sharp objects, in a solid, carefully marked container adjacent to the operative site.

HIV/AIDS

Forty million people (range, 34 to 46 million) were living with HIV/AIDS by the end of 2003 with 5 million new cases that year. It has been estimated that 20% to 25% of HIV-positive patients will require surgery during their illness.[59]

Clinical and Pathologic Features. HIV-1 is a single-strand RNA retrovirus. After entering the cell, the virus is copied by a reverse transcriptase; this enables the virus to produce double-stranded DNA, which then integrates into the host's cells. The most common mode of infection is sexual transmission through the genital mucosa. HIV may also be spread by transfusion of contaminated blood or by needle sharing or needle-stick injury.

Within 2 days the virus can be detected in the internal iliac lymph nodes, and within 5 days (range, 4 to 11 days) the virus can be cultured from the plasma. There is rapid dissemination to lymphoid tissue and the brain. The CD4+ T lymphocytes (T-helper cells) are the primary target of infection. Progression of HIV illness is defined by the decline in CD4+ cell count leading to immune deficiency and manifest by opportunistic infections and unusual neoplasia. Thus progression is followed by monitoring the cell count per cubic millimeter.

Plasma viral load (which can be quantified) is initially extremely high and then declines in the clinical latency period. This early acute infection, the seroconversion illness, is transient; symptoms include fever, fatigue, rash, headache, lymphadenopathy, pharyngitis, myalgia or arthralgia, and nausea, vomiting, and diarrhea. This may be confused with a flu-like illness.

The clinical latency period may last 7 to 12 years during which time billions of virions and CD4+ cells are destroyed each day. The T lymphocytes are replenished and immune status remains functional.

Prior to the development of "full blown AIDS" the patient enters a stage of persistent generalized lymphadenopathy. In this stage nodes of greater than 1 cm in more than two noninguinal sites are present for more than 3 months. The patient may lose weight and develop seborrheic dermatitis.

AIDS is diagnosed by a CD4+ count of less than 200 cells/µL or the presence of one or more defining illnesses (Table 12-7). The patient is at significant risk for opportunistic infections and malignancies, including toxoplasmosis, cryptococcal meningitis, progressive multifocal leukoencephalopathy, cytomegalovirus infection, herpes symplex virus infection, brain lymphomas, and tuberculosis. HIV is thus a multisystem disease (Table 12-8).

With the development of constitutional symptoms (physiologic reserve is depleted), viral load again increases and the patient becomes extremely infectious. This has significant implications for health care providers.

Anesthesia and HIV. Perioperative risk correlates well with immune function. A CD4+ cell count of less than 200 cells/µL puts the patient at significant risk for opportunistic infections and increased infectious risk associated with surgery.[60] The presence of pulmonary, cardiac, or renal disease may also lead to perioperative complications. Consequently, the patient with AIDS requires significant preoperative workup. This should include complete blood cell count, a coagulation panel, and liver and renal function tests. The patient should have an electrocardiogram and chest radiograph, regardless of age and gender. If there is a history of pulmonary disease, and the patient is undergoing major surgery, pulmonary function testing is necessary.

There are numerous airway complications of HIV/AIDS: oral candidiasis, herpes simplex ulcers (risk of transmission to the laryngoscopist), and hemorrhagic Kaposi's sarcoma lesions. Lung parenchyma may be damaged by *Pneumocystis*, histoplasmosis, cytomegalovirus, or tuberculosis, with significant impact on gas exchange. This may lead to a higher F_{IO_2} requirement intraoperatively, and prolonged postoperative mechanical ventilation.

TABLE 12–7   AIDS-Defining Illnesses

Candidiasis of bronchi, trachea, lungs, or esophagus
Invasive cervical cancer
Coccidioidomycosis, disseminated or extrapulmonary
Cryptococcosis, extrapulmonary
Cryptosporidiosis, chronic intestinal (greater than 1 month's duration)
Cytomegalovirus disease (other than liver, spleen, or nodes)
Cytomegalovirus retinitis (with loss of vision)
Encephalopathy, HIV-related
Herpes simplex: chronic ulcer(s) (greater than 1 month's duration); or bronchitis, pneumonitis, or esophagitis
Histoplasmosis, disseminated or extrapulmonary
Isosporiasis, chronic intestinal (greater than 1 month's duration)
Kaposi's sarcoma
Lymphoma, Burkitt's (or equivalent term)
Lymphoma, immunoblastic (or equivalent term)
Lymphoma, primary, of brain
Mycobacterium avium complex or *M. kansasii*, disseminated or extrapulmonary
Mycobacterium tuberculosis, any site (pulmonary or extrapulmonary)
Mycobacterium, other species or unidentified species, disseminated or extrapulmonary
Pneumocystis carinii pneumonia
Pneumonia, recurrent
Progressive multifocal leukoencephalopathy
Salmonella septicemia, recurrent
Toxoplasmosis of brain

The cardiovascular system may be affected by autonomic neuropathy (inadequate heart rate response to vasodilatory effects of anesthetic agents), cardiomyopathy, and myocardial lymphoma. If cardiac involvement is suspected, the patient should have preoperative echocardiography to determine both systolic and diastolic function. The presence of significant cardiac dysfunction is an indication for invasive perioperative monitoring.

Many neurologic problems are associated with HIV/AIDS. These include delirium, headache, localized or generalized seizures, limb weakness, and visual loss. It is important to document, preoperatively, the presence or absence of focal neurologic deficit to avoid confusion with complications of anesthesia and surgery. The presence of AIDS-related dementia may preclude the patient consenting to both surgery and anesthesia.[61]

A variety of opportunistic infections of the gastrointestinal tract manifest in HIV/AIDS. Chronic diarrhea is common and associated with hypokalemia and volume

TABLE 12–8   Complications of HIV Multiorgan Disease

Respiratory

Pneumocystis carinii

Bacterial pneumonia

Tuberculosis

Aspergillosis

Cytomegalovirus

Oral/pharyngeal candidiasis, herpetic infections

Hematologic

Leukopenia, lymphopenia

Thrombocytopenia

Anemia

Drug toxicity, bone marrow suppression

Cardiac

Pericarditis effusion

Pericarditis

Myocarditis (late stages of infection)

Dilated cardiomyopathy

Endocarditis (intravenous drug abuse)

Pulmonary hypertension

Drug-related cardiotoxicity

Thromboembolitic events

Myocardial infarction

Gastrointestinal

Infectious diarrhea, proctitis

Gastrointestinal bleeding

Acalculous cholecystitis

Vomiting, loss of appetite, cachexia

Dysphagia (*Candida albicans*, cytomegalovirus), esophagitis

Liver disease, hepatitis B and C, other infections

Neurologic Problems in AIDS Patients

Distal, symmetrical sensory neuropathy: numbness, tingling, painful dysesthesias and paresthesias

Chronic, inflammatory demyelinating polyneuropathy

AIDS encephalopathy or AIDS dementia complex: cognitive, motor, and behavioral changes

Vacuolar myelopathy: sensory disturbance, spasticity and hyperreflexia (acute or chronic progression)

Segmental (focal) myelopathy, acute or subacute (less common)

Data from Hughes SC: HIV and Anesthesia. Anesthesiol Clin North Am 2004;22:379-404.

TABLE 12–9   Antiretroviral Drug Therapy: Side Effects with Anesthetic Significance

Side Effect	Responsible Antiretroviral Drug
Neutropenia	Ganciclovir Trimethoprim/sulfamethoxazole
Thrombocytopenia	Isoniazid Phenytoin Rifampin Zidovudine
Electrolyte disturbances	Protease inhibitors Pentamidine
Hepatic dysfunction	Ethambutol Phenytoin
Peripheral neuropathy	Didanosine Lamivudine Stavudine Zalcitabine
Bronchospasm	Pentamidine
Cardiac dysrhythmias	Pentamidine

From Kuczkowski KM: Human immunodeficiency virus in the parturient. J Clin Anesth 2003;15:224-233.

depletion. Colonic perforation has been associated with cytomegalic colitis. Lymphoma has been associated with bowel obstruction, increasing the risk of aspiration pneumonitis.

Patients with HIV/AIDS have a predisposition for anemia, as a consequence of bone marrow suppression, associated with chronic disease, malnutrition (gastrointestinal involvement impairs iron, vitamin B_{12}, and folate absorption), and drug therapy (zidovudine).

Past medical/social history is of particular importance in this patient population. Substance abuse, and intravenous drug abuse in particular, remains the most significant risk factor. The concurrent presence of sexually transmitted diseases such as hepatitis B, hepatitis C (severe hepatic involvement), and syphilis (neurologic deficits in late stage) may alter anesthetic management.[62]

The current standard therapy for HIV/AIDS is highly active antiretroviral therapy (HAART), which involves combination chemotherapy. These drugs fall into four categories: nucleoside analog reverse transcriptase inhibitors, non-nucleoside analog reverse transcriptase inhibitors, protease inhibitors, and the new category of fusion inhibitors (Table 12-9).

From the anesthesiologist's perspective, protease inhibitors are the most important agents. They are potent cytochrome P450 inhibitors, thus prolonging the duration of action of hepatically metabolized drugs, such as fentanyl, midazolam, and morphine. Judicious dosing and careful titration are recommended.

The anesthesia care plan should take into account immunosuppression, systemic disease, and the risk of transmission of the virus to health care providers. There is no evidence of increased anesthesia risk in this patient population, nor is there evidence of increased complications associated with regional anesthesia.[63,64]

Specific surgical procedures associated with HIV/AIDS and anesthesia implications are described next.

Surgery and HIV.

Splenectomy. Patients with HIV may develop a variant of thrombocytopenia purpura known as HIV-associated immune thrombocytopenia purpura (HIV-ITP). This characteristically does not respond to corticosteroid therapy and may occur with HIV infection or AIDS. The treatment of choice is combination retroviral therapy; however, in refractory cases splenectomy is required.[64]

The anesthesiologist must be aware that the patient is at significantly increased risk of bleeding and that the platelet count cannot be raised by administration of corticosteroids or platelet transfusion. Consequently, epidural anesthesia should be avoided, as should the placement of large-bore intravenous catheters in noncompressible vessels.

Abdominal Surgery. Patients with HIV may develop abdominal pain for a variety of reasons, rarely requiring laparotomy. Surgery may be required for resection of neoplasm, particularly if there is bowel obstruction, drainage of intra-abdominal abscess, and appendectomy.

The presence of immunodeficiency may mask the signs (leukocytosis) of infection, leading to delayed diagnosis.[65] Moreover, these patients may mount a less dramatic SIRS response than expected, leading to dramatic development of severe sepsis without warning. Low CD4+ count independently predicts an increased incidence of postoperative sepsis.[60]

Patients with HIV are at particular risk for biliary tract disease—cholecystitis, cholangitis, and infections with opportunistic organisms such as *Salmonella*, cytomegalovirus, and *Cryptosporidium*. There is an increase risk of extrahepatic biliary obstruction caused by external compression of the common bile duct by enlarged portal lymph nodes (or lymphoma).[66] Laparoscopic cholecystectomy or choledochojejunostomy may be required.

Patients infected with HIV, or with AIDS, frequently require anorectal surgery for excision of extensive condylomata, anal fistulas, or perirectal abscesses. The patient is positioned in the prone-jackknife position. General or spinal anesthesia (assuming the patient does not have a coagulopathy) can be safely administered, as with patients who are not infected. Postoperative wound healing in patients with HIV, but not AIDS, is not impaired.[67]

Neurosurgery. Intracranial pyogenic abscess, toxoplasmosis, or lymphoma may cause neurologic symptoms in

HIV-infected patients. Infrequently, stereotactic needle biopsy is required for diagnosis. The procedure is usually carried out under monitored anesthesia care, for example with a remifentanil-propofol infusion and spontaneous ventilation.

Thoracic Surgery. The HIV-infected patient will occasionally require open lung biopsy to clarify the diagnosis in the event of respiratory failure. Opportunistic infections can usually be diagnosed by sputum examination or bronchoalveolar lavage. However, the identification, classification, and staging of lymphoma may require surgery. There is additional risk of recurrent pneumothorax and empyema, which can be managed by VATS.

It is important to assess and clarify the extent of the respiratory insult and the degree of hypoxemia in these patients before surgery. Careful attention must be placed in the ventilation strategy in the presence of hypoxemic respiratory failure. In the presence of significant parenchymal lung disease, the patient may be intolerant of one-lung anesthesia.

Obstetrics. Management of HIV-seropositive pregnant women includes attempts to minimize the infant's risk of acquired infection. Perinatal HIV transmission occurs antepartum, intrapartum, or postpartum. High maternal viral load increases the likelihood of perinatal transmission of HIV. Most perinatal HIV transmissions occur during labor and vaginal delivery. Hence obstetric care is targeted at minimizing exposure to maternal blood and genital secretions. This involves avoiding the following: percutaneous umbilical cord sampling, fetal scalp clips (when possible), fetal scalp sampling, delivery techniques that could produce abrasions in the infant's skin (e.g., vacuum or forceps), and immediate removal of maternal blood and fluids from the infant.[59] There is a relationship between the mode of delivery and risk of transmission: the risk is significantly reduced by elective cesarean section (Table 12-10).[68,69] This benefit may be lost if

TABLE 12–10 Elective Cesarean Delivery to Reduce the Transmission of HIV: Rates of Vertical Transmission

	Elective Cesarean Delivery	Other Mode of Delivery
No antiretroviral therapy	10.4%	19.0%
Antiretroviral therapy	2.0%	7.3%

From The mode of delivery and the risk of vertical transmission of human immunodeficiency virus type 1—a meta-analysis of 15 prospective cohort studies. The International Perinatal HIV Group. N Engl J Med 1999;340:977-987.

spontaneous rupture of the membranes has occurred. HIV may be transmitted through breast milk so breast feeding is discouraged.

Elective cesarean section should be performed under spinal anesthesia, as in noninfected parturients.[61,63]

HIV and the Risk to the Anesthesiologist/Health Care Worker. HIV is the most feared of all occupationally acquired diseases. It is important to note that patients with HIV/AIDS represent a reservoir of potential infectious exposures, in addition to the virus itself. The most important of these is tuberculosis. Additionally, the patient may be simultaneously infected with hepatitis B or C or both.

Universal precautions (see Table 12-5). should be employed when handling body fluids, tissue, blood, and blood products. The anesthesiologist must wear gloves at all times when in contact with the patient, the patient's blood, or tissues.[70] Where there is significant risk of exposure to the patient's body fluids—inserting arterial or central lines, performing bronchoscopy or fiberoptic intubation, or using epidural, spinal or regional anesthetic—a gown and face mask with eye protection is recommended. Contaminated needles should not be recapped by hand.

The risk of HIV transmission from a needle-stick injury with HIV-infected blood is approximately 0.32% (a far lower risk than with hepatitis C).[70] Immediately after needle-stick injury the health care worker should be treated with antiretroviral drugs (within 1 hour); this can reduce the rate of seroconversion by 80%.[1] Factors determining the risk to the exposed health care provider include type of the procedure for which needle was used, depth of needle-stick injury, the quantity of blood involved, and viral titers in the HIV-infected patient.[61]

Tuberculosis

Tuberculosis (TB) remains a major worldwide scourge. Approximately one third of the world's population has been exposed, and there are about 8 million new cases per year and 4 million deaths. Nevertheless, until the AIDS epidemic, the prevalence of TB declined dramatically from the 1950s to the 1980s. There was a 20% increase in the incidence of TB in the United States between 1985 and 1992, due principally to AIDS but also associated with immigration form countries with endemic TB, poverty, and limited health services in impoverished areas. After peaking at 25,287 cases in 1993, the number of reported cases began to fall again. In 2001, 15,989 cases of TB were reported to the U.S. Centers for Disease Control and Prevention (CDC). Three fourths of cases among foreign immigrants came from seven countries: Vietnam, the Philippines, India, China, South Korea, Mexico, and Haiti.

Mycobacterium tuberculosis is an aerobic rod that thrives in an aerobic environment, at a PO_2 of 140 mm Hg. Consequently, it preferentially infects the anterior apical segments of the lung. The bacilli are transmitted via droplet infection as a result of coughing or sneezing. TB may also be transmitted from one patient to another through anesthesia breathing systems or mechanical ventilators.

The principal site of infection of tuberculosis is the lung, but the bacterium may infect other organs, including the kidneys, brain, bones, joints, spine, and genitourinary tract.

Pulmonary TB typically presents as general malaise, anorexia, weight loss, fever, night sweats, productive cough, and hemoptysis. Diagnosis is made by serial sputum sampling for detection of acid-fast bacilli. In active primary TB, chest radiography reveals lobar pneumonia, with subsegmental atelectasis and ipsilateral hilar adenopathy. The more classic "reactivation" form of TB manifests with cavitating lesions in the posterior segment of the right upper lobe and apical segments of the lower lobes. A normal radiograph does not exclude TB, and in the presence of HIV the lesions are often atypical. If TB is suspected, respiratory isolation precautions should be instituted immediately, until the patient is deemed not to be infectious (acid-fast bacillus negative on three successive sputum samples, improving symptoms and improving chest radiograph).

Current therapeutic regimens for TB involve four-drug therapy, over 6 months:

- Initial 2 months (all oral doses)—Isoniazid (INH), 300 mg/day; rifampin (RIF), 600 mg/day; pyrazinamide (PZA), 2 g/day); and ethambutol (ETB), 2 g/day
- Final 4 months (if initial 2 months are successful by smear conversion and resolving symptoms)—INH, 300 mg/day, and RIF, 600 mg/day, or, alternatively, INH, 900 mg, and RIF, 600 mg, twice weekly.

Patients suspected of having active TB are nursed in respiratory isolation, in specially engineered negative pressure isolation rooms. Precautions can be supplemented with high-efficiency particulate air (HEPA) filters and ultraviolet irradiation devices installed near the ceiling of the room. Clear infection control guidelines must be in place and followed rigorously. The patient should wear a surgical mask when outside an isolation room.

Anesthesia Implications. A patient with active TB represents major infection risk for other patients and health care workers. Elective surgery should be avoided and postponed until the patient is no longer infections. For emergent or semi-emergent surgery, special precautions should be taken.

Contact with health care workers should be minimized; the number of staff in the operating room should be kept to a minimum. The operating room doors should be kept closed and infectious risk signs placed prominently as alerts to unwitting staff. The anesthesia breathing system should be separated from the mechanical ventilator by a HEPA filter. The breathing system should be disposed of at the end of the case.

Standard surgical face masks provide insufficient protection from droplet infection: the anesthesiologist should wear a National Institute for Occupational Safety and Health (NIOSH) N95 standard face mask and eye protection. The mask should fit snugly over the face such that all inspired air passes through it.

Extreme care should be placed in the disposal of soiled endotracheal tubes, suction tubing, and so on. If laryngeal mask anesthesia is performed, the mask should not be recycled. The patient should undergo recovery in isolation. If no isolation room is available, recovery is in the operating room or in an ICU isolation room (Table 12-11).

Prions

Prions (proteinaceous infective particles) are infectious proteins without (known) nucleic acid genomes. A number of these agents infect mammals, preferentially targeting neurologic tissue, causing spongiform encephalopathies.

TABLE 12–11   American Society of Anesthesiologist's Guidelines for Operative Care of the Patient with Tuberculosis

1. Elective operative procedures on a patient who has tuberculosis should be delayed until the patient is no longer infectious.

2. Patients should be transported to the operating room wearing surgical masks to prevent respiratory secretions from entering the air.

3. The doors of the operating room should be closed, and traffic into and out of the room should be minimized.

4. Perform the procedure at a time when other patients are not present in the operating room suite and when a minimal number of personnel are present (e.g., at the end of the day). Ideally the operating room should have an anteroom that is negative pressure to the corridor and the operating room. The anesthesiologist and other health care workers should wear a NIOSH N95 compatible face mask.

5. Exhausted air should be diverted away from hospital.

6. A bacterial filter between the anesthesia circuit and the patient's airway will prevent contamination of anesthesia equipment or discharge of tubercle bacilli into the ambient air.

7. These filters can be placed between the Y-connector and the mask, laryngeal mask, or endotracheal tube.

8. During recovery from anesthesia, the patient should be monitored and should be placed in an isolation room.

9. Alternatively, the patient should undergo recovery in the operating room or the patient's own room.

They include Creutzfeldt-Jakob disease (CJD), Gerstmann-Straussler-Scheinker syndrome, and kuru, among others in humans; scrapie in sheep; and spongiform encephalopathy in cattle (bovine spongiform encephalopathy: BSE—"mad cow disease"). These neurodegenerative diseases are universally lethal.

Recent interest in these agents followed the description, in 1996, of a new variant of CJD (known as variant CJD [vCJD]), which appears to have crossed over from BSE.[71,72] Following a cluster of reported cases in the United Kingdom, the specter of perioperative transmission of CJD and nvCJD has emerged. Moreover, emerging data suggest that these diseases may be spread by blood transfusion.[73]

Clinical and Pathologic Features. Variant CJD affects mainly young people. The average age of patients is 29 years, and the median duration of illness is 14 months. Since vCJD was first reported in the UK in 1996, there have been 151 cases of definite or probable vCJD; and 146 deaths (http://www.cjd.ed.ac.uk/figures.htm). There have been 1010 reported cases of CJD of all causes in the United Kingdom alone.

CJD causes progressive neuropsychiatric degeneration, associated with gradual reduction in consciousness, myoclonus, ataxia, chorea, or dystonia. In the late stages the patient progresses to a near catatonic state.

The prions causing vCJD are found in high concentration in the brain, spinal cord, and eye. They are also found in lymphoreticular tissue, a potential source of infectiousness.

Diagnosis of vCJD is difficult with no reliable investigation available. Diagnosis is made by a combination of clinical symptoms and signs and a positive tonsillar biopsy or by the presence of bilateral high pulvinar signal on magnetic resonance imaging (MRI).

Anesthesia Implications. Anesthesia may be required for patients with vCJD for tonsillar or brain biopsy, tracheostomy, or placement of a percutaneous endoscopic gastrostomy (PEG) feeding tube. This has significant implications for the performance of anesthesia and for the operating suite staff. Most important is the potential for transmission of disease between patients via contaminated instruments. Prions are small enough to reside in the microscopic crypts on stainless steel instruments and are not removed easily by standard washing techniques; furthermore, they are resistant to deactivation by traditional methods of decontamination. Although some novel approaches have been suggested, they have not been widely adopted.[74]

All unnecessary equipment and staff should be removed or excluded from the operating room, and warning signs placed outside. Staff must take extraordinary barrier measures such as double gloving, eye protection, aprons, and disposable liquid-repellant gowns.

Where possible, disposable equipment should be used—including laryngoscopes, face masks, and oral and laryngeal mask airways—these items should be incinerated. If the diagnosis of CJD or vCJD is confirmed, all instruments should be disposed of.[75]

In setting up the anesthetic it is preferable to use an ICU style ventilator, which can be stripped afterward and disposables incinerated. If the patient is already intubated, the ventilator from the ICU should travel with the patient. Total intravenous anesthesia can be administered. Although there are no specific contraindications to anesthesia agents, succinylcholine should be avoided when degenerative myopathy exists. Pipeline vacuum systems should not be used, and a portable machine should accompany the patient in the operating room, recovery, and ward.[76] During surgery all needles, clamps, sutures, or sharps should be directly disposed of into a suitable receptacle. Tissue matter should be carefully disposed of in clearly labeled bags.

The patient should either undergo recovery in the recovery room or be returned directly to the ICU.

INTRA-ABDOMINAL INFECTIONS AND ANESTHESIA

Intra-abdominal abscesses are walled-off collections of pus or parasites surrounded by fibrotic tissue, induced by inflammation, occurring within the abdomen. They may be located within viscera, in the peritoneum, between loops of bowel, or in the retroperitoneal space.

Intraperitoneal infections result from postsurgical anastomotic leakage, viscus perforation (e.g., a ruptured diverticulum), resolution of diffuse peritonitis into multiple small abscesses, or infection with parasites.

Pyogenic Liver Abscess

Liver abscesses are divided into pyogenic and parasitic (amebic and hydatid). The incidence of hepatic abscess is estimated as 13 to 20 cases per 100,000.[77] Most pyogenic liver abscesses are secondary to infection originating in the abdomen (Table 12-12). Cholangitis due to stones or strictures is the most common cause, followed by abdominal infection due to diverticulitis or appendicitis. In 15% of cases no cause can be found.

In the United States 80% of cases of liver abscess are pyogenic. The majority of pyogenic liver abscesses are polymicrobial infections, usually with gram-negative aerobic and anaerobic organisms. Most organisms are of bowel origin, with *Escherichia coli, Klebsiella pneumoniae,* Bacteroides, enterococci, anaerobic streptococci, and microaerophilic streptococci being most common. In approximately 50% of cases there is infection with anaerobic organisms. In patients with preexisting infections such as dental abscess or endocarditis, infection with

TABLE 12–12   Origins and Causes of Pyogenic Liver Abscess

Liver and Biliary Tract
Gallstones
Biliary strictures
Cholangiocarcinoma
Blocked biliary stent
Liver biopsy
Gallbladder empyema
Secondary infection of hepatic cyst

Extrahepatic
Appendicitis
Diverticulitis
Crohn's disease
Trauma

Abscess Extension
Perforated peptic ulcer
Subphrenic abscess

Disseminated Sepsis
Catheter-related bloodstream infection
Infective endocarditis
Dental infection

Data from Krige JEJ, Beckingham IJ: ABC of diseases of liver, pancreas, and biliary system: Liver abscesses and hydatid disease. BMJ 2001:322:537-540.

hemolytic streptococci, staphylococci, or *Streptococcus milleri* may occur. In the immunosuppressed population, such as patients undergoing chemotherapy, with AIDS, or following transplantation, opportunistic organisms or fungi may infect the liver.[78] The classic presentation of pyogenic liver abscess is with abdominal pain, swinging fever, night sweats, nausea, vomiting, anorexia, anergia, and malaise. There is usually hepatomegaly, tenderness in the right upper quadrant, and raised right hemidiaphragm (with sympathetic pleural effusion) on chest radiography. There is leukocytosis, anemia, and, in the presence of biliary tree compression due to mass effect, increased serum transaminase and alkaline phosphatase levels. Ultrasonography is the preferred imaging technique, because internal septations or daughter cysts (hydatid disease) are more clearly visualized.

Treatment is determined by the size, number, and nature of the lesions within the liver. Multiple small abscesses are treated by antimicrobial therapy alone, which must include a penicillinase-resistant penicillin, an anti–gram-negative agent, and metronidazole. In the absence of an intra-abdominal source, aspiration of the abscess under ultrasound or computed tomography (CT) can be performed. Usually a continuous drainage catheter is left in place. If an abdominal source is present, if there is a very large abscess or multilocular abscesses, or if antibiotics fail, then surgical drainage is necessary.

Amebic Liver Abscess

About 10% of the world's population is chronically infected with *Entamoeba histolytica*.[78] Amebiasis is the third most common parasitic cause of death, surpassed only by malaria and schistosomiasis. The prevalence of infection varies widely, and it occurs most commonly in tropical and subtropical climates. Overcrowding and poor sanitation are the main predisposing factors.

The parasite is transmitted through the fecal-oral route with the ingestion of viable protozoal cysts. The cyst wall disintegrates in the small intestine, releasing motile trophozoites. These migrate to the large bowel, where pathogenic strains may cause invasive disease. Mucosal invasion results in the formation of flask-shaped ulcers through which amebae gain access to the portal venous system. The abscess is usually solitary and affects the right lobe in 80% of cases. The abscess contains sterile pus and reddish brown ("anchovy paste") liquefied necrotic liver tissue. Amebae are occasionally present at the periphery of the abscess.

Clinical and Pathologic Features. Patients may have had symptoms from a few days to several weeks before presentation. Pain is a prominent feature, and the patient appears toxic, febrile, and chronically ill.

The diagnosis is based on clinical, serologic, and radiologic features. The patient is usually resident in an endemic area or has visited one recently, although there may be no history of diarrhea. Patients commonly have leukocytosis, with 70% to 80% polymorphs (eosinophilia is not a feature), a raised erythrocyte sedimentation rate, and moderate anemia. In patients with severe disease and multiple abscesses, alkaline phosphatase activity and bilirubin concentration are raised. Stools may contain cysts, or, in the case of dysentery, hematophagous trophozoites.

Chest radiography usually shows a raised right hemidiaphragm with atelectasis or pleural effusion. Ultrasonography shows the size and position of the abscess and is useful when aspiration is necessary and to assess response to treatment. Serologic tests provide a rapid means of confirming the diagnosis, but the results may be misleading in endemic areas because of previous infection. Indirect hemagglutination titers for *Entamoeba* are raised in over 90% of patients. In areas where amebiasis is uncommon, failure to consider the infection may delay diagnosis.

Serious complications occur as a result of secondary infection or rupture into adjacent structures such as pleural, pericardial, or peritoneal spaces. Two thirds of ruptures occur intraperitoneally and one third are intrathoracic.

Treatment. Ninety-five percent of uncomplicated amoebic abscesses resolve with metronidazole alone (800 mg, three times a day for 5 days). Supportive measures such as adequate nutrition and pain relief are important. Clinical symptoms usually improve greatly within 24 hours. Lower doses of metronidazole are often effective in invasive disease but may fail to eliminate the intraluminal infection, allowing clinical relapses to occur. After the amebic abscess has been treated, patients are prescribed diloxanide furoate, 500 mg, every 8 hours for 7 days, to eliminate intestinal amebae.

Patients should have ultrasonographically guided needle aspiration if serology gives negative results or the abscess is large (>10 cm), if they do not respond to treatment, or if there is impending peritoneal, pleural, or pericardial rupture. Surgical drainage is required only if the abscess has ruptured causing amebic peritonitis or if the patient has not responded to drugs despite aspiration or catheter drainage.

Anesthesia Implications of Pyogenic and Amebic Abscesses. Abnormal liver function is unusual except in the event of biliary obstruction or parenchymal compression. The presence of jaundice or raised serum transaminases likely has little effect on the conduct of anesthesia, because inherent liver metabolic function is usually intact. The patient may have evidence of low-grade or frank sepsis, in which case the guidelines established for the management of the septic patients, described earlier in the chapter, should be followed. If the patient is bacteremic, then epidural analgesia and placement of central venous catheters should be avoided, to prevent the development of catheter-related infection.

Hydatid Disease

Hydatid disease in humans is caused by the dog tapeworm *Echinococcus granulosus*. Dogs are the definitive host. Ova are shed in the feces and then infect the natural intermediate hosts such as sheep or cattle. Hydatid disease is endemic in many sheep-raising countries. Increasing migration and world travel have made hydatidosis a global problem of increasing importance. Human infection follows accidental ingestion of ova passed in dog feces. The ova penetrate the intestinal wall and pass through the portal vein to the liver, lung, and other tissues. Hydatid cysts can develop anywhere in the body, but two thirds occur in the liver and one fourth in the lungs.

Clinical and Pathologic Features. Patients with a liver hydatid may present either with liver enlargement and right upper quadrant pain due to pressure from the cyst or acutely with a complication. Complications include rupture of the cyst into the peritoneal cavity, which results in urticaria, anaphylactic shock, eosinophilia, and implantation into the omentum and other viscera. Cysts may compress or erode into a bile duct causing pain, jaundice, or cholangitis, or the cyst may become infected secondary to a bile leak.

Ultrasonography and CT will show the size, position, and number of liver cysts and any extrahepatic cysts. Classically "daughter cysts" are visualized within the main collection. Around 10% of patients with a liver cyst will also have a lung hydatid on chest radiography. The diagnosis is confirmed by hemagglutination and complement fixation tests. Aspiration of the cyst for diagnostic purposes is avoided until the diagnosis is confirmed. Biliary tree compression may increase serum bilirubin and transaminase levels. Eosinophilia is present in 40% of patients.

Surgery and Hydatid Disease. All symptomatic cysts require surgical removal to prevent complications. Radiologic cyst drainage has been described but is not widely practiced.[79] Consequently, the majority of these patients require general anesthesia.

The primary goal of surgery is careful dissection and removal of the intact cyst, avoiding spillage of its contents, which would result in the development of secondary cysts in the peritoneum. The patient is treated with albendazole for 4 weeks preoperatively, to shrink the cyst. The surgical field is carefully isolated by abdominal swabs soaked in scolicidal fluid. The cyst fluid is aspirated and replaced by a scolicidal agent such as 0.5% sodium hypochlorite, 0.5% cetrimide, 0.5% silver nitrate, 30% hypertonic saline, or sodium hydroxide. This sterilizes the cyst cavity. After decompression, the cyst and contents are carefully shelled and the cavity filled with isotonic saline or omentum and closed.

Anesthesia Implications. Liver dysfunction caused by an enlarging cyst rarely interferes with metabolic function. There may be compressive atelectasis in the lower segments of the right lung, leading to hypoxemia, that worsens after induction of anesthesia. PEEP is recommended. There is no contraindication to epidural catheter placement, although epidural infusion should be delayed until the cyst has been successfully excised. An arterial line should be placed to monitor beat-to-beat variation in blood pressure.

Two major intraoperative complications have been described: cyst rupture, leading to anaphylactic shock,[80] and hyperosmolar coma, following the administration of hypertonic saline.[81,82] Anaphylaxis is treated with intravenous fluid, epinephrine, antihistamines, and corticosteroids—all of which should be at hand in the operating room. Pretreatment with H1 and H2 antagonists may be beneficial.[83]

Splenic Abscess

Splenic abscesses are rare. There are five major causes: (1) metastatic spread from septic foci—including intravenous drug abuse, endocarditis, salmonella (in AIDS), osteomyelitis, tuberculosis, dental extractions, infected intravascular devices; (2) spread from adjacent organs—pancreatic and subphrenic abscesses, gastric and colonic perforations; (3) infection of splenic infarct—seen in hemoglobinopathies, including sickle cell disease and splenic artery embolization; (4) splenic trauma, and (5) immunocompromise.

Clinical and Pathologic Features. Patients present with fever, leukocytosis, and right upper quadrant pain. It may be associated with raised left hemidiaphragm, pleural effusion, and pain referred to the left shoulder.

Splenic abscess is most effectively diagnosed by CT or MRI. In approximately 50% of patients, blood cultures are positive. In the majority of abscesses streptococci or staphylococci are present, gram-negative rods are present in 30%, anaerobes in 12%, and mixed organisms in 25%. Antimicrobial treatment includes penicillinase-resistant β-lactam, aminoglycoside, or aztreonam and metronidazole.

Appendiceal Abscess

Appendiceal abscesses result from acute rupture of an acutely inflamed appendix. Appendicitis is the consequence of obstruction of the appendiceal lumen by a fecalith. There is increased intraluminal pressure associated with bacterial proliferation. There is venous congestion, distention of the organ, and eventually arterial compromise. Ischemia and gangrene result. In the majority of cases this results in abscess formation. However, rupture may also result in diffuse peritonitis, which represents a surgical emergency.

Clinical and Pathologic Features. Patients present with lower abdominal pain, guarding, leukocytosis, and low-grade fever.

The diagnosis is confirmed by CT. If a contrast agent is given, abscesses are well defined with rim enhancement; a phlegmon does not enhance. This will also provide information regarding the feasibility of percutaneous drainage.

Antimicrobial therapy is targeted at the polymicrobial nature of the abscess—a combination of gentamicin or amikacin plus either metronidazole or clindamycin is recommended.

There are two surgical approaches to appendix abscess: (1) immediate appendectomy with abscess drainage, the major risk of which is pus dissemination through the peritoneum due to the friability of tissues, and (2) delayed surgery—awaiting abscess organization. If the latter approach is planned, spontaneous resolution of the abscess is anticipated and appendectomy is planned at 6 to 8 weeks. However, if the abscess persists it should be drained percutaneously.

Diverticular Abscess

Diverticular abscesses form after perforation of a diverticulum. Perforation into the peritoneum leads to diffuse peritonitis, requiring immediate surgery. Often, however, the abscess may be contained by mesentery and/or local structures. The patient thus presents with malaise, pyrexia, leukocytosis, and generalized abdominal pain. The diagnosis is confirmed by CT. The most common site of diverticular disease is the sigmoid colon. The patient usually develops a colonic ileus.

Clinical and Pathologic Features. In the early stages, following perforation, when there is fecal soiling of the peritoneum, the patient may remain surprisingly well, leading to a false sense of security. This "honeymoon" period lasts 24 to 48 hours, followed by a dramatic SIRS response, fluid sequestration, and hypoxemia. This is the clinical manifestation of the proliferation of bowel bacteria in the peritoneum. Early laparotomy allows for peritoneal irrigation and colonic resection. At this stage mild to moderate vasodilatation may be present but patients rarely have overt signs of sepsis.

Diverticular abscesses are usually drained radiologically—using CT guidance. This may require sequential procedures. Once the initial inflammatory response has resolved and the source is controlled, laparotomy and bowel resection is performed.

Antimicrobial coverage should include therapy for gram-positive organisms and anaerobes and includes ampicillin/sulbactam or ampicillin, gentamicin, and metronidazole.

NECROTIZING SOFT TISSUE INFECTIONS

Necrotizing soft tissue infections (NSTIs) represent a group of diseases characterized by rapidly spreading necrotizing infection of subcutaneous tissue, fascial planes, and muscle. NSTIs are classified anatomically, determined by the depth of infection and the tissues involved (Table 12-13).[84]

The history is usually minor trauma or surgery in a vulnerable patient.[85] Often unexplained pain that increases rapidly over time is the first manifestation. The patient may develop early dramatic symptoms and signs of sepsis—confusion, delirium, tachycardia, tachypnea, hypotension, oliguria. The source may not be readily apparent. Clinical findings include erythema, edema, and induration of the tissues, occasionally with bullae formation.

Necrotizing infections have the following features in common:

- Extensive tissue destruction
- Thrombosis of blood vessels

TABLE 12–13   Classification and Risk Factors of Necrotizing Soft Tissue Infections

Classification

Infections of skin and subcutaneous tissue
   Progressive synergistic bacterial gangrene
   Chronic undermining burrowing ulcer (Meleney's ulcer)
   Idiopathic scrotal gangrene (Fournier's gangrene)
Infections involving subcutaneous tissue and fascia
   Hemolytic streptococcal gangrene
   Necrotizing fasciitis
   Gram-negative synergistic necrotizing cellulitis
   Clostridial cellulitis
Infections involving muscle
   Clostridial myonecrosis
   Streptococcal myositis

Risk Factors

Diabetes
Peripheral vascular disease
Chronic liver disease
Cancer
AIDS
Collagen vascular diseases
Chronic renal failure
Recent surgery
Penetrating trauma
Systemic sepsis (the "second hit")
Corticosteroids
Advanced age
Malnutrition
Alcoholism
Intravenous drug abuse
Postoperative infection
Morbid obesity

Data from Kuncir EJ, Tillou A, St. Hill CR, et al: Necrotizing soft tissue infections. Emerg Med Clin North Am 2003:21:1075-1087.

- Abundant bacteria spreading along fascial planes
- Relatively few acute inflammatory cells

Necrotizing Fasciitis

Necrotizing fasciitis is a deep-seated infection of the subcutaneous tissue that results in progressive destruction of fascia and fat, although it may spare the skin. It usually involves the extremities, the abdominal wall, or the perineum. There is much confusion about the nomenclature of this disease. For example, necrotizing infection of the perineum is often called Fournier's gangrene. Other names used include progressive bacterial synergistic gangrene (PBSG) and Meleney's ulcer. It is simpler to classify necrotizing fasciitis according to the type of microbes involved. There are two types of necrotizing fasciitis:

- Type 1 Polymicrobial form: This is an infection with mixed bowel organisms. Microbes may be aerobic (e.g., staphylococci, group A streptococci, *Escherichia coli*) or anaerobic (e.g., *Clostridium, Bacteroides, Peptostreptococcus*).

● Type 2 Monomicrobial form: This is caused by group A streptococci, which produces a number of cellular components and exotoxins that lead to the destruction of tissue and spread of infection.

Clinical and Pathologic Features. The patient usually presents with pain, out of proportion to apparent tissue injury, and malaise, with significant SIRS response. There may be a history of surgery, trauma, or minor injury, for example, in a diabetic patient.

Infection rapidly spreads throughout the subcutaneous tissues and along fascial planes. There may be localized thrombosis of blood vessels, which leads to loss of perfusion and necrosis/gangrene. Crepitus may be present, owing to gas production in the tissues.

The natural progression of the disease is severe sepsis, septic shock, multiorgan failure, and death. Early aggressive skin débridement is imperative, often with the patient in extremis. In addition to source control, empirical antibiotics must be administered, principally clindamycin, aminoglycosides, or third-generation cephalosporins and metronidazole. Supportive care usually involves aggressive volume resuscitation and vasopressors, which can usually be weaned with removal of necrotic tissue.

Surgical débridement of necrotic tissue is often extensive and usually involves multiple trips to the operating room. Amputation of limbs may be necessary. In addition, where anaerobic, gas-producing bacteria are involved, hyperbaric oxygen therapy may be indicated.

Anesthesia Implications. Anesthesiologists may be involved with patients with necrotizing fasciitis either during the initial presentation, where fulminant sepsis is the major manifestation, or during subsequent visits to the operating room for tissue débridement. Surgery should not be delayed by the anesthesiologist, because resuscitation and hemodynamic stabilization is usually impossible without surgical débridement. The incision is made directly over the area of skin involved or the most indurated region. The skin incision parallels the neurovascular bundles and carries down to the fascia. The underlying muscle and fascia is inspected and all necrotic tissue excised in all directions until healthy tissue is reached. Débridement is adequate when a finger can no longer easily separate the subcutaneous fat from the fascia. The wound is left exposed, without skin flaps, for subsequent assessment.

The patient may be intolerant of the vasodilatory effects of volatile agents and may require massive volume resuscitation plus vasopressor therapy as is described earlier in this chapter. Importantly, as débridement progresses, cytokine release reduces and the patient usually becomes hemodynamically more stable. In the absence of a volatile agent, ketamine is a suitable alternative to maintain hypnosis during surgery, along with fentanyl or hydromorphone for analgesia.

Clostridial Myonecrosis (Gas Gangrene)

Clostridial species are obligate anaerobes that infect devitalized tissue. Three types of clostridial infections have been identified: (1) simple wound contamination or colonization, (2) anaerobic cellulitis, and (3) clostridial gas gangrene.

Myonecrosis is caused by *Clostridium perfringens*, an exotonin-secreting and spore-forming bacterium found in the soil. This infection is often called gas gangrene, owing to the palpable crepitus caused by liberation of gas. Muscle is remarkably resistant to infection. Infection follows significant loss of barrier function, as occurs with contamination of deep-seated wounds, as occurs in trauma, knife wounds, septic abortions, immunocompromise, and surgery. The introduction of the organism is complemented by the presence of an anaerobic environment with a low oxidation-reduction potential and acid pH, which is ideal for the growth of clostridial organisms. Another form of myonecrosis, spontaneous gangrenous myositis, is caused by group A streptococci.

The toxic effects of clostridial organisms result from the release of toxins (there are 12). Alpha toxin is lecithinase (phospholipase C), which degrades lecithin in cell membranes causing lysis. In addition, *C. perfringens* produces a variety of hydrolytic enzymes—proteases, DNases, hyaluronidase and collagenases—that liquefy tissue, thus promoting spread of infection.

Clinical and Pathologic Features. The patient presents with sudden onset of malaise and painful swelling of the affected area. There may be a smelly purulent discharge and discoloration of skin. Gram stain of infected material reveals gram-positive rods. Exotoxins and proteolytics released by the organism cause fermentation of tissue carbohydrates and accumulation of gas bubbles in the subcutaneous space, resulting in crepitus.

Treatment is extensive surgical débridement of all infected tissue and intravenous antibiotics: benzylpenicillin, 2.4 g every 4 hours, plus clindamycin, 500 mg every 6 hours. Again, hyperbaric oxygen may have a role but has not been proven by prospective clinical trials.

Anesthesia Implications. Anesthesia care of the patient with myonecrosis is similar to that of the patient with necrotizing fasciitis.

Soft Tissue Infections of the Head and Neck

Soft tissue infections of the neck are of particular importance to anesthesiologists owing to the possibility of significant airway obstruction. The most common sources of life-threatening infections of the head and neck are the teeth and tonsils. The majority are polymicrobial in nature—usually oral flora (*Bacteroides, Peptostreptococcus, Actinomyces, Fusobacterium,* and microaerophilic streptococci) that become virulent. Infection spreads along facial planes to distant sites.

Clinical and Pathologic Features. The most well-known neck space infection was described by Wilhelm von Ludwig in 1836 and is known as Ludwig's angina. This is a severe cellulitis of the tissue of the floor of the mouth with involvement of the submandibular and sublingual spaces. There is edema of the neck and tongue, cellulitis, and gradual airway compromise. The source of infection is almost always the second and third mandibular molars. If the infection is allowed to continue there may be local lymphadenitis, systemic sepsis, and extension of the disease to involve deep cervical fascia with a cellulitis that extends from the clavicle to the superficial tissues of the face. The disease is almost always polymicrobial, including α-hemolytic streptococci and anaerobes such as *Peptostreptococcus, Prevotella melaninogenica,* and *Fusobacterium nucleatum.* Most patients with Ludwig's angina are young, healthy adults.

Patients usually present with mouth pain, dysphagia, drooling, and stiff neck. The patient often maintains the neck in an extended position and may have a muffled or "hot potato" voice.

Anesthesia Implications. Urgent airway control is usually advised. Traditionally, tracheostomy has been performed under local anesthesia. This, however, may be technically difficult owing to extensive edema and inflammation, and inevitable infection and inflammation of the stoma site. Incision and drainage is indicated if suppurative infection develops and if the presence of fluctuance, crepitus, and soft tissue gas mandate the need for surgical intervention. CT can be used to help identify these suppurative complications. Surgical drainage has been required in 50% of patients. This may be performed under local anesthesia or cervical block.[86] If any question of airway compromise arises, then the airway must be secured. Forty to 60 percent of patients with Ludwig's angina require tracheostomy or endotracheal intubation.[87] Conventional intravenous induction and neuromuscular blockade is unacceptable; spontaneous ventilation should be maintained. An awake fiberoptic "look see" approach appears optimal. The airway is visualized after appropriate topical preparation. If the glottis and supraglottic area are patient, the anesthesiologist proceeds to intubation. If not, awake tracheostomy is performed. An alternative approach is inhalational induction of anesthesia with sevoflurane: the major drawback of this approach is difficulty in maintaining airway patency (owing to the edematous tissues of the neck), obstruction, and hypoxemia. Cricothyroidotomy is extremely difficult in this situation. Penicillin with a β-lactamase inhibitor is the agent of choice for Ludwig's angina: ampicillin/sulbactam or piperacillin-tazobactam, with either clindamycin or metronidazole.

Epiglottitis

Acute epiglottitis is inflammation of the epiglottis secondary to bacterial infection, usually *Hemophilus influenzae,* type B. Infection results in significant edema and airway compromise, which may be life threatening. Inflammation can also occur in the arytenoid cartilage, false vocal cords, or pharyngeal wall, resulting in acute supraglottitis. The mean age at presentation ranges from 42 to 50 years, with male predominance and an association with cigarette smoking.

Clinical and Pathologic Features. Patients typically present after approximately 2 days of symptoms and sore throat and pain in swallowing (Table 12-14). Thickening of the epiglottis is the classic radiographic finding and is present on 73% to 86% of lateral neck radiographs.[88] Other radiographic findings strongly suggestive of acute epiglottitis and supraglottitis include enlargement of aryepiglottic folds, arytenoid enlargement, prevertebral soft tissue swelling, and an emphysematous epiglottitis.

Anesthesia Implications. Although generally avoided in children, laryngoscopy appears to be safe in adults and can be used to evaluate patients with a clinical suspicion of acute epiglottitis but with a negative neck radiograph. A "cherry red" epiglottitis is the classic finding, and most patients have supraglottic inflammation and edema. The need to

TABLE 12–14   Signs and Symptoms of Acute Epiglottitis and Corresponding Frequency in Adults

Sign/Symptom	Frequency (%)
Muffled voice	54-79
Pharyngitis	57-73
Fever	54-70
Pharyngitis	57-73
Tenderness of anterior neck	79
Dyspnea	29-37
Drooling	22-39
Stridor	12-27

From Bansal A, Miskoff J, Lis RJ: Otolaryngologic critical care. Crit Care Clin 2003;19:55-72.

sit upright, bacteremia, and a rapid onset of serious symptoms have been associated with the need for airway intervention: intubation or tracheostomy (5% to 20% of patients). The patient should continue to breath spontaneously while the airway is secured. Hence, awake fiberoptic intubation, or inhalational induction of anesthesia with sevoflurane, should be performed. Care should be taken with topicalization to prevent precipitation of acute airway obstruction. Intubation should be performed by the most skilled anesthesiologist, and a full airway team including an otolaryngologist, with an open tracheostomy pack, should be present.

The antimicrobial of choice is a second- or third-generation cephalosporin with activity against *H. influenzae*. Additional therapies such as the administration of racemic epinephrine or dexamethasone are of undetermined utility.[89]

INFECTIOUS AGENTS OF BIOTERRORISM

Biological weapons have been used to wage war and promote terror throughout history. One of the earliest uses of biological weapons occurred in the 6th century BC when the Assyrians poisoned enemy wells with rye ergot. In 1347, the Tartar army catapulted the bodies of bubonic plague victims over the walls of the city of Kaffa in the Crimea, leading to a plague epidemic. The Spanish, in 1495, infected French wine with blood from leprosy patients. In the mid 1600s, a Polish military general reportedly put saliva from rabid dogs into hollow artillery spheres for use against his enemies. On several occasions, smallpox was used as a biological weapon. This occurred in South America in the 15th century, during the French-Indian war, and during the Civil War. In each case, clothes from smallpox victims were given to natives or prisoners.

Horses, mules, and cattle were deliberately infected with anthrax and glanders in 1915 to infect Allied military personnel.

The Japanese extensively used aerosolized anthrax during the World War II. In 1941, the Japanese military released an estimated 150 million plague-infected fleas from airplanes over villages in China and Manchuria, resulting in several plague outbreaks. In 1942 the Soviet military used weaponized tularemia on German soldiers during the battle of Stalingrad.

From 1975 to 1983, Soviet-backed forces in Laos, Cambodia, and Afghanistan allegedly used tricothecene mycotoxins (T-2 toxins) in what was called "yellow rain." In 1979, an outbreak of pulmonary anthrax occurred in Yekaterinburg in the Russia as a result of an accidental release of anthrax in aerosol form from a Soviet bioweapons facility.

Iraq is suspected to have used bombs and scud warheads filled with *Botulinum* toxin, anthrax, and aflatoxin against Kurds in 1991. At the dawn of the 21st interest in biological weapons has increased owing to the

TABLE 12–15   Agents of Concern for Use in Bioterrorism

Highest Priority (Category A)

Microbe or Toxin	Disease
Bacillus anthracis	Anthrax
Variola virus	Smallpox
Yersinia pestis	Plague
Clostridium botulinum	Botulism
Francisella tularensis	Tularemia
Filoviruses	Ebola hemorrhagic fevers, Marburg disease
Arenaviruses	Lassa fever, South American hemorrhagic fevers
Bunyaviruses	Rift Valley fever, Congo-Crimean hemorrhagic fevers

Moderately High Priority (Category B)

Microbe or Toxin	Disease
Coxiella burnetti	Q fever
Brucella spp.	Brucellosis
Burkholderia mallei	Glanders
Alphaviruses	Viral encephalitides
Ricin	Ricin intoxication
Staphylococcus aureus enterotoxin B	Staphylococcal toxin illness
Salmonella spp., *Shigella dysenteriae*, *Escherichia coli* O 157:H7, *Vibrio cholerae*, *Cryptosporidium parvum*	Food- and water-borne gastroenteritis

Category C

Microbe or toxin	Disease
Hantaviruses	Viral hemorrhagic fevers
Flaviviruses	Yellow fever
Mycobacterium tuberculosis	Multidrug resistant tuberculosis

Miscellaneous

Genetically engineered vaccine- and/or antimicrobial-resistant category
A or B agents
HIV-1
Adenoviruses
Influenza
Rotaviruses
Hybrid pathogens (e.g., smallpox-plague, smallpox-Ebola)

rise of terror networks and the production of such weapons by "rogue states." There have been many foiled attempts by terrorists to produce bioweapons and several successful attacks; in Japan, in 1994-1995, in the United States in 1984 (salmonella), and in 2001 (anthrax).

In the fall of 2004, Viktor Yushchenko, the opposition candidate of the presidency of Ukraine, was poisoned with dioxin, leading to severe facial disfiguration, abdominal pain, and extensive ulceration of the gastrointestinal tract.

It is presumed that he consumed food poisoned by supporters of his political opponent.

In the event of a terrorist biological attack, the anesthesiologist will be intensely involved with triage and resuscitation of the injured patient. A familiarity with potential bioweapons (Table 12-15) is necessary.

An ideal biological weapon is robust, is highly infectious, is highly potent, and can be delivered as an aerosol. A vaccine should be available. In addition, the weapons should be manufactured quickly and easily. In general, the primary difficulty is not the production of the biological agent but the development of an effective method of delivering the weapon to its intended target (Table 12-16).

Anthrax

Bacillus anthracis is a gram-positive rod that primarily infects animals, particularly herbivores. Humans can contract the disease from infected animals or animal products. However, in most countries, domestic animal vaccinations have all but eliminated the disease. In an unfavorable environment anthrax endospores are formed that are highly resistant to disinfectants, temperature, and alkali. These spores have been manufactured by a number of countries as biological weapons. In the fall of 2001, letters with spores were sent from Trenton, New Jersey, to five media offices and two U.S. senators. Twenty-two individuals developed anthrax infections, mostly of the cutaneous variety. Five died of inhalation anthrax from cross contamination of the mail.

Clinical and Pathologic Features. Infection occurs with the introduction of the spore through a break in the skin, causing cutaneous anthrax, or through the mucosa of the gastrointestinal tract.

To cause pulmonary infection, weapons-grade anthrax spores must be used. The reason for this is that anthrax must be delivered as single spores, which can work their way down into to small airways, where they are phagocytosed and transported to the hilar lymph nodes where bacteria proliferate. To deliver single spores, anthrax must be treated, to "unclump" the spores by being rendered electrostatically neutral.

Proliferating bacteria produce three exotoxins: edema factor, protective antigen, and lethal factor. Protective antigen binds to cell surface receptors, facilitating entry of the two other exotoxins into the cell by the creation of a channel. Edema factor causes cell swelling. Lethal factor has protease activity, which causes cell lysis.

Anthrax is a biphasic disease. Inhalational anthrax manifests, following a 3- to 6-day incubation period, as nonspecific symptoms of pyrexia, malaise, myalgia, and dry cough. The second stage begins 2 days hence, with fulminant sepsis associated with pyrexia, dyspnea, and vasoplegic shock. Expiratory stridor, owing to tracheal compression by enlarged paratracheal nodes, may accompany other respiratory symptoms.

TABLE 12–16 Differential Diagnosis for Inhalational Anthrax

Diagnosis	Distinguishing Features
Pneumonic plague (*Yersinia pestis*)	Hemoptysis relatively common with pneumonic plague but rare with inhalational anthrax.
Tularemia (*Francisella tularensis*)	Clinical course usually indolent, lasting weeks; less likely to be fulminant.
Community-acquired bacterial pneumonia Mycoplasmal pneumonia (*Mycoplasma pneumoniae*) Pneumonia caused by *Chlamydia pneumoniae* Legionnaires' disease (*Legionella pneumophila* or other *Legionella* species) Psittacosis (*Chlamydia psittaci*) Other bacterial agents (e.g., *Staphylococcus aureus, Streptococcus pneumoniae, Haemophilus influenzae, Klebsiella pneumoniae, Moraxella catarrhalis*)	Rarely as fulminant as inhalational anthrax Legionellosis and many other bacterial agents (*S. aureus, S. pneumoniae, H. influenzae, K. pneumoniae, M. catarrhalis*) usually occur in persons with underlying pulmonary or other disease or in elderly. Bird exposure occurs with psittacosis. Gram stain of sputum may be useful. Community outbreaks caused by other etiologic agents not likely to be as explosive as pneumonic plague outbreak. Outbreaks of *S. pneumoniae* usually institutional. Community outbreaks of legionnaires' disease often involve exposure to cooling towers.
Viral pneumonia Influenza Hantavirus Respiratory syncytial virus Cytomegalovirus	Influenza generally seasonal (October-March in United States) or involves history of recent cruise ship travel or travel to tropics. Exposure to mice droppings, feces with Hantavirus. RSV usually occurs in children (although may be cause of pneumonia in elderly); tends to be seasonal (winter/spring). CMV usually occurs in immunocompromised patients.
Q fever (*Coxiella burnetii*)	Exposure to infected parturient cats, cattle, sheep, goats Severe pneumonia not prominent feature

The diagnosis of inhalational anthrax is suspected by circumstances (e.g., a mail worker with acute respiratory failure), sepsis, and respiratory failure in a patient with a widened mediastinum (i.e., adenopathy) on chest radiography.[90]

Cutaneous anthrax presents as a painless, pruritic papule on the skin up to 1 week after infection. Progression of the diseased lesion involves the development of one or more vesicles and edema surrounding the primary lesion, fever, and malaise. The vesicles subsequently rupture, revealing a necrotic ulcer and a characteristic black eschar. This dries and falls off after a week or 10 days.

The most important clinical approach to cutaneous anthrax is to avoid surgical débridement, which may be associated with bacteremia and systemic infection.[91]

Gastrointestinal anthrax is contracted by ingesting food contaminated with anthrax spores. Three to 5 days after infection the patient develops fever, malaise, nausea, vomiting, and diarrhea, associated with abdominal pain. Ulcers may develop in the intestinal mucosa, leading to profuse bleeding, mesenteric lymphadenitis, and ascites.

Definitive diagnosis is the identification of encapsulated broad gram-positive bacilli on examination of skin smears, blood, or cerebrospinal fluid.

Treatment of inhalational anthrax is ciprofloxacin plus clindamycin, rifampicin, or vancomycin.[92] For postexposure chemoprophylaxis, ciprofloxacin, doxycycline, and penicillin G have been recommended. Amoxicillin has been recommended for the treatment of cutaneous anthrax.

There is very little information available regarding hospital infection control and anthrax. There is no risk of person-to-person transmission with inhalational anthrax. If discharging skin lesions are present, contact precautions are necessary. Contaminated surfaces should be treated with sporicidal solutions.

Anesthesia Implications. The anesthesiologist may be involved with the critical care management of the patient with inhalational anthrax—for intubation and supportive care. There is no risk of person-to-person transmission (Table 12-17).

Smallpox

Smallpox is caused by the variola virus. The disease was eradicated worldwide in 1977 but exists in two known repositories, at the CDC in Atlanta and at the Institute of Viral Preparations in Moscow. It is feared that stockpiles of this virus are in the hands of others and may be used as a biological weapon.

Smallpox is spread from person to person without animal vector. The virus is inhaled into the respiratory tract and makes its way into the blood, and thence all body organs, via pulmonary lymph nodes. The incubation period is 1 to 2 weeks, during which the virus replicates in the reticuloendothelial system, followed by a prodromal syndrome (i.e., fever, backache, headaches, malaise, rigors, delirium, nausea and vomiting) after which a rash appears. At this point, and for a period of several weeks, the disease is communicable. The most prominent manifestation of smallpox is its characteristic centrifugal rash, which appears on the extremities first and then the trunk. This initially appears as a widespread macular eruption, with associated skin edema. An extensive pustular eruption follow; after 14 days these lesions rupture, necrose, and leave prominent pockmark scars.

Death from smallpox results from septic shock and MODS.

The rash of smallpox must be differentiated from that of chickenpox (varicella zoster). In varicella infection there is a shorter prodrome, lesions appear predominantly on

TABLE 12–17 Infection Control Issues for Selected Agents of Bioterrorism

Disease	Incubation Period (days)	Person-to-Person Transmission	Infection Control Precautions
Inhalational anthrax	2-43	No	Standard
Botulism	12-72 hours	No	Standard
Primary pneumonic plague	1-6	Yes	Droplet
Smallpox	7-17	Yes	Contact and airborne
Tularemia	1-14	No	Standard
Viral hemorrhagic fevers	2-21	Yes	Contact and airborne
Viral encephalitides	2-14	No	Standard
Q fever	2-14	No	Standard
Brucellosis	5-60	No	Standard
Glanders	10-14	No	Standard

From Cohen J, Powderly W: Infectious Diseases, 2nd ed. Philadelphia, Mosby, 2004, p 101.

the trunk with facial sparing, and the rash is different: the lesions in chickenpox are soft and do not scar and are at different stages of development; in smallpox the lesions progress in synchrony.

There is no known treatment for smallpox. Patients should be managed supportively, with full isolation and barrier precautions, in a negative-pressure room. Meticulous contact tracing is imperative. A vaccine is available, based on live vaccinia virus. Routine vaccination of children was abandoned in the 1960s because of the high incidence of vaccine-related complications. If the affected patient is in the early phase of the disease, he or she should be vaccinated.[93]

Tularemia

Tularemia is an acute, febrile, granulomatous, infectious zoonosis caused by the aerobic gram-negative pleomorphic bacillus *Francisella tularensis*. Its name relates to the description in 1911 of a plague-like illness in ground squirrels in Tulare County, California. The disease commonly infects rabbits and rodents, including mice, groundhogs, squirrels, and sheep.

There are 150 to 300 tularemia cases reported in the United States annually, with a majority of those from Alaska, Arkansas, Illinois, Oklahoma, Missouri, Tennessee, Texas, Utah, and Virginia.

F. tularensis was weaponized by the United States (until the 1960s) and the former Soviet Union (until the 1990s). Other countries have been or are suspected to have weaponized this bacteria. This organism can potentially be produced in either a wet or dry form and introduced by aerosolization or contamination of food and water sources.

Many routes of human exposure to the tularemia organism are known to exist. The common routes include direct contact with blood or tissue while handling infected animals, through the bite of arthropods (e.g., ticks, mosquitoes) or from handling or eating undercooked small game animals (e.g., rabbit). Less common means of transmission are drinking or swimming in contaminated water, from animal scratches or bites of animals contaminated from eating infected animals, and inhaling dust from contaminated soil or handling contaminated pelts or paws of animals. Tularemia is not directly transmitted from person to person. Laboratory workers exposed to the bacteria are at higher risk.

The clinical form of disease reflects the mode of transmission. Some authors classify the disease as typhoidal (predominance of systemic symptoms), pneumonic (pulmonary findings), or ulceroglandular (regional symptoms).

Weaponized tularemia is most likely acquired by inhalation or consumption of contaminated food. The most common form of tularemia is usually acquired through the bite of blood-sucking arthropods or from contact with infected animals. Inhalation of the organism will result in sudden chills, fever, weight loss, abdominal pain, fatigue, and headaches. Inhalation of *F. tularensis* may result in tularemic pneumonia. Patchy, ill-defined infiltrates appear in one or more lobes on chest radiography. Bilateral hilar adenopathy may be present. Bloody pleural effusions are characteristic and demonstrate a mononuclear cellular response. This may progress to ARDS. Ingestion of the organism in contaminated food or water may result in painful pharyngitis, abdominal pain, diarrhea, and vomiting. As many as 20% of patients have a rash that may begin as blotchy, macular, or maculopapular and progress to pustular lesions. Erythema nodosum and erythema multiforme rarely occur. Other systems may also be involved, leading to meningitis, pericarditis, peritonitis, and osteomyelitis.

Symptoms generally appear between 1 and 14 days, but usually within 3 to 5 days. Diagnosis is exceedingly difficult to make. It is usually based on serology (the tularemia tube agglutination test). However, there is a 12- to 14-day delay in receiving the result of this test. Treatment is with gentamicin or streptomycin. Otherwise therapy is supportive. Mortality in untreated patients is 5% to 15%; in treated patients it is 1% to 3%.

Plague

Yersinia pestis is a gram-negative bacillus that causes plague. Like anthrax, it primarily infects animals, particularly rodents. The disease is spread to humans via bites from infected rodent fleas. In this form, known as bubonic plague, approximately 10 cases per year are reported in the United States (Table 12-18).

Numerous epidemics of bubonic plague have swept the world during the course of the last 1000 years. It is believed that one third of the population of Europe succumbed in the 14th century to plague, commonly known as the "Black Death."

Plague was used as a biological weapon during World War II by the Japanese in China, when infected fleas were released. It is known that the United States and the Soviet Union developed an aerosolized version during the Cold War and maintain stockpiles to this day.

The bubonic plague typically presents 2 to 8 days after exposure, with sudden onset of fever, chills, weakness, and acutely swollen lymph nodes, termed buboes. These are usually located in the groin, axilla, or cervical regions. Buboes are egg shaped, 1 to 10 cm in length, and often exquisitely tender. The patient develops acute severe sepsis, progressing to multiorgan failure, characterized by microvascular thrombosis, over a 2-day period. Peripheral tissue necrosis, similar to that seen in meningococcemia (i.e., necrotitis fulminans) is seen. Person-to-person spread of bubonic plague does not occur.

TABLE 12–18   Clinical Presentations and Syndromic Differential Diagnoses of Selected Agents of Bioterrorism

Clinical Presentation	Disease	Differential Diagnosis
Nonspecific "flu-like" symptoms with nausea, emesis, cough with or without chest discomfort, without coryza or rhinorrhea, leading to abrupt onset of respiratory distress with or without shock, mental status changes, with chest radiographic abnormalities (wide mediastinum, infiltrates, pleural effusions)	Inhalational anthrax	Bacterial mediastinitis, tularemia, Q fever, psittacosis, legionnaires' disease, influenza, *Pneumocystis carinii* pneumonia, viral pneumonia, ruptured aortic aneurysm, superior vena cava syndrome, histoplasmosis, coccidioidomycosis, sarcoidosis
Pruritic, painless papule, leading to vesicle(s), leading to ulcer, leading to edematous black eschar with or without massive local edema and regional adenopathy and fever, evolving over 3 to 7 days	Cutaneous anthrax	Recluse spider bite, plague, staphylococcal lesion, atypical Lyme disease, orf, glanders, tularemia, rat-bite fever, ecthyma gangrenosum, rickettsialpox, atypical mycobacteria, diphtheria
Rapidly progressive respiratory illness with cough, fever, rigors, dyspnea, chest pain, hemoptysis, possible gastrointestinal symptoms, lung consolidation with or without shock	Primary pneumonic plague	Severe community-acquired bacterial or viral pneumonia, inhalational anthrax, inhalational tularemia, pulmonary infarct, pulmonary hemorrhage
Sepsis, disseminated intravascular coagulation, purpura, acral gangrene	Septicemic plague	Meningococcemia; gram-negative, streptococcal, pneumococcal or staphylococcal bacteremia with shock; overwhelming postsplenectomy sepsis; acute leukemia; Rocky Mountain spotted fever; hemorrhagic smallpox; hemorrhagic varicella (in immunocompromised patients)
Fever, malaise, prostration, headache, myalgias followed by development of synchronous, progressive papular leading to vesicular and then pustular rash on face, mucous membranes (extremities more than the trunk); the rash may become generalized, with a hemorrhagic component and systemic toxicity.	Smallpox	Varicella, drug eruption, Stevens-Johnson syndrome, measles, secondary syphilis, erythema multiforme, severe acne, meningococcemia, monkeypox (with African travel history), generalized vaccinia, insect bites, coxsackievirus infection, vaccine reaction
Nonspecific flu-like, febrile illness with pleuropneumonitis, bronchiolitis with or without hilar lymphadenopathy; variable progression to respiratory failure	Inhalational tularemia	Inhalational anthrax, pneumonic plague, influenza, mycoplasma pneumonia, legionnaires' disease, Q fever, bacterial pneumonia
Acute onset of afebrile, symmetrical, descending flaccid paralysis that begins in bulbar muscles, dilated pupils, diplopia or blurred vision, dysphagia, dysarthria, ptosis, dry mucous membranes, leading to airway obstruction with respiratory muscle paralysis. Clear sensorium and absence of sensory changes	Botulism	Myasthenia gravis, brain stem cerebrovascular accident, polio, Guillain-Barré syndrome variant, tick paralysis, chemical intoxication
Acute onset fevers, malaise, prostration, myalgias, headache, gastrointestinal symptoms, mucosal hemorrhage, altered vascular permeability, disseminated intravascular coagulation, hypotension, leading to shock, with or without hepatitis and neurologic findings	Viral hemorrhagic fever	Malaria, meningococcemia, leptospirosis, rickettsial infection, typhoid fever, borrelioses, fulminant hepatitis, hemorrhagic smallpox, acute leukemia, thrombotic thrombocytopenic purpura, hemolytic uremic syndrome, systemic lupus erythematosus

When *Yersinia* is spread by aerosolized droplets, the subsequent disease is known as pneumonic plague. It is highly contagious. This would be the route of attack by terrorists or the military.

After exposure there is an incubation period of 2 to 4 days, with sudden onset of fever, rigors, and muscular pain. Within 24 hours the patient develops hemoptysis, owing to the production of coagulase and fibrolysin by the bacterium, leading to tissue necrosis. The patient may complain of abdominal pain, chest pain, nausea, and vomiting. The disease progresses to ARDS, with severe hypoxemia, and to septic shock. Without appropriate antibiotics within 18 hours, the disease is fatal.

The diagnosis of plague may be difficult in isolated cases: the symptoms and signs may be indistinguishable from other forms of acute severe sepsis (e.g., meningococcemia or pneumococcal pneumonia). A history of hemoptysis on presentation should alert the clinician to the possibility of plague. Moreover, if a biological attack is carried out with *Yersinia,* multiple patients will begin presenting to the emergency department with symptoms of rapidly progressing pneumonia and hemoptysis. Sputum Gram stain reveals gram-negative rods. Blood cultures are usually positive, but the diagnosis is usually retrospective because, by the time the cultures emerge, without treatment the patient will be dead.

The treatment of choice for plague is streptomycin, gentamicin, doxycycline, or ciprofloxacin. These agents are not routinely used or recommended for community-acquired pneumonia. If the patient has symptoms or signs of meningitis, chloramphenicol should be used. Strict isolation with droplet precautions should be enforced for 48 hours.

Anesthesia Implications. The anesthesiologist may be involved with airway management and commencement of mechanical ventilation. Extreme precautions should be taken to avoid contact with patients' secretions. The anesthesiologist should wear a gown, mask, and eye protection because of the potential for contagion. All health care workers involved in face-to-face contact must be given chemoprophylaxis with doxycycline for at least 7 days. Patients are managed supportively in the ICU. There are no indications for surgery in the early stages. In particular, buboes should not be incised or débrided owing to the risk of spreading the infection. Peripheral necrosis requires surgical débridement or amputation, but this is delayed until the patient is in the recovery stage of the disease.

BIOLOGICAL TOXINS

Sarin

Sarin (GB) is an organophosphate nerve agent first developed by Nazi scientists in 1938. A number of similar agents exist, such as tabun (GA), soman (GD), cyclosarin (GF), and VX toxin. VX is the most potent known biotoxin. Sarin is one of the few biological weapons known to have been used in military and terrorist attacks. It is widely believed that sarin was used by the Iraqi military against Kurdish villagers in 1988 as well as during the Iraq-Iran War.[94] A Japanese terrorist cult known as Aum Shinrikyo used sarin against civilians in Japan, first in Matsumoto in 1994, killing 8 people, then in the Tokyo Subway in 1995, killing 13 and injuring hundreds.[95]

Clinical and Pathologic Features. At room temperature, sarin is a volatile liquid that can be aerosolized by explosive devices. Exposure to sarin occurs by one of two routes: topically/transdermally or inhaled into the lungs.[96] Once acquired, organophosphate nerve agents bind to and inactivate acetylcholinesterase (AchE). This leads to toxic accumulation of acetylcholine at nicotinic, muscarinic, and CNS synapses. Thus, sarin is a noncompetitive agonist at neuromuscular junctions, parasympathetic nerve terminals, and nicotinic adrenergic receptors. The result is a medley of symptoms (Table 12-19)[97]:

Initial symptoms and signs depend on the route of exposure and quantity of agent involved.[96] Transdermal poisoning causes insidious symptoms—initially vasodilatation, sweating, localized muscle fasciculations, and paralysis and then generalized muscle weakness, paralysis, and respiratory depression.

Inhalation of large quantities of nerve agent leads to acute respiratory distress, loss of consciousness, flaccid paralysis, convulsions, and coma.

TABLE 12–19 Symptoms Associated with Sarin or Organophosphate Poisoning

Respiratory: Dyspnea, cough, chest tightness, wheezing (bronchospasm)
Cardiovascular (adrenal medullary stimulation): tachycardia, hypertension
Neurologic: Headache, weakness, fasciculations, extremity numbness, decreased level of consciousness, vertigo, dizziness, convulsions
Ophthalmic: Eye pain, blurred vision, dim vision, conjunctival injection, tearing
Ear, nose, throat: Rhinorrhea
Gastrointestinal: Nausea, vomiting, diarrhea, tenesmus, fecal incontinence
Genitourinary: Urinary incontinence
Dermal: Sweating
Psychological: Agitation
General: Fatigue

Data from Lee EC: Clinical manifestations of sarin nerve gas exposure. JAMA 2003;290:659-662.

Physical signs include dyspnea, tachypnea, and wheezing. There may be tachycardia or bradycardia, reduced levels of consciousness, weakness, muscle fasciculation, flaccid paresis. Examination of the eyes reveals miosis and lacrimation.

If a sarin gas attack is suspected it is imperative that health care providers take extraordinary personal protective measures. Protective equipment includes protective suits, heavy butyl rubber gloves, and self-contained breathing apparatus. Aggressive decontamination of victims is required to prevent further exposure to them and others

Goals of decontamination are to prevent further absorption of nerve agents by victims and to prevent the spread of nerve agents to others. Decontamination is necessary only with topical exposure. The skin should be washed with an alkaline solution of soap and water or 0.5% hypochlorite solution (made by diluting household bleach 1:10). This chemically neutralizes the nerve agent.

Anesthesia Implications. The anesthesiologist's involvement in the emergency care of patients poisoned with organophosphates usually involves securing the airway, commencing mechanical ventilation, and transferring the patient to the ICU. The patient should be treated with supplemental oxygen before intubation. A hypnotic agent is administered to facilitate intubation. Succinylcholine should be avoided because it is metabolized by cholinesterase and will have a prolonged duration of action. Neuromuscular blockade is usually unnecessary. Intubation may be made more difficult because of excessive salivation and airway secretions.

Two essential antidotes are required to treat organophosphate poisoning: atropine and pralidoxime.[96] Atropine reverses the muscarinic effects of the poison, which include bronchoconstriction, abdominal pain, nausea, vomiting, and bradycardia. Pralidoxime acts by disrupting covalent bonds between nerve agent and AChE before they become permanent; thus, AChE is reactivated and skeletal muscle weakness is reversed. Convulsions are treated with benzodiazepines.[97]

Ricin

Ricin is a plant carbohydrate binding protein (lectin) found in high concentration in castor beans. Ricin is active orally or on inhalation and thus could be aerosolized or used to poison food. Ricin has relatively low potency, although it has been used as a biological weapon, most famously in the assassination of Georgi Markov in 1978 after skin perforation with the tip of an umbrella. A recent find of ricin and castor bean extraction equipment during a police raid of an apartment in the United Kingdom and in a postal facility in the United States indicates interest in this agent by terrorists.

Ricin is composed of two hemagglutinins and two toxins. The toxins, RCL III and RCL IV, are dimers of approximately 66,000 daltons. The toxins have an A and a B chain, which are polypeptides and joined by a disulfide bond. The B chain binds to cell surface glycoproteins and affects entry into the cell by an unknown mechanism. The A chain acts on the 60S ribosomal subunit and prevents the binding of elongation factor-2. This inhibits protein synthesis and leads to cell death.

Clinical and Pathologic Features. After inhalation exposure there is an incubation period of 4 to 8 hours, followed by fever, cough, dyspnea, nausea, and the development of ARDS. By the oral route there is necrosis of the gastrointestinal tract and significant bleeding. In parenteral exposure there is induration, erythema, and gradual development of systemic symptoms.

Mortality and morbidity depend on the route and amount of exposure. Therapy is supportive. The airway is secured, and ventilation is ensured. Decontamination is carried out similar to sarin infection.

Botulinum

Botulism is caused by the toxin of *Clostridium botulinum*, an aerobic, spore-forming bacterium. The bacterium occurs naturally in soil. Botulism is a neuroparalytic disease. Although manufactured as a bioweapon, botulinum toxin has never been used as such. The most likely bioterrorism dissemination scenarios include contamination of food and aerosolization.

Clinical and Pathologic Features. Following infection, the neurotoxin is absorbed through the intestinal mucosa and is widely distributed throughout the body. Initial presentation includes gastrointestinal problems that rapidly progress to cranial nerve abnormalities (e.g., diplopia, dysphagia, dysarthria) and, particularly, bulbar deficits. A progressive, bilateral, descending motor neuron flaccid paralysis ensues, followed by respiratory failure and death. The toxin combines irreversibly with peripheral cholinergic synapses, preventing acetylcholine release[98] and leading to flaccid paralysis not dissimilar to that seen with neuromuscular blocking drugs. There are no antiadrenergic effects. Blockade of neurotransmitter release at the terminal is permanent, and recovery only occurs when the axon sprouts a new terminal to replace the toxin-damaged one. Mortality is less than 5% if the infection is treated but approaches 60% if it is untreated (Table 12-20).

Anesthesia Implications. Treatment of botulism involves immediate administration of antitoxin, respiratory monitoring, and administration of mechanical ventilation. Once forced vital capacity falls below 30% of predicted,

TABLE 12–20 Differential Diagnosis of Botulism

Condition	Features that Distinguish Each Condition from Botulism
Guillain-Barré syndrome (GBS) (particularly Miller Fisher variant)	Usually an ascending paralysis, although Miller Fisher variant may be descending and may have pronounced cranial nerve involvement Abnormal cerebrospinal fluid protein 1 to 6 weeks after illness onset (although may be normal early in clinical course) Paresthesias commonly occur (often stocking/glove pattern) EMG shows abnormal nerve conduction velocity; facilitation with repetitive nerve stimulation does not occur (as with botulism) History of antecedent diarrheal illness (suggestive of *Campylobacter* infection)
Myasthenia gravis	Dramatic improvement with edrophonium chloride (although some botulism patients may exhibit partial improvement following administration of edrophonium chloride) EMG shows decrease in muscle action potentials with repetitive nerve stimulation.
Tick paralysis	Ascending paralysis Paresthesias common Careful examination reveals presence of tick attached to skin. Recovery occurs within 24 hr after tick removal. EMG shows abnormal nerve conduction velocity and unresponsiveness to repetitive stimulation. Usually does not involve cranial nerves
Lambert-Eaton syndrome	Commonly associated with carcinoma (often oat cell carcinoma of lung) Although EMG findings are similar to those in botulism, repetitive nerve stimulation shows much greater augmentation of muscle action potentials, particularly at 20-50 Hz. Increased strength with sustained contraction Deep tendon reflexes often absent; ataxia may be present. Usually does not involve cranial nerves
Stroke or CNS mass lesion	Paralysis usually asymmetrical. Brain imaging (CT or MRI) usually abnormal. Sensory deficits common. Altered mental status may be present.
Poliomyelitis	Febrile illness CSF shows pleocytosis and increased protein. Altered mental status may be present. Paralysis often asymmetrical.
Paralytic shellfish poisoning or ingestion of puffer fish	History of shellfish (i.e., clams, mussels) or puffer fish ingestion within several hours before symptom onset Paresthesias of mouth, face, lips, extremities commonly occur.
Belladonna toxicity	History of recent exposure to belladonna-like alkaloids Fever Tachycardia Altered mental status
Aminoglycoside toxicity	History of recent exposure to aminoglycoside antibiotics More likely to occur in the setting of renal insufficiency Most commonly seen with neomycin Most commonly associated with other neuromuscular blocking agents such as succinylcholine and paralytics
Other toxicities (hyper-magnesemia, organo-phosphates, nerve gas, carbon monoxide)	History of exposure to toxic agents *Carbon monoxide toxicity:* altered mental status may occur, cherry-colored skin *Hypermagnesemia:* history of use of cathartics or antacids may be present, elevated serum magnesium level *Organophosphate toxicity:* fever, excessive salivation, altered mental status, paresthesias, miosis
Other conditions	CNS infections (particularly brain stem infections) Inflammatory myopathy Hypothyroidism Diabetic neuropathy Viral infections Streptococcal pharyngitis (pharyngeal erythema and sore throat can occur in botulism owing to dryness caused by parasympathetic cholinergic blockade)

CSF, cerebrospinal fluid; EMG, electromyogram; CT, computed tomography; MRI, magnetic resonance imaging.
From Infectious Disease Society of North America. Available at http://www.cidrap.umn.edu/cidrap/content/bt/botulism/biofacts/botulismfactsheet.html

intubation is necessary. No specific interventions are required for intubation. The administration of neuromuscular blocking agents is unnecessary. Patients may require mechanical ventilation for up to 6 weeks. Full recovery may take 1 year.

References

1. Gerberding JL: Management of occupational exposures to blood-borne viruses. N Engl J Med 1995;332:444-451.
2. Braun BI, Darcy L, Divi C, et al: Hospital bioterrorism preparedness linkages with the community: Improvements over time. Am J Infect Control 2004;32:317-326.
3. Bone RC, Balk RA, Cerra FB, et al: Definitions for sepsis and organ failure and guidelines for the use of innovative therapies in sepsis. The ACCP/SCCM Consensus Conference Committee. American College of Chest Physicians/Society of Critical Care Medicine. Chest 1992;101:1644-1655.
4. Bone RC: Sir Isaac Newton, sepsis, SIRS, and CARS. Crit Care Med 1996;24:1125-1128.
5. Levy MM, Fink MP, Marshall JC, et al: 2001 SCCM/ESICM/ACCP/ATS/SIS International Sepsis Definitions Conference. Crit Care Med 2003;31:1250-1256.
6. Dellinger RP, Bone RC: To SIRS with love. Crit Care Med 1998;26:178-179.
7. Vincent JL: Dear SIRS, I'm sorry to say that I don't like you. Crit Care Med 1997;25:372-374.
8. Marshall JC: SIRS and MODS: What is their relevance to the science and practice of intensive care? Shock 2000;14:586-589.
9. Rangel-Frausto MS, Pittet D, Costigan M, et al: The natural history of the systemic inflammatory response syndrome (SIRS): A prospective study. JAMA 1995;273:117-123.
10. Alberti C, Brun-Buisson C, Goodman SV, et al: Influence of systemic inflammatory response syndrome and sepsis on outcome of critically ill infected patients. Am J Respir Crit Care Med 2003;168:77-84.
11. Kim PK, Deutschman CS: Inflammatory responses and mediators. Surg Clin North Am 2000;80:885-894.
12. Casey LC: Immunologic response to infection and its role in septic shock. Crit Care Clin. 2000;16:193-213.
13. Jackson WF: Ion channels and vascular tone. Hypertension 2000;35:173-178.
14. Quayle JM, Nelson MT, Standen NB: ATP-sensitive and inwardly rectifying potassium channels in smooth muscle. Physiol Rev 1997;77:1165-1232.
15. Landry DW, Levin HR, Gallant EM, et al: Vasopressin deficiency contributes to the vasodilation of septic shock. Circulation 1997;95:1122-1125.
16. Kumar A, Haery C, Parrillo JE: Myocardial dysfunction in septic shock. Crit Care Clin 2000;16:251-287.
17. Ince C, Sinaasappel M: Microcirculatory oxygenation and shunting in sepsis and shock. Crit Care Med 1999;27:1369-1377.
18. Hinds C, Watson D: Distributive Shock, Microcirculatory Changes. In Intensive Care, 2nd ed. Philadelphia, Saunders, 1996, pp 73-74.
19. Schrier RW, Wang W: Acute renal failure and sepsis. N Engl J Med 2004;351:159-169.
20. Fein AM, Calalang-Colucci MG: Acute lung injury and acute respiratory distress syndrome in sepsis and septic shock. Crit Care Clin 2000;16:289-317.
21. Dreyfuss D, Saumon G: From ventilator-induced lung injury to multiple organ dysfunction? Intensive Care Med 1998;24:102-104.
22. Ventilation with lower tidal volumes as compared with traditional tidal volumes for acute lung injury and the acute respiratory distress syndrome. The Acute Respiratory Distress Syndrome Network. N Engl J Med 2000;342:1301-1308.
23. Kim PK, Chen J, Andrejko KM, Deutschman CS: Intraabdominal sepsis down-regulates transcription of sodium taurocholate cotransporter and multidrug resistance-associated protein in rats. Shock 2000;14:176-181.
24. Grinnell BW, Joyce D: Recombinant human activated protein C: A system modulator of vascular function for treatment of severe sepsis. Crit Care Med 2001;29:S53-S61.
25. Marshall JC, Christou NV, Meakins JL: The gastrointestinal tract: The "undrained abscess" of multiple organ failure. Ann Surg 1993;218:111-119.
26. Annane D, Bellissant E, Bollaert PE, et al: Corticosteroids for severe sepsis and septic shock: A systematic review and meta-analysis. BMJ 2004;329:480.
27. Van den BG, de Zegher F, Baxter RC, et al: Neuroendocrinology of prolonged critical illness: Effects of exogenous thyrotropin-releasing hormone and its combination with growth hormone secretagogues. J Clin Endocrinol Metab 1998;83:309-319.
28. Faust SN, Heyderman RS, Levin M: Coagulation in severe sepsis: A central role for thrombomodulin and activated protein C. Crit Care Med 2001;29:S62-S68.
29. Bernard GR, Vincent JL, Laterre PF, et al: Efficacy and safety of recombinant human activated protein C for severe sepsis. N Engl J Med 2001;344:699-709.
30. Rivers E, Nguyen B, Havstad S, et al: Early goal-directed therapy in the treatment of severe sepsis and septic shock. N Engl J Med 2001;345:1368-1377.
31. Ernest D, Belzberg AS, Dodek PM: Distribution of normal saline and 5% albumin infusions in septic patients. Crit Care Med 1999;27:46-50.
32. Ernest D, Belzberg AS, Dodek PM: Distribution of normal saline and 5% albumin infusions in cardiac surgical patients. Crit Care Med 2001;29:2299-302
33. Schierhout G, Roberts I: Fluid resuscitation with colloid or crystalloid solutions in critically ill patients: A systematic review of randomised trials. BMJ 1998;316:961-964.
34. Choi PT, Yip G, Quinonez LG, Cook DJ: Crystalloids vs. colloids in fluid resuscitation: A systematic review. Crit Care Med 1999;27:200-210.
35. Moretti EW, Robertson KM, El Moalem H, Gan TJ: Intraoperative colloid administration reduces postoperative nausea and vomiting and improves postoperative outcomes compared with crystalloid administration. Anesth Analg 2003;96:611-617, table.
36. Gan TJ, Soppitt A, Maroof M, et al: Goal-directed intraoperative fluid administration reduces length of hospital stay after major surgery. Anesthesiology 2002;97:820-826.
37. Lang K, Boldt J, Suttner S, Haisch G: Colloids versus crystalloids and tissue oxygen tension in patients undergoing major abdominal surgery. Anesth Analg 2001;93:405-409.
38. Mythen MG, Webb AR: Perioperative plasma volume expansion reduces the incidence of gut mucosal hypoperfusion during cardiac surgery. Arch Surg 1995;130:423-429.
39. Sinclair S, James S, Singer M: Intraoperative intravascular volume optimisation and length of hospital stay after repair of proximal femoral fracture: Randomised controlled trial. BMJ 1997;315:909-912.
40. Finfer S, Bellomo R, Boyce N, et al: A comparison of albumin and saline for fluid resuscitation in the intensive care unit. N Engl J Med 2004;350:2247-2256.
41. Dellinger RP, Carlet JM, Masur H, et al: Surviving Sepsis Campaign guidelines for management of severe sepsis and septic shock. Crit Care Med 2004;32:858-873.
42. Rivers E, Nguyen B, Havstad S, et al: Early goal-directed therapy in the treatment of severe sepsis and septic shock. N Engl J Med 2001;345:1368-1377.
43. Marik PE, Mohedin M: The contrasting effects of dopamine and norepinephrine on systemic and splanchnic oxygen utilization in hyperdynamic sepsis. JAMA 1994;272:1354-1357.
44. Martin C, Saux P, Eon B, et al: Septic shock: A goal-directed therapy using volume loading, dobutamine and/or norepinephrine. Acta Anaesthesiol Scand 1990;34:413-417.
45. Hannemann L, Reinhart K, Grenzer O, et al: Comparison of dopamine to dobutamine and norepinephrine for oxygen delivery and uptake in septic shock. Crit Care Med 1995;23:1962-1970.

46. Bellomo R, Chapman M, Finfer S, et al: Low-dose dopamine in patients with early renal dysfunction: A placebo-controlled randomised trial. Australian and New Zealand Intensive Care Society (ANZICS) Clinical Trials Group. Lancet 2000;356:2139-2143.

47. Van den BG, de Zegher F, Lauwers P: Dopamine and the sick euthyroid syndrome in critical illness. Clin Endocrinol (Oxf) 1994;41:731-737.

48. Denton R, Slater R: Just how benign is renal dopamine? Eur J Anaesthesiol 1997;14:347-349.

49. Neviere R, Mathieu D, Chagnon JL, et al: The contrasting effects of dobutamine and dopamine on gastric mucosal perfusion in septic patients. Am J Respir Crit Care Med 1996;154:1684-1688.

50. Meier-Hellmann A, Reinhart K, Bredle DL, et al: Epinephrine impairs splanchnic perfusion in septic shock. Crit Care Med 1997;25:399-404.

51. Reinelt H, Radermacher P, Kiefer P, et al: Impact of exogenous beta-adrenergic receptor stimulation on hepatosplanchnic oxygen kinetics and metabolic activity in septic shock. Crit Care Med 1999;27:325-331.

52. Malay MB, Ashton RC Jr, Landry DW, Townsend RN: Low-dose vasopressin in the treatment of vasodilatory septic shock. J Trauma 1999;47:699-703.

53. Buijk SE, Bruining HA: Vasopressin deficiency contributes to the vasodilation of septic shock. Circulation 1998;98:187.

54. Goldsmith SR: Vasopressin deficiency and vasodilation of septic shock. Circulation 1998;97:292-293.

55. Reid IA: Role of vasopressin deficiency in the vasodilation of septic shock. Circulation 1997;95:1108-1110.

56. Tsuneyoshi I, Yamada H, Kakihana Y, et al: Hemodynamic and metabolic effects of low-dose vasopressin infusions in vasodilatory septic shock. Crit Care Med 2001;29:487-493.

57. Hill MK, Sanders CV: Skin and soft tissue infections in critical care. Crit Care Clin 1998;14:251-262.

58. Dreyfuss D, Saumon G: Ventilator-induced lung injury: Lessons from experimental studies. Am J Respir Crit Care Med 1998;157:294-323.

59. Hughes SC: HIV and anesthesia. Anesthesiol Clin North Am 2004;22:379-404, v.

60. Emparan C, Iturburu IM, Ortiz J, Mendez JJ: Infective complications after abdominal surgery in patients infected with human immunodeficiency virus: Role of CD4+ lymphocytes in prognosis. World J Surg 1998;22:778-782.

61. Kuczkowski KM: Human immunodeficiency virus in the parturient. J Clin Anesth 2003;15:224-233.

62. Birnbach DJ, Bourlier RA, Choi R, Thys DM: Anaesthetic management of caesarean section in a patient with active recurrent genital herpes and AIDS-related dementia. Br J Anaesth 1995;75:639-641.

63. Avidan MS, Groves P, Blott M, et al: Low complication rate associated with cesarean section under spinal anesthesia for HIV-1–infected women on antiretroviral therapy. Anesthesiology 2002;97:320-324.

64. Tyler DS, Shaunak S, Bartlett JA, Iglehart JD: HIV-1–associated thrombocytopenia: The role of splenectomy. Ann Surg 1990;211:211-217.

65. Bova R, Meagher A: Appendicitis in HIV-positive patients. Aust NZ J Surg 1998;68:337-339.

66. Bonacini M: Hepatobiliary complications in patients with human immunodeficiency virus infection. Am J Med 1992;92:404-411.

67. Buehrer JL, Weber DJ, Meyer AA, et al: Wound infection rates after invasive procedures in HIV-1 seropositive versus HIV-1 seronegative hemophiliacs. Ann Surg 1990;211:492-498.

68. The mode of delivery and the risk of vertical transmission of human immunodeficiency virus type 1—a meta-analysis of 15 prospective cohort studies. The International Perinatal HIV Group. N Engl J Med 1999;340:977-987.

69. Elective caesarean-section versus vaginal delivery in prevention of vertical HIV-1 transmission: A randomised clinical trial. The European Mode of Delivery Collaboration. Lancet 1999;353:1035-1039.

70. Kristensen MS, Sloth E, Jensen TK: Relationship between anesthetic procedure and contact of anesthesia personnel with patient body fluids. Anesthesiology 1990;73:619-624.

71. Will RG, Ironside JW, Zeidler M, et al: A new variant of Creutzfeldt-Jakob disease in the UK. Lancet 1996;347:921-925.

72. Beghi E, Gandolfo C, Ferrarese C, et al: Bovine spongiform encephalopathy and Creutzfeldt-Jakob disease: Facts and uncertainties underlying the causal link between animal and human diseases. Neurol Sci 2004;25:122-129.

73. Wilson K, Ricketts MN: Transfusion transmission of vCJD: A crisis avoided? Lancet 2004;364:477-479.

74. Fichet G, Comoy E, Duval C, et al: Novel methods for disinfection of prion-contaminated medical devices. Lancet 2004;364:521-526.

75. Estebe JP: Prion disease and anaesthesia. Ann Fr Anesth Reanimation 1997;16:955-963.

76. Farling P, Smith G: Anaesthesia for patients with Creutzfeldt-Jakob disease: A practical guide. Anaesthesia 2003;58:627-629.

77. Huang CJ, Pitt HA, Lipsett PA, et al: Pyogenic hepatic abscess: Changing trends over 42 years. Ann Surg 1996;223:600-607.

78. Krige JEJ, Beckingham IJ: ABC of diseases of liver, pancreas, and biliary system: Liver abscesses and hydatid disease. BMJ 2001;322:537-540.

79. Men S, Hekimoglu B, Yucesoy C, et al: Percutaneous treatment of hepatic hydatid cysts: An alternative to surgery. AJR Am J Roentgenol 1999;172:83-89.

80. Wellhoener P, Weitz G, Bechstein W, et al: Severe anaphylactic shock in a patient with a cystic liver lesion. Intensive Care Med 2000;26:1578.

81. Albi A, Baudin F, Matmar M, et al: Severe hypernatremia after hypertonic saline irrigation of hydatid cysts. Anesth Analg 2002;95:1806-1808, table.

82. Rakic M, Vegan B, Sprung J, et al: Acute hyperosmolar coma complicating anesthesia for hydatid disease surgery. Anesthesiology 1994;80:1175-1178.

83. Kambam JR, Dymond R, Krestow M, Handte RE: Efficacy of histamine H1 and H2 receptor blockers in the anesthetic management during operation for hydatid cysts of liver and lungs. South Med J 1988;81:1013-1015.

84. Kuncir EJ, Tillou A, St Hill CR, et al: Necrotizing soft-tissue infections. Emerg Med Clin North Am 2003;21:1075-1087.

85. Headley AJ: Necrotizing soft tissue infections: A primary care review. Am Fam Physician 2003;68:323-328.

86. Mehrotra M, Mehrotra S: Decompression of Ludwig angina under cervical block. Anesthesiology 2002;97:1625-1626.

87. Moreland LW, Corey J, McKenzie R: Ludwig's angina: Report of a case and review of the literature. Arch Intern Med 1988;148:461-466.

88. Neff SP, Merry AF, Anderson B: Airway management in Ludwig's angina. Anaesth Intensive Care 1999;27:659-661.

89. Bansal A, Miskoff J, Lis RJ: Otolaryngologic critical care. Crit Care Clin 2003;19:55-72,

90. Dixon TC, Meselson M, Guillemin J, Hanna PC: Anthrax. N Engl J Med 1999;341:815-826.

91. Swartz MN: Recognition and management of anthrax—an update. N Engl J Med 2001;345:1621-1626.

92. From the Centers for Disease Control and Prevention. Update: Investigation of bioterrorism-related anthrax and interim guidelines for exposure management and antimicrobial therapy, October 2001. JAMA 2001;286:2226-2232.

93. Breman JG, Henderson DA: Diagnosis and management of smallpox. N Engl J Med 2002;346:1300-1308.

94. Newmark J: The birth of nerve agent warfare: Lessons from Syed Abbas Foroutan. Neurology 2004;62:1590-1596.

95. Yokoyama K, Yamada A, Mimura N: Clinical profiles of patients with sarin poisoning after the Tokyo subway attack. Am J Med 1996;100:586.

96. Newmark J: Therapy for nerve agent poisoning. Arch Neurol 2004;61:649-652.

97. Lee EC: Clinical manifestations of sarin nerve gas exposure. JAMA 2003;290:659-662.

98. Arnon SS, Schechter R, Inglesby TV, et al: Botulinum toxin as a biological weapon: Medical and public health management. JAMA 2001;285:1059-1070.

CHAPTER

13 Diseases of the Endocrine System

MICHAEL F. ROIZEN, MD, and NADER M. ENANY, MD

A crucial factor in successful surgical treatment of endocrine diseases is a complete and accurate preoperative diagnosis. Sometimes the differential diagnosis is difficult, and often it requires the expertise of the endocrinologist, radiologist, and clinical pathologist. Armed with a complete and accurate diagnosis, the anesthesiologist and surgeon can offer the patient better relief of his or her symptoms and a more optimistic prognosis. Perioperative outcome in many of these conditions involves an understanding by the anesthesiologist of what the surgeon is trying to accomplish and, equally important, the end organ effect of the endocrine disorder. For example, diabetics often have renal and cardiac disease and peripheral and autonomic neuropathies. Understanding these consequences of diabetes and optimizing their treatment is crucial to the perioperative management of the diabetic, more so than is the finesse of managing insulin requirements by one of the many schemes available.

PARATHYROID GLANDS

Physiology

Total (bound and free) serum calcium concentration is maintained at the normal level of 9.5 to 10.5 mg/dL by the effects of parathyroid hormone (PTH), calcitonin, and vitamin D.[1] When the ionized calcium concentration decreases or the serum phosphate level rises, release of PTH is stimulated. PTH is secreted by the four parathyroid glands, which are usually located posterior to the upper and lower poles of the thyroid gland.[2] PTH increases tubular reabsorption of calcium and decreases tubular reabsorption of phosphate to raise the serum calcium concentration. A renal phosphate leak is the result of excessive PTH secretion. Calcitonin (produced in the C cells of the thyroid gland) antagonizes the effects of PTH and is released in response to high serum ionized calcium. Approximately 50% of the serum calcium is bound to serum proteins (albumin). Forty percent of the serum calcium is ionized, and the remaining 10% is bound to such chelating agents as citrate. If the serum protein concentration decreases, the total serum calcium concentration will also decrease. The rule of thumb is that for every 1-g decrement in albumin, a 0.8-mg/dL decrement in total serum calcium concentration occurs. Likewise, if the serum proteins increase (as in myeloma), total serum calcium level will increase. Acidosis tends to increase the ionized calcium, whereas alkalosis tends to decrease it. There may be a slight tendency for the serum calcium level to decrease with age, with a concomitant elevation of the serum PTH, perhaps contributing to the osteoporosis associated with the aging process.[3]

Vitamin D plays an important role in calcium homeostasis. Cholecalciferol is synthesized in the skin by the effects of ultraviolet light. Cholecalciferol is hydroxylated in the liver to form 25-hydroxycholecalciferol. The 25-hydroxy derivative is further hydroxylated in the kidney to form 1,25-dihydroxycholecalciferol (1,25$[OH]_2D_3$). The 1,25-dihydroxy derivative is by far the most potent vitamin D compound yet discovered. 1,25$(OH)_2D_3$ stimulates absorption of both calcium and phosphorus from the gastrointestinal tract.[4] Thus, vitamin D provides the substrates for the formation of mineralized bone. 1,25$(OH)_2D_3$ may also directly enhance mineralization of newly formed osteoid matrix in bone. Vitamin D derivatives also seem to work synergistically with PTH in bringing about increased resorption of bone. Clinically, this is an important point because immobilization alone increases bone reabsorption, and if the patient is receiving a vitamin D derivative, bone reabsorption may be increased further. Evidence now indicates that the hydroxylation of 25-hydroxycholecalciferol is controlled in the kidney by PTH and the phosphorus level. Elevated PTH and hypophosphatemia tend to accentuate the synthesis of 1,25$(OH)_2D_3$, whereas low levels of PTH and high levels of phosphate turn off the synthesis of 1,25$(OH)_2D_3$ in the kidney. PTH maintains a normal calcium level in blood by increasing calcium reabsorption from bone and by promoting synthesis of 1,25$(OH)_2D_3$, which in turn enhances calcium reabsorption from the gut. Finally, PTH directly increases calcium reabsorption from the renal tubule.

Thus, PTH accelerates the breakdown of bone by a complex mechanism that includes a fast component and a slow component (involving protein synthesis and cellular proliferation). In addition, PTH has an anabolic effect on bone formation, and in tissue culture it increases the number of active osteoblasts, the maturation of cartilage, and osteoid formation within the bone shaft.

Hypercalcemia

Patients with hypercalcemia present with a variety of symptoms that are often nonspecific because calcium is important to many functions: free intracellular calcium initiates and/or regulates muscle contraction, release of neurotransmitters, secretion of hormones, enzyme action, and energy metabolism. The level of blood calcium is frequently related to the degree and severity of symptoms. With calcium levels above 14 mg/dL, signs and symptoms such as anorexia, nausea, vomiting, abdominal pain, constipation, polyuria, tachycardia, and dehydration may occur.[1,5] Psychosis and obtundation are usually the end results of severe and prolonged hypercalcemia. Band keratopathy is a most unusual physical finding. Patients with hyperparathyroidism occasionally present with a history of calcium-containing kidney stones or peptic ulcers. Nephrolithiasis occurs in 60% to 70% of patients with hyperparathyroidism. Sustained hypercalcemia can result in tubular and glomerular disorders. Polyuria and polydipsia are common complaints. Bone disease in hyperparathyroidism, such as subperiosteal resorption, can also be seen in radiographs of the teeth and hands.[6] Severe bone disease in hyperparathyroidism, such as osteitis fibrosa cystica, is only very rarely seen and usually only in older patients who have had long-standing (perhaps up to 20 years) disease. The older patient with severe osteopenia, and perhaps vertebral compression fractures, should prompt suspicion of hyperparathyroidism. Many patients with hyperparathyroidism can tolerate blood calcium levels of 12 mg/dL without many symptoms.[5] This situation, often found by multiphasic screening, presents the dilemma of whether to operate on asymptomatic patients. The risk-benefit ratio is not clear at this point, and advocates of no treatment but watchful waiting appear to have the outcome data to at least present a reasonable argument.[5] Although surgical removal of a parathyroid adenoma is usually curative in asymptomatic patients and can be done safely in the very elderly, patients with mild, uncomplicated primary hyperparathyroidism may be followed medically if the serum calcium levels are less than 11.5 mg/dL and bone density and renal function are normal. Such patients should have quarterly check-ups of blood pressure, bone density, and renal function. Complications may be prevented by avoiding dehydration, thiazide diuretics, and immobilization. Parathyroid hyperplasia, usually involving all four parathyroid glands, may be a major cause of the hyperparathyroid syndrome. Carcinoma of the parathyroid glands is extremely rare. It is conceivable that all adenomas begin as hyperplasia[7]; therefore, for any one patient, exactly where in the natural history of the disease an operation occurs may determine whether hyperplasia or an adenoma is found.

Patients with hyperparathyroidism have elevated calcium and low serum phosphate levels. Very mild hyperchloremic acidosis may be present. The PTH level is usually elevated but is certainly elevated for the level of calcium concentration, and PTH reduction is the hallmark of successful surgery.[5,8,9] The only two situations in which hypercalcemia would be associated with a high PTH level are hyperparathyroidism and the ectopic PTH syndrome (usually secondary to a tumor of the lung or kidney that produces a biologically active fragment of PTH).[1] All other causes of hypercalcemia are associated with either normal or, more appropriately, low levels of PTH. When a patient presents with an extremely high blood calcium level (above 14 mg/dL), more likely than not, the patient has a distant cancer rather than hyperparathyroidism. Overall, about 50% of all cases of hypercalcemia are due to cancer invading bone. In these cases, prognosis is poor: more than 50% of patients die within 6 months. Treating hypercalcemia does not prolong survival but usually improves quality of life.[10,11] The technetium diphosphonate bone scan is positive in a large percentage of cancers that have metastasized to bone. Myeloma is another important cancer that is associated with hypercalcemia. The isotope bone scan is sometimes normal in this disease.

A number of other anomalies have to do with excessive absorption of calcium from the gastrointestinal tract. These abnormalities include (1) milk-alkali syndrome, which is usually due to excessive ingestion of calcium-containing antacids; (2) vitamin D intoxication; and (3) sarcoidosis, which is associated with hypersensitivity of the gastrointestinal tract to vitamin D. Hyperthyroidism is occasionally associated with increased bone resorption, and hypercalcemia may be present. Many patients with hyperthyroidism also have hyperparathyroidism. Some patients become hypercalcemic during treatment with thiazide diuretics. Thiazides increase renal tubular reabsorption of calcium and may even enhance the PTH effects on the renal tubule. Most patients who have significant hypercalcemia associated with thiazide diuretics have hyperparathyroidism. An important cause of increased bone reabsorption, and occasionally of mild hypercalcemia, is prolonged immobilization. Immobilization in any situation that is already associated with increased bone reabsorption, such as Paget's disease or ingestion of large quantities of vitamin D, can result in exaggerated hypercalcemia and excessive bone reabsorption. Cancer may produce hypercalcemia by at least three mechanisms: (1) metastasis to bone with increased bone reabsorption, (2) production by the cancer of a biologically active fragment of PTH, and (3) production of a prostaglandin that causes bone reabsorption. Table 13-1 lists the different causes of hypercalcemia and laboratory studies that differentiate them. In addition to obtaining the blood calcium and phosphate levels, determination of the bony fraction of the alkaline phosphatase, creatinine level, electrolyte values, and urinary calcium level is done, as well as obtaining the appropriate skeletal radiographs and isotope bone scan, by endocrinologists to aid diagnosis.

Severe hypercalcemia (especially above levels of 14 to 16 mg/dL) constitutes a medical emergency, and often treatment must be begun before the diagnosis is complete. There is no way to relate the signs and symptoms any one patient experiences to the level of blood calcium. In an extreme situation it is possible to have one patient who is almost asymptomatic, with a total blood calcium level of 14 mg/dL, whereas another who has an identical blood calcium level has severe polyuria, tachycardia, dehydration, and even psychosis. Age seems to be a factor; that is, for any given calcium level, the older patient is more likely to be symptomatic than a younger one. Tachydysrhythmias, including sinus tachycardia, are extremely common and usually out of proportion to the degree of volume depletion. Occasionally heart block results. Extreme care must be exercised in the use of digitalis derivatives for patients with hypercalcemia. Digitalis intoxication occurs quite readily in the presence of hypercalcemia. Digitalis toxicity dysrhythmias are extremely common in this setting.

Other measures decrease reabsorption of bone and include pamidronate sodium (90 mg intravenously), salmon calcitonin (100 to 400 units) or plicamycin hydration; and, in general, any patient with a calcium level of 16 mg/dL should be considered a medical emergency and treated with saline hydration (with careful attention to the risk of precipitating congestive heart failure [CHF]) and furosemide. Salmon mithramycin (or human, if a patient is allergic), corticosteroids, intravenous phosphates, or indomethacin can also be used.[11] A few patients with calcium levels of 14 mg/dL (especially older patients) also qualify for emergency treatment.

Preoperative Considerations for Patients with Hyperparathyroidism

Patients with moderate hypercalcemia who have normal renal and cardiovascular function present no special preoperative problems. Electrocardiographic (ECG) findings can be examined preoperatively and intraoperatively for shortened PR or QT interval.[12] Because severe hypercalcemia can result in hypovolemia, normal intravascular volume and electrolyte status should be restored before anesthesia and surgery are begun.

Management of hypercalcemia can include increasing urinary calcium excretion by means of hydration and diuresis.[11] Complications of these interventions include hypomagnesemia and hypokalemia.

Phosphate should be given to correct hypophosphatemia, because hypophosphatemia decreases calcium uptake into bone, increases calcium absorption from the intestine, stimulates breakdown of bone, and can result in CHF or pump failure.[13] Hydration and diuresis, accompanied by phosphate repletion, suffice as management for most hypercalcemic patients. If additional intervention is

TABLE 13–1   Differential Diagnosis of Hypercalcemia

	Serum Phosphorus	Serum Alkaline Phosphatase	Creatinine	Urinary Calcium	Blood Parathyroid Hormone	Comments
Cancer (metastatic)	N	↑	N	↑	N or ↑	Osteolytic lesion bone scan is +
Ectopic PTH production	↓	N or ↑	N	↑	↑ or N	Cancer of lung and kidney common
Myeloma	N	N or ↑	↑	↑	↓	Plasma protein ↑
Hyperparathyroidism	↓	N or ↑	N	N or ↑	↑	Subperiosteal resorption, kidney stones
Milk-alkali syndrome	N	N	↑	N	↓	Alkalosis; history of calcium intake
Vitamin D intoxication	↑	N or ↑	↑	↑	↓	Vitamin D levels ↑
Hyperthyroidism	N	N or ↑	N	↑	↓	T_4 or T_3 levels ↑
Sarcoid	N	N or ↑	N	↑	↓	Plasma proteins ↑
Thiazides	N or ↓	N or ↑	N	N or ↓	N or ↑	Coexistent hyperparathyroidism often
Adrenal insufficiency	N	N	N or ↑	N	↓	Hyponatremia, hyperkalemia
Immobilization	N	N	N	↑	N	If fracture, alkaline phosphatase ↑
Paget's disease	N	↑↑	N	↑	N	Bone scan is +

↑, elevated; ↑↑, markedly elevated; ↓, decreased; N, normal.

needed, glucocorticoids, pamidronate sodium (90 mg intravenously), plicamycin, or salmon calcitonin (100 to 400 units) may be given. Corticosteroids inhibit further gastrointestinal calcium absorption. Consultation with an endocrinologist or oncologist is advisable before mithramycin is given, because it has a narrow therapeutic-to-toxic ratio.

Calcitonin lowers serum calcium levels through direct inhibition of bone resorption. It can decrease serum calcium levels within minutes after intravenous administration. Calcitonin is less effective than phosphate or plicamycin, however, for patients with hypercalcemia caused by hyperparathyroidism. Side effects include urticaria and nausea.

It is especially important to know whether hypercalcemia has been chronic, because serious abnormalities in the cardiac, renal, or central nervous system may have resulted. Hypercalcemia associated with severe renal failure often can be treated successfully only by peritoneal dialysis or hemodialysis, with a low calcium concentration in the dialysis bath.

Finally, there are a few additional preanesthetic considerations. Aspiration precautions must be taken because the hypercalcemic patient with altered mental status may have a full stomach or be unable to protect the airway. The possibility of lytic or pathologic fractures warrants careful positioning. Radiographs of the cervical spine should be taken to rule out lytic lesions when hypercalcemia results from cancer.[14] Laryngoscopy in a patient with an unstable cervical spine may result in quadriplegia.

Intraoperative and Postoperative Considerations for Patients with Hyperparathyroidism

No controlled study has demonstrated clinical advantages of any one anesthetic drug over others. A review of cases at the University of California, San Francisco, and another at the University of Chicago from 1968 to 1982 revealed that virtually all anesthetic techniques and agents have been employed without adverse effects that could have been even remotely attributable to either the agent or the technique.

Maintenance of anesthesia usually presents little difficulty. No special intraoperative monitoring for patients with these conditions is required; a blood pressure cuff, lead II and/or MCL$_5$ electrocardiogram, temperature probe, and esophageal stethoscope typically are used. Because of the proximity of surgical retraction to the face, meticulous care is taken to protect the eyes. Response to neuromuscular blocking agents may be unpredictable when calcium levels are elevated[15]; reversal of the effects may be difficult.[14]

Failure to remove all the lesions at the first operation at times necessitates a second or third or even additional operation. Sestamibi scanning and venous sampling of PTH levels in thyroidal venous beds at times provide useful information to the surgeon at reoperation.[16] Unusual sites of parathyroid adenoma include areas behind the esophagus, in the mediastinum, and within the thyroid.

Of the many possible postoperative complications (nerve injuries, bleeding, and metabolic abnormalities), bilateral recurrent nerve trauma and hypocalcemic tetany are feared most. Bilateral recurrent laryngeal nerve injury (by trauma or edema) causes stridor and laryngeal obstruction as a result of unopposed adduction of the vocal cords and closure of the glottic aperture. Immediate endotracheal intubation is required in such cases, usually followed by tracheostomy to ensure an adequate airway. This rare complication occurred only once in more than 30,000 operations at the Lahey Clinic. Unilateral recurrent nerve injury often goes unnoticed because of compensatory overadduction of the uninvolved cord. Because bilateral injury is rare and clinically obvious, laryngoscopy after thyroid or parathyroid surgery need not be performed routinely; however, one can easily test vocal cord function after surgery by asking the patient to say "e" or "moon." Unilateral nerve injury is characterized by hoarseness, and bilateral nerve injury is characterized by aphonia. Selective injury of adductor fibers of both recurrent laryngeal nerves leaves the abductor muscles relatively unopposed, and pulmonary aspiration is a risk. Selective injury of abductor fibers, on the other hand, leaves the adductor muscles relatively unopposed, and airway obstruction can occur.

Bullous glottic edema is edema of the glottis and pharynx, which occasionally follows parathyroid surgery. This is an additional cause of postoperative respiratory compromise; it has no specific origin, and there is no known preventive measure.

Unintended hypocalcemia during surgery for parathyroid disease occurs in rare cases, usually from the lingering effect of vigorous preoperative treatment. This effect is especially important for patients with advanced osteitis because of the calcium affinity of their bones. After parathyroidectomy, magnesium or calcium ions may be redistributed internally (into "hungry bones"), thus causing hypomagnesemia, hypocalcemia, or both.

Management after parathyroid surgery should include serial determinations of serum calcium, inorganic phosphate, magnesium, and PTH levels.[13,17-21] Serum calcium levels should fall by several milligrams per deciliter in the first 24 hours. The lowest level usually is reached within 4 or 5 days. In some patients, hypocalcemia may be a postoperative problem. Causes include insufficient residual parathyroid tissue, operative trauma or ischemia, postoperative hypomagnesemia, and delayed recovery of function of normal parathyroid gland tissue. It is particularly important to correct hypomagnesemia in patients with hypocalcemia because PTH secretion is diminished in the presence of hypomagnesemia.[18,19] Potentially lethal complications of severe hypocalcemia include laryngeal spasm and hypocalcemic seizures.

In addition to monitoring total serum calcium or ionized calcium postoperatively, one can test for Chvostek's and Trousseau's signs. Because Chvostek's sign is present in 10% to 20% of individuals who do not have hypocalcemia, an attempt should be made to elicit this sign preoperatively. Chvostek's sign is a contracture of the facial muscles produced by tapping the ipsilateral facial nerves at the angle of the jaw. Trousseau's sign is elicited by application of a blood pressure cuff at a level slightly above the systolic pressure for a few minutes. The resulting carpopedal spasm, with contractions of the fingers and inability to open the hand, stems from the increased muscle irritability in hypercalcemic states, which is aggravated by ischemia produced by the inflated blood pressure cuff. Because postoperative hematoma can compromise the airway, the neck and wound dressings should be examined for evidence of bleeding before a patient is discharged from the recovery room.

Hypophosphatemia may also occur postoperatively. It is particularly important to correct this deficiency in patients with congestive heart failure. In a group of patients with severe hypophosphatemia, correction of serum phosphate concentration from 1.0 to 2.9 mg/dL led to significant improvement in left ventricular contractility at the same preload.[13] Other complications of hypophosphatemia include hemolysis, platelet dysfunction, leukocyte dysfunction (depression of chemotaxis, of phagocytosis, and of bactericidal activity), paresthesias, muscular weakness, and rhabdomyolysis.[19] In patients with both hypocalcemia and hypomagnesemia, correction of the hypomagnesemia may cause markedly increased PTH secretion, resulting in dramatic hypophosphatemia. Serum phosphate levels should be monitored closely in such patients.[18,19]

Hypomagnesemia may occur postoperatively. Clinical sequelae of magnesium deficiency include cardiac dysrhythmias (principally ventricular tachydysrhythmias), hypocalcemic tetany, and neuromuscular irritability that is independent of hypocalcemia (tremors, twitching, asterixis, and seizures).[17] Both hypomagnesemia and hypokalemia augment the neuromuscular effects of hypocalcemia. Often, just restoring the magnesium deficit corrects the hypocalcemia. It is preferable to use oral calcium (1 or 2 g four times daily of calcium gluconate) when the patient is able to take oral fluids.

During the first week or 10 days after surgery, vitamin D derivatives are avoided to allow the suppressed parathyroid tissue (if present) to function. Vitamin D derivatives are always started if the patient has significant hypocalcemia 2 weeks after surgery. The older vitamin D derivatives include vitamin D_2 (ergocalciferol) and vitamin D_3 (cholecalciferol). Of these derivatives, 40,000 units is equal to approximately 1 mg. Therapy in the patient with permanent hypoparathyroidism is begun with 40,000 units daily of either vitamin D_2 or D_3. The dosage is increased by 20,000 units every 2 weeks until the desired calcium level is attained. Vitamin D is fat soluble, and the significant fat stores in adipose tissue, muscle, and liver must first be saturated before a therapeutic level is achieved.

Patients with surgical hypoparathyroidism sometimes require huge quantities of vitamin D derivatives (200,000 to 300,000 units or 5 to 7 mg daily) and thus appear to have an end organ resistance to its effects. In the hypoparathyroid patient it is best to aim for a calcium level of 8.5 to 9.0 mg/dL. While these patients have a urinary calcium leak because of the absence of PTH, in general it is best to keep the urinary calcium level below 300 mg/24 hr. If the urinary calcium level is above 300 mg/24 hr, the vitamin D dose should be dropped back by 25% of the patient's initial dose. .Another vitamin D derivative is dihydrotachysterol (Dygratyl). Doses of 250 to 2000 μg of dihydrotachysterol are required to control the hypocalcemia in hypoparathyroidism. The compound 25-hydroxycholecalciferol is 15 times more potent than the parent vitamin D_2, and $1,25(OH)_2D_3$ is about 1500 times more potent.

The management of hypoparathyroidism is not easy, and careful follow-up of patients is mandatory. Blood calcium and urinary calcium should be checked every 6 months after surgery. Vitamin D intoxication is an ever-present danger.

Hypocalcemia

Probably the most common cause of hypocalcemia is hypoalbuminemia, followed by surgical removal of the parathyroids. However, the differential diagnosis of hypocalcemia should also include chronic renal insufficiency, malabsorption syndrome, pseudohypoparathyroidism, hypomagnesemia, osteoblastic metastasis to bone, pancreatitis, and the rare autoimmune abnormality of deficiency in multiple endocrine glands. A very rare cause of hypocalcemia is thymic hypoplasia associated with hypoparathyroidism (DiGeorge syndrome). In true hypocalcemia (i.e., when free calcium is low), myocardial contractility is often affected. Table 13-2 lists the differential diagnosis of hypocalcemia and some tests used to differentiate these cases. Measurement of PTH is not nearly as useful in differentiating the hypocalcemic states as it is in the hypercalcemic disorders. The vitamin D deficiency

of the malabsorption syndrome, osteomalacia (in the adult) and rickets (in the child), is associated with a low serum phosphorus concentration. In all other causes of hypocalcemia the serum phosphorus value tends to be elevated. It is disproportionately elevated in chronic renal failure. Cataracts and basal ganglion calcification are seen in both hypoparathyroidism and pseudohypoparathyroidism. Subperiosteal resorption (the hallmark of excessive PTH secretion) is seen mainly in chronic renal failure associated with secondary hyperparathyroidism and in some forms of pseudohypoparathyroidism. Most of the clinical manifestations of hypoparathyroidism are attributable to hypocalcemia. Hypocalcemia occurs because of a fall in the equilibrium level of the blood-bone calcium relationship, in association with a reduction in renal tubular reabsorption and gastrointestinal absorption of calcium. PTH inhibits renal tubular reabsorption of phosphate and bicarbonate; hence, serum phosphate and bicarbonate levels are elevated in patients with hypoparathyroidism.

Pseudohypoparathyroidism is an unusual entity associated with short stature, round facies, and short metacarpals, as well as parathyroid hyperplasia. It represents in part as end organ resistance to the action of PTH. $1,25(OH)_2D_3$ levels are low in pseudohypoparathyroidism, and replacement of this vitamin D derivative can partially reverse the end organ resistance. Hypomagnesemia impairs PTH release and thus can cause profound hypocalcemia.[17,19] Hypomagnesemia is common in patients with alcoholism, malnutrition, or chronic severe malabsorption states. The calcium level may be restored by replacing magnesium. Relative parathyroid insufficiency may account for the persistent hypocalcemia observed in patients with acute pancreatitis.

The acute manifestations of acute hypoparathyroidism have already been discussed with postoperative management of hypercalcemia.

A nerve exposed to low calcium concentration has a reduced threshold of excitation, responds repetitively to a single stimulus, and has impaired accommodation and continuous activity. Tetany usually begins with paresthesias of the face and extremities, which increase in severity. Spasms of the muscles in the face and extremities follow. Pain in the contracting muscle may be severe. Patients often hyperventilate, and the resulting hypocapnia worsens the tetany. Spasm of laryngeal muscles can cause the vocal cords to be fixed at the midline, and this leads to stridor and cyanosis.

Chvostek's and Trousseau's signs (see earlier) are two classic signs of latent tetany. Manifestations of spasm distal to the inflated blood pressure cuff should occur within 2 minutes (see earlier).

Hypocalcemia delays ventricular repolarization, thus increasing the QT_c interval (normal, 0.35 to 0.44). With electrical systole thus prolonged, the ventricles may fail to respond to the next electrical impulse from the SA node,

TABLE 13–2　Differential Diagnosis of Hypocalcemia

	Serum Phosphorus	Serum Alkaline Phosphatase	Creatine	PTH	Comments
Hypoparathyroidism (usually surgical)	↑	N	N	↓ or 0	Cataracts; basal ganglia calcification; other endocrine gland hypofunction
Chronic renal disease (secondary hyperparathyroidism)	↑↑	↑	↑↑	↑↑	Impaired renal 1,25(OH)$_2$D synthesis
Malabsorption syndrome (vitamin D deficiency)	↓↓	↑	N	N or ↓	Vitamin D malabsorption or deficiency (osteomalacia or rickets)
Pseudo-hypoparathyroid variants	↑	N	N	↑	Metastatic calcification, cataracts, short stature
Hypomagnesemia	↑	N	N	N or ↑	Malnutrition, alcoholism, and malabsorption
Osteoblastic metastasis	N	N or ↑	N	N or ↑	X-ray skeletal, seen in prostatic cancer
Acute pancreatitis	N	N or ↑	N	N or ↓	Mechanism unknown
Low plasma proteins	N	N	N or ↑	N	Ionized calcium may be normal; malnutrition nephrosis

↑, Elevated; ↑↑, markedly elevated; ↓, decreased; N, normal.

causing 2:1 heart block. Prolongation of the QT interval is a moderately reliable ECG sign of hypocalcemia, not for the population as a whole but for individual patients.[20,22] Thus, following the QT interval as corrected for heart rate (Fig. 13-1) is a useful but not always accurate means of monitoring hypocalcemia. CHF may also occur with hypocalcemia, but this is rare. Because CHF in patients with coexisting heart disease is reduced in severity when calcium and magnesium ion levels are restored to normal, these levels should be normal before surgery. Sudden decreases in blood levels of ionized calcium (as with chelation therapy) can result in severe hypotension.[18]

Patients with hypocalcemia may have seizures. These may be focal, jacksonian, petit mal, or grand mal in appearance, indistinguishable from such seizures in the absence of hypocalcemia. Patients may also have a type of seizure called *cerebral tetany*, which consists of generalized tetany followed by tonic spasms. Therapy with standard anticonvulsants is ineffective and may even exacerbate these seizures (by an anti–vitamin D effect). In long-standing hypoparathyroidism, calcifications may appear above the sella, representing deposits of calcium in and around small blood vessels of the basal ganglia. These may be associated with a variety of extrapyramidal syndromes.

Other common clinical signs of hypocalcemia are clumsiness, depression, muscle stiffness, paresthesias, dry scaly skin, brittle nails and coarse hair, and soft tissue calcifications. Patients with long-standing hypoparathyroidism sometimes adapt to the condition well enough to be asymptomatic.

The symptoms related to tetany seem to correlate best with the level of the ionized calcium. If alkalosis is present, it is possible for the total calcium level to be normal but the ionized calcium low, and symptoms of neuromuscular irritability may result (i.e., hyperventilation syndrome). With slowly developing chronic hypocalcemia the symptoms may be very mild despite severe hypocalcemia, and this may in part be due to adaptive changes in the level of the ionized calcium. Even with calcium levels of 6 to 7 mg/dL, minor muscle cramps, fatigue, and mild depression may

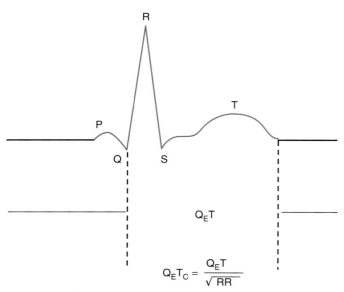

FIGURE 13–1 The QT_C interval (properly termed Q_ET_C, to indicate that it begins with the start of the Q wave, lasts for the entire QT interval, ends with the end of the T wave, and is corrected for heart rate) is measured as illustrated. RR, RR interval in seconds. *(From Hensel P, Roizen MF: Patients with disorders of parathyroid function. Anesthesiol Clin North Am 1987;5:294.)*

be the only symptoms. Many patients with a calcium level of 6 to 6.5 mg/dL are totally asymptomatic aside from some mild depression of intellectual function.

Vitamin D derivatives are used in the management of hypoparathyroidism (see preceding section), chronic renal insufficiency with secondary hyperparathyroidism, pseudohypoparathyroidism, the malabsorption syndromes, and other vitamin D deficiency states. Malabsorption syndrome associated with fat malabsorption may require an intramuscular preparation of vitamin D (2000 to 4000 units/day) if adequate oral therapy fails. A high-calcium diet (2 g elemental calcium) is indicated whenever a vitamin D preparation is used for this purpose. A low-phosphorus diet (including use of aluminum hydroxide) is useful in chronic renal failure, but a high-phosphate diet (calcium phosphate preparation may be used) is useful in patients with malabsorption syndrome and other vitamin D deficiency states (rickets and osteomalacia). In chronic renal disease the bone abnormalities due to excessive PTH levels (subperiosteal reabsorption) are essentially reversed by 1 or 2 μg of $1,25(OH)_2D_3$ (Rocaltrol); however, the osteomalacic changes in chronic renal disease may not be totally reversed by this potent vitamin D derivative. Pseudohypoparathyroidism and hypoparathyroidism are managed essentially in the same fashion (see earlier). Phenothiazines should be used with caution in patients with hypocalcemia (especially hypoparathyroidism), because they may precipitate dystonic reactions or dysrhythmias. Furosemide may decrease calcium levels more in patients with hypoparathyroidism.

Perioperative Considerations for Patients with Hypoparathyroidism

Because treatment of hypoparathyroidism is not surgical, hypoparathyroid patients who come to the operating room are those who require surgery for an unrelated condition. Their calcium, phosphate, and magnesium levels should be measured both preoperatively and postoperatively. Patients with symptomatic hypocalcemia should be treated with intravenous calcium gluconate before surgery. Initially, 10 to 20 mL of 10% calcium gluconate may be given at a rate of 10 mL/min. The effect on serum calcium levels is of short duration, but a continuous infusion with 10 mL of 10% calcium gluconate in 500 mL of solution over 6 hours may help to maintain adequate serum calcium levels.

The objective of therapy is to have symptoms under control before surgery and anesthesia. In patients with chronic hypoparathyroidism, the objective is to maintain the serum calcium level in at least the lower half of the normal range. A preoperative electrocardiogram can be obtained and the QT_C interval calculated. The QT_C value may be used as a guide to the serum calcium level if a rapid laboratory assessment is not possible. No special choice of anesthetic agents or techniques is indicated, with the exception of avoidance of respiratory alkalosis, because this tends to further decrease levels of ionized calcium.

Summary

Physiologic derangements in patients with disorders of parathyroid function are caused principally by inappropriate serum calcium levels. Preoperative evaluation of these patients commonly includes determination of calcium, phosphate, and magnesium levels. An electrocardiogram with calculation of the QT_C interval can be obtained preoperatively and can be followed intraoperatively. The patient's volume status may be affected, because both hypercalcemia and its treatment may lead to hypovolemia. Other measures to decrease calcium such as with other anticancer agents and with calcitonin may need other measures of side effects.

There is no evidence supporting any particular anesthetic technique. In addition to the QT_C interval, the free calcium level can be checked intraoperatively, if possible. Muscle relaxant dose and timing may be a special concern.[21] Calcium, phosphate, and magnesium levels often vary postoperatively. The patient should be observed closely for evidence of nerve injury, hematoma, or hypocalcemic tetany.

THYROID GLAND

Perhaps no endocrine organ has contributed as much to the development of surgery as a specialty as has the thyroid gland. The Cleveland Clinic and the clinics of such prominent surgeons as Lahey, Crile, and the Mayo brothers had their beginnings as centers for the traditional "steal" of the hyperthyroid patient and for the safe removal of enlarged thyroid glands. These clinics were located in regions where the soil was deficient in iodine. As a result, both water and food contained less than optimal amounts of iodine, thus contributing to the development of endemic goiter.

As with many other endocrinopathies, two themes emerge when anesthesia for patients with thyroid disease is discussed: (1) The organ system that most affects the anesthetic management of patients having any endocrinopathy is the cardiovascular system. (2) In almost all emergency situations, and certainly in all elective situations, any endocrine abnormality affecting the patient's preoperative state that can be stabilized may improve outcome. It is the task of the anesthesiologist to educate the primary care physician and surgeon about the hazards of not optimizing endocrine function preoperatively.[22-24]

Physiology

Thyroid hormone biosynthesis involves five steps.[25,26] They are as follows: (1) iodide trapping, (2) oxidation of iodide and iodination of tyrosine residues, (3) hormone storage in the colloid of the thyroid gland as part of the large thyroglobulin molecule, (4) proteolysis and release of hormones, and (5) conversion of less active prohormone thyroxine to more potent hormone 3,5,3-triiodothyronine. The first four steps are regulated by pituitary thyroid-stimulating hormone (TSH). Proteolysis of stored hormone in the colloid is inhibited by iodide.

The major thyroid products are the prohormone thyroxine (T_4, a product of the thyroid gland) and the more potent hormone 3,5,3-triiodothyronine (T_3, a product of both the thyroid and the extrathyroidal enzymatic deiodination of thyroxine). Approximately 85% of T_3 is produced outside the thyroid gland. Production of thyroid hormones is maintained by secretion of TSH by the pituitary gland, which in turn is regulated by secretion of thyrotropin-releasing hormone (TRH) in the hypothalamus. The production of thyroid hormone is initiated by absorption of iodine from the gastrointestinal tract, where the iodine is reduced to an iodide and released into plasma. It is then concentrated up to 500-fold by the thyroid gland.

Once in the gland, the iodide is oxidized by a peroxidase to iodine (organification) and then bound to tyrosine, forming either monoiodotyrosine or diiodotyrosine. Both of these are then coupled enzymatically to form T_4 or T_3. The T_3 and T_4 are bound to the protein thyroglobulin and stored as colloid in the gland. A proteolytic enzyme releases T_3 and T_4 from the thyroglobulin as the prohormones pass from the cell to the plasma. T_3 and T_4 are transported through the bloodstream on thyroxine-binding globulin and thyroxine-binding prealbumin. The plasma normally contains 4 to 11 µg of T_4 and 0.1 to 0.2 µg of T_3 per 100 mL. Secretion of TSH and TRH appears to be regulated by T_3 in a negative-feedback loop. Most of the effects of thyroid hormones are mediated by T_3; T_4 is both less potent and more protein bound, thus having lesser biologic effect, and is now considered a prohormone.[26]

In peripheral tissues there exists a ubiquitous deiodinase that converts T_4 to T_3. Thus, T_4 appears to be a prohormone for T_3. Monodeiodinations can remove either the iodine at the 5' position to yield T_3 or the iodine at the 5 position to yield reverse T_3 (rT_3). Reverse T_3 is totally inactive biologically. In general, when T_3 levels are depressed, rT_3 levels are elevated. In a number of circumstances, rT_3 levels are increased, such as during gestation, malnutrition, chronic disease, and surgical stress (Fig. 13-2).[27] A feedback circuit exists between the pituitary gland and the circulating thyroid hormones. High levels of thyroid hormones reduce release of pituitary TSH, whereas low levels result in more TSH release (Fig. 13-3).

Energy-dependent transport systems move T_3 across the target cell membrane into the cytoplasm. It then diffuses to receptors in the cell nucleus, where its binding to high-affinity nuclear receptors (TR α and TR β) alters the production of specific messenger-RNA sequences that result in physiologic effects. Thyroid hormone has anabolic effects, promotes growth, and advances normal brain and organ development. Thyroid hormone also increases the concentration of adrenergic receptors,[28] which may account for many of its cardiovascular effects.

The diagnosis of thyroid disease is confirmed by one of several biochemical measurements: levels of free T_4, total serum concentration of T_4, or estimate of free T_4. The estimate is obtained by multiplying total T_4 (T_4-RIA) by the thyroid-binding ratio (formerly called the resin T_3 uptake).[26,29]

Thyroid Function Tests

Total Thyroxine

Serum Thyroxine by Radioimmunoassay (T_4-RIA). The normal plasma range of the total T_4 is 4.5 to 10 µg/dL. The T_4 is high in hyperthyroidism and low in hypothyroidism. Most of the T_4 is bound to a plasma protein known as thyroid-binding globulin (TBG). Changes in TBG can affect the total T_4 level. Estrogens, infectious hepatitis, and genetic factors can elevate the level of the TBG and thus secondarily raise total T_4. Androgens, nephrosis, hypoproteinemia, and genetic factors can lower the TBG and thus secondarily lower the total T_4.

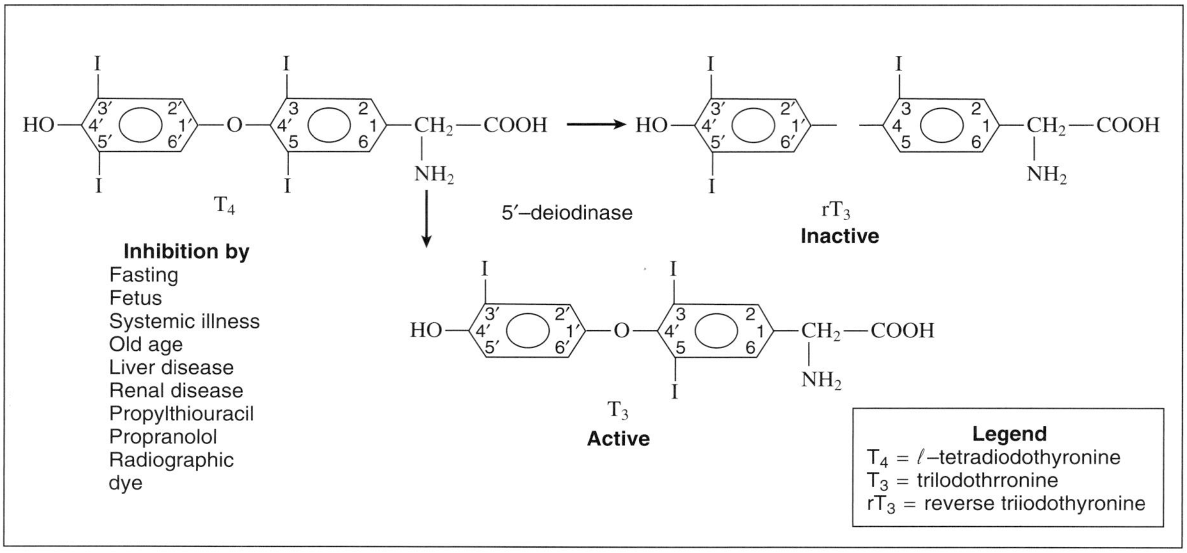

Inhibition by
Fasting
Fetus
Systemic illness
Old age
Liver disease
Renal disease
Propylthiouracil
Propranolol
Radiographic
dye

Legend
$T_4 = l-$tetradiodothyronine
$T_3 = $ trilodothrronine
$rT_3 = $ reverse triiodothyronine

FIGURE 13–2 Peripheral deiodination of T_4.

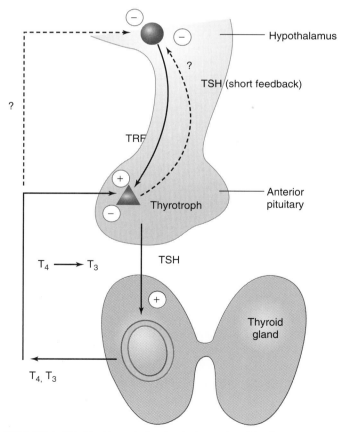

FIGURE 13–3 Hypothalamic pituitary thyroid axis. TRF, thyrotropin-releasing factor; TSH, thyroid-stimulating hormone; T_3, triiodothyronine; T_4, 1-tetraiodothyronine; +, stimulation; −, inhibition.

Thyroid-Binding Ratio

Resin Triiodothyronine Uptake (RT₃U). This important in-vitro test depends on the binding of a tracer amount of radioactive T_3 to an artificial resin. The amount of binding to resin is inversely proportional to the unoccupied binding sites of TBG. If the T_4 level is high because there is an excess of TBG (i.e., after estrogen administration), there will be an increase in the number of unoccupied binding sites and the thyroid-binding ratio will be low. The thyroid-binding ratio varies in different laboratories but the average is 20% to 25%. If the ratio is multiplied by total T_4, an index is achieved. This index is usually called the "free T_4 estimate." The free T_4 estimate corrects the total T_4 level for any changes in TBG concentration or in unoccupied binding sites on the TBG molecule. It is very difficult to assay the free T_4 level directly, because it amounts to only about 0.5% of the total T_4 (approximately 1 to 2 ng/dL). The free T_4 estimate correlates directly with the metabolic status of the patient.

Free Serum Triiodothyronine by Radioimmunoassay (T₃-RIA). This extremely potent hormone normally is present in a concentration range of 75 to 200 ng/dL. It is important to note that the upper limit of normal tends to drop with each decade of life. Thus, a 20-year-old patient with a level of 190 ng/dL may be euthyroid whereas an 80-year-old patient with the same level may be hyperthyroid.

Serum Thyroid-Stimulating Hormone. In patients with primary hypothyroidism, the TSH level is high for the level of T_4 or T_3 in blood. Often serum concentrations of thyroid hormone are in the normal range, and only serum TSH levels are elevated.[29]

Radioactive Iodine Uptake. The radioactive iodine uptake (RAIU) is measured as the percentage of a tracer that is taken up by the thyroid in 24 hours. The normal range is 10% to 25%. Patients with hyperthyroidism have values above 25%. The major use of this test is to confirm the diagnosis of hyperthyroidism; however, patients with subacute thyroiditis can be hyperthyroid but have essentially no uptake. If a patient has used inorganic iodides or dyes (e.g., for gallbladder scans or intravenous pyelography) the RAIU may be low.

Ultrasound Radioactive, MRI and Thin-Slice CT Thyroid Scan

These scans all have uses in diagnosis and treatment. Functioning thyroid nodules are rarely malignant, whereas "cold" or hypofunctioning nodules have a greater probability of malignancy.

Other Tests

The diagnosis of pituitary or hypothalamic disease can be quite complicated. The procedure is often aided by the use of TRH. This tripeptide is the hypothalamic factor that brings about release of TSH from the pituitary. It may also be used to confirm the diagnosis of hyperthyroidism. Thyroid antibodies (antithyroglobulin and antimicrosomal) are useful in arriving at the diagnosis of Hashimoto's thyroiditis. Serum thyroglobulin levels tend to be elevated in patients with thyrotoxicosis. Painless thyroiditis is associated with transient hyperthyroidism. This latter entity is a lymphocytic thyroiditis associated with low RAIU.

Measurement of the α subunit of TSH has been helpful in identifying the rare patients who have a pituitary neoplasm and who usually have increased α-subunit concentrations. Some patients are clinically euthyroid in the presence of elevated levels of total T_4 in serum. Certain drugs, notably gallbladder dyes, corticosteroids, and amiodarone, block the conversion to T_3 to T_4, thus elevating T_4 levels. Severe illness also slows the conversion of T_4 to T_3. Levels of TSH are often high when the rate of this conversion is decreased. In hyperthyroidism, cardiac function and responses to stress are abnormal; return of normal cardiac function parallels the return of TSH levels to normal values.

Pathophysiology of Thyroid Disease

Hyperthyroidism

Hyperthyroidism is usually caused by multinodular diffuse enlargement of the gland in Graves' disease that is also associated with disorders of the skin and eyes.[30] Hyperthyroidism can be associated with pregnancy,[31] thyroiditis (with or without neck pain), thyroid adenoma, choriocarcinoma, or TSH-secreting pituitary adenoma. Five percent of women have been reported to suffer thyrotoxic effects 3 to 6 months post partum, and they tend to have recurrences with subsequent pregnancies.[31]

Major manifestations of hyperthyroidism are weight loss, diarrhea, warm moist skin, weakness of large muscle groups, menstrual abnormalities, nervousness, intolerance of heat, tachycardia, cardiac dysrhythmias, mitral valve prolapse,[32] and heart failure. When the thyroid is functioning abnormally, the system threatened most is the cardiovascular system. Severe diarrhea can lead to dehydration, which can be corrected before a surgical procedure is undertaken. Mild anemia, thrombocytopenia, increased serum alkaline phosphatase, hypercalcemia, muscle wasting, and bone loss frequently occur in patients with hyperthyroidism. Muscle disease usually involves proximal muscle groups; it has not been reported to cause respiratory paralysis. In the apathetic form of hyperthyroidism (seen most commonly in persons over 60 years of age), cardiac effects dominate the clinical picture.[33,34] The signs and symptoms include tachycardia, irregular heartbeat, atrial fibrillation, heart failure, and occasionally papillary muscle dysfunction.[33-36] In fact, the presence of atrial fibrillation of unknown origin indicates the need to be concerned about apathetic hyperthyroidism. This concern is more than academic because "thyroid storm" can occur in such patients when they undergo operations for other diseases.

Although β-adrenergic receptor blockade can control heart rate, its use is fraught with hazards in a patient who is already experiencing CHF. However, decreasing the heart rate may improve the cardiac pump function. Thus, hyperthyroid patients who have high ventricular rates, who have CHF, and who require emergency surgery are given propranolol in doses guided by changes in pulmonary artery wedge pressure and the overall clinical condition. If slowing the heart rate with a small dose of esmolol (50 μg/kg) does not aggravate heart failure, more esmolol (50 to 500 μg/kg) is administered. The aim is to avoid imposing surgery on any patient whose thyroid function is clinically abnormal. Therefore, only "life-or-death" emergency surgery should preclude making the patient pharmacologically euthyroid, a process that can take 2 to 6 weeks.

Preparation of the Hyperthyroid Patient for Surgery. Nevertheless, 200,000 thyroid and parathyroid operations are performed annually in the United States. In general, the patients still considered appropriate for surgery are children, adolescents, women whose pregnancy is associated with Graves' disease, women of child-bearing age, and patients who have extremely large thyroid glands. A number of patients refuse radioactive iodine treatment, thereby becoming candidates for surgery. The traditional method for making the patient euthyroid involves giving one of the antithyroid drugs for 2 to 3 months before surgery to inhibit thyroid hormone synthesis. The drug that is still (after 30 years) most used is propylthiouracil, because it inhibits both thyroid hormone synthesis and the peripheral conversion of T_4 to T_3. The usual dosage is 300 mg daily in divided doses. Most patients will be euthyroid in 2 to 3 months on this dosage. If the patient is severely hyperthyroid or has an unusually large gland, larger doses may be used (up to 1 g daily). In general, the smaller the gland, the shorter the interval necessary to achieve euthyroidism. An alternative drug is methimazole (Tapazole). Doses of 30 to 60 mg daily are comparable to the above doses of propylthiouracil. About 10 days before surgery it is common to give the patient a potassium iodide solution (10 drops daily of a saturated solution) to decrease gland vascularity and block release of stored hormone. Lithium carbonate (300 mg four times daily) may be given in lieu of iodide, especially if there is a known allergy to iodine. Lithium carbonate, like iodide, blocks the proteolysis and release of stored thyroid hormone.

Published reports indicate a trend toward preoperative preparation with propranolol and iodides alone.[37-39] This approach is less time consuming (i.e., 7 to 14 days vs. 2 to 6 weeks); it causes the thyroid gland to shrink, as does the more traditional approach; and it treats symptoms, but abnormalities in left ventricular function may not be corrected.[34,36,38,39] Regardless of the approach used, antithyroid drugs should be administered both chronically and on the morning of surgery. If emergency surgery is necessary before the euthyroid state is achieved or if the hyperthyroidism gets out of control during surgery, intravenous administration of 50 to 500 µg/kg of esmolol can be titrated for restoration of a normal heart rate (assuming that CHF is absent; see previous discussion). Larger doses may be required, and in the absence of better data, the return of a normal heart rate and the absence of CHF serve as guides to therapy. In addition, intravascular fluid volume and electrolyte balance should be restored. It should be kept in mind that administering propranolol does not invariably prevent "thyroid storm."[38-41]

Management of Thyrotoxicosis During Pregnancy

The management of the thyrotoxicosis of Graves' disease during pregnancy presents some special problems. Radioactive iodine therapy is usually considered contraindicated because it crosses the placenta. The physician has a choice between antithyroid drugs and surgery. Antithyroid drugs also cross the placental barrier and can cause fetal hypothyroidism. This problem may theoretically be obviated by the simultaneous administration of L-thyroxine or T_3. However, most of the evidence indicates that neither T_4 nor T_3 crosses the placental barrier. The occurrence of

fetal hypothyroidism when small doses of antithyroid drugs alone are used is quite unusual as long as the mother remains euthyroid. It is usually better to err on the side of undertreatment than overtreatment with antithyroid drugs. Small amounts of propylthiouracil (50 to 100 mg/day or even every other day) are often sufficient. Chronic use of iodide in the mother is usually contraindicated because fetal goiter and hypothyroidism may result. The use of propranolol during pregnancy is controversial. There have been case reports that infants whose mothers had received propranolol experienced intrauterine growth retardation and low Apgar ratings. Bradycardia and hypoglycemia also have been described in these infants. The thyrotoxicosis of pregnancy tends to be quite mild and often improves in the second and third trimester. Surgery is an acceptable alternative to treatment (this surgery is usually postponed until neural development and organogenesis of the first trimester are complete).[42]

After pregnancy, it is impossible to predict the thyroid status of the mother. Whereas some patients remain hyperthyroid, some become hypothyroid after delivery. Approximately 5% of women suffer transient thyrotoxic effects 3 to 6 months post partum, and these mothers tend to have recurrences with subsequent pregnancies.[31]

The status of the neonate after delivery needs attention. Either hypothyroidism or hyperthyroidism may be present. Neonatal hypothyroidism is characterized by a low total T_4 (below 7 µg/dL) and an elevated TSH. At times the T_4 may be perfectly normal and only the TSH elevated. Amniotic fluid reverse T_3 levels tend to be low in the hypothyroid fetus in the third trimester, and likewise the blood reverse T_3 concentration is low after birth if hypothyroidism exists.

Management of neonatal hypothyroidism consists of the immediate replacement with L-thyroxine in the dose range of 9 µg/kg/day. This dose is relatively large, but it is often required to normalize the TSH level and T_4 concentration. Normally the total T_4 level (8 to 15 µg/dL) tends to be high in the first year of life and slowly but progressively drops until after puberty. Likewise, thyroid hormone replacement doses tend to be higher than in the average adult until puberty is complete.

Neonatal hyperthyroidism is most unusual and is always associated with high levels of thyroid-stimulating immunoglobulins. These immunoglobulins cross the placental barrier and are probably the cause of fetal hyperthyroidism. Consequently, it is common to measure these immunoglobulins in thyrotoxic women in the third trimester. Controlling maternal hyperthyroidism seems to prevent the development of hyperthyroidism in infants.

Thyroid storm refers to the clinical diagnosis of a life-threatening illness in a patient whose hyperthyroidism has been severely exacerbated by illness or operation. It is manifested by hyperpyrexia, tachycardia, and striking alterations in consciousness.[40,41] No laboratory tests are diagnostic of thyroid storm, and the precipitating (nonthyroidal) cause is the major determinant of survival. Therapy usually includes blocking the synthesis of thyroid hormones by administration of antithyroid drugs, blocking release of preformed hormone with iodine, meticulous attention to hydration and supportive therapy, and correction of the precipitating cause. In fact, survival is directly related to the success of treatment of the underlying cause. Blocking of the sympathetic nervous system with α- and β-receptor antagonists may be exceedingly hazardous and requires skillful management and constant monitoring of the critically ill patient. More than 10% of patients treated with the antiarrhythmic agent amiodarone develop thyroid dysfunction, either hyperthyroidism or hypothyroidism.[24] Approximately 35% of the drug's weight is iodine, and a 200-mg tablet releases about 20 times the optimal daily dose of iodine. This iodine can lead to reduced synthesis of thyroxine or to increased synthesis. In addition, amiodarone inhibits the conversion of T_4 into the more potent T_3.

Patients receiving amiodarone might be considered in need of special attention preoperatively, and even may require special attention to anesthesia, not just due to the arrhythmia that led to such therapy but also to ensure no perioperative dysfunction or surprises due to unsuspected thyroid hyperfunction or hypofunction.[24] Many patients with amiodarone thyrotoxicosis receive corticosteroids for a period of time, another area of questioning that might be triggered by the use of amiodarone by a preoperative patient.

Hypothyroidism

Hypothyroidism is a common disease, occurring in 5% of a large adult population in Great Britain, in 3% to 6% of a population of healthy elderly individuals in Massachusetts, and in 4.5% of a medical clinic population in Switzerland.[43,44] The apathy and lethargy that often accompany hypothyroidism often delay its diagnosis, so that the perioperative period may be the first place to spot many such hypothyroid patients. However, usually hypothyroidism is subclinical, serum concentrations of thyroid hormones are in the normal range, and only serum TSH levels are elevated.[25,45] The normal range of TSH being 0.03 to 4.5 mU/L, TSH values of 5 to 15 mU/L are characteristic of this entity.[35] In such cases, hypothyroidism may have little or no perioperative significance. However, a retrospective study of 59 mildly hypothyroid patients found that more hypothyroid patients than control subjects required prolonged postoperative intubation (9 of 59 vs. 4 of 59) and had significant electrolyte imbalances (3 of 59 vs. 1 of 59) and bleeding complications (4 of 59 vs. 0 of 59).[46] Because only a small number

of charts were examined, these differences did not reach statistical significance. In another study, a high percentage of patients with a history of subclinical hypothyroidism later developed overt hypothyroidism. Many women with postpartum thyroiditis develop hypothyroidism, which is often mistaken for postpartum depression.

Hypofunction of the thyroid gland can be caused by surgical ablation, radioactive iodine administration, irradiation to the neck (e.g., for Hodgkin's disease), iodine deficiency or toxicity, genetic biosynthetic defects in thyroid hormone production, antithyroid drugs such as propylthiouracil, amiodarone pituitary tumors, or hypothalamic disease. Perhaps the most common cause of primary thyroid hypofunction is a form of thyroiditis, often chronic lymphocytic thyroiditis or Hashimoto's thyroiditis. The gland is usually enlarged, nontender, and extremely firm and indurated. A variety of antithyroid antibodies are found in the serum, including antithyroglobulin and antimicrosomal antibodies in high titer. Hypothyroidism seems to be the most common consequence of Hashimoto's thyroiditis and, indeed, is the most common cause of hypothyroidism in adults.[45] Patients with Hashimoto's thyroiditis are extremely susceptible to iodides and to antithyroid drugs, and overt severe hypothyroidism can be exacerbated by these maneuvers. Usually, symptoms of hypothyroidism are subclinical, serum concentrations of thyroid hormones are in the normal range, and only serum TSH levels are elevated.[25,45,46]

In the less frequent cases of overt hypothyroidism, the deficiency of thyroid hormone results in slow mental functioning, slow movement, dry skin, intolerance to cold, depression of the ventilatory responses to hypoxia and hypercarbia,[47] impaired clearance of free water, slow gastric emptying, and bradycardia. In extreme cases, cardiomegaly, heart failure, and pericardial and pleural effusions are manifested as fatigue, dyspnea, and orthopnea.[48] Hypothyroidism is often associated with amyloidosis, which may cause enlargement of the tongue, abnormalities of the cardiac conduction system, and renal disease. The tongue may be enlarged in the hypothyroid patient even in the absence of amyloidosis, and this may hamper intubation.[49] Full-blown myxedema presents as a variety of symptoms, including cold intolerance, apathy, hoarseness, constipation, retarded movement, anemia, hearing loss, and bradycardia.

Preparation of the Hypothyroid Patient for Surgery. Hypothyroidism decreases anesthetic requirements slightly.[50] Ideal preoperative management of hypothyroidism consists of restoring normal thyroid status: the normal dose of T_3 or T_4 should be administered routinely on the morning of surgery, even though these drugs have long half-lives (1.4 to 10 days). The usual daily replacement dose in adults is 0.1 to 0.2 mg of L-thyroxine (Synthroid).

The T_4 level itself can be used as a guide to therapy. Both the T_4 and TSH serum levels are usually in the normal range in adequately treated patients.

Myxedema coma is a rare complication that is associated with profound hypothyroidism. It is associated with extreme lethargy, severe hypothermia, bradycardia, and alveolar hypoventilation with hypoxia and is occasionally accompanied by pericardial effusion and CHF. Hyponatremia associated with marked decrease in free water clearance by the kidney is also often part of the syndrome. This is the one single indication for intravenous T_4 therapy. For patients in myxedema coma who require emergency surgery, T_3 or T_4 can be given intravenously (with the risk of precipitating myocardial ischemia, however) while supportive therapy is undertaken to restore normal intravascular fluid volume, body temperature, cardiac function, respiratory function, and electrolyte balance. L-Thyroxine is given in a single intravenous dose of 300 to 500 µg. Intravenous T_3 (Cytomel) may also be given in the dose range of 25 to 50 µg every 8 hours until the blood level of T_3 is normal. Intravenous T_3 probably is superior to intravenous T_4, because T_3 is the most physiologically active form of thyroid hormone therapy and because it bypasses the normal T_4 to T_3 peripheral conversion pathway, which tends to be markedly depressed in patients with serious systemic illnesses. The intravenous preparations should always be prepared fresh before use.

Hypothyroid Patients with Coronary Artery Disease

Treating hypothyroid patients who have symptomatic coronary artery disease poses special problems and may require compromises in the general practice of preoperatively restoring euthyroidism with drugs.[24,51,52] Although both T_4 and esmolol may be given, adequate amelioration of both ischemic heart disease and hypothyroidism may be difficult to achieve. The need for thyroid therapy must be balanced against the risk of aggravating anginal symptoms. One review suggests early consideration of coronary artery revascularization.[51] It advocates initiating thyroid replacement therapy in the intensive care unit soon after the patient's arrival from the operating room after myocardial revascularization surgery. However, several deaths resulting from dysrhythmias and CHF as well as cardiogenic shock with infarction have occurred while patients who were not given thyroid therapy were awaiting surgery. Thus, there is a need to consider "truly" emergency coronary artery revascularization in patients who have both severe coronary artery disease and significant hypothyroidism. In fact, several large medical centers consider the presence of both disease to be as important an indicator for immediate surgery as is left main coronary artery disease with unstable angina for immediate coronary revascularization.

In the presence of hypothyroidism, respiratory control mechanisms do not function normally.[48] However, the response to hypoxia and hypercarbia and the clearance of free water become normal with thyroid replacement therapy. Drug metabolism has been reported anecdotally to be slowed, and awakening times after administration of sedatives were found to be prolonged during hypothyroidism. However, no formal study of the pharmacokinetics and pharmacodynamics of sedatives or anesthetic agents in patients with hypothyroidism has been published. These concerns disappear when thyroid function is normalized preoperatively.

Addison's disease (with its relative steroid deficiency) is more common in hypothyroid than in euthyroid individuals, and some endocrinologists routinely treat patients who have noniatrogenic hypothyroidism by giving stress doses of corticosteroids perioperatively. The possibility that this steroid deficiency exists should be considered if the patient becomes hypotensive perioperatively.

Thyroid Nodules and Carcinoma

Identifying malignancy in a solitary thyroid nodule is a difficult and important procedure. Fine-needle aspiration biopsy has become a standard tool.[53] Males and patients with previous radiation to the head and neck have an increased likelihood of malignant disease in their nodules.[54] Twenty-seven percent of all irradiated patients develop nodules. Often, needle biopsy and scanning are sufficient for the diagnosis, but occasionally an excisional biopsy is needed. If a cancer is found at surgery it is usually routine to do total thyroidectomy. Instead of starting these patients on exogenous thyroid immediately after surgery, this decision should be temporarily postponed until a decision is made as to whether massive amounts of radioactive ^{131}I therapy are indicated. A week after 50 to 100 mCi of ^{131}I is given, exogenous replacement thyroid therapy can be instituted. Some internists prefer to start exogenous thyroid immediately after surgery, because it may have a cancer-suppressing effect.[55] However, before a radioactive iodine scan or definitive therapy with radioactive iodine can be accomplished, exogenous thyroid hormone must be stopped for at least 6 weeks. Papillary carcinoma accounts for more than 60% of all carcinomas. Simple excision of lymph node metastases appears to be as efficacious for patient survival as are radical neck procedures.[56]

Medullary carcinoma is the most aggressive form of thyroid carcinoma. It is associated with familial incidence of pheochromocytoma, as are parathyroid adenomas. For this reason, a history should be obtained for patients who have a surgical scar in the thyroid and parathyroid region, so that the possibility of occult pheochromocytoma can be ruled out.

Intraoperative Anesthetic Considerations and Postoperative Problems in Patients with Thyroid Disease

The major considerations regarding anesthesia for patients with disorders of the thyroid are (1) attainment of a euthyroid state preoperatively, (2) preoperative preparation and attention to the characteristics of the diseases mentioned previously, and (3) normalization of cardiovascular function and temperature perioperatively.

No controlled study has demonstrated clinical advantages of any one anesthetic drug over another for surgical patients who are hyperthyroid. Thus, there are no data on human subjects to imply that the choice of anesthetic affects patient outcome in the presence of thyroid disease. Furthermore, although some authors have recommended that anticholinergic drugs (especially atropine) be avoided because they interfere with the sweating mechanism and cause tachycardia, atropine has been given as a test for adequacy of antithyroid treatment. Because patients are now subjected to operative procedures only when they are euthyroid, the traditional "steal" of the heavily premedicated hyperthyroid patient to the operating room has vanished.

A patient who has a large goiter and an obstructed airway can be treated like any other patient whose airway management is problematic. Preoperative medication need not include "deep" sedation, and an airway can be established, often with the patient awake. A firm armored endotracheal tube is preferable and should be passed beyond the point of extrinsic compression. It is most useful to examine computed tomographic (CT), magnetic resonance imaging (MRI), or ultrasound scans of the neck preoperatively to determine the extent of compression. Maintenance of anesthesia usually presents little difficulty. Body heat mechanisms are inadequate in hypothyroid patients, and temperature can be monitored and maintained, especially in patients who require emergency surgery before the euthyroid state is attained.[44] Because there is an increased incidence of myasthenia gravis in hyperthyroid patients, it may be advisable to use a twitch monitor to guide muscle relaxant administration.

Postoperatively, extubation should be performed under optimal circumstances for reintubation, in case the tracheal rings have been weakened and the trachea collapses. Possible postoperative complications are those for hyperparathyroidism (see earlier).

Summary

Preoperative normalization of thyroid function helps ensure that the patient with thyroid disease is at little additional risk of experiencing perioperative complications. The organ system most threatened by thyroid disease is the cardiovascular system. In apathetic hyperthyroidism, a rapid heart rate or idiopathic atrial fibrillation may be the only clue to such a diagnosis. Patients with hypothyroidism and myocardial ischemia also pose problems for perioperative management. No particular anesthetic techniques or agents have proved more beneficial or successful than others. Securing the airway and checking for nerve palsies, hematoma formation, hypothermia, and hypocalcemia must not be overlooked perioperatively. If a patient has a neck scar, the medical history should probably be reviewed because of the possibility of associated pheochromocytoma.

PITUITARY GLAND

Physiology

The pituitary gland is divided into an anterior and a posterior portion that have substantially different organizations. The anterior pituitary is connected to the hypothalamus via a complex portal vascular system. Hypothalamic releasing or inhibitory factors are synthesized in the hypothalamus, are secreted into the portal system, and reach the anterior pituitary gland in very high concentrations. Functional activity in the posterior pituitary has a different organization: specialized neurons in the hypothalamus synthesize vasopressin and oxytocin. These two hormones are then secreted through specialized axons down the stalk of the pituitary gland and are stored in the posterior pituitary gland.

Each pituitary hormone has a specific releasing factor associated with it—and in some cases a specific inhibitory factor. Except for the positive effect of TRH on both TSH and prolactin secretion and for disease states, generally there is no overlap in function of the hypothalamic hormones. For instance, in acromegaly, both somatotropin-releasing factor and thyrotropin-releasing factor can bring about release of growth hormone (GH). In the normal state this would not occur. Specific hypothalamic-releasing hormones have been defined for TSH, adrenocorticotropic hormone (ACTH), and the gonadotropins (both luteinizing hormone [LH] and follicle-stimulating hormone [FSH]). Both a releasing and an inhibitory hypothalamic factor have been discovered for GH. Prolactin is primarily associated with an inhibitory hypothalamic factor (probably the neurotransmitter dopamine). An additional factor involving hypothalamic control of the pituitary is the pulsatile periodic operation of the hypothalamus. Probably the most important biologic rhythm is the sleep or light-dark pattern. For instance, GH and ACTH show specific nocturnal bursts in males. Prolactin also tends to increase in concentration in the blood immediately after sleep begins. LH shows a sleep pattern especially during puberty.

The three monoamine neurotransmitters—dopamine, norepinephrine, and serotonin—can profoundly affect hypothalamic function and are found in high concentration in major hypothalamic centers. There is essentially no blood-brain barrier in either the pituitary or the hypothalamus, and target organ products such as estrogen, testosterone, thyroid, and adrenal hormones can exert feedback at either the hypothalamic or pituitary level (Fig. 13-4).

Diseases of the Anterior Pituitary Gland

Hypofunction of the Pituitary Gland

All or several of the trophic hormones may be involved in hypopituitary states. The causes of hypopituitarism include chromophobe adenoma, Rathke's pouch cysts or craniopharyngioma in children, necrosis following circulatory collapse due to hemorrhage after delivery (Sheehan's syndrome), surgical hypophysectomy, irradiation to the skull or brain, granulomatous diseases, other infectious diseases, surgical or other trauma, and hemochromatosis.[56-58] Metastatic disease (especially from breast cancer) is only rarely seen. Destruction of the gland by tumor (i.e., chromophobe adenoma) is probably the most common cause of hypopituitarism. One third to one half of all patients with chromophobe adenoma secrete excessive quantities of the hormone prolactin. Excessive secretion of prolactin may be associated with galactorrhea and amenorrhea (gonadotropin deficiency).[57] GH deficiency in a child results in severe growth failure. Loss of TSH or ACTH function usually occurs later in life, when variable features related to thyroid deficiency or cortisol lack inevitably manifest themselves. If a tumor exists, it may grow above the sella (suprasellar extension), and headaches and visual field defects, notably bitemporal hemianopsia, will occur. Single isolated deficiencies of specific pituitary hormones have been described. The most common is gonadotropin deficiency. A well-known syndrome is gonadotropin deficiency associated with loss of the sense of smell (Kallmann's syndrome). This interesting hypothalamic entity is caused by failure of gonadotropin-releasing factor to function appropriately. Although depression might be expected to decrease ACTH response, it did not do so in a recent controlled study.[59]

It is possible to measure by radioimmunoassay virtually all of the hormones of the anterior pituitary gland. This includes measurements of GH, TSH, LH, FSH, prolactin, and ACTH. Low LH and FSH associated with estrogen deficiency in a female or low testosterone in a male points to a hypothalamic or pituitary deficiency even of ACTH.[60] Likewise low TSH with a low T_4 by radioimmunoassay also indicates either hypothalamic or pituitary deficiency. An elevated prolactin level is commonly associated with chromophobe adenomas.

An evaluation of the hypothalamic-pituitary-adrenal axis, however, can be quite difficult. The metapyrone test has long been a standard test for determination of the

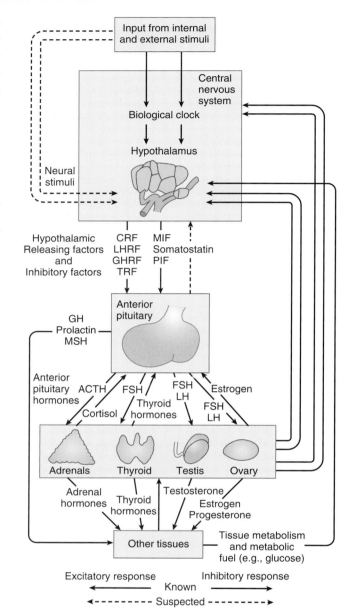

Pituitary Hormone	Hypothalamic Regulatory Hormones
Adrenocorticotropic hormone (ACTH)	Corticotropin releasing factor (CRF)
Thyroid stimulating hormone (TSH)	Thyrotropin releasing factor (TRF)
Follicle stimulating hormone (FSH) and luteinizing hormone (LH)	Gonadotropin releasing factor (GHRF)
Growth hormone (GH)	Growth hormone releasing factor (GHRF), somatostatin (inhibitory)
Prolactin	Prolactin inhibitory factor (PIF)

FIGURE 13–4 Basic feedback mechanisms in the neuroendocrine system. *(From Hosp Pract 1975;10:60.)*

pituitary-adrenal axis. Metapyrone blocks the conversion of 11-deoxycortisol to cortisol. Normally, 11-deoxycortisol is not measurable. The metapyrone test consists of giving a single oral dose of metapyrone (3 g) at midnight and measuring plasma cortisol and 11-deoxycortisol concentrations the following morning. If the 11-deoxycortisol level is greater than 10 μg/mL, ACTH stimulation must have occurred and the patient has a normal pituitary-adrenal axis. If both 11-deoxycortisol and cortisol are low, this means that ACTH was not stimulated and the patient has little or no ACTH pituitary reserve. The test can also be performed using the measurement of urinary 17-hydroxycorticoids while 750 mg of metapyrone is given every 4 hours for six doses.

Hypoglycemia induced by giving 0.1 unit of insulin per kilogram of body weight intravenously can also be used to test not only ACTH reserve but also GH reserve. Hypoglycemia (blood glucose concentration less than 50 mg/dL) should result in significant rises in both plasma cortisol and GH if the pituitary gland is functioning normally. Failure of the plasma cortisol level to rise after intravenous insulin is an indication that ACTH reserve is low.

Hyperfunction of the Pituitary Gland

There are three major hyperfunctioning pituitary gland tumors: (1) prolactin-secreting chromophobe adenoma, (2) an ACTH-secreting tumor associated with Cushing's disease (see section on adrenal disease), and (3) acromegaly associated with excessive GH secretion. Gonadotropin- and thyrotropin-secreting pituitary tumors are extraordinarily rare.

Acromegaly is a syndrome that presents as characteristic facies, weakness, enlargement of the hands (often to the point of rendering the usual oximeter probes difficult to use) and feet, thickening of the tongue (often to the point of making endotracheal intubation difficult), and enlargement of the nose and mandible with spreading of the teeth (often to the point of requiring larger than normal laryngoscope blades).[60-63] The patient may even appear myxedematous. Other findings include abnormal glucose tolerance, carpal tunnel syndrome, and osteoporosis. The most specific test for acromegaly is measurement of GH before and after glucose administration. The typical acromegalic has very elevated fasting levels of GH (usually above 10 mg/mL), and the levels do not change appreciably after oral glucose is administered. In the normal state, glucose markedly suppresses the GH level. A few patients with active acromegaly have normal levels of fasting GH that are not suppressed after glucose is given. The drug L-dopa, which normally causes an elevation of GH in healthy subjects, in the acromegalic either has no effect or lowers GH levels. Therapy for acromegaly includes the options of pituitary irradiation (heavy particle or implants) and transsphenoidal hypophysectomy.[64-66] If suprasellar extension exists, conventional transfrontal hypophysectomy is often employed. The dopaminergic agonist bromocriptine can lower GH levels, but long-term follow-up has not shown that this therapy is definitive.

Prolactin has been one of the most interesting markers for identifying patients with pituitary tumors.[57] Elevated prolactin levels are often (but not invariably) associated with galactorrhea. Females commonly have amenorrhea, and males have impotence. Optimal therapy for prolactin-secreting tumors is still being evaluated: the dopamine agonist bromocriptine can be extremely effective in controlling the prolactin level and restoring gonadotropin function; however, in females who wish to get pregnant, the concern that pregnancy will cause rapid growth of these tumors may make a surgical procedure more desirable. Pituitary irradiation has not been uniformly successful.

Multiple Endocrine Adenomatosis Syndrome

Pituitary tumors are sometimes associated with multiple endocrine adenomatosis syndrome (MEA). Pituitary tumors are found more commonly in the MEA I syndrome where adenomas of the parathyroid glands and islets of the pancreas along with the Zollinger-Ellison syndrome may be associated.

Anesthetic Considerations for Patients with Abnormal Anterior Pituitary Function

The basic approach of rendering normal all abnormal endocrine functions before surgery holds for endocrine abnormalities originating in the pituitary as well as in the end organ. These considerations are dealt with in the individual sections in this chapter on thyroid and adrenal disorders and on conditions with abnormal glucose metabolism or control, and, as noted earlier, acromegalic patients can be difficult to intubate.[60-62] One special area—that of operations on the pituitary itself—deserves note here, however. The most common approach is now transsphenoidal hypophysectomy, performed on more than 30,000 patients in the United States each year.[63,66] For the patient undergoing craniotomy, the concerns common to any craniotomy, such as provision of patent airway, adequate pulmonary ventilation, control of circulating blood volume, inhibition of increase in brain size, and effective constant monitoring for adverse complications associated with posture, anesthesia, and operation are appropriate. Premedication, use of anesthetic agents and techniques, and monitoring indicated for operations on the pituitary gland are essentially measures that the individual anesthesiologist prefers for operations on other parts of the brain. The effects of anesthetic agents on secretion of pituitary hormones do not constitute an important factor in the selection of agents for use during operation on the pituitary gland.[64,65] Disorders arising from this surgery include temperature deregulation and abnormalities of endocrine function, including the need for immediate treatment of steroid deficiency, hypoglycemia, and excessive or deficient secretion of vasopressin (also called antidiuretic hormone [ADH]). Even for operations done under local anesthesia, the risk of carotid artery injury may necessitate the participation of an anesthesiologist[67]; placement of a nasal endotracheal tube can be hazardous in the patient who has had prior transsphenoidal surgery.[68] An exaggerated response on extubation to epinephrine infiltration for transsphenoidal hypophysectomy has been reported,[69,70] even without the drugs that sensitize the myocardium to epinephrine.

Disorders of the Posterior Pituitary Gland

Deficiency of vasopressin synthesis results in the disease known as diabetes insipidus. Clinically, it is characterized by the excretion of a large volume of hypotonic urine, which in turn necessitates the intake of equally large amounts of fluid or prevention of hyperosmolarity of body fluids and dehydration.[71] Other causes of diabetes insipidus include compulsive water drinking and nephrogenic resistance to the action of vasopressin (Table 13-3).

The classic test to distinguish patients with diabetes insipidus from compulsive water drinkers and patients with nephrogenic diabetes insipidus is the water deprivation test.[71] Following dehydration, patients with diabetes insipidus can only minimally concentrate their urine. When the serum osmolarity rises to 295 mOsm/L (osmotic threshold), all normal patients release vasopressin into the blood and concentrate their urine to conserve water. Simultaneous measurements of urine and plasma osmolarity are made as water deprivation continues. Once the urine and plasma osmolarity have stabilized (usually with a 3% to 5% loss in body weight), the patient is given an injection of vasopressin. If vasopressin is being maximally secreted by the posterior pituitary, then exogenous pitressin or vasopressin will have no effect. The patient with vasopressin deficiency never quite reaches stable plasma osmolarity, and the urine osmolarity rarely gets much above 500 mOsm/L. Moreover, even after severe dehydration, exogenous pitressin or vasopressin causes a significant increase in urine osmolarity only in patients with true diabetes insipidus. Thus, this sensitive test even distinguishes patients who have partial diabetes insipidus.

Compulsive water drinkers may at times present a diagnostic problem, because they often cannot concentrate their urine well, and the water deprivation test must be carried out until the osmotic threshold is reached. Tests employing hypertonic saline as a physiologic stimulus to ADH are cumbersome and difficult to interpret. Adrenocortical insufficiency can mask the polyuria of

---

TABLE 13–3 Causes of Diabetes Insipidus
Vasopressin Deficiency (Neurogenic Diabetes Insipidus)
Acquired
Idiopathic
Trauma (accidental, surgical)
Tumor (craniopharyngioma, metastasis, lymphoma)
Granuloma (sarcoid, histiocytosis)
Infections (meningitis, encephalitis)
Vascular (Sheehan's syndrome, aneurysm, aortocoronary bypass)
Familial (autosomal dominant)
Excessive Water Intake (Primary Polydipsia)
Acquired
Idiopathic (resetting of the osmostat)
Psychogenic
Familial (?)
Vasopressin Insensitivity (Nephrogenic Diabetes Insipidus)
Acquired
Infectious (pyelonephritis)
Postobstructive (prostatic, ureteral)
Vascular (sickle cell disease, trait)
Infiltrative (amyloid)
Cystic (polycystic disease)
Metabolic (hypokalemia, hypercalcemia)
Granuloma (sarcoid)
Toxic (lithium, demeclocycline, methoxyflurane)
Solute overload (glucosuria, postobstructive)
Familial (X-linked recessive)

---

partial diabetes insipidus, because it lowers the osmotic threshold for vasopressin release. Institution of corticosteroid therapy in such patients unmasks the diabetes insipidus, and severe polyuria may result.

A number of drugs have been shown to alter the release and action of ADH. The sulfonylurea agents, notably chlorpropamide, have been shown to augment release of ADH and are used in the treatment of patients with partial nephrogenic diabetes insipidus. Likewise, clofibrate, carbamazepine (Tegretol), vincristine, and cyclophosphamide all either release ADH or potentiate its action on the renal tubule. Ethanol as well as phenytoin (Dilantin) and chlorpromazine inhibit the action of ADH and its release. Lithium, a drug widely used to treat manic-depressive disorders, can inhibit the formation of cyclic adenosine monophosphate (AMP) in the renal tubule and probably even inhibit its synthesis of ADH directly and thus can result in a diabetes insipidus–like picture.

The treatment of diabetes insipidus usually consists of replacement of ADH. The preparation of ADH for intramuscular use is pitressin tannate in oil, 5 units/mL, given intramuscularly every 48 hours. A synthetic lysine vasopressin, Diodid (50 units/mL in isotonic saline), is also used as a nasal spray. This agent is short acting and is given as an adjunct to pitressin tannate. A longer-acting nasal preparation, desmopressin (1-deamino-8-D-arginine vasopressin [DDAVP]), is most commonly used.

For patients with incomplete diabetes insipidus, a trial of thiazide diuretics or chlorpropamide can increase the renal adenyl cyclase response to low levels of ADH, and this can be used for control of urinary flow. Other agents used for incomplete diabetes insipidus are carbamazepine (Tegretol) and clofibrate.

Management of the patient with complete diabetes insipidus during surgery usually does not present difficult problems. A very small amount of aqueous vasopressin (10 to 20 units per ampule) can be given as a continuous intravenous infusion. Just before surgery, the patient is given an intravenous bolus of 100 mU aqueous vasopressin and then a constant intravenous infusion of 100 to 200 mU of vasopressin per hour. In this situation isotonic fluids such as normal saline may be given safely, and there is little danger of water depletion or hypernatremia. The plasma osmolarity can be monitored during surgery and in the immediate postoperative period. The normal range for plasma osmolarity is 283 to 285 mOsm/L. Serum osmolarity can be calculated from the following formula:

$$\text{Osmolarity} = 2\,(\text{Na}+[\text{mEq/L}]) + \frac{\text{Glucose (mg/dL)}}{20}$$
$$+ \frac{\text{Blood urea nitrogen (mg/dL)}}{3}$$

When blood glucose and blood urea nitrogen are normal, the plasma osmolarity may be calculated by multiplying the serum sodium concentration by 2. If the plasma osmolarity comes up much above 290 mOsm/L, then hypotonic fluids should be considered and the amount of aqueous vasopressin given intravenously should be increased above 200 mU/hr. In patients who have only partial vasopressin or ADH insufficiency, nonosmotic stimuli such as volume depletion or the stress of surgery may stimulate large quantities of ADH, and it probably is not necessary to use aqueous vasopressin unless there is a demonstrated rise in plasma osmolarity above 290 mOsm/L during surgery or immediately postoperatively. Pitressin tannate in oil (5 to 10 units daily) may be given intramuscularly or desmopressin given intranasally in the immediate postoperative period until the long-acting intranasal preparations can be used.

Hypersecretion of Vasopressin

As first described by Bartter and Schwartz in 1967, excessive secretion of ADH (syndrome of inappropriate secretion of ADH [SIADH]) is a disorder characterized by hyponatremia that results from water retention, which in turn is due to ADH release that is inappropriately high for

the plasma osmolality or serum sodium concentration.[71] Because patients with this syndrome are unable to excrete dilute urine, ingested fluids are retained and expansion of extracellular fluid volume without edema occurs. The hallmark of SIADH is hyponatremia in the presence of urinary osmolality that is higher than plasma osmolality.

The most common cause of SIADH is production of ADH by neoplasms. The ADH produced by neoplasms is identical to the arginine vasopressin secreted by the normal neurohypophysis. The most common of the neoplasms producing ADH are small cell and oat cell carcinomas of the lungs. SIADH is also associated with various nonmalignant and inflammatory conditions of the lungs and central nervous system (CNS). Any patient suspected of having SIADH should be screened for possible adrenal insufficiency or hypothyroidism.[71] The diagnosis is essentially one of exclusion. A wide variety of drugs can bring about hypersecretion or augmentation of ADH and result in the syndrome of inappropriate secretion. The most common drugs that cause inappropriate secretion of ADH are chlorpropamide, clofibrate, psychotropics, thiazides, and the antineoplastic agents vincristine, vinblastine, and cyclophosphamide.

Most of the clinical features associated with SIADH are related to hyponatremia and the resulting brain edema; these features include weight gain, weakness, lethargy, mental confusion, obtundation, and disordered reflexes and may progress, finally, to convulsions and coma. This form of edema rarely leads to hypertension.

SIADH should be suspected when any patient with hyponatremia excretes urine that is hypertonic relative to plasma. The following laboratory findings further support the diagnosis:

- Urinary sodium greater than 20 mEq/L
- Low blood urea nitrogen and serum levels of creatinine, uric acid, and albumin
- Serum sodium less than 130 mEq/L
- Plasma osmolality less than 270 mOsm/L
- Hypertonic urine relative to plasma

The response to water loading is a useful means of evaluating the patient with hyponatremia. Patients with SIADH are unable to excrete dilute urine, even after water loading. Assay of ADH in blood can confirm the diagnosis.

Patients with mild to moderate symptoms of water intoxication can be treated with restriction of fluid intake to 500 to 1000 mL/day. Patients with severe water intoxication and CNS symptoms may need vigorous treatment, with intravenous administration of 200 to 300 mL of 5% saline solution over several hours, followed by fluid restriction.

Treatment should be directed at the underlying problem. If SIADH is drug induced, the drug should be withdrawn. Inflammation should be treated with appropriate measures, and neoplasms should be managed with surgical resection, irradiation, or chemotherapy, whichever is indicated.

At present, no drugs are available that can suppress release of ADH from the neurohypophysis or from a tumor. Phenytoin (Dilantin) and narcotic antagonists such as naloxone and butorphanol have some inhibiting effect on physiologic ADH release but are clinically ineffective in SIADH. Drugs that block the effect of ADH on renal tubules include lithium, which is rarely used because its toxicity often outweighs its benefits, and demethylchlortetracycline in doses of 900 to 1200 mg/day. The last drug interferes with the ability of the renal tubules to concentrate urine, causing excretion of isotonic or hypotonic urine and thus lessening hyponatremia. Demethylchlortetracycline can be used for ambulatory patients with SIADH in whom it is difficult to accomplish fluid restriction.

Anesthetic Considerations for Patients with ADH Abnormalities

The abnormalities of ADH function that affect perioperative management are those of either a relative or an absolute lack of ADH or an excess of ADH. No matter what the cause of the ADH disorder, the perioperative management problems can be grouped into situations with *inadequate ADH* and situations with *excess ADH*.[71] This categorization or emphasis is not meant to minimize the importance of the diverse causes of perioperative management. Moreover, the cause of the ADH disorder should be sought and the potential perioperative problems evaluated; however, the focus in the remainder of this chapter is on "how to" and "why to" manage the ADH disorder perioperatively.

Inadequate ADH

Diabetes insipidus, and thus an inadequate ADH level, is a significant problem in children undergoing posterior fossa craniotomy[72] and is the most significant complication after hypophysectomy. The severity and duration of diabetes insipidus depend on the degree of injury to the adjacent hypothalamus. The majority of patients who develop diabetes insipidus after hypophysectomy recover within a few days to 6 months. Patients with diabetes insipidus secondary to head trauma or surgery usually recover after a short period. Those who continue to have symptoms, and patients with a long history of diabetes insipidus who require surgery, present a challenge for the anesthesiologist with regard to perioperative management.

Perioperative management of patients with diabetes insipidus is based on the extent of the ADH deficiency. Management of a patient with complete diabetes insipidus and a total lack of ADH usually does not present any major problems as long as side effects of the drug are avoided and as long as that status is known before surgery.

Just before surgery, such a patient is given the usual dose of desmopressin intranasally or an intravenous bolus of 100 mU of aqueous vasopressin, followed by constant infusion of 100 to 200 mU/hr. All of the intravenous fluids given intraoperatively should be isotonic, so that the risk of water depletion and hypernatremia is reduced. Plasma osmolality should be measured every hour, both intraoperatively and in the immediate postoperative period. If the plasma osmolality goes well above 290 mOsm/L, hypotonic fluids should be administered; the rate of the intraoperative vasopressin infusion should be increased to more than 200 mU/hr.

In patients who have a partial deficiency of ADH, it is not necessary to use aqueous vasopressin perioperatively unless the plasma osmolality rises above 290 mOsm/L. Nonosmotic stimuli (e.g., volume depletion, stress of surgery) usually cause release of large quantities of ADH in the perioperative period. Consequently, these patients require only frequent monitoring of plasma osmolality during this period.

Because of the side effects, the dose of vasopressin should be limited to that necessary for control of diuresis.[72,73] This limit is applicable especially to patients who are pregnant or who have coronary artery disease, because of the oxytocic and coronary artery–constricting properties of vasopressin.[72] Another problem for anesthesiologists is the care for patients who come to the operating room with a pitressin drip for treatment of bleeding from esophageal varices. Although this situation is rare, the vasoconstrictive effect of vasopressin on the splanchnic vasculature is being used to decrease bleeding. Such patients are often volume depleted and may have concomitant coronary artery disease. Because vasopressin has been shown to markedly decrease oxygen availability, primarily because of a decreased stroke volume and heart rate, monitoring of tissue oxygen delivery may be useful. In 1982, Nikolic and Singh[74] reported on a patient with a history of angina pectoris who received a combination of cimetidine and vasopressin for esophageal varices and who developed bradyarrhythmias and atrioventricular block, requiring a pacemaker. Cessation of either of these drugs alleviated the symptoms on two occasions. This indicates that the combination of cimetidine and vasopressin could be deleterious to patients because of the combined negative inotropic and dysrhythmogenic effects of the two drugs.

Excessive ADH

Patients with SIADH resulting from malignancy have the usual problems present in malignancy, such as anemia and malnutrition, and often they have an imbalance of fluids and electrolytes.[71-75] Perioperatively, they usually have low urine output, high urine osmolality, low serum osmolality, and delayed awakening from anesthesia or awakening with mental confusion.

When a patient with SIADH comes to the operating room for any surgical procedure, fluids are managed by measuring the central volume status by central venous pressure or pulmonary artery lines, by transesophageal echocardiography, and by frequent assays of urine osmolarity, plasma osmolarity, and serum sodium, often into the immediate postoperative period. Despite the common impression that SIADH is frequently seen in elderly patients in the postoperative period, studies have shown that the patient's age and the type of anesthetic have no bearing on the postoperative development of SIADH. It is not unusual to see many patients in the neurosurgical intensive care unit suffering from this syndrome. The diagnosis is usually one of exclusion. Patients with SIADH usually require only fluid restriction; very rarely is hypertonic saline needed.

Summary

There have been no controlled studies on the risks and benefits of various types of perioperative management for patients with either inadequate or excessive ADH.[75] Nevertheless, increasing knowledge of the pathophysiology of these endocrine aberrations and the use of pharmacologic treatment probably have led to improved clinical results. Inadequate levels of ADH secretion lead to a diabetes insipidus state, with production of large amounts of hypotonic urine, hypernatremia, and a resulting intravascular volume deficit (dehydration). Perioperative treatment consists of replacement of vasopressin by infusion or nasal spray. Because vasopressin causes vasoconstriction of arteriolar beds, monitoring of tissue oxygen delivery and of myocardial ischemia is commonly used. Excess levels of ADH lead to SIADH, which is manifested by low urine output, high urine osmolality, low serum osmolality, hyponatremia, and disordered nervous system functioning (ranging from confusion and delayed awakening from anesthesia to seizures). The perioperative procedures used for SIADH consist of fluid management with a central volume monitor (I tend to restrict fluids and administer normal saline) and frequent assays for serum sodium level and osmolality and for urine volume and osmolality.

ADRENAL CORTEX

Physiology

Cholesterol in the adrenal gland is converted to Δ^5-pregnenolone. This compound is changed either to progesterone or to 17-hydroxypregnenolone. Progesterone can be converted to aldosterone, the principal mineralocorticoid, only in the zona glomerulosa of the adrenal cortex. In the zona fasciculata and zona reticularis, progesterone is made into 11-deoxycortisol and finally to cortisol, the

principal glucocorticoid. Sex hormones are also synthesized in the adrenal cortex. Testosterone is the most potent sex hormone synthesized; dehydroisoandrosterone and $^4\Delta$-androstenedione are weaker androgens but at times can contribute significantly to the androgen pool. Under certain circumstances, even estradiol, the female sex hormone, can be synthesized from its precursor hormone testosterone. Thus, three major classes of hormones—glucocorticoids, mineralocorticoids, and androgens—are secreted by the adrenal cortex. An excess or a deficiency of each of these is associated with a characteristic clinical syndrome.[76-80] Medical use of corticosteroids, now widespread, may render the adrenal cortex incapable of responding normally to the demands placed on it by surgical trauma and subsequent healing.

More than 100 years ago, Brown-Séquard first demonstrated that bilateral adrenalectomy caused premature death. Over the past century, the central role of adrenal hormones in the maintenance of hemodynamic and metabolic homeostasis by regulation of volume and electrolytes has been defined.

Glucocorticoids

The principal glucocorticoid cortisol is an essential regulator of carbohydrate, protein, lipid, and nucleic acid metabolism.[78] Cortisol exerts its biologic effects by a sequence of steps initiated by its binding to stereospecific, intracellular cytoplasmic receptors. This bound complex stimulates nuclear transcription of specific messenger RNAs. These messenger RNAs are then translated to give rise to proteins that mediate the ultimate effects of these hormones.[78]

Most cortisol is bound to corticosteroid-binding globulin (CBG, transcortin). It is the relatively small amounts of unbound cortisol that enter cells to induce actions or to be metabolized.[78] Conditions that induce changes in the amount of CBG include liver disease and nephrotic syndrome, both of which result in decreased circulating levels of CBG, and estrogen administration and pregnancy, which result in increased CBG production. Total serum cortisol levels may become elevated or depressed under these conditions that alter the amount of bound cortisol and yet the unbound, active form of cortisol is present in normal amounts. The most accurate measure of cortisol activity is the level of urinary cortisol, that is, the amount of unbound, active cortisol filtered by the kidney.[78]

The serum half-life of cortisol is 80 to 110 minutes; however, because cortisol acts through intracellular receptors, pharmacokinetics based on serum levels is not a good indicator of cortisol activity. After a single dose of glucocorticoid, the serum glucose level is elevated for 12 to 24 hours; improvements in pulmonary function in patients with bronchial asthma can still be measured

24 hours after glucocorticoid administration.[79,80] Treatment schedules for glucocorticoid replacement are based, therefore, not on the measured serum half-life but on the well-documented, prolonged end-organ effect of these steroids. In the past, hospitalized patients who required chronic glucocorticoid replacement therapy were usually treated twice daily, with a slightly higher dose in the morning than in the evening to simulate the normal diurnal variations in cortisol levels.[81,82] For patients who require parenteral "steroid coverage" during and after surgery (see later), administration of glucocorticoid every 8 to 12 hours seems appropriate.[83-85] Relative potencies of glucocorticoids are listed in Table 13-4. Cortisol is inactivated primarily in the liver and is excreted as 17-hydroxycorticosteroid. Cortisol is also filtered and excreted unchanged into the urine.

The synthetic glucocorticoids vary in their binding specificity in a dose-related manner. When given in supraphysiologic doses (more than 30 mg/day), cortisol and cortisone bind to mineralocorticoid receptor sites and cause salt and water retention and loss of potassium and hydrogen ions.[86,87] When these steroids are administered in maintenance doses of 30 mg/day or less, patients require a specific mineralocorticoid for electrolyte and volume homeostasis. Many other steroids do not bind to mineralocorticoid receptors, even in large doses, and have minimal mineralocorticoid effect (see Table 13-4).[87]

Control of Glucocorticoid Secretion. The hypothalamic-pituitary-adrenal axis is shown in Figure 13-4. Secretion of glucocorticoids is regulated exclusively by pituitary ACTH.[76,88] ACTH is synthesized from a precursor molecule (preopiomelanocortin) that breaks down to form an endorphin (β-lipoprotropin) and ACTH. ACTH secretion has a diurnal rhythm; it is normally greatest during the early morning hours in men (afternoon in women) and is regulated at least in part by sleep-wake cycles.[78]

Its secretion is stimulated by release of corticotropin-releasing factor (CRF) from the hypothalamus.[76] Cortisol and other glucocorticoids exert negative feedback at both pituitary and hypothalamic levels to inhibit secretion of ACTH and CRF.

Overproduction of glucocorticoids can be caused by adrenal tumors (primary Cushing's disease)[89] or by overstimulation of normal adrenal glands by elevated levels of ACTH from pituitary microadenomas (secondary Cushing's disease). Inappropriately low levels of glucocorticoids may result from destruction or atrophy of the adrenal gland itself (primary adrenal insufficiency) or from diminished levels of ACTH in pituitary dysfunction (secondary adrenal insufficiency).[90]

Mineralocorticoids

Aldosterone, the major mineralocorticoid secreted in humans, comes from the zona glomerulosa of the adrenal cortex, causes reabsorption of sodium and secretion of potassium and hydrogen ions, and thus contributes to electrolyte and volume homeostasis. This action is most prominent in the distal renal tubules, but it also occurs in salivary and sweat glands. The main regulator of aldosterone secretion is the renin-angiotensin system.[91] Juxtaglomerular cells in the cuff of the renal arterioles are sensitive to decreased renal perfusion pressure or volume and consequently secrete renin. Renin splits the precursor angiotensinogen (from the liver) into angiotensin I, which is further converted by converting enzyme, primarily in the lung, to angiotensin II. Mineralocorticoid secretion is increased by increased levels of angiotensin.

Androgens

Androstenedione and dehydroepiandrosterone, which are weak androgens arising from the adrenal cortex,

---

TABLE 13–4   Relative Potencies and Biologic Half-Lives of Cortisol and Its Synthetic Analogues

Common Name	Other Name	Estimated Potency		Biologic Half-Life (hr)
		Glucorticoid	Mineralocorticoid	
Cortisol	Compound F, hydrocortisone	1	1	8-12
Cortisone	Cortone	0.8	0.8	8-12
Prednisone		4	0.25	12-36
Methylprednisolone	Medrol	5	0.25	12-36
Triamcinolone	Aristocort, Kenacort	5	0.25	12-36
Dexamethasone	Decadron	20-30	±	26-54
Fluorohydrocortisone	Florinef	5	200	—
Desoxycorticosterone	Percorten	0	15	—

constitute major sources of androgens in women[75] (and have gained prominence for their use or abuse by baseball players seeking to hit more home runs). These androgens are converted outside the adrenal glands to testosterone, a potent virilizing hormone.[75,92] Excess secretion of androgen in women causes masculinization, pseudopuberty, or female pseudohermaphroditism. Some tumors convert this androgen to an estrogenic substance, in which case feminization results. Some congenital enzyme defects that cause abnormal levels of androgens in blood also result in glucocorticoid and mineralocorticoid abnormalities. The altered sexual differentiation in the presence of such defects requires no specific modification of anesthetic technique. All syndromes related to abnormal androgen levels are associated with cortisol deficiency. In patients who have associated alterations in glucocorticoid or mineralocorticoid activity, anesthetic plans should be modified as outlined in the following sections.

Excessive Adrenocortical Hormones: Hyperplasia, Adenoma, Carcinoma

Sex Hormone–Secreting Tumors of the Adrenal Glands

Hirsutism in females may be due to either adrenal or ovarian tumor. Adrenal virilizing tumors are almost always associated with markedly elevated 17-ketosteroid urinary excretion, whereas functioning ovarian tumors tend to produce very potent androgens such as testosterone or dihydrotestosterone, which are not measured as part of the 17-ketosteroids. Rarely, adrenal tumors produce only testosterone and are stimulated by human chorionic gonadotropin. Similarly, some androgen-producing ovarian tumors have been shown to respond to dexamethasone suppression. A common cause of hirsutism in females is polycystic ovarian disease, which is associated with bilaterally enlarged ovaries.[77] Extreme feminization in males can occasionally be due to an estrogen-producing tumor of the adrenal gland. Functioning sex hormone–producing tumors of the adrenal gland almost always tend to be unilateral. Pelvic B-mode ultrasonography, CT, and MRI are very useful modalities for localizing lesions. Most patients do not have to be managed with glucocorticoids during or after surgery. The only exception is the patient who has associated Cushing's syndrome with cortisol excess; in this instance management should be as outlined later for tumors of the adrenal gland.

Adrenal genital syndrome should be ruled out as a possible cause of hirsutism. These patients are not surgical candidates. Generally, in addition to high 17-ketosteroid levels in the urine, these patients have very high urinary pregnanetriol levels and elevated 17-OH progesterone blood levels. They are usually managed with mildly suppressive doses of corticosteroids.

Excessive Glucocorticoids

Glucocorticoid excess (Cushing's syndrome), resulting from either endogenous oversecretion or long-term treatment with large doses of glucocorticoids, produces a characteristic appearance and a predictable complex of disease states (Table 13-5). The individual appears moon faced and plethoric, having a centripetal distribution of fat and thin extremities because of muscle wasting. The heart and diaphragm apparently are spared the effects of muscle wasting.[78] The skin is thin and easily bruised, and striae are often present. Hypertension (because of increases in renin substrate and vascular reactivity caused by glucocorticoids) and fluid retention are present in 85% of patients.[78,91] Nearly two of every three patients also have hyperglycemia resulting from inhibition of peripheral glucose use with concomitant stimulation of gluconeogenesis. These patients often have osteopenia as a result of decreased bone matrix formation and impaired calcium absorption. One third of the patients have pathologic fractures.

Special preoperative considerations for patients with Cushing's syndrome include regulating diabetes and hypertension and ensuring that intravascular fluid volume and electrolyte concentrations are normal.[92,93] Ectopic ACTH production from sites other than the pituitary may cause marked hypokalemic alkalosis.[78] Treatment with the aldosterone antagonist spironolactone arrests the potassium loss and helps mobilize excess fluid. Because of the high incidence of severe osteopenia and the risk of fractures, meticulous attention to patient positioning is necessary.[76] In addition, glucocorticoids are lympholytic and immunosuppressive, perhaps increasing the patient's susceptibility to infection.[94-96] The tensile strength of healing wounds decreases in the presence of glucocorticoids, an effect at least partially reversed by topical administration of vitamin A.[97]

Specific considerations pertain to the surgical approach for each cause of Cushing's syndrome. For example, nearly three fourths of the cases of spontaneous Cushing's disease result from a pituitary adenoma that secretes ACTH.[78] Perioperative treatment for patients who have Cushing's disease and a pituitary microadenoma differs from that for patients who have a pituitary adenoma associated with amenorrhea and galactorrhea. The Cushing's syndrome patient tends to bleed more easily and (based on anecdotal evidence) tends to have a higher central venous pressure. Thus, during transsphenoidal tumor resection in such patients, we routinely monitor central venous pressure or end-diastolic left ventricular volume on transesophageal echocardiography and maintain pressure and/or volume in the low end of the normal range. Such monitoring is needed only infrequently in other cases of transsphenoidal resection of microadenoma.[78]

TABLE 13–5 Clinical Features of Hyperadrenalism (Cushing's Syndrome) and Hypoadrenalism	
Cushing's Syndrome	**Hypoadrenalism**
Central obesity	Weight loss
Proximal muscle weakness	Weakness, fatigue, lethargy
Osteopenia at a young age and back pain	Muscle and joint pain
Hypertension	Postural hypotension and dizziness
Headache	Headache
Psychiatric disorders	Anorexia, nausea, abdominal pain, constipation, diarrhea
Purple stria	
Spontaneous ecchymoses	Hyperpigmentation
Plethoric facies	Hyperkalemia, hyponatremia
Hyperpigmentation	Occasional hypoglycemia
Hirsutism	Hypercalcemia
Acne	Prerenal azotemia
Hypokalemic alkalosis	
Glucose intolerance	
Kidney stones	
Polyuria	
Menstrual disorders	
Increased leukocyte count	

From Miller RD (ed): Miller's Anesthesia, 6th ed. Philadelphia, Churchill Livingstone, 2005, with permission.

Ten to 15 percent of patients with Cushing's syndrome have adrenal overproduction of glucocorticoids (adrenal adenoma or carcinoma). If either unilateral or bilateral adrenal resection is planned, I normally begin administering glucocorticoids at the start of the tumor resection, normally giving 100 mg of hydrocortisone phosphate intravenously every 24 hours.[93] This amount is reduced over the next 3 to 6 days until a maintenance dose of 20 to 30 mg/day in divided doses is reached. Beginning on about day 3, 9α-fluorocortisone (a mineralocorticoid) is also given, 0.05 to 0.1 mg/day. Both steroids may require several adjustments in some patients. This therapy is continued for patients who have undergone bilateral adrenal resection. For patients who have had unilateral resection, therapy is individualized, based on the status of the remaining adrenal gland.

Patients with Cushing's syndrome who require bilateral adrenalectomy have a high incidence of postoperative complications. The incidence of pneumothorax approaches 20% with adrenal carcinoma resection, and it is sought and treatment begun before the wound is closed. Ten percent of patients with Cushing's syndrome who undergo adrenalectomy are found to have an undiagnosed pituitary tumor. After reduction of high levels of cortisol by adrenalectomy, the pituitary tumor enlarges (Nelson's syndrome).[98] These pituitary tumors are potentially invasive and may produce large amounts of ACTH and melanocyte-stimulating hormone, thus increasing pigmentation.

Adrenal tumors are at least 85% incidentomas, that is, discovered incidentally during screening (and largely unindicated) CT scans. Nonfunctioning adrenal adenomas are found in as many as 10% of autopsies.[99-101]

Adrenal adenomas are usually treated surgically, and often the contralateral gland will resume functioning after several months. Frequently, however, the effects of carcinomas are not cured by surgery. In such cases, administration of inhibitors of steroid synthesis such as metyrapone or o, p'-DDD[2,2-bis-(2-chlorophenyl-4-chlorophenyl)-1,1-dichloroethane] may ameliorate some symptoms but may not improve survival. These drugs and the aldosterone antagonist spironolactone may alleviate symptoms in the case of ectopic ACTH secretion if the primary tumor proves unresectable. Patients given these adrenal suppressants are also given chronic glucocorticoid replacement therapy (with the goal of complete adrenal suppression). These patients should be considered to have suppressed adrenal function, and glucocorticoid replacement should be increased perioperatively as discussed earlier.

Excessive Mineralocorticoids

Excess mineralocorticoid activity leads to sodium retention, potassium depletion, hypertension, and hypokalemic alkalosis.[102-108] These symptoms constitute primary hyperaldosteronism, or Conn's syndrome (a cause of low-renin hypertension, because renin secretion is inhibited by the effects of the high aldosterone levels).

Primary hyperaldosteronism is present in 0.5% to 1% of hypertensive patients who have no other known cause of hypertension. Primary hyperaldosteronism is most often the result of a unilateral adenoma, although 25% to 40% of patients may have bilateral adrenal hyperplasia. Intravascular fluid volume, electrolyte concentrations, and renal function should be restored to within normal limits preoperatively by treatment with spironolactone. The effects of spironolactone are slow to appear and increase for 1 to 2 weeks. In addition, patients with Conn's syndrome have a high incidence of ischemic heart disease and hemodynamic monitoring appropriate for their degree of cardiovascular impairment should be undertaken. A retrospective anecdotal study indicated that intraoperative stability, with preoperative control of blood pressure and electrolytes, was better with spironolactone than with other antihypertensive agents.[103] The efficacy for patient outcome of optimizing the preoperative status of patients with disorders of glucocorticoid or mineralocorticoid secretion, however, has not been clearly established.

Adrenocortical Hormone Deficiency

Glucocorticoid Deficiency

Withdrawal of steroids or suppression of their adrenal synthesis by steroid therapy is the leading cause of underproduction of corticosteroids.[76] The management of this type of glucocorticoid deficiency is discussed below (see Patients Taking Corticosteroids for Medical Conditions). Fewer cases of this potential problem are expected, in part because of a change from systemic corticosteroids to inhaled ones for treatment of asthma.[79] Other causes of adrenocortical insufficiency include destruction of the adrenal gland by cancer (including AIDS), tuberculosis, hemorrhage, or an autoimmune mechanism; some forms of congenital adrenal hyperplasia (see previous discussion); and administration of cytotoxic drugs.

Primary adrenal insufficiency (Addison's disease) is caused by a local process within the adrenal gland that leads to destruction of all zones of the cortex and causes both glucocorticoid and mineralocorticoid deficiency if the insufficiency is bilateral. Autoimmune disease is the most common cause of primary (nonendogenous) bilateral ACTH deficiency.[76,90] Autoimmune destruction of the adrenals may be associated with other autoimmune disorders, such as Hashimoto's thyroiditis. Enzymatic defects in cortisol synthesis also cause glucocorticoid insufficiency, compensatory elevations of ACTH, and congenital adrenal hyperplasia.

Adrenal insufficiency usually develops slowly. Patients with Addison's disease can develop marked pigmentation (because excess ACTH is present to drive an unproductive adrenal gland) and cardiopenia (apparently secondary to chronic hypotension).

Secondary adrenal insufficiency occurs when ACTH secretion is deficient, often because of a pituitary or hypothalamic tumor. Treatment of pituitary tumors by surgery or radiation may result in hypopituitarism and consequent adrenal failure.

If glucocorticoid-deficient patients are not stressed, they usually have no perioperative problems.[93] However, acute adrenal (addisonian) crisis can occur when even a minor stress (e.g., upper respiratory tract infection) is present.[104] In the preparation of such a patient for anesthesia and surgery, hypovolemia, hyperkalemia, and hyponatremia can be treated. Because these patients cannot respond to stressful situations, it was traditionally recommended that they be given a maximum stress dose of glucocorticoids (i.e., hydrocortisone, 300 mg/70 kg/day) perioperatively. Symreng and colleagues[105] gave 25 mg of hydrocortisone phosphate intravenously to adults at the start of the operative procedure, followed by 100 mg intravenously over the next 24 hours. Because using the minimal drug dose that will cause an appropriate effect is desirable, this latter regimen seems attractive. Evidence is accumulating that less steroid supplementation does not cause problems, and I recommend giving hydrocortisone phosphate intravenously in a dose of 100 mg/70 kg/24 hr.[104,105]

Udelsman and colleagues[104] studied glucocorticoid replacement in primates. In that study, adrenalectomized primates and sham-operated controls were maintained on physiologic doses of steroids for 4 months. The animals were then randomized to receive subphysiologic (one tenth the normal cortisol production), physiologic, and supraphysiologic (10 times the normal cortisol production) doses of cortisol for 4 days before abdominal surgery (cholecystectomy). Hemodynamic variables were measured with arterial and pulmonary artery catheters. The animals were maintained on their randomized dosing schedules during and after surgery. The group receiving subphysiologic doses of steroid perioperatively had a significant increase in postoperative mortality. The death rates in the physiologic and supraphysiologic replacement groups were the same and did not differ from that for sham-operated controls. Death in the subphysiologic replacement group was related to severe hypotension associated with a significant decrease in systemic vascular resistance and a reduced left ventricular stroke work index. The filling pressures of the heart were unchanged, as compared with those in control animals. There was, therefore, no evidence of hypovolemia or severe CHF. Despite the low systemic vascular resistance, the animals did not become tachycardic. All of these responses are compatible with the previously documented interaction of glucocorticoids and catecholamines, suggesting that glucocorticoids mediate catecholamine-induced increases in cardiac contractility and maintenance of vascular tone.

The investigators used a sensitive measure of wound healing by studying hydroxyproline accumulation. All treatment groups, including that which received supraphysiologic doses of glucocorticoids, had the same capacity for wound healing. Furthermore, there were no adverse metabolic consequences of supraphysiologic corticosteroid doses given perioperatively.[104]

This well-conducted study confirms several "old wives' tales" about patients who have inadequate adrenal function, either from underlying disease or secondary to exogenous steroids. Inadequate replacement of corticosteroids perioperatively can lead to addisonian crisis and death. Administration of supraphysiologic doses of corticosteroids for a short time perioperatively caused no discernible complications. It is clear that inadequate corticosteroid coverage can cause death. What is not so clear is what dose of corticosteroid for replacement therapy should be recommended.

Mineralocorticoid Deficiency

Hypoaldosteronism, a condition less common than glucocorticoid deficiency, can be congenital or can occur after unilateral adrenalectomy or prolonged administration of heparin.[106] It may also be a consequence of long-standing diabetes and renal failure. Nonsteroidal inhibitors of prostaglandin synthesis may also inhibit renin release and exacerbate this condition in patients with renal insufficiency.[107] Levels of plasma renin activity are below normal and fail to rise appropriately in response to sodium restriction or diuretics. Most of the patients have low blood pressure; rarely, however, a patient may be normotensive or even hypertensive. Most symptoms are due to hyperkalemic acidosis rather than hypovolemia. Patients with hypoaldosteronism can have severe hyperkalemia, hyponatremia, and myocardial conduction defects. These defects can be treated successfully with mineralocorticoids (9α-fluorocortisone, 0.05 to 0.1 mg/day) preoperatively. Doses must be carefully titrated and monitored so that increasing hypertension can be avoided.

Patients Taking Corticosteroids for Medical Conditions

Perioperative Stress and the Need for Corticoid Supplementation[77]

Many reports (mostly anecdotal) concerning normal adrenal responses during the perioperative period and responses of patients taking steroids for other diseases indicate the following:

1. Perioperative stress is related to the degree of trauma and the depth of anesthesia. Deep general or regional anesthesia causes the usual intraoperative glucocorticoid surge to be postponed to the postoperative period.
2. Few patients who have suppressed adrenal function have perioperative cardiovascular problems if they do not receive supplemental steroids perioperatively.[108]
3. Occasionally, a patient who habitually takes steroids will become hypotensive perioperatively, but this event has only rarely been documented sufficiently to implicate glucocorticoid or mineralocorticoid deficiency as the cause.
4. Although it occurs rarely, acute adrenal insufficiency can be life threatening.
5. There is little risk in giving these patients high-dose corticosteroid coverage perioperatively.

What dose of corticosteroids should one give and to whom? A definitive answer is not available; however, the recommendation of 100 mg/70 kg/24 hr stands until a prospective, randomized, double-blind trial in patients receiving physiologic doses of corticosteroids is performed. A smaller dose probably can be used. In any case, I never supplement perioperatively with a dose lower than that the patient has already been receiving.

If in doubt, how can one determine a patient's need for perioperative supplementation with glucocorticoids? Because the risk is low, I normally provide supplementation for every patient who has received corticosteroids, including inhaled corticosteroids, at any time during the previous year. It has been shown that topical application of corticosteroids (even without the use of occlusive dressings) can suppress normal adrenal responses for as long as 9 months or a year.[109]

How can one determine whether the patient's adrenal responsiveness has returned to normal? The morning plasma cortisol level does not reveal whether the adrenal cortex has recovered sufficiently to ensure that cortisol secretion increases enough to meet the demands under stress. Insulin-induced hypoglycemia has been advocated as a sensitive test of pituitary-adrenal competence (see Anterior Pituitary Disease), but its use is impractical and probably more dangerous than simply administering glucocorticoids. If plasma cortisol is measured during acute stress, a value greater than 25 µg/dL assuredly indicates, and more than 15 µg/dL probably indicates, normal pituitary-adrenal responsiveness.

The most sensitive test of adrenal reserve is the ACTH stimulation test. To test pituitary-adrenal sufficiency, one determines the baseline plasma cortisol level. Then 250 µg of synthetic ACTH (cosyntropin) is given, and the plasma cortisol is measured 30 to 60 minutes later. An increment in plasma cortisol of 7 to 20 µg/dL or more is normal.

A normal response indicates a recovery of pituitary-adrenal axis function. A lesser response usually indicates pituitary-adrenal insufficiency, possibly requiring perioperative supplementation with corticosteroids.

Usually, laboratory data defining pituitary-adrenal adequacy are not available before surgery. However, rather than delay surgery or test most patients, it is assumed that any patient who has taken corticosteroids at any time in the preceding year has pituitary-adrenal suppression and will require perioperative supplementation.

Under perioperative conditions, the adrenal glands secrete 116 to 185 mg of cortisol daily. Under maximum stress, they may secrete 200 to 500 mg daily. A good correlation between the severity and duration of the operation and the response of the adrenal gland was shown during major surgery that included procedures such as colectomy and minor surgery procedures such as herniorrhaphy. In one study, the mean maximal plasma cortisol level during major surgery in 20 patients was 47 µg/dL (range, 22 to 75 µg/dL). Values remained above 26 µg/dL for a maximum of 72 hours after operation. The mean maximal plasma cortisol level during minor surgery was 28 µg/dL (range, 10 to 44 µg/dL).[84]

Although the precise amount of glucocorticoid required has not been established, I usually administer one third of the maximal amount that the body manufactures in response to maximal stress; that is, about 200 mg/70 kg/day of intravenous hydrocortisone phosphate. For minor procedures, I usually give hydrocortisone phosphate, 25 to 50 mg/70 kg/day intravenously. Unless infection or some other perioperative complication develops, this is decreased by approximately 25% per day until oral intake can be resumed. At this point, the usual maintenance dose of glucocorticoids can be employed.

Risks of Supplementation

Rare potential risks of perioperative supplementation with steroids include aggravation of hypertension, hyperglycemia, fluid retention, the induction of stress ulcers, and psychiatric disturbances. Two risk factors associated with glucocorticoid administration to surgical patients have been described and reviewed[94]: abnormal wound healing and an increased rate of infection. However, the evidence is inconclusive because it relates to acute glucocorticoid administration and not to chronic administration of glucocorticoids with increased doses at times of stress. For example, in rats wounded before and after topical application of cortisone, delayed wound closure was found secondary to inhibition of granulation tissue and decreased proliferation of fibroblasts and of new blood vessels. Ehrlich and Hunt[97] found that moderate to large doses of steroids exerted their morphologic effects maximally within 3 days after injury, and they postulated that the inhibition of the early inflammatory process by steroids after wounding was responsible for delayed

healing. Vitamin A protected somewhat against delayed healing, presumably because of its effect in stabilizing lysosomes. In contrast to these studies that suggest a deleterious effect of perioperative glucocorticoid administration on wound healing in rats, a study on primates suggests that large doses of glucocorticoids, administered perioperatively, did not impair sensitive measures of wound healing.[104] An overall assessment of these results suggests that short-term perioperative steroid treatment has a small but definite deleterious effect on wound healing that is perhaps partially reversed by topical administration of vitamin A.

Information on the risk of infection as a result of perioperative supplement with glucocorticoids is also unclear. Winstone and Brook[96] reported four cases of septicemia among 18 surgical patients given perioperative supplementation with glucocorticoids but no similar complications in 17 others who also took glucocorticoids but were not given perioperative supplementation. In a controlled study of 100 patients who received perioperative supplementation with glucocorticoids, there were 11 wound infections in the steroid-treated group and only one in the control group.[94] Test subjects and controls were not matched for underlying disease, however. In contrast, Jensen and Elb[110] found no change in the incidence of wound infections or other infections in an uncontrolled series of 419 patients subjected to surgery and perioperative supplementation with glucocorticoids. Oh and Patterson[111] found only one minor suture abscess among a group of 17 corticosteroid-dependent asthmatic patients undergoing 21 surgical procedures. Thus, these data are inadequate to show that perioperative supplementation with corticosteroids increases the risk of infection.

Summary

Abnormalities in adrenal cortical function can be manifested as deficiencies or excesses of androgens, mineralocorticoids, or glucocorticoids. Deficiency of androgens is often accompanied by deficiency of the other hormones. Excess androgens result in no unusual perioperative problems for the anesthetist. Mineralocorticoid abnormalities can be associated with blood volume, electrolyte, and cardiac disturbances. I routinely seek and treat these abnormalities preoperatively as well as intraoperatively and postoperatively.

Abnormal levels of glucocorticoids often cause mineralocorticoid disturbances, as well as suppressing healing and the capacity to combat infection. It is probably better to give supplemental corticosteroids to any patient who has received exogenous steroids in the previous year. The dose that provides the greatest benefit-risk ratio for supplementation appears to be declining (I now use 100 mg/70 kg/day of hydrocortisone phosphate intravenously). Etomidate suppresses adrenal cortical steroid synthesis, and its use probably should be accompanied by steroid supplementation.[112] No controlled studies indicate that any one anesthetic practice or choice of drugs is better than any other for patients with adrenal disease. As with most other endocrinopathies, the focus of complications resides in the cardiovascular system.

ADRENAL MEDULLA: PHEOCHROMOCYTOMA

Cells of neural crest origin are capable of developing into catecholamine-secreting tumors. Indeed, pheochromocytomas, or catecholamine tumors, have been reported in neural-crest sites ranging from the neck to the inguinal ligament. Pheochromocytomas have been reported as part of the multiple endocrine adenomatosis syndrome and in association with neuroectodermal dysplasias, including neurofibromatosis, tuberous sclerosis, Sturge-Weber syndrome, and von Hippel-Lindau disease. Although pheochromocytomas cause fewer than 0.1% of all cases of hypertension, they are important to the anesthesiologist. Twenty-five to 50 percent of hospital deaths of patients with pheochromocytoma occur during induction of anesthesia or during operative procedures for other disorders.[113]

Three issues are important in considering pheochromocytoma[24,114-121]: (1) the organ system that most influences the anesthetic management of patients with pheochromocytoma is the cardiovascular system; (2) major reductions in morbidity associated with resection of pheochromocytoma occurred when the anesthetist was adequately informed about this disorder and when the patient had received adequate α-adrenergic blockade; and (3) no controlled studies have been done on almost any aspect of the diagnosis or treatment of pheochromocytoma; thus this summary is based on conclusions derived from the many published anecdotal studies.

Physiology and Diagnosis

The physiologic transmitters (catecholamines) are released from the terminals of the postganglionic sympathetic nervous system. Synthesis of catecholamines begins in the postganglionic nerve cell bodies when tyrosine is hydroxylated in the rate-limiting step to dopa; dopa is decarboxylated to dopamine; and, in most cells, dopamine is hydroxylated to norepinephrine. In the adrenal, in rare parts of the CNS, and at some ganglia, this norepinephrine can be converted by phenyl-ethanolamine-N-transferase to epinephrine. The release of dopamine, norepinephrine, and epinephrine occurs both basally and in response to physiologic and pharmacologic stressors such as hypotension (through baroreceptors), low tissue perfusion, hypoxia, hypoglycemia, anger, determination, fear, and anxiety. Such release from the sympathetic nervous system can be generalized or localized. Most pheochromocytomas are independent of these physiologic stressors, however.

Some pheochromocytomas are under neurogenic control, with increased release of catecholamines stimulated by physiologic and pharmacologic stressors. However, much of the release of catecholamines from pheochromocytomas is not controlled by neurogenic influence. This lack of neurologic control is utilized in the clonidine suppression test for pheochromocytoma (see later).[122]

Painful or stressful events such as intubation often cause an exaggerated catecholamine response in a less than perfectly anesthetized patient with pheochromocytoma. This response is caused by release of catecholamines from nerve endings that are "loaded" by the reuptake process. Stresses may cause catecholamine levels of 200 to 2000 pg/mL in normal patients. For the patient with pheochromocytoma, even simple stresses can lead to blood catecholamine levels of 2000 to 20,000 pg/mL. Squeezing the tumor, however gently, or infarction of the tumor with release of products onto peritoneal surfaces can result in blood levels of 200,000 to 1 million pg/mL, a potentially disastrous situation that should be anticipated and avoided. The physician should ask for a temporary stay of surgery, if at all possible, during which the rate of nitroprusside infusion will be increased.

It has been found in several studies that the triad of paroxysmal sweating, hypertension, and headache is more sensitive and specific than any laboratory test for the diagnosis of pheochromocytoma. These are the symptoms that one experiences when given an infusion of epinephrine.[123] Physical examination of a patient with pheochromocytoma is usually unrewarding unless the patient is observed during an attack. Occasionally, palpation of the abdomen causes the bladder or rectum to rub against the tumor and stimulates release of catecholamines; however, the laboratory measurement of catecholamines or their metabolites has been the standard method of diagnosis.

Half of all patients with pheochromocytoma have continuous hypertension with occasional paroxysms, and another 40% have paroxysmal hypertension. Labile hypertension or the triad of hypertension, headache, and sweating usually is an indication for urine testing.

In more than 85% of cases, pheochromocytomas are sporadic tumors of unknown cause that are localized in the medulla of one adrenal gland; however, these vascular tumors can occur anywhere. They are found in the right atrium, the spleen, the broad ligament of the ovary, or the organs of Zuckerkandl at the bifurcation of the aorta. Malignant spread, which occurs in fewer than 15% of cases of pheochromocytoma, usually proceeds via venous and lymphatic channels, with a predilection for the liver. Occasionally, this tumor is a familial autosomal-dominant trait. It may be a part of the pluriglandular-neoplastic syndrome known as multiple endocrine adenoma type IIa or type IIb. Type IIa consists of medullary carcinoma of the thyroid, parathyroid adenoma or hyperplasia, and pheochromocytoma. Type IIb consists of medullary carcinoma of the thyroid, a marfanoid appearance, mucosal neuromas, and pheochromocytoma. Often, bilateral tumors are present in the familial form.

Urine tests have become a mainstay of diagnosis. The usual urine tests used measure 3-methoxy-4-hydroxymandelic acid, or metanephrines, or native catecholamines per milligram of creatine secreted. If the results of three 24-hour collections of urine are normal, the patient is considered not to have a pheochromocytoma.[114,115,121]

Although urine testing has been the standard for diagnosis, many more patients are found at autopsy to have had pheochromocytoma and to have died of its complications (often during operations for other problems) than have pheochromocytoma diagnosed while they are alive. If urine test results are normal, but the suspicion is strong enough, provocative tests with glucagon to promote catecholamine release by the tumor can be used, and the diagnosis is based on the blood pressure response and plasma catecholamine elevation. Catecholamine levels in urine and plasma are diagnostic when elevated to three times the normal median value. If plasma catecholamine levels are above normal, but below three times the normal median, a clonidine suppression test is recommended. Clonidine, by its α_2-adrenergic agonist activity in the brainstem, suppresses neurogenically controlled peripheral catecholamine release. Because most pheochromocytomas are not under neurogenic control, catecholamine release in patients with pheochromocytoma will not be suppressed and the plasma level will remain elevated.[122]

Once the diagnosis of pheochromocytoma is made, the tumor must be localized and pretreated before surgical resection. The protocol for localizing these often small tumors has undergone radical revision. Plain radiographs or intravenous pyelograms that show lateral displacement of a kidney are a first approach. MRI has replaced CT, which itself replaced urography and venous sampling. When such techniques do not yield definitive results, scanning with [129]I-metaiodobenzylguanidine (a guanethidine analog) can be tried.

Anesthetic Considerations for Patients With Pheochromocytoma

There are many published reports on perioperative morbidity and mortality associated with pheochromocytoma, but little is known about the factors that affect the rates of morbidity and mortality.[116,124-127] Although no controlled, randomized, prospective clinical study has been done on the value of adrenergic blocking drugs, the preoperative use of these drugs for patients with pheochromocytoma is recommended because these α blockers are likely to reduce the incidence of the perioperative complications of hypertensive crisis, wide fluctuations in blood pressure during intraoperative manipulation of the tumor (especially until the venous drainage is obliterated), and perioperative myocardial dysfunction.[118,122-127] Perioperative mortality associated with the excision of pheochromocytoma was reduced from 13% to 45% to 0% to 3% when α-adrenergic blockade was introduced as preoperative therapy and when it was recognized that these patients often had hypovolemia preoperatively (Table 13-6).[127,128]

The presence of hyperglycemia preoperatively reflects the metabolic effects of catecholamines, resolves with tumor resection, and usually does not require insulin therapy preoperatively or perioperatively. Persistently elevated catecholamine levels may result in catecholamine myocarditis. This cardiomyopathy appears to pose an extra

TABLE 13–6 Perioperative Mortality for Pheochromocytoma Resection

Year	Investigator(s)	Mortality (%)	No. of Patients in Study
1951	Apgar (review)	45	91
1951	Apgar	33	12
1963	Stackpole, et al.	13	100
Before 1960	Mayo Clinic	0-26?	101?
After 1960	Mayo Clinic Modlin, et al.	2.9?	44?
Before 1967	No alpha blockade	18	17
After 1967	Alpha blockade	2	41
1976	Scott, et al.	3	33
1976-1985	Roizen, et al.	0	38

Data abstracted from Roizen MF: Anesthetic implications of concurrent diseases. In Miller RD (ed): Anesthesia. New York, Churchill Livingstone, 1994, vol 1, pp 903-1014.

risk for patients,[129] but it can be treated successfully by α-adrenergic blockade preoperatively (see later). Mortality for patients with pheochromocytoma is usually the result of myocardial failure, myocardial infarction, or hemorrhage (hypertensive) into the myocardium or brain. The incidence of all of these catastrophic situations appears to be reduced with α-adrenergic blockade.

Preoperative therapy consisting of α-adrenergic blockade with phenoxybenzamine, prazosin, or labetalol alleviates the patient's symptoms, favors a successful fetal outcome (i.e., in patients whose pheochromocytoma is discovered during pregnancy),[119,120,124] and allows reexpansion of intravascular plasma volume by eradicating the vasoconstrictive effects of high levels of catecholamines. This reexpansion of fluid volume is often accompanied by a decreased hematocrit. Because some patients are sensitive to phenoxybenzamine, it should initially be administered in doses of 10 to 20 mg orally two or three times a day. Most patients require 60 to 250 mg/day. The efficacy of the therapy is judged by the reduction of symptoms (especially sweating) and by stabilization of blood pressure. For patients with catecholamine myocarditis as evidenced by often localized ST and T wave ECG changes, preoperative, long-term administration of α-adrenergic blockade (for 15 days to 6 months) has been shown to be effective in resolving the clinical and ECG alterations.[124]

β-Adrenergic receptor blockade with concomitant administration of phenoxybenzamine is suggested for patients who have persistent dysrhythmias or tachycardia. It is recommended that β-adrenergic receptor blockade not be used without α-adrenergic blockade, however, lest the vasoconstrictive effects of the latter go unopposed and produce dangerous hypertension. The latter complication has been reported only rarely, however, and perhaps no firm rules are necessary.

To date, no one has investigated the optimal duration of preoperative phenoxybenzamine therapy. Most patients require treatment for 10 to 14 days, as determined by the time needed for stabilization of blood pressure and amelioration of symptoms. If the patient does not complain of nasal stuffiness, he or she is not ready for surgery. Because pheochromocytomas spread slowly, little is lost by waiting until the patient's preoperative condition has been optimized by means of medical therapy. The following criteria for an optimal preoperative condition are recommended:

1. No "in-hospital" blood pressure reading higher than 160/90 mm Hg should be evident for 24 hours before surgery. I normally measure the blood pressure in each patient (as an outpatient) every minute for an hour in a recovery room setting during preoperative visits. This setting is most stressful to the medically naive and thus a good test of inhibition of responses to sympathetic stimulation. If no blood pressure reading higher than 160/90 mm Hg is recorded, the patient is scheduled for surgery, assuming the following three criteria are also met.

2. Orthostatic hypotension, with readings above 80/45 mm Hg, should be present.

3. The electrocardiogram should be free of ST-T abnormalities for at least a week; if abnormalities are persistent, two-dimensional echocardiography should reveal no evidence of global or regional dysfunction that cannot be attributed to a permanent deficit.

4. The patient should have no more than one premature ventricular contraction every 5 minutes.

Although specific anesthetic drugs have been recommended for patients with pheochromocytoma, optimal preoperative preparation, careful and gradual induction of anesthesia, and good communication between surgeon and anesthesiologist are most important. I usually give phenoxybenzamine in one half to two thirds of its normal dose immediately preceding surgery. Virtually all anesthetic agents, muscle relaxants, and techniques have been used successfully for patients with pheochromocytoma, and all are associated with a high rate of transient intraoperative dysrhythmias.[125] Although some agents may have advantages or disadvantages in theory, they have not been demonstrated clinically. For example, one might wish to avoid histamine release, because it can stimulate catecholamine release. Yet neither curare nor morphine has been associated with poor patient outcome. Case reports of hypertension after small doses of droperidol have appeared, but no study comparing variation in blood pressure after droperidol and after saline has been published. And it is very evident, on placement of an arterial line, that patients with pheochromocytoma have wide variations in blood pressure. In our randomized studies, use of Innovar (which contains droperidol) was not associated with greater blood pressure fluctuations than the other three agents tested.[125] (Patients with pheochromocytoma tend to be particularly sensitive to pain; we often have much more difficulty than in normal cases placing arterial and venous lines in such patients.)

Because both are easy to administer, phenylephrine or dopamine is used for treatment of hypotension, whereas nitroprusside is preferable when hypertension occurs.[24] Phentolamine, previously a mainstay of intraoperative therapy, has too long a period of onset and duration of action. After the venous supply has been secured, and if the intravascular volume is normal (as measured by pulmonary artery wedge pressure), the blood pressure usually becomes normal. I usually do not treat abnormal blood pressure in α-adrenergically blocked patients unless it is below 75/40 mm Hg; however, some patients become hypotensive after tumor removal and occasionally require a relatively large infusion of catecholamines. On rare occasions, patients remain hypertensive intraoperatively.

Postoperatively, about 50% of patients have hypertension for 1 to 3 days and have markedly elevated but declining plasma catecholamine levels. After 3 to 10 days, all but 25% become normotensive. Catecholamine levels do not return to normal for 10 days; therefore, early measurement of urine concentrations of catecholamines is usually not helpful in ensuring that all catecholamine has been removed from tissue.

Because pheochromocytomas may be hereditary, it is important to screen other family members and advise them that, should they require surgery in the future, they should inform the anesthesiologist about the potential for such disease.

Summary

A lack of controlled studies precludes definitive statements about anesthetic management of patients with pheochromocytoma. It is known that the symptoms of paroxysmal hypertension, sweating, and headache are highly suggestive of the diagnosis. It appears that mortality can be reduced by preoperative α-adrenergic receptor blockade with progressively increasing doses of a blocking agent for 10 days to 2 months for treatment of symptoms, by treatment of myocarditis, and by restoration of intravascular volume. In fact, the largest decrease in mortality of patients after pheochromocytoma resection occurred with the introduction of preoperative α-adrenergic receptor blockade. I believe that knowledge on the part of the anesthetist about the pathophysiology of pheochromocytoma, preoperative patient preparation, and communication between surgeon and anesthetist are more important to patient outcome than is the choice of the anesthetic or muscle-relaxing agent.

PANCREAS

Physiology

Pancreatic islets are composed of at least three cell types: alpha cells that secrete glucagon, beta cells that secrete insulin, and delta cells that contain secretory granules. Insulin is first synthesized as proinsulin, converted to insulin by proteolytic cleavage, and then packaged into granules within the beta cells. A large quantity of insulin, normally about 200 units, is stored in the pancreas, and continued synthesis is stimulated by glucose. There is basal, steady-state release of insulin from the beta granules and additional release that is controlled by stimuli external to the beta cell. Basal insulin secretion continues in the fasted state and is of key importance in the inhibition of catabolism and ketoacidosis. Glucose and fructose are the primary and most important regulators of insulin release. Other stimulators of insulin release include amino acids, glucagon, gastrointestinal hormones (gastrin, secretin,

cholecystokinin-pancreozymin, and enteroglucagon), and acetylcholine. Epinephrine and norepinephrine inhibit insulin release by stimulating α-adrenergic receptors, and they stimulate its release at β-adrenergic receptors.

A normal plasma glucose level requires adequate endogenous substrate for glucose production, normal enzymatic mechanisms capable of converting glycogen and other substrates to glucose, and normal hormonal modulation of gluconeogenesis.[130] The rise in glucose levels after a meal causes release of insulin from beta cells in the pancreas. The magnitude of the insulin response is governed in part by the action of other gastrointestinal hormones that are secreted after food intake. The action of these other hormones accounts for the greater rise in insulin levels after oral than after parenteral administration of glucose. Release of insulin can also be triggered by β-adrenergic stimuli that are believed to act by increasing cyclic AMP levels. Insulin release is inhibited by α-adrenergic stimuli. The action of insulin tends to return the levels of plasma glucose to normal within 1 to 2 hours after completion of a meal.

When endogenous nutrients are not available, plasma glucose levels are maintained by hepatic glycogenolysis and then gluconeogenesis.[130] In these situations, insulin levels are low and glucagon, GH, cortisol, and catecholamines play important roles in gluconeogenesis. Insulin is normally secreted from the pancreas in response to elevated levels of blood glucose as a prohormone (proinsulin). This hormone is rapidly cleaved into C-peptide and insulin in the portal vein. Patients with insulinoma tend to have high levels of proinsulin (more than 20% of total insulin) in plasma and levels of C-peptide that parallel insulin levels.

Hypoglycemia and Hyperinsulinism (Islet Cell Tumors of the Pancreas)

Almost all of the signs and symptoms in patients with insulinomas are directly related to prolonged hypoglycemic states. The word "hypoglycemia" means different things to different people. Hypoglycemia is a clinical syndrome that may have a variety of causes and that results in plasma glucose levels sufficiently low to promote secretion of catecholamines and to impair the function of the CNS.[131] The diagnosis of hypoglycemia requires the presence of three findings: (1) symptomatic hypoglycemia (confusion, abnormal behavior, amnesia for the episode of hypoglycemia), (2) a plasma glucose level in the hypoglycemic range (less than 40 mg/dL for females and less than 45 mg/dL for males), and (3) amelioration of symptoms when plasma glucose is restored to normal levels.

The two major classifications of hypoglycemia can be distinguished by the relationship of symptoms to meals: (1) reactive, that is, if the hypoglycemia occurs within 2 to 4 hours after ingestion of food and is associated primarily with adrenergic symptoms, and (2) fasting, that is, if the hypoglycemia occurs more than 6 hours after a meal, is precipitated by exercise, and is often associated with CNS symptoms. Insulinomas usually cause fasting hypoglycemia.[130,132]

Reactive hypoglycemia can be caused by alimentation, impaired glucose tolerance, or functional causes. *Alimentary hypoglycemia* is associated with low levels of plasma glucose 2 to 3 hours after ingestion of food by patients who have rapid gastric emptying, for example, after subtotal gastrectomy, vagotomy, or pyloroplasty. It is postulated that rapid gastric emptying and rapid absorption of glucose may result in excessive release of insulin, falling glucose levels, and reactive hypoglycemia. *Impaired glucose tolerance* resulting in hypoglycemia, an early symptom of diabetes, usually occurs 4 to 5 hours after ingestion of food. *Functional hypoglycemia*, on the other hand, usually occurs 3 to 4 hours after ingestion of food and is associated with adrenergic symptoms.

Because the brain is extremely sensitive to glucose utilization, CNS effects are often manifest. Most patients show CNS symptoms that included visual disturbances, dizziness, confusion, epilepsy, lethargy, transient loss of consciousness, and coma. Perhaps because of these many CNS manifestations of insulinomas, many patients with these tumors have been misdiagnosed as suffering from psychiatric illness.

Less frequent but nevertheless important manifestations of insulinomas involve the cardiovascular system. More than 10% of insulinoma patients have palpitations, tachycardia, or hypertension, or all three. These symptoms are probably related to catecholamine release secondary to hypoglycemia, and about 9% of the patients have either severe hunger or gastrointestinal upset, including cramping, nausea, and vomiting. Other investigators have noted obesity or weight gain as a symptom. The symptoms of hypoglycemia due to insulinoma may occur at a particular time of day that is associated with a low blood glucose level, especially 6 hours or more after eating, after fasting for a time, or in the early morning.

Fasting hypoglycemia results from inadequate hepatic glucose production or from overutilization of glucose in the peripheral tissues. The causes of inadequate production of glucose during the fasting state may be hormone deficiencies, enzyme defects, inadequate substrate delivery, acquired liver disease, or drugs. Overutilization of glucose may occur in the presence of either elevated or appropriate insulin levels.

To define the diagnosis of insulinomas, Whipple introduced a triad of diagnostic criteria, which have been modified to include (1) symptoms of hypoglycemia brought on by fasting and exercise; (2) blood glucose levels, while symptoms are present, of less than 40 mg/dL in females and less than 45 mg/dL in males; and (3) relief of these symptoms by administration of glucose, either orally or

intravenously. If an insulinoma is suspected and Whipple's triad is confirmed, several tests may be done with which one can differentiate insulinoma from other causes of hypoglycemia.

In recent years, because it has been possible to determine insulin levels as well as glucose levels, the diagnosis has been made with even more certainty.[131] During a prolonged fast, in patients with insulinoma, hypoglycemia develops because of a relative underproduction of glucose by the liver rather than because of increased glucose utilization.[131] High levels of C-peptide and proinsulin levels greater than 20% of total insulin measured in blood are also helpful.

Selective celiac CT angiography or MRI of the pancreatic region is often used for localization of tumors before surgical exploration.

Medical management of insulin-secreting tumors is often difficult but has been simplified before and during surgery and in cases in which surgery fails to remove all of the tumor(s), by somatostatin.

Surgical treatment of insulin-secreting islet cell tumors involves their removal, usually from the pancreas, where they are most often located. In 13% of cases more than one adenoma has been present. Most insulinomas are benign; approximately one third of those that are malignant are found at laparotomy to have metastasized to the liver.

Anesthetic Considerations for Patients with Hypoglycemia

Most patients who come to surgery with the diagnosis of reactive or fasting hypoglycemia do not require special intraoperative care other than frequent assays of blood glucose levels and adequate infusion of dextrose. The variations in plasma glucose levels are exaggerated in patients with functional islet cell adenoma, and the frequency of procedures to remove insulinomas has increased.[132-134]

A rise in blood glucose during operation, which is sometimes quite striking, is thought to be evidence of tumor removal.[133-134] Therefore, two other methods of intraoperative glucose management have been designed not to mask this hyperglycemic rebound. In the first of these, glucose infusion is stopped approximately 2 hours before surgery. Blood glucose is monitored frequently, but no glucose is administered unless the level drops below a certain value, usually below 40 to 50 mg/dL. A bolus of glucose is then given that is calculated to return the level in blood to more than 50 mg/dL, and constant glucose infusion is also started so that the blood glucose level is maintained at more than 50 mg/dL.

The second method makes use of the "artificial beta cell," or feedback-controlled dextrose infusion, during surgery. The artificial beta cell can be used either solely for monitoring of glucose or for monitoring and administering both glucose and insulin. A printout of the blood glucose level, amount of glucose infused, and amount of insulin infused can be obtained. This allows for frequent (every 60 seconds) determinations of the glucose level, so that any decrease in glucose requirement (the hyperglycemia response) can be observed.

Administration of insulin to hyperglycemic patients during and after surgery is aimed at short-term control of glucose levels. Intraoperatively, I treat blood glucose levels above 300 to 400 mg/dL by administering regular insulin intravenously. Frequent monitoring of glucose is continued, and more insulin is given every 60 to 90 minutes if the hyperglycemia persists. Postoperatively, hyperglycemia, especially ketosis, is also treated with insulin. Blood glucose levels of 250 to 400 mg/dL may be treated by subcutaneous administration of insulin while blood glucose is monitored at fairly frequent intervals. Blood glucose levels higher than this are treated more aggressively, not with additional insulin (10 units/70 kg/hr) but with more frequent glucose monitoring, intravenous administration of insulin (either as a bolus or as a continuous infusion), and repletion of fluid, potassium, and phosphate.

Blood glucose also is monitored in the postoperative period because hyperglycemia and its complications can occur. Hyperglycemic rebound has been used as a diagnostic tool by several authors but may not be as effective as was once thought. Muir and coworkers[132] reviewed 39 patients who underwent surgery for insulinoma. After tumor removal, all patients but one had an increase in plasma glucose concentration. That patient subsequently proved to be cured, whereas a patient who had a hyperglycemic response was later shown not to be cured. Furthermore, in 6 patients whose blood glucose concentration increased after tumor resection, the rise was less sharp than that before tumor removal.

Whether the perioperative control of glucose levels is aimed at euglycemia, with either glucose infusion or an artificial beta cell, or at slight hypoglycemia, one should try to keep the blood glucose level higher than the level at which the patient becomes symptomatic while awake. This aim is achieved more easily with euglycemic methods. Furthermore, although a hyperglycemic response is useful diagnostically when it occurs, it is not a substitute for careful exploration of the pancreas. Also, citrate-phosphate-dextrose (CPD) preservative or acid-citrate-dextrose (ACD) blood contains dextrose, which may create a rise in blood glucose that could be confused with a hyperglycemic response.

Summary

The signs and symptoms of insulinomas are the signs and symptoms of hypoglycemia, which have predominantly CNS manifestations. The symptoms of hyperglycemia

and hypoglycemia are masked by general anesthesia, but their deleterious systemic effects are not prevented. It is important to monitor blood glucose levels frequently in the perioperative period because either hyperglycemia or hypoglycemia may develop. Hypoglycemia is more dangerous, particularly because of its effects on the CNS. Hyperglycemia is deleterious because hyperosmolar coma and ketoacidosis may occur. A hyperglycemic response does not invariably occur after successful tumor resection, nor is it always diagnostic of cure. When hyperglycemia does occur postoperatively, it is treated with insulin until euglycemic levels are restored.

Diabetes Mellitus

Clinicians primarily think about diabetes in relation to glucose and the importance of its level chronically and in patients requiring intensive care.[135-141] Recent data indicate that the end organ disease that diabetes creates or with which it is associated should also be considered. This accent on problems other than hyperglycemia may seem strange at a time when lifelong tight control of blood glucose is being debated. The concern for the end organ manifestations of diabetes originates in recent epidemiologic studies of surgical mortality.

Surgical mortality rates for the diabetic population are on average five times higher than those for the nondiabetic population.[142-144] However, in epidemiologic studies in which diabetes itself was segregated from the complications of diabetes (including cardiac and vascular disease) and old age, this finding was questioned.[143-147] Similarly, if diabetics undergoing major vascular surgery are compared with nondiabetics matched for type of surgery, age, sex, weight, and complicating diseases, there is no difference in the mortality rate or the number of postoperative complications,[145] as long as the diabetic does not need to be cared for in an intensive care unit for longer than 24 hours.

Diabetes mellitus is a heterogeneous group of disorders (present in more than 5% of the population of developed countries) that have the common feature of a relative or absolute deficiency of insulin. Diabetes can be divided into two very different diseases, which share end organ abnormalities.[148,149] Type I diabetes is associated with autoimmune diseases and has a concordance rate of 40% to 50% (i.e., if one of a pair of monozygotic twins has diabetes, the likelihood that the other twin also will have it is 40% to 50%). In type I the patient is insulin deficient, has inadequate basal and stimulated insulin secretion, and is prone to ketoacidosis if exogenous insulin is withheld. Treatment with immunolytic agents once a viral infection has occurred appears to decrease the rate of development of type I diabetes.[149] For type II (non-insulin-dependent) diabetes, the concordance rate is 100% (i.e., the genetic material is both necessary and sufficient for the development of type II diabetes). Type II patients are not prone to develop ketoacidosis in the absence of insulin, and they have peripheral insulin resistance.

Type I and type II diabetes differ in other ways as well. Type I formerly was termed "juvenile-onset diabetes." The term may be a misnomer, because many older patients also fall into the same category. Most children and adolescents who are diabetic have type I diabetes; that is, they require insulin to prevent ketoacidosis. The maturity-onset diabetic is usually older and tends to be overweight; however, a younger person can develop type II and an older person can develop type I diabetes.

Type II diabetics tend to be elderly, overweight, relatively resistant to ketoacidosis, and prone to the development of a hyperglycemic, hyperosmolar, nonketotic state. Plasma insulin levels are normal or elevated but are low relative to the level of blood glucose.

Currently, therapy for type II diabetes usually begins with exercise and dietary management. A diet rich in fiber and less saturated fat, and daily physical activity of 30 minutes, is often associated with normalization of fasting blood glucose and delay of glucose intolerance by more than 50% of subjects. The next stage of therapy is use of oral hypoglycemic medications that act by stimulating release of insulin by pancreatic beta cells and by improving the tissue responsiveness to insulin by reversing the postbinding abnormality. The common orally administered drugs are tolazamide (Tolinase), tolbutamine (Orinase), and the newer sulfonylureas glyburide (Micronase), glipizide (Glucotrol), and glimperide. These last drugs have a longer blood glucose-lowering effect, which persists for 24 hours or more, and fewer drug-drug interactions. Oral hypoglycemic drugs may produce hypoglycemia for as long as 50 hours after intake (chlorpropamide [Diabinese] has the longest half-life). Other drugs include metformin, which decreases hepatic glucose output and may increase peripheral responsiveness to glucose (and is associated with lactic acidosis if the patient becomes dehydrated); acarbose, which decreases glucose absorption; and the thiaolidinediones (rosiglitazone and pioglitizone), which increases peripheral responsiveness to insulin. Troglitazone, another drug of this latter class, has been taken off the market because of 61 cases of acute renal failure after its use. Progressively, physicians advocating tight control of blood sugar levels give insulin to "maturity onset" insulin-dependent diabetic patients twice a day, or even more frequently.

Acute complications for the diabetic patient include hypoglycemia, diabetic ketoacidosis, and hyperglycemic, hyperosmolar, nonketotic coma. Diabetic patients also are subject to a series of long-term complications from cataracts, retinopathy, neuropathy, nephropathy, and angiopathy that lead to considerable morbidity and premature mortality. Many of these complications bring the diabetic patient to surgery. In fact, over 50% of all diabetics come to surgery at some time in their disease.

Hyperglycemic, hyperosmolar, nonketotic diabetic coma[150] is characterized by elevated serum osmolality (over 330 mOsm/L) and an elevated blood glucose level (over 600 mg/dL) without acidosis. Blood glucose level, in milligrams per deciliter, divided by 18 yields the contribution of glucose to osmolality. Trauma or infection in type II diabetes patients usually leads to this state rather than to ketoacidosis.[150] Hyperglycemia induces marked osmotic diuresis and dehydration, enhancing the hyperosmolar state; this can result in failure to emerge from anesthesia and persistent coma. Serum electrolyte values are often normal, although a widened anion gap ($Na^+[HCO_3]$ − $[Cl^-]$ = 16) may point to lactic acidosis or a uremic state.

The evidence that hyperglycemia itself accelerates complications or that tight control of blood sugar levels decreases the rate of progression of microangiopathic disease is now definitive.[135-140] Glucose itself may be toxic because high levels can promote nonenzymatic glycosylation reactions, leading to formation of abnormal proteins that may decrease elastance—responsible for the stiff joint syndrome (and fixation of the atlantooccipital joint, making intubation difficult)—and wound-healing tensile strength. Glucose elevations may increase production of macroglobulins by the liver, increasing blood viscosity, and may promote intracellular swelling by favoring production of nondiffusable, large molecules (like sorbitol). Newer drug therapies aim to decrease intracellular swelling by inhibiting formation of such large molecules, and surgical nerve compartment splitting is aimed at reducing the effect of such swelling. Glucose can also inhibit the phagocytic function.

Glycemia disrupts autoregulation.[151-161] Glucose-induced vasodilatation prevents target organs from protecting against increases in systemic blood pressure. Glycosylated hemoglobin of 8.1% is the threshold above which risk of microalbuminuria increases logarithmically. A person with type I diabetes with greater than 29 mg/day of microalbuminuria has an 80% chance of developing renal insufficiency. The threshold for glycemic toxicity is different for different vascular beds. The threshold for retinopathy is a glycosylated hemoglobin value of 8.5% to 9.0% (12.5 mmol/L or 225 mg/dl); for cardiovascular disease it is an average blood glucose value of 5.4 mmol/L (96 mg/dL). Thus, different degrees of hyperglycemia may be required before different vascular beds are damaged or certain degrees of glycemia are associated with other risk factors for vascular disease. Another view is that perhaps severe hyperglycemia and microalbuminuria are simply concomitant effects of a common underlying cause. Diabetics who develop microalbuminuria are more resistant to insulin; insulin resistance is associated with microalbuminuria in first-degree relatives of patients with type II diabetes; and persons with normoglycemia who subsequently develop clinical diabetes have atherogenic risks before onset of disease.

Because of the known glucotoxicities, how tightly blood sugar levels should routinely be controlled was once controversial. It is now known that chronic tight control is a benefit. The controversy centers on whether attempts to attain normal blood sugar levels or levels that result in glycosylated hemoglobin values of less than 8.1% in diabetic patients are of greater benefit than risk.

Perioperative management of the diabetic patient may affect surgical outcome. Physicians who advocate tight control of blood glucose levels point to the evidence of increased wound healing tensile strength and decreased wound infections in animal models of (type I) diabetes under tight control. Insulin is necessary in the early stages of the inflammatory response but seems to have no effect on collagen formation after the first 10 days. Healing epithelial wounds exhibit minimal leukocyte infiltration and, unlike deep wounds, are not dependent on collagen synthesis for the integrity of the tissue. Thus, simple epithelial repair is not inhibited in the diabetes patient whereas the repair of deeper wounds is impaired with respect to collagen formation and defense against bacterial growth.

Infections account for two thirds of postoperative complications and about 20% of perioperative deaths in diabetic patients. Experimental data suggest many factors that may make diabetics vulnerable to infection. Many alterations in leukocyte function have been demonstrated in hyperglycemic diabetics, including decreased chemotaxis and impaired phagocytic activity of granulocytes, as well as reduced intracellular killing of pneumococci and staphylococci. When diabetic patients are treated aggressively and blood glucose levels are maintained below 250 mg/dL (13.7 mmol/L), the phagocytic function of granulocytes is improved and intracellular killing of bacteria is restored to nearly normal levels. It has been thought that diabetic patients experience more infections in clean wounds than do nondiabetics. In a review of 23,649 surgical patients, the rate of wound infection in clean incisions was found to be 10.7% for diabetics, as compared with 1.8% for nondiabetics; however, when age is accounted for, the difference in the incidence of wound infection in diabetic and nondiabetic surgical patients is not statistically significant.

Recent information on the relationship between blood glucose and neurologic recovery after a global ischemic event may have important implications for perioperative diabetes management. In a study of 430 consecutive patients resuscitated after out-of-hospital cardiac arrest, mean blood glucose levels were found to be higher in patients who never awakened (341 ± 13 mg/dL) than in those who did (262 ± 7 mg/dL). Among patients who awakened, those with persistent neurologic deficits had higher mean glucose levels (286 ± 15 mg/dL) than did those without deficits (251 ± 7 mg/dL). These results are consistent with the finding that hyperglycemia during a stroke is associated with poorer short- and long-term neurologic outcomes. The possibility that blood glucose is a determinant of brain damage after global ischemia is supported by studies of global and focal CNS ischemia. Data are accumulating that suggest that a major effect of glycemia is to disrupt autoregulation, making arteries and arterioles (macrovessels and microvessels) vulnerable to the force disruption caused by increased blood pressure.[155-161] Glycemia appears to disrupt autoregulation by enhancing activation of protein kinase C.[151,161] This activation may occur in anyone whose glucose level exceeds 96 mg/dL (5.7 mmol/L) and is a major factor in arterial degeneration (aging). Before long, we may all want to tightly control our glucose levels, not only perioperatively but throughout our lives. Until better data are available, most recommend that the diabetic patient about to undergo surgery in which hypotension or reduced cerebral flow may occur should have a blood glucose level below 225 mg/dL during the period of cerebral ischemia. Two other special situations can also affect how tightly one should manage the patient's glucose level: (1) surgery requiring cardiopulmonary bypass and (2) surgery in pregnant patients or in patients already suffering from diabetic ketoacidosis.

Perioperative Considerations for Patients with Diabetes

Before surgery, assessment and optimization of treatment of the potential end organ effects of diabetes are at least as important as an assessment of the diabetic's current overall metabolic status. Special emphasis should be placed on history; autonomic, cardiovascular, renal, and drug therapy; and the status of skin care.[135-147,162-165] Basic laboratory examinations might include determination of fasting blood sugar and blood urea nitrogen or creatinine levels and an electrocardiogram.

Patients with severe diabetic autonomic neuropathy are at increased risk for gastroparesis and consequent aspiration and for intraoperative and postoperative cardiorespiratory arrest. Recent data indicate that diabetics who exhibit signs of autonomic neuropathy, such as early satiety, lack of sweating, lack of pulse rate change with inspiration or orthostatic maneuvers, and impotence, have a very high incidence both of painless myocardial ischemia and gastroparesis.[144,163-165]

Measuring the degree of sinus arrhythmia or beat-to-beat variability provides a simple, accurate test for significant autonomic neuropathy. The difference between maximal and minimal heart rate on deep inspiration, normally 15 beats per minute, was found to be five or less in all diabetic patients who previously sustained cardio-respiratory arrest.[163,164]

Other characteristics of patients with autonomic neuropathy include postural hypotension with a drop of more than 30 mm Hg, resting tachycardia, nocturnal diarrhea, and dense peripheral neuropathy. Diabetics with significant autonomic neuropathy may have impaired respiratory responses to hypoxia and are particularly susceptible to the action of drugs that have depressant effects. Such patients may warrant very close, continuous cardiac and respiratory monitoring for 12 to 24 hours postoperatively, although such logical treatment has not yet been tested in a rigorous, controlled trial.

Approach to Perioperative Management

There may be a relationship between blood glucose and neurologic recovery after a global ischemic nervous system event that has important implications for perioperative diabetic management.[152,166] In a study of 430 consecutive patients resuscitated after out-of-hospital cardiac arrest, mean blood glucose levels were found to be higher in patients who never awakened (341 ± 13 mg/dL) than in those who did (262 ± 7 mg/dL).[166] Among patients who awakened, those with persistent neurologic deficits had higher mean glucose levels (286 ± 15 mg/dL) than those without deficits (251 ± 7 mg/dL). These results are consistent with the finding in experimental models that hyperglycemia is associated with poorer short- and long-term neurologic outcomes.[152] If high glucose levels predispose to poor outcomes, the mechanism for the association of hyperglycemia with ischemic brain damage is not known. Until better data are available, there will be those who argue that the diabetic patient about to undergo surgery in which hypotension or reduced cerebral flow may occur should have a blood glucose level below 225 mg/dL during a period of cerebral ischemia; however, the risk of undetected hypoglycemia is much greater during surgery than while the patient is awake, because the normal physiologic responses are impaired and masked. Only frequent intraoperative monitoring of glucose levels can protect the patient. A popular approach, continuous insulin infusion for strict control of blood sugar during major surgery, has been highly recommended in some publications and is demonstrated to result in better outcome in those requiring intensive care for more than 24 hours.[135-141,167,168] This method does result in lower blood glucose levels but carries the risk of significant hypoglycemia in patients receiving 2 or more units of insulin per hour.

There are various methods of managing diabetes during surgery. The key to success includes individualized decision making for each patient, with the frequency of intraoperative monitoring appropriate to the tightness of control desired and with tailoring of insulin therapy to periodically measured blood glucose levels. The basic objectives of the perioperative management of diabetics include:

1. Achieving good control of blood glucose level with correction of any acid/base, fluid, or electrolyte abnormalities before surgery
2. Providing an adequate amount of carbohydrate to inhibit catabolic proteolysis, lipolysis, and ketosis (this requires an average of 100 to 150 g of glucose per day for a 70-kg person during the operative period)
3. Providing insulin adequate to prevent hyperglycemia, glycosuria, and ketoacidosis while also avoiding hypoglycemia
4. Keeping in mind problems associated with diabetes that require special perioperative attention or predispose to iatrogenic complications
5. Remembering that the tighter the desired control of blood glucose, the more frequently blood glucose must be measured

Non–Insulin-Dependent Diabetes. Insulin is usually not required for minor surgery on patients whose diabetes is controlled by diet or small doses of oral agents. Short-acting oral hypoglycemic agents are omitted on the day of surgery, and long-acting agents are discontinued 2 days before surgery. Insulin may be required during and after surgery for major thoracic or abdominal operations or during prolonged parenteral alimentation. Given the potential of developing insulin allergy with intermittent insulin exposure, some physicians advocate the use of human insulin in this perioperative setting.

Insulin-Dependent Diabetes and Minor Surgery. There are many methods for managing insulin-dependent diabetics during surgery, but few comparisons of efficacy and safety have been published. Regular insulin given subcutaneously begins to act within 30 minutes, reaches peak effect in 2 to 4 hours, and has a duration of action of 6 to 8 hours. Intermediate-acting insulin (NPH or Lente) given subcutaneously begins to act within 100 to 120 minutes, reaches a peak effect in 6 to 12 hours, and has an 18- to 24-hour duration of action. The conventional preoperative therapy for the well-controlled, fasting diabetic consists of administration of half of the dose of insulin the patient usually takes. This insulin is given subcutaneously on the morning of surgery with a 5% dextrose infusion at 100 to 150 mL/hr. Regular insulin is then given as a supplement to the intermediate-acting insulin when the need is indicated by blood glucose levels. The recommendations on whether a diabetic patient should be a morning admittance patient versus an outpatient for minor surgery are listed in Table 13-7.

Insulin-Dependent Diabetes and Major Surgery. Continuous intravenous insulin therapy similar to that used in the treatment of ketoacidosis is often administered to "brittle

TABLE 13–7 Should a Diabetic be an Outpatient or a Morning-Admittance Patient?	
Outpatient If:	**Morning Admittance Patient If:**
Can evaluate history in advance	Cannot evaluate history
End organ disease does not require monitoring	End organ disease requires invasive monitoring
Prehydration is available or is unnecessary	Needs careful prehydration
No central nervous system ischemia or planned cardiopulmonary bypass	Central nervous system ischemia is present or cardiopulmonary bypass is planned
Not pregnant	Pregnant
Patient or vested caregiver can determine blood glucose level	Patient cannot determine blood glucose level
Has vested individual to provide care	No vested individual to provide care
Can take temperature or look for "red" wound	Cannot take temperature or look for "red" wound
Plan higher admit rate (no data)	Social care network is unsuitable

From Miller RD (ed): Miller's Anesthesia, 6th ed. Philadelphia, Churchill Livingstone, 2005, with permission.

diabetics" during major surgery. Several methods of intravenous insulin therapy have been studied. Taitelman and coworkers compared constant intravenous insulin infusion with conventional subcutaneous administration of insulin in patients before orthopedic procedures.[168] They used 500 mL/hr of 5% dextrose for the first hour, followed by 125 mL/hr plus 1 or 2 units per hour of regular insulin (0.16 or 0.32 unit of insulin per gram of infused glucose) in one group of patients. They compared the outcome with that for a group of patients who were given two thirds of their daily maintenance dose of insulin subcutaneously immediately before surgery. The two methods resulted in equivalent diabetic control. At 2 units/hr, or 0.32 unit of insulin per gram of infused glucose, euglycemic levels were more readily achieved, but hypoglycemia requiring treatment occurred in several patients.

Guidelines for Continuous Intravenous Insulin Administration

The amounts of insulin and glucose that are administered need to be correlated. There is some argument about whether 5% or 10% dextrose should be used. Infusion of 10% dextrose provides more calories, thus favoring anabolism, but may lead to venous irritation and thrombosis. Concentrations of infused insulin vary from 0.2 to 0.4 unit per gram of glucose (equal to 1 to 2 units/100 mL of 5% dextrose in water) under normal conditions. Higher levels of insulin may be required under certain circumstances, for example, in patients with liver disease, marked obesity, or severe infection, and in patients undergoing corticosteroid therapy or coronary artery bypass surgery. Cessation of intravenous insulin may rapidly cause hyperglycemia, because insulin has a

serum half-life of only 4 minutes and a biologic half-life of 20 minutes. Because it may be necessary to adjust the amount of insulin or glucose independently, these solutions should be kept in separate bottles, with one line "piggybacked" into the other. Separation of the intravenous line that contains the insulin and dextrose from all other intravenous fluids (these other fluids should contain no dextrose or lactate) reduces the risk of hypoglycemia or excessive hyperglycemia (Table 13-8).

Renal Transplant Surgery. The effectiveness of continuous intravenous administration of insulin has been compared with that of subcutaneous insulin in diabetics undergoing renal transplant surgery.[167] In this comparison, patients on intravenous insulin received 5% dextrose in

TABLE 13–8   Intravenous Insulin Regimen for "Brittle" Diabetic Undergoing Major Surgery
1. Obtain plasma glucose and potassium STAT on morning of surgery.
2. Begin intravenous infusion of 5% dextrose in water at 100 to 150 mL/hr and maintain dextrose infusion until the patient is taking oral nutrition.
3. "Piggyback" to above an IV infusion of 50 units of regular insulin in 500 mL of 0.9% normal saline by using infusion pump; flush 60 mL to saturate insulin-binding sites of tubing.
4. Set infusion rate at: Insulin (U/hr) = Last plasma glucose (mg/dL) ÷ 150. (Divide by 100 instead of 150 if patient is on corticosteroids, is markedly obese, or has infection.)
5. Determine glucose level every 2 o 3 hours; make appropriate insulin adjustments to obtain plasma glucose level of 80 to 150 mg/dL.

water, with the hourly dose of insulin controlled by an infusion pump according to the following equation:

$$\text{Hourly insulin (U)} = \text{Plasma glucose value}/100$$

(divided by 150 instead of 100 if the patient is thin or is not taking corticosteroids). Low-dose continuous insulin infusion maintained blood glucose levels at between 100 and 200 mg/dL and was more effective than endogenous control, on the average, in nondiabetics. Conventional subcutaneous insulin therapy was found to be grossly inadequate for maintenance of acceptable glucose levels in diabetic patients undergoing renal transplantation.

Cardiopulmonary Bypass Operations. For diabetics undergoing cardiopulmonary bypass surgery, the closed-loop "artificial pancreas" has been used in some studies for aggressive control of blood glucose level. Elliott and colleagues compared the use of Biostator, a closed-loop glucose-controlled system for infusion of insulin during open-heart surgery, with simpler, open-loop, constant intravenous administration of insulin.[169] A closed loop is characterized by automatic sensing and feedback control of insulin and glucose infusion. One intravenous line samples blood glucose levels by withdrawing blood at a rate of 1 mL/min, while insulin or glucose is infused through the other intravenous line as dictated by this measurement. An open-loop requires physician-directed regulation of insulin and glucose infusion. With both methods, no glucose infusion was given during the procedure, and blood glucose concentration was maintained at between 100 and 180 mg/mL throughout surgery. Insulin requirements increased during some phases of the operation, including cardiopulmonary bypass, transfusion of ACD stored blood, the rewarming phase, and injection of inotropic agents. A peak infusion rate of 20 units/hr was required during rewarming.

Mechanical problems were encountered postoperatively with the use of the Biostator. These included difficulties caused by peripheral vasoconstriction, movement of the patient, and nursing procedures that resulted in interruptions in feedback and led to elevations in blood glucose. Open-loop systems currently remain superior to closed-loop techniques because of cost and mechanical problems.[170,171]

Emergency Surgery and Ketoacidosis

Many diabetics who need emergency surgery for trauma or infection have significant metabolic decompensation, including ketoacidosis.[172] Often little time is available for stabilization of the patient, but even a few hours may be sufficient for correction of fluid and electrolyte disturbances that are potentially life threatening. It is futile to delay surgery in an attempt to eliminate ketoacidosis completely if the underlying surgical condition will lead to further metabolic deterioration. The likelihood of intraoperative cardiac dysrhythmias and hypotension resulting from ketoacidosis will be reduced if volume depletion and hypokalemia are at least partially treated.

Insulin therapy is initiated with a 10-unit intravenous bolus of regular insulin, which is followed by continuous insulin infusion. The actual amount of insulin administered is less important than regular monitoring of glucose, potassium, and pH. Because the number of insulin-binding sites is limited, the maximum rate of glucose decline is fairly constant, averaging 75 to 100 mg/dL per hour, regardless of the insulin dose.[150,173] During the first 1 to 2 hours of fluid resuscitation, the glucose level may fall more precipitously. When the serum glucose concentration reaches 250 mg/dL, I usually add 5% dextrose to the intravenous fluid.

The volume of fluid required for therapy varies with overall deficits; it ranges from 3 to 5 L, but it can be as high as 10 L. Despite losses of water in excess of losses of solute, sodium levels are generally normal or reduced. Factitious hyponatremia caused by hyperglycemia or hypertriglyceridemia may result in this seeming contradiction. The plasma sodium concentration decreases by about 1.6 mEq/L for every 100 mg/dL increase in plasma glucose concentration above normal. Initially, normal saline is infused at the rate of 250 to 1000 mL/hr, depending on the degree of volume depletion and on the cardiac status. Some measure of left ventricular volume should be monitored in diabetics who have a history of myocardial dysfunction. About one third of the estimated fluid deficit is corrected in the first 6 to 8 hours, and the remaining two thirds is corrected over the next 24 hours.

The degree of acidosis is determined by measurement of arterial blood gases and an increased anion gap $[Na^+ - (Cl^- + HCO_3^-)]$. Acidosis with an increased anion gap (at least 16 mEq/L) in an acutely ill diabetic may be caused by ketones in ketoacidosis, lactic acid in lactic acidosis, increased organic acids from renal insufficiency, or all three. In ketoacidosis, the plasma levels of acetoacetate, β-hydroxybutyrate, and acetone are increased. Plasma and urinary ketones are measured semiquantitatively with the Ketostix and Acetest tablets. The role of bicarbonate therapy in diabetic ketoacidosis is controversial. Myocardial function and respiration are known to be depressed at a blood pH below 7.0 to 7.10; yet rapid correction of acidosis with bicarbonate therapy may result in alterations in CNS function and structure. The alterations may be caused by (1) paradoxical development of cerebrospinal fluid and CNS acidosis resulting from rapid conversion of bicarbonate to carbon dioxide and diffusion of the acid across the blood-brain barrier, (2) altered CNS oxygenation with decreased cerebral blood flow, and (3) development of unfavorable osmotic gradients. After treatment with fluids and insulin, β-hydroxybutyrate levels decrease rapidly, whereas acetoacetate levels may remain stable or even increase before declining. Plasma acetone levels remain elevated for 24 to 42 hours, long after blood glucose, β-hydroxybutyrate, and acetoacetate levels have returned to normal; the result is continuing ketonuria.[150] Persistent ketosis, with a serum bicarbonate level of less than 20 mEq/L in the presence of a normal glucose level, represents a continued need for intracellular glucose and insulin for reversal of lipolysis.

The most important electrolyte disturbance in diabetic ketoacidosis is depletion of total body potassium. The deficits range from 3 mEq/kg up to 10 mEq/kg. Rapid declines in serum potassium level occur, reaching a nadir within 2 to 4 hours after the start of intravenous insulin administration. Aggressive replacement therapy may be required. The potassium administered moves into the intracellular space with insulin as the acidosis is corrected. Potassium is also excreted in the urine with the increased delivery of sodium to the distal renal tubules that accompanies volume expansion. Phosphorus deficiency in ketoacidosis caused by tissue catabolism, impaired cellular uptake, and increased urinary losses may result in significant muscular weakness and organ dysfunction. The average phosphorus deficit is approximately 1 mmol/kg. Replacement may be needed if the plasma concentration falls below 1.0 mg/dL.[150]

Summary

Management of the diabetic surgical patient includes careful preoperative assessment, prevention of infection,[173] frequent glucose and electrolyte monitoring, and, above all, administration of adequate amounts of insulin and glucose based on that monitoring. The sine qua non of tight control is frequent determination of blood glucose levels. With good control of glucose levels, many of the metabolic problems associated with surgery in diabetics can be prevented or alleviated. However, such tight control may not be worth the risk incurred. Epidemiologic evidence indicates that the major risk factor for the diabetic is not the blood glucose level but the end organ effects of diabetes. Autonomic neuropathy often is associated with painless myocardial ischemia and gastroparesis. These problems, as well as myocardial and renal dysfunction, may need special perioperative treatment or monitoring. Whether tight control of blood glucose levels is warranted remains to be determined in future studies. As with most of the other endocrinopathies dealt with in this chapter, it is not the endocrinopathy per se that is associated with morbidity but its cardiovascular and/or autonomic end organ effects that appear crucial to patient outcome. Little is known about how the choice of anesthetic or anesthetic adjuvant drug(s) affects outcome; consequently, attention might be directed to the cardiovascular and/or autonomic end organ effects to optimize outcome.

Acknowledgements

Parts of this chapter have been revised from Pender JW, Basso LV: Diseases of the endocrine system. In Katz J, Benumof J, Kadis L (eds): Anesthesia and Uncommon Diseases, 2nd ed. Philadelphia, WB Saunders, 1981, p 155. Other parts have been adapted from Roizen MF (ed): Anesthesia for Patients with Endocrine Disease. Anesthesiol Clin North Am 1987;5:245.

References

1. Hensel P, Roizen MF: Patients with disorders of parathyroid function. Anesthesiol Clin North Am 1987;5:287.
2. Aurbach GD, Marx SJ, Spiegel AM: Parathyroid hormone, calcitonin, and the calciferols. In Wilson JD, Foster DW (eds): Williams' Textbook of Endocrinology, 8th ed. Philadelphia, WB Saunders, 1992, p 8.
3. Kebebew E, Duh QY, Clark OH: Parathyroidectomy for primary hyperparathyroidism in octogenarians and nonagenarians: A plea for early surgical referral. Aaarch Surg 2003;138;867-871.
4. Parsons JA, Zanelli JM, Gray D, et al: Double isotope estimates of intestinal calcium absorption in rats: Enhancement by parathyroid hormone and 1,25 dihydroxycholecalciferol. Calcif Tissues Res 1977;22(Suppl):127.
5. Gallagher SF, Denham DW, Murr MM, Norman JG: The impact of minimally invasive parathyroidectomy on the way endocrinologists treat primary hyperparathyroidism. Surgery 2000;134:910-917.
6. Crocker EF, Jellins J, Freund J: Parathyroid lesions localized by radionuclide subtraction and ultrasound. Radiology 1979;130:215.
7. Brennan MF, Brown EM, Marx SJ, et al: Recurrent hyperparathyroidism from an autotransplanted parathyroid adenoma. N Engl J Med 1978;299:1057.
8. Kao PC, van Heerden JA, Taylor RL: Intraoperative monitoring of parathyroid procedures by a 15 minute parathyroid hormone immunochemiluminometric assay. Mayo Clin Proc 1994;69:532.
9. Mihai R, Farndon JR: Parathyroid disease and calcium metabolism. Br J Anaesth 2000;85;29-43.
10. Bilezikian JP: Clinical review 51: Management of hypercalcemia. J Clin Endocrinol Metab 1993;77:1445.
11. Nussbaum SR: Pathophysiology and management of severe hypercalcemia. Endocrinol Metab Clin North Am 1993;22:343.
12. Yu PNG: The electrocardiographic changes associated with hypercalcemia and hypocalcemia. Am J Med Sci 1952;224:413.
13. Knochel JP: The pathophysiology and clinical characteristics of severe hypophosphatemia. Arch Intern Med 1977;137:203.
14. Braunfeld M: Hypercalcemia. In Roizen MF, Fleisher LA (eds): Essence of Anesthesia Practice. Philadelphia, WB Saunders, 1997, p 167.
15. Nahrwold ML, Mantha S: Hyperparathyroidism. In Roizen MF, Fleisher LA (eds): Essence of Anesthesia Practice. Philadelphia, WB Saunders, 1997, p 174.
16. Allendorf J, Kim L, Chabot J: The impact of sestamibi scanning on the outcome of parathyroid surgery. J Clin Endocrinol Metab 2003;88:3015-3018.
17. Anast CS, Mohs JM, Kaplan SL, et al: Evidence for parathyroid failure in magnesium deficiency. Science 1972;177:606.
18. Zaloga GP, Chernow B: Hypocalcemia in critical illness. JAMA 1986;256:1924.
19. Rude RK: Magnesium metabolism and deficiency. Endocrinol Metab Clin North Am 1993;22:377.
20. Rumancik WM, Denlinger JK, Nahrwold ML, et al: The QT interval and serum ionized calcium. JAMA 1978;240:366.
21. Muir MA, Jaffar M, Arshad M, et al: Reduced duration of muscle relaxation with rocuronium in a normocalcemic hyperparathyroid patient. Can J Anaesth 2003;50;558-561.
22. Farling PA: Thyroid disease. Br J Anaesth 2000;85:15-28.

23. Roizen MF, Hensel P, Lichtor JL, et al: Patients with disorders of thyroid function. Anesthesiol Clin North Am 1987;5:277.

24. Loh KC: Amiodarone-induced thyroid disorders: A clinical review. Postgrad Med J 2000;76:133-140.

25. Woeber KA: Update on the management of hyperthyroidism and hypothyroidism. Arch Intern Med 2000;160:1067-1071.

26. Larsen PR, Ingbar SH: The thyroid gland. In Wilson JD, Foster DW (eds): Williams' Textbook of Endocrinology, 8th ed. Philadelphia, WB Saunders, 1992, pp 414-445.

27. Chopra IJ: Reciprocal changes in serum concentrations of reverse T_3 and T_4 in systemic illness. J Clin Endocrinol Metab 1975;41:1043.

28. Williams LT, Lefkowitz RJ, Watanabe AM, et al: Thyroid hormone regulation of β-adrenergic receptor number. J Biol Chem 1977;252:2787.

29. Larsen PR, Alexander NM, Chopra IJ, et al: Revised nomenclature for tests of thyroid hormones and thyroid-related proteins in serum. J Clin Endocrinol Metab 1987;64:1089.

30. Roizen MF: Hyperthyroidism. In Roizen MF, Fleisher LA (eds): Essence of Anesthesia Practice. Philadelphia, WB Saunders, 1997, p 177.

31. Amino N, Morik H, Iwatani Y, et al: High prevalence of transient postpartum thyrotoxicosis and hypothyroidism. N Engl J Med 1982;306:849.

32. Channick BJ, Adlin EV, Marks AD, et al: Hyperthyroidism and mitral-valve prolapse. N Engl J Med 305:497, 1981.

33. Davis PJ, Davis FB: Hyperthyroidism in patients over the age of 60 years: Clinical features in 85 patients. Medicine 1974;53:161.

34. Forfar JC, Miller HC, Toft AD: Occult thyrotoxicosis: A correctable cause of "idiopathic" atrial fibrillation. Am J Cardiol 1979;44:9.

35. Toft AD, Irvine WJ, Sinclair I, et al: Thyroid function after surgical treatment of thyrotoxicosis: A report of 100 cases treated with propranolol before operation. N Engl J Med 1978;298:643.

36. Symons G: Thyroid heart disease. Br Heart J 1979;41:257.

37. Forfar JC, Muir AL, Sawers SA, et al: Abnormal left ventricular function in hyperthyroidism: Evidence for a possible reversible cardiomyopathy. N Engl J Med 1982;307:1165.

38. Eriksson M, Rubenfeld S, Garber AJ, et al: Propranolol does not prevent thyroid storm. N Engl J Med 1977;296:263.

39. Trench AJ, et al: Propranolol in thyrotoxicosis: Cardiovascular changes during thyroidectomy in patients pretreated with propranolol. Anaesthesia 1978;33:535.

40. Roizen MF, Becker CE: Thyroid storm: A review of cases at the University of California, San Francisco. Calif Med 1971;115:5.

41. Burch HB, Wartofsky L: Life-threatening thyrotoxicosis: Thyroid storm. Endocrinol Metab Clin North Am 1993;22:263.

42. Zuckerman R: Pregnant surgical patient. In Roizen MF, Fleisher LA (eds): Essence of Anesthesia Practice, 2nd ed. Philadelphia, WB Saunders, 2002, p 449.

43. Sawin CT, Castelli WP, Hershman JM, et al: The aging thyroid: Thyroid deficiency in the Framingham Study. Arch Intern Med 1985;145:1386.

44. Butterworth J: Hypothyroidism. In Roizen MF, Fleisher LA (eds): Essence of Anesthesia Practice. Philadelphia, WB Saunders, 1997, p 185.

45. Singer PA: Thyroiditis: Acute, subacute, and chronic. Med Clin North Am 1991;75:61.

46. Weinberg AD, Brennan MD, Gorman CA, et al: Outcome of anesthesia and surgery in hypothyroid patients. Arch Intern Med 1983;143:893.

47. Bough EW, Crowley WF, Ridgway EC, et al: Myocardial function in hypothyroidism: Relation to disease severity and response to treatment. Arch Intern Med 1978;138:1476.

48. Zwillich CW, Pierson DJ, Hofeldt FD, et al: Ventilatory control in myxedema and hypothyroidism. N Engl J Med 1975;292:662.

49. Abbott TR: Anaesthesia in untreated myxedema. Br J Anaesth 1967;35:510.

50. Babad AA, Eger EI II: The effects of hyperthyroidism and hypothyroidism on halothane and oxygen requirements in dogs. Anesthesiology 1968;29:1087.

51. Levine HD: Compromise therapy in the patient with angina pectoris and hypothyroidism: A clinical assessment. Am J Med 1980;69:411.

52. Paine TD, Rogers WJ, Baxley WA, et al: Coronary arterial surgery in patients with incapacitating angina pectoris and myxedema. Am J Cardiol 1977;40:226.

53. Gharib H: Fine-needle aspiration biopsy of thyroid nodules: Advantages, limitations, and effect. Mayo Clin Proc 1994;69:44.

54. National Cancer Institute: Information for physicians on irradiation-related thyroid cancer. Cancer 1976;26:150.

55. Gharib H, James EM, Charboneau JW, et al: Suppressive therapy with levothyroxine for solitary thyroid nodules: A double-blind controlled clinical study. N Engl J Med 1987;317:70.

56. Jenkins JS, Gilbert CJ, Ang V: Hypothalamic pituitary function in patients with craniopharyngiomas. J Clin Endocrinol Metab 1976;43:394.

57. Molitch ME: Pathologic hyperprolactinemia. Endocrinol Metab Clin North Am 1992;21:877.

58. Jordan RM, Kendall JW: The primary empty sella syndrome. Am J Med 1977;62:569.

59. Cohen KL: Metabolic, endocrine and drug-induced interference with pituitary function tests: A review. Metabolism 1977;26:1165.

60. Karga HJ, Papapetrou PD, Karpathios SE, et al: L-Thyroxine therapy attenuates the decline in serum triiodothyronine in nonthyroidal illness induced by hysterectomy. Metabolism 2003;52:1307-1312.

61. Schmitt H, Buchfelder M, Radespiel-Troger M, Fahlbusch R: Difficult intubation in acromegalic patients: Incidence and predictability. Anesthesiology 2000;93;110-114.

62. Southwick JP, Katz J: Unusual airway difficulty in the acromegalic patient: Indications for tracheostomy. Anesthesiology 1979;51:72.

63. Wall RT III: Acromegaly. In Roizen MF, Fleisher LA (eds): Essence of Anesthesia Practice. Philadelphia, WB Saunders, 1997, p 6.

64. Dougherty TB, Cronau LH Jr: Anesthetic implications for surgical patients with endocrine tumors. Int Anesthesiol Clin 1998;36:31-44.

65. Molitch EM: Diagnosis and treatment of prolactinomas. Adv Intern Med 1999;44:117-153.

66. Berkow L: Transsphenoidal surgery. In Roizen MF, Fleisher LA (eds): Essence of Anesthesia Practice, 2nd ed. Philadelphia, WB Saunders, 2002, p 477.

67. Robertson GL: Thirst and vasopressin function in normal and disordered states of water balance. J Lab Clin Med 1983;101:351.

68. Cannon JF: Diabetes insipidus: Clinical and experimental studies with consideration of genetic relationship. Arch Intern Med 1955;96:215.

69. Bartter FC, Schwartz WB: The syndrome of inappropriate secretion of antidiuretic hormone. Am J Med 1967;42:790.

70. Carlson DE, Gann DS: Effect of vasopressin antiserum on the response of adrenocorticotropin and cortisol to haemorrhage. Endocrinology 1984;114:317.

71. Newfield P: Syndrome of inappropriate antidiuretic hormone secretion (SIADH). In Roizen MF, Fleisher LA (eds): Essence of Anesthesia Practice, 2nd ed. Philadelphia, WB Saunders, 1997, p 303.

72. Berardi RS: Vascular complication of superior mesenteric artery infusion with pitressin in treatment of bleeding esophageal varices. Am J Surg 1974;127:757.

73. Corliss RJ, McKenna DH, Sialers S, et al: Systemic and coronary hemodynamic effects of vasopressin. Am J Med Sci 1968;256:293.

74. Nikolic G, Singh JB: Cimetidine, vasopressin, and chronotropic incompetence. Med J Aust 1982;2:435.

75. Malhotra N, Roizen MF: Patients with abnormalities of vasopressin secretion and responsiveness. Anesthesiol Clin North Am 1987;5:395.

76. Lampe GH, Roizen MF: Anesthesia for patients with abnormal function at the adrenal cortex. Anesthesiol Clin North Am 1987;5:245.

77. Derksen J, Negesser SK, Meinders AE, et al: Identification of virilizing adrenal tumors in hirsute women. N Engl J Med 1994;331;968-973.

78. Tyrell JB: Cushing's syndrome. In Wyngaarden JB, Smith LH, Bennett JC (eds): Cecil Textbook of Medicine, 19th ed. Philadelphia, WB Saunders, 1992, pp 1284-1288.

79. Cornbridge TC, Hall JB: The assessment and management of adults with status asthmaticus. Am J Respir Crit Care Med 1995;151:1296.

80. Ellul-Micallef R, Borthwick RC, McHardy GJR: The time-course of response to prednisolone in chronic bronchial asthma. Clin Sci 1974;47:105.

81. Moore-Ede MC, Czeisler CA, Richardson GS: Circadian time-keeping in health and disease: I. Basic properties of circadian pacemakers. N Engl J Med 1983;309:469.

82. Goldmann DR: The surgical patient on steroids. In Goldmann DR, Brown FH, Levy WK, et al (eds): Medical Care of the Surgical Patient: A Problem-Oriented Approach to Management. Philadelphia, JB Lippincott, 1982, pp 113-125.

83. Hume DM, Bell CC, Bartter F: Direct measurement of adrenal secretion during operative trauma and convalescence. Surgery 1962;52:174.

84. Plumpton FS, Besser GM, Cole PV: Corticosteroid treatment and surgery: An investigation of the indications for steroid cover. Anaesthesia 1969;24:3.

85. Sampson PA, Brooke BN, Winstone NE: Biochemical confirmation of collapse due to adrenal failure. Lancet 1961;1:1377.

86. Avioli LV: Effects of chronic corticosteroid therapy on mineral metabolism and calcium absorption. Adv Exp Biol Med 1984;171:80.

87. Axelrod L: Glucocorticoid therapy. Medicine 1976;55:39.

88. Taylor AL, Fishman LM: Corticotropin-releasing hormone. Med Progr 1988;319:213.

89. Cook DM: Adrenal mass. Endocrinol Metab Clin North Am 1997;26:829-852.

90. Werbel SS, Ober KP: Acute adrenal insufficiency. Endocrinol Metab Clin North Am 1993;22:303.

91. Hollenberg NK, Williams GH: Hypertension, the adrenal and the kidney: Lessons from pharmacologic interruption of the renin-angiotensin system. Adv Intern Med 1980;25:327.

92. Lampe GH: Cushing's syndrome. In Roizen MF, Fleisher LA (eds): Essence of Anesthesia Practice, 2nd ed. Philadelphia, WB Saunders, 2002, p 102.

93. Symreng T: Steroids. In Roizen MF, Fleisher LA (eds): Essence of Anesthesia Practice. Philadelphia, WB Saunders, 1997, p 545.

94. Engquist A, Backer OG, Jarnum S: Incidence of post-operative complications in patients subjected to surgery under steroid cover. Acta Chir Scand 1974;140:343.

95. Dale DC, Fauci AS, Wolff SM: Alternate-day prednisone: Leukocyte kinetics and susceptibility to infections. N Engl J Med 1974;291:1154.

96. Winstone NE, Brook BN: Effects of steroid treatment on patients undergoing operation. Lancet 1961;1:973.

97. Ehrlich HP, Hunt TK: Effects of cortisone and vitamin A on wound healing. Ann Surg 1968;167:324.

98. Moore TJ, Dluhy RG, Williams GH, et al: Nelson's syndrome: Frequency, prognosis, and effect of prior pituitary irradiation. Ann Intern Med 1976;8:731.

99. Mantero F, Masini AM, Opocher G et al: On behalf of the National Italian Study Group on Adrenal Tumors: Adrenal incidentaloma: An overview of hormonal data from the National Italian Study Group. Horm Res 1997;47:284.

100. Sandburg N: Time relationship between administration of cortisone and wound healing in rats. Acta Chir Scand 1964;127:446.

101. Moore TJ, Dluhy RG, Williams GH, et al: Nelson's syndrome: Frequency, prognosis, and effect of prior pituitary irradiation. Ann Intern Med 1976;8:731.

102. Miller MK: Hyperaldosteronism (secondary). In Roizen MF, Fleisher LA (eds): Essence of Anesthesia Practice, 2nd ed. Philadelphia, WB Saunders, 2002, p 171.

103. Hanowell ST, Hittner KC, Kim YD, et al: Anesthetic management of primary aldosteronism. Anesthesiol Rev 1982;9:30.

104. Udelsman R, Ramp J, Gallucci WT, et al: Adaptation during surgical stress: A re-evaluation of the role of glucocorticoids. J Clin Invest 1986;77:1377.

105. Symreng T, Karlberg BE, Kagedal B: Physiologic cortisol substitution of long-term steroid-treated patients undergoing major surgery. Br J Anesthesiol 1981;53:949.

106. Schambelan M, et al: Prevalence, pathogenesis and functional significance of aldosterone deficiency in hyperkalemic patients with chronic renal insufficiency. Kidney Int 1980;17:89.

107. Zusman RM: Prostaglandins and water excretion. Ann Rev Med 1981;32:359.

108. Cassinello Ogea C, Giron Nombiela JA, Ruiz Tramazaygues J, et al: Severe perioperative hyptension after nephrectomy with adrenalectomy. Rev Esp Anestesiol Reanimacion 2002;49:213-217.

109. Rabinowitz IN, Watson W, Farber EM: Topical steroid depression of the hypothalamic-pituitary-adrenal axis in psoriasis vulgaris. Dermatologica 1977;154:321.

110. Jensen JK, Elb S: Per-og postoperative komplikationer hos tigligere kortikosteroid behandlede patienter. Nord Med 1966;76:975-978.

111. Oh SH, Patterson R: Surgery in corticosteroid asthmatics. J Allergy Clin Immunol 1974;53:345.

112. Wagner RL, White PF, Kan PB, et al: Inhibition of adrenal steroidogenesis by the anesthetic etomidate. N Engl J Med 1984;310:1415.

113. St. John Sutton MG, Sheps SG, Lie JT: Prevalence of clinically unsuspected pheochromocytoma: Review of a 50-year autopsy series. Mayo Clin Proc 1981;56:354.

114. Witteles RM, Kaplan EL, Roizen MF: Sensitivity of diagnostic and localization tests for pheochromocytoma in clinical practice. Arch Intern Med 2000;160:2521-2524.

115. Pauker SG, Kopelman RI: Interpreting hoofbeats: Can Bayes help clear the haze? N Engl J Med 1992;327:1009.

116. Lucon AM, Pereira MAA, Mendonca BB, et al: Pheochromocytoma: Study of 50 cases. J Urol 1997;157:1208.

117. Brown IE, Milshteyn M, Kleinman B, et al: Case 3-2002 Pheochromocytoma presenting as a right intra-atrial mass. J Cardiothorac Vasc Anesth 2002;16:370-373.

118. Roizen MF, Schreider BD, Hassan SK: Anesthesia for patients with pheochromocytoma. Anesthesiol Clin North Am 1987;5:269.

119. Roizen MF: Pheochromocytoma. In Roizen MF, Fleisher LA (eds): Essence of Anesthesia Practice. Philadelphia, WB Saunders, 1997, p 251.

120. Roizen MF: Adrenalectomy for pheochromocytoma. In Roizen MF, Fleisher LA (eds): Essence of Anesthesia Practice. Philadelphia, WB Saunders, 1997, p 339.

121. Gifford RW Jr, Manger WM, Bravo EL: Pheochromocytoma. Endocrinol Metab Clin North Am 1994;23:387.

122. Bravo EL, Tarazi RC, Fovad FM, et al: The clonidine suppression test: A useful aid in the diagnosis of pheochromocytoma. N Engl J Med 1981;305:623.

123. Jensen JA, Jansson K, Goodson WH III, et al: Epinephrine lowers subcutaneous wound oxygen tension. Curr Surg 1985;42:472.

124. Roizen MF, Hunt TK, Beaupre PN, et al: The effect of alpha-adrenergic blockade on cardiac performance and tissue oxygen delivery during excision of pheochromocytoma. Surgery 1983;94:941.

125. Roizen MF, Horrigan RW, Koike M, et al: A prospective randomized trial of four anesthetic techniques for resection of pheochromocytoma. Anesthesiology 1982;57:A43.

126. Cooperman LH, Engelman K, Mann PEG: Anesthetic management of pheochromocytoma employing halothane and beta adrenergic blockade. Anesthesiology 1967;28:575.

127. Desmonts JM, Le Houelleur J, Remond P, et al: Anaesthetic management of patients with phaeochromocytoma: A review of 102 cases. Br J Anaesth 1977;49:991.

128. Smith DS, Aukberg SJ, Levitt JD: Induction of anesthesia in a patient with undiagnosed pheochromocytoma. Anesthesiology 1978;49:368.

129. Schaffer MS, Zuberbuhler P, Urlson G, et al: Catecholamine cardiomyopathy: An unusual presentation of pheochromocytoma in children. J Pediatr 1981;99:276.

130. Service FJ: Hypoglycemia. Med Clin North Am 1995;79:1.

131. Rizza RA, Haymond MW, Verdonk CA, et al: Pathogenesis of hypoglycemia in insulinoma patients, suppression of hepatic glucose production by insulin. Diabetes 1981;30:377.

132. Muir JJ, Enders SM, Offord K, et al: Glucose management in patients undergoing operation for insulinoma removal. Anesthesiology 1983;59:371.

133. Reubi J-C, Laissue JA: Multiple actions of somatostatin in neoplastic disease. Trends Pharmacol Sci 1995;16:110.

134. Muir JJ: Insulinoma. In Roizen MF, Fleisher LA (eds): Essence of Anesthesia Practice. Philadelphia, WB Saunders, 1997, p 191.

135. Finney SJ, Zekveld C, Elia A, Evans TW: Glucose control and mortality in critically ill patients. JAMA 2003;2910:2041-2047.

136. Krinsley JS: Association between hyperglycemia and increased hospital mortality in a heterogeneous population of critically ill patients. Mayo Clin Proc 2003;78:1471-1478.

137. Retinopathy and nephropathy in patients with type I diabetes four years after a trial of intensive therapy. The Diabetes Control and Complications Trial/Epidemiology of Diabetes Interventions and Complications Research Group. N Engl J Med 2000;342:381-389.

138. UK Prospective Diabetes Study Group: Tight blood pressure control and risk of macrovascular and microvascular complications in type II diabetes. BMJ 1998;317:703-713.

139. Tuomilehto J, Lindstrom J, Erridsson JG, et al: Finnish diabetes prevention study group. Prevention of type 2 diabetes mellitus by changes in lifestyle among subjects with impaired glucose tolerance. N Engl J Med 2001;344;1343-1350.

140. Narayan KM, Boyle JP, Thomson TJ, et al: Lifetime risk for diabetes mellitus in the United States. JAMA 2003;290:1884-1890.

141. Van den Berghe G, Wouters P, Weekers F, et al: Intensive insulin therapy in critically ill patients. N Engl J Med 2004;345:1359-1367.

142. Walsh DB, Eckhauser FE, Ramsburgh SR, et al: Risk associated with diabetes mellitus in patients undergoing gallbladder surgery. Surgery 1982;91:254.

143. Fowkes FGR, Lunn JN, Furow SC, et al: Epidemiology in anesthesia: III. Mortality risk in patients with coexisting physical disease. Br J Anaesth 1982;54:819.

144. Burgos LG, Ebert TJ, Asiddao C, et al: Increased intraoperative cardiovascular morbidity in diabetes with autonomic neuropathy. Anesthesiology 1989;70:591.

145. Hjortrup A, Rasmussen BF, Kehlet H: Morbidity in diabetic and nondiabetic patients after major vascular surgery. BMJ 1983;287:1107.

146. Douglas JS, King SB, Craver JM, et al: Factors influencing risk and benefit of coronary bypass surgery in patients with diabetes mellitus. Chest 1981;80:369.

147. Ransohoff DF, Miller GL, Forsythe SB, et al: Outcome of acute cholecystitis in patients with diabetes mellitus. Ann Intern Med 1987;106:829.

148. Creutzfeldt W, Kabberling J, Neel JV: The Genetics of Diabetes Mellitus. New York, Springer-Verlag, 1976.

149. Campbell PJ, Bolli GB, Cryer PE, et al: Pathogenesis of the dawn phenomenon in patients with insulin-dependent diabetes mellitus. N Engl J Med 1985;312:1473.

150. Kreisberg RA: Diabetic ketoacidosis: New concepts and trends in pathogenesis and treatment. Ann Intern Med 1978;88:681.

151. Porte D Jr, Schwartz MW: Diabetic complications: Why is glucose potentially toxic? Science 1996;272:699.

152. Wass CT, Lanier WL: Glucose modulation of ischemic brain injury: Review and clinical recommendations. Mayo Clin Proc 1996;71: 801-812.

153. Walters DP, Gatling W, Houston AC, et al: Mortality in diabetic subjects: An eleven-year follow-up of community-based population. Diabet Med 1994;11:968.

154. Bagdade JD, Root RK, Bulger RJ: Impaired leukocyte function in patients with poorly controlled diabetes. Diabetes 1974;23:9.

155. Clark CM Jr, Lee DA: Prevention and treatment of the complications of diabetes mellitus. N Engl J Med 1995;332:1210.

156. Brenner BM: Hemodynamically mediated glomerular injury and the progressive nature of kidney disease. Kidney Int 1983;23:647.

157. Forsblom CM, Eriksson JG, Ekstrand AV, et al: Insulin resistance and abnormal albumin excretion in non-diabetic first-degree relatives of patients with NIDDM. Diabetologia 1995;38:363.

158. Krolewski AS, Laffel LMB, Krolewski M, et al: Glycosylated hemoglobin and the risk of microalbuminuria in patients with insulin-dependent diabetes mellitus. N Engl J Med 1995;332:1251.

159. Lanier WL: Glucose management during cardiopulmonary bypass: Cardiovascular and neurologic implications. Anesth Analg 1991;72:423.

160. Viberti G, Mogensen CE, Groop LC, et al: Effect of captopril on progression to clinical proteinuria in patients with insulin-dependent diabetes mellitus and microalbuminuria. JAMA 1994;271:275.

161. Ishii H, Jirousek MR, Koya D, et al: Amelioration of vascular dysfunction in diabetic rats by an oral PKG beta inhibitor. Science 1996;272:728.

162. Brenner WI, Lansky Z, Engelman RM, et al: Hyperosmolar coma in surgical patients: An iatrogenic disease of increasing incidence. Ann Surg 1973;178:651.

163. Page MMcB, Watkins PJ: Cardiorespiratory arrest and diabetic autonomic neuropathy. Lancet 1978;1:14.

164. Charlson ME, MacKenzie CR, Gold JP: Preoperative autonomic function abnormalities in patients with diabetes mellitus and patients with hypertension. J Am Coll Surg 1994;179:1.

165. Wright RA, Clemente R, Wathen R: Diabetic gastroparesis: An abnormality of gastric emptying of solids. Am J Med Sci 1985;289:240.

166. Longstreth WT, Inui TS: High blood glucose level on hospital admission and poor neurological recovery after cardiac arrest. Ann Neurol 1984;15:59.

167. Meyer EJ, Lorenzi M, Bohannon NV, et al: Diabetic management by insulin infusion during major surgery. Am J Surg 1979; 137:323.

168. Taitelman U, Reece EA, Bessman AN: Insulin in the management of the diabetic surgical patient; continuous intravenous infusion vs subcutaneous administration. JAMA 1977;237:658.

169. Elliott MJ, Gill GV, Home PD, et al: A comparison of two regimens for the management of diabetes during open-heart surgery. Anesthesiology 1984;60:364.

170. Johnson WD, Pedraza PM, Kayser KL: Coronary artery surgery in diabetics: 261 consecutive patients followed four to seven years. Am Heart J 1982;104:823.

171. Alberti KG, Thomas DJ: The management of diabetes during surgery. Br J Anaesth 1979;51:693.

172. Molitch ME, Reichlin S: The care of the diabetic patient during emergency surgery and postoperatively. Orthop Clin North Am 1978;9:811.

173. Ammon JR: Diabetic ketoacidosis (DKA). In Roizen MF, Fleisher LA (eds): Essence of Anesthesia Practice, 2nd ed. Philadelphia, WB Saunders, 2002.

14 Mitochondrial Diseases

RICHARD J. LEVY, MD, and STANLEY MURAVCHICK, MD, PHD

The terms *mitochondrial myopathy* or *inherited mitochondrial encephalomyopathy* originally encompassed a grouping of pediatric neurologic syndromes produced by maternally inherited mitochondrial genetic defects. However, it is now clear that respiratory chain deficiencies undermine metabolic energy production, produce excessive levels of "free radical" reactive oxygen species (ROS), and may generate almost any symptom, in any organ system, at any stage of life. Therefore, the scope of human disease attributable to the inherited, acutely acquired, or insidious onset of impaired mitochondrial function may be far more broad than previously believed.

In addition to the energy production essential for life, the hundreds of mitochondria found in every cell also provide a wide variety of metabolic and cell regulatory functions. For example, hepatic mitochondria provide detoxification of ammonia. In neurons, they are essential for neurotransmitter synthesis. Therefore, mitochondrial dysfunction is emerging as a pivotal factor in the etiology of sepsis, neurodegenerative disorders, diabetes, arteriosclerotic disease, and even normal human aging.[1,2] In this chapter we provide an overview of current concepts of the perioperative assessment and anesthetic management of pediatric and adult patients with uncommon mitochondrial-based syndromes. In addition, we discuss more familiar disease states that are now thought to be manifestations of organ system dysfunction attributable to disruption or depression of aerobic metabolism or other aspects of mitochondrial function.

BACKGROUND

Mitochondria produce adenosine triphosphate (ATP) by oxidative phosphorylation via an electron transport chain composed of five enzyme complexes located on the inner mitochondrial membrane (Fig. 14-1). Reduction of molecular oxygen is coupled to phosphorylation of adenosine diphosphate (ADP), resulting in ATP synthesis.[3] The reduced cofactors nicotinamide adenine dinucleotide (NADH) and flavin adenine dinucleotide ($FADH_2$), generated by the Krebs cycle and by fatty acid oxidation, donate electrons to complex I (NADH dehydrogenase) and complex II (succinate dehydrogenase). Electrons are then transferred to coenzyme Q and subsequently to complex III. From complex III, reduced cytochrome c donates its electrons to complex IV (cytochrome c oxidase), resulting in the reduction of molecular oxygen to water. Complexes I, III, and IV actively pump hydrogen ions across the inner membrane of the mitochondrion into the intermembrane space, creating an electrochemical gradient. Influx of protons back into the mitochondrial matrix through complex V results in ATP synthesis.[4] This process of

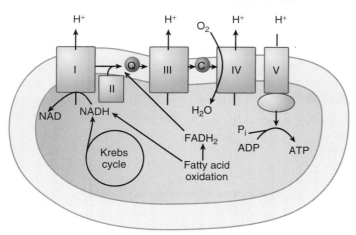

FIGURE 14-1 The electron transport chain needed for oxidative phosphorylation is located on complexes I to V on the inner mitochondrial membrane. The Krebs cycle and fatty acid oxidation yield NADH and $FADH_2$, which initiate electron transfer to the respiratory chain. Coenzyme Q (Q) and cytochrome c (C) transport electrons to complex III and complex IV, respectively. Complex V uses the hydrogen ion gradient (H+) created by hydrogen pumps within complexes I, III, and IV to phosphorylate adenosine diphosphate (ADP) to synthesize adenosine triphosphate (ATP).

oxidative phosphorylation is the major intracellular source of the free radicals (O_2^-, H_2O_2, and OH^-) that are generated as byproducts of the interaction between excess electrons and oxygen.

The enzymes, membranes, and other molecular components of these five major enzyme/protein complexes needed for mitochondrial oxidative phosphorylation are encoded in a complementary manner by the circular genome found within the mitochondrion itself, as well as by the much larger nuclear genome of the host cell. The mitochondrial genome encodes for 13 essential subunits of the electron transport chain, two types of ribosomal ribonucleic acid (rRNA), and 22 forms of transfer RNA (tRNA). Each mitochondrion contains multiple copies of mitochondrial deoxyribonucleic acid (mtDNA). Nuclear DNA (nDNA) encodes an additional 900 proteins that are needed for normal mitochondrial function.

The complementary relationship between two genomes within each cell and the putative evolution of the mitochondrion from a free-living organism into an organelle within the cell have been known and discussed by cell biologists only within the past three or four decades. The implications of this biologic curiosity with regard to our understanding of embryology, evolution, aging, and even the mechanism of death itself may be profound. The mitochondrion, through a central role in the modulation of bioenergetics and cellular apoptosis (see later), may also serve as both a "biosensor" for oxidative stress and as the final determinant of cellular viability.

The most severe inherited mitochondrial disease syndromes become clinically apparent during infancy, but a few were eventually described in which symptoms did not appear until early adulthood. The original descriptions of the mitochondrial diseases of childhood assumed that there was maternal transmission of mitochondria and of both normal ("wild type") and mutant mtDNA. Because mutant mtDNA coexists with wild-type mtDNA, variability in the severity of all these inherited conditions is thought to reflect *heteroplasmy,* the random differences in the proportion of mutant mtDNA distributed throughout the target tissues during embryogenesis. For the mitochondrial disorders of adult onset, variability in disease severity and an exceptionally wide range of phenotypic symptom patterns are thought to reflect both heteroplasmy and the markedly different and progressively changing metabolic demands of different target tissues during adulthood. Hundreds of mtDNA mutations have already been identified in detail and classified as mitochondrial myopathies, encephalomyopathies, or cytopathies.[5,6]

A recent report of a patient with mutated mtDNA of paternal origin, however, suggests that some paternal mtDNA also survives in the zygote and therefore may also contribute to the mtDNA pool.[7] The important role of defects in nDNA in disorders characterized by declining mitochondrial bioenergetics has also been clarified, reflecting the fact that the interaction of nuclear and mitochondrial genomes has become better understood.[8] It is now clear that there are subunits of the electron transport chain not encoded by mtDNA that arise from nDNA. Diseases caused by nuclear genes that do not encode subunits but affect mtDNA stability are an especially interesting group of mitochondrial disorders. In these syndromes, a primary nuclear gene defect causes secondary mtDNA information loss or deletion, which leads to subsequent tissue dysfunction in the form of disrupted oxidative phosphorylation. Therefore, there are some genetically determined defects in oxidative phosphorylation that follow classic mendelian patterns of dominant-recessive genetic transmission, rather than the maternal patterns usually associated with mtDNA defects.

EFFECT OF ANESTHETICS ON MITOCHONDRIAL FUNCTION

The effects of anesthetics on mitochondrial function were first investigated in the 1930s. Although the mechanisms of action are still not all established, it is now clear that virtually all volatile, local, and intravenous anesthetics have significant depressant effects on mitochondrial energy production. These effects are believed to occur primarily at the level of the electron transport chain on the inner membrane of mitochondria. Early studies reported inhibition of the oxidation of glucose, lactate, and pyruvate by narcotics; and more recent work explores the mechanism of reduced oxygen consumption in the brain after treatment with barbiturates.[9] A common final pathway of depressed bioenergetic activity, possibly through a variety of intracellular or mitochondrial mechanisms, may, at least in part, also explain the primary anesthetic effects of these drugs.[10] There is, however, need for caution with regard to the interpretation of the available data on this subject because much of the work examining anesthetic-induced mitochondrial dysfunction has been done in vitro, in isolated mitochondria, not in functioning cells. Furthermore, the anesthetic concentrations used to inhibit mitochondrial function experimentally have been up to 10-fold higher than concentrations used clinically, although it appears that anesthetics inhibit mitochondria in a dose-dependent fashion. These are major limitations in this field of investigation and should be taken into consideration when reviewing the subject.

Inhalational and Local Anesthetics

Nitrous oxide and the potent inhalational agents have significant effects on mitochondrial respiration.[11-14] In cardiac mitochondria, halothane, isoflurane, and sevoflurane have all been shown to inhibit complex I of the electron transport chain.[12] At concentrations equal to 2 MAC (minimal alveolar concentration), complex I activity is reduced by 20% following exposure to halothane and isoflurane, and by 10% following exposure to sevoflurane. Oxidative phosphorylation in liver mitochondria is also measurably disrupted after exposure to halothane. Concentrations of 0.5% to 2% halothane lead to reversible inhibition of complex I (NADH: ubiquinone oxidoreductase) in the electron transport chain. Halothane-induced mitochondrial inhibition in the liver is further exacerbated by the addition of nitrous oxide.[13] Local anesthetics have also been shown to disrupt oxidative phosphorylation[14,15] and significantly degrade bioenergetic capacity in mitochondrial isolates.

Barbiturates and Propofol

Barbiturate effects have been well studied in the brain, heart, and liver. Like the inhalational agents, barbiturates inhibit complex I of the electron transport chain. This inhibition, however, occurs at serum levels that far exceed those required to produce the anesthetic effect. Propofol disrupts electron transport in the respiratory chain.[16] Decreased oxygen consumption and inhibited electron flow have been demonstrated in cardiac mitochondria exposed to propofol.[17] Similarly, work with mitochondria from the liver has demonstrated that propofol inhibits complex I of the electron transport chain.[18] Table 14-1 is a summary of the effect of various anesthetic agents on mitochondrial function.

TABLE 14–1 Effect of Anesthetics on Mitochondrial Function
Volatile agents inhibit complex I.
Barbiturates inhibit complex I.
Propofol inhibits complex I and slows electron transport of respiratory chain.
Local anesthetics disrupt oxidative phosphorylation by unknown mechanisms.

Other Effects

Exposure to the volatile anesthetics has also been shown to alter the ability of the mitochondrion to respond to rising levels of ROS, a "preconditioning" effect that may protect the cell if it is subsequently exposed to periods of hypoxia or ischemia. Although the mechanism of "anesthetic preconditioning" remains speculative, anesthetic agents appear to disrupt mitochondrial bioenergetics sufficiently that they produce the low levels of oxidative stress that induce short-term genetic expression of heat shock protein (HSP) or other protective substances. HSP can also be induced by brief, sublethal episodes of ischemia or hypoxia, suggesting that the prophylactic administration of HSP or similar interventions may have potential therapeutic value for cardiac protection and neuroprotection during major surgery, during which tissue perfusion or oxygenation is disrupted.[19]

Therefore, anesthetics may not only depress bioenergetic activity but may also affect other functions of the mitochondrion, such as the role of this organelle as a "biosensor" for oxidative stress or perhaps the role of the mitochondrion as an effector organelle for cellular apoptosis. Accumulation of ROS increases outer membrane permeability of the mitochondrion and leads to the ingress of potassium and ionized calcium and to the release of cytochrome c and other "pro-apoptotic" soluble proteins. Leakage of cytochrome c from mitochondria not only rapidly degrades the bioenergetic capacity of the cell by removing a key component of the respiratory chain but also appears to trigger the release of caspases, which are cysteine-containing protease enzymes. They, in turn, activate other enzymes that digest nDNA, the final step in "cell suicide," or apoptosis.

INHERITED DISORDERS WITH CHILDHOOD ONSET

Mitochondrial diseases with childhood onset often present in the newborn period. The clinical features may be quite variable because a single organ system or multiple organ systems may be affected. The organ systems most often involved are the central (CNS) and peripheral nervous systems, liver, heart, kidneys, muscle, gastrointestinal tract, skin, and a number of endocrine glands. Nonspecific signs include lethargy, irritability, hyperactivity, and poor feeding. The presentation can be very abrupt and dramatic, with acute onset of hypothermia or hyperthermia, cyanosis, seizures, emesis, diarrhea, or jaundice. Some of the more insidious signs and symptoms of mitochondrial disease in the newborn are listed in Table 14-2.

MtDNA depletion syndrome (MDS) is a severe disease of childhood characterized by liver failure and neurologic abnormalities, in which tissue-specific loss of mtDNA is seen. MDS is thought to be caused by a putative nuclear gene that controls mtDNA replication or stability.[20] Similarly, children with mitochondrial neurogastrointestinal encephalomyopathy (MNGIE) may have multiple mtDNA deletions and/or mtDNA depletion that results from an nDNA mutation.[21] Although nonspecific gastrointestinal and hepatic symptoms are commonly found in most mitochondrial disorders, they are among the cardinal manifestations of primary mitochondrial diseases such as MDS and MNGIE.

CNS manifestations of mitochondrial disorders include encephalopathy, a cardinal feature of Leigh's syndrome. Seizures and ataxia also occur with myoclonic epilepsy with ragged-red fibers (MERRF). Dementia and stroke-like symptoms are a major feature of mitochondrial encephalomyopathy with lactic acidosis and stroke-like episodes (MELAS). When the peripheral nervous system is involved there may be axonal sensory neuropathies. Cardiac involvement with pediatric mitochondrial disease may produce hypertrophic cardiomyopathy, seen with MELAS, or dilated cardiomyopathy, heart block, and pre-excitation syndrome, features of Leber's hereditary optic neuropathy (LHON). Impaired renal bioenergetics produce tubular acidosis; muscle abnormalities present largely as myopathies. Hepatic failure, dysphagia, pseudo-obstruction, and constipation all suggest gastrointestinal

impairment. Vision and hearing are often impaired by ophthalmoplegia, ptosis, cataracts, optic atrophy, pigmentary retinopathy, and sensorineural deafness. Endocrine organ involvement manifests as diabetes mellitus, hypoparathyroidism, hypothyroidism, and gonadal failure. Typical symptoms and signs of the most well-known mtDNA-related syndromes are listed in Table 14-3.

INHERITED DISORDERS WITH ADULT-ONSET AND ACQUIRED MITOCHONDRIAL DYSFUNCTION

Inherited Disorders

Inherited neurologic/metabolic syndromes produced by genetic defects that disrupt mitochondrial energy production are typically seen during infancy, or they may first be apparent only many years later. They can appear during the early-to-middle adult years in the form of declining organ system reserve in tissues such as brain and retina that require maintenance of relatively high rates of metabolic activity for normal functioning. Symptoms include progressive motor weakness and lethargy, decreased color or night vision, and ataxia. Like those of most syndromes of infancy, adult mitochondrial syndromes such as NARP are caused by maternally transmitted mutations of mtDNA. The acronym NARP reflects the fundamental clinical stigmata of that disorder, that is, sensory neuropathy, ataxia, and retinitis pigmentosa. In NARP, a point mutation at base pair position 8993 of mtDNA produces defects in ATPase. Consequently, reduced enzymatic activity and lower rates of ATP production are found in mitochondrial isolates of lymphoblastoid cell lines obtained from NARP patients, and there are increased brain levels of phosphocreatine and inorganic phosphate in NARP patients compared with age- and sex-matched control subjects, suggesting generalized impairment of the efficiency of oxidative metabolic pathways.[22] The specific genetic defects that produce NARP and several other mitochondrial disorders have been identified (Fig. 14-2).

Some of the pathognomonic features of adult-onset mitochondrial disorders may also occur long after the syndrome itself is established by secondary characteristics. For example, stroke-like episodes may not appear until decades after initial clinical onset of MELAS.[23] A progressive decrease in cardiac, muscle, and nervous system functional reserve probably begins long before the appearance of overt signs or symptoms but can usually be confirmed by careful and detailed review of the patient's history and ability to accomplish the normal activities of daily life.

Even when the focus of mitochondrial disease was limited to the inherited disorders of childhood, it was suspected that mtDNA missense mutations could play

---

TABLE 14–2   Differential Diagnosis of Signs and Symptoms of Mitochondrial Disorders in the Newborn Period

Unexplained sepsis or recurrent severe infection
Organic acidemias such as maple syrup urine disease and methylmalonic aciduria
Urea cycle defects such as ornithine transcarbamylase deficiency
Carbohydrate disorders such as galactosemia or hereditary fructose intolerance
Aminoacidopathies such as homocystinuria, tyrosinemia, and nonketotic hyperglycemia
Endocrinopathies such as congenital adrenal hyperplasia and congenital diabetes

TABLE 14–3   Symptoms and Signs of Mitochondrial Disorder

Disease	Mutation	Inheritance	Symptoms and Signs
Kearns-Sayre syndrome	Large-scale mtDNA deletion	Sporadic	Ataxia, peripheral neuropathy, muscle weakness, ophthalmoplegia, ptosis, pigmentary retinopathy, sideroblastic anemia, diabetes mellitus, short stature, hypoparathyroidism, cardiomyopathy, conduction defects, sensorineural hearing loss, Fanconi syndrome, lactic acidosis, ragged-red fibers on muscle biopsy
Progressive external ophthalmoplegia	Large-scale mtDNA deletion	Sporadic	Muscle weakness, ophthalmoplegia, ptosis, lactic acidosis, ragged-red fibers on muscle biopsy
Pearson's syndrome	Large-scale mtDNA deletion	Sporadic	Ophthalmoplegia, sideroblastic anemia, pancreatic dysfunction, Fanconi syndrome, lactic acidosis, ragged-red fibers on muscle biopsy
Myoclonic epilepsy with ragged-red fibers (MERRF)	mtDNA point mutation, tRNA abnormality	Maternal	Seizures, ataxia, myoclonus, psychomotor regression, peripheral neuropathy, muscle weakness, short stature, sensorineural hearing loss, lactic acidosis, ragged-red fibers on muscle biopsy
Mitochondrial encephalopathy, lactic acidosis, and stroke-like episodes (MELAS)	mtDNA point mutation, tRNA abnormality	Maternal	Seizures, ataxia, myoclonus, psychomotor regression, abnormality hemiparesis, cortical blindness, migraine, dystonia, peripheral neuropathy, muscle weakness, diabetes mellitus, short stature, cardiomyopathy, conduction defects, intestinal pseudo-obstruction, sensorineural hearing loss, Fanconi syndrome, lactic acidosis, ragged-red fibers on muscle biopsy
Aminoglycoside-induced deafness	tRNA abnormality		Cardiomyopathy, sensorineural hearing loss
Neuropathy, ataxia, and retinitis pigmentosa (NARP)	mtDNA point mutations, mRNA abnormality	Maternal	Ataxia, peripheral neuropathy, muscle weakness, pigmentary retinopathy, optic atrophy, sensorineural hearing loss
Maternally inherited Leigh's syndrome	mtDNA point mutation, mRNA abnormality	Maternal	Seizures, ataxia, psychomotor regression, dystonia, muscle weakness, abnormality pigmentary retinopathy, optic atrophy, cardiomyopathy, lactic acidosis
Leber's hereditary optic neuropathy	Multiple mtDNA point mutations, mRNA abnormality	Maternal	Dystonia, optic atrophy, conduction defects

an etiologic role in a wide range of neurodegenerative disorders.[24] Among the adult neurodegenerative diseases, a mitochondrial focus has now been clearly established for Parkinson's disease,[25] Alzheimer's dementia, and amyotrophic lateral sclerosis.[26] More recently, the spinal cord atrophy of multiple sclerosis has been attributed to inflammation that may be controlled by a mitochondrion-driven, genetically determined mechanism similar to that of other neurodegenerative disorders.[27] However, there are other important processes implicated in neurodegenerative disorders, several of which involve degradation of proteins or compromise of the mechanisms by which damaged proteins are cleared from within neurons. Oxidative modification of proteins, perhaps by increased levels of ROS, causes them to become dysfunctional and makes them targets for selective destruction by the proteolytic machinery of the proteasomal system. This system is distributed in the cytosol, nucleus, and endoplasmic reticulum of the neuron and contains a multicatalytic protease complex and various regulatory and control elements.[28]

Several adult-onset clinical syndromes associated with multiple mtDNA deletions have been characterized, the most frequently described being autosomal dominant

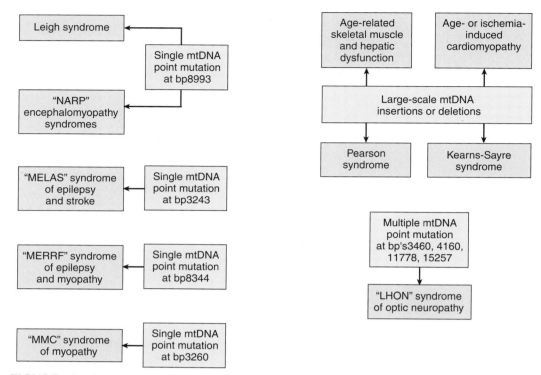

FIGURE 14–2 Inherited mitochondrial syndromes and disorders can reflect single-point, multiple-point, or large-scale errors in mitochondrial DNA (mtDNA).

progressive external ophthalmoplegia (adPEO). Alper's syndrome, Pearson's marrow-pancreas syndrome,[29] and Navajo neuropathy are all proven or suspected primary mitochondrial hepatopathies, although there are even less well-described secondary mitochondrial hepatopathies in which mitochondrial dysfunction is due to alcohol abuse, drugs, or other hepatotoxins. Mitochondrial defects are now also associated with predispositions to two types of inherited neoplasia syndromes.[30] There is growing evidence that mitochondrial dysfunction plays a pivotal, if not necessarily etiologic, role in renal disease, adult-onset diabetes, and perhaps a wide variety of cardiomyopathies. The most frequent renal symptom is proximal tubular dysfunction, usually as de Toni-Debré-Fanconi syndrome, and, less often, renal tubular acidosis, Bartter's syndrome, chronic tubulointerstitial nephritis, or nephrotic syndrome.[31]

Examination of mitochondrial respiration in the skeletal muscle of patients with occlusive peripheral arterial disease suggests that mitochondrial respiratory activity is abnormal. Impaired bioenergetics may be a pathophysiologic component of this group of disorders.[32] Similarly, an increase in oxidative stress is now believed to contribute to the pathology of vascular disease in stroke, hypertension, and diabetes.[33] A 40% reduction in oxidative phosphorylation as assessed in vivo by magnetic resonance spectroscopy suggests that age-associated decline in mitochondrial function contributes to the reduced insulin-stimulated muscle glucose metabolism that characterizes insulin resistance in the elderly.[34] This insulin resistance appears to reflect an inherited defect of fatty acid metabolism.[35]

Acquired Mitochondrial Disorders— Acute Onset

Cardiac mitochondria are obviously essential to myocardial energy production and ionic homeostasis, but they also control myocardial cell viability. Most drugs used to treat myocardial ischemia may exert their cardioprotective effects via their actions on cardiac mitochondrial function.[36] Accumulating evidence also suggests that ROS play an important role in the development and progression of heart failure, regardless of the etiology.[37] Under pathophysiologic conditions, ROS have the potential to cause cellular damage and dysfunction. Recent experimental studies have suggested a possible causal role for increased ROS in the development of contractile dysfunction after myocardial infarction.[38] Whether the effects of increasing myocardial ROS are beneficial or harmful will depend on site, source, and amount of ROS produced and on the overall metabolic status of the myocyte. In addition to direct effects on cellular, enzymatic, and protein function, ROS have been implicated in the development of agonist-induced cardiac hypertrophy, cardiomyocyte apoptosis, and the subsequent remodeling of the failing myocardium. These alterations in phenotype are driven by metabolically sensitive gene expression, and in this way ROS may act as potent intracellular second messengers.

Another example of an acquired mitochondrial disorder of acute onset is overwhelming infection. Sepsis, the systemic inflammatory response syndrome (SIRS), and multiple organ dysfunction syndrome (MODS) are the leading causes of morbidity and mortality in critically ill surgical patients. Despite improvements in monitoring and therapy, as well as advances in our understanding of the pathophysiology of sepsis, mortality rates remain between 40% and 60%.[39] Pulmonary impairment manifests early as acute lung injury and acute respiratory distress syndrome (ARDS). Acute-onset cardiovascular, hepatic, and renal dysfunction are common, and most organs develop multiple abnormalities in their metabolic pathways and enzyme systems. Some studies have demonstrated decreased ATP levels during prolonged sepsis, suggesting that impaired bioenergetics may play a role in diffuse cellular and organ dysfunction under these circumstances.[40] However, other investigators have demonstrated normal ATP levels in various tissues during sepsis, although this does not necessarily imply normal mitochondrial bioenergetics because cells and organ systems are capable of reducing their energy requirements during sepsis. Therefore, review of the sepsis literature with regard to bioenergetics can be confusing.

A potentially unifying concept regarding the role of mitochondria in sepsis is that of "cytopathic hypoxia," the inability of cells to use molecular oxygen to produce ATP.[41] In effect, pathologically impaired bioenergetic capacity would be masked by decreased ATP demand due to downregulation. Cytopathic hypoxia may reflect altered enzyme function because of inhibition of any or all of the five complexes of the electron transport chain. It may also be caused by abnormalities in genetic transcription or translation or by changes in electron chain enzyme kinetics. Messenger RNA (mRNA) synthesis could be disrupted by abnormalities of either nuclear or mitochondrial transcription, since the subunits of the five respiratory chain enzymes arise from both nDNA and mtDNA. Errors in translation, the process of protein synthesis from mRNA, could also result in decreased electron chain function. Finally, the kinetic activity of each enzyme is dependent on pH and temperature. Therefore, sepsis-related abnormalities in pH, temperature, or the presence of inhibitors or conformational changes in enzyme structure could disrupt oxidative metabolism and explain the appearance of cytopathic hypoxia during sepsis.[42]

There are, in fact, clinical data to support the concept of cytopathic hypoxia in sepsis. Cytochrome oxidase subunit I mRNA and protein levels are decreased in the heart and in macrophages in both sepsis and sepsis-related disorders.[43] In addition, decreased cardiac cytochrome oxidase subunit IV and complex II protein levels have been demonstrated, as well as impaired function of each of the enzymes of the electron transport chain.[44] Myocardial cytochrome oxidase is reversibly inhibited early in sepsis but appears to become irreversibly inhibited during the later phase of sepsis.[45] Possible causes of mitochondrial enzyme inhibition during sepsis include nitric oxide (NO), peroxynitrite, ROS, and carbon monoxide. NO is produced by the enzyme nitric oxide synthase and is a reversible inhibitor of complex IV.[46] Peroxynitrite, a reactive nitrogen species, is formed when NO reacts with ROS and it inhibits complex I, II, and V and irreversibly inhibits cytochrome oxidase.[47] ROS cause lipid peroxidation, damaging membranes and mtDNA and irreversibly inhibiting complex IV.[48] Carbon monoxide, produced when heme is broken down by heme oxygenase, is an irreversible inhibitor of cytochrome oxidase. In fact, all of these potential inhibitors are produced in various tissues during sepsis and may contribute to sepsis-associated mitochondrial dysfunction.

Acquired Mitochondrial Disorders—Gradual Onset

Within the past two decades, loss of mitochondrial bioenergetic capacity has become a highly plausible and intriguing explanation for the ubiquitous and insidious deterioration of organ system functional reserve that characterizes normal human aging.[1] Because it is a universal phenomenon, the declining bioenergetics that characterize the middle to late adult years should be viewed as a physiologic process rather than an age-related disease. Oxidative stress, in general terms, describes the progressive accumulation of ROS within or around mitochondria and implies disruption of the equilibrium among the mediators of oxidative metabolism and mitochondrial integrity. Mitochondrial DNA is thought to be exposed to progressively increasing levels of ROS throughout adulthood, and it becomes increasingly vulnerable to oxidative damage and mutation during these years of exposure, as scavenging and repair mechanisms become less effective.[49] At higher "oxidative stress" levels, free radicals such as superoxide are also believed capable of damaging or destroying membranes and other cellular and organelle microarchitecture directly. This may lead to a decline in bioenergetic capacity, as well as impaired synthesis of protective enzymes such as superoxide dismutase that scavenge ROS from the cytosol. In effect, cellular aging may be a "vicious cycle" of progressive bioenergetic failure in the mitochondria and rising levels of ROS (Fig. 14-3).

Currently, therefore, biogerontologists have focused on the role of long-term oxidative stress[50] as a cause of the increasing damage to mitochondrial DNA and intracellular protein[51] that is believed to explain the decline in

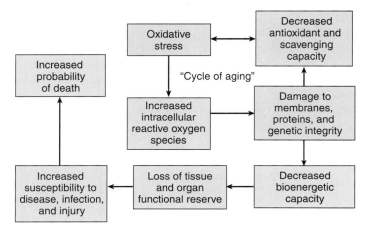

FIGURE 14–3 Schematic representation of the mitochondrial "cycle of aging" and the link between bioenergetics and the increased risk of perioperative morbidity and mortality in a geriatric population.

functional reserve that characterizes aging mammalian tissues.[52] There is a growing body of experimental and observational data to support the concept that aging is, in effect, a complex expression of chronic oxygen toxicity. More than two dozen mutations of mtDNA have been observed in the somatic tissues of aged human individuals. Although these mutations are present at relatively low levels, they accumulate exponentially with increasing age in skeletal muscle, cardiac muscle, and other human tissues as normal mtDNA declines.[53] Accelerated aging syndromes such as Down, Werner's, and the Hutchinson-Gilford syndromes are characterized not only by shortened life span but also by symptoms and disorders associated with increased oxidative stress.[54]

Because ROS are ephemeral and present in minute quantities, they have yet to be measured within organelles directly. Therefore, it may be premature to state that they are the primary etiologic factor in processes of aging. Nevertheless, if years of vigorous aerobic metabolism and ROS production inevitably lead to progressive failure of a genetically predetermined capacity of human cells to scavenge free radicals and to clear the random damage to mtDNA caused by ROS, this concept is extremely attractive because it is compatible with both stochastic (random "wear and tear") and nonstochastic ("programmed") theories of aging.

Apoptosis and Death

Apoptosis, programmed cell death, and the related concept of mitochondrial self-destruction ("mitoptosis") may be the physiologic links between the progressive decline in organ system functional reserve inevitably associated with mammalian aging and the equally inevitable onset of death. As currently envisioned, rising levels of

oxidative stress eventually outstrip intrinsic mechanisms for scavenging ROS and for repairing ROS-induced damage to organelles, proteins, and nucleotides. As the stress levels rise, the mitochondrion undergoes an increase in outer membrane permeability that leads to release of "pro-apoptotic" substances. At low intracellular concentrations, NO appears to inhibit or suppress apoptosis. At higher levels, however, ROS and NO may actually function as "death messengers" in the presence of elevated intracellular or intramitochondrial calcium.

Many pro-apoptotic molecules act to increase mitochondrial membrane permeability and release the soluble proteins from the mitochondrial intermembrane space that can precipitate rapid cell destruction. Leakage of cytochrome c from mitochondria, for example, not only rapidly degrades the bioenergetic capacity of the cell by removing a key component of the respiratory chain but also appears to trigger the release of caspases, which are cysteine-containing proteases. Caspases, in turn, activate nucleases, enzymes that digest nDNA, the final step of "cell suicide." Therefore, despite their fundamental and life-long value as the energy sources within each cell, once the process of apoptosis has been activated, mitochondria are rapidly converted into what have been called "killer organelles."[55]

There may be other pathways for apoptosis that do not require caspase activation, primarily via apoptosis-inducing factor (AIF), a flavoprotein normally sequestered in the intermembrane region of the mitochondrion. AIF normally stabilizes mitochondrial membrane permeability, but once released into the cytosol, it can damage both nuclear and mitochondrial DNA. In addition, there is evidence that, under conditions of extreme oxidative stress, ROS can directly trigger an apoptotic response independent of both the cytochrome-caspase mechanism and the pathway utilized by AIF. Cytokines such as HSP help to protect cellular integrity during sepsis[56] and can be induced by ischemic or hypoxic preconditioning. HSP appears to interfere specifically with the AIF-mediated apoptotic pathway and may have great therapeutic potential for cardiac protection and neuroprotection.[57]

As the complexity of mitochondrial function and apoptosis unfolds, it has become clear that understanding this process may be essential, not only to understand aging and death, but also to understand mechanisms of both inherited and acquired disease. Carcinogenesis may reflect an unbalancing of the dynamic equilibrium between pro-apoptotic and anti-apoptotic forces. Propagation of viruses probably requires suppression of apoptosis, and it is unlikely that cellular development and tissue specialization during embryogenesis could occur without short-term suppression of apoptosis. Because caspases are involved in most apoptotic processes, understanding the source and mechanism of endogenous and exogenous caspase inhibitors may also be key to learning about, and eventually altering, these events.

PREOPERATIVE EVALUATION

Owing to the heteroplasmy of mitochondria in tissues, as discussed earlier, patients with mitochondrial disorders may present with a wide variety of symptoms, many of them extremely vague or subtle, even if a defined mtDNA mutation is involved. Mitochondrial cytopathy should be included in the differential diagnosis whenever clinical signs and symptoms include persistent muscle pain associated with weakness or fatigue,[58] or if there is diffuse multisystem involvement that does not clearly fit an established pattern of conventional disease.[59] Subclinical hepatic and renal involvement is common, but the diagnosis of a mitochondrial-based respiratory chain deficiency is rarely entertained even when renal symptoms are present, unless they are associated with evidence of skeletal muscle weakness or encephalopathy.

If a mitochondrial myopathy is suspected, diagnostic investigations should include screening for increased lactate/pyruvate and ketone body molar ratios and measurement of serum and cerebrospinal fluid lactate. With a very high index of suspicion, skeletal muscle biopsy may confirm the presence of characteristic "ragged-red fibers," which reflect accumulations of defective mitochondria, excess glycogen granules, and cytochrome c oxidase–deficient cells. The biopsy can also provide material for genetic analysis and subsequent genetic counseling. Because mitochondrial cytopathies involve enzymatic defects in ATP production that lead to organ dysfunction, common sequelae are lactic acidosis and abnormalities in glucose metabolism. For pediatric patients, initial investigation to confirm the diagnosis involves blood and urine testing, although normal lactate and glucose do not necessarily rule out the presence of mitochondrial disease. Table 14-4 lists the most common laboratory tests used to detect mitochondrial disorders.[60] As in adults, confirmatory diagnostic studies include skin or muscle biopsies for microscopic evaluation and mtDNA analysis.

To define the extent to which declining mitochondrial energy production has produced clinical compromise in patients with adult-onset mitochondrial disease, extensive preoperative assessment of organ system functional reserve is more useful rather than traditional preoperative tests used to screen for the presence of specific disease entities. Unique concerns regarding comorbidity include decreased anesthetic requirement and susceptibility to prolonged drug-induced nervous system depression because of impaired neuronal bioenergetics, even when overt encephalopathy has not yet developed, as well as intrinsic skeletal muscle hypotonia and cardiomyopathy with increased risk of sudden death from conduction abnormalities. Skeletal muscle weakness may produce a general decrease in aerobic work capacity that may compromise postoperative ventilation following upper abdominal or thoracic surgery,[61] and subclinical erosion of hepatorenal reserve may further predispose these patients to prolonged drug effects and delayed recovery from anesthesia, muscle relaxants, and opioids.

Many of these clinical concerns may be exacerbated by acute or sustained stress (Table 14-5). Many neurologists recommend a diet and nutritional supplements rich in antioxidants, as well as treatment with vitamins and various cofactors such as coenzyme Q (Table 14-6), although there are little data supporting this approach as a mandatory preoperative regimen. Therefore, optimization of the patient's physical status and treatment of the stigmata of acquired or adult-onset mitochondrial diseases remains supportive. Preoperative therapy should focus on serious overt clinical manifestations such as cardiac dysrhythmias,[62] muscle weakness, and postural imbalance and endocrinopathy.

TABLE 14–4 Initial Laboratory Investigation for Suspected Mitochondrial Disorders

Glucose
Electrolytes with anion gap
Complete blood cell count
Blood urea nitrogen
Lactate, pyruvate, and lactate/pyruvate ratio
Ammonia
Creatinine kinase
Biotinidase level
Blood and urine amino acids
Blood and urine organic acids
Acyl carnitines
Skin and muscle biopsies

TABLE 14–5 Questions to Ask Primary Physician, Neurologist, or Metabolic Specialist

Any existing comorbidities involving:
Central nervous system?
Heart?
Lungs?
Skeletal muscle?
Hepatorenal systems?
Any abnormalities with glucose regulation?
Any recent illnesses, infection, or sustained stress?
Any previous adverse drug reactions and allergies?
Any prior anesthetic exposure or complications? Obtain anesthesia records.

TABLE 14–6 Possible Concurrent Therapy for Patients with Mitochondrial Disorders
Coenzyme Q,
L-Carnitine
Riboflavin (vitamin B_2)
Acetyl-L-carnitine
Thiamine (vitamin B_1)
Nicotinamide (vitamin B_3)
Vitamin E
Vitamin C
Lipoic acid
Selenium
Beta-carotene
Biotin
Folic acid
Calcium, magnesium, phosphorous
Vitamin K
Succinate
Creatine
Citrates
Prednisone

TABLE 14–7 Intraoperative Management
Consider intensive care unit for postoperative ventilation or monitoring.
Use glucose-containing intravenous fluid.
Maintain normal temperature and pH.
Avoid natural airway or prolonged spontaneous ventilation during anesthesia.
Consider adding arterial cannula for arterial blood gases, glucose, and lactate to routine monitors.
Have dantrolene or malignant hyperthermia cart available.
Consider total intravenous anesthetic with avoidance of malignant hyperthermia "triggers."

ANESTHETIC MANAGEMENT

Surgical patients with mitochondrial disease should be considered at significant increased risk of adverse outcome compared with the general population. Perioperative adverse events in these patients include stroke, deterioration of neurologic status, coma, seizures, respiratory failure, arrhythmias, and death. Therefore, informing the patients and their families of these risks is an important part of the preoperative evaluation. Although patients with inherited mitochondrial encephalomyopathies have been exposed to many different general anesthetic regimens without apparent adverse consequences,[63,64] it still remains unclear whether there is a "safe" or "best" anesthetic for these patients. There is continuing controversy regarding whether the anesthetic plan should, or should not, include neuromuscular blockade, especially in children (Table 14-7).

Susceptibility to malignant hyperthermia (MH) or myasthenia-like sensitivity to neuromuscular blockade are issues typically considered for patients with more familiar muscular dystrophies and neurogenic myopathies, but these concerns are probably not crucial for most forms of inherited mitochondrial encephalopathy and myopathy.[65,66] Nevertheless, there is one report suggesting increased sensitivity to nondepolarizing blockade[67] and many discussions of anesthesia for mitochondrial disease that nevertheless recommend MH precautions.[68] Only the

very rare mitochondrial myopathies with "multicore" or "minicore" histology may actually be associated with MH.[69] Avoidance of depolarizing muscle relaxants may further reduce the possibility of MH, but the residual effects of nondepolarizing agents in patients with compromised hepatorenal function may exacerbate intrinsic muscle weakness. Therefore, anesthetic techniques requiring spontaneous intraoperative ventilation that offer an opportunity for airway obstruction intraoperatively should probably be avoided. Muscle weakness may also increase the risk of ventilatory failure postoperatively. Endotracheal intubation with positive-pressure ventilation will prevent intraoperative ventilatory failure, but the anesthesiologist must decide if the patient should be extubated immediately after surgery or remain intubated and receive prolonged recovery in an intensive care unit. "Late-onset mitochondrial myopathy" may be age-related and yet still reflect primary mitochondrial dysfunction owing to the clonal expansion of different mtDNA deletions in individual fiber segments. Although the origin of these mtDNA mutations is not clear, the phenotype seems to represent an exaggerated form of what is observed in the normal aging process.[70]

Patients with mitochondrial cytopathy are usually instructed not to fast for long durations and to eat small frequent meals, a regimen that can be problematic in the setting of perioperative NPO guidelines. To avoid metabolic crisis in children, an intravenous infusion of glucose should be initiated during the period of preoperative fasting. Choice of intravenous fluids may also be important intraoperatively, with most anesthesiologists choosing to avoid Ringer's solution because of the lactate load. Monitoring and controlling normal blood glucose, body temperature, and acid-base values is crucial intraoperatively and postoperatively, and as with any anesthetic, an electrocardiogram should be monitored along with blood pressure, pulse-oximetry, temperature, and exhaled gas concentrations. In addition, arterial catheterization should be considered to facilitate frequent sampling for blood glucose, arterial blood gases, and serum lactate levels.

There are few reports that describe the anesthetic treatment of adult-onset or acquired mitochondrial encephalomyopathy,[71] and only one, for example, dealing with NARP syndrome.[72] Clinical reports suggest that patients with other mitochondrial disorders "do well" with regional anesthetics, despite the fact that these agents, like those used for general anesthesia, depress mitochondrial bioenergetics. In addition, there is reason to suspect that some of the effects of anesthetics on mitochondria may be beneficial in the event of tissue hypoxia or ischemia. It is now clear that the phenomenon of anesthetic preconditioning, in which prior exposure to volatile anesthetics reduces tissue injury after an ischemic or hypoxic episode, is mediated through their effects on the mitochondria, either directly or via several possible signaling pathways.[73]

The nervous system may play a particularly prominent role in our understanding of the consequences of altered mitochondrial function, whether inherited or acquired. Consciousness is the most complex manifestation of nervous system function. Because cortical neurons and deeper nervous system tissues with high rates of neurotransmitter synthesis have very high rates of oxygen utilization, depression of mitochondrial bioenergetics or organelle injury due to oxidative stress usually compromises nervous system function before other tissues appear to be affected. Therefore, resistance to loss of consciousness, one possible definition of anesthetic requirement, could provide the clinician with a metric for assessing remaining nervous system functional reserve. Recent preliminary data, in fact, suggest that extreme sensitivity to anesthetics may reflect greatly reduced reserve and a high risk of susceptibility to neurodegenerative disorders, postoperative cognitive decline, and even long-term mortality in elderly patients.[74] Increasing age and deeper levels of anesthesia are also independently but significantly predictive of increased mortality within 1 year of surgery.[75]

Basic genetic manipulation in subprimates confirms a direct link between mitochondrial genetics and anesthetic requirement.[76] Children with inherited mitochondrial disorders have been shown to have significantly increased sensitivity to volatile anesthetics.[77] In addition, a general relationship between declining anesthetic requirement and increasing age has been unequivocally established for adults in the general population (Fig. 14-4).

CONCLUSION

Mitochondrial dysfunction may be fundamental to a very broad spectrum of human disease, both inherited and acquired, and perhaps even to aging and death itself. Full understanding of the status of mitochondrial bioenergetics

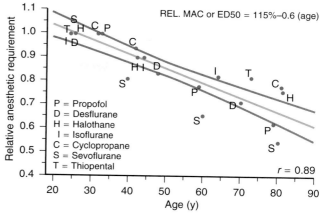

FIGURE 14–4 The progressive decline in relative anesthetic requirement (MAC or ED50) that occurs during adulthood is a consistent characteristic reported for a wide variety of inhaled and injectable anesthetic agents. This phenomenon, shown here as a graphic representation of data from nonsedated human subjects, probably reflects a generalized process within the central nervous system that may involve declining mitochondrial bioenergetics.

may eventually play a life-critical role in caring for patients with mitochondrial disorders, in anticipating the responses of children and adults to anesthetics, and in avoiding perioperative ischemic or hypoxic injuries. At the present time, however, the basic principles of anesthetic management of children and adults with genetically transmitted mitochondrial disorders include awareness of the decreased bioenergetic capacity of major organ systems and special attention to the clinical implications of generalized weakness and myopathy, cardiac arrhythmias and dysfunction, sensorineural compromise, and impaired hepatorenal function.

References

1. Linnane AW, Marzuki S, Ozawa T, et al: Mitochondrial DNA mutations as an important contributor to ageing and degenerative diseases. Lancet 1989;1:642-651.
2. Hattori K, Tanaka M, Sugiyama S, et al: Age-dependent decrease in mitochondrial DNA in the human heart: Possible contributory factor to presbycardia. Am Heart J 1991;121:1735-1742.
3. Wallace DC: Mitochondrial diseases in man and mouse. Science 1999;283:1482-1488.
4. DiMauro S, Schon EA: Mitochondrial respiratory-chain diseases. N Engl J Med 2003;348:2656-2668.
5. Wei YH: Mitochondrial DNA mutations and oxidative damage in aging and diseases: An emerging paradigm of gerontology and medicine. Proc Natl Sci Council (China)—Part B 1998;22:55-67
6. Schmiedel J, Jackson S, Schafer J, et al: Mitochondrial cytopathies. J Neurol 2003;250:267-277.
7. Schwartz M, Vissing J: New patterns of inheritance in mitochondrial disease. Biochem Biophys Res Comm 2003;310:247-251.
8. Kagaway, Hamamoto T, Endo H, et al: Genes of human ATP synthase: Their roles in physiology and aging. Biosci Report 1997;17:115-146.
9. Cohen PJ: Effect of anesthetics on mitochondrial function. Anesthesiology 1973;39:153-164.
10. Nahrwold ML, Clark CR, Cohen PJ: Is depression of mitochondrial respiration a predictor of in-vivo anesthetic activity? Anesthesiology 1974;40:566-570.

11. Lee SL, Alto LE, Dhalla NS: Subcellular effects of some anesthetic agents on rat myocardium. Can J Physiol Pharmacol 1979;57:65-71.

12. Hanley PJ, Ray J, Brandt U, et al: Halothane, isoflurane and sevoflurane inhibit NADH:ubiquinone oxidoreductase (complex I) of cardiac mitochondria. J Physiol 2002;544:687-693.

13. Nahrwold ML, Cohen PJ: Additive effect of nitrous oxide and halothane on mitochondrial function. Anesthesiology 1973;39:534-536.

14. Garlid KD, Nakashima RA: Studies on the mechanism of uncoupling by amine local anesthetics: Evidence for mitochondrial proton transport mediated by lipophilic ion pairs. J Biol Chem 1983;258:7974-7980.

15. Tarba C, Cracium C: A comparative study of the effects of procaine, lidocaine, tetracaine, and dibucaine on the functions and ultrastructure of isolated rat liver mitochondria. Biochem Biophys Acta 1990;1019:19-28.

16. Stevanato R, Momo F, Marian M, et al: Effects of nitrosopropofol on mitochondrial energy-converting system. Biochem Pharmacol 2002;64:1133-1138.

17. Schenkman KA, Yan S: Propofol impairment of mitochondrial respiration in isolated perfused guinea pig hearts determined by reflectance spectroscopy. Crit Care Med 2000;28:172-177.

18. Rigoulet M, Devin A, Averet N, et al: Mechanisms of inhibition and uncoupling of respiration in isolated rat liver mitochondria by the general anesthetic 2,6-diisopropylphenol. Eur J Biochem 1996;241:280-285.

19. Raeburn CD, Cleveland JC Jr, Zimmerman MA, et al: Organ preconditioning. Arch Surg 2001;136:1263-1266.

20. Treem WR, Sokol RJ: Disorders of the mitochondria. Semin Liver Dis 1998;18:237-253.

21. Suomalainen A, Kaukonen J: Diseases caused by nuclear genes affecting mtDNA stability. Am J Med Genet 2001;106:53-61.

22. Tatuch Y, Robinson BH: The mitochondrial DNA mutation at 8993 associated with NARP slows the rate of ATP synthesis in isolated lymphoblast mitochondria. Biochem Biophys Res Comm 1993;192:124-128.

23. Minamoto H, Kawabata K, Okuda B, et al: Mitochondrial encephalomyopathy with elderly onset of stroke-like episodes. Intern Med 1996;35:991-995.

24. Wallace DC, Lott MT, Shoffner JM, et al: Diseases resulting from mitochondrial DNA point mutations. J Inherit Metabol Dis 1992;15:472-479.

25. Beal MF: Mitochondria, oxidative damage, and inflammation in Parkinson's disease. Ann NY Acad Sci 2003;991:120-131.

26. Jordan J, Cena V, Prehn JH: Mitochondrial control of neuron death and its role in neurodegenerative disorders. J Physiol Biochem 2003;59:129-141.

27. Kalman B, Leist TP: A mitochondrial component of neurodegeneration in multiple sclerosis. Neurol Mol Med 2003;3:147-158.

28. Stolzing A, Grune T: The proteasome and its function in the ageing process. Clin Exp Dermatol 2001;26:566-572.

29. Gillis LA, Sokol RJ: Gastrointestinal manifestations of mitochondrial disease. Gastroenterol Clin North Am 2003;32:789-817.

30. Eng C, Kiuru M, Fernandez MJ, et al: A role for mitochondrial enzymes in inherited neoplasia and beyond. Nat Rev Cancer 2003;3:193-202.

31. Rotig A: Renal disease and mitochondrial genetics. J Nephrol 2003;16:286-292.

32. Pipinos II, Sharov VG, Shepard AD, et al: Abnormal mitochondrial respiration in skeletal muscle in patients with peripheral arterial disease. J Vasc Surg 2003;38:827-832.

33. Yorek MA: The role of oxidative stress in diabetic vascular and neural disease. Free Radical Res 2003;37:471-480.

34. Petersen KF, Befroy D, Dufour S, et al: Mitochondrial dysfunction in the elderly: Possible role in insulin resistance. Science 2003;300:1140-1142.

35. Petersen KF, Dufour S, Befroy D, et al: Impaired mitochondrial activity in the insulin-resistant offspring of patients with type 2 diabetes. N Engl J Med 2004;350:664-671.

36. Monteiro P, Oliveira PJ, Concalves L, et al: Pharmacological modulation of mitochondrial function during ischemia and reperfusion. Rev Port Cardiol 2003;22:407-429.

37. Corral-Debrinski M, Stepien G, Shoffner M, et al: Hypoxemia is associated with mitochondrial DNA damage and gene induction: Implications for cardiac disease. JAMA 1991;266:1812-1816.

38. Byrne JA, Grieve DJ, Cave AC, et al: Oxidative stress and heart failure. Arch Mal Coeur Vaisseaux 2003;96:214-221.

39. Davies MG, Hagen PO: Systemic inflammatory response syndrome. Br J Surg 1997;84:920-935.

40. Budinger GR, Duranteau J, Chandel NS, et al: Hibernation during hypoxia in cardiomyocytes: Role of mitochondria as the O_2 sensor. J Biol Chem 1998;273:3320-3326.

41. Fink MP: Bench-to-bedside review: Cytopathic hypoxia. Crit Care 2002;6:491-499.

42. Bruemmer-Smith S, Stuber F, Schroeder S: Protective functions of intracellular heat-shock protein (HSP) 70-expression in patients with severe sepsis. Intens Care Med 2001;27:1835-1841.

43. Watts JA, Kline JA, Thornton LR, et al: Metabolic dysfunction and depletion of mitochondria in hearts of septic rats. J Mol Cell Cardiol 2004;36:141-150.

44. Gellerich FN, Trumbeckaite S, Hertel K, et al: Impaired energy metabolism in hearts of septic baboons: Diminished activities of complex I and complex II of the mitochondrial respiratory chain. Shock 1999;11:336-341.

45. Levy RJ, Vijayasarathy C, Raj NR, et al: Competitive and noncompetitive inhibition of myocardial cytochrome C oxidase in sepsis. Shock 2004;21:110-114.

46. Brunori M, Giuffre A, Sarti P, et al: Nitric oxide and cellular respiration. Cell Mol Life Sci 1999;56:549-557.

47. Sharpe MA, Cooper CE: Interaction of peroxynitrite with mitochondrial cytochrome oxidase: Catalytic production of nitric oxide and irreversible inhibition of enzyme activity. J Biol Chem 1998;273:30961-30972.

48. Luft R: The development of mitochondrial medicine. Proc Natl Acad Sci U S A 1994;91:8731-8738.

49. Barja G, Herrero A: Oxidative damage to mitochondrial DNA is inversely related to maximum life span in the heart and brain of mammals. FASEB J 2000;14:312-318.

50. Sohal RS, Weindruch R: Oxidative stress, caloric restriction, and aging. Science 1996;273:59-63.

51. Stadtman ER: Protein oxidation in aging and age-related diseases. Ann NY Acad Sci 2001;928:22-38.

52. Ozawa T: Genetic and functional changes in mitochondria associated with aging. Physiol Rev 1997;77:425-464.

53. Hattori K, Tanaka M, Sugiyama S, et al: Age-dependent decrease in mitochondrial DNA in the human heart: Possible contributory factor to presbycardia. Am Heart J 1991;121:1735-1742.

54. Knight JA: The biochemistry of aging. Adv Clin Chem 2000;35:1-62.

55. Ravagnan L, Roumier T, Kroemer G: Mitochondria, the killer organelles and their weapons. J Cell Physiol 2002;192:131-137.

56. Chen HW, Hsu C, Lu TS, et al: Heat shock pretreatment prevents cardiac mitochondrial dysfunction during sepsis. Shock 2003;20:274-279.

57. Sheth K, De A, Nolan B, et al: Heat shock protein 27 inhibits apoptosis in human neutrophils. J Surg Res 2001;99:129-133.

58. Griggs RC, Karpati G: Muscle pain, fatigue, and mitochondriopathies. N Engl J Med 1999;341:1077-1078.

59. Walker UA, Collins S, Byrne E: Respiratory chain encephalomyopathies: A diagnostic classification. Eur Neurol 1996;36:260-267.

60. Cohen BH: Mitochondrial cytopathies: A primer. Mitochondrial cytopathies 2000. [online publication, June 2000]. Available at http://www.umdf.org/pdf/MITOCYTO.PDF

61. Grattan-Smith PJ, Shield LK, Hopkins IJ, et al: Acute respiratory failure precipitated by general anesthesia in Leigh's syndrome. J Child Neurol 1990;5:137-141.

62. Lauwers MR, Van Lersberghe C, Camu F: Inhalation anaesthesia and the Kearns-Sayre syndrome. Anaesthesia 1994;49:876-878.

63. Maslow A, Lisbon A: Anesthetic considerations in patients with mitochondrial dysfunction. Anesth Analg 1993;76:884-886.

64. Matsuno S. Hashimoto H. Matsuki A: Neuroleptanesthesia for a patient with mitochondrial encephalomyopathy. Masui 1994; 43:1038-1040. In Japanese.

65. Wiesel S, Bevan JC, Samuel J, et al: Vecuronium neuromuscular blockade in a child with mitochondrial myopathy. Anesth Analg 1991;72:696-699.

66. D'Ambra MN, Dedrick D, Savarese JJ: Kearns-Sayre syndrome and pancuronium-succiny1choline induced neuromuscular blockade. Anesthesiology 1979;51:343-345.

67. Naguib M, el Dawlatly AA, Ashour M, et al: Sensitivity to mivacurium in a patient with mitochondrial myopathy. Anesthesiology 1996;84:1506-1509.

68. Itaya K, Takahata O, Mamiya K, et al: Anesthetic management of two patients with mitochondrial encephalopathy, lactic acidosis and stroke-like episodes (MELAS). Masui 1995;44:710-712. In Japanese.

69. Figarella-Branger D, Kozak-Ribbens G, Rodet L, et al: Pathological findings in 165 patients explored for malignant hyperthermia susceptibility. Neuromusc Dis 1993;3:553-556.

70. Johnston W, Karpati G, Carpenter S, et al: Late-onset mitochondrial myopathy. Ann Neurol 1995;37:16-23.

71. Sabate S, Ferrandiz M, Paniagua P, et al: Anesthesia in Kearns-Sayre syndrome mitochondrial myopathy. Rev Esp Anestesiol Reanimacion 1996;43:255-257. In Spanish.

72. Ciccotelli KK, Prak EL, Muravchick S: An adult with inherited mitochondrial encephalomyopathy: Report of a case. Anesthesiology 1997;87:1240-1242.

73. Tanaka K, Ludwig LM, Kersten JR, et al: Mechanisms of cardioprotection by volatile anesthetics. Anesthesiology 2004;100:707-721.

74. Lennmarken C, Lindholm, M-L, Greenwald S, et al: Confirmation that low intraoperative BIS™ levels predict increased risk of post-operative mortality. Anesthesiology 2003;99:A303.

75. Weldon BC, Mahla ME, van der Aa MT, et al: Advancing age and deeper intraoperative anesthetic levels are associated with higher first year death rates. Anesthesiology 2002;96:A1097.

76. Kayser EB, Morgan PG, Sedensky MM: GAS-1: A mitochondrial protein controls sensitivity to volatile anesthetics in the nematode *Caenorhabditis elegans*. Anesthesiology 1999;90:545-554.

77. Morgan PG, Hoppel CL, Sedensky MM: Mitochondrial defects and anesthetic sensitivity. Anesthesiology 2002;96:1268-1270.

15 Behavioral and Psychiatric Disorders

ALAN D. KAYE, MD, PhD, DABPM, JASON M. HOOVER, MD,
ROBERT A. ERTNER, MD, and PATRICIA B. SUTKER, PhD

Mental illnesses, or mental, personality, and cognitive disorders that interfere seriously with life activities and abilities to function, constitute a pervasive and prevalent health problem among varied American population subsets, including the young and the elderly. The presence of mental disorders, associated symptoms, possible concomitant pathology, and prescribed medications are of significance to all health care providers and not simply those in the field of mental health. Against the backdrop of rates and patterns of ill health and disability, the burden of mental disorders on health care utilization and effectiveness has become a topic of worldwide interest.[1] Beyond concerns about treatment adequacy for mental illnesses globally and in the United States there are considerations regarding management of the seriously mentally ill in emergency care and inpatient treatment situations, general medicine, family practice and pain clinics, and the surgical theater.[2] Important to anesthesiologists managing patient care is knowledge about patient mental and physical illnesses; histories of alcohol, drug, and tobacco use; the abuse and use of prescription medications, over-the-counter drugs, and herbal products; previous physical and mental traumas; and potential areas of cognitive impairment or compromise before, during, and after surgical procedures and in other treatment circumstances. It is important that anesthesiologists recognize the factors involved in determining the presence of the true mental disorder, because certain medical conditions can mimic psychiatric disturbances (Table 15-1).[3]

The presence of mental disorders and the associated use of psychotropic medications, including antidepressants, anxiolytic drugs, major tranquilizers, and anticonvulsants and mood stabilizers introduce neurochemical, behavioral, cognitive, and emotional factors that increase the complexity of medical or surgical tasks. For example, patients with mental disorders may not communicate well about their diseases, symptoms, medications, and history; may present with difficult behaviors; and often bring a background of polypharmacy that requires unraveling.[4] The use of psychotropic medications has increased over each decade, with psychiatrists and family practice physicians prescribing tranquilizers, neuroleptics, and antidepressants, even among youth.[5-7] In the case of depression alone complexities have been described in prescribing medications and understanding side effect and adverse effect profiles, as well as drug interactions with other

TABLE 15–1   Medical Conditions That Can Mimic Psychiatric Disorders

Endocrine Abnormalities
Hypothyroidism
Cushing's syndrome

Alcohol and Drug Abuse
Neurologic Disorders
Seizure
Head trauma
Demyelinating disease
Central nervous system tumors
Encephalitis

Toxic and Metabolic Disorders
Vitamin B_{12} or folate deficiency
Anticholinergic toxicity
Drug-induced toxicity

Collagen Vascular Diseases

Adapted from Derrer SA, Helfaer MA: Evaluation of the psychiatric patient. In Rogers MC, Tinker JH, Covino BG, Longnecker DE (eds): Principles and Practice of Anesthesiology. St. Louis, Mosby, 1993, pp 567-574.

medications prescribed for mental and physical problems. In this chapter we review the major types of mental disorders, describe disorder epidemiology and characteristics, and outline issues and concerns that face anesthesia care providers in planning case management. Specifically, information is provided concerning appropriate perioperative management of patients with mental disorders undergoing surgical procedures requiring anesthetic intervention.

EPIDEMIOLOGY OF MENTAL DISORDERS

For more than two decades, scientists have applied detailed, structured lay interviews to diagnose mental disorders in community surveys and to determine the incidence and prevalence of serious mental illnesses. A landmark project collecting data from 1980 to 1985, called the Epidemiologic Catchment Area (ECA) study, interviewed more than 20,000 adults aged 18 years or older in five surveys, yielding data from 18,571 households and 2,290 institutionalized residents. The maximum combined sample size was 20,291 adults who were interviewed directly at wave 1, and 12 months later in wave 2, using the Diagnostic Interview Schedule and 1-month recall to determine psychiatric diagnoses.[8-10] Findings revealed that 15.7% of those surveyed suffered a mental or addictive disorder during the past month and 6.6% developed one or more new disorders after being assessed as having no previous lifetime diagnosis at wave 2, with an estimated annual mental or addictive disorder prevalence rate of 28.1%. Using application to the 1980 U.S. adult population, the

researchers estimated that 44.7 million persons were affected by one or more mental or addictive disorders and 35.1 million by a nonaddictive mental disorder in the 1-year interval. Looking at the data differently, Bourdon and colleagues determined that in any 6-month period, 19.5% of the adult population, or one in five individuals, suffer a diagnosable mental disorder.[11]

Mandated by the U.S. Congress, the National Comorbidity Study (NCS) included administration of a structured psychiatric interview to a representative sample of noninstitutionalized persons aged 15 to 54 years in the 48 contiguous states and a survey of campus-housing students. Data were collected between 1990 and 1992 in 8,089 respondents. The study purpose was to assess comorbidity of substance use disorders and non-substance psychiatric disorders using a modified version of the Composite International Diagnostic Interview.[12] Morbidity rates were found to be higher than ECA estimates, possibly owing to methodologic and illness-defining differences in study implementation. Nevertheless, results were impressive toward developing an understanding of mental disorder prevalence and comorbidity. Nearly 50% of respondents reported at least one lifetime disorder, and almost 30% at least one 12-month disorder, the most common being a major depressive episode, alcohol dependence, social phobia, and simple phobia. Morbidity was concentrated in approximately one sixth of the population who evidenced history of three or more comorbid disorders.[13] Factors of age, race, socioeconomic status, gender, and geographic region influenced prevalence trends. For example, women were found to have elevated rates of affective and anxiety disorders compared with men, who showed higher rates of substance use disorders and antisocial personality. The majority of individuals with psychiatric disorders failed to obtain professional treatment, suggesting that patients with mental disorders may not be identified readily by medical health care providers.

Calling attention to the strong association between reduced health-related quality of life, diminished productivity, and high health care utilization, Hoge and colleagues studied hospitalizations among active-duty military personnel from 1990 to 1999 and ambulatory visits from 1996 to 1999.[14] Rates of hospitalization and ambulatory visits were examined over these 10- and 4-year periods across the entire military. As many as 4,815,864 active-duty personnel were studied, with women accounting for 12%. Considering that the military represents approximately 1% of the adult working U.S. population between the ages of 18 and 45, these data have particular interest. Mental disorder diagnoses were involved in 13% of hospitalizations, accounting for nearly a fourth of inpatient bed days. In a 1-year cohort of personnel, 47% of those hospitalized for the first time for a mental disorder left military service within 6 months, a rate different from that of 12% after hospitalization for any of 15 other disease categories. More than 6% of the entire active-duty population were reported to have received outpatient treatment for a mental disorder annually in 1998 and 1999. Data showed that the most common primary diagnoses were alcohol- and substance-related, adjustment, mood, and personality disorders. Researchers concluded that mental disorders represent the most important source of military medical and occupational morbidity, underscoring that mental disorders are common, disabling, and costly to individuals and society.

CHARACTERIZATION OF MENTAL DISORDERS

Definition of mental disorders is taken from the *Diagnostic and Statistical Manual of Mental Disorders,* fourth edition (DSM-IV), in which each of the disorders is conceptualized as a clinically significant behavioral or psychological syndrome associated with present distress or disability, or perhaps with significantly increased risk of suffering death, pain, disability, or loss of freedom.[15] As such, a disorder is a manifestation of a behavioral, psychological, or biologic dysfunction. Mental disorders in individuals constitute an enormous public health problem, interfering with life activities and functions and afflicting 5.4% of the U.S. adult population each year.[2] As stated by Wang and associates, Public Law 102-321 defines serious mental illness as the presence of any DSM mental disorder, substance use disorder, or developmental disorder that leads to "substantial interference" with "one or more major life activities." In this framework, mood and anxiety disorders and nonaffective psychoses are characterized, in addition to substance abuse disorders, difficult-to-define personality disorders, and disorders affecting development and life course phenomena, such as those identified in infancy or childhood (e.g., mental retardation) and/or associated with physical trauma leading to organic brain syndrome, and cognitive disorders, such as dementia of mid to late life stages.

Other disorders of interest to the practicing clinician are mental disorders resulting from a general medical condition, somatoform disorders, and disorders of eating, sleep, impulse control, and adjustment. Attention has also been directed toward clarifying the clinical status of primary care patients with symptoms of mental distress that fall below the threshold criteria for a mental disorder. Olfson and coworkers found that in primary care patients, the morbidity of subthreshold symptoms was often explained by confounding mental, physical, or demographic factors.[16] Yet depressive symptoms and panic symptoms tended to be disabling, and patients with these symptoms were suggested to be at increased risk for development of major depression, even though they were a heterogeneous group.

GENERAL APPROACHES TO PREOPERATIVE EVALUATION OF PATIENTS WITH MENTAL DISORDERS

Regardless of the pathologic process or processes with which patients present, assessment of patients with mental disorders presents unique challenges to clinical anesthesiologists. Many of these patients will not communicate well with anesthesiologists either because they choose not to (e.g., embarrassment, hostility) or because they are unable to do so (e.g., profound psychosis, delirium, memory disturbances). It may be difficult to establish rapport with such patients even if they seem otherwise cooperative. There are also issues involving patients' abilities to consent or refuse certain medical interventions.[3] Most often, when anesthesiologists are confronted with patients, they find it easy to obtain data from medical records concerning the patients' medical history, medications being taken, and previous medical interventions. In the case of patients with mental disorders, for the just-stated reasons, it is often more difficult to obtain this information. However, only in a minority of cases will patients with mental disorders present without clinicians having access to their medical records. When patient medical records are available, clinicians must review these records carefully and be prepared to measure the information obtained from them against patient-reported history. Often, patients' records provide more accurate information than can be obtained otherwise. Likewise, physicians may trust the objective data obtained from a careful physical examination more than the history obtained.[3]

In some cases, it is possible to obtain direct consultation with primary care physicians or psychiatrists in charge of care for patients with mental disorders. If this is possible, concerns that anesthesiologists may have concerning the care of patients in the perioperative period can be addressed directly. However, despite possible interactions that may exist between caretakers, an earnest attempt to establish rapport with patients must be sought, because the potential exists to minimize emotional trauma that might present itself within the operating theater.[3] In this regard, the role of anesthesiologists as consultants cannot be overstated. In some instances, patients may present for surgery with a disease entity that mimics psychopathology but has not been diagnosed. Appropriate history-taking skills, physical examination, and laboratory tests may reveal one of these disorders. Furthermore, many substances, including both illicit drugs and legal pharmaceuticals, may produce signs and symptoms that mimic psychiatric disease. Any organic cause for symptoms must be eliminated fastidiously before subjecting patients to anesthesia, because there is potential for adverse outcomes arising from inappropriate management of such disorders.[3]

MOOD DISORDERS

Major Depression

In the *DSM-IV,* disorders of mood are classified in terms of episodes, such as depressive and manic episodes, depressive disorders including major depression and dysthymia, bipolar disorders, and mood disorders associated with general medical conditions and/or substance abuse.[15] Specifiers can be added to describe severity, other features such as postpartum onset, and course of recurrent episodes. Among the mood disorders, major depression has been studied most often and found to be a frequent and disabling psychiatric disorder in the United States. The prevalence of major depression has been shown to be 14.9% for lifetime and 8.6% for 12 months, and a predominance of women to men has been demonstrated in both lifetime and 12-month cases.[17] As many as 74% of NCS respondents with lifetime depression showed one or more disorders, with anxiety (58%) and substance abuse (38%) disorders found to be most common. The prevalence of depression in cancer patients has been found to be two to three times the rate documented in the general population, and as many as 25% of extended care facility patients may suffer from major depression.[5,18,19] Major depression appears to have increased, reaching younger age persons, yet often going undetected and undiagnosed in all age groups.

In the 2001-2002 National Comorbidity Survey Replication (NCS-R), Kessler and colleagues reported the prevalence and correlates of major depression using *DSM-IV* criteria in 9,090 household residents aged 18 years and older.[20] They calculated a prevalence of lifetime major depression of 16.2% and of 6.6% for a 12-month period, estimated to affect 32 to 35 million and 13 to 14 million adults, respectively. Among other results, risk seemed to be low until the early teens, but depressive disorders occur throughout the life cycle. Factors associated with risk were female gender, homemaker status, unemployed or disabled, never having married, lower education, and living in or near poverty levels; and major depression was highly comorbid with other mental disorders. As many as 72% of respondents with lifetime major depression met criteria for at least one other disorder, such as anxiety disorder at 59%, substance abuse disorder at 24%, and impulse-control disorder at 30%. Approximately 90% of 12-month major depression cases were classified as moderate, severe, or very severe. Depression has also been associated with physical illnesses, affecting multiple domains of functioning and well-being; and patients with depressive conditions have been shown to have poorer mental, emotional, and social functioning than even those with chronic medical conditions.[21,22] For example, depressed patients may report higher levels of fatigue and fatigue-related interferences than cancer patients.[23]

Characteristics of depressive mood disorders include feelings of sadness, hopelessness, and discouragement, but sadness may be bypassed with complaints of somatic problems, persistent anger or increased irritability, disinterest or lack of pleasure in activities, changes in appetite and sleep patterns, and altered psychomotor behaviors, such as agitation. Decreased energy, tiredness, and fatigue are common, as are feelings of worthlessness and guilt. There may be concentration problems, difficulties in decision making, thoughts of death and suicide, and varied degrees of social and work impairment. In many cases, depressed persons present with tearfulness, irritability, ruminations, anxiety, phobias, concern over physical health, pain complaints, and brooding. Major depression is usually differentiated from mood disorder due to a general medical condition, substance abuse–induced mood disorder, dementia, and adjustment disorder with depressed mood and simple bereavement. Turning to the opposite end of the spectrum, manic episodes are characterized by inflated self-esteem or grandiosity, decreased need for sleep, pressured speech, flight of ideas, distractibility, increased involvement in goal-directed activities, and psychomotor agitation. Expansiveness and unwarranted optimism coupled with poor judgment may lead to imprudent excesses, as discussed later.

Selective Serotonin Reuptake Inhibitors

Depressed patients prescribed psychotropic medications rose from 44.6% in 1987 to 79.4% in 1997, an increase attributed primarily to a class of medications unavailable in 1987, the selective serotonin reuptake inhibitors (SSRIs) (Table 15-2).[24-30] Psychopharmacologic research and discovery have altered depression treatment protocols, particularly over the past 20 years, and use of antidepressants has increased from 1988 to 1994 threefold to fivefold among youth younger than 20 years of age.[31] Noting that primary care physicians initiate more antidepressant pharmacotherapy than psychiatrists, the literature addresses issues involved in recognition and management of depression in primary care settings, clearly outlining that the pharmacology of depression treatment and its effects constitute a multifactorial challenge for physicians who must take into account medication side effects, adverse drug effects, and drug-drug interactions, as well as patient specific factors such as gender, age, and other illnesses.[5]

Antidepressants have a multitude of receptor and neurochemical modulating effects (Table 15-3).[32] The SSRIs, as previously stated, are the most frequently prescribed antidepressants encountered by practicing anesthesiologists. As their name implies, they selectively potentiate the transmission of central nervous impulses along serotonergic pathways while having little effect on other neuroendocrine pathways, such as those involving norepinephrine or acetylcholine. As such, they tend to cause nausea, diarrhea,

TABLE 15–2 Depressive Disorder Medications

Class	Generic Name (Trade Name)
Tricyclic antidepressants (TCAs)	Amitriptyline (Elavil, Endep, Entrofen, Loroxyl, Tryptizol)
	Amoxapine (Asendin)
	Clomipramine (Anafranil)
	Desipramine (Norpramin, Pertofran)
	Doxepin (Adapin, Sinequan)
	Imipramine (Norfranil, Tofranil, Tipramine)
	Maprotiline (Ludiomil)
	Nortriptyline (Aventyl, Noratren, Pamelor)
	Protriptyline (Vivactil)
	Trimipramine (Surmontil)
Selective serotonin reuptake inhibitors (SSRIs)	Citalopram (Celexa, Cipram, Cipramil, Serostat)
	Escitalopram (Lexapro)
	Fluoxetine (Prozac, Sarafem)
	Fluvoxamine (Dumirox, Feverin, Floxyfral, Luvox)
	Paroxetine (Paxil)
	Sertraline (Zoloft)
Monoamine oxidase inhibitors (MAOIs)	Deprenyl (Eldepryl, Selegiline)
	Isocarboxazid (Marplan)
	Moclobemide (Aurorix)
	Phenelzine (Nardil)
	Tranylcypromine (Parnate)
Atypical medications	Amisulpride (Deniban, Solian, Sulamid)
	Bupropion (Wellbutrin, Zyban)
	Duloxetine (Cymbalta)
	Milnacipran (Ixel)
	Mirtazapine (Remeron)
	Nefazodone (Dutonin, Serzone)
	Reboxetine (Edronax, Vestra)
	Trazodone (Desyrel, Trazon, Trialodine)
	Venlafaxine (Effexor)
	Viloxazine (Vivalan, Vivarint)
Herbal and natural remedies	Ginkgo biloba
	Ginseng
	Hypericum perforatum (St. John's Wort)
	S-adenosine-L-methionine (SAMe)
	Valeria officinalis (Valerian)

PERTINENT SIDE EFFECTS OF THESE MEDICATIONS: antiadrenergic effects, anticholinergic effects, blurred vision, constipation, decreased cardiac conduction, drowsiness, dry mouth, dysuria, hepatotoxicity, hyponatremia, orthostatic hypotension, sedation, seizures, tremors, urinary retention.

headache, sexual dysfunction, agitation, and despite some mild sedative effects, insomnia. They lack many of the side effects associated with other classes of antidepressants. However, side effects are noted and SSRIs such as escitalopram, possibly associated with hyponatremia, and sertraline, possibly linked to dry mouth, are reactions that should be recognized when present.

Notable among the SSRIs is fluoxetine, because it is a potent inhibitor of the cytochrome p450 2D6 isoenzyme.[33] The implication of this inhibition is a rise in the plasma concentration of drugs that depend on hepatic metabolism for clearance. Generally, other drugs used to treat coexisting diseases such as β blockers, benzodiazepines, and some cardiac antidysrhythmic drugs are affected. The most obvious results of this inhibition derive from treatment of the patients' depression itself, because patients may be treated with several antidepressants from different classes. Concomitant treatment of depressed patients with both fluoxetine and a tricyclic drug may result in substantial rises in plasma concentrations of the latter. Combination with monamine oxidase inhibitors (MAOIs), with the pharmacology discussed later, may precipitate serotonin syndrome, which is similar to neuroleptic malignant syndrome both in its presentation and its mortality and is marked by flushing, restlessness, anxiety, chills, ataxia, insomnia, and hemodynamic instability. Combining fluoxetine with the mood stabilizers carbamazepine or lithium may also precipitate this syndrome. There has been an ongoing debate as to whether SSRIs may increase the risk of suicide in a small subgroup of depressed patients. On this last point, however, evidence is lacking.

From the perspective of anesthesia, the SSRIs represent little additional challenge to administration of general anesthesia. Some care must be taken to limit drugs that depend on the cytochrome system for metabolism such as barbiturates, benzodiazepines, and certain neuromuscular blocking drugs. It is also of note that there is no effect of SSRIs on seizure threshold. This is an important point to remember during administration of general anesthesia to patients with coexisting seizure disorder or for patients undergoing electroconvulsive therapy (ECT) for the treatment of depression or other psychiatric disorders.

Tricyclic Antidepressants

Prior to the introduction of the SSRIs to clinical practice, the tricyclic antidepressants (TCAs) were the most widely used drugs used to treat clinical depression. They are so named because their chemical structure is composed of three conjoined rings. If the nitrogen atom on the center ring is a tertiary amine, the drug belongs to the first-generation TCAs; if it is a secondary amine, the drug is a second-generation tricyclic. Most of the side effects discussed below are more pronounced with the first-generation TCAs. It is generally believed that the TCAs are equally potent with regard to treatment of depression. On the other hand, all of the TCAs cause some anticholinergic symptoms, orthostatic hypotension, cardiac dysrhythmia, and sedation. However, they do so in varying degrees when compared with their efficacy as antidepressants.

TABLE 15–3   Pharmacology of Antidepressants*

	Antimuscarinic Activity[†]	Antihistamine Activity (H1)[†]	Anti-α1-Adrenergic Activity	Reuptake Inhibition		Elimination Half-Life (hr)
				NE	5-HT	
Amitriptyline	3	3	3	2	4	32-40
Doxepin	2	4	3	1	2	8-25
Imipramine	2	1	1	2	4	6-20
Trimipramine	2	4	3	1	1	9
Desipramine	1	0	1	4	3	12-54
Nortriptyline	1	1	2	2	3	15-90
Protriptyline	3	½	1	3	3	54-92
Amoxapine	1	1	2	2	2	8-30
Maprotiline	1	2	1	2	1	27-58
Trazodone	0	½	2	0	3	3-9
Fluoxetine	½	0	0	1	4	168-210
Bupropion	0	0	0	0	0	8-24

NE, norepinephrine; 5-HT, 5-hydroxytryptamine (serotonin).
*Relative scale of 1 to 4 with 1 = least effect.
[†]Relative agents: atropine = 4 (antimuscarinic activity), diphenhydramine = 2 (antihistamine activity, phentolamine = 4 (anti-α$_1$-adrenergic activity).
From Haddox JD, Chapkowski SL: Neuropsychiatric drug use in pain management. In Raj PP (ed): Practical Management of Pain, 3rd ed. St. Louis, Mosby, 2000, pp 489-512.

This differing side effect profile serves as the basis for much of the strategy employed by practitioners prescribing these drugs. For example, a drug that causes a greater degree of sedation might be chosen preferentially for patients experiencing insomnia as part of their symptomatology. Similarly, practitioners might avoid drugs that have greater anticholinergic activity in patients who have glaucoma or reflux disease, for example.

The degree of cardiac dysrhythmia potential is essentially the same for TCAs, and they should be avoided in patients with known cardiac conduction abnormalities such as second-degree atrioventricular block. It has been shown that despite their potential for causing cardiac dysrhythmias, they may paradoxically show some antidysrhythmic activity.[34] Also of note is the fact that despite the electrocardiographic (ECG) changes that occur with these drugs, the changes tend to dissipate with ongoing treatment, implying some sort of tolerance on the part of the cardiac conduction system to these effects.[35] However, these changes are of particular concern during the early phase of treatment of depressed patients with suicidal ideations. This concern arises from the fact that a frequently chosen method of suicide is overdose, and the medications chosen are those in possession of patients, in this case, possibly their antidepressants. Overdose with TCAs may be achieved by ingesting as little as 5 to 10 times the daily dosage, resulting in fatal arrhythmia or resistant myocardial depression. Despite these facts, overdose with TCAs typically presents as central nervous system (CNS)

depression, including seizures, hypoventilation, and coma. Anticholinergic symptoms are also present and may confuse diagnosis. Normally, when patients present to the operating theater, these problems are not present. However, in the setting of trauma, there may be need for concern if acute drug ingestion is present as part of a suicide attempt or abuse of these drugs.

Considerations regarding the administration of general anesthesia to patients undergoing treatment of depression with TCAs revolve around the side effects of these medications and their interactions with other drugs. The mechanism of action of TCAs involves enhancement of serotonergic and noradrenergic activity. They also cause inhibition of histaminergic, cholinergic, and α$_1$-adrenergic activity as well. This inhibition is responsible for many of the side effects of the drugs. Most of the anesthetic considerations affected by patients being treated with a TCA involve the cardiovascular system and are brought about by the interaction of the drug with a specific neurotransmitter, such as norepinephrine. Administration of TCAs causes an increase of this neurotransmitter to be stored in noradrenergic nerve terminals. Thus, administration of indirect-acting vasopressors such as ephedrine may cause an exaggerated response. This effect is most pronounced with acute treatment and gradually dissipates after the first 2 to 3 weeks. Caution is therefore advised with regard to using drugs with sympathomimetic effects on patients receiving TCAs.

Another neurotransmitter system that is of particular concern to the anesthesiologist is the cholinergic system. Many of the drugs used by anesthesiologists are anticholinergics or have anticholinergic effects. Preoperatively, some anesthesiologists employ scopolamine for its sedative, anxiolytic, and antisialogogic properties. Intraoperatively, glycopyrrolate and atropine are both used for their anticholinergic properties. Pancuronium, which has significant anticholinergic effects, is still used for procedures requiring a long period of muscle relaxation, especially cardiac surgery. Atropine and glycopyrrolate have been noted to have increased muscarinic activity in the presence of TCAs, and administration of pancuronium has been documented to precipitate tachydysrhythmias in a sample of patients studied.[36] Furthermore, there is the possibility that preoperative treatment with scopolamine may increase the incidence of emergence delirium, although there are no studies to support this suspicion.

Overall, the increased amount of neurotransmitters available in the CNS due to treatment with SSRIs is responsible for increasing the minimal alveolar concentration (MAC) of inhalational agents.[37] Also, in general, owing to the sensitization of the sympathetic nervous system by TCAs, there is the possibility that ketamine might have a similar effect to pancuronium, although evidence is lacking. Finally, halothane and the epinephrine used to extend the length of action of centrally or peripherally administered nerve blockade also have the theoretical potential to cause dysrhythmias, although evidence to support this concern is lacking.

Monoamine Oxidase Inhibitors

The monoamine oxidase inhibitors (MAOIs) represent a third class of antidepressants. As their name implies, they inhibit the enzyme monamine oxidase, which is responsible for the oxidative deamination of several biogenic amines, among them norepinephrine. As a consequence, they act to extend the effect of norepinephrine at the nerve terminals. Whereas their use has declined over the past several decades, largely owing to the advent of more specific drug therapies, these drugs are still available. MAOIs are reserved primarily for the treatment of patients who have failed treatment with other antidepressants. The MAOIs are devoid of many of the side effects of the earlier-mentioned drugs. The principal side effect is the ability to precipitate profound hypertension when foods are consumed that contain the substance tyramine, most commonly wines or cheeses, or when combined with drugs with intrinsic sympathomimetic effects such as certain β blockers. Tyramine and sympathomimetic drugs stimulate the release of norepinephrine from noradrenergic nerve terminals, and owing to the mechanism of the drug, the α-adrenergic effects of the neurotransmitter become pronounced. Other side effects of the drug include orthostatic hypotension, sedation, blurry vision, and peripheral neuropathy.

In addition to the just-mentioned side-effects, perhaps the greatest reason that MAOIs have fallen out of favor as first-line therapy for the treatment of depression is their tendency to interact with an extensive list of other drugs, including both prescription and over-the-counter medications, such as meperidine and the herbal medicine St. John's Wort. The manifestations of these reactions include but are not limited to the previously mentioned hypertensive crisis, serotonin syndrome, and, in many cases, exaggerated effects of many of the medications with which the MAOI interacts. This interaction profile severely limits the utility of this class of drugs. When patients who are being treated with MAOIs present for surgery there are several things for anesthesiologists to consider. In the past, it was suggested that MAOIs be discontinued 2 to 3 weeks before any elective procedure involving general anesthesia. This precaution is no longer encouraged or practical for many procedures, because discontinuation of the drug may acutely place patients at greater risk for suicide.[38]

As with the TCAs, the MAC is conceivably elevated in patients undergoing treatment with MAOIs, although this elevation has never been delineated. Furthermore, serum cholinesterase activity may be impaired, requiring the dose of succinylcholine to be reduced.[39] Liver function indices may become elevated during treatment with MAOIs; and, as such, halothane should probably be avoided owing to its potential to cause hepatic dysfunction. As with TCAs, indirect-acting vasopressors as well as epinephrine-containing local anesthetics should be avoided because of their potential to cause severe hypertension. Finally, because MAOIs are known to interact with opioids, their use should be limited by necessity. Meperidine is the most commonly implicated of the narcotics, but, with the exception of fentanyl, they all have the possibility of precipitating a hyperpyrexic response that can be confused with malignant hyperthermia and carries a similar potential for mortality.[40] Postoperative pain control can be achieved with minimal use of opioids and employment of alternatives such as NSAIDs and regional anesthesia, when possible.

Second-Generation Drugs

A final pharmacologic option for the treatment of depression is the use of alternative second-generation drugs such as venlafaxine, trazodone, bupropion, and mirtazapine. The methods of action of many of these drugs are currently being elucidated but remain poorly understood. Like the MAOIs, these drugs are most likely chosen by practitioners for the treatment of patients who have failed pharmacologic management of their depression with other drugs such as the SSRIs. Most often, the drug's side effect profile acts as guide for which drug is chosen. For example, venlafaxine may be linked to seizures and constipation as two side effects. Another drug in this class, trazodone, is the most sedating of the second-generation antidepressants and might be chosen to treat patients who suffer from insomnia. Unlike the TCAs, these alternative agents possess almost no anticholinergic effects and do not cause potential for cardiac dysrhythmias. For patients receiving more than one drug as part of their therapy, avoidance of MAOIs in patients undergoing therapy with a second-generation antidepressant is recommended.

Caution is warranted regarding St. John's Wort *(Hypericum perforatum),* used by many people in an attempt to treat themselves for what they feel is depression. Many of these individuals have never been diagnosed by a psychologist or psychiatrist as having depression but may still treat themselves nonetheless. Recent studies indicate St. John's Wort is no more effective than placebo in the treatment of major depressive disorder.[41] Its efficacy for less severe cases is disputed. However, there are still patients encountered in the scope of clinical practice who take this nutraceutical agent. The side effect profile is extensive, but the only major concern for anesthesiologists is the similarity that this drug bears to the MAOIs in their potential for precipitation of hypertension and hyperpyrexia by the aforementioned mechanisms.

Scher and Anwar reported that the proportion of surgery patients taking antidepressants is 35%.[42] Furthermore, the investigators found that a large percentage of such patients did not reveal the use of these drugs on routine preanesthetic assessment. In this regard, a similar percentage of patients, roughly one third, admitted to taking one or more nutraceuticals (herbal agents). However, 70% did not disclose this information on preanesthetic assessment, and many of these agents possess neurobehavioral effects and can interact with anesthetics.[43,44] In addition to the potential effects of depressive psychopathology on patient reporting of illness, behaviors before and after surgery, and recovery outcomes, antidepressant medications may interact with anesthetics and influence behavior or cognitive functioning postoperatively. One such complication is the risk of developing acute confusional states, which is thought to be elevated in depressed patients taking antidepressants.

One group of researchers compared 80 depressed patients with 50 control patients undergoing orthopedic surgery and found that cortisol response to surgery is associated with postoperative confusion and that the use of fentanyl during anesthesia decreases the incidence of postoperative confusion, related to the inhibition of cortisol secretion by fentanyl.[45] Another study evaluated 80 patients ages 35 to 63 years with major depression who underwent anesthesia during orthopedic surgery, divided into those who continued or discontinued antidepressants 72 hours before surgery.[46] Depressed patients were taking imipramine, clomipramine, maprotiline, and mianserin. Results revealed a low incidence of intraoperative hypotension and arrhythmias in depressed patients whether antidepressant treatment was ceased preoperatively or not, but that discontinued use of antidepressants was associated with increased incidence of delirium, confusion, and depressive symptoms. In another investigation, Kudoh and colleagues observed temperature regulation during anesthesia and postoperative shivering in chronically depressed patients undergoing orthopedic surgery who were taking imipramine, clomipramine, maprotiline, or mianserin for more than 1 year compared to a control sample. The intraoperative core temperature and incidence of shivering in the depressed group were significantly higher.[47]

Dysthymic Disorder

The *DSM-IV* defines dysthymia as a chronically depressed mood that occurs for most of the day, more days than not, for at least 2 years.[15] The disorder can be found in children who may exhibit irritability rather than depression, or in addition to sadness. When depressed mood prevails, at least two additional symptoms may be present, such as poor appetite or overeating, insomnia or hypersomnia, low energy or fatigue, low self-esteem, difficulties concentrating or making decisions, and feelings of hopelessness. Often, patients with dysthymia see their symptoms as characterizing their personality over time. The lifetime prevalence is approximately 6% according to the *DSM-IV,* and it is noted that dysthymia is often marked by early, insidious onset and a chronic course.[15] Dysthymia may be superimposed on major depression; and in many cases, patients are prescribed medications similar to those used for major depression. Loss of interest, feelings of guilt or brooding about the past, excessive anger, and decreased activity, effectiveness, and productivity may be common; and with time the disorder may be associated with multiple physical illnesses or coexist with such illnesses.

Bipolar Disorders

When individuals exhibit bouts or episodes characterized as manic, often in sequence with depressive episodes, they are characterized within this category. A manic episode is seen as a distinct period marked by abnormally, persistently elevated, expansive, or irritable mood accompanied by such additional symptoms as inflated self-esteem or grandiosity, decreased need for sleep, pressured speech, flight of ideas, distractibility, and increased involvement in goal-directed activities with high potential for painful consequences. The disturbance is sufficiently severe to cause marked impairments in social or occupational functioning and may include psychotic features. Mood in manic episodes may be seen as euphoric, unusually cheerful, or high; and the expansive quality is described as unceasing and indiscriminate, particularly in interpersonal, sexual, or occupational interactions. Uncritical self-acceptance may hold firm, and individuals may not recognize that they are ill and resist efforts to be treated. Mood may shift rapidly to anger or depression. Depending on the length, severity, and course of symptom complexes over time, individuals may be diagnosed as bipolar I or bipolar II disorder. Bipolar I disorder is characterized by one or more manic or mixed episodes, usually with major depressive episodes. The diagnosis of bipolar II disorder suggests recurrent depressive episodes and at least one hypomanic episode. Among the specifiers to designate subtypes within the bipolar spectrum are those reflecting severity, psychosis, remission, catatonic features, and postpartum onset. Seasonal patterns and the nature of cycling (rapid or not) are also considered, and thus the history of current and past episodes determines diagnosis of actual mood disorder.

The phenomenology of bipolar symptoms is multifaceted across and within individuals over time, taking into account both symptom severity and variability.[48] Studying the prevalence and disability of bipolar spectrum disorders in the United States and adding investigation of subthreshold cases, Judd and Akiskal found a combined community prevalence of 6.4%.[49] Subthreshold cases were at least five times more prevalent than *DSM*-defined core syndromal diagnoses, cited at about 1%. These researchers emphasized that bipolar disorders are associated with significant service utilization and psychosocial impairment. Among the pharmacologic treatments for bipolar disorders are drugs used to treat mood disorders generally, including antidepressants, lithium salts, and other medications. Lithium carbonate was the first and is still the most important antimanic agent (Table 15-4).[25-30] For cases refractory to treatment with pharmacologic agents, ECT may be used as an intervention of last resort.

The use of lithium carbonate to treat mania began after an Australian psychiatrist, John Cade, noticed the calming effect that the salt had on laboratory animals. For many years the soft drink 7Up contained lithium and was marketed as having a calming effect. While the mechanism of action of lithium is still not precisely known, it is widely distributed throughout the CNS, where it is believed to have a variety of effects. It is known that lithium interacts with many neurotransmitter systems, increasing the synthesis of serotonin while decreasing norepinephrine release, and these effects are thought to be responsible for its clinical effect.

Despite its efficacy in the treatment of mania, lithium has a very narrow therapeutic index and plasma levels of the drug must be monitored routinely. A serum concentration of 0.6 to 0.8 mEq/L is considered therapeutic for the treatment of stable mania. Slightly higher levels up to 1.2 mEq/L are accepted for treatment of acute episodes. Levels of 2.0 mEq/L are considered toxic and require withdrawal of the drug and aggressive hydration with sodium-containing solutions or administration of osmotic diuretics such as mannitol.[50] Lithium toxicity is evidenced by weakness, sedation, ataxia, and widening of the QRS complexes on the electrocardiogram. These symptoms in patients receiving lithium demand drug withdrawal and testing of serum lithium levels, because with greater toxicity, atrioventricular blockade, cardiovascular instability, seizures, and death may result.

Besides the possibility of toxicity, lithium also has long-term effects that require periodic monitoring. Lithium is known to inhibit the release of thyroid hormones, resulting in hypothyroidism in as many as 5% of patients receiving the drug. It may also cause nephrogenic diabetes insipidus that does not respond to treatment with vasopressin. In a small number of patients, leukocytosis may develop, noted as a white blood cell count between 10,000 and 14,000 cells/ mm³. All of these effects resolve with withdrawal of the drug but mandate periodic testing of patients' thyroid levels, urine osmolality, and white blood cell count. In patients with known sinus nodal dysfunction, it may be prudent first to place a permanent pacemaker secondary to possible disturbances of the cardiac conduction system by lithium treatment.

Lithium ions are freely filtered in the glomerulus and then reabsorbed in the proximal convoluted tubule. The amount of reabsorption is inversely proportional to the concentration of sodium ions present in the ultrafiltrate. In patients receiving loop or thiazide diuretics, the increase in the concentration of sodium ions in the ultrafiltrate causes a subsequent increase in lithium reabsorption. Coupled with the relative decrease in extracellular fluid, lithium ion concentration may rise by as much as 50% and toxicity may ensue. Therefore, a reduced lithium dose along with more careful monitoring of lithium levels is recommended in patients receiving diuretic therapy with either of these agents. Besides the just-mentioned considerations, lithium interacts with several classes of

TABLE 15–4 Bipolar/Cyclothymic Disorder Medications

Carbamazepine (Tegretol)
Valproic acid (Depakote)
Gabapentin (Neurontin)
Lamotrigine (Lamictal)
Topiramate (Topamax)
Lithium carbonate (Eskalith, Lithium, Lithobid)

PERTINENT SIDE EFFECTS OF THESE MEDICATIONS: ataxia, confusion, convulsions, lithium toxicity, nephrogenic diabetes insipidus, sedation, tremors.

anesthetic agents. Specifically, the length of action of several nondepolarizing neuromuscular blocking drugs is prolonged because of lithium's ability to replace sodium in propagation of action potentials.[51] In addition, the MAC is reduced in patients receiving lithium because of lithium's blockage of brain stem epinephrine and norepinephrine release; thus, emergence may be prolonged.[52] Nutraceuticals and herbal agents have also been used to treat mood disorders, and evaluation for these agents is necessary for anesthesiologists. In this regard, fish oils have had positive results in bipolar disorder and can affect the coagulation cascade.[53]

Electroconvulsive Therapy

An often-questioned treatment procedure for depression and other mental disorders, ECT remains within the arsenal of weapons to impact the symptoms of major depression and bipolar disorder.[54] It may also be applied in cases of schizophrenia, particularly when patients do not respond to other therapeutic efforts.[55] It is thought that the therapeutic mechanism of ECT is related to the generalized seizures it induces, and there are potentially important interactions between psychotropics, anesthetics, and ECT, necessitating effective cooperation between the medical disciplines involved in its administration. Several clinician researchers have explored combinations of anesthetics to facilitate favorable outcomes.[56] In general, ECT is thought of as a treatment of last resort, applied when either other treatments have failed or if patients develop suicidal ideations acutely.[57] At present, the mechanism of ECT is unknown. Until recently, most practitioners have touted the theory that seizure duration is the most important factor relating to treatment efficacy.[58] However, newer studies cast doubt on this theory.[59] The only absolute contraindications to ECT are elevated intracranial pressure and pheochromocytoma. Relative contraindications include recent cerebrovascular accident, aortic disease, cerebral aneurysms, cardiac conduction disturbances, and certain high-risk pregnancies.

Usually, once an electrical stimulus has been applied to the brain, a grand-mal seizure is induced. A brief initial tonic phase is followed by a more prolonged clonic phase that lasts on the order of 30 seconds to several minutes. Another technique is to induce three seizures at one sitting and use intubation with hyperventilation to decrease carbon dioxide. By hyperventilating and decreasing carbon dioxide levels, the seizure threshold can be lowered. On the average, approximately eight treatments are necessary to treat most patients with a response rate of close to 75%. Over the course of the treatments, the only significant side effect that develops is memory loss. To minimize this complication, the stimulus can be applied to the nondominant hemisphere only. However, efficacy is reduced by this maneuver.

During ECT treatments there are several physiologic consequences that mandate close monitoring of patients. Initially, a substantial vagal discharge is noted with consequent bradycardia and hypotension. This is immediately followed by a much longer period of time during which sympathetic activity predominates, resulting in hypertension and tachycardia. During this time, cardiac ischemia or significant tachydysrhythmias may develop. In fact, the most frequent cause of mortality in patients receiving ECT is myocardial infarction.[60] Several treatments have been suggested to address these side effects, including short-acting β blockers, narcotics, and nitrates. Careful consideration must be given to such agents, because profound bradycardia and asystole have been reported after their administration.[61]

Clinicians who administer anesthesia for ECT need to be aware of untoward physiologic responses and be prepared to treat them. In addition, they need to be aware of the effects that different agents used for anesthesia have on the administration of the therapy. In the past, traditional wisdom has suggested that methohexital was superior to other agents because of its ability to decrease seizure threshold. More recent research has indicated, however, that etomidate provides a longer window of seizure activity than does either methohexital or propofol.[62] Until agreement is reached concerning the exact mechanism of action of ECT, which agent is superior remains unknown. Ketamine, with its ability to lower seizure threshold, may seem to provide some benefit, but studies have not shown this to be the case.[63]

Given the tonic-clonic nature of seizure, muscle relaxation is essential, and because of the ultra-short duration of action, succinylcholine is an almost perfect agent for this purpose, because it may be administered as a single bolus or via infusion. However, there is potential to cause mild vagal blockade, and careful attention must be paid to its potential to amplify the initial vagal phase of the induced seizure. The administration of glycopyrrolate preprocedurally may help circumvent this complication. Mivacurium has also been used for this purpose but has the disadvantage of causing prolonged relaxation and increasing the total anesthetic requirements.

In addition to the standard monitors used for general anesthesia, electromyography (EMG) and electroencephalography (EEG) are also employed by most practitioners to monitor the length of induced seizure activity both peripherally and centrally. The inflation of a tourniquet on the limb used to monitor EMG before administration of the muscle relaxant helps to augment the efficacy of this monitoring modality. Intubation of the trachea is usually not required unless there is a history of gastroesophageal reflux or hiatal hernia, but ventilation must be supported during the procedure owing to the need for muscle relaxation. Thus, the antisialogogic effect of glycopyrrolate is an additional benefit of pretreatment with this medication.

Patients undergoing ECT are often receiving treatment with other psychotropic medications. These medications may have an impact on the physiologic implications of ECT, as well as possible interactions with medications used to anesthetize patients during ECT. For example, the aforementioned effects of TCAs on the sympathetic nervous system and on the cardiac conduction system may predispose patients receiving ECT to a more significant risk of profound hypertension and dysrhythmias. Patients taking MAOIs may find themselves at a similarly increased risk of hypertension. Lithium treatment may prolong the effect of benzodiazepines or barbiturates used for induction of general anesthesia while increasing the likelihood of treatment-induced cognitive side effects. Also, preprocedural treatment with centrally acting anticholinergic medications may increase the likelihood of postprocedural delirium. Clearly, the anesthetic record must be complete. This includes descriptions of which drugs are administered and in what quantities, especially drugs used to treat hemodynamic fluctuations. The induction stimulus, length of the induced seizure, and length of time to recovery must be assiduously documented. This is particularly important because ECT is administered repeatedly over a course of several weeks and the events of the previous treatment can serve to guide modifications of future treatments.

ANXIETY DISORDERS

Generalized Anxiety Disorder

Studies over the past two decades have shown anxiety disorders as a whole to be the most prevalent of mental disorders, affecting as many as one in four individuals in American society at some time in their lives.[13] Although differing by subtype and among the most diverse, anxiety disorders are more often found among women, the more poorly educated, the unmarried, and the childless.[64] Leon and colleagues estimated that 30 million Americans may have suffered from an anxiety disorder, and Lépine called attention to the prevalence of the anxiety disorders and their cost to society.[65,66] Among these disorders are generalized anxiety disorder, thought to hold current prevalence rates from 1.2% to 2.8%, and 4.0% to 6.6% for lifetime estimates.[66] Generalized anxiety disorder is a persistent and troublesome condition with high degrees of comorbidity, making it a consequence of and risk factor for other disorders. According to the *DSM-IV*, the essential features are excessive anxiety and uncontrolled worry about varied activities and events occurring over a period of 6 months.[15] Anxiety and worry are accompanied by additional symptoms, including restlessness, fatigue, concentration problems, irritability, muscle tension, and disturbed sleep. The intensity, duration, and amount of anxiety are disproportionate to the actual likelihood or impact of the feared event, and persons affected have difficulty changing their thought patterns from incessant worry. Many patients suffering generalized anxiety disorder seek treatment from their primary care providers.

Social Phobia

Another of the anxiety disorders is social phobia, a relatively common disorder, although prevalence estimates differ depending on measurement instruments, time period under consideration, and other methodologic features. Nevertheless, estimates of lifetime prevalence range from 0.5% to 16% in one report and 3% to 13% in the *DSM-IV*.[15,67] The essential feature is marked and persistent fear of social or performance situations leading to possible embarrassment, and exposure to the threatening situation provokes an immediate anxiety response such as panic attack. In most cases, individuals avoid the feared situations and the disorder interferes significantly with normal routines, academic or occupational functioning, and social activities, and relationships. Social phobia is common, associated with significant impairment in a number of life areas, and has been identified in 2.9% to 7.0% of primary care patients.[68] In this arena, patients are often women with a mean age at onset of 15.1 years, tend to be younger and less educated than others with anxiety disorders, and may hold poorer views of their health and physical function, with common suicidal ideation. The disorder may be unrecognized by medical providers across settings, particularly when patients present for surgery.

Obsessive-Compulsive Disorder

Other anxiety disorders are panic disorder, agoraphobia, specific phobia, and obsessive-compulsive disorder. Disorders involving great fearfulness, behavioral agitation, somatic involvement, and avoidance of important life activities or situations are perhaps more obvious, such as panic disorder, agoraphobia, and specific phobia. Obsessive-compulsive disorder, however, may be difficult to identify, particularly among high-functioning, intelligent adults. The disorder is one of the most severe and chronic of the anxiety disorders, with essential features of recurrent obsessions or compulsions that are time consuming and distressing. Obsessions are commonly about themes of contamination, dirt, or illness; needs for orderliness; and somatic and religious ideation. Compulsions may include washing, checking, and repeating rituals, either behavioral or cognitive.[69] Although previously thought to be relatively rare in the general population, recent community studies have estimated a lifetime prevalence of 2.5% and 1-year prevalence of 1.5% to 2.1%.[15] In many instances, obsessive-compulsive disorder afflicts persons of higher intelligence and functioning capacity;

therefore, the symptomatology may be masked by the appearance of productivity. Some degree of success in treatment has been achieved with use of the SSRIs.

Post-traumatic Stress Disorder

Receiving considerable attention with the rise of domestic violence and civil unrest, the occurrence of natural disasters such as hurricane, acts of terrorism, and exposure to war and other traumatic events, post-traumatic stress disorder (PTSD) was first described in 1980.[15] Mental health professionals recognized officially what psychoanalysts postulated in the past century, that traumatic events may have long-lasting effects on the human psyche, with implications for mental and physical functioning, particularly as stressful events are prolonged, severe, life-threatening, and gruesome. Trauma exposure is a necessary condition for diagnosis in the *DSM-IV*, and the critical determinant is individual cognitive and affective reactivity to the trauma, with the event eliciting severe and incapacitating psychological distress, such as feelings of "intense fear, helplessness, or horror."[15] Symptoms include high levels of anxiety; distressing thoughts, feelings, and images that recapitulate the trauma; avoidance of stimuli associated with the event; emotional numbing of responsiveness; restricted range of affect; sense of foreshortened future; interpersonal anomalies; and stress-related symptoms of distress, arousal, fear, and irritability. Data from a variety of studies suggest that traumatic events are not unusual and that the average American is likely to suffer one or multiple exposures.[70] PTSD may occur following a wide range of stressful events, including participating in war, torture, rape, and other criminal victimization; air and motor vehicle accidents; industrial accidents; and devastating acts of nature, such as hurricane and earthquake.

Given the epidemiology of traumatic events, it is not surprising that lifetime prevalence for PTSD in the community may vary from 1% to 14%, depending on the population sampled and study methodology.[15] Research focusing on special groups at high risk, such as survivors of natural disaster, combat veterans, former prisoners of war (POWs), and soldiers assigned graves registration duties in the war zone reveal highly variable rates, depending on the severity and nature of the stressful experience and, to a lesser degree, individual difference factors. Three examples are illustrative. Results of the National Vietnam Readjustment Study showed that among men, 15% and 30% met criteria for current and lifetime PTSD.[71] The figures for women were 9% and 27%, respectively. Sutker and colleagues found current rates of PTSD as high as 48% in a small sample of Gulf War veterans who performed graves registration duties in the war zone and as high as 70% and 86% for current PTSD in former POWs held by the Japanese during World War II and by the Koreans and Chinese in the Korean War.[72-74]

Treatment for PTSD has often incorporated a variety of medications, including antidepressants such as the SSRIs, TCAs, and MAOIs. Inhibitors of adrenergic activity such as clonidine, propranolol, and the diazepines have been used. Thus, patients suffering PTSD, and possibly other comorbid disorders, such as dysthymia, other anxiety disorders, and substance abuse disorders, may present for medical treatment and surgery with a complex array of prescription medications for anesthesiologists to understand. Behavioral complications of the disorder may pose barriers to effective communication and cooperation with physicians, and patients suffering PTSD may become irritable, anxious, confused, and belligerent under conditions where they experience misunderstandings, lack of control, and potential exposure to life-threatening stress. Medical intervention outcomes may be diminished by the direct effects of PTSD psychopathology.

Panic Attacks

Common to the anxiety disorders overall, panic attacks represent a feature of psychopathology that bears consideration in evaluating patients for surgery and anesthesia. According to the *DSM-IV*, panic attacks involve a period of fear or anxiety distinguished by physiologic and cognitive symptoms.[15] These attacks seem to present unexpectedly and are often associated with phobic avoidance of situations in which they have occurred. Therefore, individuals who associate medical treatments and illnesses with panic attacks may be particularly vulnerable to suffer such attacks in a medical situation or in anticipation of such. Barlow found that panic disorder is less prevalent than some other anxiety disorders but is one of the most common found in outpatient treatment programs.[75] Patients with a history of panic attacks may describe use of TCAs, MAOIs, SSRIs, and benzodiazepines. Table 15-5 lists the medications commonly used to treat anxiety disorders.[76-78]

It is not surprising that patients suffering from anxiety as the fundamental symptom of their mental disorder may experience heightened fear, worry, and anxiety before anesthesia and surgery, associated with high levels of circulating catecholamines, behavioral and autonomic agitation, and fearful behaviors. Heart palpitations and peripheral vasoconstriction may be evidenced. Sedgwick and coworkers wrote that the treatment of choice is with benzodiazepines and β blockers continued throughout the operative period.[4] They pointed to the need for careful preoperative consultation and appropriate premedications using benzodiazepines or opiates and suggested that anesthetic requirements may be increased owing to increased level of circulating catecholamines with the risk of cardiac dysrhythmias. Benzodiazepines and barbiturates may be used in treatment of anxiety as premedicants, with the caution that patients taking barbiturates may suffer withdrawal phenomena and may have increased

TABLE 15–5	Anxiety Disorder Medications
Class	**Generic Name (Trade Name)**
Benzodiazepines and other anxiolytic medications	Alprazolam (Xanax) Barbiturates β Blockers Brotizolam (PIM 919) Buspirone (BuSpar) Chlordiazepoxide (Librium) Clobazam (Frisium, Mystan) Clonazepam (Klonopin) Clonidine (Catapress) Clorazepate (Tranxene) Diazepam (Valium) Estazolam (ProSom) Flunitrazepam (Rohypnol) Flurazepam (Dalmane) Loprazolam (Triazulenone) Lorazepam (Ativan) Lormetazepam (Loramet, Lormetazepam, Noctamid) Meprobamate (Miltown) Midazolam (Versed) Monamine Oxidase Inhibitors (MAOIs) Nitrazepam (Nitrazepam, Mogadon) Oxazepam (Serax) Prazepam (Centrex) Quazepam (Doral) Selective serotonin reuptake inhibitors (SSRIs) Temazepam (Restoril) Triazolam (Halcion)
Tricyclic antidepressants (TCAs)	
Sedative-hypnotic medications	Chloral hydrate (Noctec) Diphenhydramine (Benadryl) Doxylamine (Unisom Nighttime Sleep-Aid) Estazolam (ProSom) Flurazepam (Dalmane) Hydroxyzine (Atarax, Vistaril) Mirtazapine (Remeron) Nefazodone (Dutonin, Serzone) Quazepam (Doral) Temazepam (Restoril) Trazodone (Desyrel, Trazon, Trialodine) Triazolam (Halcion) Zaleplon (Sonata) Zopiclone (Imovane) Zolpidem (Ambien)
Herbal and natural remedies	Kava Kava Melatonin Valeria officinalis (Valerian)

PERTINENT SIDE EFFECTS OF THESE MEDICATIONS: abuse potential, aggression, amnestic syndromes, cognitive impairment, drowsiness, intoxication, respiratory problems, withdrawal symptoms such as diaphoresis, rebound insomnia, and tremor.

tolerance to some of the intravenous induction agents, such as thiopentone.

With over 29,000 herbal products, many have been tried for various anxiety states.[43,44] For example, kava extracts are likely effective for short-term treatment of anxiety disorders. Multiple clinical trials have demonstrated positive results compared with placebo and low-dose benzodiazepines. However, dozens of case reports linking kava to hepatic failure have been reported worldwide, thus requiring anesthesiologists to obtain a detailed history and high index of suspicion. The mechanism for kava-induced hepatic dysfunction appears to be linked to the kava alkaloid pipermethystin, which has a strong negative effect on liver cell cultures. Furthermore, four alkaloids with similar structures to pipermethystin are known cytotoxic agents. It is thought that epoxidation of pipermethystin may lead to hepatotoxic products. Herb-drug interactions may also be linked to kava toxicity, because it is rarely administered alone and is typically taken with other supplements or drugs. There are case reports and theoretical considerations that warrant concern regarding kava intake with alcohol, certain herbal agents, alprazolam, fluoxetine, paroxetine, acetylsalicylic acid, oral contraceptives, celecoxib, omeprazole, paracetamol, and others with either reported or associated side effects, examples of such being potential hepatotoxicity and CNS depression. Finally, genetic polymorphism of the CYP2D6 enzyme may play a role in kava-induced liver toxicity. Different ethnicities have varying frequency of deficiency of this metabolizer of kavalactones. Roughly 10% or more of whites have a deficiency in this enzyme, whereas the Polynesian population (which has not reported kava-induced liver failure) does not demonstrate this enzyme deficiency.[79-82] Clinical anesthesiologists should link signs of liver failure with a history of kava intake and request additional laboratory investigation.

NONAFFECTIVE PSYCHOSES

Schizophrenia

A clinically complex and heterogeneous disorder, schizophrenia is defined by disturbances in emotional, behavioral, and cognitive arenas manifested in almost every aspect of life functioning, including sense of well being, social adaptation, health, and self-sufficiency.[83] With a community prevalence rate at about 1%, schizophrenia takes its toll on thinking, attention, language, communication, behavioral monitoring, affect, hedonic capacity, motivation, and general productivity in thought, speech, emotion, and behavior.[15] Symptoms have been classified into three broad categories: positive, negative, and cognitive. Positive symptoms reflect an excess or distortion of normal functions, particularly referring to sensory and perceptual experiences, thoughts, and behaviors that include hallucinations, delusions, and bizarre, strange, or grossly disorganized behaviors. Negative symptoms reflect diminution or loss of normal functions, or absence of emotions and behaviors ordinarily present, such as anhedonia, apathy, social withdrawal, and blunted affect. Negative symptoms also include restrictions in thought productivity and speech and in initiation of goal-directed activities. A third category of symptoms is impairment in attention, information processing, and memory. A thoughtful review of the biopsychologic aspects of schizophrenia reveals the heterogeneity of schizophrenia and the complexities in unraveling its components.[84] Although disturbances of language and, by inference, perception and thought are probably the most salient clinical phenomena, research summaries reveal comorbid problems with depression, anxiety, and PTSD.[83] Treatment advances have resulted from increased understanding of the multifactorial nature of the disease and its various presentations and subtypes, bolstered by a voluminous body of research in psychopharmacology, neuropsychiatry, neuropsychology, and neurobiology.

Kane described the gains resulting from research and development that yielded a new generation of antipsychotics that have been associated with less negative side-effect profiles.[85] He observed that the first three decades of widespread antipsychotic use, dating from the 1950s, were marked by major deficiencies, such as elevated incidence of acute and chronic neurologic effects, frequently poor or only partial outcome responses, and high rates of noncompliance. He emphasized that the introduction of clozapine helped to set the stage for new perspectives on antipsychotic drug treatment and development as well as outcome assessment (Table 15-6).[86-89] The success of clozapine in some refractory patients led to renewed interest in developing better treatment strategies, particularly for patients thought to be "poor responders." Some treatment options have included adjunctive lithium, benzodiazepines, anticonvulsants, and ECT; however, the second-generation antipsychotics such as risperidone and olanzapine, marketed initially in 1994 and 1996, respectively, and quetiapine offer new hope for patients with schizophrenia.

Patients with a history of schizophrenia, or schizophrenic-like disorders, such as schizoaffective disorder, require careful workup for medications taken over time as well as tactful and thoughtful management in the medical situation. Stressful events of all types may exacerbate symptoms of distrust, disorganization, and fears among these patients, and diagnosis of medical illnesses and prospects of surgery may trigger symptom exacerbation. This point is underscored by Pollard, Brook, and Shafer in a case report of a 40-year-old man treated for schizophrenia who underwent podiatric surgery with an ankle block regional technique.[90] In this event, the patient threatened violence to his wife and father when sedative effects were decreasing and necessitated appropriate management and psychiatric

TABLE 15–6	Nonaffective Psychoses Medications
Class	**Generic Name (Trade Name)**
Antipsychotic medications	Acetophenazine (Tindal)
	Carphenazine (Proketazine)
	Chlorpromazine (Thorazine)
	Chlorprothixene (Taractan)
	Clozapine (Clozaril)
	Droperidol (Inapsine)
	Fluphenazine (Permitil, Prolixin)
	Haloperidol (Haldol)
	Loxapine (Loxitane)
	Mesoridazine (Serentil)
	Molindone (Lidone, Moban)
	Olanzapine (Zyprexa)
	Perphenazine (Trilafon)
	Pimozide (Orap)
	Piperacetazine (Quide)
	Prochlorperazine (Compazine)
	Quetiapine (Seroquel)
	Risperidone (Risperdal)
	Sertindole (Serdolect)
	Thioridazine (Mellaril)
	Thiothixene (Navane)
	Trifluoperazine (Stelazine)
	Triflupromazine (Vesprin)
	Ziprasidone (Geodon)
	Zotepine (Nipolept)

PERTINENT SIDE EFFECTS OF THESE MEDICATIONS: acute and late-onset (tardive) extrapyramidal side effects, agranulocytosis, anticholinergic effects, disturbances of cardiac rhythm, dry mouth, dysregulation of temperature, hypersalivation, orthostatic hypotension, sedation, seizures, thromboembolism, tremors, withdrawal symptoms.

consultation. In an investigation of the relationship between postoperative confusion and plasma norepinephrine and cortisol response to surgery in patients with schizophrenia compared with a control sample, higher rates of postoperative confusion 72 hours after surgery in schizophrenic (28%) compared to control (6%) patients have been reported.[45] The researchers concluded that the occurrence of confusion in patients with schizophrenia was associated with an increase in plasma norepinephrine and cortisol levels during and after surgery.

Raised incidence of potential abnormal behaviors, including threats of violence and confusion postoperatively, have been observed to be of concern to anesthesiologists and surgeons.[6] Studies have pointed to the chronic administration of antipsychotic agents as being associated with other anomalies, such as alterations in autonomic functioning and pituitary-adrenal activity after surgery, as well as abnormal secretion of vasopressin, aldosterone, and atrial natriuretic peptide during anesthesia.[91,92] These and other difficulties result from the multiple potential adverse effects of the antipsychotic agents in and of themselves, such as behavioral toxicity, motor aberrations, cardiovascular and autonomic nervous systems effects, and hepatotoxicity, as examples. There are also disturbances in autonomic nervous system functions, ECG abnormalities, and onset of diseases such as diabetes arising in association with long-term use of antipsychotics. Beyond the effects of the antipsychotic medications themselves, there are problems with drug-drug interactions between certain psychotropic drugs and anesthetic agents (Table 15-7).[3] Additionally, it is notable that there is a dose-response relationship between number of physical problems and the risk of self-harm, necessitating physicians to consider the possibility of suicidal ideation in patients with physical illnesses complicated by schizophrenia, depression, and other mental disorders.[93]

The method of action of all antipsychotics is direct interference with the centrally located dopaminergic neurotransmitter system. Furthermore, they have been shown to stimulate the parasympathetic nervous system and to block the effects of α-adrenergic stimulation of the sympathetic nervous system. This implies the possibility for cardiovascular side effects, including hypotension, tachycardia, prolongation of the QT interval on the ECG, and, although very rare, ventricular fibrillation and torsades de pointes. Owing to the functional hypovolemia induced during general or regional anesthesia, or to blood loss and fluid shifts for acutely injured and septic patients, respectively, these concerns become heightened intraoperatively. It should be noted as well that most antipsychotics are metabolized by the cytochrome P450 enzyme system, most notably the 2D6 isoenzyme. Several of the newer drugs are metabolized by several of the cytochrome isoenzymes concurrently, including the 1A2 and 3A4 subsystems.

The incidence of extrapyramidal side effects is higher with older, more potent agents such as haloperidol. With the advent of clozapine, the incidence of these side effects has decreased markedly. However, they still occur and can be life threatening. One such reaction that is seen rarely is laryngospasm, requiring treatment with an anticholinergic medication or diphenhydramine. More frequently seen are acute dystonic reactions such as oculogyric crisis, torticollis, or tremor. One of the more tragic dystonic reactions is tardive dyskinesia, which is characterized by involuntary choreoathetoid movements of the neck and face. Once these movements have begun, they may never resolve, even with withdrawal of the medication responsible. Nearly every neuroleptic medication may cause tardive dyskinesia, with clozapine posing the least risk.

Perhaps the most feared complication of treatment with antipsychotics is neuroleptic malignant syndrome (NMS).[94] NMS is very similar to malignant hypothermia (MH) and may share a similar etiologic mechanism. This syndrome most often occurs within the first several weeks of treatment with or a significant dosage increase of antipsychotic medications. It manifests as increased body temperature, skeletal muscle rigidity, and sympathetic nervous system instability (blood pressure fluctuations, diaphoresis, and tachydysrhythmias). Often liver function tests are abnormal, although the mechanism for this abnormality is uncertain. Because of the severe muscle rigidity, creatinine kinase levels may be elevated and the kidneys may become damaged from myoglobinuria. If these concerns become significant, muscle relaxation with a nondepolarizing neuromuscular blocking drug and subsequent mechanical ventilation of the lungs may become necessary. Treatment of this disorder requires withdrawal of the offending agent and initiation of bromocriptine or dantrolene therapy. Of these two therapies, dantrolene is preferred by some practitioners because of bromocriptine potentially precipitating hypotension. ECT may also have a therapeutic effect on these patients as well. Additional treatments are

TABLE 15–7 Interactions Between Psychotropic Medications and Anesthetic Agents		
Psychotropic Medication	**Anesthetic Agent**	**Interaction**
Tricyclic antidepressants (TCAs)	Halothane and pancuronium Anticholinergics Sympathomimetics	Tachydysrhythmias Exaggerated anticholinergic responses Hypertension
Monoamine oxidase inhibitors (MAOIs)	Meperidine Sympathomimetics	Hypertension, seizures, hyperpyrexia Hypertension
Phenothiazines	Enflurane and isoflurane	Hypotension
Lithium	Barbiturates Nondepolarizing relaxants Depolarizing relaxants	Prolonged somnolence Prolonged blockade Prolonged blockade
Donepezil	Depolarizing relaxants	Prolonged blockade

Adapted from: Derrer SA, Helfaer MA: Evaluation of the psychiatric patient. In Rogers MC, Tinker JH, Covino BG, Longnecker DE (eds): Principles and Practice of Anesthesiology. St. Louis, Mosby, 1993, pp 567-574.

supportive and include antipyretics, intravenous hydration, and dialysis, in addition to those measures just described. Mortality in untreated cases can be as high as 20%. If the patient survives, further treatment with antipsychotics is usually not suggested secondary to the possibility of recurrence. In these patients, alternative therapies like lithium or ECT are advocated.

Anesthesia personnel must be aware of the similarity of NMS and MH and especially vigilant when providing care to persons with a documented history of the former because of the possibility, although unproven, that these patients may be predisposed to the development of the latter. Despite this possibility, it has been shown that administration of succinylcholine to patients receiving ECT as treatment for NMS is safe.[95] Intuitively, it would seem that because of the similarity of the two syndromes, they may, as previously stated, share a similar molecular mechanism. Although evidence to support this supposition is lacking, caution is advised when administering general anesthesia to patients with a history of NMS and more broadly to anyone receiving treatment with neuroleptics.

Delusional Disorder

Among other psychotic disorders are schizophreniform and schizoaffective disorders, both sharing features in common with schizophrenia and depression, psychotic disorders judged to be a direct physiologic consequence of a general medical condition, and the unusual but interesting delusional disorder. The notion of delusion is plagued by conceptual confusion, but the *DSM-IV* calls attention to a condition characterized by the presence of one or more non-bizarre delusions that persist for at least 1 month but not in the context of an history of schizophrenia.[15] Apart from the direct impact of the delusions, psychosocial functioning is not markedly impaired and behavior may not be seen as odd or bizarre. In this disorder, the following themes are often found: erotomanic, grandiose, jealous, persecutory, and somatic.[95] Thus, patients may maintain unusual beliefs about romantic love or idealized spiritual union or hold a view of themselves as having great but unrecognized talents or insights. Persecutory delusions may be found, with the central delusional theme involving beliefs that one is being cheated, spied upon, or conspired against. Although such disorders are uncommon in clinical settings, they may appear unexpectedly to anesthesiologists or surgeons, particularly in adult patients in mid to late life. Evaluation of delusions is difficult, especially in the absence of obvious, marked psychopathology, and relationships with affective disorders, schizophrenia, and organic brain disorders, such as epilepsy, and a range of other disorders must be considered. In the case of somatic delusions, reported cases include patients suffering from temporal lobe epilepsy, narcolepsy, Huntington's chorea, cerebral malaria, multiple sclerosis, encephalitis, chronic liver disease, pellagra, disorders of the thyroid, and others.[95]

SUBSTANCE-RELATED DISORDERS

Included in the *DSM-IV* are a variety of substance-related disorders having to do with side effects of medications, toxin exposure, and use and abuse of prescription and illicit drugs, as well as alcohol.[15] The substances are classified in 11 categories: alcohol, amphetamine or similarly acting sympathomimetics, caffeine, cannabis, cocaine, hallucinogens, inhalants, nicotine, opioids, phencyclidine or similarly acting arylcyclohexylamines, and sedatives, hypnotics, or anxiolytics. Use of substances may be seen as "abuse" or "dependence" depending on behavioral and psychologic characteristic use patterns, and assessment of features of both tolerance and dependence are critical in defining abuse and dependence. Problems resulting from substance intoxication, or recent ingestion of or exposure to a substance, may arise in evaluation of patients for anesthesia. Indicating the seriousness of such problems, Smothers and colleagues reported the first national prevalence estimates of *DSM-IV* alcohol use disorders among 2,040 inpatient admissions to 90 acute care, nonfederal U.S. general hospitals.[15,96] These researchers found an estimated 1.8 million annual admissions met criteria for current alcohol use disorder, with an overall prevalence of 7.4%. Moreover, among current-drinking admissions, estimated prevalence was 24%.[96]

Although alcohol is one of the substances that might have been ingested by patients over time, possibly concomitant with hospital admission or preoperative evaluations, the potential complications to health and medical treatment associated with alcohol effects are enormous. Primary health care providers are often faced with patients who abuse substances of extreme variety, and when patients present for anesthesia and surgery there is a mandate to detect manifest mental problems, as well as covert substance use patterns that may impact response to anesthetic agents and the surgical procedure. Although beyond the scope of this chapter, it is necessary to call attention to the need for comprehensive anesthesia screening procedures to uncover patterns of alcohol use and abuse, as well as use of other drugs, many of which represent illegalities and thus may be glossed over by patients. Wu and associates reported that 2% of adults responding to the 1997 National Household Survey on Drug Abuse reported using services for alcohol or drug problems in the previous year.[97] One approach is application of the Alcohol Use Disorders Identification Test (AUDIT) for anesthesia screening. This 10-item measure was developed from a six-country collaborative project as a screening instrument for hazardous and harmful alcohol consumption and provides a simple method of detection for anesthesia screening.[98]

Clearly, there is a need for comprehensive but efficient screening for all possible drugs of use and abuse that may impact response to anesthesia and surgery. Identification of addiction and issues in pain management are critical to the safe and effective clinical management of anesthesia in surgical situations, as well as in the management of pain problems more generally. However, detailed consideration of those issues is beyond the scope of this chapter.

DELIRIUM, DEMENTIA, AND OTHER COGNITIVE DISORDERS

Delirium

Delirium is a disturbance of consciousness accompanied by changes in cognition of multiple causes. The disturbance develops over the course of the day and may fluctuate during the day and over time. Awareness of the environment, ability to reason, and clarity of expression and thought are compromised. Disorientation, memory impairments, rambling speech, and perceptual distortions can occur. The range and type of disorders leading to delirium states are broad and beyond the scope of this chapter, yet delirium is considered because postoperative delirium is a major problem in many patients undergoing surgery, particularly among the elderly or patients with multiple illnesses or debilitation. An acute disorder of attention and cognition, delirium after surgery may be found in 28% to 50% of patients undergoing hip fracture repair.[99] Zahriya and coworkers reported that an inability to mount a stress response or lack of increase in white blood cell count and abnormal serum sodium levels were risk factors for occurrence of postoperative delirium in elderly patients undergoing hip fracture repair. Other conditions thought to be associated with acute confusional states and altered mental states include dementia, alcoholism, severe medical illness, vision or hearing impairments, advanced age, institutionalization, and depression, to name a few (Fig. 15-1).[99,100]

Dementia

The *DSM-IV* defines dementia as characterized by multiple cognitive deficits that include memory impairment.[15] Classification is often determined by presumed etiology, such as dementia of the Alzheimer's type, vascular dementia, and dementia due to other general medical conditions, head trauma, Parkinson's disease, and Huntington's disease, to name some examples. In addition to memory impairment, symptoms of dementia may include aphasia, apraxia, agnosia, or executive function disturbances or deficit. Problems with judgment and insight are common, and patients with dementia may exhibit little or no awareness of memory loss or cognitive abnormalities. Motor disturbances leading to falls, neglect of personal hygiene, misplaced possessions, disinhibited behavior, and disregard of societal conventions may be observed. Because physical and mental stressors may exacerbate symptomatology, diagnosis of medical illness and receiving medical, surgical, and anesthesia treatments can be particularly stressful and disorganizing. Community studies reveal a 1-year prospective prevalence of almost 3% with severe cognitive impairment, and it is estimated that 2% to 4% of the population older than 65 are afflicted with Alzheimer's disease, a disorder that increases with age.[15]

Medical care of patients with limited and declining cognitive resources and adaptability as a result of an ongoing dementia is impacted adversely by patient difficulties in expression, language, and memory. Problems may result from individuals being unable to describe past and present illnesses to complete inability to communicate, or mutism. Physicians must rely on reports of significant others and family members to provide information pertinent to physical status or the basic data of the history and physical examination. Patients with dementia may become irritable, behaviorally agitated, and difficult to manage before surgical procedures and may be afflicted with delirium, postoperative confusion, and other impediments to recovery after procedures. Patients in the early stages of dementia may be taking anti-dementia medications such as donepezil. Clinical anesthesiologists should be aware that this agent is a cholinesterase inhibitor and can potentially exacerbate succinylcholine-induced muscle relaxation. Cholinesterase inhibitors may have vagotonic effects and cholinomimetic effects (Table 15-8).[101,102] The complete picture of presentation therefore is complicated and requires additional time and effort to work toward safe and effective delivery of anesthetic agents.

Regarding new medications for the treatment of Alzheimer's disease, recent investigations on the safety and efficacy of memantine, a noncompetitive *N*-methyl-D-aspartate (NMDA) receptor antagonist, have shown promising results.[103] A randomized, double-blind, placebo-controlled clinical trial of 404 patients, already receiving donepezil, and with moderate to severe Alzheimer's disease, revealed significant improvement in cognition, activities of daily living, global outcome, and behavior after memantine administration. Thus, the use of memantine to treat patients with moderate to severe Alzheimer's disease may represent a novel pharmacologic approach to this dreaded disease.[103] Drugs on the horizon, such as alzamed, currently in phase 3 trials, may also show promise in providing yet another defense for patients against Alzheimer's disease.

Other Cognitive Disorders

Mild to moderate cognitive impairments can occur as a result of head injury, specific medical conditions, and CNS dysfunction, but these deficits may not be sufficiently severe to meet criteria for dementia. For example,

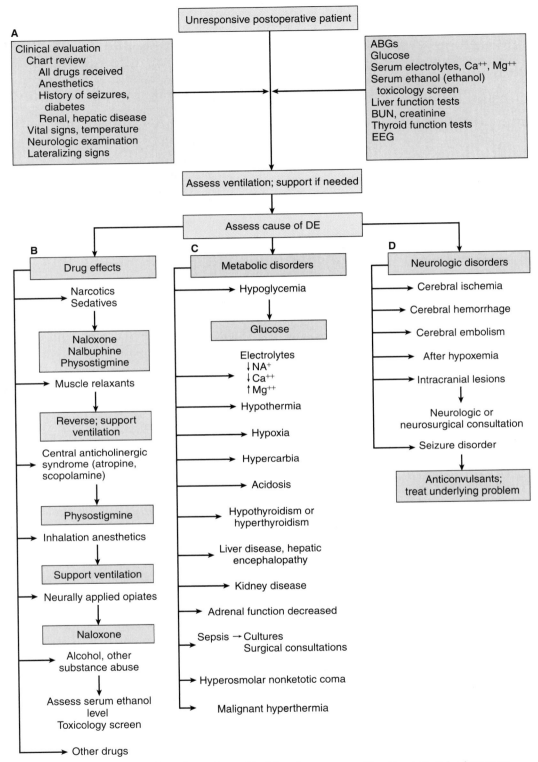

FIGURE 15–1 Approach to the patient with delayed emergence. *(From Bready LL: Delayed emergence. In Bready LL, Smith RB [eds]: Decision Making in Anesthesiology, 2nd ed. St. Louis, Mosby, 1992, pp 364-365.)*

TABLE 15-8   Delirium, Dementia, and Other Cognitive Disorder Medications

Class	Generic Name (Trade Name)
Attention deficit disorder medications	D-Amphetamine (Dexedrine, Dexedrine Spansule, DextroStat) Methylphenidate (Ritalin)
Central nervous system (CNS) stimulants	D-Amphetamine (Dexedrine, Dexedrine Spansule, DextroStat) Methylxanthines (Caffeine, Theobromine, Theophylline)
Memory enhancers	Donepezil (Aricept) Galanthamine (Reminyl) Physostigmine (Antilirium) Rivastigmine (Exelon) Tacrine (Cognex)
Herbal and natural remedies	Ginkgo biloba

PERTINENT SIDE EFFECTS OF THESE MEDICATIONS: addiction potential, bradycardia, cardiac arrhythmias, circulatory collapse, diaphoresis, hypertension, reflex hyperactivity, skeletal muscle paralysis, vertigo.

neuropsychological assessment may reveal evidence of weaknesses in executive functions, working memory, and semantic processing associated with head trauma or other CNS insult. Patients with cognitive disorders require identification and special attention in preoperative and postoperative conditions, because cognitive deficits place them at risk for confusion, behavioral agitation, depression, and other problems before and after surgery or after administration of anesthetics. There is also the possibility of increased vulnerability to anesthetic damage or drug interaction with anesthetic agents.

Clinicians and researchers have observed that anesthesia may provoke persistent alterations in cognitive performances in individuals at risk, including those with multiple illnesses, the elderly, and patients with dementia who have neuronal changes that may exacerbate pharmacotoxic effects. It is important that anesthesiologists recognize that acute and intermediate psychiatric problems may be associated with surgery or hospitalization.[104] For example, patients may experience delirium with psychotic elements as a result of the surgical or medical condition and may experience anxiety as a result of the imminent operation. Another source of stress for patients and anesthesiologists in the perioperative period is "intensive care unit (ICU) psychosis."[104] The ICU setting may be linked to delirium in perioperative or very ill patients as a result of decreased sleep, increased arousal, social isolation, and mechanical ventilation.[104]

Regarding the postoperative period, in an assessment of 140 patients older than age 64 who completed a battery of cognitive tests before and at 9 days and 3 months after surgery, Ancelin and associates found a decline in performance 9 days postoperatively in 5.8% to 70.3% of patients, depending on the cognitive domain explored.[105]

Twenty-nine percent of patients showed no significant alteration on any test score after 9 days, and 44% showed no deficit after 3 months. The greatest degree of impairment tended to be among the most elderly, least educated, and those having a history of cognitive deterioration. Type of anesthesia was found to be the most significant determinant of decline in verbal fluency, semantic prompt, visuospatial analysis, and implicit memory scores. Researchers concluded that anesthesia and orthopedic surgery are related to long-term (3-month) postoperative decline in the elderly, with secondary and implicit memory and visuospatial and linguistic tasks most frequently impacted. Among high risk factors were age older than 75, less education, high levels of depressive symptoms, and recent history of cognitive impairment. The influence of the stress of surgery and the effects of pain could not be evaluated, although they may play a role in cognitive decline. Other research has showed cognitive decline after major noncardiac operations, with impairment most notable immediately after surgery but sometimes persisting. Grichnik and colleagues studied 29 patients who had thoracic and vascular procedures preoperatively and 6 to 12 weeks postoperatively.[106] They found the incidence of cognitive deficit to be 44.8%, with severity of decline being an average of 15%.

The incidence of cognitive decline seems to be most notable in patients subsequent to cardiac surgeries, where it is well recognized and often studied. One investigation evaluated 127 patients undergoing coronary artery bypass grafting preoperatively and at 1 month and 1 year across several cognitive domains.[107] At 1 year, less than one third of patients showed significant cognitive change compared with baseline performance, and change was associated with both medical and surgical variables, pointing to multiple causes such as the nonspecific effects of anesthesia and prolonged surgery interacting with the specific effects of the surgical procedure itself. Among the medical history variables, diabetes was associated with short- and long-term change in executive functions and psychomotor speed. Interest in pharmacologic cerebral protection for cardiac patients has been high, with some evidence that lidocaine infused at induction of anesthesia and continued for 48 hours may have protective effects. One group found cerebral protection by lidocaine unrelated to any effect on depression or anxiety and at a level noticed by patients.[108] Similarly, Wang and colleagues showed a reduction in cognitive dysfunction in patients treated with lidocaine in the early postoperative period.[109] Exploration of possible protective agents to work against cognitive decline or impairments associated with the stress of surgery or anesthetic agents and their delivery is of high priority, particularly for patients who are at risk by reason of various vulnerabilities. Butterworth and Hammon concluded that although controversy persists among those who study cardiac surgery outcomes, there are data that lidocaine may have neuroprotectant effects in focal neurologic injury and in reducing adverse neurobehavioral outcomes.[110]

DISORDERS IDENTIFIED IN DEVELOPMENTAL STAGES

Mental Retardation

Mental retardation is characterized by significantly subaverage general intellectual functioning with limitations in adaptive functioning, such as in communication, self-care, home living, interpersonal skills, and self-direction. Many causes and different levels of severity can be found, but patients are markedly limited in their abilities to manage the exigencies of life. In all cases, patients require custodial care at some level of supervision and generally are managed by a guardian or family member. Although many patients with mental retardation do not pose extreme behavioral problems, preparing them for surgery and anesthesia demands special precautions. For example, Chan and Chilvers described inducing anesthesia in a combative, intellectually impaired adult whose needs suggested that anesthesia induction in the home was helpful to facilitate essential surgery.[111] This adult, with a history of escalating violence toward hospital personnel, was administered an anesthetic in his home before hospital transfer for surgery, illustrating an innovative approach to improving response to treatment. This is but one example of the problems possibly encountered in treating medical illnesses and symptoms in individuals with mental retardation or other intellectually impairing conditions. Although rarer, autistic disorder may also be identified, a disorder marked by abnormal and impaired development in social interaction and communication and often associated with moderate mental retardation.

Attention-Deficit/Hyperactivity Disorder

Often diagnosed when children are young, and now frequently in adults, attention-deficit/hyperactivity disorder (ADHD) is characterized by persistent patterns of inattention and/or hyperactivity and impulsivity greater than might be expected, typically appearing before age 7. The *DSM-IV* estimated disorder prevalence at 3% to 5% in school-aged children, and diagnosis requires evidence of problems in social, academic, or occupational functioning.[15] Inattention may be exhibited as failing to notice details, sustain attention, or persist with tasks to completion, and affected children may not follow through on requests, may be disorganized, and may avoid activities that require sustained self-application and mental effort. Frequent shifts in conversation, not listening, and failures to listen and follow rules may be seen. Impulsivity and hyperactivity may present as impatience, difficulty delaying responses, interrupting others, being constantly on the go, fidgeting and squirming, and avoiding sedentary activities. Found in a variety of contexts and thought to be familial, these behaviors are usually seen in two settings, such as home and school. In many instances, primary care physicians identify ADHD using reports of parents and teachers; and over time there has been increased treatment of symptoms with antidepressants and/or stimulants (see Table 15-8).[101,102]

Although ADHD is a significant health complication, mental health disorders more generally constitute a common cause of disability and distress among both children and adolescents. One group reported that 20% of outpatients age 18 and younger met criteria for psychiatric diagnosis in a given year and that psychotropic medications accounted for a substantial, increasing fraction of outpatient costs.[112] In light of multiple psychotropic pharmacotherapy among children and adolescents in various settings, the need for careful screening of minors for medications as part of anesthesia evaluation is obvious. In such instances, discussions with parents and children may be necessary to develop a full picture of medication and perhaps even other drug use. In this regard, numerous nutraceuticals, or herbal agents, have been utilized and have had some positive results with ADHD.[113,114]

Problem Behaviors in Late Life

Aggressive and inappropriate behaviors in older people have been linked to varied physical and psychological conditions and associated with added risks in the event of medical treatments and surgeries. Behavior problems pose complex challenges for caregivers in the home and in medical settings. Although these behaviors are often reported in clinical or nursing home settings, or when patients are afflicted with dementia, a growing literature describes problem behaviors as common in the last year of life in older people.[115] Studying 6,748 decedents, Bedford and colleagues discovered that 20% exhibited problem behaviors in the last year of life, with risks being higher for those with dementia, mental illness, alcohol abuse, and bronchitis or emphysema. Such problems as violent threats and destroyed property were identified as relatively common, with implications for health care providers in general and anesthesiologists and surgeons more particularly.

CONCLUSION

Patients of all ages and with diverse mental and physical conditions may present for anesthesia under many, and unexpected, circumstances. Mental and cognitive disorders may disrupt normal communication between physicians and patients and contribute to difficulties in deciding on the best medications and strategies for anesthesia. The information presented on mental disorders provides convincing evidence that thorough screening is required for all patients and that special care is demanded when there are mental or physical handicaps, complex histories of drug use, mental disorder symptoms, and other risk factors for anesthesia delivery and recovery from surgery. Of great concern are the potential interactions between drugs used during anesthesia and those prescribed for treatment of mental disorders, and anesthesiologists need also be aware of the behaviors that signify and characterize mental illness. Studies have shown that a high number of patients scheduled for surgical procedures take psychiatric medications or agents that possess potential neurobehavioral effects. Inasmuch as these studies indicate poor self-disclosure to health care providers, anesthesiologists are required to assess each patient carefully and thoroughly. In this regard, many psychiatric drugs can alter MAC requirements, affect sedation levels, and influence anesthetic techniques, such as successful delivery of regional anesthesia.

References

1. Murray CJL, Lopez AD: Alternative projections of mortality and disability by cause 1990-2020: Global Burden of Disease Study. Lancet 1997;349:1498-1504.
2. Wang PS, Demler O, Kessler RC: Adequacy of treatment for serious mental illness in the United States. Am J Public Health 2002;92:92-98.
3. Derrer SA, Helfaer MA: Evaluation of the psychiatric patient. In Rogers MC, Tinker JH, Covino BG, Longnecker DE (eds): Principles and Practice of Anesthesiology. St. Louis, Mosby–Year Book, 1993, pp 567-574.
4. Sedgwick JV, Lewis IH, Linter SPK: Anesthesia and mental illness. Int J Psychiatry Med 1990;20:209-225.
5. Barkin RL, Schwer WA, Barkin SJ: Recognition and management of depression in primary care: A focus on the elderly: A pharmacotherapeutic overview of the selection process among the traditional and new antidepressants. Am J Ther 1999;7:205-226.
6. Tsuji Y, Ohue H, Ikuta H, et al: Surgical treatment of patients with psychiatric disorders: A review of 21 patients. Jpn J Surg 1997;27:387-391.
7. Martin A, Van Hoof T, Stubbe D, et al: Multiple psychotropic pharmacotherapy among child and adolescent enrollees in Connecticut Medicaid managed care. Psychiatr Serv 2003;54:72-77.
8. Regier DA, Narrow WE, Rae DS, et al: The de facto US mental and addictive disorders service system: Epidemiologic catchment area prospective 1-year prevalence rats of disorders and services. Arch Gen Psychiatry 1993;50:85-94.
9. Robins LN, Helzer JE, Croughan J, et al: National Institute of Mental Health diagnostic interview schedule: Its history, characteristics, and validity: Arch Gen Psychiatry 1981;38:381-389.
10. Rogler LH, Malgady RG, Tryon WW: Evaluation of mental health: Issues of memory in the diagnostic interview schedule. J Nerv Ment Dis 1992;180:215-222.
11. Bourdon KH, Rae DS, Locke BZ, et al: Estimating the prevalence of mental disorders in U.S. adults from the Epidemiologic Catchment Area Survey. Public Health Rep 1992;107:663-668.
12. Robins LN, Wing J, Wittchen HU, et al: The composite international diagnostic interview: An epidemiologic instrument suitable for use in conjunction with different diagnostic systems and in different cultures. Arch Gen Psychiatry 1988;45:1069-1077.
13. Kessler RC, McGonagle, KA, Zhao S, et al: Lifetime and 12-month prevalence of DSM-III-R psychiatric disorders in the United States: Results from the national comorbidity survey. Arch Gen Psychiatry 1994;51:8-19.
14. Hoge CW, Lesikar SE, Guevara R, et al: Mental disorders among U.S. military personnel in the 1990s: Association with high levels of health care utilization and early military attrition. Am J Psychiatry 2002;159:1576-1583.
15. American Psychiatric Association: Diagnostic and Statistical Manual of Mental Disorders, 4th ed. Washington, DC, APA, 1994.
16. Olfson M, Broadhead WE, Weissman MM, et al: Subthreshold psychiatric symptoms in a primary care group practice. Arch Gen Psychiatry 1996;53:880-886.
17. Kessler RC, Nelson CB, McGonagle KA, et al: Comorbidity of DSM-III-R major depressive disorder in the general population: Results from the US national comorbidity survey. Br J Psychiatry 1996;168(suppl 30):17-30.
18. Pirl WF, Roth AC: Diagnosis and treatment of depression in cancer patients. Oncology 1999;13:1293-1301.
19. Rothschild AJ: The diagnosis and treatment of late-life depression. J Clin Psychiatry 1996;57(suppl 5):5-11.
20. Kessler RC, Berglund P, Demler O, et al: The epidemiology of major depressive disorder: results from the national comorbidity survey replication (NCS-R). JAMA 2003;289:3095-3105.
21. Hays RD, Wells KB, Sherbourne CD, et al: Functioning and well-being outcomes of patients with depression compared with chronic general medical illnesses. Arch Gen Psychiatry 1995;52:11-19.
22. Wells KB, Sherbourne CD: Functioning and utility for current health of patients with depression or chronic medical conditions in managed care practices. Arch Gen Psychiatry 1999;56:897-904.
23. Anderson KO, Getto CJ, Mendoza TR, et al: Fatigue and sleep disturbance in patients with cancer, patients with clinical depression, and community-dwelling adults. J Pain Symptom Manage 2003;25:307-318.
24. Olfson M, Marcus SC, Druss B, et al: National trends in the outpatient treatment of depression. JAMA 2002;287:203-209.
25. Rehm LP, Wagner AL, Ivens-Tyndal C: Mood disorders: Unipolar and bipolar. In Sutker PB, Adams HE (eds): Comprehensive Handbook of Psychopathology, 3rd ed. New York, Kluwer Academic/Plenum Publishers, 2001, pp 277-308.
26. Barkin RL, Schwer WA, Barkin SJ: Recognition and management of depression in primary care: A focus on the elderly. A pharmacotherapeutic overview of the selection process among the traditional and new antidepressants. Am J Ther 7:205-226, 1999.
27. Mischoulon D, Fava M: Role of S-adenosyl-L-methionine in the treatment of depression: A review of the evidence. Am J Clin Nutr 2002;76:1158S-1161S.
28. Mycek MJ, Harvey RA, Champe PC: Antidepressant drugs. In Harvey RA, Champe PC (eds): Pharmacology, 2nd ed. Philadelphia, Lippincott Williams & Wilkins, 2000, pp 119-126.

29. Janicak PG, Davis JM, Preskorn SH, Ayd FJ Jr: Treatment with antidepressants. In Harvey RA, Champe PC (eds): Principles and Practice of Psychopharmacotherapy, 3rd ed. Philadelphia, Lippincott Williams & Wilkins, 2001, pp 215-326.

30. Stahl SM: Classical antidepressants, serotonin selective reuptake inhibitors, and noradrenergic reuptake inhibitors. In: Essential Psychopharmacology: Neuroscientific Basis and Practical Applications, 2nd ed. Cambridge, Cambridge University Press, 2000, pp 199-244.

31. Zito JM, Safer DJ, dosReis S, et al: Rising prevalence of antidepressants among US youth. Pediatrics 2002;109:721-727.

32. Haddox JD, Chapkowski SL: Neuropsychiatric drug use in pain management. In Raj PP, Abrams BM, Benzon HT, et al (eds): Practical Management of Pain, 3rd ed. St. Louis, Mosby, 2000, pp 489-512.

33. Stevens JC, Wrighton SA: Interaction of the enantiomers of fluoxetine and norfluoxetine with human liver cytochrome P450. J Pharmacol Exp Ther 1993;266:964-971.

34. Veith RC, Raskind MA, Caldwell JH, et al: Cardiovascular effects of tricyclic antidepressants in depressed patients with chronic heart disease. N Engl J Med 1982;306:954-959.

35. Thompson TL, Moran MG, Nies AS: Psychotropic drug use in the elderly. N Engl J Med 1983;308:194-198.

36. Edwards RP, Miller RD, Roizen MF, et al: Cardiac responses to imipramine and pancuronium during anesthesia with halothane or enflurane. Anesthesiology 1979;50:421-425.

37. Miller RD, Way WL, Eger EI: The effects of alpha-methyldopa, reserpine, guanethidine and iproniazid on minimum alveolar anesthetic requirement (MAC). Anesthesiology 1968;29:1153-1158.

38. El-Ganzouri AR, Ivankovich AD, Braverman B, et al: Monoamine oxidase inhibitors: Should they be discontinued preoperatively? Anesth Analg 1985;64:592-596.

39. Wong KC: Preoperative discontinuation of monoamine oxidase inhibitor therapy: An old wives' tale. Semin Anesthiol 1986;5:145-148.

40. Browne B, Linter S: Monoamine oxidase inhibitors and narcotic analgesics: A critical review of the implications for treatment. Br J Psychiatry 1987;151:210-212.

41. Hypericum Depression Trial Study Group: Effect of *Hypericum perforatum* (St. John's wort) in major depressive disorder: A randomized, controlled trial. JAMA 2002;287:1807-1814.

42. Scher CS, Anwar M: The self-reporting of psychiatric medications in patients scheduled for elective surgery. J Clin Anesth 1999;7:619-621.

43. Kaye AD, Sabar R, Clarke R, et al: Herbal medications and anesthetics: A review on current concepts. Am J Anesth 2000;27:467-471.

44. Kaye AD, Clarke R, Sabar R, et al: Herbal medicines: Current trends in anesthesiology practice—a hospital survey. J Clin Anesth 2000;12:468-471.

45. Kudoh A, Takahira Y, Katagai H, et al: Schizophrenic patients who develop postoperative confusion have an increased norepinephrine and cortisol response to surgery. Neuropsychobiology 2002;46:7-12.

46. Kudoh A, Katagai H, Takazawa T: Antidepressant treatment for chronic depressed patients should not be discontinued prior to anesthesia. Can J Anesth 2002;49:132-136.

47. Kudoh A, Takase H, Takazawa T: Chronic treatment with antidepressants decreases interoperative core hypothermia. Anesth Analg 2003;97:275-279.

48. Rehm LP, Wagner AL, Ivens-Tyndal C: Mood disorders: Unipolar and bipolar. In Sutker PB, Adams HE (eds): Comprehensive Handbook of Psychopathology, 3rd ed. New York, Kluwer Academic/Plenum Publishers, 2001, pp 277-308.

49. Judd LL, Akiskal HS: The prevalence and disability of bipolar spectrum disorders in the US population: Re-analysis of the ECA database taking into account subthreshold cases. J Affect Disord 2003;73: 123-131.

50. Stoelting RK, Dierdorf SF: Psychiatric disease and substance abuse. In: Anesthesia and Co-existing Disease, 4th ed. Philadelphia, Churchill Livingstone, 2002, pp 629-654.

51. Hill GE, Wong KC, Hodges MR: Lithium carbonate and neuromuscular blocking agents. Anesthesiology 1977;46:122-126.

52. Lichtor JL: Anesthesia for ambulatory surgery. In Barash PG, Cullen BF, Stoelting RK (eds): Clinical Anesthesia, 4th ed. Philadelphia, Lippincott Williams & Wilkins, 2001, pp 1217-1238.

53. Stoll AL, Severus WE, Freeman MP, et al: Omega 3 fatty acids in bipolar disorder: A preliminary double-blind, placebo-controlled trial. Arch Gen Psychiatry 1999;56:407-412.

54. Naguib M, Koorn R: Interactions between psychotropics, anesthetics and electroconvulsive therapy: Implications for drug choice and patient management. CNS Drugs 2002;16:229-247.

55. Benatov R, Sirota P, Megged S: Neuroleptic-resistant schizophrenia treated with clozapine and ECT. Convuls Ther 1996;12:117-121.

56. Conca A, Germann R, König P: Etomidate vs. thiopentone in electroconvulsive therapy. Pharmacopsychiatry 2003;36:94-97.

57. Selvin BL: Electroconvulsive therapy—1987. Anesthesiology 1987;67:367-385.

58. American Psychiatric Association Committee on Electroconvulsive Therapy: The Practice of Electroconvulsive Therapy: Recommendations for Treatment, Training, and Privileging, 2nd ed. Washington, DC, APA, 2001.

59. Sackeim HA, Devanand DP, Prudic J: Stimulus intensity, seizure threshold, and seizure duration: Impact on the efficacy and safety of electroconvulsive therapy. Psychiatr Clin North Am 1991;14:803-843.

60. Gerring JP, Shields HM: The identification and management of patients with a high risk for cardiac dysrhythmias during modified ECT. J Clin Psychiatry 1981;43:140-143.

61. Wulfson HD, Askanazi J, Finck AD: Propranolol prior to ECT associated with asystole. Anesthesiology 1984;60:255-256.

62. Trzepacz PT, Weniger FC, Greenhouse J: Etomidate anesthesia increases seizure duration during ECT: A retrospective study. Gen Hosp Psychiatry 1993;15:115-120.

63. Rasmussen KG, Jarvis MR, Zorumski CF: Ketamine anesthesia in electroconvulsive therapy. Convuls Ther 1996;12:217-223.

64. Greenberg PE, Sisitsky T, Kessler RC, et al: The economic burden of anxiety disorders in the 1990s. J Clin Psychiat 1999;60:427-435.

65. Leon AC, Portera L, Weissman MM: The social costs of anxiety disorders. Br J Psychiatry 1995;166(suppl 27):19-22.

66. Lépine J-P: The epidemiology of anxiety disorders: Prevalence and societal costs. J Clin Psychiat 2002;63(suppl 14):4-8.

67. Furmark T, Tillfors M, Everz P-O, et al: Social phobia in the general population: Prevalence and sociodemographic profile. Soc Psychiatry Psychiatr Epidemiol 1999;34:416-424.

68. Lang AJ, Stein MB: Social phobia: Prevalence and diagnostic threshold. J Clin Psychiatry 2001;62(suppl 1):5-10.

69. Turner SM, Beidel DC, Stanley MA, et al: Obsessive-compulsive disorder. In Sutker PB, Adams HE (eds): Comprehensive Handbook of Psychopathology, 3rd ed. New York, Kluwer Academic/Plenum Publishers, 2001, pp 151-182.

70. Kessler RC, Sonnega A, Bromet E, et al: Posttraumatic stress disorder in the national comorbidity survey. Arch Gen Psychiatry 1995;52: 1048-1060.

71. Kulka RA, Schlenger WE, Fairbank JA, et al: Trauma and the Vietnam War Generation: Report of Findings from the National Vietnam Veterans Readjustment Study. New York, Brunner/Mazel, 1990.

72. Sutker PB, Uddo M, Brailey K, et al: Psychopathology in war-zone deployed and nondeployed Operation Desert Storm troops assigned graves registration duties. J Abn Psychol 1994;103:383-390.

73. Sutker PB, Allain AN, Winstead DK: Psychopathology and psychiatric diagnoses of World War II Pacific theater prisoner of war survivors and combat veterans. Am J Psychiatry 1993;150:240-245.

74. Sutker PB, Winstead DK, Galina ZH, et al: Cognitive deficits and psychopathology among former prisoners of war and combat veterans of the Korean conflict. Am J Psychiatry 1991;148:67-72.

75. Barlow DH: Anxiety and Its Disorders: The Nature and Treatment of Anxiety and Panic. New York, Guilford, 1988.

76. Christ D: Central neuropharmacology. In: High-Yield Pharmacology, 2nd ed. Philadelphia, Lippincott Williams & Wilkins, 2004, pp 50-71.

77. Mycek MJ, Harvey RA, Champe PC: Anxiolytic and hypnotic drugs. In Harvey RA, Champe PC (eds): Pharmacology, 2nd ed. Philadelphia, Lippincott Williams & Wilkins, 2000, pp 89-98.

78. Stahl SM: Anxiolytics and sedative-hypnotics. In: Essential Psychopharmacology: Neuroscientific Basis and Practical

Applications, 2nd ed. Cambridge, Cambridge University Press, 2000, pp 297-334.

79. Woelk H, Kapula O, Lehrl S, et al: Comparison of kava special extract WS 1490 and benzodiazepines in patients with anxiety. Allg Med 1993;69:271-277.

80. Pittler MH, Ernst E: Efficacy of kava extract for treating anxiety: Systematic review and meta-analysis. J Clin Psychopharmacol 2000;20:84-89.

81. Volz HP, Kieser M: Kava-kava extract WS 1490 versus placebo in anxiety disorders—a randomized placebo-controlled 25-week outpatient trial. Pharmacopsychiatry 1997;30:1-5.

82. Lehman E, Kinzler E, Friedemann J, et al: Efficacy of a special kava extract (piper methysticum) in patients with states of anxiety, tension, and excitedness of non-mental origin—a double-blind placebo-controlled study of four weeks treatment. Phytomedicine 1996;3:113-119.

83. Pratt SI, Mueser KT: Schizophrenia. In Antony MM, Barlow DH (eds): Handbook of Assessment and Treatment Planning for Psychological Disorders. New York, Guilford, 2002, pp 375-414.

84. Maher BA, Deldin PJ: Schizophrenia: Biological aspects. In Sutker PB, Adams HE (eds): Comprehensive Handbook of Psychopathology, 3rd ed. New York, Kluwer Academic/Plenum Publishers, 2001, pp 341-370.

85. Kane JM: Pharmacologic treatment of schizophrenia. Biol Psychiatry 1999;46:1396-1408.

86. Gibson RL, Burch EA: Emotional disorder and medical illness. In Sutker PB, Adams HE (eds): Comprehensive Handbook of Psychopathology, 3rd ed. New York, Kluwer Academic/Plenum Publishers, 2001, pp 797-811.

87. Mycek MJ, Harvey RA, Champe PC: Neuroleptic drugs. In Harvey RA, Champe PC (eds): Pharmacology, 2nd ed. Philadelphia, Lippincott Williams & Wilkins, 2000, pp 127-132.

88. Janicak PG, Davis JM, Preskorn SH, Ayd FJ Jr: Treatment with antipsychotics. In: Principles and Practice of Psychopharmacotherapy, 3rd ed. Philadelphia, Lippincott Williams & Wilkins, 2001, pp 83-192.

89. Stahl SM: Antipsychotic agents. In: Essential Psychopharmacology: Neuroscientific Basis and Practical Applications, 2nd ed. Cambridge, Cambridge University Press, 2000, pp 401-458.

90. Pollard JB, Brook MW, Shafer A: Patient threats present an ethical dilemma for the anesthesiologist. Anesth Analg 2001;93:1544-1545.

91. Kudoh A, Kudo M, Ishihara H: Depressed pituitary-adrenal response to surgical stress in chronic schizophrenic patients. Neuropsychobiology 1997;36:112-116.

92. Kudoh A, Kudo M, Ishihara H, et al: Increased plasma vasopressin and atrial natriuretic peptide in chronic schizophrenic patients during abdominal surgery. Neuropsychobiology 1998;37:169-174.

93. Goodwin RD, Marusic A, Hoven CW: Suicide attempts in the United States: The role of physical illness. Soc Sci Med 2003;56:1783-1788.

94. Geiduschek J, Cohen SA, Khan A, Cullen BF: Repeated anesthesia for a patient with neuroleptic malignant syndrome. Anesthesiology 1988;68:134-137.

95. Maher BA: Delusions. In Sutker PB, Adams HE (eds): Comprehensive Handbook of Psychopathology, 3rd ed. New York, Kluwer Academic/Plenum Publishers, 2001, pp 308-339.

96. Smothers BA, Yahr HT, Sinclair MD: Prevalence of current DSM-IV alcohol use disorders in short-stay, general hospital admissions, United States, 1994. Arch Intern Med 2003;163:713-719.

97. Wu L-T, Ringwalt CL, Williams CE: Use of substance abuse treatment services by persons with mental health and substance use problems. Psychiatr Serv 2003;54:363-369.

98. Saunders JB, Aasland OG, Babor TF, et al: Development of the alcohol use disorders identification test (AUDIT): WHO collaborative project on early detection of persons with harmful alcohol consumption: II. Addiction 1993;88:791-804.

99. Zakriya KJ, Christmas C, Wenz JF, et al: Preoperative factors associated with postoperative change in confusion assessment method score in hip fracture patients. Anesth Analg 2002;94:1628-1632.

100. Bready LL: Delayed emergence. In Bready LL, Smith RB (eds): Decision Making in Anesthesiology, 2nd ed. St. Louis, Mosby–Year Book, 1992, pp 364-365.

101. Mycek MJ, Harvey RA, Champe PC: CNS stimulants. In Harvey RA, Champe PC (eds): Pharmacology, 2nd ed. Philadelphia, Lippincott Williams & Wilkins, 2000, pp 99-106.

102. Stahl SM: Cognitive enhancers. In: Essential Psychopharmacology: Neuroscientific Basis and Practical Applications, 2nd ed. Cambridge, Cambridge University Press, 2000, pp 459-498.

103. Tariot PN, Farlow MR, Grossberg GT, et al: Memantine treatment in patients with moderate to severe Alzheimer disease already receiving donepezil: A randomized controlled trial. JAMA 2004;291:317-324.

104. Eisendrath SJ, Lichtmacher JE: Psychiatric disorders. In Tierney LM Jr, McPhee SJ, Papadakis MA (eds): Current Medical Diagnosis and Treatment. New York, Lange Medical Books/McGraw-Hill, 2004, pp 1001-1061.

105. Ancelin M-L, De Roquefeuil G, Ledésert B, et al: Exposure to anesthetic agents, cognitive functioning and depressive symptomatology in the elderly. Br J Psychiatry 2001;178:360-366.

106. Grichnik KP, Ijsselmuiden AJJ, D'Amico TA, et al: Cognitive decline after major noncardiac operations: A preliminary prospective study. Ann Thorac Surg 1999;68:1786-1791.

107. Selnes OA, Goldsborough MA, Borowitz LM Jr, et al: Determinants of cognitive change after coronary artery bypass surgery: A multifactorial problem. Ann Thorac Surg 1999;67:1669-1676.

108. Mitchell SJ, Pellett O, Gorman DF: Cerebral protection by lidocaine during cardiac operations. Ann Thorac Surg 1999;67:1117-1124.

109. Wang D, Wu X, Li J, et al: The effect of lidocaine on early postoperative cognitive dysfunction after coronary artery bypass surgery. Anesth Analg 2002;95:1134-1141.

110. Butterworth J, Hammon JW: Lidocaine for neuroprotection: More evidence of efficacy. Anesth Analg 2002;95:1131-1133.

111. Chan WP, Chilvers CR: Induction of anesthesia in the home. Anesth Intensive Care 2002;30:809-812.

112. Martin A, Leslie D: Psychiatric inpatient, outpatient, and medication utilization and costs among privately insured youths, 1997-2000. Am J Psychiatry 2003;160:757-764.

113. Stordy BJ: Dark adaptation, motor skills, docosahexaenoic acid, and dyslexia. Am J Clin Nutr 2000;71(suppl 1):323S-326S.

114. Kaye AD, Kucera I, Sabar R: Perioperative anesthesia clinical considerations of alternative medicines. Anesthesiol Clin North Am 2004;22:125-139.

115. Bedford S, Melzer D, Guralnik J: Problem behavior in the last year of life: Prevalence, risks, and care receipt in older Americans. J Am Geriatr Assoc 2001;49:590-595.

16 Patients on Herbal Medications

Alan D. Kaye, MD, PhD, DABPM, and Jason M. Hoover, MD

The use of herbal medications or nutraceutical agents in the form of herbal remedies has increased significantly in the United States in recent years. The majority of consumers of herbal agents are white middle-aged women with some college education.[1] A recent study of 567 rural women found that 59.1% of the participants used herbal medications.[2] Currently, evidence is lacking regarding the effectiveness of certain herbal medications, their potential interactions with over-the-counter (OTC) or prescribed medications, and the potential side effects of herbal medications when used alone or in conjunction with OTC or prescribed medications. In addition, there seems to be an increasing trend toward the reimbursement of herbal medications by managed care organizations and insurance companies.[3]

The medical community, in general, and the anesthesiologist, in particular, should be cognizant of what data and information are available regarding herbal medications. For example, the medical community may not be aware that approximately 30% of all modern conventional therapeutic agents are derived from plants.[4] Furthermore, the clinical anesthesiologist might be interested in a recent survey of 752 patients scheduled for elective surgery that was conducted within the Department of Anesthesiology at Texas Tech University in Lubbock. The results of this study revealed that, of those surveyed, 32% were actively using at least one herbal agent and 70% of these patients did not inform their anesthesiologist of such use during the routine preoperative assessment.[5] Knowing that herbal medications can have effects on the central nervous, respiratory, cardiovascular, and gastrointestinal systems, to name a few, the importance of education in the form of

a brief history and thorough examination of selected herbal medications cannot be overlooked.

The use of herbal medications, in some capacity, has occurred for centuries throughout the world. In the United States, herbal medicine use began in the early colonial days when health care was, for the most part, provided in the home. By the 19th century, the advancement of scientific methods allowed for the practice of conventional medicine to flourish and the subsequent decrease in the use of herbal medications.[3] It was not until the 1960s that herbal agents began to return in popularity, and in 1992 the Office of Alternative Medicines was established by the National Institutes of Health in Bethesda, Maryland, thus reflecting the prevalence of herbal use.

Many herbal agents are not regulated strictly as to their quality assurance and, therefore, consumers must rely on manufacturer labels.[6] Unfortunately, patients often do not consider herbal compounds to be medications and, as mentioned previously, do not convey the use of such agents during the preoperative assessment.[5] Furthermore, one estimate concluded that as many as 20% of the adult U. S. population take prescription drugs along with herbal medications.[7,8] Herbal medications are recognized under the Dietary Supplement Health and Education Act, and this act has served to limit the regulation of such substances by the U. S. Food and Drug Administration (FDA).[1] For example, in contrast to prescription medication, the FDA must first demonstrate that an herbal agent is unsafe before it is removed from the market.[6] With savvy advertisement by herbal manufacturers, word-of-mouth popularity, and a relatively lax standardization policy by the FDA regarding these herbal compounds, the herbal industry has become a multibillion dollar industry.[3] Finally, the medical community has observed patients dissatisfied with the cost or effectiveness of their prescription medications searching for the easily obtainable and relatively inexpensive panacea of herbal medications.

A survey from 1996 of 163 health food retail stores in the United States indicated the top selling herbal medications were echinacea (*Echinacea purpurea, Echinacea pallida,* and *Echinacea angustifolia*), garlic (*Allium sativum*), goldenseal (*Hydrastis canadenis*), ginseng (*Asian Panax ginseng* and *American Panax quinquefolius*), gingko (*Gingko biloba*), saw palmetto (*Serenoa repens*), aloe (*Aloe* species), ma huang (*Ephedra sinica*), and Siberian ginseng (*Eleutherococcus senticosus*).[6,9] Data from 1998 revealed that St. John's wort (*Hypericum perforatum*), valerian (*Valeriana officinalis*), and feverfew (*Tanacetum parthenium*) were also gaining in popularity.[3] To support such conclusions, a survey of 755 patients scheduled to undergo outpatient surgery from 2000 found garlic, gingko biloba, and St. John's wort to be among the top herbal agents self-administered by patients (Fig. 16-1).[10]

With the recent federal ban on ma huang (*Ephedra sinica*) the use of that herbal may decrease; but with the seemingly infinite number of herbal medications, it is certain that another agent will take its place. The anesthesiologist should recognize the prevalence of these compounds and their physiologic effects on the patient. For example, some herbal medications have the potential to decrease platelet aggregation and inhibit clotting (Table 16-1), and their use should be included in the differential of perioperative bleeding. The risks of bleeding remain dependent on the dose and preparation of the herbal in question. The American Society of Anesthesiologists (ASA) has suggested that anyone taking an herbal medication

TABLE 16–1   Herbal Medications Associated with Bleeding Abnormalities
Bilberry
Bromelain
Chamomile
Dandelion root
Dong quoi
Fenugreek
Feverfew
Fish oil
Flax seed oil
Garlic
Ginger
Gingko biloba
Ginseng
Grape seed extract
Horse chestnut
Kava kava
Meadowsweet
Motherworth
Red clover
Tamarind
Turmeric
Willow

should desist ingestion for at least 2 to 3 weeks before a surgical procedure to ensure that the herbal medication is no longer in the system. It takes five half-lives for a drug (or herbal medication) to clear the system; given the variability in the preparation and bioavailability of herbal medications, the 2- to 3-week guideline is a general estimate to cover all preparations. Furthermore, there are herbal agents that cause alteration of the cytochrome P450 system and herbal medications that are associated with hepatotoxicity and/or nephrotoxicity (Tables 16-2 and 16-3). Finally, some herbal agents may potentiate the depressant effects of central nervous system anesthetics and, in the case of ginseng, inhibit the analgesic effect of opioids (Tables 16-4 and 16-5).[11] In this chapter, we review popular herbal medications, their intended use, physiologic

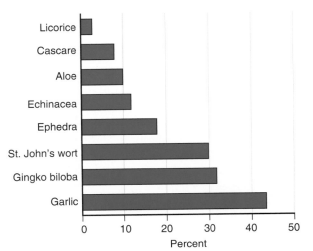

FIGURE 16-1 Percentage of patients self-administering herbal medications. (*Adapted from Kaye AD, Clarke RC, et al: Herbal medicines: Current trends in anesthesiology practice—a hospital survey. J Clin Anesth 2000;12:468-471, with permission.*)

TABLE 16–2   Herbal Medications Associated with Serum Medication Concentration Abnormalities
Echinacea
Garlic
Kava kava
St. John's wort

TABLE 16–3   Herbal Medications Associated with Liver and/or Renal Dysfunction
Echinacea
Kava kava
Meadowsweet
Willow

TABLE 16–4   Herbal Medications Associated with Excessive CNS Depression During Anesthesia
Chamomile
Hops
Kava kava
Passion flower
Valerian

effects, side effects, and potential interactions with anesthetic agents.

ECHINACEA

The *Echinacea* are members of the daisy family and grow widely throughout North America. There are nine species of *Echinacea,* and the medicinal preparations are primarily derived from three of these: *Echinacea pallida* (pale purple coneflower), *Echinacea purpurea* (purple coneflower), and *Echinacea angustifolia* (narrow leaved coneflower).[12-14] This herbal medication accounts for more than $300 million in sales each year. The recommended use of echinacea is as a prophylactic and as a treatment agent for upper respiratory tract infections, although evidence is lacking to support the former.[6] It has alkylamide and polysaccharide constituents that possess significant in-vitro and in-vivo immunostimulation properties, owing to enhanced phagocytosis and nonspecific T-cell stimulation.[15]

The consumption of echinacea at the onset of symptoms has been clinically shown to decrease both the severity and duration of the cold and flu. Investigations utilizing quantitative polymerase chain reaction to identify in-vivo alterations in the expression of immunomodulatory genes in response to echinacea have been performed.[16] Studies conducted on in-vivo gene expression within peripheral

TABLE 16–5 Common Herbal Medications, Adverse Effects, and Anesthetic Considerations		
Herbal Medication	**Adverse Effects**	**Anesthetic Considerations**
Echinacea	Unpleasant taste, tachyphylaxis, cytochrome P450 alterations, potential hepatotoxicity	May potentiate barbiturate toxicity
Ephedra	Hypertension, tachycardia, cardiomyopathy, CVA, cardiac arrhythmias	May interact with volatile anesthetics, i.e., halothane, and cause ? fatal cardiac dysrhythmias. Profound intraoperative hypotension controlled with phenylephrine and not pseudoephedrine.
Feverfew	Aphthous ulcers, gastrointestinal irritability, headache	Increased risk of intraoperative bleeding; discontinue 2 to 3 weeks before surgery.
Garlic	Halitosis, prolongation of bleeding time, hypotension, cytochrome P450 alterations	Increased risk of intraoperative bleeding
Ginger	Prolongation of bleeding time	Increased risk of intraoperative hemodynamic instability
Gingko biloba	Platelet dysfunction	Increased intraoperative and postoperative bleeding tendencies. May decrease effectiveness of intravenous barbiturates
Ginseng	Hypertension, prolonged bleeding time, hypoglycemia, insomnia, headache, vomiting, epistaxis	Increased risk of intraoperative hemodynamic instability
Kava kava	Characteristic ichthyosiform dermopathy, cytochrome P450 alterations, potential hepatotoxicity	May potentiate the effect of barbiturates/benzodiazepines, thereby resulting in excessive sedation
St. John's wort	Dry mouth, dizziness, cytochrome P450 alterations, constipation, nausea	Pseudoephedrine, MAOIs, and SSRIs should be avoided

CVA, cerebrovascular accident; MAOIs, monoamine oxidase inhibitors; SSRIs, selective serotonin reuptake inhibitors.
Adapted from Kaye AD, Clarke RC, Sabar R, et al: Herbal medicines: Current trends in anesthesiology practice—A hospital survey. J Clin Anesth 2000;12:468-471.

leukocytes were evaluated in six healthy nonsmoking subjects (18 to 65 years of age). Blood samples were obtained at baseline and on days 2, 3, 5, and 12 after consumption of a commercially blended echinacea product. The overall gene expression pattern at 48 hours to 12 days after taking echinacea was consistent with an anti-inflammatory response. The expression of interleukin-1β, intracellular adhesion molecule, tumor necrosis factor-α (TNF-α), and interleukin-8 was modestly decreased up through day 5 and returned to baseline by day 12. In addition, the expression of interferon-alfa consistently increased through day 12, indicating an antiviral response. Thus, the initial data yielded a gene expression response pattern consistent with the reported ability of echinacea to decrease both the intensity and the duration of cold and flu symptoms.[16]

Although different preparations of E. purpurea have been investigated for their potential to augment immune function, primarily through the activation of the innate immune responses, there are few studies available that have examined the ability for enhancement of humoral immunity. However, a study using female Swiss mice as the model found support for the acute use of E. purpurea, as suggested by anecdotal reports, and demonstrated the potential for enhancement of humoral immune responses in addition to innate immune responses.[17] Despite the anecdotal reports and immunostimulatory data associated with echinacea, the use of E. purpurea, as dosed in one study, was not effective in treating upper respiratory tract infections and related symptoms in pediatric patients, ages 2 to 11. Furthermore, the consumption of E. purpurea was associated with an increased risk of rash.[18]

Echinacea is often well tolerated, with the most common side effect being its unpleasant taste.[6,19] Extended use of echinacea for more than 2 months may lead to tachyphylaxis.[20] Anaphylaxis has also been reported with a single dose of this herbal agent.[12] Furthermore, echinacea use has been associated with hepatoxicity if taken with other anesthetic or nonanesthetic hepatotoxic agents such as anabolic steroids, amiodarone, ketoconazole, and methotrexate.[21] Flavonoids from E. purpurea can affect the hepatic cytochrome P450 and sulfotransferase systems.[22,23] For example, one investigation found that echinacea decreased the oral clearance of substrates of the cytochrome P450 1A2 system but not the oral clearance of substrates of the 2C9 and 2D6 isoenzymes in vivo. The herbal agent also selectively modulates the activity of the cytochrome P450 P3A isoenzyme at both hepatic and intestinal sites. The researchers, therefore, urged caution when echinacea is combined with medications dependent on the cytochrome P450 3A or 1A2 systems for elimination.[24] Finally, echinacea use should not last longer than 4 weeks, and it should not be used in patients with systemic and autoimmune disorders, patients who are pregnant, and patients who are immunocompromised.[6,25]

Anesthesia Implications. The immunostimulatory effects of echinacea may antagonize the immunosuppressive actions of corticosteroids and cyclosporine. Because the herb can cause inhibition of the hepatic microsomal enzymes, its concomitant use with drugs such as phenytoin, rifampin, and phenobarbital, which are metabolized by the hepatic microsomal enzymes, should be avoided, because echinacea can precipitate toxicity of these drugs.

EPHEDRA

As previously mentioned, the recent federal ban on ephedra, also known as ma huang, may lead to a decline in its use. However, patients may still present for perioperative assessment with a history or present use of ephedra. Ma huang, an ephedra-based alkaloid, is similar in structure to amphetamines and is traditionally indicated for the treatment of various respiratory disorders, such as the common cold, flu, allergies, bronchitis, and nonrespiratory conditions such as appetite suppression.[6] Other indications are hypotension, fever, arthritis, and fluid retention. Ma huang acts as a sympathomimetic agent and exhibits potent positive inotropic and chronotropic responses. In addition to its antitussive actions, ma huang may also possess bacteriostatic properties.[26] As a cardiovascular and respiratory sympathomimetic, it utilizes an α- or β-adrenergic sensitive pathway.[27] Furthermore, recent laboratory data using the feline pulmonary vascular bed indicate that ma huang–mediated pulmonary hypertension is dependent on an α_1-adrenoreceptor sensitive pathway.[28]

The appetite suppressant and metabolic enhancer effects of ma huang made it a potent ingredient of various OTC weight loss compounds. However, before the federal ban on ma huang, many herbal manufacturers advertised ephedra-free supplements as a result of its numerous reported adverse effects.

Deleterious effects of ma huang administration include hypertension, tachycardia, cardiomyopathy, cardiac dysrhythmias, myocardial infarction, stroke, seizures, psychosis, tremors, and/or death.[6] Numerous complications have been linked to the use of this herbal agent, and these outcomes have been attributed to a lack of standardization in its formulation.[29,30] Before the federal ban of ma huang, approximately 16,000 cases of adverse events and 164 deaths had been reported to the FDA since 1994.[31] Furthermore, the Bureau of Food and Drug Safety of the Texas Department of Health reported eight fatalities, during a 21-month period between 1993 and 1995, associated with ephedra-containing compounds. Seven of these deaths were secondary to myocardial infarction or stroke.[8] Patients who are pregnant or have hypertension, coronary vascular disease, a seizure history, glaucoma, anxiety, and mania are at significant risk for ephedra-induced side effects.[6]

Anesthesia Implications. The use of ephedrine-containing OTC products is highly relevant to the perioperative period. The possibility of hypertension causing myocardial ischemia or stroke needs to be considered. Ephedra can potentially interact with volatile general anesthetic agents (e.g., halothane, isoflurane, desflurane) and cardiac glycosides (e.g., digitalis) to cause cardiac dysrhythmias. Patients taking ephedra for prolonged periods of time can deplete peripheral catecholamine stores. Thus, under general anesthesia, these patients can potentially have profound intraoperative hypotension, which can be controlled with a direct vasoconstrictor (e.g., phenylephrine) instead of ephedrine. Use of ephedra with phenelzine or other monoamine oxidase inhibitors may result in insomnia, headache, and tremulousness. Concomitant use with oxytocin has been shown to cause hypertension.[32]

FEVERFEW

The herbal agent feverfew is used to treat headache and fever, prevent migraines, and treat menstrual abnormalities.[33] The word is derived from the Latin word *febrifugia*, which means "fever reducer."[26] Although feverfew is commonly used for migraine headaches, the literature is not conclusive with regard to its effectiveness.[34,35] For example, one investigation sought to review evidence from double-blind randomized controlled trials to evaluate the clinical efficacy of feverfew versus placebo for migraine prophylaxis. The researchers concluded that there was insufficient evidence from the trials to suggest a benefit of feverfew over placebo for the prevention of migraine.[36] Like most herbal compounds, analyses of feverfew-based products have yielded significant variations in the parthenolide contents, a proposed active ingredient, between feverfew products.[37]

Regarding the effects of the anti-inflammatory lactone parthenolide, one German study has indicated that parthenolide may support T-cell survival by down-regulating the CD95 system. The CD95 system is a critical component of the apoptotic, or programmed cell death, pathway of activated T cells. The investigators concluded that parthenolide may have some therapeutic potential as an anti-apoptotic substance against the activation-induced cell death of activated T cells.[38]

Feverfew also has demonstrated inhibition of serotonin release from aggregating platelets. This mechanism may be related to the inhibition of arachidonic acid release via a phospholipase pathway.[39-41] Furthermore, feverfew has effectively decreased 86% to 88% of prostaglandin production without exhibiting inhibition of cyclooxygenase.[42]

Adverse reactions to feverfew include aphthous ulcers, abdominal pain, flatulence, nausea, vomiting, and rebound headache with an abrupt stoppage of the herb.[26,33] This herbal may be better tolerated than other conventional migraine medications because in clinical trials feverfew caused no change in heart rate, blood pressure, body weight, or blood chemistry like conventional migraine drugs.[33] As with many herbal agents, feverfew is not recommended in the pediatric population or pregnant or nursing patients.[43] Finally, a condition known as "post-feverfew syndrome" can occur in chronic users of feverfew and manifests as anxiety, headaches, insomnia, arthralgias, muscle and joint stiffness, and fatigue.[33,44]

Anesthesia Implications. Because feverfew can inhibit platelet activity, it is reasonable to avoid the concomitant use of this herb in patients taking medications such as heparin, warfarin, nonsteroidal anti-inflammatory agents (NSAIDs), aspirin, and vitamin E.[45,46] For patients with perioperative bleeding abnormalities, the use of feverfew should be considered in the differential diagnosis. Furthermore, tannin-containing herbs like feverfew can interact with iron preparations, thereby reducing the bioavailability of such preparations.[21]

GARLIC

Garlic is a popular herbal medication that is available in powdered, dried, and fresh forms.[6] Allicin, the main active ingredient in garlic, contains sulfur. Crushing the garlic clove activates the enzyme allinase, which results in the conversion of alliin to allicin.[12]

Recommended use has centered on treating hypercholesterolemia, hypertension, and cardiovascular disease.[6] Thus, recent studies have targeted its hypocholesterolemic and vasodilatory effects.[47-51] Investigations have concluded that garlic may cause inhibition of the HMG-CoA reductase and 14α-demthylase enzyme systems to exert its lipid-lowering effect.[6] Additionally, garlic derivatives may be used for their antiplatelet, antioxidant, and fibrinolytic actions.[47,52,53] Decreased platelet aggregation has been reported with the use of garlic in conjunction with its use for hyperlipidemia.[48-51] However, there is minimal evidence corroborating the use of garlic for hypertension, because its depressor effects on systolic and diastolic blood pressure appear to range from minimal to modest.[6,12]

Long-term oral consumption of garlic has been reported to augment the endogenous antioxidants of the heart.[54] A recent investigation hypothesized that garlic-induced cardiac antioxidants may provide protection against acute doxorubicin (Adriamycin)-induced cardiotoxicity. Using rats as the model, the researchers found in the doxorubicin group increased oxidative stress, as evidenced by a significant increase in myocardial thiobarbituric acid reactive substances (TBARS) and a decrease in myocardial superoxide dismutase (SOD), catalase, and glutathione peroxidase activity. However, in the garlic-treated rats, an increase in myocardial TBARS and a decrease in endogenous antioxidants by doxorubicin was significantly prevented.

Thus, the investigators concluded that chronic garlic administration may prevent acute doxorubicin-induced cardiotoxicity.[54]

Regarding the effects of allicin in the lung vasculature, data have revealed that allicin has significant vasodilator activity in the pulmonary vascular bed of the rat and cat.[55]

Furthermore, although allicin has been found to lower blood pressure, insulin, and triglyceride levels in fructose-fed rats, it has also been considered important to investigate its effect on the weight of animals. One group of researchers used male Sprague-Dawley rats and found that the control group that was fed a diet enriched by only fructose continued to have an increase in weight. However, those groups fed allicin did not have weight gain.[56]

Evidence indicates that garlic may also be an effective treatment against methicillin-resistant *Staphylococcus aureus* (MRSA) infection. Using mice as the model, investigators demonstrated that the garlic extracts diallyl sulfide and diallyl disulfide exhibited protective functions against MRSA infection. Such conclusions, coupled with further study, may result in the employment of these extracts in the treatment of MRSA infection.[57]

Side effects of garlic are minimal, with odor and gastrointestinal distress being the most commonly reported.[6] However, there is a reported case of spontaneous spinal/epidural hematoma in an 87-year-old man that was thought to be associated with platelet dysfunction as a result of excessive ingestion of garlic.[58] Finally, induction of the cytochrome P450 system may occur, as evidenced by reduction of serum levels of the medication saquinavir.[6]

Anesthesia Implications. The clinical anesthesiologist should be aware that garlic may augment the effects of warfarin, heparin, NSAIDs, and aspirin and may result in an abnormal bleeding time, which can lead to an increased risk of intraoperative or postoperative bleeding.[59] In addition, an investigation on the effects of garlic dialysate on diastolic blood pressure (DBP), heart rate (HR), and electrocardiographic (ECG) readings in anesthetized dogs, and its effects on frequency and tension of isolated rat atria was conducted.[60] The garlic dialysate led to a decrease in DBP and HR in a dose-dependent manner, and the ECG readings revealed a regular sinus bradycardic rhythm. Furthermore, the addition of garlic dialysate to isolated left rat atria resulted in a decrease in tension development in a dose-dependent manner. Finally, the results revealed that the positive chronotropism and inotropism induced by the addition of isoproterenol were partially antagonized by preincubation of the rat atria with the garlic dialysate. The investigators concluded that these findings may be explained by a depressant effect on automaticity and tension development in the heart, thus suggesting a β-adrenergic antagonist action modulated by garlic dialysate.[60]

GINGER

Ginger *(Zingiber officinale)* has been used for the treatment of nausea, vomiting, motion sickness, and vertigo.[25] The effects of ginger on study subjects with vertigo found that none of the study subjects experienced nausea after caloric stimulation of the vestibular system. This finding was in contrast to those receiving the placebo.[61] Furthermore, ginger may be superior to the agent dimenhydrinate in decreasing motion sickness.[62]

A randomized, double-blind, controlled trial compared the efficacy of ginger to vitamin B_6 for the treatment of nausea and vomiting during pregnancy. The investigators found the nausea score and number of vomiting episodes were significantly reduced after ginger and vitamin B_6 therapy. Comparing the efficacy of ginger and vitamin B_6, the researchers concluded there was no significant difference between them when used for the treatment of nausea and vomiting during pregnancy.[63] Ginger has also been effective in abating the symptoms associated with hyperemesis gravidarum.[64]

Regarding the effects of ginger on coagulation, it has exhibited potent inhibition of thromboxane synthetase. Such inhibition in activity results in a prolonged bleeding time.[65] The ability of ginger constituents and related substances to inhibit arachidonic acid-induced platelet activation in human whole blood has been studied. The data from that investigation revealed that ginger compounds and derivatives are more potent antiplatelet agents than aspirin under conditions employed in the study. Specifically, [8]-paradol, a natural constituent of ginger, was identified as the most potent antiplatelet aggregation agent and cyclooxygenase-1 inhibitor.[66]

Regarding treatment using ginger in type I diabetic rats, there was a significant increase in insulin levels and a decrease in fasting glucose levels in the rats. Administration of ginger also caused a decrease in blood pressure, serum cholesterol, and serum triglycerides in diabetic rats. The data from this investigation suggest a potential antidiabetic activity of ginger in type I diabetic rats.[67]

Side effects of ginger include bleeding abnormalities, and its use is contraindicated in patients with coagulation dysfunction or those on anticoagulant medications such as NSAIDs, aspirin, heparin, and warfarin.[25]

Anesthesia Implications. Ginger may increase bleeding risk, enhance barbiturate effects, and, as a result of an inotropic effect, interfere with cardiac medication therapy. Large quantities of ginger may also cause cardiac arrhythmias and central nervous system depression.

GINGKO BILOBA

Numerous active compounds are present in gingko, such as the flavonoid glycosides, terpenoids, and organic acids.

The physiologic effects of the compounds vary.[6,12] For example, the flavonoids have exhibited antioxidant activity and the terpenoids have demonstrated antagonistic ability to platelet-activating factor.[6] The extract that has received the most investigation is EGB761.

As a result of its effects, gingko is used to treat intermittent claudication, enhance memory, and treat diseases associated with free-radical production and vertigo.[8] Subjects using this herbal agent have reported decreased pain in the affected lower extremities and increased symptom-free walking distance. In addition to the inhibition of platelet-activating factor, gingko may also mediate nitric oxide release and decrease inflammation.[6,68-73] A recent investigation of 187 cardiology patients found that 106 of the subjects used supplements and that one of them was gingko. However, the data reported that the average low-density lipoprotein (106 vs. 108 mg/dL), average hemoglobin (Hb) A1c (8.7% vs. 7.7%), and average blood pressure (132/77 vs. 138/78 mm Hg) were not significantly different between users and nonusers of the supplements.[74]

To test the effects of gingko on dementia, a double-blind and placebo-controlled randomized trial of EGB761 was performed. The researchers found that this extract had the potential to stabilize and modestly improve cognitive performance and social functioning.[6,75] Furthermore, the modest improvement in cognition was comparable to the effect of donepezil on dementia.[6] The beneficial effect on cognition and memory attributed to gingko may be related to its activation of the cholinergic neurotransmitter system. The data are inconclusive regarding the ability of gingko to improve memory in healthy subjects.[6]

Regarding the effects of gingko on induced-acute pancreatitis, investigators have found that prophylactic treatment of EGB761 in Sprague-Dawley rats has a significant beneficial effect on the course of acute pancreatitis.[76] Although the pathogenesis of acute pancreatitis is not well understood, there are numerous data that suggest a role for oxygen free radicals in the progression and complications of pancreatitis. Therefore, the positive influence of EGB761 on acute pancreatitis may be linked to the free radical scavenger effect of this extract.[76]

At the recommended dose, gingko is well tolerated in the healthy adult population for approximately 6 months.[6] The side effects associated with its use may be limited to mild gastrointestinal discomfort and headache.[25] However, as a potential result of gingko's anti–platelet activating factor effect, gingko biloba–induced spontaneous hyphema (bleeding from iris and the anterior chamber of the eye), spontaneous bilateral subdural hematomas, and subarachnoid hemorrhage have been reported.[6,77-80] Therefore, the use of anticoagulants and gingko should be closely monitored, if not avoided.[6] Regarding the effects of gingko on pharmacokinetics, an open-labeled and randomized crossover trial was conducted on eight healthy human volunteers to determine if ginkgo alters the pharmacokinetics of digoxin. The investigators concluded that the concomitant use of orally administered gingko and digoxin did not appear to have any significant effect on the pharmacokinetics of digoxin in healthy volunteers.[81]

Anesthesia Implications. Concomitant use of gingko biloba with aspirin, or any NSAIDs, and anticoagulants such as warfarin and heparin is not recommended because gingko may increase the potential for bleeding in these patients. It would also be appropriate to avoid its concomitant use with anticonvulsant drugs (e.g., carbamazepine, phenytoin, phenobarbital) because gingko may decrease the effectiveness of these agents.[21] In addition, it has been recommended that gingko should be avoided in patients taking tricyclic antidepressant agents, because it might potentiate the seizure threshold-lowering action of these drugs.[21]

GINSENG

There is a significant variation in the components of this herb. There are three main groups of ginseng that are classified based on their geographic origin.[6] These are *Panax ginseng* (Asian ginseng), *Panax quinquefolius* (American ginseng), and *Eleutherococcus senticosus* (Siberian ginseng), which belongs to a different genus.[6,8] The active ingredients in ginseng are the ginsenosides.[6,26]

Asian and American ginseng have been used for their adaptogenic properties, which allow for increased resistance to environmental stress, as a diuretic, digestion aid, immune system stimulant, and hypoglycemic agent.[82,83] Asian ginseng may be effective in improving cognitive function when combined with gingko.[83] American ginseng has been examined for its potential to stimulate human TNF-α production in cultured human peripheral blood monocytes.[84] Direct stimulation of mononuclear cell TNF-α production in vitro occurred, as demonstrated by TNF-α mRNA gene expression, as early as 6 hours into cell incubation with ginseng. Thus, one may conclude that in-vitro immunostimulating activity of ginseng occurs when using TNF-α production as an index, and further in-vivo studies are warranted.[84] American ginseng may also possess hypoglycemic properties.[85,86] Such effects have been observed in both normal and diabetic subjects and may be attributed to the ginsenoside Rb2 and panaxans I, J, K, and L ingredients of ginseng.[87-91]

Although generally well tolerated, adverse effects of ginseng use are hypertension, bleeding abnormalities secondary to antiplatelet activity, insomnia, headache, vomiting, Stevens-Johnson syndrome, abnormal vaginal bleeding, and epistaxis.[92-98] Drug interactions between Asian ginseng and calcium channel blockers, warfarin, phenelzine, and digoxin have been reported.[6] Therefore, it is recommended that ginseng be avoided in patients who are pregnant or breastfeeding, the pediatric population, and patients with cardiovascular disease.[8,21]

Anesthesia Implications. Ginseng should be avoided with patients on anticoagulant medications such as warfarin, heparin, NSAIDs, and aspirin. Because ginseng can cause hypertension, the clinical anesthesiologist should be focused on the clinical consequences of long-term use of this agent. Long-standing hypertension can cause end-organ damage, volume depletion, and autonomic instability. Furthermore, because many anesthetic agents can cause generalized vasodilatory effects, hemodynamic variability can be seen, including profound intraoperative hypotension. Concomitant use of ginseng with monoamine oxidase inhibitors (e.g., phenelzine sulfate) should be avoided, because manic episodes have been reported with routine use of ginseng.[99,100] As a result of its potential to exert hypoglycemic effects, ginseng should be used cautiously in diabetic patients on insulin or oral hypoglycemic medications. It would therefore follow that the anesthesiologist would need to have appropriate evaluation of blood glucose levels perioperatively for applicable patients.

KAVA KAVA

Kava kava, an extract of the plant *Piper methysticum,* is used as an anxiolytic, antiepileptic, antidepressant, antipsychotic, sedative, and muscle relaxant.[101-103] Active ingredients of kava kava include the kava lactones or kava pyrones, kawain, methysticin, dihydrokawain, dihydromethysticin, along with others.[104,105] The kava extracts that are available commercially are formulated to contain between 30% and 70% kava lactones.[104]

The extract WS 1490 has been investigated in clinical studies to determine the effectiveness of kava kava for treatment of anxiety disorders.[104] WS 1490 has proved to be an effective treatment alternative to benzodiazepines and tricyclic antidepressants, without the associated tolerance problems with the latter two classes, in anxiety disorders.[106] Peak therapeutic effect may take as many as 4 weeks, and data have indicated treatment for 1 to 8 weeks to obtain significant improvement.[104,107] Regarding the effects of kava kava on vasculature in the feline lung, vasodepressor effects were demonstrated and shown to be mediated or modulated by both γ-aminobutyric acid (GABA) and L-type calcium channel sensitive pathways.[108] An important side effect associated with kava kava use is hepatic dysfunction. Patients who experience hepatic adverse reactions are known as "poor metabolizers," or those patients with a deficiency in the cytochrome P450 2D6 isozyme.[104] Therefore, it is recommended that patients who use kava kava receive routine liver function tests such as aspartate aminotransferase (AST), alanine aminotransferase (ALT), alkaline phosphatase, gamma-glutamyltransferase (GGT), lactate dehydrogenase (LDH), and total and conjugated bilirubin to monitor for the development of hepatotoxicity.[104] Furthermore, there have been 24 documented cases of hepatotoxicity after use of this herbal agent; and in some cases, death or liver transplant occurred after only 1 to 3 months of use.[104] In countries such as Germany and Australia, kava kava use longer than 3 months is not recommended.[107] Other side effects of kava kava use include visual changes, a pellagra-like syndrome with characteristic ichthyosiform dermopathy, and hallucinations.[3,104,109]

The kava pyrones have demonstrated competitive inhibition of the monoamine oxidase B.[104] Inhibition of this enzyme may result in the psychotropic effects related to kava kava use.[110] However, the exact mechanism of its effects on the central nervous system is largely unknown.[104] Regarding drug interactions, kava kava may react adversely with alprazolam, central nervous system depressants, statins, rifampin, alcohol, and levodopa.[104,111] Finally, kava kava may also affect platelets in an antithrombotic fashion by inhibiting cyclooxygenase, therefore decreasing production of thromboxane.[104]

Anesthesia Implications. Antinociceptive effects produced by kava kava may be similar to local anesthetic responses and appear to be mediated through a non–opiate-dependent pathway.[112,113] Ethanol can increase the hypnotic effects of kava kava.[114] It should be avoided in patients with endogenous depression and can potentiate the effect of barbiturates and benzodiazepines and cause excessive sedation.[115]

SAW PALMETTO

The herbal agent known as saw palmetto is used primarily for benign prostatic hyperplasia.[6] The key ingredients are the free fatty acids and sterols.[6] Although the mechanism of action is currently unknown, data exist that demonstrate antagonism at the androgen receptor for dihydrotestosterone and at the 5α-reductase enzyme.[6] Furthermore, biopsies have demonstrated decreases in the transitional zone epithelia (17.8% to 10.7%) in the prostates of men treated with saw palmetto compared with placebo, although prostate size and prostate-specific antigen level are not decreased by this herbal agent.[6] Compared with the 5α-reductase inhibitor finasteride, saw palmetto has demonstrated increased urine flow and decreased side effects.[6] One prospective, randomized, open-label investigation has sought to evaluate the safety and efficacy of saw palmetto compared with finasteride in patients with prostatitis/chronic pelvic pain syndrome.[116] The study found that at the end of the trial more patients wanted to continue finasteride treatment rather than saw palmetto treatment. The researchers concluded that in patients with this condition, saw palmetto had no considerable long-term improvement, and, with the exception of voiding, the patients on finasteride therapy had significant improvement in all examined parameters.[116]

Adverse reactions to saw palmetto are rare, with occasional reports of mild gastrointestinal symptoms and headaches.[6] Finally, there are few, if any, herbal-drug interactions in the literature regarding this herbal agent.[6] Results of one investigation indicated that recommended doses of saw palmetto are not likely to alter the pharmacokinetics of coadministered medications dependent on the cytochrome P450 isoenzymes CYP2D6 or CYP3A4, such as dextromethorphan (CYP2D dependent) and alprazolam (CYP3A4 dependent).[117]

Anesthesia Implications. Although no detailed studies have been done with regard to the anesthetic interactions, caution should be used if the patient is using benzodiazepines (e.g., alprazolam) or medications such as dextromethorphan because saw palmetto can alter pharmacokinetics of these medications. Elaborate clinical trials on anesthetic-herb interactions are warranted.

ST. JOHN'S WORT

St. John's wort is used in the treatment of anxiety, mild to moderate depression, and sleep-related disorders.[6,25] It has also been employed in the treatment of cancer, fibrositis, migraine headache, obsessive-compulsive disorder, and sciatica.[118] The active compounds include the naphthodihydrodianthrones hypericin and pseudohypericin, the flavonoids quercitrin, rutin, and hyperin, and the xanthones.[6,8]

It is speculated that extracts of St. John's wort, such as WS 5570, are widely and effectively used to treat mild to moderate depression.[119,120] The extracts are standardized based on the hypericin content and have demonstrated effectiveness superior to placebo and potentially as effective as selective serotonin reuptake inhibitors and low-dose tricyclic antidepressants.[118]

The exact mechanism of action of St. John's wort remains controversial. The herbal medication exhibits irreversible inhibition of monoamine oxidase in vitro; however, such inhibition has yet to be observed in vivo.[121] In the feline lung vasculature, St. John's wort exhibited a vasodepressor effect that was mediated or modulated by both a GABA receptor and an L-type calcium channel sensitive mechanism.[122] Studies performed in vitro have demonstrated GABA receptor inhibition by *Hypericum*. This mechanism may indicate that a GABA inhibitory mechanism is the cause of the antidepressant effect.[123,124] However, other theorized pathways have included inhibition of serotonin, dopamine, and norepinephrine reuptake in the central nervous system.[6]

St. John's wort is typically well tolerated.[6] Associated side effects may include photosensitivity, restlessness, dry mouth, dizziness, fatigue, constipation, and nausea.[6,25] Two noteworthy side effects of St. John's wort include its induction of the cytochrome P450 system (CYP 34A), which may affect serum levels of cyclosporine post organ transplantation, and the association with serotonergic syndrome in patients concurrently taking prescription antidepressants.[6] The serotonergic syndrome is characterized by hypertonicity, myoclonus, autonomic dysfunction, hallucinosis, tremors, hyperthermia, and, potentially, death.[12,125]

Anesthesia Implications. The concomitant use of St. John's wort is not recommended with photosensitization drugs (e.g., piroxicam, tetracycline), monoamine oxidase inhibitors, β-sympathomimetic amines (e.g., ma huang, pseudoephedrine), or selective serotonin reuptake inhibitors. There are no data regarding the multitude of potential interactions between anesthetics and St. John's wort.

ALTERNATIVE MEDICINE

Although beyond the scope of this chapter, it is important that the anesthesiologist recognize the presence of other forms of medicine such as homeopathy, chiropractic treatment, and massage therapy, to name a few. For example, reductions in blood pressure and heart rate have been observed after massage therapy (Kaye, unpublished data). Such alterations in cardiovascular function indicate potential autonomic mechanisms that may contribute to erroneously low vital signs readings in the perioperative assessment. Therefore, as emphasized in the herbal medications section, it is necessary to obtain a complete history from the patient to identify current and past treatment with alternative medicine.

CONCLUSION

The growing use of herbal medications in the United States warrants a better, more comprehensive understanding of these agents by the medical community. One role the anesthesiologist is charged with is regulating the patient's physiologic functions during various operative procedures. As demonstrated in this chapter, the use of herbal compounds may alter heart rate, respiratory rate, and the pharmacokinetics of various medications. Such medications may include chosen anesthetics employed during the stages of anesthesia. Thus, it is recommended that a thorough investigation be undertaken by the anesthesiologist to identify the prescribed, OTC, and herbal medications taken by the adult and pediatric patient. Furthermore, education of patients regarding the serious potential drug-herbal interactions should be a daily part of the preoperative assessment. The ASA recommends all herbal medications be discontinued 2 to 3 weeks before elective surgery.

Due to lax regulations, herbal medications are poorly categorized and not adequately standardized. This results in a high risk of adverse effects when used by uninformed/misinformed patients and the general public. There is also a lack of motivation for herbal manufacturers to conduct randomized, placebo-controlled, double-blinded safety and efficacy trials on such agents because of the lack of federal regulation. Within the past few decades, hundreds of deaths have been linked to the use of herbal medications. Furthermore, evidence suggests less than 1% of adverse effects associated with herbal supplements are reported. Such tragic outcomes may serve as the impetus for tighter standards and guidelines. However, the federal ban of ma huang may serve as a much-needed first step toward stricter regulations.

References

1. Abebe W: An overview of herbal supplement utilization with particular emphasis on possible interactions with dental drugs and oral manifestations. J Dent Hyg 2003;77:37-46.
2. Glover DD, Rybeck BF, Tracy TS: Medication use in a rural gynecologic population: Prescription, over-the-counter, and herbal medicines. Am J Obstet Gynecol 2004;190:351-357.
3. Winslow LC, Kroll DJ: Herbs as medicines. Arch Intern Med 1998;158:2192-2199.
4. Kleiner SM: The true nature of herbs. Phys Sports Med 1995;23:13-14.
5. Kaye AD, Sabar R, Clarke R, et al: Herbal medications and anesthetics: A review on current concepts. Am J Anesth 2000;27:467-471.
6. Hughes EF, Jacobs BP, Berman BM: Complementary and alternative medicine. In Tierney LM Jr, McPhee SJ, Papadakis MA (eds): Current Medical Diagnosis and Treatment. New York, Lange Medical Books/McGraw-Hill, 2004, pp 1681-1703.
7. Eisenberg DM, Davis RB, Ettner SL, et al: Trends in alternative medicine use in the United States, 1990-1997. JAMA 1998;280:1569-1575.
8. Leak JA: Herbal medicine: Is it an alternative or an unknown? A brief review of popular herbals used by patients in a pain and symptom management practice setting. Curr Rev Pain 1999;3:226-236.
9. Brevoort P: The U.S. botanical market: An overview. Herbal Gram 1996;36:49-57.
10. Kaye AD, Clarke RC, Sabar R, et al: Herbal medicines: Current trends in anesthesiology practice—a hospital survey. J Clin Anesth 2000;12:468-471.
11. Abebe W: Herbal medication: Potential for adverse interactions with analgesic drugs. J Clin Pharm Ther 2002;27:391-401.
12. Ness J, Sherman FT, Pan CX: Alternative medicine: What the data say about common herbal therapies. Geriatrics 1999;54:33-43.
13. Bauer R, Khan IA: Structure and stereochemistry of new sesquiterpene esters from E. purpurea. Helv Chim Acta 1985;68:2355-2358.
14. Melchart D, Walther E, Linde K, et al: Echinacea root extracts for the prevention of upper respiratory tract infections: A double-blind, placebo-controlled, randomized trial. Arch Fam Med 1998;7:541-545.
15. Grimm W, Muller HH: A randomized controlled trial of the effect of fluid extract of Echinacea purpurea on the incidence and severity of colds and respiratory infections. Am J Med 1999;106:138-143.
16. Randolph RK, Gellenbeck K, Stonebrook K, et al: Regulation of human immune gene expression as influenced by a commercial blended Echinacea product: Preliminary studies. Exp Biol Med (Maywood) 2003;228:1051-1056.
17. Freier DO, Wright K, Klein K, et al: Enhancement of the humoral immune response by Echinacea purpurea in female Swiss mice. Immunopharmacol Immunotoxicol 2003;25:551-560.
18. Taylor JA, Weber W, Standish L, et al: Efficacy and safety of echinacea in treating upper respiratory tract infections in children: A randomized controlled trial. JAMA 2003;290:2824-2830.
19. Parnham MJ: Benefit-risk assessment of the squeezed sap of the purple coneflower (E. purpurea) for long-term oral immunostimulation. Phytomedicine 1996;3:95-102.
20. Blumenthal M, Gruenwald J, Hall T, et al (eds): German Commission E Monographs: Therapeutic Monographs on Medicinal plants for Human Use. Austin, American Botanical Council, 1998.
21. Miller LG: Herbal medicinals. Arch Intern Med 1998;158:2200-2211.
22. Eaton EA, Walle UK, Lewis AJ, et al: Flavonoids, potent inhibitors of the human P-form of phenolsulfotransferase: Potential role in drug metabolism and chemoprevention. Drug Metab Dispos 1996;24:232-237, 1996.
23. Schubert W, Eriksson U, Edgar B, et al: Flavonoids in grapefruit juice inhibit the in-vitro hepatic metabolism of 17 beta-estradiol. Eur J Drug Metab Pharmacokinet 1995;20:219-224.
24. Gorski JC, Huang SM, Pinto A, et al: The effect of echinacea (Echinacea purpurea root) on cytochrome P450 activity in vivo. Clin Pharmacol Ther 2004;75:89-100.
25. Kaye AD, Sabar R, Vig S, et al: Neutraceuticals—current concepts and the role of the anesthesiologist. Am J Anesthesiol 2000;27:405-407.
26. Kaye AD, Sabar R, Vig S, et al: Neutraceuticals—current concepts and the role of the anesthesiologist. Am J Anesthesiol 2000;27:467-471.
27. Tinkleman DG, Avner SE: Ephedrine therapy in asthmatic children: Clinical tolerance and absence of side effects. JAMA 1977;237:553-557.
28. Fields AM, Kaye AD, Richards TA, et al: Pulmonary vascular responses to ma huang extract. J Altern Complement Med 2003;9:727-733.
29. Gurley BJ, Gardner SF, White LM, et al: Ephedrine pharmacokinetics after ingestion of nutritional supplements containing ephedra sinica (ma huang). Ther Drug Monit 1998;20:439-445.
30. MMWR Morb Mortal Wkly Rep 1996;45:689-693.
31. Jurgensen K, Stevens C (eds): Finally, a ban on ephedra. USA Today, April 13, 2004, p 22A.
32. Gruenwald J, Brendler T, Jaenicke C, et al: PDR for Herbal Medicines. Montvale, NJ, Medical Economics, 1998, pp 826-827.
33. Jellin JM, Gregory PJ, Batz F, et al (eds): Feverfew. In: Natural Medicines: Comprehensive Database, 5th ed. Stockton, CA: Therapeutic Research Faculty, 2003, pp 541-543.
34. Murphy J, Heptinstall S, Mitchell JR, et al: Randomized double-blind, placebo-controlled trial of feverfew in migraine prevention. Lancet 1988;2:189-192.
35. De Weerdt C, Bootsma H, Hendricks H: Herbal medicines in migraine prevention: Randomized double-blind, placebo-controlled crossover trial of a feverfew preparation. Physomed 1996;3:225-230.
36. Pittler M, Ernst E: Feverfew for preventing migraine. Cochrane Database Syst Rev 2004;1:CD002286.
37. Nelson MH, Cobb SE, Shelton J: Variations in parthenolide content and daily dose of feverfew products. Am J Health Syst Pharm 2002;59:1527-1531.
38. Li-Weber M, Giaisi M, Baumann S, et al: The anti-inflammatory sesquiterpene lactone parthenolide suppresses CD95-mediated activation–induced cell death in T cells. Cell Death Differ 2002;9:1256-1265.
39. Marles RJ, Kaminski J, Arnason JT, et al: A bioassay of inhibition of serotonin release from bovine platelets. J Nat Prod 1992;55:1044-1056.
40. Fozard JR: 5-Hydroxytryptamine in the pathophysiology of migraine. In Bevan JA (ed): Vascular Neuroeffector Mechanisms. Amsterdam, Elsevier, 1985, pp 321-328.
41. Makheja AN, Bailey JM: A platelet phospholipase inhibitor from the medicinal herb feverfew (Tanacatum parthenium). Prostaglandins Leukot Med 1982;8:653-660.
42. Collier HO, Butt NM, McDonald-Gibson WJ, et al: Extract of feverfew inhibits prostaglandins biosynthesis. Lancet 1980;2:922-923.
43. Drug information, U.S. Pharmacopoeia: U.S. Pharmacopoeia Consumer Information. Feverfew. Rockville, MD, U.S. Pharmacopoeia Convention, 1998.

44. Baldwin CA, Anderson LA, Phillipson JD, et al: What pharmacists should know about feverfew. J Pharm Pharmacol 1987;239: 237-238.

45. Heptinstall S, Groenwegen WA, Spangenberg P, et al: Extracts of feverfew may inhibit platelet behavior neutralization of sulphydryl groups. J Pharm Pharmacol 1987;39:459-465.

46. Makheja AN, Bailey J: The active principle in feverfew [letter]. Lancet 1981;2:1054.

47. Jain AK, Vargas R, Gotzowsky S, et al: Can garlic reduce levels of serum lipids? A controlled clinical study. Am J Med 1993;94:632-635.

48. Silagy CA, Neil HAW: A meta-analysis of the effect of garlic on blood pressure. J Hypertension 1994;12:463-468.

49. Neil HAW, Silagy CA, Lancaster T, et al: Garlic powder in the treatment of moderate hyperlipidemia: A controlled trial and meta-analysis. J R Coll Physician 1996;30:329-334.

50. Berthold HK, Sudhop T, von Bergmann K: Effect of a garlic oil preparation on serum lipoproteins and cholesterol metabolism: A randomized controlled trial. JAMA 1998;279:1900-1902.

51. Cooperative group for essential oil of garlic: The effect of essential oil of garlic on hyperlipidemia and platelet aggregation: An analysis of 308 cases. J Tradit Chin Med 1986;6:117-120.

52. Reuter HD: *Allium sativum* and *Allium ursinum*: II. Pharmacology and medicinal applications. Phytomedicine 1995;2:73-91.

53. Beaglehole R: Garlic for flavor, not cardioprotection. Lancet 1996;348:1186-1187.

54. Mukherjee S, Banerjee SK, Maulik M, et al: Protection against acute Adriamycin-induced cardiotoxicity by garlic: Role of endogenous antioxidants and inhibition of TNF-alpha expression. BMC Pharmacol 2003;3:16.

55. Kaye AD, Nossaman BD, Ibrahim IN, et al: Analysis of responses of allicin, a compound from garlic, in the pulmonary vascular bed of the cat and in the rat. Eur J Pharmacol 1995;276:21-26.

56. Elkayam A, Mirelman D, Peleg E, et al: The effects of allicin on weight in fructose-induced hyperinsulinemic, hyperlipidemic, hypertensive rats. Am J Hypertens 2003;16:1053-1056.

57. Tsao SM, Hsu CC, Yin MC: Garlic extract and two diallyl sulphides inhibit methicillin-resistant *Staphylococcus aureus* infection in BALB/cA mice. J Antimicrob Chemother 2003;52:974-980.

58. Rose KD, Croissant PD, Parliament CF, et al: Spontaneous spinal epidural hematoma with associated platelet dysfunction from excessive garlic consumption: A case report. Neurosurgery 1990;26:880-882.

59. Bordia A: Effect of garlic on human platelet aggregation in vitro. Atherosclerosis 1978;30:355-360.

60. Martin N, Bardisa L, Pantoja C, et al: Experimental cardiovascular depressant effects of garlic *(Allium sativum)* dialysate. J Ethnopharmacol 1992;37:145-149.

61. Grontved A, Hentzer E: Vertigo-reducing effect of ginger root. J Otolaryngol 1986;48:282-286.

62. Holtmann S, Clarke AH, Scherer H, et al: The anti-motion sickness mechanism of ginger. Acta Otolaryngol (Stockh) 1989;108: 168-174.

63. Sripramote M, Lekhyananda N: A randomized comparison of ginger and vitamin B_6 in the treatment of nausea and vomiting of pregnancy. J Med Assoc Thai 2003;86:846-853.

64. Fischer-Rasmussen W, Kjaer SK, Dahl C, et al: Ginger treatment of hyperemesis gravidarum. Eur J Obstet Gyn Rep Biol 1990;38:19-24.

65. Backon J: Ginger: Inhibition of thromboxane synthetase and stimulation of prostacyclin: Relevance for medicine and psychiatry. Med Hypoth 1986;20:271-278.

66. Nurtjahja-Tjendraputra E, Ammit AJ, Roufogalis BD, et al: Effective antiplatelet and COX-1 enzyme inhibitors from pungent constituents of ginger. Thromb Res 2003;111:259-265.

67. Akhani SP, Vishwakarma SL, Goyal RK: Anti-diabetic activity of *Zingiber officinale* in streptozotocin-induced type I diabetic rats. J Pharm Pharmacol 2004;56:101-105.

68. Bauer U: Six-month double-blind randomized clinical trial of gingko biloba extract versus placebo in two parallel groups in patients suffering from peripheral arterial insufficiency. Arzneimittelforschung 1984;34:716-720.

69. Peters H, Kieser M, Holscher U: Demonstration of the efficacy of gingko biloba special extract EGB 761 on intermittent claudication—a placebo-controlled, double-blind multicenter trial. Vasa 1998;27: 106-110.

70. Braquet P: BN 52021 and related compounds: A new series of highly specific PAF-acether receptor antagonists isolated from gingko biloba. Blood Vessels 1985;16:559-572.

71. Braquet P, Bourgain RH: Anti-anaphylactic properties of BN 52021: A potent platelet activating factor antagonist. Adv Exp Med Biol 1987;215:215-233.

72. Marcocci L: The nitric oxide scavenging properties of gingko biloba extract Egb761: Inhibitory effect on nitric oxide production in the macrophage cell line RAW 264.7. Biochem Pharmacol 1997;53:897-903.

73. Kobuchi H, Ldroy-Lefaix MT, Christen Y, et al: Gingko biloba extract (Egb 761): Inhibitory effect on nitric oxide production in macrophage cell line RAW 264.7. Biochem Pharmacol 1997;53:897-903.

74. Stys T, Stys A, Kelly P, et al: Trends in use of herbal and nutritional supplements in cardiovascular patients. Clin Cardiol 2004; 27:87-90.

75. LeBars PL, Katz MM, Berman N, et al: A placebo-controlled, double-blind, randomized trial of an extract of gingko biloba for dementia. JAMA 1997;278:1327-1332.

76. Zeybek N, Gorgulu S, Yagci G, et al: The effects of gingko biloba extract (EGb 761) on experimental acute pancreatitis. J Surg Res 2003;115:286-293.

77. Rosenblatt M, Mindel J: Spontaneous hyphema associated with ingestion of gingko biloba extract [letter]. N Engl J Med 1997;336:1108.

78. Rowin J, Lewis SL: Spontaneous bilateral subdural hematomas associated with chronic gingko biloba ingestion have also occurred. Neurology 1996;46:1775-1776.

79. Gilbert GJ: Gingko biloba [commentary]. Neurology 1997;48:1137.

80. Vale S: Subarachnoid hemorrhage associated with gingko biloba [letter]. Lancet 1998;352:36.

81. Mauro VF, Mauro LS, Kleshinski JF, et al: Impact of ginkgo biloba on the pharmacokinetics of digoxin. Am J Ther 2003;10:247-251.

82. Ng TB, Li WW, Yeung HW: Effects of ginsenosides, lectins and *Momordica charantia* insulin like peptide on corticosterone production by isolated rat adrenal cells. J Ethnopharm 1987;21:21-29.

83. Jellin JM, Gregory PJ, Batz F, et al (eds): Ginseng, American, ginseng, Panax. In: Natural Medicines: Comprehensive Database, 5th ed. Stockton, CA, Therapeutic Research Faculty, 2003, pp 614-619.

84. Zhou DL, Kitts DD: Peripheral blood mononuclear cell production of TNF-alpha in response to North American ginseng stimulation. Can J Physiol Pharmacol 2002;80:1030-1033.

85. Jie YH, Cammisuli S, Baggiolini M, et al: Immunomodulatory effects of *Panax* ginseng: CA Meyer in the mouse. Agents Actions Suppl 1984;15:386-391.

86. Sotaniemi EA, Haapakkoski E, Rautio A, et al: Ginseng therapy in non–insulin dependent diabetic patients. Diabetes Care 1995;18: 1373-1375.

87. Yokozawa T, Kobayashi T, Oura H, et al: Studies on the mechanism of hypoglycemic activity of ginsenoside-Rb2 in streptozotocin-diabetic rats. Chem Pharm Bull 1985;33:869-872.

88. Oshima Y, Kkonno C, Hikono H: Isolation and hypoglycemic activity of panaxans I, J, K and L, glycans of *Panax* ginseng roots. J Ethnopharm 1985;14:255-259.

89. Konno C, Murakami M, Oshima Y, et al: Isolation and hypoglycemic activity of panaxans Q, R, S, T and U, glycans of *Panax* ginseng roots. J Ethnopharm 1985;14:69-74.

90. Konno C, Sugiyama K, Oshima Y, et al: Isolation and hypoglycemic activity of panaxans A, B, C, D and E glycans of *Panax* ginseng roots. Planta Med 1984;50:436-438.

91. Tokmoda M, Shimada K, Konno M, et al: Partial structure of panax A: A hypoglycemic glycan of *Panax* ginseng roots. Planta Med 1984;50:436-438.

92. Baldwin CA: What pharmacists should know about ginseng. Pharm J 1986;237:583-586.

93. Hammond TG, Whitworth JA: Adverse reactions to ginseng [letter]. Med J Aust 1981;1:492.

94. Dega H, Laporte J, Frances C, et al: Ginseng a cause of Stevens-Johnson syndrome [letter]? Lancet 1996;347:1344.

95. Greenspan EM: Ginseng and vaginal bleeding [letter]. JAMA 1983;249:2018.

96. Hopkins MP, Androff L, Benninghoff AS, et al: Ginseng face cream and unexpected vaginal bleeding. Am J Obstet Gynecol 1988;159:1121-1122.

97. Palmer BV, Montgomery AC, Monterio JC, et al: Ginseng and mastalgia. BMJ 1978;1:1284.

98. Kuo SC, Teng CM, Lee JG, et al: Antiplatelet components in *Panax* ginseng. Planta Med 1990;56:164-167.

99. Shader RI, Greenblatt DJ: Phenelzine and the dream machine—ramblings and reflections [editorial] J Clin Psychopharmacol 1985;5:65.

100. Jones BD, Runikis AM: Interactions of ginseng with phenelzine. J Clin Psychopharmacol 1987;7:201-202.

101. Nowakowska E, Ostrowicz A, Chodera A: Kava kava preparations—alternative anxiolytics. Pol Merkuriusz Lek 1998;4:179-180a.

102. Skidmore-Roth L: Kava. In: Mosby's Handbook of Herbs and Natural Supplements. St. Louis, Mosby, 2001, pp 486-490.

103. Uebelhack R, Franke L, Schewe HJ: Inhibition of platelet MAO-B by kava pyrone–enriched extract from *Piper methysticum* Forster (kava-kava). Pharmacopsychiatry 1998;31:187-192.

104. Jellin JM, Gregory PJ, Batz F, et al (eds): Kava. In: Natural Medicines: Comprehensive Database, 4th ed. Stockton, CA, Therapeutic Research Faculty, 2002, pp 759-761.

105. Abourashed EA, Khan IA: Microbial transformation of kawain and methysticin. Chem Pharmaceutical Bull 2000;48:1996-1998.

106. Volz HP, Kieser M: Kava kava extract WS 1490 versus placebo in anxiety disorders: A randomized placebo-controlled 25-week outpatient trial. Pharmacopsychiatry 1997;30:1-5.

107. Forget L, Goldrosen J, Hart JA, et al (eds): Herbal Companion to AHFS DI. Bethesda, MD, American Society of Health-System Pharmacists, 2000.

108. Hoover JM, Kaye AD, Ibrahim IN, et al: Analysis of responses to kava kava in the feline pulmonary vascular bed. Journal of Medicinal Food, in press, 2005.

109. Garner LF, Klinger JD: Some visual effects caused by the beverage kava. J Ethnopharm 1985;13:307-311.

110. Seitz U, Schule A, Gleitz J: [3H]-monoamine uptake inhibition properties of kava pyrones. Planta Med 1997;63:548-549.

111. Jellin JM, Gregory PJ, Batz F, et al (eds). Kava. In: Natural Medicines: Comprehensive Database, 5th ed. Stockton, CA, Therapeutic Research Faculty, 2003, pp 788-791.

112. Jamieson DD, Duffield PH: The antinociceptive actions of kava components in mice. Clin Exp Pharmacol Physiol 1990;17:495-507.

113. Singh YN: Effects of kava on neuromuscular transmission and muscular contractility. J Ethnopharm 1983;7:267-276.

114. Jamieson DD, Duffield PH: Positive interaction of ethanol and kava resin in mice. Clin Exp Pharmacol Physiol 1990;17:509-514.

115. Gruenwald J, Brendler T, Jaenicke C, et al: PDR for Herbal Medicines. Montvale, NJ, Medical Economics, 1998, pp 1043-1045.

116. Kaplan SA, Volpe MA, Te AE: Prospective, 1-year trial using saw palmetto versus finasteride in the treatment of category III prostatitis/chronic pelvic pain syndrome. J Urol 2004;171:284-288.

117. Markowitz JS, Donovan JL, Devane CL, et al: Multiple doses of saw palmetto (*Serenoa repens*) did not alter cytochrome P450 2D6 and 3A4 activity in normal volunteers. Clin Pharmacol Ther 2003;74:536-542.

118. Jellin JM, Gregory PJ, Batz F, et al (eds): St. John's wort. In: Natural Medicines: Comprehensive Database, 4th ed. Stockton, CA, Therapeutic Research Faculty, 2002, pp 1180-1184.

119. Hostanska K, Reichling J, Bommer S, et al: Aqueous ethanolic extract of St. John's wort (*Hypericum perforatum* L.) induces growth inhibition and apoptosis in human malignant cells in vitro. Pharmazie 2002;57:323-331.

120. Lecrubier Y, Clerc G, Didi R, et al: Efficacy of St. John's wort extract WS 5570 in major depression: A double-blind, placebo-controlled trial. Am J Psychiatry 2002;159:1361-1366.

121. Staffeldt B, Kerb R, Brockmoller J, et al: Pharmacokinetics of hypericin and pseudohypericin after local intake of the *Hypericum perforatum* extract LI160 in healthy volunteers. J Geriatr Psych Neurol 1994;7:S47-S53.

122. Hoover JM, Kaye AD, Ibrahim IN, et al: Analysis of responses to St. John's wort in the feline pulmonary vascular bed. J Herbal Pharmacother 2004;4(4):47-62.

123. Cott JM: In vitro receptor binding and enzyme inhibition by *Hypericum perforatum* extract. Pharmacopsychiatry 1997;30:108-112.

124. Cott JM, Misra R: Medicinal plants: A potential source of new psychotherapeutic drugs. In Kanba S, Richelson SE (eds): New Drug Development from Herbal Medicines in Neuropharmacology, vol 5. New York, Brunner/Mazel, 1998.

125. Czekalla J, Gastpar M, Hubner WD, et al: The effect of *Hypericum* extract on cardiac conduction as seen in the electrocardiogram compared to that of imipramine. Pharmacopsychiatry 1997;30:86-88.

17 Trauma and Acute Care

RICHARD P. DUTTON, MD, MBA, and THOMAS E. GRISSOM, MD

BASIC CONSIDERATIONS

Trauma—disruption of anatomy and physiology due to application of external energy—is the leading cause of death in Americans younger than 45 years old and the leading cause of lost years of life.[1] Anesthesiologists see trauma patients in the emergency department (ED), in the operating room (OR), in the intensive care unit (ICU), and in the pain clinic. Specialists in trauma anesthesia are rare, but every anesthesiologist will see trauma patients at times and must be aware of the specific medical issues associated with this challenging population. This chapter begins with an overview of issues common to most trauma patients—team organization, multi-trauma priorities, emergency airway management, and fluid resuscitation—and then presents a discussion of specific types of patients and injuries.

Team Organization and Multi-Trauma Priorities

Trauma care is a team sport, where outcomes depend as much on the coordination of services as on the quality of each individual practitioner. A number of studies have shown that the more organized and experienced a trauma service is, the better the outcomes it achieves.[2,3] Practicing anesthesiologists must understand how the local trauma service is organized and how anesthesia personnel are expected to participate.

Trauma is considered a surgical disease, and seriously injured patients are usually managed by a trauma general surgeon. The surgeon will have responsibility for the sequencing of diagnostic and therapeutic procedures and for resource allocation among multiple patients. The anesthesiologist may be involved in initial airway management and hemodynamic resuscitation and will certainly be involved in the timing and extent of any surgery. Close communication with the surgeon is essential to the appropriate allocation of scarce operating room resources. As the gatekeeper to the OR, the anesthesiologist is required to determine how trauma cases will be accommodated in a busy elective schedule. Understanding surgical priorities is essential to this process.

Table 17-1 is an outline of trauma case priorities.[4] *Emergent* cases must reach the OR as soon as possible. While surgical airway access and resuscitative thoracotomy usually occur in the ED, immediate follow-up in the OR will be necessary if the patient survives. Also considered emergent are any exploratory surgeries (laparotomy or thoracotomy) in a hemodynamically unstable patient and craniotomy in a patient with a depressed or deteriorating mental status. Limb-threatening orthopedic and vascular injuries should undergo surgical exploration as soon as the necessary diagnostic studies have been performed and interpreted. *Urgent* cases are not immediately life threatening but require surgery as soon as possible to reduce the incidence of subsequent complications. Examples include exploratory laparotomy in stable patients with free abdominal fluid; irrigation, débridement, and initial stabilization of open fractures; and repair of contained rupture of the thoracic aorta. Early fixation of closed fractures, especially spine and long-bone fractures,

TABLE 17–1 Surgical Priorities in Trauma Patients

Priority	Procedure
Immediate Available OR or at bedside	Airway access Thoracotomy or laparotomy to control hemorrhage Evacuation of epidural or subdural hematoma
Urgent First available OR	Perforated viscus Unstable spine with no deficit or a partial deficit Decompressive craniotomy Decompressive laparotomy Fasciotomy or limb salvage procedure
As soon as possible Next unscheduled OR	Open fractures Irrigation and débridement of soft tissue wounds Open globe injury or entrapped ocular muscle Isolated closed long-bone fracture
Elective Next scheduled OR	Small bone fractures: wrist, ankle, hand, foot Facial surgery "Second-look" laparotomy or thoracotomy Acetabular reconstruction Fixation of stable spinal fractures Plastic surgery and wound reconstruction Repeat irrigation and débridement of open wounds

has been shown to benefit trauma patients by reducing the incidence of subsequent pulmonary complications. Definitive repair within 24 hours is recommended in otherwise stable and non–brain-injured patients. *Nonurgent* cases are those that can be safely delayed until a scheduled OR time is available. Face, wrist, and ankle fracture fixation are not time dependent: early surgery will shorten the patient's length of stay but may be technically more difficult due to swelling and distortion of the surrounding tissue. These surgeries are commonly postponed and may be undertaken days to weeks after injury, when tissue edema has resolved and the patient's condition is otherwise stable.

In addition to facilitating timely surgery in those patients who require it, the anesthesiologist and surgeon working together must often determine the extent of surgery to be permitted. The concept of "damage control" has revolutionized surgical thinking in the past decade, limiting initial therapeutic procedures to those required for hemostasis while delaying reconstructive procedures until adequate resuscitation has been achieved.[5] In a typical example, the surgeon treating an unstable patient with blunt trauma might perform an exploratory laparotomy, rapid splenectomy, staple resection of injured bowel (without attempt at reanastomosis), ligation of bleeding large vessels, and packing of all four abdominal quadrants. The abdomen would be left open under a sterile watertight dressing and the patient taken to the ICU. Angiographic embolization might be used to facilitate hemostasis in the liver and retroperitoneum. After resolution of shock, warming, and normalization of laboratory values, the patient would return to the OR in 24 to 48 hours for débridement of nonviable tissue, reconstruction of the

bowel, placement of enteral feeding access, and abdominal closure. The concept of damage control may also be applied to orthopedic injuries: initial external fixation of the pelvis and long bones is adequate for temporary stabilization of fractures, without imposing the additional physiologic burdens of intramedullary nailing or open fixation.[6] While objective indicators of the need for damage control have not been established, this approach should be considered in any patient with persistent hypoperfusion, elevated lactate, or transfusion requirement in excess of one blood volume.

Airway Management

The first priority in the care of any trauma patient is assurance of a patent airway and adequate oxygenation and ventilation.[7] Anesthesiologists are the acknowledged experts for airway management in most hospitals, including those in which trauma patients are managed initially by Emergency Medicine physicians. Whether in the ED or the OR, the ability to swiftly and safely intubate injured patients may be lifesaving.

Pathophysiology. Indications for intubation of the trauma patient are shown in Table 17-2. Hypoxemia may be the result of impaired respiratory effort, obstruction of the upper airway, aspiration of blood or gastric contents, mechanical disruption of the chest cavity, or severe hemorrhagic shock. Traumatic brain injury (TBI) and intoxication with alcohol or other drugs contribute to impaired effort, upper airway obstruction, and aspiration, whereas direct trauma to the face, neck, or chest may

TABLE 17–2   Indications for Intubation

Apnea

Traumatic brain injury
Intoxication
Medication effect

Hypoxemia

Pulmonary injury
    Contusion
    Hemothorax/pneumothorax
    Aspiration
Cardiac contusion/ischemia with pulmonary edema
Neurologic injury with decreased cough or respiratory effort
Carbon monoxide poisoning

Airway Obstruction

Traumatic brain injury
Intoxication
Upper airway injury or hemorrhage
Airway burn

Need for Anesthesia

Painful injuries
Urgent surgical procedures
Combative or uncooperative patient

---

cause bleeding, anatomic disruption of the airways, or pneumothorax.

Ventilatory failure is common in trauma patients, both at initial presentation and in the days immediately following. Pulmonary contusion, with subsequent consolidation of alveolar space, may take hours to develop and may not be obvious until after fluid resuscitation and initial surgeries have been completed. Ventilatory failure may also be due to exacerbation of underlying chronic cardiac or pulmonary disease or to pulmonary embolus (PE). Trauma patients are at very high risk for PE, and this condition should be suspected in any patient with an abrupt decline in respiratory status. Multiply injured patients are likely to develop the systemic inflammatory response syndrome (SIRS), manifested by progressive respiratory compromise, recurrent sepsis, and multiple organ system failure.

All trauma patients are considered to have full stomachs, both because obtaining an accurate history in the injured patient is difficult and because trauma itself will lead to an immediate cessation of gastrointestinal motility, with ileus persisting for hours to days after injury.[8] Trauma patients are also at risk for aspiration of blood from open fractures or penetrating wounds of the face. Impaired mental status due to TBI or intoxication makes aspiration more likely, particularly when combined with the use of sedative or analgesic drugs given to facilitate diagnostic procedures (such as computed tomography [CT]) or minor surgical procedures (such as reducing a fracture or suturing a laceration).

Impairment of mental status is also the leading cause of combative or uncooperative behavior. Although it may be possible through history taking and physical examination to determine which patients have suffered a TBI and which are simply intoxicated, the similarities between the two conditions make absolute knowledge impossible before CT. Successful treatment of TBI is highly time dependent, meaning that the patient with impaired mental status must be treated as if an epidural hematoma is present, until proven otherwise.

Evaluation. Assessment of the patient before airway management is no different than assessment of an elective surgery patient, but it must be adjusted for the urgency of the situation. A thorough history and physical examination of the face, neck, and chest is appropriate when possible. Any suggestion that intubation will be difficult should suggest the need for additional equipment or personnel and a modification of the usual rapid-sequence protocol. When the urgency of the situation does not allow for a thorough assessment, the anesthesiologist must gather what information is immediately available from other providers and a quick look at the patient and then proceed as necessary. Factors predicting a difficult airway are summarized in Table 17-3, in approximate order of importance.

The need for intubation in the combative or uncooperative patient is controversial, and the provider must carefully assess the risks and benefits of intervention. On the one hand, induction of anesthesia will allow for immediate diagnostic studies, and thus more rapid identification of life-threatening conditions such as epidural

TABLE 17–3   Factors Predicting a Difficult Intubation

Emergency setting

Presence of hypoxemia

Prior history of a difficult intubation (may be noted on a Medic-Alert bracelet)

Obesity

History of sleep apnea

Presence of a cervical collar and backboard

Soft tissue injury to the neck or face

Known cervical spine injury (possibility of prevertebral edema)

Limited mouth opening

Limited neck extension (ankylosing spondylitis, previous cervical fusion)

Upper airway hemorrhage

Tongue injury

Foreign bodies in the airway

Previous attempts at intubation

hematoma or splenic rupture. Induction and intubation may also prevent the patient from injuring himself or others and allow for deeper and safer levels of sedation during diagnostic studies. On the other hand, induction can precipitate hemodynamic instability and technical complications of rapid sequence intubation may be difficult to justify in the uninjured patient. Early intubation, diagnostic imaging, and rapid extubation of the intoxicated patient without significant trauma are possible in some settings but a substantial economic burden in others. Ultimately, the trauma team, including the anesthesiologist, must evaluate the potential for life-threatening trauma, the patient's ability to tolerate CT (with or without additional sedation), and the likely ease of intubation when deciding how to proceed with this sort of patient. No matter what course is elected, close monitoring of the patient's neurologic status and respiratory effort is required.

Preoperative Preparation. Sufficient trained personnel must be on hand to physically manage the airway, administer induction drugs, provide cricoid pressure, and stabilize the cervical spine. The anesthesiologist must coordinate this process and must ensure that all participants are clear on their roles. When appropriate, the plan of care should be discussed with the patient and family ahead of time and any questions answered. Preoxygenation with a tight-fitting face mask (if tolerated) or assisted bag-valve-mask ventilation should be provided while preparations are underway. A high-flow suction device should be immediately available. All necessary intubating equipment, including emergency medications, should be close at hand and in good working order. Figure 17-1 is a picture of the trauma resuscitation unit intubating box used at the R. Adams Cowley Shock Trauma Center, provided as an example.

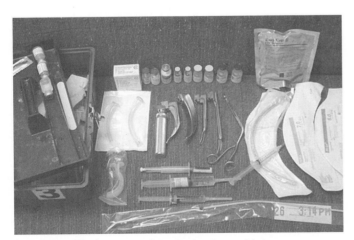

FIGURE 17–1 A typical intubation box, with its contents. Everything required for immediate emergent intubation is available, including a laryngoscope handle and blades, endotracheal tubes, an intubating stylet, a carbon dioxide detector, and prefilled syringes of sodium thiopental, succinylcholine, and lidocaine.

Patient positioning can greatly facilitate intubation and is often overlooked in the emergent situation. The bed or stretcher should be placed at a convenient height for the anesthesiologist and enough space provided at the head of the bed to allow room for unhindered motion. Ergonomic design of the trauma bay has been shown to improve the process of emergency intubation.[9]

The presence of cervical spine instability will be a possibility in most trauma victims requiring emergent intubation, because the exclusion of this condition requires a conscious, cooperative, pain-free patient who has undergone a number of diagnostic studies (see later). The traditional "sniffing position" is thus contraindicated, whereas the presence of a rigid cervical collar and the maintenance of in-line cervical stabilization also contribute to the difficulty of intubation.[10] Whereas some have advocated the routine use of fiberoptic intubation for all trauma patients with the potential for cervical instability, this approach is time and resource intensive. Direct laryngoscopy with manual in-line stabilization is unlikely to aggravate an existing cervical spine injury and has been judged safe and appropriate for the majority of trauma patients.[11]

Preprocedure preparation should include the availability of a device to facilitate intubation of an anterior larynx (e.g., a trigger tube or gum elastic bougie), rescue devices for impossible intubation (e.g., the laryngeal mask airway or Combitube), and an understanding of when cervical spine protection should be abandoned in favor of achieving a successful intubation. The likelihood of an anterior larynx argues for the routine use of a stylet in the endotracheal tube. Capnometry should be available to confirm endotracheal placement of the tube and adequacy of ventilation. Equipment should also be on hand for emergent cricothyroidotomy in the worst case.

Intraoperative Considerations. A rapid-sequence intubation (RSI) technique is recommended, with the use of cricoid pressure from induction until confirmation of endotracheal tube placement. Although the consistency with which the Sellick maneuver prevents the aspiration of gastric contents has been called into question,[12] cricoid pressure is also beneficial in moving the larynx into a more posterior position, thus facilitating the laryngoscopic view of the vocal cords. If excessive pressure is distorting airway anatomy or preventing passage of the endotracheal tube, then it should be abandoned. Aspiration is unlikely during direct visualization of the airway, with a suction catheter immediately at hand.

Advantages and disadvantages of various induction drugs are shown in Table 17-4. While agents that lack a negative inotropic effect (e.g., ketamine or etomidate) are more likely to preserve cardiovascular function in the euvolemic patient, any induction drug—and even the change to positive-pressure ventilation alone—can precipitate hemodynamic instability in the patient in shock.

TABLE 17–4	Medications Used During Emergency Airway Management	
Medication	**Class**	**Comments**
Sodium thiopental	Sedative	Fast, inexpensive, negative inotrope and vasodilator
Etomidate	Sedative	Fast, expensive, fewer cardiovascular effects, may cause transient myoclonus
Propofol	Sedative	Fast, expensive, easily titrated, negative inotrope and vasodilator
Ketamine	Sedative	Fast, inexpensive, positive inotrope, may cause "bad dreams" or dysphoric reactions
Lidocaine	Sedative/analgesic	Blunts airway reactivity, negative inotrope
Midazolam	Sedative	Expensive, slower onset, negative inotrope and vasodilator, may cause retrograde amnesia
Fentanyl	Analgesic	Blunts airway reactivity, does not produce amnesia
Morphine	Analgesic	Slower onset and longer half-life than fentanyl, may cause histamine release, has a euphoric effect
Succinylcholine	Paralytic	Most rapid onset, produces fasciculations, will cause potassium release in vulnerable patients (burns, spinal cord injury)
Vecuronium	Paralytic	Slower onset and longer duration, no hemodynamic side effects
Rocuronium	Paralytic	Intermediate onset and duration, but less predictable than vecuronium, no hemodynamic side effects

Note that any sedative or analgesic medication will reduce the endogenous catechol response and may precipitate hemodynamic instability.

This is because the hypovolemic patient is relying on a high serum level of catecholamines to support the blood pressure. Any sedative or analgesic agent may impair the adrenal response to hemorrhage and "unmask" hypovolemia. Because internal hemorrhage may not be readily apparent at the time of induction, and because vital signs are only a crude indicator of fluid volume status, care should be used with any anesthetic agent. The use of smaller than normal doses, with titration against the patient's response, is recommended.

Succinylcholine is the standard paralytic agent for rapid-sequence intubation and is recommended in the absence of obvious contraindications (previous neuromuscular disease, known or suspected hyperkalemia, burn or spinal cord deficit occurring more than 24 hours previously). High doses of rocuronium or vecuronium can be used in place of succinylcholine and will provide adequate intubating conditions in the majority of cases, at the cost of prolonged paralysis thereafter.

The administration of positive-pressure breaths by bag-valve-mask during RSI is controversial. In routine OR cases, in which RSI is undertaken in a cooperative, preoxygenated patient in a good sniffing position, positive-pressure ventilation is avoided because of concern that it will distend the stomach and increase the likelihood of aspiration. In the emergent setting, however, ventilation throughout RSI should be strongly considered. Preoxygenation may be difficult in the combative patient, anatomic positioning is not optimal, and even transient hypoxemia is dangerous to the patient with TBI or hemorrhagic shock. In the not-uncommon situation that the anesthesiologist is supervising a less skilled provider, the provision of a positive-pressure breath of 100% oxygen before laryngoscopy will allow for a longer and safer intubation effort.

With trained providers, RSI of the trauma patient is successful on the first attempt about 90% of the time. In the remaining cases, knowledge of the local difficult airway algorithm becomes essential. Providers vary in their skills, institutions vary in the available equipment, and the time pressure of an emergent intubation makes creative thought difficult, which is why it is incumbent on every anesthesiologist to pre-plan for the steps he or she intends to follow if a given intubation proves challenging. It is assumed that every anesthesiologist is acquainted with the difficult airway algorithm of the American Society of Anesthesiologists (ASA),[13] which should be followed in most cases. The algorithm for emergent intubations is considerably simpler, because waking the patient up is not usually a viable option. Figure 17-2 is the algorithm used at the R. Cowley Shock Trauma Center, as one example.

Successful intubation, by whatever route, must be confirmed by detection of CO_2 in exhaled breaths. In areas where intubation and mechanical ventilation are common, such as the ED trauma bay, continuous waveform capnometry is highly recommended. For other areas a disposable CO_2 detector should be part of the emergency intubation setup. Patients with no cardiac output may not exhale CO_2, even with cardiopulmonary resuscitation in progress. In these cases, successful intubation should be confirmed by direct laryngoscopic inspection or by observation of lung motion if the chest has been opened.

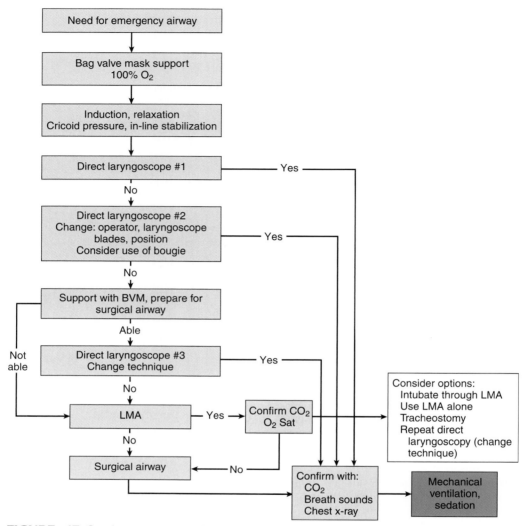

FIGURE 17–2 The emergency intubation algorithm of the R. Adams Cowley Shock Trauma Center. The algorithm assumes that oxygenation and/or ventilation are already failing and that airway access and mechanical ventilation are absolutely required. BVM, bag-valve-mask ventilation; LMA, laryngeal mask airway.

After confirmation of successful intubation, the anesthesiologist is responsible for assessment of hemodynamic stability after induction, for initial ventilator settings, and for ongoing sedation and analgesia. Undesired patient awareness during mechanical ventilation is a significant problem in most EDs, particularly when paralytic agents are used to facilitate diagnostic studies or minor procedures. Even if not directly involved in this phase of care, the anesthesiologist can contribute substantially to the recognition of this problem and to the education of nursing and medical personnel.

Fluid Resuscitation

Airway and breathing are the first priorities in trauma care, followed closely by assessment of the circulation—the ABCs.[7] The anesthesiologist may share responsibility for hemodynamic management in the ED with other members of the trauma team, but in the OR this becomes a primary task.

Pathophysiology. Tissue injury causes disruption of blood vessels, and hemorrhage is a hallmark of trauma. While bleeding associated with some injuries stops spontaneously, in other cases active intervention is required to prevent exsanguination. Life-threatening hemorrhage occurs into one of five compartments, summarized in Table 17-5.[4] Trauma is a surgical disease because early diagnosis and treatment of ongoing hemorrhage are essential. What is less obvious, but equally true, is the importance of nonsurgical hemorrhage control and ongoing resuscitation.

TABLE 17–5 Sites of Exsanguinating Hemorrhage: Diagnostic and Therapeutic Options

Site	Diagnostic Mechanism	Therapeutic Options
Chest	Auscultation Chest radiograph CT	Tube thoracostomy Exploratory thoracotomy
Abdomen	FAST CT	Nonoperative management Angiographic embolization Exploratory laparotomy
Retroperitoneum	CT Angiography	Pelvic stabilization Angiographic embolization
Thigh or thighs	Physical examination Radiograph Angiography	Fracture reduction Fracture fixation Vascular exploration
"The street" (outside the body)	Physical examination Paramedic report	Direct pressure Surgical closure

CT, computed tomography; FAST, focused assessment by sonography for trauma.

Shock is the term used to describe the complex pathophysiology that arises from inadequate systemic oxygen delivery. Symptoms of shock are listed in Table 17-6. Shock was first described in trauma patients because hemorrhage is a common and obvious cause.[14] Trauma patients may also be in shock from mechanical impairment of blood flow (tension pneumothorax or cardiac tamponade), cardiac dysfunction, spinal cord injury, ingestion of toxins, or a mixture of causes, but hemorrhage is considered to be the source until it is definitively ruled out. Much of the Advanced Trauma Life Support (ATLS) curriculum is devoted to this important diagnostic and therapeutic process.[7] Figure 17-3 is a rough algorithm for management of the trauma patient with active hemorrhage.

Hemorrhage reduces circulating blood volume, leading to decreased preload and reduced cardiac output. Vasoconstriction and increased inotropy mediated by the sympathetic nervous system allow for continued blood flow to vital organs in the presence of blood loss as severe as 40% of normal intravascular volume (2 of 5 L in a 70-kg male). Acute blood loss in excess of this amount causes a critical reduction of perfusion to the heart and brain, manifesting as coma, pulseless electrical activity, and death. Blood loss less than this amount may also be lethal, because reduced perfusion leads to anaerobic metabolism and accumulation of lactic acid and other toxins. Individual cells react to ischemia by hibernation (reduction of all nonessential activities), apoptosis ("programmed cell death"), or outright necrosis, depending on the organ system in question.[15] Many ischemic cells—especially gut and muscle cells—react to ischemia by absorption of extracellular fluid.[16] The resulting tissue edema is both locally and systemically disruptive by clogging capillary pathways (the no-reflow phenomenon) and further

depleting intravascular volume. Ischemic cells also release inflammatory mediators, triggering a chemical cascade that perpetuates the pathophysiology of shock long after adequate circulation is restored (Fig. 17-4).[17] The "dose" of shock absorbed by the body, a summation of the depth of hypoperfusion and its duration, largely determines the patient's clinical outcome, ranging from a mild inflammatory response to organ system failure to death. The typical young male trauma patient has an enormous compensatory

TABLE 17–6 Symptoms of Shock

Patient Appearance
Pallor
Diaphoresis
Prolonged capillary refill
Poor skin turgor

Mental Status
Agitation, then progressive obtundation
Thirst

Vital Signs
Hypotension (automated devices may be inaccurate)
Narrowed pulse pressure
Tachycardia
Tachypnea
Diminished or absent pulse oximeter signal

Laboratory Signs
Metabolic acidosis
Elevated serum osmolarity
Elevated serum lactate
Decreased hematocrit (takes time to develop)
Coagulopathy

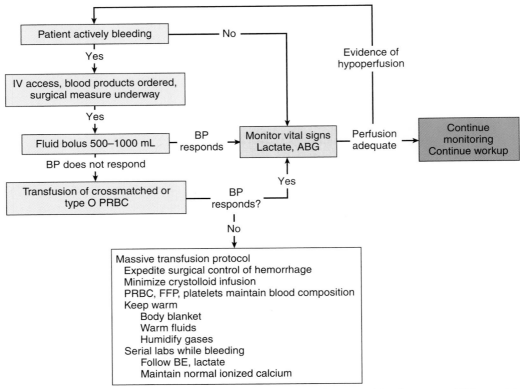

FIGURE 17–3 Algorithm for management of active hemorrhage. BP, blood pressure; ABG, arterial blood gases; PRBC, packed red blood cells; FFP, fresh frozen plasma; BE, base excess.

reserve and may achieve normal pulse and blood pressure while still significantly fluid depleted and highly vasoconstricted. This phenomenon, known as the occult hypoperfusion syndrome, is associated with a high incidence of organ system failure if not recognized and corrected.[18]

Isotonic crystalloid infusion increases preload and produces an immediate increase in cardiac output and blood pressure. Crystalloid therapy is a double-edged sword, however. Increased blood pressure leads to increased bleeding from open vessels and rebleeding from previously hemostatic injuries, due in part to decreased blood viscosity and relaxation of compensatory vasoconstriction.[19] Aggressive crystalloid infusion dilutes red cell mass and clotting factor concentration and leads to hypothermia in most prehospital and ED settings. Studies of uncontrolled hemorrhagic shock in rats,[20] swine,[21] sheep,[22] and dogs[23] have all demonstrated improved survival when initial fluid therapy is titrated to a lower than normal systolic blood pressure (70 to 80 mm Hg). This finding is supported by two human trials conducted within the past decade.[24,25]

Dilution of red cell mass is inevitable during early resuscitation, because losses to hemorrhage are compounded by intravascular recruitment of extracellular fluid and exogenous crystalloid administration. A hematocrit measured soon after hemorrhagic trauma may show little change, because whole blood is being lost and the percentage of

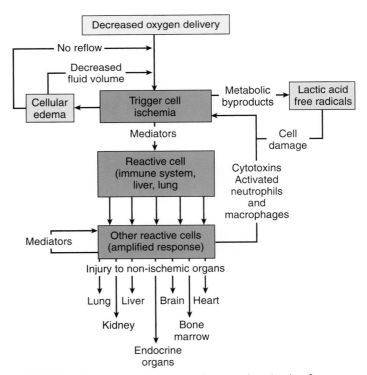

FIGURE 17–4 The shock cascade. A single episode of hypoperfusion can trigger a prolonged systemic response.

red cells in the remaining volume does not change. The longer hemorrhage and resuscitation persist, however, the more the hematocrit will fall. Loss of red cells leads to decreased blood viscosity, allowing for more rapid flow of blood. Below a hematocrit of about 30%, however, this rheologic improvement in blood flow is overbalanced by the decrease in carrying capacity, and tissue oxygen delivery begins to decrease.

Evaluation. The diagnostic characteristics of hemorrhagic shock are listed in Table 17-6. Control of bleeding is the first priority in treatment, and nothing must interfere with the indicated diagnostic or therapeutic procedures shown in Table 17-5. Relevant patient physiology is assessed by continuous measurement of vital signs (facilitated by early placement of an arterial pressure catheter) and by immediate and repeated measurement of arterial blood gases, complete blood chemistry, clotting function, and serum lactate determination. Toxicology screening and electrocardiography may help to diagnose underlying intoxication or cardiac disease.

Response to fluid therapy will provide important diagnostic information. Most patients in shock will demonstrate an improvement in vital signs after bolus fluid administration. In those who have achieved spontaneous hemostasis (e.g., those with lung injury or peripheral orthopedic injuries), the improvement in vital signs will be sustained. In those with ongoing hemorrhage (e.g., abdominal visceral trauma, pelvic fracture) the response to fluid will be transient. These are the patients most in need of urgent diagnostic studies and therapeutic procedures. Those patients who do not respond at all to an initial fluid bolus either have a nonhemorrhagic source of shock (e.g., spinal cord injury, cardiac disease) or are bleeding very rapidly.

Preparation. Resuscitation of the actively hemorrhaging patient requires large-bore, high-flow intravenous access through at least two separate catheters. Warmed intravenous fluids are highly recommended, especially early in resuscitation. Commercial fluid warming technology is highly effective and should be used as commonly (or more so) in the trauma bay as in the operating room. Rapid infusion systems are designed to warm and actively administer large fluid volumes quickly and may be lifesaving in the patient with rapid and uncontrolled hemorrhage.

The ability to rapidly administer uncrossmatched type O blood may be lifesaving. Many trauma center blood banks and emergency departments maintain a supply on hand for just this purpose. Crossmatched blood, plasma, and platelets should be requested at the earliest moment that a massive transfusion seems likely. OR nursing and anesthesia resources should be mobilized to allow for extra personnel to facilitate the early stages of emergency surgery and resuscitation.

Intraoperative Considerations. Resuscitation must be carried out simultaneously with diagnostic and therapeutic procedures to control hemorrhage, in such a way that tissue perfusion is supported without making bleeding worse. Recent understanding of the potential for rebleeding and dilution has led to a change away from the traditional ATLS approach of rapid crystalloid infusion to one of deliberate, controlled fluid administration, titrated to specific physiologic end points (Table 17-7).

Replacement of red cells is essential to limiting the depth and duration of shock after hemorrhage. Packed red blood cells should be administered early in the resuscitative process, using uncrossmatched type O units if necessary. Adverse reaction to this therapy is extremely unlikely: more than 100,000 units of uncrossmatched blood were administered during the Vietnam War without a single documented case of fatal transfusion reaction, as compared with the nine cases that occurred in the 600,000 crossmatched transfusions.[26] Immediate transfusion of type O blood is sufficiently safe and beneficial that it should be considered for any patient presenting in extremis from hemorrhagic shock. The most appropriate target hematocrit

TABLE 17–7	Goals for Fluid Resuscitation During Active Hemorrhage	
Total Fluids	Adequate to prevent worsening of shock (increasing lactate or base deficit)
Vital Signs	Systolic blood pressure 80-100 mm Hg Heart rate < 120 beats per minute Pulse oximeter functioning
Blood Content	Hematocrit 20%-30%; higher if risk factors for ischemic coronary disease Normal prothrombin and partial thromboplastin time Platelet count > 50,000/mm³ Normal serum ionized calcium
Temperature	Core > 35°C
Anesthetic Depth	Fluid therapy to allow appropriate anesthetic and analgesic depth
Overly aggressive resuscitation must be weighed against the risk of exacerbating hemorrhage.	

for resuscitation must be individualized on the basis of age, specific injury pattern, preexisting disease, and the potential for further hemorrhage. In previously healthy patients, 20% is an absolute minimum during resuscitation whereas 30% is an appropriate maximum value.

Coagulopathy due to acute consumption of coagulation factors is likely in any patient losing more than a single blood volume (5 L) or receiving more than 10 units of red blood cells.[27] Because coagulopathy is more easily prevented than treated, early administration of plasma to any patient who has lost or will lose this amount of blood is highly recommended. Plasma should be ordered from the blood bank for any patient presenting emergently to the OR with symptoms of acute hemorrhagic shock. A ratio of 1:1 replacement of red cells and plasma is appropriate for any patient who has lost or will lose more than a blood volume but should be guided when possible by both laboratory and clinical assessment. The same is also true of thrombocytopenia. Platelet count will usually remain adequate longer than coagulation factor concentration, and platelet therapy is thus less commonly required than plasma therapy. Transfused platelets have a very short functional life span in the circulation and represent a strong immune stimulus. For these reasons platelet therapy should be reserved for those trauma patients with both a platelet count of less than 50,000/mm^3 and clinical evidence of bleeding. Coagulation factor concentrates and cryoprecipitate do not offer a benefit beyond that of plasma infusion in the hemorrhaging trauma patient, unless fluid overload is a significant risk (as in the coagulopathic elderly patient) or the patient is known to have a specific factor deficiency. Use of human factor VIIa may represent an exception to this principle, however, as recent anecdotal reports have described rapid resolution of traumatic coagulopathy after administration of 20 to 100 µg/kg.[28] Because of the expense of this therapy and the lack of prospectively collected safety data in trauma patients, however, it cannot be recommended unless conventional therapy has failed and exsanguination is likely.

Electrolyte abnormalities are common during resuscitation from hemorrhage. Hyperosmolarity may result from alcohol ingestion, dehydration, hypovolemia, or administration of normal saline. Mild hyperglycemia secondary to high circulating catecholamine levels is expected. Neither of these conditions mandates specific treatment during resuscitation, because both will resolve with restoration of adequate intravascular volume. Hyperchloremic metabolic acidosis is a significant risk of over-resuscitation, especially with mildly hypertonic solutions such as normal saline,[29] and can be managed with the titrated addition of hypotonic fluids. Hypocalcemia arises from chelation of circulating calcium by the citrate or adenosine additives found in banked blood products. Intravenous administration of calcium is indicated in patients with low serum ionized calcium levels, particularly in the presence of

hemodynamic instability. Serum bicarbonate levels will be lower than normal in the hemorrhaging patient, owing to increased lactic acidosis and impaired renal blood flow. Administration of bicarbonate solutions has been recommended by some to increase systemic pH in very acidotic patients, to enhance the functioning of important protein systems, including coagulation and catecholamine receptors.[30] The clinical utility of this therapy has never been proven, however. Adequate fluid resuscitation remains the primary therapy for restoration of normal acid-base status.

Paradoxically, while early resuscitation has evolved toward less aggressive fluid administration, resuscitation after control of hemorrhage (usually in the ICU) has moved in the opposite direction. Late resuscitation is characterized by the need to completely restore and support perfusion. To do so requires the practitioner to look beyond the vital signs for a more direct measure of tissue perfusion. Placement of invasive monitoring or a transesophageal echocardiographic probe and administration of fluid until the cardiac output is maximized is one approach. Close observation of chemical markers is another. The speed with which serum lactate level normalizes after shock is strongly associated with the risk of death from organ system failure.[31] Those patients who do not show a significant downward trend in lactate after resolution of hemorrhage require more aggressive fluid therapy and closer monitoring.

SPECIFIC CONDITIONS

Traumatic Brain Injury

Traumatic brain injury causes at least half of all deaths from trauma.[1] As with hemorrhagic shock, the pathophysiology of TBI consists of both the primary injury, in which tissue is disrupted by mechanical force, and a secondary physiologic response. Because prevention of secondary injury is critical to outcome, the anesthesiologist plays an important role in managing these patients both in the OR and in the ICU.

Pathophysiology. Traumatic brain injury is classified as mild, moderate, or severe, depending on the Glasgow Coma Scale (GCS) score on admission. *Mild* TBI (GCS 13 to 15) is the most common. Although mild TBI does not usually necessitate intensive treatment, patients may be significantly debilitated by postconcussive symptoms, including headaches, sleep and memory disturbances, and mood swings.[32] Progression of mild TBI is rare but may be catastrophic.

Moderate TBI (GCS 9 to 12) is more likely to be associated with intracranial lesions that require surgical evacuation. These patients have a higher potential for deterioration and are more susceptible to secondary insult if not carefully managed.

Severe TBI (GCS < 9) is a highly lethal condition, almost always associated with intraparenchymal or intraventricular hemorrhage or evidence of diffuse axonal injury on cranial CT. Patients with severe TBI are usually unable to maintain airway patency and may evidence diminished or absent respiratory drive, with inability to protect the airway from aspiration. Most patients presenting to the OR for surgical treatment will have severe TBI, with elevation of intracranial pressure (ICP) due to hemorrhage (epidural, subdural, or intraparenchymal), edema, or both. Failure to promptly relieve elevated ICP will lead to herniation of brain tissue, loss of brain blood flow, and death. The goal of surgical therapy is the resolution of increased ICP and the control of any active hemorrhage.

Evaluation. The neurologic examination is the most important component of preoperative assessment in the patient with TBI. Recovery from TBI is a gradual process, and the sedative effects of anesthetic medications may be exaggerated, meaning that the trauma patient will seldom improve immediately at the conclusion of cranial decompression. It is important to know when a deterioration has occurred, however, so that follow-up studies and appropriate ICU management can commence.

More controversial is the timing of noncranial surgery in the patient with TBI. Transient hypotension or hypoxemia associated with orthopedic surgery may lead to worsening of neurologic injury, whereas delay in repair of fractures increases the risk of pulmonary complications and sepsis.[33] Although no definitive prospective study has been conducted, more recent retrospective work suggests that early surgery with meticulous anesthetic care does not necessarily worsen TBI.[34]

Preoperative Preparation. Early intubation of the TBI patient may be required owing to combative or agitated behavior, the need for diagnostic studies before reaching the OR, and the potentially catastrophic consequences of respiratory depression or pulmonary aspiration. In fact, most patients with moderate or severe TBI will present to the OR having been already intubated in the field or ED.

Arterial pressure monitoring is required for any intracranial procedure, because dramatic swings in the blood pressure can occur throughout the case. Large-bore intravenous access is necessary, because blood loss can become excessive, particularly in patients with severe TBI and early onset of coagulopathy. Supplemental medications likely to be needed include mannitol and/or hypertonic saline solution, phenytoin, and thiopental.

Intraoperative Management. Patients with mild TBI pose few additional anesthetic risks but are more susceptible to the effects of sedative medication. Benzodiazepines should be used with care in the preoperative period.

The anesthesiologist should strive to have the patient's sensorium as clear as possible as rapidly as possible after any anesthetic. Any change from the patient's preoperative mental status not attributable to anesthetic drugs is an indication for immediate repeat cranial tomography and neurosurgical reassessment.

The care of patients with moderate TBI consists of serial assessment of neurologic function, with repeat CT at regular intervals. If close monitoring is not possible, owing to the need for general anesthesia or sedating medications, then continuous invasive measurement of cerebral perfusion pressure (CPP) is indicated.[35] An ICP monitor is recommended in any patient with moderate or severe TBI undergoing noncranial surgery likely to last longer than 2 hours.

Patients with severe TBI represent a substantial anesthetic challenge. Early, rapid management focused on restoration of systemic homeostasis and perfusion-directed care of the injured brain is required to produce the best possible outcomes. The occurrence of hypoxemia (PaO_2 < 60 mm Hg) or hypotension (systolic blood pressure < 90 mm Hg) in patients with severe TBI is associated with a significant increase in mortality.[36] Management requires a highly skilled facility, close cooperation among providers, and a stepwise implementation of therapies as shown in Figure 17-5.

Aggressive restoration of intravascular volume is indicated to maintain intracranial perfusion, especially if associated pulmonary injuries necessitate the use of high mean airway pressures to support oxygenation. Hyperventilation therapy, long a mainstay in the management of patients with TBI, is no longer an appropriate treatment, unless there are signs of imminent herniation. This is because hyperventilation lowers ICP by reduction of blood flow, putting ischemic brain tissue at further risk for necrosis or apoptosis. Hyperventilation is indicated only for those patients who present with strong lateralizing signs who are en route to CT and emergent decompressive surgery.

Patients with severe TBI should be maintained at a mean arterial pressure (MAP) greater than 90 mm Hg until invasive ICP monitoring is instituted and CPP (MAP − ICP) can be directly calculated. Placement of a ventriculostomy allows both continuous monitoring of CPP and therapeutic drainage of cerebrospinal fluid (CSF), and this approach is preferred over other invasive ICP monitors.[37] Current guidelines suggest maintenance of CPP at a minimum of 70 mm Hg *at all times.* Contrary to practice in the past, the patient with severe TBI should be maintained in a *euvolemic* state. Fluid resuscitation is the mainstay of therapy, followed by vasoactive infusions as needed. If surgery is indicated, care should be taken with the ventriculostomy drain; both failure of drainage and excessive loss of CSF can occur during transport. Familiarity is also beneficial for the more advanced monitors of jugular bulb and brain tissue oxygenation that are now coming into use.

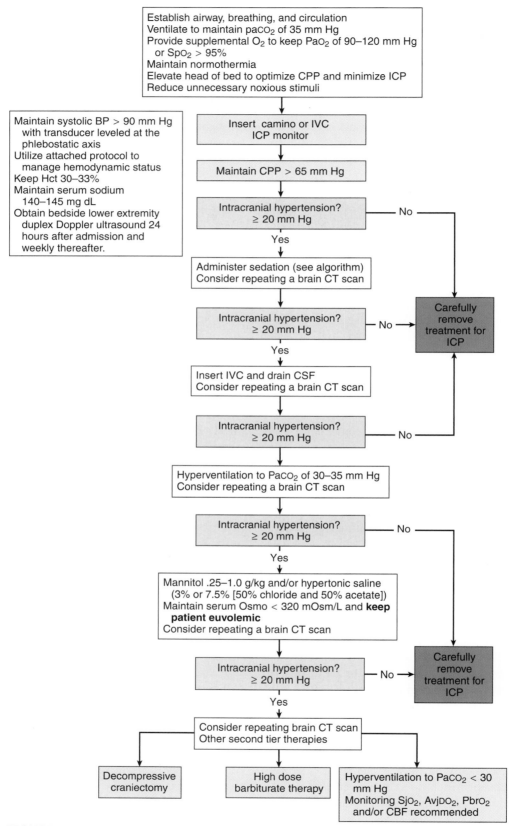

FIGURE 17–5 Critical pathway for treatment of cerebral perfusion pressure (CPP) for patients with severe traumatic brain injury. BP, blood pressure; Hct, hematocrit; ICP, intracranial pressure; IVC, intravenous catheter; CT, computed tomography; CSF, cerebrospinal fluid; CBF, cerebral blood flow.

Positional therapy is used in almost every case of severe TBI. Elevation of the head facilitates venous and CSF drainage from the cranium, lowering ICP and improving CPP as long as the patient is euvolemic. Pulmonary ventilation-perfusion ($\dot{V}/\dot{Q}$) matching may also improve in this position, making maintenance of cerebral oxygen delivery easier. The patient should be transported to the OR in this position and maintained with the head up during surgery if at all possible.

Analgesics are indicated for treatment of pain arising from coexisting injuries. Sedatives are useful for control of elevated ICP but may make serial examination difficult. Propofol is popular because it offers the most rapid return of neurologic function when discontinued, but the clinician must use this drug cautiously. Large doses of propofol sustained over days to weeks have recently been associated with the development of lethal rhabdomyolysis (the propofol infusion syndrome).[38] The use of sedatives to decrease ICP frequently mandates the use of vasoactive drugs to maintain MAP. Invasive hemodynamic monitoring with a pulmonary artery catheter and frequent assessment of lactate and base deficit may be necessary to maintain an appropriate intravascular volume in the presence of confounding pharmacologic agents and ongoing mechanical ventilation.

Osmotic diuretic agents are common first-line therapy for severe TBI. Mannitol decreases ICP by drawing edema fluid out of brain tissue and into the circulation and may have secondary benefit as a scavenger of free radicals and other harmful inflammatory compounds. Hypertonic saline has a similar osmotic effect and may also act as a beneficial immunologic agent. Use of either drug will lead to increased diuresis, necessitating greater attention to adequate volume replacement so that euvolemia can be maintained. Use of osmotic agents to reduce elevated ICP is usually titrated to a serum osmolarity of 310 to 230 mOsm/L.

Invasive physiologic monitoring, positional therapy, sedation, and osmotic diuresis will be applied to most patients with severe TBI.[35] The next tier of therapy is reserved for the subset of patients with intractable elevations of ICP. A small percentage may respond to *barbiturate coma*. In addition to lowering the cerebral metabolic rate, barbiturates have been shown to decrease excitatory neurotransmitters.[39] Management of barbiturate coma necessitates exquisite management of intravascular volume, usually requiring a pulmonary artery catheter, and the use of vasoactive and inotropic agents to maintain CPP.

Decompressive craniectomy is a surgical procedure that is gaining popularity in the management of intractable ICP elevations. Relieving pressure by removal of a piece of cranium and use of a dural patch may improve mortality and morbidity in patients who might not otherwise survive.[40] *Decompressive laparotomy* may also be indicated in patients with severe TBI, if coexisting injuries or vigorous volume infusion have increased intra-abdominal compartment pressure to greater than 20 mm Hg.[41] Elevated abdominal pressure causes elevated intrathoracic pressure, higher ventilator pressures, and increased ICP.

Although vigorous control of fever is an undisputed recommendation, deliberate hypothermia to reduce the cerebral metabolic rate remains controversial[42] and is not currently recommended. Corticosteroid therapy for severe TBI has not been proven beneficial and is now contraindicated owing to the high potential for deleterious side effects. A number of other drugs, monitors, and therapies for severe TBI are under investigation, offering the promise that the next decade will see significant improvement in outcomes from this challenging disease.

Spinal Cord Injury

Pathophysiology. Spinal cord injury with complete or partial neurologic deficit occurs in approximately 8,000 Americans a year.[43] High energy falls or motor vehicle crashes cause the majority of serious spinal cord injuries. Incomplete deficits—known as "stingers"—commonly resolve within hours to days. Complete deficits represent a total disruption of the spinal cord and are much less likely to improve over time. Cervical spine injuries causing quadriplegia are accompanied by significant hypotension, owing to inappropriate vasodilatation and loss of cardiac inotropy (neurogenic shock). Autonomic functioning of the lower cord will return over days to weeks, with restoration of vascular tone but absence of sensory or motor transmission. Patterns of spinal cord injury are described in Table 17-8.

Evaluation. Early intubation is almost universally required for patients with cervical spine fracture and quadriplegia. Ventilatory support is absolutely required for patients with a deficit above C4, who will lack diaphragmatic function. Patients with levels from C4 to C7 are also likely to require early intubation, because of lost chest wall innervation, paradoxical respiratory motion, and the inability to clear secretions. Atelectasis will develop quickly and may lead to rapid, progressive desaturation. Recurrent pneumonia is a common complication that will lead to tracheostomy in half of all patients with complete deficits at the C5 to C7 level.

Preoperative Preparation. The urgency of surgery to stabilize the spine is determined by the neurologic status of the patient and the anatomic presentation. A patient with a partial deficit and visible impingement of the spinal canal is considered an emergency because of the potential for regaining neurologic function after decompression. Patients with no deficit or complete deficit may require surgical stabilization to facilitate mobilization but are less urgent cases. Surgery is more commonly required for

TABLE 17–8   Types of Spine Fracture

Type	Description
Upper cervical spine (occiput to C2)	Usually fatal; considered to be unstable in survivors; Jefferson, hangman's, and odontoid fractures
Lower cervical spine (C3 to T1)	Flexion with axial loading produces vertebral body compression fractures with possible displacement of fragments; often with ligamentous injury; involvement with posterior elements can cause unilateral or bilateral jumped facets
Thoracic spine (T2-T10)	Flexion-extension injuries most common; with axial loading can produce burst fracture; displacement of fragments into canal frequently associated with complete cord injury secondary to smaller canal
Lumbar spine (T11-L1)	Classified by mechanism-compression fracture with flexion, burst fracture with axial loading, transverse process fracture, flexion-distraction injury, shear injury
Lower lumbar and sacral spine	Uncommon injuries; can occur with hyperflexion and axial loading; longitudinal sacral fracture may have radiculopathy while horizontal fracture is associated with injury to cauda equina
Ligamentous injury without bony injury	Plain radiographs with no evidence of bony injury do not preclude ligamentous injury; may be unstable and produce subsequent neurologic injury

cervical lesions, whereas supportive bracing of the torso is more common for thoracic and lumbar fractures.

Determining cervical spine stability can be difficult, and many trauma patients will present to the OR with a rigid cervical collar still in place. Protocols to rule out instability of the cervical spine are controversial and may vary substantially between centers. These protocols include plain films, CT, flexion-extension radiography, magnetic resonance imaging (MRI), and examination by orthopedic or neurosurgical specialists and may take days to complete.[44] Insistence on definitive clearance of cervical spine injury before proceeding with urgent or semiurgent surgery is not reasonable. The risk of pulmonary complications posed by delaying needed orthopedic procedures greatly outweighs the risk of worsening an unsuspected spine injury during intubation and anesthesia. For lower-risk patients and for patients who are uncooperative or hemodynamically unstable the preferred approach is an RSI with maintenance of manual inline axial stabilization throughout the procedure. The safety record of this approach is impressive.[11]

Intraoperative Management. For the cooperative patient with a known or highly probable injury (existing deficit, suspicious radiographs, or substantial neck pain), maintaining the patient in a rigid collar or cervical traction while performing an awake fiberoptic intubation is the safest approach. When awake intubation is elected, the nasal route is usually easier. Oral intubation is more challenging technically but will be of greater value if the patient remains intubated postoperatively, because of a lower risk for sinusitis. Blind nasal intubation, transillumination with a lighted stylet, use of an intubating laryngeal mask airway or Bullard laryngoscope, and any of a variety of other instrument systems for indirect laryngoscopy are acceptable. The clinician is advised to use the equipment and

techniques that are most familiar. The goal is to achieve tracheal intubation with the least possible motion of the cervical spine, while preserving the ability to assess neurologic function after intubation and patient positioning.

Hemodynamic instability may complicate urgent and emergent spinal surgery. Hypotension from neurogenic shock is characterized by bradycardia due to loss of cardiac accelerator function and unopposed parasympathetic tone but can still be difficult to distinguish from hypotension due to acute hemorrhage. Aggressive fluid administration is indicated, subject to the end points of resuscitation outlined earlier. Once hemorrhage has been ruled out or treated, some data exist that support maintenance of an elevated MAP greater than 85 mm Hg for 7 days after spinal cord injury, although this approach is highly controversial.[45] Fluid administration will help to expand the vascular volume and counter the effects of inappropriate vasodilatation but may produce an added strain on the heart. Any patient with a poor response to initial volume loading, particularly an elderly one, should receive pulmonary artery catheterization to guide subsequent resuscitation.

Almost all patients with a persistent deficit after spinal cord injury will be treated with high doses of methylprednisolone in the days after surgery.[46] Although this therapy is highly controversial, and the expected benefit to most patients is slight, no other alternatives are presently available. Corticosteroid infusions should be continued during operative interventions, and the clinician should be wary of the development of corticosteroid-related side effects, including adrenocortical insufficiency, gastric ulceration, and occult infections.

Autonomic hyperreflexia develops in 85% of patients with a complete injury above T5, owing to the loss of inhibitory control of vascular reflexes.[47] This condition mandates general or conduction anesthesia for any subsequent surgery in a quadriplegic or high-paraplegic patient, even if the planned procedure is in an insensate region.

Ocular Trauma

Ocular trauma, both penetrating and nonpenetrating, is an important cause of visual loss and disability, with up to 90,000 injuries per year resulting in some degree of visual impairment.[48] Many of the patients with severe ocular injuries have concomitant head and neck trauma that delay initial recognition and evaluation of these problems. With current diagnostic methods, surgical techniques, and rehabilitation, vision can be salvaged in many patients. Despite a better understanding of anesthetic, medical, and surgical management, penetrating eye trauma continues to be a complicated and challenging condition.

Pathophysiology. Types of ocular trauma are listed in Table 17-9. Severe concussive injury to the globe and orbit can cause damage to all of the ocular tissue. Force directed against the eye pushes the globe back into the orbit. The resulting compression of the eye stretches the softer tissues lining the eye, producing significant stretching vectors. Additionally, the thin bony medial wall and floor of the orbit are prone to movement, producing a "blowout" fracture. These fractures typically do not require

TABLE 17-9 Types of Ocular Trauma
Periocular
Ecchymosis
Lid laceration
Orbital
Facial fracture
Retrobulbar hemorrhage
Traumatic optic neuropathy
Superficial Ocular
Corneal abrasion
Foreign body
Chemical injury
Thermal injury
Infection
Closed-Globe
Iritis
Iris injury
Retinal damage
Traumatic cataract
Subchoroidal hemorrhage
Lens subluxation
Open-Globe
Globe rupture
Laceration
Penetrating foreign body

emergent surgery unless visual impairment or globe injury is present. With penetrating injuries of the eye, closure of the laceration is the primary surgical goal due to concerns of infection and loss of intraocular contents, particularly from the posterior segment. Prognosis for penetrating eye injuries is related to a number of factors, including initial visual acuity, type and extent of injury, presence of retinal detachment, and presence of foreign bodies.

Evaluation. Preoperative documentation of prior visual function and the degree of visual loss is important and may affect subsequent decisions and the timing of surgery. The documented examination should be as complete as possible, but any further injury to the globe should be avoided. Because many ocular injuries are associated with head and neck trauma, a thorough secondary survey should be accomplished, including CT for the evaluation of both intraocular and periocular structures. Also, CT may show whether a patient has sustained an intracranial injury, such as subdural hemorrhage. Although CT provides a helpful adjunct in penetrating ocular trauma, it may not be sensitive enough to be relied on as the sole means of evaluating a potential open globe injury.

Preoperative Preparation. Once a known or suspected globe injury has been identified, it becomes important to avoid significant increases in intraocular pressure (IOP) such as may occur during coughing, bucking, straining, or a Valsalva maneuver. This may require the judicious use of sedatives and narcotics in the preoperative period. In general, most of these agents will lower IOP and can be used if not contraindicated by other considerations. Additionally, the open globe should be protected with a shield and a broad-spectrum antibiotic may be administered to prevent infection. Optimal timing for surgical interventions is based on a number of factors, including concomitant injuries, coexisting disease, and operative factors (Table 17-10). Because a large number of open globe injuries occur in children, pediatric considerations will frequently be required in their management.[49]

Intraoperative Considerations. While general anesthesia is used most commonly in the repair of penetrating eye injuries, local or regional anesthesia can be used safely with cooperative patients in the setting of limited corneal lacerations where the potential for extrusion of intraocular tissue is minimal. General anesthesia is indicated for cases of severe lacerating injuries, pediatric patients, or patients who are uncooperative because of alcohol or drug intoxication. This provides an immobile eye and eliminates the need for patient cooperation, while allowing for the control of factors affecting IOP. Care must be taken during anesthetic induction not to apply direct pressure to the globe with the face mask.

TABLE 17–10	Timing of Intervention in Various Forms of Ocular Trauma
Timing	**Condition**
Absolute emergency	Chemical injury (alkali > acid)
	Threat of gas gangrene
	Orbital abscess
	Expulsive choroidal hemorrhage extruding intraocular tissues through the open wound
	Vision loss because of expanding orbital hemorrhage
Urgent	Endophthalmitis
	High-risk IOFB
Within 24 hours	Open wounds requiring surgical closure
	IOFB
Within a few days (24-72 hours preferred)	Thick submacular hemorrhage
Within 2 weeks	IOFB
	Secondary reconstruction if retina is detached
	Media opacity in the amblyopic age group

IOFB, intraocular foreign body.
Adapted from Kuhn F: Strategic thinking in eye trauma management. Ophthalmol Clin North Am 2002;15:171-177.

With the use of general anesthesia for the management of patients with potential or known open globe injuries, the management objectives include (1) overall patient safety, (2) avoidance of elevated IOP, (3) provision of a stable operative field, (4) avoidance of external ocular pressure, and (5) minimized bleeding. With most trauma patients, the anesthesiologist must assume that the stomach is full, making an RSI the technique of choice. As long as a deep level of anesthesia is provided during induction, any intravenous agent with the exception of ketamine is acceptable.

The choice of muscle relaxant for use in induction has been surrounded by controversy. Succinylcholine, which can cause contraction of extraocular muscles and choroidal congestion, has been shown to transiently increase IOP to a small degree. When given without intravenous or inhalational anesthetics, the IOP rise can be as high as 18 mm Hg.[50] Typically, however, the increase is 2 to 5 mm Hg with a high of 10 mm Hg with appropriate induction.[51] A recent review looking at the published studies and recommendations regarding the use of succinylcholine and open globe injuries cited only anecdotal reporting of vitreous loss associated with its use.[52] Several case series and animal studies have failed to demonstrate the extrusion of vitreous with the use of succinylcholine when used with a nondepolarizing pretreatment, although there is a lack of randomized controlled trials.[53,54] Currently, it appears that the use of succinylcholine should be dictated by the need for rapid onset or termination of muscle relaxation rather than concerns about loss of ocular contents. Pretreatment with a small dose of a nondepolarizing muscle relaxant should precede the use of succinylcholine to blunt the expected increase in IOP. The use of intravenous lidocaine, β blockers,

and short-acting narcotics may be useful at induction to blunt the hypertensive response to laryngoscopy and intubation, which are also associated with increases in IOP.[55,56]

After induction and intubation, deep anesthesia with a combination of narcotics, inhalational anesthesia, and muscle relaxants will allow for the avoidance of extraocular pressure and choroidal congestion by eliminating coughing, straining, or movement. Although occurring infrequently during repair of eye lacerations, the oculocardiac reflex may occur during manipulation of the globe. Whereas use of a retrobulbar block will abolish or prevent this reflex, it should not be used with a potential open globe injury. If possible, maintenance of a head-up position will facilitate venous drainage.

During emergence from anesthesia, an increase in IOP is possible. While the concern for loss of intraocular contents is lessened, straining, emesis, coughing, and agitation may increase the risk of bleeding and affect the surgical outcome. Appropriate antiemetic therapy is indicated along with the use of narcotics for pain management. Shivering should also be avoided and can be treated with small doses of meperidine.

Complex Facial Injuries

Although frequently distracting in appearance, severe maxillofacial trauma is not often life threatening unless there is involvement of the airway or, rarely, severe hemorrhage. The face and head are exposed to a broad range of physical trauma (Table 17-11). An estimated 3 million patients require hospital treatment for facial injuries every year from motor vehicle crashes alone.[57] Life-threatening airway and bleeding problems; severe ocular, nasal, or jaw dysfunction; and significant cosmetic deformities

TABLE 17–11   Major Causes of Facial Injuries

Vehicle crash: motorized and nonmotorized
Pedestrian accident
Industrial accident
Violence
Blunt force such as fist or club
Penetrating such as knife or gunshot
Sports
Falls
Thermal injury
Chemical injury

are the potential consequences of facial trauma. The anesthesiologist must be familiar with these injuries to ensure appropriate initial management, to facilitate emergent treatment, and to support surgical correction.

Pathophysiology. The type and severity of injury is determined by several factors, including the mechanism of injury, extent, direction and duration of force, and characteristics of the impacted facial structures. Significant bone trauma can coexist with only modest soft tissue injury; similarly, dramatic soft tissue injury may occur in the absence of facial fractures.

Each of the major mechanisms of injury produces not only distinctive patterns of injury but also necessitates a search for likely associated trauma. Blunt trauma typically has a greater effect on the facial skeleton than soft tissue. In cases of interpersonal violence or sports-related blunt trauma, edema and hematoma may be the only soft tissue findings with significant underlying facial fractures. Patients involved in motor vehicle crashes presenting with significant facial trauma should be presumed to have traumatic brain and cervical injury[58] until proven otherwise. With penetrating trauma from close range (e.g., shotguns, rifles, and high-velocity projectiles), there may be significant loss of soft tissue with massive facial destruction. Burns are associated with progressive cutaneous and mucosal edema, necessitating early management of a potentially compromised airway.

The direction of force applied to the facial structures determines the fracture location. Given the lower force requirements to produce fracture of the nasal bones, zygoma, frontal sinus, and mandibular ramus compared with other facial bones, these are the more common sites of injury.[59,60] As would be expected with blunt trauma, the greater the change of velocity at the time of impact, the greater the severity of the resultant fracture. With penetrating trauma from gunshot wounds, the damage potential is directly related to the velocity of the projectile on impact. Fortunately, the structure of the midfacial skeleton provides some buttressing and protection for the thinner,

laminar bones in this area. This allows for dispersal of traumatic forces and may prevent fracture of low-resistance facial bones and reduced energy transmission to the base of the skull.[61,62]

The face can be divided into three anatomic regions. The lower third contains the mandible and includes the temporomandibular joint and coronoid process. The middle third comprises the maxilla, nasal bones, orbits, and zygomatic arch. The upper third contains the frontal bone, frontal sinuses, frontozygomatic process, and nasoethmoidal complex. A summary of signs, symptoms, and long-term complications associated with these fractures is found in Table 17-12. Along with soft tissue injuries, this provides a framework for classification of facial injuries.

Soft tissue injuries range from minor to severe, including contusions, abrasions, punctures, lacerations, avulsion flaps, and frank tissue loss. Early management usually consists of débridement, conversion of unfavorable to favorable wounds, and meticulous closure. Careful examination should be performed to evaluate for injury to other important structures such as the facial nerve, parotid gland, and the lacrimal apparatus. Lacerations in the vicinity of the zygomatic arch may include injury to the frontal branch of the facial nerve. Large hematomas, particularly involving the nasal septum and auricular cartilage, may require drainage to prevent subsequent cosmetic deformity.[63]

Mandibular fractures are the second most common form of facial fracture after the nasal bones. Because greater than 50% of mandibular fractures occur in two or more locations, a second fracture site should almost always be suspected when evaluating a patient.[63] The strong musculature attached to the mandible has a tendency to produce displacement of fractured bones along with malocclusion and asymmetry. In some cases this may produce compromise of the airway affecting surgical and anesthetic management.

Midface fractures include nasal, Le Fort, orbital, and zygomatic arch fractures. The nasal bones are the most commonly injured facial bones. Disruption of the nasal septum may result in airway obstruction and lead to significant hemorrhage. The classic midface fractures were described by Rene Le Fort in 1902 and were named Le Fort I, II, and III. Le Fort I is a dentoalveolar horizontal fracture that separates the maxillary alveolus from the midface. Le Fort II is a pyramidal or triangular fracture separating the maxilla from the zygoma, with the fracture lines demarcating a central fragment involving the maxillary alveolus, the medial portion of the orbit, and the nose. A Le Fort III fracture is a complete dislocation of the facial skeleton from the cranial skeleton running parallel to the skull base. This fracture involves the ethmoid bones and can extend into the cribriform plate, allowing a communication with the anterior fossa. Thus, the presence of rhinorrhea could signal the presence of a CSF leak.

TABLE 17–12   Types of Facial Fractures

Type	Signs and Symptoms	Long-Term Complications
Nasal	Pain, obstruction, crepitus, swelling, epistaxis	Malunion, obstruction
Naso-orbital, ethmoid	Pain, visual change, epistaxis, swelling, telecanthus	Malunion, telecanthus
Frontal sinus	Pain, epistaxis	Mucopyocele
Zygomatic arch	Lateral pain, trismus, asymmetry, lateral depression	Unstable, recurrent depression
Zygoma	Numb cheek and/or lip, visual change, swelling entrapment, scleral hemorrhage, epistaxis, step-off, enophthalmos, associated globe injury	Asymmetry, entrapment, enophthalmos
Orbital blowout	See Zygoma; rarely, numbness, epistaxis, and step-off	Entrapment, enophthalmos
LeFort	Malocclusion, trismus, numbness, visual changes, massive swelling, epistaxis, scleral hemorrhage, midface mobility	Malocclusion, malunion, dental loss, asymmetry, lacrimal obstruction
Mandible	Lower lip numbness, trismus, pain referred to ear, crepitus, malocclusion, open bite	Malocclusion, malunion, osteomyelitis, ankylosis, dental loss, nerve injury

Adapted from Darian VB: Maxillofacial trauma. In Trunkey DD, Lewis FR (eds): Current Therapy of Trauma, 4th ed. St. Louis, Mosby, 1999.

The absence of rhinorrhea, however, does not rule out the possibility of disruption of the cribriform plate and a skull base fracture. While useful in describing elements of a midface fracture, rarely are the classic patterns identified in isolation. Le Fort fractures are rarely bilateral and may be seen in combination with other facial fractures and soft tissue injury.

Zygomatic arch fractures are caused by blows to the lateral aspect of the midface. Trismus may occur due to swelling from hematoma or edema within the masseter muscle or direct mechanical impingement of the bone fragments of the arch onto the coronoid process of the mandible. Fractures of the zygoma and orbital walls may affect eye movement through entrapment of periorbital soft tissue, including extraocular muscles. Direct globe trauma may also occur and should be included in the initial evaluation.

Fractures involving the upper third of the facial structure include frontal sinus and frontal bone fractures. Concomitant nasoethmoidal, supraorbital, zygomatic, and cranial base fractures are commonly seen and may involve the anterior cranial fossa. Thus, particular attention must be paid to assessing for frontal lobe contusion, CSF rhinorrhea, and pneumocephalus.

Evaluation. Because facial trauma frequently occurs in the multiply injured patient, initial evaluation should focus on life-threatening problems and complete assessment of more emergent injuries. Upper and occasionally lower airway obstruction can occur with facial trauma, necessitating a detailed evaluation of the airway and potential for subsequent compromise. Patients with multiple mandibular fractures or combined maxillary, mandibular, and nasal fractures are more likely to experience early

airway obstruction.[64,65] The arch configuration of the mandible suspends the tongue anteriorly such that posterior displacement from a complex mandibular fracture allows the floor of the mouth to fall backward, causing airway obstruction. Obstruction of the nasopharynx may occur with some midface fractures. Although this will not produce complete airway compromise in the presence of mouth breathing, impaired consciousness with posterior collapse of oral structures can lead to severe obstruction. Alternatively, swelling of the tongue, pharynx, palate, or floor of the mouth from trauma, burns, or penetrating injuries may produce progressive airway occlusion.

The diagnosis of facial injuries is generally made by physical examination and radiographic analysis. Careful observation for soft tissue injuries, facial symmetry, gross deformities, eye movements, and alterations in muscle tone should be documented exactly. Palpation of the face may reveal pain, crepitus, numbness, and deformity suggestive of facial injury. Malocclusion is a very important sign of maxillofacial fracture. The ability of the patient to open the mouth should be ascertained, including the presence or absence of pain with opening. In the setting of limited mouth opening, it is important to determine if the cause is mechanical obstruction or pain/spasm. Anesthetics and muscle relaxants can relieve muscle spasm or trismus; however, their use in a patient with a mechanical obstruction may lead to loss of the airway and inability to perform direct laryngoscopy. Finally, a thorough airway examination should include an evaluation of the oral cavity to note the presence of loose or missing teeth, tongue mobility, and source of hemorrhage, if present.

Blunt trauma causing extensive facial injury should alert one to the possibility of concomitant *cervical spine* and/or closed-head injury.[58,59] Extreme care needs to be taken with these patients in regard to subsequent airway management to avoid spinal cord injury. Radiographic analysis, including plain films and CT, are essential in evaluating the extent of facial injuries but will also provide information on associated injuries.

Preoperative Preparation. The majority of penetrating facial injuries will require urgent exploration and surgical management. The timing of surgical repair of blunt facial injuries, however, is determined by many factors, including associated injuries, extent of soft tissue damage, edema, and overall patient condition. Definitive repair of these injuries is sometimes undertaken shortly after the time of injury, particularly if associated injuries require operative intervention. Many facial fractures can wait 7 to 10 days for definitive repair provided that soft tissue injuries are treated and intermaxillary fixation is applied, if necessary.

Airway management in the patient with significant facial trauma is the principal task of the anesthesiologist during the preoperative management phase. Decisions regarding airway management depend on many factors, including the significance of airway compromise, state of consciousness, etiology and type of injuries sustained, condition and anatomic distortion of the airway, identifiable or known premorbid conditions, and need for medical or surgical intervention. Partial airway obstruction is common for the reasons just described, and placement of an oral or nasal airway may alleviate the problem. A nasal airway is less likely to stimulate gagging if airway reflexes are present but should not be used in the presence of a nasal or skull base fracture.[66] Patients with severely distorted airway anatomy may be best managed with an elective tracheotomy, with or without first securing the airway through other means.

Preoperative preparation for emergent surgery should proceed as with any other traumatized patient, paying close attention to establishing adequate respiration and circulation while maintaining cervical spine immobilization. For cases of delayed surgical repair, attempts should be made to clear the cervical spine of injury to facilitate subsequent intraoperative management. Judicious use of sedatives and analgesics is indicated and may help with spasm of muscles associated with fractures through the temporomandibular joint, provided mechanical obstruction is ruled out.

Intraoperative Considerations. Mask ventilation has only limited use in facial trauma; there are constant problems attaining appropriate seal and adequate airway opening without applying pressure to fracture sites or extending the cervical spine. In patients with a compromised but stable airway, an awake intubation technique may be the best choice for airway management. To optimize access to

the surgical field, procedures involving the lower face, including the mandible, are best managed with nasal intubation if not contraindicated by other injuries or conditions. Conversely, procedures involving the midface are best managed with oral intubation or a surgical airway. The risks and benefits of approaching the airway with alternative blind techniques, either orally or nasally, must be strongly weighed.

Choice of anesthetic technique should take into consideration that facial reconstructions are long cases, have intermittent intervals of intense stimulation, and may involve significant blood loss. Surgeons will demand unencumbered access to the face and neck and may request controlled hypotension at times. In addition, monitoring of facial nerve function may be necessary.

After completion of surgery, postsurgical edema may further affect airway patency. Patients should be awake with intact reflexes before extubation. In cases of soft tissue edema, dexamethasone, 4 to 8 mg intravenously, may help reduce the tissue swelling, although the effect is not immediate. If intermaxillary fixation is applied, wire cutters should be available at the bedside and remain with the patient in the event of airway obstruction or hemorrhage.

Penetrating Trauma

While fortunately rare in most hospitals, knife and gunshot wounds cause up to 30% of all admissions to busy urban trauma centers. Penetrating injuries can affect any region of the body, and considerations for the anesthetic care of penetrating trauma victims are not substantially different than for the victims of blunt trauma. When initially assessing the patient it is important to establish the trajectory and energy transmission of the injury, so as to estimate the organ systems at risk. Gunshot wounds, particularly from high-velocity weapons such as rifles, may cause concussive damage to organs in the proximity of the bullet path even in the absence of direct penetration. Patient intoxication with alcohol or narcotics may mask signs of pain, whereas youthful physiology and use of cocaine may lead to underestimation of blood loss.

Patients who are hemodynamically unstable after penetrating trauma should be taken immediately to the OR and undergo direct exploration, the only exception being patients with limited thoracic penetration who respond promptly to tube thoracostomy. Damage control principles are applied, with the goal of controlling hemorrhage as rapidly as possible, completing resuscitation, and then returning for definitive reconstruction after 24 to 48 hours of stability in the ICU. Patients who are initially stable may undergo diagnostic testing with plain radiographs, CT, and ultrasound. The number of hemodynamically stable penetrating trauma patients who require diagnostic surgery is decreasing in recent years, because of the increasing capability of diagnostic modalities such as

CT and angiography to exclude operative injury. Exploration of neck wounds, the diagnostic pericardial window, and exploratory laparotomy for flank wounds are all performed less commonly today. Noninvasive technology is still not sufficiently sensitive to reliably exclude diaphragmatic or bowel penetration, however, and a penetrating wound that is likely to have violated the peritoneum is still a strong indicator for urgent exploratory laparotomy.

Traumatic Aortic Injury

Pathophysiology. Any high-injury blunt trauma resulting in sudden acceleration or deceleration of the torso may result in a traumatic injury to the aorta, with catastrophic consequences for the patient. Shear forces are typically concentrated at the aortic isthmus, where the relatively free-floating heart and aortic arch are tethered to the descending thoracic aorta by the ligamentum arteriosum. The spectrum of anatomic injury ranges from "cracking" of the intima with creation of a small intravascular flap all the way to complete transection. Many patients with the latter condition are found dead at the scene of injury, but survival to hospital admission is not uncommon owing to the tamponading effect of the surrounding pleura and pericardium. These patients have a very high risk of free rupture and exsanguination during the hours immediately after injury. The natural history of small intimal flaps is unknown, although some of these patients go on to form pseudoaneurysms that may become symptomatic years after the initial injury.[67] Patients with underlying atherosclerotic disease may experience proximal or distal dissection of the aorta arising from the site of injury.

Evaluation. Diagnosis of aortic injury begins with a high degree of suspicion in any patient who has suffered a high-speed frontal or lateral impact motor vehicle collision (particularly when no airbag is present), any pedestrian struck by a motor vehicle, any motorcyclist, and any patient who has fallen more than 10 feet. Symptoms of aortic injury are nonspecific, consisting mainly of back pain in the thoracic region. The blood pressure is commonly labile, with exaggerated peaks and troughs in response to hemorrhage from other injuries, painful stimulation, and sedating medications. Common coexisting injuries include fractured ribs or sternum, left hemothorax, humeral fracture, splenic rupture, and left-sided femur or acetabular fracture, although none of these is a highly sensitive marker for aortic trauma. Chest radiography is indicated but often not discriminatory. If the aortic contour is normal and well visualized, the chance of aortic injury is small, but a confident interpretation of the anteroposterior chest radiograph is possible in less than 50% of patients at risk. Visible disruption of the aortic contour or other unusual shadowing of the mediastinal structures is caused by injury to small vessels in the vicinity of the aorta and is a strong indication for further diagnostic assessment. The traditional gold standard for aortic clearance is contrast aortography. Chest CT is gaining in resolution and accuracy for aortic injury and is now the standard in large centers with experienced radiographers.[68] Transesophageal echocardiography is also highly sensitive and specific and is an appropriate diagnostic approach when an experienced operator is available.

Preoperative Preparation. Transfer of the patient to a trauma center with experience in aortic surgery is highly desirable if it can be expeditiously arranged. β-Blocker therapy is indicated in the presurgical interval to reduce sheer-force stresses on the proximal aorta. Large-bore intravenous access, right radial arterial pressure monitoring, and assessment of central pressures by pulmonary artery catheterization or transesophageal echocardiography are strongly indicated.

Intraoperative Management. Surgical treatment of traumatic aortic injury is indicated in any patient who can tolerate the procedure. Angiographically guided vascular stenting is an investigational therapy at this time, although likely to play a larger role in the near future.[69] Aortic surgery should be approached on an urgent basis, following only emergent procedures such as damage control laparotomy or evacuation of intracranial hemorrhage. Intraoperative anesthetic management requires double lumen intubation to facilitate surgical exposure of the left pleural cavity. Partial cardiac bypass is commonly used to support systemic perfusion. A full description of this technique is beyond the scope of this chapter but can be found in an excellent paper by Read and associates.[70]

Orthopedic Injuries

Orthopedic trauma produces life- and limb-threatening musculoskeletal injuries, including hemorrhage from wounds and fractures, infections from open fractures, limb loss from vascular damage and compartment syndrome, and loss of function from spinal or peripheral neurologic injuries. The management of these cases presents a wide variety of challenges for the anesthesiologist. Musculoskeletal injuries comprise the most common indication for operative management in most trauma centers. Because many procedures might be appropriately managed under regional anesthesia, familiarity with regional anesthetic techniques is essential. In addition to a familiarity with an array of regional anesthetic procedures, the anesthesiologist may need skill with fiberoptic intubation, hypotensive anesthesia, hemodilution, intraoperative cell saver techniques for minimizing intraoperative blood loss, and invasive hemodynamic and evoked potential monitoring. The length of many procedures, particularly with the presence of multiple extremity injuries, necessitates attention to body positioning, maintenance of normothermia, fluid balance, and preservation of peripheral blood flow, especially in reimplantation procedures.

Pathophysiology. For the past 15 years, the emphasis in trauma management of the multiply injured patient has included early stabilization of long bone, spine, pelvic, and acetabular fractures. Failure to do so results in increased morbidity, pulmonary complications, and length of hospital stay.[71,72] In one study only 2% of patients with femoral shaft fractures stabilized within the first 24 hours of injury had pulmonary complications, as compared with 38% of patients in whom fracture stabilization was delayed for more than 48 hours.[73] Thus, the clinical picture, treatment plan, and anesthetic management of orthopedic trauma must be focused on early entry into the operating room.

Classification of orthopedic injuries takes into account the mechanism of injury, site, type of fracture, soft tissue involvement, vascular or nerve injury, and whether the fracture is open. The anticipated rate of and severity of fracture-related complications such as need for amputation, infection, nonunion, and prognosis are linked with the classification of open fractures (Table 17-13). The mechanism of injury for a given site can predict potential complications that would affect or alter the anesthetic plan. For instance, approximate blood loss from fracture hemorrhage varies from 500 mL with a closed tibia fracture up to life-threatening hemorrhage with a pelvic fracture.

Extremity injuries include fractures, dislocations, soft tissue damage, or a combination of these findings. An understanding of anatomy and the mechanism of injury can be helpful in predicting associated injuries such as nerve and vascular damage. For instance, displaced intracapsular femoral neck fractures have a high risk of avascular necrosis, and posterior dislocation of the knee is associated with popliteal vessel injury.

Pelvic fractures occur as the result of substantial force and can be associated with significant morbidity and mortality from direct pelvic trauma combined with other injuries. They can be classified as having anteroposterior compression, lateral compression injury, or vertical shear patterns. The mechanism of injury is important because the relative risk of hemorrhage from the internal iliac artery or posterior pelvic venous plexus damage is increased with anteroposterior compression and vertical shear injuries.[73] Early stabilization of the fracture with the use of external compressive devices or external fixation and/or angiography with selective embolization may be needed before operative repair while addressing other life-threatening injuries. In addition to significant hemorrhage, other direct injuries include nerve injury, rectal or vaginal laceration, bladder rupture, and urethral injury.

Damage to the spinal column is common in traumatic injury and is frequently associated with neurologic dysfunction. The level of injury is most commonly cervical (55%), with 30% at the thoracic level and 15% in the lumbar region.[74] The most basic classification of spinal cord injuries delineates complete or partial loss of function at a given level. A complete injury is defined as a total loss of sensory and motor function lasting for more than 48 hours in areas innervated more than two levels below the level of bony injury.[75] Late injury may still occur if stability has been compromised. Mechanism and site of injury produce typical fracture patterns and frequently determine the need for surgical stabilization (see Table 17-8). A more complete discussion of spinal cord injury can be found in Chapter 8.

Evaluation. During evaluation of the orthopedic trauma patient, initial attention should be paid to the adequacy of the patient's airway, quality of ventilation, and status of perfusion, just as in any injured patient. Once these areas have been addressed and appropriate therapies initiated, subsequent evaluation should focus on the identification and treatment of associated injuries. In the multiply injured patient, this requires prioritization of the injuries and coordination of the care with the anesthetic team. Many orthopedic injuries require emergent intervention to attempt limb salvage, control of hemorrhage, nerve repair, or prevent infection.

A thorough history and examination is always vital. Time course of the injury is important because many

TABLE 17–13   Classification of Open Fracture Wounds

Type	Description
I	Clean wound less than 1 cm long
II	Laceration > 1 cm without extensive soft tissue damage, skin flaps, or avulsions
IIIA	Extensive soft tissue lacerations or flaps with adequate soft tissue coverage of bone; result of high-energy trauma
IIIB	Extensive soft tissue loss with periosteal stripping and bony exposure; usually contaminated
IIIC	Arterial injury requiring repair regardless of size of soft tissue wound

orthopedic surgeons believe all open fractures require surgical débridement within 6 hours of the initial trauma. A history inconsistent with the extent of injury may suggest either a pathologic fracture or the possibility of abuse. After the initial assessment, a secondary examination should include documentation of a thorough neurologic examination with attention to function and sensation in injured extremities. This may be particularly important if regional anesthesia is chosen, because postoperative deficits may be inadvertently attributed to the anesthetic technique. Distal perfusion should also be well documented by assessment of distal pulses. Capillary refill is not, by itself, adequate clinical evidence of intact perfusion and does not exclude the presence of a compartment syndrome or vascular injury.

Preoperative Preparation. The initial management of patients with orthopedic trauma is not substantially different from that of any injured patient. Airway management remains the highest priority. Consideration should be given to early definitive management in patients with multiple extremity fractures, serious pelvic injury, and high spine injuries with deficit. The evaluation process will often include multiple trips to remote locations such as the radiology suite, CT, and angiography, where there may not be suitable provisions for emergent airway management. Additionally, early intubation is frequently needed to allow for manipulation of fractures, treatment of dislocation, or placement of fixation pins. Ongoing assessment of adequacy of ventilation and oxygenation must be maintained throughout the evaluation process.

Maintaining adequate circulation becomes the next highest priority. Intravenous access should be established with large-bore peripheral catheters if possible, but extremities with known injuries should be avoided. Use of central venous lines may be necessary, although femoral or lower extremity cutdowns should be avoided with suspected pelvic injuries owing to the potential for pelvic venous injury. In addition, it is important to anticipate the need for blood products.[76] The mean 24-hour requirements in patients admitted with clear signs of shock is over 5 units, and approximately 20% of these patients will require more than 15 units.

Intraoperative Considerations. Choice of anesthetic technique will depend on a multitude of factors, including associated injuries, ability to cooperate with the anesthetic plan, hemodynamic stability, coexisting disease, and patient preference. Because patients present with a continuum of injury severity, no anesthetic technique is clearly superior for all patients. Presentations range from minor injuries that can be managed with infiltration of a local anesthetic, to injuries that could be treated with a peripheral nerve or subarachnoid block, and finally to injuries that

require general anesthesia with invasive monitoring. Typically, general anesthesia is the technique of choice for patients with multiple injuries. While regional anesthesia may seem attractive because it produces less interaction with the patient's cardiopulmonary function and avoids airway manipulation, patients with serious trauma benefit from endotracheal intubation and mechanical ventilation and are unlikely to cooperate with lying still during prolonged surgery. The use of neuraxial blockade can interfere with compensation for hemorrhage and produce hemodynamic instability. Thus, regional anesthesia is most useful for isolated limb trauma, for example, brachial plexus block for a hand fracture.

There are some specific considerations for the intraoperative management of patients requiring surgery for orthopedic trauma, including positioning, temperature management, use of tourniquets, potential for fat embolism, and development of deep venous thrombosis (DVT). Optimal outcome for an unstable multiply injured patient is achieved if all injuries can be corrected at the time of initial surgery. The victim of blunt trauma with multiple fractures especially benefits from early fracture fixation that reduces ongoing hemorrhage, intravascular release of bone marrow, and postoperative complications of immobilization.[71,72] During prolonged surgery, the anesthesiologist must closely monitor electrolytes, coagulation abnormalities, fluid balance, and the adequacy of ventilation/oxygenation.

Positioning. Many orthopedic surgical procedures require a nonsupine position. Care should be taken to ensure ventilation is not compromised, and positioning should allow for adequate diaphragmatic excursion and thoracic expansion without producing excessive airway pressure. All extremities should be placed in positions of comfort, preventing torsion or traction on neurovascular bundles, particularly the brachial plexus. All pressure points should be padded, especially where nerves are placed in the dependent position. The eyes, ears, nose, breasts, and genitalia should be protected when the patient is lateral or prone.

Temperature. Hypothermia is a real risk in trauma patients, particularly those with multiple injured extremities. Many patients enter the trauma center with low body temperature resulting from environmental exposure. Further exposure to a cold operating room, evaporative heat loss from the respiratory tract, infusion of cold fluids, and loss of heat production secondary to shock can produce a further drop in core temperature or reduce the effectiveness of warming efforts. With recent therapy being directed toward early fracture stabilization and definitive repair, patients with multiple extremity fractures will have long operations and large fluid volume requirements. All skin surfaces not in the surgical field should be covered to reduce convective and radiant heat loss. The addition of forced-air warming should be used where possible. Humidification of inspired gases through the use of heat-moisture exchange units reduces evaporative heat loss from the lung. The use of active heating and saturation of inspired gases can produce active warming of the patient. Only warmed intravenous fluids should be used, and in situations where large volumes of fluid or blood will be used, heat exchangers capable of warming fluids to 37°C at very rapid infusion rates should be employed. Hypothermia is a potentially life-threatening condition in these patients owing to increased susceptibility to cardiac dysrhythmias, coagulopathies, central nervous system (CNS) depression, and altered liver and kidney function.

Tourniquet Problems. Tourniquets are frequently used in extremity surgery to reduce blood loss and improve surgical visualization. When used for excessive durations or at excessive pressure tourniquets can cause injury to underlying nerves, muscle, and blood vessels, as well as producing systemic effects. Effects can be seen with initial inflation, during prolonged inflation, and on tourniquet deflation. Inflation of the tourniquet and exsanguination of the limb typically produces only small increases in central venous or arterial pressures. The application of bilateral lower extremity cuffs, however, may result in significant elevation of central venous pressure.[77] Forty-five to 60 minutes after tourniquet inflation patients under general anesthesia may develop systemic hypertension.[78] The mechanism for this elevated blood pressure is not clearly understood, and the hypertension does not always respond to deepening anesthetic depth. Deflation of the tourniquet with reperfusion of the ischemic limb may be associated with significant decreases in central venous and arterial pressures. The sudden reduction in peripheral vascular resistance with blood pooling in the extremity and the circulatory effects of ischemic metabolites most likely account for these changes.[79] Finally, awake patients undergoing regional anesthesia may complain of tourniquet pain despite an otherwise adequate block. Use of small doses of intravenous narcotics or transient deflation (10 to 15 minutes) may relieve the discomfort.

Recommended levels are 100 mm Hg above systolic pressure for thigh cuffs and 50 mm Hg above systolic pressure for upper extremity cuffs.[80] Duration of cuff inflation should generally not exceed 120 minutes.[81,82] Anesthesiologists who use regional anesthesia may be implicated when postoperative nerve injuries are identified when in fact they are secondary to tourniquet injury.

Fat Embolism. After long-bone fractures, some lung dysfunction occurs in almost all patients, ranging from minor laboratory abnormalities to full-blown fat embolism syndrome. A lack of universally accepted diagnostic criteria combined with concomitant pulmonary and cardiovascular dysfunction accounts for the varying incidences reported in the literature. Most studies suggest clinically significant fat embolism syndrome occurs in 3% to 10% of patients, although the presence of multiple long-bone fractures is associated with the higher incidence. Patients with coexisting lung injury are at additional risk of fat embolism. Signs include hypoxia, tachycardia, mental status changes, and petechiae on the upper portions of the body, including the axillae, upper arms and shoulders, chest, neck, and conjunctivae. Fat embolism syndrome should be considered whenever the alveolar-arterial oxygen gradient deteriorates in conjunction with loss of pulmonary compliance and CNS deterioration. Under general anesthesia, the CNS changes will be lost but may present as failure to wake up after surgery. If central hemodynamic monitoring is available, pulmonary artery pressures are elevated, often accompanied by decreases in cardiac index. Efforts to surgically correct fractures early and minimize trauma to the bone marrow lessen the degree of fat/bone marrow embolism, although extensive reaming of the medullary canals can contribute to perioperative morbidity and the severity of fat embolism syndrome.

Diagnosis in the operating room is largely based on the clinical presentation and ruling out other treatable causes of hypoxemia. Fat globules in the urine are nondiagnostic, but lung infiltrates seen on chest radiograph confirm the presence of lung injury and the need for appropriate ventilatory management.[83,84]

Treatment includes early recognition, oxygen administration, and judicious fluid management. A change in the orthopedic procedure may be indicated, such as converting "rodding" of the femur to external fixation. Pulmonary arterial catheter monitoring may be necessary to optimize hemodynamics because maintenance of intravascular volume is critical. Acute right-sided heart failure due to elevated pulmonary pressures is possible and requires close attention to avoid fluid overload. Finally, the use of corticosteroids has been advocated early after fat embolism syndrome.[85-87] Although clinical evidence supports improved outcomes, corticosteroids are probably not necessary in most cases.

Deep Venous Thrombosis. Deep venous thrombosis is a common problem after orthopedic trauma, with pulmonary embolism being a major contributor to postoperative mortality. The incidence of DVT varies by site and type of operative procedure (Table 17-14). The thrombosis can form during surgery with periods of venous stasis in the presence of surgical trauma. Thus, it is important to institute preventive measures starting in the operating room and continuing into the postoperative period.

Mechanical nonpharmacologic prophylaxis methods, such as intermittent pneumatic compression devices and foot pumps, increase the speed of venous flow and the volume of blood returned from the extremity to the heart.

TABLE 17–14   Incidence of Deep Venous Thrombosis (DVT) by Fracture Site or Operative Procedure

Fracture Site	Rate of DVT (%)
Knee arthroscopy	3
Total hip replacement	30-50
Total knee replacement	40-60
Tibial plateau	43
Femoral shaft	40
Tibial shaft	22
Distal tibia	13

They also produce endothelial-induced changes that decrease the risk of thromboembolic phenomenon. Because they do not affect the coagulation system, they should be used in all patients undergoing orthopedic procedures unless prevented by the presence of injury.

Epidural or spinal anesthesia reduces DVT rates after total-knee replacement by 20%[88] and after total-hip replacement by approximately 40%,[89] although postoperative epidural analgesia does not appear to provide additional benefit in reducing DVT rates.[90] Postoperative epidural analgesia may still be beneficial by allowing for earlier ambulation.

Current guidelines suggest that a low-molecular-weight heparin (LMWH) such as enoxaparin provides the best prophylaxis for venous thromboembolism in the high-risk trauma patient.[91] Once therapy has been started, LMWH should be withheld for 12 hours before surgery, if possible, and restarted a minimum of 3 hours after surgery. Recent guidelines for the use of neuraxial anesthesia and thromboprophylaxis have been published and provide clear guidance for timing of the anesthetic technique and the various agents used for thromboprophylaxis.[92] In very high-risk cases or when postoperative prophylaxis is contraindicated, vena cava filters may be placed perioperatively.

Near Drowning

As an expert in airway management and pulmonary support, the anesthesiologist may be consulted in the care of patients who present with asphyxia secondary to near drowning. Prompt intubation and restoration of normal oxygen saturation is the obvious starting point. Subsequent management is symptomatic and consists of frequent assessment of arterial blood gases with ongoing titration of mechanical ventilation to achieve adequate recruitment of collapsed lung units with the lowest possible peak airway pressure. Laryngoconstrictive reflexes are among the strongest, and many near-drowning victims do not actually aspirate significant quantities of water. Those who do have evidence of aspiration have likely reached more significant levels of hypoxia. A significant pulmonary aspiration will both remove surfactant from the lungs and contaminate the alveoli, leading to significant acute lung injury and fluid volume loss.[93] Ventilatory support is indicated and may be required for hours to days after the acute event. Because the return of normal pulmonary function is likely, long-term outcomes are driven by the patient's neurologic status, secondary to the initial period of hypoxia.

Smoke Inhalation and Carbon Monoxide Poisoning

Pathophysiology.   Patients exposed to fire and toxic gases may be hypoxic from any of three mechanisms: thermal injury to the upper airway, with edema and stricture of the larynx; particulate inhalation with subsequent bronchoconstriction; and carboxyhemoglobin formation secondary to carbon monoxide (CO) poisoning. Pulse oximetry may not accurately reflect tissue oxygen delivery because oximeters cannot discriminate carboxyhemoglobin from normal oxyhemoglobin. Because the former compound does not actually transport oxygen, significant tissue hypoxia can occur. Early arterial blood gas sampling, with specific co-oximetric measurement of the fraction of carboxyhemoglobin, is essential.

Evaluation.   While soot staining of the mucosa is common, patients with visible burns of the soft palate (blistering or erythema) should be promptly intubated, as should any patient with laryngeal edema, indicated by stridor or a progressive change in voice. Hypoxia may also be indicated by agitation or lethargy; any burn or CO-poisoning patient with an altered mental status should be intubated and mechanically ventilated until diagnostic studies have been completed. For less severely injured patients humidified oxygen and nebulized bronchodilator therapy will contribute to clearance of soot particles from the airways.

Perioperative Management.   Initial management follows the ABCs of trauma. CO poisoning is managed by administration of high concentrations of oxygen, which will competitively displace CO from hemoglobin. At an FIO_2 of 1.0, the half-life of carboxyhemoglobin is approximately 90 minutes. For patients without neurologic symptoms, face mask therapy is generally adequate. For neurologically impaired patients or those with special risk factors (pregnant, pediatric, elderly, comorbid conditions) intubation may be useful simply to increase the FIO_2. Hyperbaric therapy is indicated for severe CO poisoning cases and will significantly shorten the half-life of carboxyhemoglobin.[94]

The Pregnant Trauma Patient

Trauma to the pregnant patient presents unique problems for the anesthesiologist and resuscitation team. Significant alterations in physiologic demand associated with pregnancy may confuse and complicate the evaluation, treatment, and management of these patients. Trauma has become the leading cause of maternal death in the United States, with 3 to 4 per 1000 pregnancies requiring hospital admission for trauma.[95,96] Even minor trauma poses a significant risk to the fetus and requires extra vigilance during the most routine cases. The primary focus of resuscitation and early management is the mother, because there can be no fetal survival without maternal survival. Therefore, stabilization of the mother's condition takes priority over concerns about the fetus. One possible exception occurs during the third trimester, in the rare case in which the maternal prognosis is poor and immediate cesarean section may possibly save the fetus.

Pathophysiology. Physiologic changes associated with pregnancy alter the responses seen in traumatic injury. Table 17-15 summarizes the significant changes seen in the pregnant patient and their implications as related to trauma. During pregnancy, maternal plasma volume expands by 40% to 50% by the end of the first trimester and peaks by 30 to 34 weeks' gestation. Because red cell mass expands to a lesser degree, a dilutional anemia, referred to as the physiologic anemia of pregnancy, occurs with a normal hemoglobin range of 10.5 to 12.9 mg/dL, depending on individual variation and weeks of gestation. As a result of intravascular volume expansion, mild to moderate blood loss associated with traumatic injury may appear to be well tolerated by the mother. Subsequent alterations in uteroplacental circulation due to compensatory mechanisms, however, may have a significant impact on the fetus. Other hemodynamic alterations that may impact evaluation and management decisions include changes to baseline blood pressure and cardiac output. By 28 weeks, normal maternal blood pressure decreases by 15% to 20% owing to reductions in peripheral vascular resistance. At the same time, cardiac output increases by 35% to 50% above baseline, with a 17% increase in heart rate and a moderate increase in stroke volume. The increase in cardiac output has been attributed to a functional 20% to 30% arteriovenous shunt produced by the low-resistance placental circulation.

An additional hemodynamic effect that may have significant impact on the pregnant trauma patient is the hypotensive effect from compression of the inferior vena cava secondary to the gravid uterus. By 24 weeks' gestation, the uterus is sufficiently enlarged to produce mechanical compression of the vena cava when the patient is in a supine position. This can be manifested by as much as a 25% effective reduction of cardiac output. In the case of significant hemorrhage or cardiac arrest, hemodynamic instability due to caval compression may become an acute problem. All efforts should be made to avoid supine positioning of the severely traumatized pregnant patient during the third trimester. This can be accomplished using the left lateral decubitus position. When the patient cannot be placed on the side due to injuries, a right hip wedge, manual displacement of the uterus laterally by hand, or lateral tilt of backboard or exam table/bed can be effective.

TABLE 17–15 Physiologic Changes of Pregnancy

Organ System	Change	Implications
Cardiovascular	Decreased peripheral vascular resistance	Reduced baseline blood pressure
	Increased cardiac output	
	Increased heart rate	Resting tachycardia
	Aortocaval compression	Supine hypotension
Hematopoietic	Increased plasma volume	Dilutional anemia
	Hypercoagulable state	Thromboembolism
	Increased leukocyte count	
Respiratory	Increased minute ventilation	Respiratory alkalosis
	Decreased residual capacity	
	Elevated diaphragm	Abnormal chest radiograph
Gastrointestinal	Decreased motility	Aspiration
	Decreased lower esophageal sphincter tone	Aspiration
Renal	Increased filtration rate	
	Dilated collection system	Hydroureter, hydronephrosis
Musculoskeletal	Pelvic ligament laxity	Widened pubic symphysis
	Increased venous volume	Bleeding with fractures

Beyond the cardiovascular changes associated with pregnancy, significant respiratory changes should also be anticipated. Minute ventilation is increased by almost 50%, secondary to an increase in tidal volume. The increase in effective ventilation produces a compensated respiratory alkalosis with a reduction in buffering capacity. A "normal" blood gas in a pregnant patient should prompt an evaluation of respiratory function. Because functional residual capacity is reduced by 15% to 20% at term and oxygen consumption is significantly elevated, pregnant patients are less tolerant of apnea.

During pregnancy, capillary engorgement of the mucosa occurring throughout the respiratory tract can produce edema in the nasopharynx, oropharynx, larynx, and trachea. Manipulation of the airway requires extra care, because further injury may worsen the underlying edema and lead to airway obstruction. Endotracheal intubation with a small, cuffed endotracheal tube (6.5 to 7.0 mm) is reasonable owing to the probability for moderate supraglottic edema.

Gastrointestinal function is also affected by pregnancy, and the risk of gastric reflux is increased in the gravid patient. While alterations in gastric motility are most prominent during labor, a decrease in lower esophageal sphincter tone and increased secretion of gastric acid suggest that the risk of aspiration is increased in any pregnant patient near term.

Physiologic changes of note include increased renal blood flow and creatinine clearance. A mild physiologic hydronephrosis of pregnancy may also be present and should be considered when evaluating the patient with abdominal or pelvic trauma. Hematologic function is altered by an estrogen-influenced increase in hepatic production of coagulation factors. Pregnancy places women at increased risk for thromboembolic disease caused by increased venous stasis, vessel wall injury, and changes in the coagulation cascade that lead to hypercoagulability. Fibrinogen is also increased by 50%, such that a normal level in a pregnant patient (300 mg/dL) may suggest an abnormal consumptive process. Finally, a moderate leukocytosis is normal in pregnancy and does not by itself suggest the presence of an inflammatory or infective process.

In addition to understanding the impact of maternal physiology on the response to trauma, the anesthesiologist must also consider the effects on the fetus. The consequences of trauma on pregnancy depend on the gestational age of the fetus, the type and severity of the trauma, and the extent of disruption of normal uterine and fetal relationships. Fetal survival depends on adequate uterine perfusion and delivery of oxygen. Because autoregulation is lacking in uterine circulation, uterine blood flow is related directly to maternal systemic blood pressure. Once the mother approaches a state of hypovolemic shock, further maternal vasoconstriction will compromise uterine perfusion.

Once clinically measurable shock develops in the mother, the chances of saving the fetus are about 20%.

Fetal bradycardia or tachycardia, a decrease in baseline heart rate variability, absence of normal accelerations of fetal heart rate, or repetitive decelerations suggest that fetal oxygenation and/or perfusion have been compromised by trauma. An abnormal fetal heart rate may be the first indication of an important disruption in fetal homeostasis. Finally, direct or indirect uterine trauma can also injure the myometrium and lead to uterine contractions, with the possibility of inducing premature labor. When the maternal injuries are not lethal, placental abruption is the most common cause of fetal demise.[97] Because placental abruption can occur with low energy impacts, all patients with moderate blunt trauma should undergo fetal heart rate monitoring and close observation.[96,98]

Evaluation. Involvement of anesthesia personnel in the care of the injured pregnant patient potentially requiring surgery should begin with the initial evaluation. Immediate consultation with an obstetrician or maternal-fetal specialist will allow for better coordination of care. The primary goal in treating a pregnant trauma victim is to stabilize the mother's condition. During the primary survey, the priorities for treatment of an injured pregnant patient remain the same as those for the nonpregnant patient. Given the increased risk of aspiration, decreased tolerance for apnea, and fetal distress associated with hypoxia, endotracheal intubation should be considered early. This must be balanced against the potential for encountering a difficult airway, particularly in the later stages of pregnancy. Although tachypnea is present at baseline in the pregnant patient, other causes of respiratory compromise should be sought. Assessment of perfusion and interpretation of all vital signs should take into consideration pregnancy-related changes. With a baseline elevation of 10 to 15 beats per minute above baseline, maternal heart rate may be difficult to correlate with volume status. Assessment of central and peripheral pulses, capillary refill, skin color and temperature, and mental status are still useful tools, although significant hypovolemia can be present with minimal change in these markers.

After initiation of lifesaving measures, a more thorough secondary survey of the stable pregnant patient must include some form of fetal assessment. If possible, a pregnancy history should be obtained with attention to determining the estimated gestational age, prenatal care, and complications, including diabetes or hypertension. Estimated gestational age and viability should be determined quickly, because the fetus is considered to be viable at 24 weeks' gestation. If the mother is unable to provide a history, the ability to palpate the uterine fundus at 3 to 4 cm above the umbilicus correlates with a viable gestational age. Cardiotocographic monitoring (CTM) should be initiated as early as possible. Fetal bradycardia is a sensitive indicator of maternal perfusion and can be the first measurable change in the presence of significant maternal hypovolemia. Uterine irritability and contractions monitored through CTM are sensitive in detecting placental abruption.[99,100] The American College of Obstetricians and Gynecologists (ACOG) recommends that any pregnant woman sustaining trauma beyond 22 to 24 weeks' gestation should undergo fetal monitoring for a minimum of 24 hours.[99] In the presence of ruptured membranes, bleeding, fetal arrhythmia, fetal heart rate deceleration, or more than four contractions per hour, the patient should be admitted with continuous fetal monitoring for at least 24 hours.

Laboratory evaluation should include hemoglobin, hematocrit, type and crossmatch, urinalysis, coagulation parameters, lactate determination, and blood gas analysis. Interpretation of the results should take pregnancy-related changes into consideration. Physiologic anemia may be confused with that produced by hemorrhage in the pregnant trauma patient. A normal fibrinogen level may be an early indicator of disseminated intravascular coagulation due to placental abruption. Additionally, a normal or elevated $Paco_2$ level may suggest pending respiratory failure. Use of lactate levels as a marker of resuscitation is not affected by the pregnant state.

In the Rh-negative patient, a Kleihauer-Betke test may be ordered to assess for Rh isoimmunization. Administration of Rh_O (D) immune globulin is indicated in the presence of fetomaternal hemorrhage in this subset of patients.

Preoperative Preparation. Careful attention must be paid to the perioperative volume status of the gravid trauma patient to avoid decreases in fetal perfusion. As with all trauma patients, large-bore intravenous access is required. When large volumes of crystalloid are necessary, normal saline should be avoided because it may lead to maternal and fetal hyperchloremic acidosis. Coagulation defects should be corrected before surgery, keeping in mind pregnancy-related changes, including an elevated fibrinogen level. Prophylactic measures to reduce gastric pH and volume are warranted, because aspiration of gastric contents during general anesthesia is a major cause of maternal morbidity and mortality.

Intraoperative Considerations. The choice of anesthetic technique in the traumatized pregnant patient will be determined by the operative procedure, concomitant injuries, preexisting conditions, and maternal preference. When feasible, regional anesthesia offers some advantages to general anesthesia, although there is no direct evidence showing a reduction in mortality. A decrease in the administration of systemic medications and subsequent reduction in fetal exposure is desirable. Additionally, the avoidance of airway manipulation reduces the risk of airway loss and maternal morbidity.

Nonetheless, general anesthesia will still be a necessity for many pregnant trauma patients requiring operative procedures. Preoxygenation before anesthetic induction must be accomplished for more than 3 minutes with 100% oxygen to blunt the rapid onset of hypoxia seen with apnea in these patients.[100] This is usually accomplished in conjunction with an RSI due to the increased risk of aspiration. Left uterine displacement must be continued throughout the induction and operative periods. Invasive hemodynamic monitoring is used as dictated by maternal conditions. Maternal arterial CO_2 should be kept at 33 to 36 mm Hg. Further degrees of hyperventilation may be detrimental to fetal perfusion. Intraoperative fetal CTM can supplement other available information regarding maternal perfusion, although operative considerations may prohibit its use. CTM should be continued into the postoperative period to monitor for premature labor.

Concerns about the effects of anesthetic agents on the growth and development of the human fetus should be factored into the anesthetic plan. A more comprehensive review of pharmacologic considerations and potential teratogenicity is provided elsewhere in this text (see Chapter 19). Agents and techniques that have been widely used and evaluated should be employed for the care of the pregnant trauma patient whenever possible.

Geriatric Trauma

Outcomes from trauma are dramatically worse in elderly patients, with significantly higher in-hospital morbidity and mortality rates after identical anatomic injuries.[101] Reasons for this difference are multifactorial but may include a decreased basal metabolic rate, limited cardiopulmonary reserve, impaired wound healing, and increased susceptibility to sepsis. Elderly patients are more likely than younger ones to have coexisting medical disease, such as diabetes or atherosclerosis, that contribute to delayed healing. Preexisting neurologic impairment, including untreated depression, is common in older trauma patients. For many elderly patients it is a traumatic event that signifies the transition from independent living to a requirement for chronic nursing care or assisted living.

For the anesthesiologist, close attention to detail is required to achieve the best possible results. This may include modalities such as nutritional support, continuous insulin infusion, and perioperative β blockade. The surgical procedures required by elderly patients are similar to those in other trauma patients, but determining the optimal timing for surgery may be more challenging. Bed-bound elderly trauma patients will suffer a predictable and progressive loss of pulmonary function owing to atelectasis and pneumonia, even in the presence of attentive nursing care, meaning that delaying surgery in an effort to improve ventilation or perform further diagnostic studies may be counterproductive. Similarly, the need for urgent operative repair of long bone fractures and open wounds should limit the pursuit of specialty consultation and risk stratification studies (e.g., stress cardiac imaging) to those situations in which there is a high likelihood of a change in management. Patients with active myocardial ischemia or cardiac dysrhythmias may benefit from angioplasty or electrophysiologic intervention before an orthopedic surgery, but in most other situations the patient will benefit more from prompt surgical correction of the traumatic injury.[33]

In general, the anesthesiologist is advised to assume the worst about the patient with an unclear history or unknown cardiac risk. Anesthetic medications, including induction agents, should be chosen with the intention of maintaining cardiovascular stability and should be carefully titrated to the patient's response. Many elderly patients will exhibit prolonged sedation and disorientation after intravenous anxiolysis, frequently necessitating postoperative mechanical ventilation. Invasive arterial pressure monitoring and frequent laboratory assessment of tissue perfusion should be considered in any patient likely to experience more than a minimal blood loss. Pulmonary artery catheterization and direct assessment of myocardial performance and fluid volume status may be beneficial,[102] although this technique is cumbersome in the operating room. Transesophageal echocardiography and newer noninvasive technologies may be more appropriate for elderly patients undergoing moderate risk procedures.

Prehospital Anesthetic Care

The role of the anesthesiologist extends beyond the walls of a medical facility when he or she becomes involved in prehospital medical care. Many large trauma centers have established relationships with their local emergency medical service (EMS) to provide a field response or "Go Team" that is capable of providing extended medical support in the event of a disaster or accident where their services may be necessary for lifesaving or limb-saving interventions.[103] Physician involvement in prehospital management of trauma is limited to consultation and occasional scene response in North America, although Israel, Germany, France, and other countries have mobile ICUs staffed by anesthesiologists and other physicians.[104,105]

Inclusion on a "Go Team" brings with it certain training requirements for the unique conditions found with medical disaster response. An effective approach to the challenges of disaster response is to break the response down to recognizable tasks (Table 17-16). Although physicians involved in the response to a disaster scene will not be responsible for the majority of these tasks, familiarity with them will make their integration into the team smoother and establish a framework for their own unique skills. Individuals assigned to a "Go Team" must be

TABLE 17–16 Disaster Response Tasks

Scene Assessment
Scene description
Scene safety
Patient conditions

Incident Management
Command and control
Communications

Victim Care
Search and rescue
Primary assessment and triage
Transport
Definitive care

familiar with a number of areas, including working with hazardous materials, use of personal protective gear, maintaining scene control, decontamination, use of rescue equipment, understanding of aeromedical considerations, and basic emergency medicine training.

The most common scenario for "Go Team" response is entrapment after a motor vehicle crash or building collapse. Field amputation is occasionally required to safely extract the patient. A familiarity with intravenous anesthesia and alternative airway techniques are essential for these types of cases. In addition, the "Go Team" usually has the ability to administer blood products as well as higher degrees of sedation than are possible under most EMS protocols.

References

1. Fingerhut LA, Warner M: Injury Chartbook. Health, United States, 1996-97. Hyattsville, MD, National Center for Health Statistics, 1998.
2. West JG, Cales RH, Gazzaniga AB: Impact of regionalization—the Orange County experience. Arch Surg 1983;118:740.
3. Resources for optimal care of the injured patient: 1998. Chicago, American College of Surgeons, 1998.
4. Dutton RP, Scalea TM, Aarabi B: Prioritizing surgical needs in the multiply injured patient. In Prough DS, Fleisher L (eds): Problems in Anesthesia. Trauma Care 2002;13(3).
5. Rotondo MF, Schwab CW, McGonigal MD et al: "Damage control": An approach for improved survival in exsanguinating penetrating abdominal injury. J Trauma 1993;35:375-382.
6. Scalea TM, Boswell SA, Scott JD, et al: External fixation as a bridge to intramedullary nailing for patients with multiple injuries and with femur fractures: Damage control orthopedics. J Trauma 2000;48:613-621.
7. Committee on Trauma, American College of Surgeons: Advanced Trauma Life Support Program for Doctors. Chicago, American College of Surgeons, 1997.
8. Thierbach AR, Lipp MDW: Airway management in trauma patients. Anesth Clin North Am 1999;17:63-81.
9. Xiao Y, Hunter WA, Mackenzie CF, et al: Task complexity in emergency medical care and its implications for team coordination. Hum Factors 1996;38:636-645.
10. Todd MM, Hindman BJ, Brian JE: Cervical Spine Anatomy and Physiology for Anesthesiologists. ASA Refresher Courses in

Anesthesiology. Chicago, American Society of Anesthesiologists, 2003, pp 189-202.

11. Talucci RC, Shaikh KA, Schwab CW: Rapid sequence induction with oral endotracheal intubation in the multiply injured patient. Am Surg 1988;54:185-187.

12. Brimacombe JR, Brain AIJ, Berry AM: Anatomical implications. In Brimacombe JR, Brain AIJ (eds): The Laryngeal Mask Airway: A Review and Practical Guide. Philadelphia, WB Saunders, 1997, pp 14-26.

13. Practice guidelines for management of the difficult airway. An updated report by the American Society of Anesthesiologists Task Force on Management of the Difficult Airway. Anesthesiology 2003;98:1269-1277.

14. Crile GW: An Experimental Research into Surgical Shock. Philadelphia, JB Lippincott, 1899.

15. Peitzman AB: Hypovolemic shock. In Pinsky MR, Dhainaut JFA (eds): Pathophysiologic Foundations of Critical Care. Baltimore, Williams & Wilkins, 1993, pp 161-169.

16. Shires GT, Cunningham N, Baker CRF et al: Alterations in cellular membrane function during hemorrhagic shock in primates. Ann Surg 1972;176:288-295.

17. Dutton RP: Management of traumatic shock. In Prough DS, Fleisher L (eds): Problems in Anesthesia. Trauma Care 2002;13(3).

18. Blow O, Magliore L, Claridge JA, et al: The golden hour and the silver day: Detection and correction of occult hypoperfusion within 24 hours improves outcome from major trauma. J Trauma 1999;47:964-969.

19. Stern A, Dronen SC, Birrer P, Wang X: Effect of blood pressure on haemorrhagic volume in a near-fatal haemorrhage model incorporating a vascular injury. Ann Emerg Med 1993;22:155-163.

20. Capone A, Safar P, Stezoski SW, et al: Uncontrolled hemorrhagic shock outcome model in rats. Resuscitation 1995;29:143-152.

21. Riddez L, Johnson L, Hahn RG: Central and regional hemodynamics during fluid therapy after uncontrolled intra-abdominal bleeding. J Trauma 1998;44:1-7.

22. Sakles JC, Sena MJ, Knight DA, Davis JM: Effect of immediate fluid resuscitation on the rate, volume, and duration of pulmonary vascular hemorrhage in a sheep model of penetrating thoracic trauma. Ann Emerg Med 1997;29:392-399.

23. Burris D, Rhee P, Kaufmann C, et al: Controlled resuscitation for uncontrolled hemorrhagic shock. J Trauma 1999;46:216-223.

24. Bickell WH, Wall MJ, Pepe PE, et al: Immediate versus delayed resuscitation for hypotensive patients with penetrating torso injuries. N Engl J Med 1994;331:1105-1109.

25. Dutton RP, Mackenzie CF, Scalea TM: Hypotensive resuscitation during active hemorrhage: Impact on in-hospital mortality. J Trauma 2002;52:1141-1146.

26. Camp, FR, Conte NF, Brewer JR: Military Blood Banking 1941-1973. Fort Knox, KY, U.S. Army Medical Research Laboratory, 1973, p 20.

27. Lorentz A, Frietsch T: Transfusion medicine. N Engl J Med 2002;347:538-539.

28. Martinowitz U, Kenet G, Segal E, et al: Recombinant activated factor VII for adjunctive hemorrhage control in trauma. J Trauma 2001; 51:1-9.

29. Prough DS, Bidani A: Hyperchloremic metabolic acidosis is a predictable consequence of intraoperative infusion of 0.9% saline. Anesthesiology 1999;90:1247.

30. Otto CW: Cardiopulmonary resuscitation. In Barash PG, Cullen BF, Stoelting RK (eds): Clinical Anesthesia, 4th ed. Philadelphia, Lippincott-Raven, 2001, pp 1498-1499.

31. Abramson D, Scalea TM, Hitchcock R, et al: Lactate clearance and survival following injury. J Trauma 1993;35:584-588.

32. Evans RW: The postconcussion syndrome and the sequelae of mild head injury. Neurol Clin 1992;10:815-847.

33. Dunham CM, Bosse MJ, Clancy TV, et al: Practice management guidelines for the optimal timing of long-bone fracture stabilization in polytrauma patients: The EAST practice management guidelines work group. J Trauma 2001;50:958-967.

34. Kalb DC, Ney AL, Rodriguez JL, et al: Assessment of the relationship between timing of fixation of the fracture and secondary brain injury in patients with multiple trauma. Surgery 1998;124:739-744.

35. Guidelines for the management of severe traumatic brain injury. Brain Trauma Foundation, American Association of Neurological Surgeons, Joint Section on Neurotrauma and Critical Care. J Neurotrauma 2000;17:451-627.

36. Chestnut RM, Marshall LF, Klauber MR, et al: The role of secondary brain injury in determining outcome from severe head injury. J Trauma 1993;134:216-222.

37. Kerr EM, Marion D, Sereika MS, et al: The effect of cerebrospinal fluid drainage on cerebral perfusion in traumatic brain injured adults. J Neurosurg Anesthesiol 2000;12:324-333.

38. Cremer OL, Moons KG, Bouman EA, et al: Long-term propofol infusion and cardiac failure in adult head-injured patients. Lancet 2001;357:117-118.

39. Masuzawa M, Nakao S, Miyamoto E, et al: Pentobarbital inhibits ketamine-induced dopamine release in the rat nucleus accumbens: A microdialysis study. Anesth Analg 2003;96:148-152.

40. Soukiasian HJ, Hui T, Avital I, et al: Decompressive craniectomy in trauma patients with severe brain injury. Am Surg 2002;68:1066-1071.

41. Joseph D, Dutton RP, Aarabi B, Scalea TM: Decompressive laparotomy to reduce intracranial pressure in patients with severe traumatic brain injury. J Trauma 2004; 57:687-693.

42. Clifton GL, Emmy RM, Choi SC, et al: Lack of effect of induction of hypothermia after acute brain injury. N Engl J Med 2001;344:556-563.

43. Kiwerski JE: Neurological outcome from conservative treatment of cervical spinal cord injured patients. Paraplegia 1993;31:192-196.

44. EAST Practice Parameter Workgroup for Cervical Spine Clearance: Practice Management Guidelines for Identifying Cervical Spine Injuries Following Trauma. Eastern Association for the Surgery of Trauma 1998. Available at http://east.org/tpg.html.

45. American Association of Neurological Surgeons: Guidelines for the management of acute spinal cervical spine and spinal cord injuries. Neurosurgery 2002;59:S58.

46. Bracken MB, Shepard MJ, Holford TR, et al: Administration of methylprednisolone for 24 or 48 hours or tirilazad mesylate for 48 hours in the treatment of acute spinal cord injury: Results of the third National Acute Spinal Cord Injury Study. JAMA 1997;277:1597-1604.

47. Kewelramani LS: Autonomic dysreflexia in traumatic myelopathy. Am J Phys Med 1980;59:1.

48. Zagelbaum BM, Tostanoski JR, Kerner DJ, Hersh PS: Urban eye trauma: A one-year prospective study. Ophthalmology 1993;100: 851-856.

49. Blomdahl S, Norell S: Perforating eye injury in the Stockholm population: An epidemiological study. Acta Ophthalmol (Copenh) 1984;62:378-390.

50. Cunningham AJ, Barry P: Intraocular pressure—physiology and implications for anaesthetic management. Can Anaesth Soc J 1986;33:195-208.

51. Pandey K, Badola RP, Kumar S: Time course of intraocular hypertension produced by suxamethonium. Br J Anaesth 1972;44: 191-196.

52. Vachon CA, Warner DO, Bacon DR: Succinylcholine and the open globe: Tracing the teaching. Anesthesiology 2003;99:220-223.

53. Libonati MM, Leahy JJ, Ellison N: The use of succinylcholine in open eye surgery. Anesthesiology 1985;62:637-640.

54. Moreno RJ, Kloess P, Carlson DW: Effect of succinylcholine on the intraocular contents of open globes. Ophthalmology 1991;98:636-638.

55. Drenger B, Pe'er J, BenEzra D, et al: The effect of intravenous lidocaine on the increase in intraocular pressure induced by tracheal intubation. Anesth Analg 1985;64:1211-1213.

56. Stirt JA, Chiu GJ: Intraocular pressure during rapid sequence induction: Use of moderate-dose sufentanil or fentanyl and vecuronium or atracurium. Anaesth Intensive Care 1990;18:390-394.

57. Karlson TA: The incidence of hospital-treated facial injuries from vehicles. J Trauma 1982;22:303-310.

58. Hackl W, Hausberger K, Sailer R, et al: Prevalence of cervical spine injuries in patients with facial trauma. Oral Surg Oral Med Oral Pathol Oral Radiol Endod 2001;92:370-376.

59. Luce EA, Tubb TD, Moore AM: Review of 1,000 major facial fractures and associated injuries. Plast Reconstr Surg 1979;63:26-30.

60. Lee KF, Wagner LK, Lee YE, et al: The impact-absorbing effects of facial fractures in closed-head injuries: An analysis of 210 patients. J Neurosurg 1987;66:542-547.

61. Capan LM, Miller SM, Glickman R: Management of facial injuries. In Capan LM, Miller SM, Turndorf H (eds): Trauma Anesthesia and Intensive Care. Philadelphia, JB Lippincott, 1991, pp 385-408.

62. Krohner RG: Anesthetic considerations and techniques for oral and maxillofacial surgery. Int Anesthesiol Clin 2003;41:67-89.

63. Shepherd SM, Lippe MS: Maxillofacial trauma: Evaluation and management by the emergency physician. Emerg Med Clin North Am 1987;5:371-392.

64. Rohrich RJ, Shewmake KB: Evolving concepts of craniomaxillofacial fracture management. Clin Plast Surg 1992;19:1-10.

65. Gruss JS: Complex craniomaxillofacial trauma: Evolving concepts in management: A trauma unit's experience—1989 Fraser B. Gurd lecture. J Trauma 1990;30:377-383.

66. Martin JE, Mehta R, Aarabi B, et al: Intracranial insertion of a nasopharyngeal airway in a patient with craniofacial trauma. Milit Med 2004;169:496-497.

67. Petty SM, Parker LA, Mauro MA, et al: Chronic posttraumatic aortic pseudoaneurysm. Postgrad Med 1991;89:173-178.

68. Mirvis SE, Shanmuganathan K, Miller BH: Traumatic aortic injury: Diagnosis with contrast-enhanced thoracic CT-five year experience at a major trauma center. Radiology 1996;200:413.

69. Dunham MB, Zygun D, Petrasek P, et al: Endovascular stent grafts for acute blunt aortic injury. J Trauma 2004;56:1173-1178.

70. Read RA, Moore EE, Moore FA, Haenel JB: Partial left heart bypass for thoracic aortic repair. Arch Surg 1993;128:746.

71. Johnson KD, Cadambi A, Seibert GB: Incidence of adult respiratory distress syndrome in patients with multiple musculoskeletal injuries: Effect of early operative stabilization of fractures. J Trauma 1985;25:375-384.

72. Bone LB, Johnson KD, Weigelt J, Scheinberg R: Early versus delayed stabilization of femoral fractures: A prospective randomized study. J Bone Joint Surg Am 1989;71:336-340.

73. Dalal SA, Burgess AR, Siegel JH, et al: Pelvic fracture in multiple trauma: Classification by mechanism is key to pattern of organ injury, resuscitative requirements, and outcome. J Trauma 1989;29:981-1000.

74. Burney RE, et al: Incidence, characteristics, and outcome of spinal cord injury at trauma centers in North America. Arch Surg 1993;128:596-599.

75. Rothman RH, Simeone FA (eds): The Spine. Philadelphia, WB Saunders, 1992.

76. Klein SR, Saroyan RM, Baumgartner F, Bonegard FS: Management strategy of vascular injuries associated with pelvic fractures. J Cardiovasc Surg (Torino) 1992;33:349-357.

77. Bradford EM: Haemodynamic changes associated with the application of lower limb tourniquets. Anaesthesia 1969;24:190-197.

78. Kaufman RD, Walts LF: Tourniquet-induced hypertension. Br J Anaesth 1982;54:333-336.

79. Kahn RL, Marino V, Urquhart B, Sharrock NE: Hemodynamic changes associated with tourniquet use under epidural anesthesia for total knee arthroplasty. Reg Anesth 1992;17:228-232.

80. Klenerman L: Tourniquet time—how long? Hand 1980;12:231-234.

81. Heppenstall RB, Scott R, Sapega A, et al: A comparative study of the tolerance of skeletal muscle to ischemia: Tourniquet application compared with acute compartment syndrome. J Bone Joint Surg Am 1986;68:820-828.

82. Sapega AA, Heppenstall RB, Chance B, et al: Optimizing tourniquet application and release times in extremity surgery: A biochemical and ultrastructural study. J Bone Joint Surg Am 1985;67:303-314.

83. Hutchins PM, Macnicol MF: Pulmonary insufficiency after long bone fractures: Absence of circulating fat or significant immunodepression. J Bone Joint Surg Br 1985;67:835-839.

84. Lindeque BG, Schoeman HS, Dommisse GF, et al: Fat embolism and the fat embolism syndrome: A double-blind therapeutic study. J Bone Joint Surg Br 1987;69:128-131.

85. Kallenbach J, Lewis M, Zaltman M, et al: Low-dose corticosteroid prophylaxis against fat embolism. J Trauma 1987;27:1173-1176.

86. Schonfeld SA, Ploysongsang Y, Dilisio R, et al: Fat embolism prophylaxis with corticosteroids: A prospective study in high-risk patients. Ann Intern Med 1983;99:438-443.

87. Alho A, Saikku K, Eerola P, et al: Corticosteroids in patients with a high risk of fat embolism syndrome. Surg Gynecol Obstet 1978;147:358-362.

88. Williams-Russo P, Sharrock NE, Haas SB, et al: Randomized trial of epidural versus general anesthesia: Outcomes after primary total knee replacement. Clin Orthop 1996;331:199-208.

89. Prins MH, Hirsh J: A critical review of the evidence supporting a relationship between impaired fibrinolytic activity and venous thromboembolism. Arch Intern Med 1991;151:1721-1731.

90. Sharrock NE, Hargell MJ, Urquhart B, et al: Factors affecting deep vein thrombosis rate following total knee arthroplasty under epidural anesthesia. J Arthroplasty 1993;8:133-139.

91. Rogers FB, Cipolle MD, Velmahos G, Rozycki G: Practice Management Guidelines for the Management of Venous Thromboembolism in Trauma Patients. Atlanta, The Eastern Association for the Surgery of Trauma, 1999.

92. Horlocker TT, Wedel DJ, Berzon H, et al: Regional anesthesia in the anticoagulated patient: Defining the risks (the second ASRA Consensus Conference on Neuraxial Anesthesia and Anticoagulation). Reg Anesth Pain Med 2003;28:172-197.

93. Orlowski JP, Abulleli MM, Phillips JM: Effects of tonicities of saline solutions on pulmonary injury in drowning. Crit Care Med 1987;1:126.

94. Weaver LK, Hopkins RO, Chan KJ, et al: Hyperbaric oxygen for acute carbon monoxide poisoning. N Engl J Med 2002;347:1057-1067.

95. Connolly AM, Katz VL, Bosh KL, et al: Trauma and pregnancy. Am J Perinatol 1997;14:331-336.

96. Pearlman MD, Tintinalli JE: Evaluation and treatment of the gravida and fetus following trauma during pregnancy. Obstet Gynecol Clin North Am 1991;18:371-381.

97. Dahmus MA, Sibai BM: Blunt abdominal trauma: Are there any predictive factors for abruptio placentae or maternal-fetal distress? Am J Obstet Gynecol 1993;169:1054-1059.

98. Pak LL, Reece EA, Chan L: Is adverse pregnancy outcome predictable after blunt abdominal trauma? Am J Obstet Gynecol 1998;179:1140-1144.

99. American College of Obstetricians and Gynecologists: Obstetric Aspects of Trauma Management. ACOG educational bulletin No. 251. Washington, DC, ACOG, 2000.

100. Archer GW, Marx GF: Arterial oxygen tension during apnoea in parturient women. Br J Anaesth 1974;46:358-360.

101. Osler T, Hales K, Baack B, et al: Trauma in the elderly. Am J Surg 1988;156:537.

102. Scalea TM, Simon HM, Duncan AO, et al: Geriatric blunt multiple trauma: Improved survival with early imaging and monitoring. J Trauma 1990;30:129.

103. Jaslow D, Barbera JA, Desai S, Jolly BT: An emergency department–based field response team: Case report and recommendations for a "go team." Prehosp Emerg Care 1998;2:81-85.

104. Einav S, Donchin Y, Weisman C, et al: Anesthesiologists on ambulances: Where do we stand? Curr Opin Anaesthesiol 2003;16:585-591.

105. Benitez FL, Pepe PE: Role of the physician in prehospital management of trauma: North American perspective. Curr Opin Crit Care 2003;8:551-558.

18 Burns

SANJAY M. BHANANKER, MD, and BRUCE F. CULLEN, MD

Perioperative management of patients with severe burn injuries offers significant challenges to the anesthesiologist. It is estimated that every year approximately 1.25 million burn injuries are treated in the United States, up to 100,000 of which require hospitalization. Over 6,500 patients succumb to their thermal injuries.[1] A better understanding of the pathophysiology of burn injuries, coupled with advances in burn resuscitation, critical care, and surgical practice, has resulted in improved survival in severely burned patients over the past 3 decades.[2-5]

An expert task force of the American Burn Association (ABA) has developed a set of evidence-based guidelines for the management of acute burn injury. These guidelines summarize the current scientific basis of the clinical practice for the management of acute burn injury and have been published as a special supplement to the May/June 2001 issue of *Journal of Burn Care & Rehabilitation.*[6]

Modern care for the severely burned patient can be divided into four overlapping phases: (1) initial evaluation and resuscitation, (2) initial excision and biologic closure, (3) definitive wound closure, and (4) rehabilitation and reconstruction.[7] The anesthesiologist's services may be called on for airway management, intravenous access, and fluid resuscitation, in addition to providing sedation and analgesia in the acute phase. Administration of analgesia and sedation for wound care and provision of anesthesia for excision and grafting are even more challenging tasks.

Reconstructive surgery poses special challenges due to development of contractures, making airway management and positioning difficult.

PATHOPHYSIOLOGY

The primary determinants of severity of burn injury are the size and depth of the burn. However, patient age, body part burned, presence of preexisting disease, and associated non-burn injuries have an important impact on the outcome.[3-5] The size of the burn is most commonly estimated in adults by using the "rule of nines" and expressed as percentage of total body surface area (%TBSA) (Fig. 18-1).[8,9] The burn depth is classified into superficial, partial thickness, and full thickness (Table 18-1). First-degree (superficial) burns affect only the epidermis and are characterized by erythema and edema of the burned areas without blistering or desquamation. These are treated with daily dressing and wound care until epithelialization occurs. Second-degree (partial-thickness) burns involve the epidermis and a portion of the dermis. In most cases, these wounds can be expected to spontaneously heal in 1 to 4 weeks, although surgical treatment may be necessary for extensive or deep second-degree burns. Pain is characteristic of partial-thickness burns. Third-degree (full-thickness) burns extend entirely through both the epidermis and dermis and will not heal spontaneously.[10]

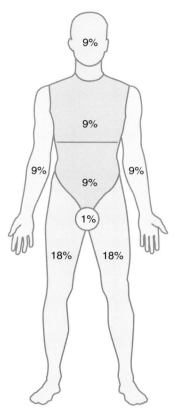

FIGURE 18–1 Rule of nines to estimate the percentage of body surface area.

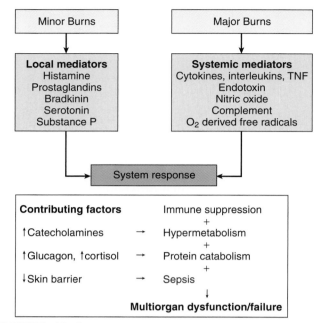

FIGURE 18–2 Pathophysiology of burns.

Mediators of Inflammation

Severe burn injury results in release of circulating mediators that evoke a physiologic response (systemic inflammatory response syndrome [SIRS]) throughout the body (Fig. 18-2).[11] These mediators include histamine,[12] serotonin,[13] cytokines,[14] tumor necrosis factor-α,[15] endotoxin,[16-18] oxygen-derived free radicals,[19-21] nitric oxide,[22] and complement.[23,24]

Cardiovascular Changes

There is an increase in capillary permeability and "third spacing" of fluid in tissues surrounding the burn. Interstitial edema and organ dysfunction in distant

organs result from combination of the vasoactive mediators and hypoproteinemia in severe burns.[25,26] Increased capillary permeability is seen in the burned tissue for more than 72 hours and in the non-burned tissue for up to 24 hours.[27] Tumor necrosis factor-α, oxygen free radicals, and endothelin-1 exert a negative inotropic effect and reduce the cardiac output acutely. The cardiovascular response to both endogenous and exogenous catecholamines is attenuated owing to decreased adrenergic receptor affinity and decreased production of second messenger. Systemic vascular resistance increases in the initial post-burn period.

Later, following successful resuscitation, in the hypermetabolic phase the cardiovascular response is an increased cardiac output and reduced systemic vascular resistance.

Metabolic Changes

Up to a 10-fold increase in circulating levels of catecholamines has been demonstrated after severe

TABLE 18-1	Classification of Burn Depth	
Classification	**Burn Depth**	**Outcome**
Superficial (first degree)	Epidermis only	Heal spontaneously
Partial thickness (second degree)	Epidermis and dermis	
Full thickness		
Third degree	Destruction of epidermis and dermis	Wound excision and grafting necessary
Fourth degree	Fascia, muscle, bone burned	Complete excision required, functional limitation likely

burn injury.[28,29] These, along with wound-released mediators, hormones, and bacterial products from the gut and wound result in SIRS, manifested as hyperdynamic circulation and large increases in basal energy expenditure (hypermetabolic response).[7,27,29] The secretion of glucagon and cortisol are increased and, together with post-injury insulin resistance, result in the use of amino acids to fuel production, with consequent muscle wasting and nitrogen imbalance.[25] The supraphysiologic thermogenesis is associated with resetting of the core temperature to higher levels, proportional to the size of the burns.[30,31] Damaged skin is no longer able to retain heat and water, and the vasomotor thermoregulatory responses are impaired. Consequently, large evaporative losses ensue.[31,32] Loss of barrier function of skin and blunting of immune response result in increased susceptibility to infection and bacterial overgrowth within the eschar.[26,31,33,34] Adequate pain control, alleviation of anxiety, maintenance of a thermoneutral environment, and treatment of infection are important steps in limiting catecholamine secretion and thus hypermetabolism.

Hematologic Changes

Hematologic and coagulation factor changes after burn injury depend on the magnitude of burn injury and time from injury. Hematocrit is typically maintained early in the post-burn period but drops during the weeks of care as erythrocyte half-life is reduced.[27,35] Platelet count diminishes as a result of formation of microaggregates in the skin and smoke-damaged lung, although this is rarely a clinical problem. Both the thrombotic and fibrinolytic mechanisms are activated after major burns.[35,36] Clinically, hypercoagulability may be a problem in late post-burn injury period and patients should receive thromboembolism prophylaxis.

Renal Function

The incidence of acute renal failure in burn patients ranges from 0.5% to 38%, depending on the severity of burns.[37,38] In the early post-burn period, the renal blood flow is reduced as a result of hypovolemia and decreased cardiac output. In addition, increased levels of catecholamines, angiotensin, vasopressin, and aldosterone contribute to renal vasoconstriction.[39] Myoglobinuria and sepsis can also aggravate renal dysfunction. Despite an increase in the renal blood flow during the hypermetabolic phase of burn injury, tubular function and creatinine clearance may be reduced and renal function may be variable.

Pharmacologic Changes

Burn injury also affects the pharmacodynamic and pharmacokinetic properties of many drugs. A decreased level of serum albumin in these patients leads to increased free fraction of acidic drugs such as thiopental or diazepam, whereas an increased level of α-acid glycoprotein results in decreased free fraction of basic drugs (with pKa > 8) such as lidocaine or propranolol.[31] Renal and hepatic functions may be impaired in patients with large burns, and this may impair the elimination of some drugs, whereas increases in renal blood flow and glomerular filtration rate in the hyperdynamic phase of burns may enhance the renal excretion of drugs. It has been shown that some drugs such as gentamicin may be lost through the open wounds.[40] The response to muscle relaxants (other than mivacurium) is altered owing to proliferation of acetylcholine receptors away from the synaptic cleft of the neuromuscular junction (see later). Pharmacokinetics of morphine are unchanged after burn injury.[41] Although lorazepam has an increased volume of distribution, increased clearance, and a reduced half-life,[42] the elimination half-life of diazepam is significantly prolonged in burn patients.[43]

Inhalation Injury

Most airway inhalation injuries are due to inhalation of smoke. A history of closed space exposure to hot gases, steam or smoke, singed nasal vibrissae, carbonaceous sputum, or elevated levels of carboxyhemoglobin or cyanide all point toward the clinical diagnosis.[6,26] Inhalation injury is a predictor of increased morbidity and mortality in burn victims.[44-46]

Upper Airway Injury

Direct thermal injury to the subglottic airway is rare, unless superheated air or steam is inhaled. The severity of inhalation injury depends on the fuels burned, intensity of combustion, duration of exposure, and confinement. Unless steam is involved, heat injury to the airway is supraglottic, causing swelling of the posterior pharynx and supraglottic regions, leading to potential upper airway obstruction. The natural history of upper airway inhalation injury is edema formation that narrows the airway over the initial 12 to 48 hours. Early tracheal intubation is recommended in patients who present with stridor, wheeze, or voice changes. Burns to the face and neck can result in tight eschar formation, which when combined with pharyngeal edema can cause difficult airway management.

Lower Airway Injury (Smoke Inhalation Injury)

Lower airway or pulmonary parenchymal damage results from inhalation of the chemical constituents of smoke, usually becoming apparent 24 to 72 hours after the injury. Findings include dyspnea, rales, rhonchi, and wheezing. Gas phase constituents of smoke include carbon monoxide (CO), cyanide, hydrochloric acid, aldehyde gases, and oxidants. These can cause direct damage to mucociliary function and bronchial vessel permeability, as well as produce bronchospasm, alveolar destruction, and pulmonary edema. Small airway occlusion results from endobronchial sloughing and resultant debris, whereas alveolar, interstitial, and chest wall edema may cause intrapulmonary shunting and reduction in compliance.[26,47] The risk of pulmonary infection and barotrauma is also increased. The clinical picture is identical to that of acute respiratory distress syndrome (ARDS). Delayed ARDS (6 to 10 days post burn) may also develop in the absence of inhalation injury in burn victims.[48] Bronchoscopy reveals carbonaceous endobronchial debris and/or mucosal ulceration.[49,50] The usefulness of serial chest radiographs or of radioisotope scanning with xenon or technetium for diagnosis and predicting prognosis is questionable.[6,51,52] Meticulous pulmonary toilet is the cornerstone of early care. Tracheal secretions are often very viscous and may contain carbonaceous particles and pieces of mucous membrane.

Carbon Monoxide and Cyanide Poisoning

Carbon monoxide has a high affinity for hemoglobin (250 times more than oxygen) and can interfere with oxygen delivery to the tissues at higher concentrations. Administration of 100% oxygen reduces the half-life of carboxyhemoglobin from 2.5 hours to 40 minutes and facilitates the elimination of CO.[53] Hyperbaric oxygen therapy has limited indications owing to the logistical challenges presented by transport of patients with concomitant burns to such chambers.[54,55] Cyanide causes tissue hypoxia by uncoupling oxidative phosphorylation in mitochondria. Treatment with sodium nitrite, sodium thiosulfate, hydroxocobalamin, or dicobalt edetate should be considered for cyanide poisoning in patients with unexplained severe metabolic acidosis associated with elevated central venous O_2 (therefore patients are clinically not cyanotic), normal arterial O_2 content, and low carboxyhemoglobin.[56]

Signs such as hyperthermia, tachycardia, leukocytosis, and tachypnea cannot be used to diagnose sepsis in burn victims. Other identifiers, such as thrombocytopenia,[57] enteral feeding intolerance,[58] and hyperglycemia have been used instead.

PREOPERATIVE PREPARATION

The preoperative evaluation of burn patients should take into account the continuum of pathophysiologic changes due to burns. Patient age, %TBSA burned, depth of burns, time after injury, sites and extent of planned excision and donor areas, presence of infection, other injuries (especially inhalation injury), and the presence and extent of comorbidities should all be assessed.

Careful assessment of airway should be made using the usual bedside tests. Mallampati class, thyromental distance, head, neck and jaw mobility, presence of facial or airway burns (or edema), and contractures of face and neck should be looked for and used to plan the perioperative airway management technique. When there is potential for airway complications, a difficult airway cart containing a range of various-sized endotracheal tubes, Eschmann stylet, laryngeal mask airways (LMAs), Fastrach LMA, fiberoptic bronchoscope, and fiberoptic stylets should be available.

Fluid Resuscitation

The widely quoted Baxter (Parkland) formula for initial fluid resuscitation of burn victims is 4 mL of Ringer's lactate per kilogram of body weight per %TBSA burned, with one half to be given during the first 8 hours after injury and the rest in the next 16 hours.[59] Hypertonic saline may be useful in early shock,[60,61] and colloids are most effective when used in the 12- to 24-hour period of resuscitation.[6,62] It is widely believed that the Parkland formula underestimates resuscitation volumes, particularly when concomitant smoke inhalation is present.[59,63] Repeated bedside observations and clinical evaluations are useful to judge the adequacy of resuscitation. Normal mentation, stable vital signs, and urine output of 30 to 50 mL/hr can be used as end points,[6] whereas use of core-periphery temperature gradient may be unreliable.[64] However, several studies have shown advantages to invasive hemodynamic monitoring (with pulmonary artery catheter) in adults with serious burns who do not respond as expected to fluid resuscitation.[65,66] Serial lactate levels,[67] monitoring the base deficit,[68,69] and optimization of intrathoracic blood volumes (ITBV)[70] have also been shown to be useful guides to successful resuscitation (Table 18-2).

TABLE 18–2 Critical Questions to Ask Patients and/or Primary Medical Doctor

Mechanism of injury, % body surface area burned and depth of burns
Closed space confinement, black sputum
Elapsed time from injury
Adequacy of resuscitation
Extent of planned excision, location of burn areas to be excised and donor areas
Surgical position, need for intraoperative change of positions
Pain scores, 24-hour analgesic requirements
Associated injuries
Coexisting diseases

Fasting Requirements

Metabolic complications in burn patients are directly related to extent of burn. Thermal injury leads to hypermetabolism and protein hypercatabolic state. Early postpyloric enteral feeding, which can be continued in the perioperative period, is recommended by the evidence-based guidelines of the ABA.[6] Early institution of enteral feeding in these patients decreases infections and sepsis,[71] improves wound healing and nitrogen balance,[72,73] and reduces stress ulceration and duration of hospitalization.[74,75] Gastric emptying may not be delayed in burn patients,[76] and gastric acid production may actually be reduced in the early post-burn period.[77] The safety and advantages of perioperative enteral feedings have been reported by Jenkins and colleagues.[78] At our institution, we continue enteral feedings throughout the perioperative period in patients who come to the operating room intubated. In nonintubated patients, shorter fasting times (typically 2 to 4 hours) may be acceptable.[27,79]

INTRAOPERATIVE CONSIDERATIONS

Burn patients could present for five types of surgical procedures: (1) decompression procedures such as escharotomy or laparotomy, (2) excision and biologic closure of burn wounds, (3) definitive closure procedures, (4) burn reconstructive procedures, or (5) general supportive procedures such as gastrostomy or line placement.[80]

Surgical Procedure

The need and timing for surgery is determined primarily by the size of injury. The objective is to identify, excise, and achieve biologic closure of all full-thickness burns. The advantages of early excision and grafting (within 1 to 5 days after burn injury) include reduction in incidence of septic episodes, reduced hospital stay, and increased survival rates.[81-86] Extensive burns may need staged excision to limit the physiologic insult of one massive surgery and to allow autologous skin grafts to be available. Excision and grafting involves "tangential excision" of the second-degree burn wound, in which the eschar is shaved off from the burn until a plane of viable tissue is reached, followed by covering the excised wound with a split-thickness skin graft, allogeneic skin from cadavers, or skin substitutes such as Integra.[87] Excision of third-degree burns requires "fascial excision," where the overlying burned skin and subcutaneous fat are excised down to muscle fascia.

Anesthetic Technique

General anesthesia, with the combination of an opioid, muscle relaxant, and a volatile agent, is the most widely used technique for burn excision and grafting.[27] Succinylcholine administration to patients more than 24 hours after burn injury is unsafe, owing to the risk of hyperkalemic ventricular dysrhythmias.[88] The time frame during which succinylcholine must be avoided after a burn begins 48 hours after the event.[89] Patients who have been bedridden because of severity of illness or concomitant disease or injury, or those receiving prolonged muscle relaxant therapy to facilitate mechanical ventilation, may be particularly vulnerable.[90] The exact period of risk is unknown, but a duration of 6 months can be considered the absolute minimum.[91] This is because of proliferation and spread of acetylcholine receptors (AChR) throughout the skeletal muscle membrane under the burn and at sites distant from the burn injury.[92] The upregulation of acetylcholine receptors, along with altered protein binding, especially to α_1-glycoprotein, makes patients with thermal injury resistant to the action of nondepolarizing muscle relaxants.[93-95] In these patients, larger doses of nondepolarizing muscle relaxants may be required to achieve a given degree of neuromuscular blockade, the onset of paralysis may take longer, and the duration of paralysis may be shorter. The resistance is usually seen in patients with greater than 30% TBSA burns; it develops after the first week of injury and peaks at 5 to 6 weeks post injury.[94,96] Mivacurium may be immune to this resistance, possibly as a result of decreased metabolism of the drug from depressed pseudocholinesterase activity in burn patients.[97,98]

Airway Management

Airway management in burn patients can be challenging. Mask ventilation may be a problem with facial burns. Successful use of an LMA for burn surgery has been reported.[99,100] However, major procedures in critically ill patients, with frequent intraoperative changes in patient position, are best done with endotracheal intubation. Awake fiberoptic intubation may be indicated if difficulties for intubation and/or ventilation are identified preoperatively. Inhalation induction, maintenance of spontaneous respirations, and intubation with fiberoptic guidance or Fastrach LMA may be advocated in uncooperative patients.

Location of burns and donor skin sites indicate the need for special positioning, for repositioning the patient during operation, or both. Fixing the endotracheal tube for prone positioning in the presence of facial burns is best achieved by wiring it to the teeth or stitching it to the nares.[101] We commonly use dental floss to tie the tube to the teeth or tie the tube to an oronasal loop of rubber catheter. A combination of prolonged prone positioning and relatively high fluid volume administration may cause significant airway swelling. It is best to wait until an air leak is present around the endotracheal tube before tracheal extubation, because this indicates resolution of edema, especially in older children.[102,103] If there is still no air leak and the patient is deemed ready for tracheal extubation, direct laryngoscopy may be necessary to determine the extent of residual edema. Once extubated, the patient should be closely monitored for progressive airway obstruction during the subsequent 24 to 48 hour.

Depending on the age of the burns, edema, scarring, or contractures may narrow the mouth opening and limit the neck movements. Surgical release of neck contractures to facilitate intubation has been described in both elective and emergency settings.[104,105]

Analgesia

Severe pain is an inevitable consequence of a major burn injury, and perioperative analgesic requirements are frequently underestimated.[106,107] Anxiety and depression are common components in a major burn and can further decrease the pain threshold. Perioperative pain management should be based on an understanding of the types of burn pain (acute or procedure-related pain versus background or baseline pain), frequent patient assessment by an acute pain service team, and the development of protocols to address problems such as breakthrough pain.

High-dose opioids are needed to manage pain associated with burn procedures, and morphine is currently the most widely used drug.[108] The pharmacokinetics of morphine are similar in burned patients and control subjects.[41] It has been shown that provision of adequate analgesia using morphine reduces the risk of post-traumatic stress syndrome.[109] Most burned patients rapidly develop tolerance to opioids. There is an interindividual variation in response to morphine, so "titration to effect" and frequent reassessment are important.

Fentanyl is also a useful analgesic perioperatively. Continuous infusion of fentanyl in the preoperative period may induce a rapid tolerance in burn patients.[110]

Methadone has the advantage of N-methyl-D-aspartate (NMDA) receptor antagonist activity, which helps in preventing the development of central sensitization, secondary hyperalgesia, and neuropathic pain.[10] In addition, the long duration of action helps in achieving postoperative analgesia and it can be administered orally in the postoperative period.

Nonsteroidal anti-inflammatory agents reduce pain perception and modify the systemic inflammatory response through inhibition of cyclooxygenase. The incidence of gastric ulceration, increased operative blood loss, and exacerbation of asthma is reduced with the use of selective cyclooxygenase-2 inhibitors. However, potential for renal tubular dysfunction does exist. These drugs have not yet been systematically evaluated in burn patients.

Acetaminophen is a useful adjunctive analgesic in combination with opioids. Its antipyretic action is particularly useful in burn patients. Doses of 15 mg/kg can be given orally or rectally every 6 hours to a maximum of 4 g/day. Liver function tests and acetaminophen levels should be checked weekly in patients receiving long-term therapy.

Tumescent local anesthesia with maximal dose of 7 mg/kg lidocaine has been shown to be safe and to be the sole possible effective locoregional anesthesia technique for the surgical treatment of pediatric burns.[111] Postoperative pain from split-skin donor sites is often more intense than the pain at the grafted site. Addition of bupivacaine or lidocaine to the "Pitkin solution" (subcutaneous crystalloid injection) can provide analgesia for pain originating from the donor areas.[112,113] A continuous fascia iliaca compartment block can also be used to reduce the pain at the thigh donor site.[114] Intravenous lidocaine (1 mg/kg) has been reported to provide significant postoperative analgesia for up to 3 days.[115]

Ventilation

Mechanical ventilation is necessary for patients with respiratory complications, inhalation injury, or large burns. Hypermetabolic state after burn injury increases the carbon dioxide production, and these patients need higher minute ventilation to maintain normocapnia. In patients who have acute lung injury and need high levels of positive end-expiratory pressure (PEEP > 15 cm H_2O) or peak inspiratory pressure (PIP > 50 cm H_2O) to maintain gas exchange, use of sophisticated intensive care ventilator and anesthesia maintenance using total intravenous anesthesia technique (TIVA) may be warranted.

Regional Anesthesia

Regional anesthesia alone or in combination with general anesthesia can be used in patients with small burns or for reconstructive procedures. For procedures on lower extremities, lumbar epidural or caudal catheters can be used to provide intraoperative and postoperative analgesia. The greatest limitation to the use of regional techniques is the extent of surgical field; most patients with major burns have a wide distribution of injuries and/or need skin harvesting from areas too large to be blocked by a regional technique. The presence of a coagulopathy or systemic or local infection may also contraindicate regional anesthetic techniques in these patients.

Monitoring

Monitoring for burn surgery should be based on knowledge of the patient's medical condition and the extent of surgery. Standard electrocardiographic electrodes may not adhere to burned surfaces. Needle electrodes or alligator clips attached to skin staples may be effective alternatives. If skin sites for pulse oximetry monitoring are limited, the ear, nose, tongue, or penis can be used with standard probes.[116] The alternative is to use reflectance pulse oximetry.

Arterial line placement allows repeated blood sampling for estimation of gas tensions, hematocrit, electrolytes, lactate, and coagulation profiles, in addition to continuous blood pressure monitoring. The decision to use invasive monitoring such as a central venous or pulmonary artery catheter should be based on coexisting medical conditions or burn-related complications. Core temperature (bladder or esophageal), urine output, and degree of neuromuscular blockade should be routinely monitored.

Hypothermia is a common complication of excision and grafting and often delays extubation. Body temperature is best maintained by a thermoneutral environment (room temperature of 28° to 32°C) with the additional use of an over-bed warming shield and warming of intravenous fluids.[85] Dry-air warmers used directly over the burn wound can cause tissue desiccation. Forced air warming devices are less effective in these patients because of the significant area of burned and donor skin sites that must remain exposed. Use of "space blankets" (aluminum foil coverings on nonexposed areas), plastic sheets over the head and face, heat and moisture exchangers in the breathing system, and low fresh gas flow with circle absorber can also help to reduce the heat loss.[31]

Blood Loss and Transfusion Requirements

Burn excision can result in massive and sudden blood loss[117] that increases with delay to primary burn excision, with a peak at 5 to 12 days after burn injury.[118,119] Other factors that correlate with increased blood loss include older age, male sex, and larger body size; area of full-thickness (third-degree) burn; high wound bacteria counts (derived from quantitative tissue cultures); total wound area excised; and operative time.[118] A mean blood loss of 2.6% to 3.4% of a patient's blood volume for each %TBSA excised has been reported in the literature.[120,121]

Several techniques have been used to reduce blood loss during primary burn excision. Intraoperative tourniquet use on burned extremities reduces overall blood loss.[122-124] Postexcision compression dressings and topical epinephrine have been used to reduce blood loss during excision and grafting procedures. Application of bandages soaked in 1:10,000 epinephrine after excision of burned skin and/or use of thrombin spray, fibrin sealant, or platelet gel is effective in producing a bloodless surface for placement of skin grafts.[85,125,126] Extremely high levels of catecholamines in the blood have been measured after the use of this technique. Sinus tachycardia and/or hypertension are common, and hence heart rate and blood pressure cannot be used to reliably titrate anesthetic or analgesic agents. Serious dysrhythmias are fortunately rare.[127,128]

Subcutaneous crystalloid is injected in generous amounts using pressure-bags and Pitkin syringes (tumescent technique) to facilitate donor skin harvesting and reduce blood loss. Epinephrine and/or local anesthetics such as bupivacaine or lidocaine may be added to this.[112,126,129,130]

Quantifying blood loss is typically difficult in burn patients,[121] and transfusion is best guided by serial hematocrit estimations. Adequate venous access is a prerequisite to burn excision and grafting procedures. At least two intravenous access routes should be established (peripheral or central), and these lines should be sutured securely to prevent accidental dislodgment while positioning. Blood products should be readily available before excision begins. Femoral venous catheters placed through burned skin have been shown to be safe,[131] although this issue has been questioned.[132] The decision to transfuse blood products should be individualized by carefully weighing the risks of transfusion, including immunosuppression, versus the benefits of correcting anemia in the setting of hypermetabolism and increased oxygen demands. If blood loss is excessive, it is prudent to rule out coagulation abnormalities. Burned patients have a consumption coagulopathy that, in combination with hemodilution during operation, results in a clinically significant deficiency of coagulation factors II, VII, and X, in spite of reactive elevation of coagulation factor VIII and fibrinogen.[133] Platelets or coagulation factors may need to be replaced, guided by the coagulation profile.

Although infrequently used in current clinical practice, intraoperative blood salvage in excisional burn surgery, using a cell saver, has been shown to recover more than 40% of shed red blood cells with acceptable levels of bacterial contamination and inflammatory mediators.[134,135]

A list of things to prepare for burn excision and grafting is presented in Table 18-3. The agent suxamethonium is contraindicated in a patient with burns.

SPECIAL CONSIDERATIONS FOR PEDIATRIC BURNS

Nearly one third of burn admissions and burn deaths occur in children below 15 years of age. Burns are second only to motor vehicle crashes as the leading cause of death

TABLE 18–3 Things to Prepare for Burn Excision and Grafting

Difficult airway cart, umbilical tape, dental floss, wire for suturing tube
Operating room warmed to 28° to 32°C, fluid warmer, radiant heat warmer
Availability of blood products
Adequate intravenous access; consider invasive monitoring

in children older than 1 year. Flame burns account for about a third of pediatric burns, are often more severe, and frequently involve concomitant inhalation injury. Children younger than 2 years of age have high surface area to body mass ratios, extremely thin skin, and minimal physiologic reserves, causing higher morbidities and mortalities than in the older age groups. The possibility of child abuse must always be considered in this age group.

The disproportionate ratio of head to body size makes the rule of nines (to estimate TBSA) not applicable in small children. Lund-Browder or Berkow charts divide TBSA into smaller units and make age-appropriate corrections (Table 18-4).[9,26] When calculating fluid resuscitation volumes, allowances should be made for daily maintenance fluids in infants and toddlers. Adequate resuscitation is reflected by normal mentation, stable vital signs, and a urine output of 1 to 2 mL/kg/hr. Infants should be monitored for signs of fluid overload and hyponatremia/hypernatremia, because their immature kidneys may not be able to handle excessive fluid and electrolyte load. Blood glucose levels should be monitored, and glucose-containing solutions added as necessary, in infants.

In children requiring high inspiratory pressures during mechanical ventilation, a cuffed endotracheal tube may be a better choice. The small internal diameter of pediatric airway and endotracheal tubes increases the risk of obstruction by the thick secretions or edema, especially in the presence of inhalation injury. Frequent suctioning helps in clearing the mucus and debris from the tracheal tree, and a high index of suspicion should be maintained for plugging of the tracheal tube. A substantial portion of subcutaneous crystalloid fluid injected for tumescent technique to harvest skin graft may be absorbed into the circulation and may cause hypervolemia in small children. Thermal maintenance is critical in young children, especially those with burns of more than 10% TBSA.

Procedural Sedation

Procedures such as dressing changes, wound care, and physical therapy frequently require sedation and analgesia in pediatric burn patients. These procedures are often performed on a daily basis on the burn ward, making involvement of an anesthesiologist impractical.

Nurse-administered opioids (intravenous, oral, or transmucosal), alone or in combination with benzodiazepine anxiolysis, is the typical regimen. However, when wound care procedures are extensive, particularly in children, more potent anesthetic agents may be of benefit. Patient monitoring must be appropriate to the level of sedation, as required by the Joint Commission on the Accreditation of Healthcare Organizations and described by the American Society of Anesthesiologists guidelines for sedation monitoring.

TABLE 18–4	Berkow Chart for Estimating TBSA Burned in Various Age Groups					
Area	1 Yr	1-4 Yr	5-9 Yr	10-14 Yr	15 Yr	Adult
Head	19	17	13	11	9	7
Neck	2	2	2	2	2	2
Anterior trunk	13	13	13	13	13	13
Posterior trunk	13	13	13	13	13	13
Right buttock	2.5	2.5	2.5	2.5	2.5	2.5
Left buttock	2.5	2.5	2.5	2.5	2.5	2.5
Genitalia	1	1	1	1	1	1
Right upper arm	4	4	4	4	4	4
Left upper arm	4	4	4	4	4	4
Right lower arm	3	3	3	3	3	3
Left lower arm	3	3	3	3	3	3
Right hand	2.5	2.5	2.5	2.5	2.5	2.5
Left hand	2.5	2.5	2.5	2.5	2.5	2.5
Right thigh	5.5	6.5	8	8.5	9	9.5
Left thigh	5.5	6.5	8	8.5	9	9.5
Right leg	5	5	5.5	6	6.5	7
Left leg	5	5	5.5	6	6.5	7
Right foot	3.5	3.5	3.5	3.5	3.5	3.5
Left foot	3.5	3.5	3.5	3.5	3.5	3.5
Total	100	100	100	100	100	100

Oral transmucosal fentanyl citrate lozenges have been shown to be safe and effective for pediatric burn wound care.[136] The starting dose for fentanyl lozenges is 10 μg/kg. Peak effect occurs after 20 to 30 minutes. About 25% of the total dose is systemically available after buccal absorption. The remaining 75% is swallowed and is slowly absorbed from the gastrointestinal tract. Up to a third of this (25% of total dose) avoids hepatic first-pass metabolism and is systemically available.[137]

Ketamine offers the advantage of stable hemodynamics and analgesia and has been used extensively as the primary agent for both general anesthesia and analgesia for burn dressing changes.[138-140] Nitrous oxide with oxygen has been used effectively for analgesia during burn wound dressing changes.[140,141] However, scavenging of the gas when administered outside of an operating room is problematic. Combination of nitrous oxide with opioids may induce a state of general anesthesia with profound respiratory depression. The efficacy of general anesthesia administered by an anesthesiologist for procedures on a burn intensive care unit has been well documented.[142]

Analgesics such as acetaminophen can be used for their opioid-sparing effect and are combined with generous administration of oral opioids.[106,143] Nonsteroidal anti-inflammatory drugs have antiplatelet effects and may not be appropriate for patients who require extensive excision and grafting procedures. In addition, burn patients can also manifest the nephrotoxic effects of nonsteroidal anti-inflammatory drugs. Music therapy,[144] hypnotherapy,[145-147] massage, a number of cognitive and behavioral techniques,[106] and, more recently, virtual reality techniques[148-150] have been successfully used to reduce pain during débridement and wound care.

CONCLUSION

Patients with severe burn injury are a challenge for the anesthesiologist. Recent advances in burn care and burn surgery have led to an improved survival of these patients. Early excision and grafting is becoming a standard practice. Effective anesthetic management of these patients requires knowledge of the continuum of pathophysiologic changes, proper planning, and a team effort.

References

1. Herndon DN, Spies M: Modern burn care. Semin Pediatr Surg 2001;10:28-31.
2. Zhou YP, Ren JL, Zhou WM, et al: Experience in the treatment of patients with burns covering more than 90% TBSA and full-thickness burns exceeding 70% TBSA. Asian J Surg 2002;25:154-156.
3. Ryan CM, Schoenfeld DA, Thorpe WP, et al: Objective estimates of the probability of death from burn injuries. N Engl J Med 1998;338: 362-366.
4. Sheridan RL, Hinson MI, Liang MH, et al: Long-term outcome of children surviving massive burns. JAMA 2000;283:69-73.
5. Tompkins RG, Remensnyder JP, Burke JF, et al: Significant reductions in mortality for children with burn injuries through the use of prompt eschar excision. Ann Surg 1988;208:577-585.
6. Practice guidelines for burn care. J Burn Care Rehabil 2001;22:S1-S69.
7. Sheridan RL. Burn care: Results of technical and organizational progress. JAMA 2003;290:719-722.
8. Livingston EH, Lee S: Percentage of burned body surface area determination in obese and nonobese patients. J Surg Res 2000;91: 106-110.
9. Miller SF, Finley RK, Waltman M, et al: Burn size estimate reliability: A study. J Burn Care Rehabil 1991;12:546-559.
10. Monafo WW: Initial management of burns. N Engl J Med 1996;335: 1581-1586.
11. Gibran NS, Heimbach DM: Mediators in thermal injury. Semin Nephrol 2003;13:344-358.
12. Leape LL: Initial changes in burns: Tissue changes in burned and unburned skin of rhesus monkeys. J Trauma 1970;10:488-492.
13. Holliman CJ, Meuleman TR, Larsen KR, et al: The effect of ketanserin, a specific serotonin antagonist, on burn shock hemodynamic parameters in a porcine burn model. J Trauma 1983;23:867-871.
14. Maass DL, White J, Horton JW: IL-1beta and IL-6 act synergistically with TNF-alpha to alter cardiac contractile function after burn trauma. Shock 2002;18:360-366.
15. Maass DL, Hybki DP, White J, et al: The time course of cardiac NF-kappaB activation and TNF-alpha secretion by cardiac myocytes after burn injury: Contribution to burn-related cardiac contractile dysfunction. Shock 2002;17:293-299.
16. Yao YM, Yu Y, Sheng ZY, et al: Role of gut-derived endotoxaemia and bacterial translocation in rats after thermal injury: Effects of selective decontamination of the digestive tract. Burns 1995;21:580-585.
17. Yao YM, Sheng ZY, Tian HM, et al: The association of circulating endotoxaemia with the development of multiple organ failure in burned patients. Burns 1995;21:255-258.
18. Dijkstra HM, Manson WL, Blaauw B, et al: Bacterial translocation in D-galactosamine-treated rats in a burn model. Burns 1996;22:15-21.
19. Basadre JO, Sugi K, Traber DL, et al: The effect of leukocyte depletion on smoke inhalation injury in sheep. Surgery 1988;104:208-215.
20. Horton JW, White DJ: Role of xanthine oxidase and leukocytes in postburn cardiac dysfunction. J Am Coll Surg 1995;181:129-137.
21. Horton JW: Free radicals and lipid peroxidation mediated injury in burn trauma: The role of antioxidant therapy. Toxicology 2003;189: 75-88.
22. Rawlingson A: Nitric oxide, inflammation and acute burn injury. Burns 2003;29:631-640.
23. Gelfand JA, Donelan M, Hawiger A, et al: Alternative complement pathway activation increases mortality in a model of burn injury in mice. J Clin Invest 1982;70:1170-1176.
24. Gelfand JA, Donelan M, Burke JF: Preferential activation and depletion of the alternative complement pathway by burn injury. Ann Surg 1983;198:58-62.
25. Youn YK, LaLonde C, Demling R: The role of mediators in the response to thermal injury. World J Surg 1992;16:30-36.
26. Sheridan RL: Comprehensive treatment of burns. Curr Probl Surg 2001;38:657-756.
27. MacLennan N, Heimbach DM, Cullen BF: Anesthesia for major thermal injury. Anesthesiology 1998;89:749-770.
28. Goodall M, Stone C, Haynes BW, Jr: Urinary output of adrenaline and noradrenaline in severe thermal burns. Ann Surg 1957;145:479-487.
29. Wilmore DW, Aulick LH, Pruitt BA Jr: Metabolism during the hypermetabolic phase of thermal injury. Adv Surg 1978;12:193-225.
30. Caldwell FT Jr, Wallace BH, Cone JB: The effect of wound management on the interaction of burn size, heat production, and rectal temperature. J Burn Care Rehabil 1994;15:121-129.
31. Woodson LC, Sherwood ER, Morvant EM, et al: Anesthesia for burned patients. In Herndon DN (ed): Total Burn Care. Philadelphia, WB Saunders, 2002, pp 183-206.
32. Moserova J, Behounkova-Houskova E: Evaporative water loss in partial skin loss in the first 24 hours. Scand J Plast Reconstr Surg 1979;13: 49-51.

33. Schwacha MG, Chaudry IH: The cellular basis of post-burn immunosuppression: Macrophages and mediators. Int J Mol Med 2002;10:239-243.

34. Alexander M, Chaudry IH, Schwacha MG: Relationships between burn size, immunosuppression, and macrophage hyperactivity in a murine model of thermal injury. Cell Immunol 2002;220:63-69.

35. Lawrence C, Atac B: Hematologic changes in massive burn injury. Crit Care Med 1992;20:1284-1288.

36. Kowal-Vern A, Gamelli RL, Walenga JM, et al: The effect of burn wound size on hemostasis: A correlation of the hemostatic changes to the clinical state. J Trauma 1992;33:50-57.

37. Schiavon M, Di Landro D, Baldo M, et al: A study of renal damage in seriously burned patients. Burns Incl Therm Inj 1988;14:107-112.

38. Davies MP, Evans J, McGonigle RJ: The dialysis debate: Acute renal failure in burns patients. Burns 1994;20:71-73.

39. Aikawa N, Wakabayashi G, Ueda M, et al: Regulation of renal function in thermal injury. J Trauma 1990;30:S174-S180.

40. Glew RH, Moellering RC Jr, Burke JF: Gentamicin dosage in children with extensive burns. J Trauma 1976;16:819-823.

41. Perreault S, Choiniere M, du Souich PB, et al: Pharmacokinetics of morphine and its glucuronidated metabolites in burn injuries. Ann Pharmacother 2001;35:1588-1592.

42. Martyn JA, Greenblatt DJ. Lorazepam conjugation umimpaired in burn patients. Anesthesiology 1985;63:A113.

43. Martyn JA, Greenblatt DJ, Quinby WC: Diazepam kinetics in patients with severe burns. Anesth Analg 1983;62:293-297.

44. Shirani KZ, Pruitt BA Jr, Mason AD Jr: The influence of inhalation injury and pneumonia on burn mortality. Ann Surg 1987;205:82-87.

45. Herndon DN, Gore D, Cole M, et al: Determinants of mortality in pediatric patients with greater than 70% full-thickness total body surface area thermal injury treated by early total excision and grafting. J Trauma 1987;27:208-212.

46. Saffle JR, Davis B, Williams P: Recent outcomes in the treatment of burn injury in the United States: A report from the American Burn Association Patient Registry. J Burn Care Rehabil 1995;16:219-232; discussion 288-289.

47. Sheridan RL: Airway management and respiratory care of the burn patient. Int Anesthesiol Clin 2000;38:129-145.

48. Dancey DR, Hayes J, Gomez M, et al: ARDS in patients with thermal injury. Intensive Care Med 1999;25:1231-1236.

49. Moylan JA, Adib K, Birnbaum M: Fiberoptic bronchoscopy following thermal injury. Surg Gynecol Obstet 1975;140:541-543.

50. Masanes MJ, Legendre C, Lioret N, et al: Fiberoptic bronchoscopy for the early diagnosis of subglottal inhalation injury: Comparative value in the assessment of prognosis. J Trauma 1994;36:59-67.

51. Teixidor HS, Rubin E, Novick GS, et al: Smoke inhalation: Radiologic manifestations. Radiology 1983;149:383-387.

52. Lin WY, Kao CH, Wang SJ: Detection of acute inhalation injury in fire victims by means of technetium-99m DTPA radioaerosol inhalation lung scintigraphy. Eur J Nucl Med 1997;24:125-129.

53. Gorman D, Drewry A, Huang YL, et al: The clinical toxicology of carbon monoxide. Toxicology 2003;187:25-38.

54. Weaver LK, Hopkins RO, Chan KJ, et al: Hyperbaric oxygen for acute carbon monoxide poisoning. N Engl J Med 2002;347:1057-1067.

55. Sheridan RL, Shank ES: Hyperbaric oxygen treatment: A brief overview of a controversial topic. J Trauma 1999;47:426-435.

56. Borron SW, Baud FJ: Acute cyanide poisoning: Clinical spectrum, diagnosis, and treatment. Arh Hig Rada Toksikol 1996;47:307-322.

57. Housinger TA, Brinkerhoff C, Warden GD: The relationship between platelet count, sepsis, and survival in pediatric burn patients. Arch Surg 1993;128:65-67.

58. Wolf SE, Jeschke MG, Rose JK, et al: Enteral feeding intolerance: An indicator of sepsis-associated mortality in burned children. Arch Surg 1997;132:1310-1314.

59. Warden GD: Burn shock resuscitation. World J Surg 1992;16:16-23.

60. Caldwell FT, Bowser BH: Critical evaluation of hypertonic and hypotonic solutions to resuscitate severely burned children: A prospective study. Ann Surg 1979;189:546-552.

61. Monafo WW: The treatment of burn shock by the intravenous and oral administration of hypertonic lactated saline solution. J Trauma 1970;10:575-586.

62. Demling R: Fluid resuscitation. In Boswick JR (ed): The Art and Science of Burn Care. Rockville, MD, Aspen, 1987, pp 189-202.

63. Cartotto RC, Innes M, Musgrave MA, et al: How well does the Parkland formula estimate actual fluid resuscitation volumes? J Burn Care Rehabil 2002;23:258-265.

64. Renshaw A, Childs C: The significance of peripheral skin temperature measurement during the acute phase of burn injury: An illustrative case report. Burns 2000;26:750-753.

65. Dries DJ, Waxman K: Adequate resuscitation of burn patients may not be measured by urine output and vital signs. Crit Care Med 1991;19:327-329.

66. Schiller WR, Bay RC, Garren RL, et al: Hyperdynamic resuscitation improves survival in patients with life-threatening burns. J Burn Care Rehabil 1997;18:10-16.

67. Holm C, Melcer B, Horbrand F, et al: Haemodynamic and oxygen transport responses in survivors and non-survivors following thermal injury. Burns 2000;26:25-33.

68. Cartotto R, Choi J, Gomez M, et al: A prospective study on the implications of a base deficit during fluid resuscitation. J Burn Care Rehabil 2003;24:75-84.

69. Choi J, Cooper A, Gomez M, et al: The 2000 Moyer Award. The relevance of base deficits after burn injuries. J Burn Care Rehabil 2000;21:499-505.

70. Holm C, Melcer B, Horbrand F, et al: Intrathoracic blood volume as an end point in resuscitation of the severely burned: An observational study of 24 patients. J Trauma 2000;48:728-734.

71. Mainous MR, Block EF, Deitch EA: Nutritional support of the gut: How and why. New Horiz 1994;2:193-201.

72. Chiarelli A, Enzi G, Casadei A, et al: Very early nutrition supplementation in burned patients. Am J Clin Nutr 1990;51:1035-1039.

73. Schroeder D, Gillanders L, Mahr K, et al: Effects of immediate postoperative enteral nutrition on body composition, muscle function, and wound healing. J Parenter Enteral Nutr 1991;15:376-383.

74. Taylor S: Early enhanced enteral nutrition in burned patients is associated with fewer infective complications and shorter hospital stay. J Hum Nutr Dietit 1999;12:85-91.

75. Garrel DR, Davignon I, Lopez D: Length of care in patients with severe burns with or without early enteral nutritional support: A retrospective study. J Burn Care Rehabil 1991;12:85-90.

76. Hu OY, Ho ST, Wang JJ, et al: Evaluation of gastric emptying in severe, burn-injured patients. Crit Care Med 1993;21:527-531.

77. Zapata-Sirvent RL, Greenleaf G, Hansbrough JF, et al: Burn injury results in decreased gastric acid production in the acute shock period. J Burn Care Rehabil 1995;16:622-666.

78. Jenkins ME, Gottschlich MM, Warden GD: Enteral feeding during operative procedures in thermal injuries. J Burn Care Rehabil 1994;15:199-205.

79. Pearson KS, From RP, Symreng T, et al: Continuous enteral feeding and short fasting periods enhance perioperative nutrition in patients with burns. J Burn Care Rehabil 1992;13:477-481.

80. Sheridan RL, Schulz JT, Ryan CM, et al: Case records of the Massachusetts General Hospital. Weekly clinicopathological exercises. Case 6-2004: A 35-year-old woman with extensive, deep burns from a nightclub fire. N Engl J Med 2004;350:810-821.

81. Gray DT, Pine RW, Harnar TJ, et al: Early surgical excision versus conventional therapy in patients with 20 to 40 percent burns: A comparative study. Am J Surg 1982;144:76-80.

82. Herndon DN, Barrow RE, Rutan RL, et al: A comparison of conservative versus early excision: Therapies in severely burned patients. Ann Surg 1989;209:547-553.

83. Janzekovic Z: A new concept in the early excision and immediate grafting of burns. J Trauma 1970;10:1103-1108.

84. Engrav LH, Heimbach DM, Reus JL, et al: Early excision and grafting vs. nonoperative treatment of burns of indeterminant depth: A randomized prospective study. J Trauma 1983;23:1001-1004.

85. Muller MJ, Ralston D, Herndon D: Operative wound management. In Herndon DN (ed): Total Burn Care. Philadelphia, WB Saunders, 2002, pp 170-182.

86. Xiao-Wu W, Herndon DN, Spies M, et al: Effects of delayed wound excision and grafting in severely burned children. Arch Surg 2002;137:1049-1054.

87. Heimbach D, Luterman A, Burke J, et al: Artificial dermis for major burns: A multi-center randomized clinical trial. Ann Surg 1988;208:313-320.

88. Schaner PJ, Brown RL, Kirksey TD, et al: Succinylcholine-induced hyperkalemia in burned patients. Anesth Analg 1996;48:764-770.

89. Martyn JA: Succinylcholine hyperkalemia after burns. Anesthesiology 1999;91:321-322.

90. Yanez P, Martyn JA: Prolonged d-tubocurarine infusion and/or immobilization cause upregulation of acetylcholine receptors and hyperkalemia to succinylcholine in rats. Anesthesiology 1996;84: 384-391.

91. Yentis SM: Suxamethonium and hyperkalaemia. Anaesth Intensive Care 1990;18:92-101.

92. Ward JM, Rosen KM, Martyn JA: Acetylcholine receptor subunit mRNA changes in burns are different from those seen after denervation: The 1993 Lindberg Award. J Burn Care Rehabil 1993;14:595-601.

93. Martyn J: Clinical pharmacology and drug therapy in the burned patient. Anesthesiology 1986;65:67-75.

94. Dwersteg JF, Pavlin EG, Heimbach DM: Patients with burns are resistant to atracurium. Anesthesiology 1986;65:517-520.

95. Martyn JA, Abernethy DR, Greenblatt DJ: Plasma protein binding of drugs after severe burn injury. Clin Pharmacol Ther 1984;35:535-539.

96. Martyn JA, Liu LM, Szyfelbein SK, et al: The neuromuscular effects of pancuronium in burned children. Anesthesiology 1983;59:561-564.

97. Martyn JA, Goudsouzian NG, Chang Y, et al: Neuromuscular effects of mivacurium in 2- to 12-yr-old children with burn injury. Anesthesiology 2000;92:31-37.

98. Martyn JA, Chang Y, Goudsouzian NG, et al: Pharmacodynamics of mivacurium chloride in 13- to 18-yr-old adolescents with thermal injury. Br J Anaesth 2002;89:580-585.

99. McCall JE, Fischer CG, Schomaker E, et al: Laryngeal mask airway use in children with acute burns: Intraoperative airway management. Paediatr Anaesth 1999;9:515-520.

100. Karam R, Ibrahim G, Tohme H, et al: Severe neck burns and laryngeal mask airway for frequent general anesthetics. Middle East J Anesthesiol 1996;13:527-535.

101. Achauer BM, Mueller G, Vanderkam VM: Prevention of accidental extubation in burn patients. Ann Plast Surg 1997;38:280-282.

102. Kemper KJ, Benson MS, Bishop MJ: Predictors of postextubation stridor in pediatric trauma patients. Crit Care Med 1991;19:352-355.

103. Mhanna MJ, Zamel YB, Tichy CM, et al: The "air leak" test around the endotracheal tube, as a predictor of postextubation stridor, is age dependent in children. Crit Care Med 2002;30:2639-2643.

104. Kreulen M, Mackie DP, Kreis RW, et al: Surgical release for intubation purposes in postburn contractures of the neck. Burns 1996;22: 310-312.

105. Waymack JP, Law E, Park R, et al: Acute upper airway obstruction in the postburn period. Arch Surg 1985;120:1042-1004.

106. Gallagher G, Rae CP, Kinsella J: Treatment of pain in severe burns. Am J Clin Dermatol 2000;1:329-335.

107. Stoddard FJ, Sheridan RL, Saxe GN, et al: Treatment of pain in acutely burned children. J Burn Care Rehabil 2002;23:135-156.

108. Martin-Herz SP, Patterson DR, Honari S, et al: Pediatric pain control practices of North American Burn Centers. J Burn Care Rehabil 2003;24:26-36.

109. Saxe G, Stoddard F, Courtney D, et al: Relationship between acute morphine and the course of PTSD in children with burns. J Am Acad Child Adolesc Psychiatry 2001;40:915-921.

110. Abdi S, Zhou Y: Management of pain after burn surgery. Curr Opin Anaesthesiol 2002;15:563-567.

111. Bussolin L, Busoni P, Giorgi L, et al: Tumescent local anesthesia for the surgical treatment of burns and postburn sequelae in pediatric patients. Anesthesiology 2003;99:1371-1375.

112. Beausang E, Orr D, Shah M, et al: Subcutaneous adrenaline infiltration in paediatric burn surgery. Br J Plast Surg 1999;52: 480-481.

113. Jellish WS, Gamelli RL, Furry PA, et al: Effect of topical local anesthetic application to skin harvest sites for pain management in burn patients undergoing skin-grafting procedures. Ann Surg 1999;229:115-120.

114. Cuignet O, Pirson J, Boughroup J, et al: The efficacy of continuous fascia iliaca compartment block for pain management in burn patients undergoing skin grafting procedures. Anesth Analg 2004;98:1077-1081.

115. Jonsson A, Cassuto J, Hanson B: Inhibition of burn pain by intravenous lignocaine infusion. Lancet 1991;338:151-152.

116. Cote CJ, Daniels AL, Connolly M, et al: Tongue oximetry in children with extensive thermal injury: Comparison with peripheral oximetry. Can J Anaesth 1992;39:454-457.

117. Brown RA, Grobbelaar AO, Barker S, et al: A formula to calculate blood cross-match requirements for early burn surgery in children. Burns 1995;21:371-373.

118. Hart DW, Wolf SE, Beauford RB, et al: Determinants of blood loss during primary burn excision. Surgery 2001;130:396-402.

119. Desai MH, Herndon DN, Broemeling L, et al: Early burn wound excision significantly reduces blood loss. Ann Surg 1990;211: 753-762.

120. Housinger TA, Lang D, Warden GD: A prospective study of blood loss with excisional therapy in pediatric burn patients. J Trauma 1993;34:262-263.

121. Budny PG, Regan PJ, Roberts AHN: The estimation of blood loss during burns surgery. Burns 1993;19:134-137.

122. Marano MA, O'Sullivan G, Madden M, et al: Tourniquet technique for reduced blood loss and wound assessment during excisions of burn wounds of the extremity. Surg Gynecol Obstet 1990;171: 249-250.

123. O'Mara MS, Goel A, Recio P, et al: The use of tourniquets in the excision of unexsanguinated extremity burn wounds. Burns 2002;28:684-687.

124. Mann R, Heimbach DM, Engrav LH, et al: Changes in transfusion practices in burn patients. J Trauma 1994;37:220-222.

125. Cartotto R, Musgrave MA, Beveridge M, et al: Minimizing blood loss in burn surgery. J Trauma 2000;49:1034-1039.

126. Robertson RD, Bond P, Wallace B, et al: The tumescent technique to significantly reduce blood loss during burn surgery. Burns 2001;27:835-838.

127. Cartotto R, Kadikar N, Musgrave MA, et al: What are the acute cardiovascular effects of subcutaneous and topical epinephrine for hemostasis during burn surgery? J Burn Care Rehabil 2003;24: 297-305.

128. Ford SA, Cooper AB, Lam-McCulloch J, et al: Systemic effects of subcutaneous and topical epinephrine administration during burn surgery. Can J Anaesth 2002;49:529-530.

129. Sheridan RL, Szyfelbein SK: Staged high-dose epinephrine clysis is safe and effective in extensive tangential burn excisions in children. Burns 1999;25:745-748.

130. Gomez M, Logsetty S, Fish JS: Reduced blood loss during burn surgery. J Burn Care Rehabil 2001;22:111-117.

131. Goldstein AM, Weber JM, Sheridan RL: Femoral venous access is safe in burned children: An analysis of 224 catheters. J Pediatr 1997;130:442-446.

132. Ramos GE, Bolgiani AN, Patino O, et al: Catheter infection risk related to the distance between insertion site and burned area. J Burn Care Rehabil 2002;23:266-271.

133. Niemi T, Svartling N, Syrjala M, et al: Haemostatic disturbances in burned patients during early excision and skin grafting. Blood Coagul Fibrinolysis 1998;9:19-28.

134. Jeng JC, Boyd TM, Jablonski KA, et al: Intraoperative blood salvage in excisional burn surgery: An analysis of yield, bacteriology, and inflammatory mediators. J Burn Care Rehabil 1998;19:305-311.

135. Samuelsson A, Bjornsson A, Nettelblad H, et al: Autotransfusion techniques in burn surgery. Burns 1997;23:188-189.

136. Sharar SR, Bratton SL, Carrougher GJ, et al: A comparison of oral transmucosal fentanyl citrate and oral hydromorphone for inpatient pediatric burn wound care analgesia. J Burn Care Rehabil 1998;19:516-521.
137. Murphy KD, Lee JO, Herndon DN: Current pharmacotherapy for the treatment of severe burns. Exp Opin Pharmacother 2003;4:369-384.
138. Kronenberg RH: Ketamine as an analgesic: Parenteral, oral, rectal, subcutaneous, transdermal and intranasal administration. J Pain Palliat Care Pharmacother 2002;16:27-35.
139. Escarment J, Cantais E, Le Dantec P, et al: [Propofol and ketamine for dressing in burnt patients]. Cah Anesthesiol 1995;43:31-34.
140. Pal SK, Cortiella J, Herndon D: Adjunctive methods of pain control in burns. Burns 1997;23:404-412.
141. Gall O, Annequin D, Benoit G, et al: Adverse events of premixed nitrous oxide and oxygen for procedural sedation in children. Lancet 2001;358:1514-1515.
142. Dimick P, Helvig E, Heimbach D, et al: Anesthesia-assisted procedures in a burn intensive care unit procedure room: Benefits and complications. J Burn Care Rehabil 1993;14:446-449.
143. Rae CP, Gallagher G, Watson S, et al: An audit of patient perception compared with medical and nursing staff estimation of pain during burn dressing changes. Eur J Anaesthesiol 2000;17:43-45.
144. Fratianne RB, Prensner JD, Huston MJ, et al: The effect of music-based imagery and musical alternate engagement on the burn débridement process. J Burn Care Rehabil 2001;22:47-53.
145. Frenay MC, Faymonville ME, Devlieger S, et al: Psychological approaches during dressing changes of burned patients: A prospective randomised study comparing hypnosis against stress reducing strategy. Burns 2001;27:793-799.
146. Van der Does AJ, Van Dyck R, Spijker RE: Hypnosis and pain in patients with severe burns: A pilot study. Burns Incl Therm Inj 1988;14:399-404.
147. Patterson DR, Everett JJ, Burns GL, et al: Hypnosis for the treatment of burn pain. J Consult Clin Psychol 1992;60:713-717.
148. Hoffman HG, Patterson DR, Magula J, et al: Water-friendly virtual reality pain control during wound care. J Clin Psychol 2004;60:189-195.
149. Patterson DR, Tininenko JR, Schmidt AE, et al: Virtual reality hypnosis: A case report. Int J Clin Exp Hypn 2004;52:27-38.
150. Hoffman HG, Patterson DR, Carrougher GJ: Use of virtual reality for adjunctive treatment of adult burn pain during physical therapy: A controlled study. Clin J Pain 2000;16:244-250.

19 Pregnancy and Complications of Pregnancy

DAVID HEPNER, MD, BHAVANI SHANKAR KODALI, MD, and SCOTT SEGAL, MD

Pregnancy is neither uncommon nor a disease. One study in a well-defined, continuously screened female population between 18 and 44 years of age found a pregnancy rate of over 10% per year.[1] The routine anesthetic care of pregnant women is certainly not an uncommon situation. Given that 1% to 2% of pregnant women will undergo nonobstetric surgery during their pregnancies,[2,3] even this clinical scenario would not qualify as "uncommon." Even unrecognized pregnancy in outpatients occurs in about 1 in 300 women.[4] Why, then, is a chapter on pregnancy included in this book?

The challenge of care of the obstetric patient lies in the physiologic changes of pregnancy and their interaction with anesthetic drugs and techniques. In addition, the urgency of care is often intensified by the presence of a viable fetus. In this chapter we explore some of the more unusual clinical challenges, both in obstetric anesthesia and analgesia, as well as in the anesthetic care of the pregnant patient undergoing nonobstetric procedures.

PHYSIOLOGIC CHANGES OF PREGNANCY

Administration of safe anesthesia for any pregnant woman necessitates a clear understanding of the physiologic changes that are associated with pregnancy. Thorough reviews of physiologic changes are beyond the scope of this chapter. Nonetheless, it should be emphasized that there are several important physiologic changes that have direct bearing on anesthetic management of obstetric patients (Table 19-1).[5,6] They are (1) airway changes in pregnancy that could pose intubation difficulties; (2) changes in the metabolic and respiratory system, resulting expeditiously in hypoxemia during apnea; (3) changes in the gastrointestinal system, predisposing the parturient to regurgitation and aspiration; (4) the pressure of the growing uterus on the aorta and inferior vena cava; and (5) mechanical, hormonal, and biochemical factors that can result in increased spread of intrathecal and epidural local anesthetic agents in pregnancy.

The implications of these physiologic changes on the coexisting disease, or vice versa, must be evaluated in every pregnant woman presenting with a coexisting disease or a complication of pregnancy. A coexisting disease, such as a cardiovascular lesion or a pulmonary condition, can translate physiologic changes into a morbidly pathologic state, thereby contributing to an increasing morbidity and mortality. In addition, pharmacokinetic and pharmacodynamic profiles are altered in pregnancy, and drug administration must be titrated carefully to the desired effect. With the increase in blood volume there is a greater volume of distribution; the low albumin and increased α glycoprotein can also alter the free drug concentrations. Issues of fetal well-being, such as maintenance of uteroplacental blood flow and oxygenation, prevention of fetal asphyxia, avoidance of teratogenic drugs, and prevention

TABLE 19–1 Physiologic Changes of Pregnancy	
Respiratory System	
Minute ventilation	↑ 50%
Functional residual capacity	↓ 20%
Oxygen consumption	↑ 20%
Carbon dioxide production	↑ 20%
Apneic desaturation	Faster
$PaCO_2$	32 mm Hg
$PaCO_2 - PETCO_2$	−1 to 0.75 mm Hg
Cardiovascular System	
Cardiac output	↑ 50%
Stroke volume	↑ 25%
Heart rate	↑ 25%
Systemic vascular resistance	No change
Blood pressure	No change at term gestation
Gastrointestinal System	
Barrier pressure	↓
Gastric emptying time	No change
Renal system:	
Plasma creatinine	↓
Brain	
Minimal alveolar concentration	↓
Metabolic	
Free drug availability	↑
Plasma cholinesterase activity	↓

Data from Farraghar R, Bhavani Shankar K: Obstetric anesthesia. In Healy TEJ (ed): Wylie and Churchill Davidson's A Practice of Anesthesia, 7th ed. London, Arnold, 2003, pp 923-940; and Chang B: Physiological changes of pregnancy. In Obstetric Anesthesia: Principles and Practice. Philadelphia, Elsevier, 2004, pp 15-36.

TABLE 19–2 General Considerations for Nonobstetric Surgery in Pregnancy
Maternal Safety
Respiratory system
Fragility of nasal mucosa
Upper airway edema
↑ Risk of difficult intubation
↑ Risk of desaturation
Gastrointestinal system
↑ Risk aspiration (? Timing in gestation)
Cardiovascular system
Expansion of blood volume (normal filling pressures)
Elevated cardiac output
Physiologic anemia of pregnancy
Fetal Safety
Direct effects of anesthesia
Maternal hypoxia and hypotension→fetal acidosis
Avoid uteroplacental vasoconstrictors (?alpha agonists, vasopressin, ketamine, high systemic local anesthetic concentrations)
Teratogenicity of drugs
No specific link to any anesthetic drug
Caution with nitrous oxide
Inhalation anesthetics may cause "behavioral teratogenicity" (behavioral abnormalities without structural defects)
Avoidance of preterm labor

of pre-term labor, are essential to consider when taking care of the pregnant patient. Maintenance of uteroplacental blood flow is essential to fetal well-being.

NONOBSTETRIC SURGERY IN PREGNANCY

General Considerations

The anesthetic management of pregnancy patients undergoing nonobstetric procedures has been extensively reviewed in major textbooks of obstetric anesthesiology, as well as several reviews. The principal considerations are maternal safety, fetal physiologic well-being, avoidance of teratogenicity, and prevention of preterm labor (Table 19-2).

Maternal Safety

Maternal safety requires understanding of the altered physiology of pregnancy. The most important changes affecting the anesthetic management of these patients are the respiratory, gastrointestinal, and cardiovascular systems.

Although there is considerable controversy regarding the physiology of gastric emptying and gastric acid production in pregnancy, it seems prudent whenever practical to consider pregnant patients beyond the late second trimester to be at a somewhat elevated risk of aspiration. The cardiovascular changes of greatest interest are the expansion of blood volume (but normal central venous pressure [CVP] and pulmonary capillary wedge pressure [PCWP]), elevated cardiac output, physiologic anemia of pregnancy, and aortocaval compression. Respiratory system changes affecting anesthetic management most notably include the increased fragility of the respiratory mucosa, upper airway edema, more difficult mask ventilation, a tenfold increase in the risk of difficult intubation, functional residual capacity and oxygen consumption changes that predispose to desaturation during apnea, and chronic respiratory alkalosis.[6]

In addition, general anesthesia in pregnant patients must take into consideration the altered response to anesthetic drugs. Minimal alveolar concentration (MAC) decreases in pregnancy, well before endorphins increase during labor.[7] Indeed, increased sensitivity to intravenous and inhalation anesthetics occurs during the first trimester. There is increased sensitivity to succinylcholine,[8] and patients receiving magnesium sulfate for preterm labor or preeclampsia are more sensitive to nondepolarizing neuromuscular blocking drugs as well.[9] Decreased protein binding due to lower concentrations of plasma proteins, as well as increased volume of distribution due to increased blood volume and weight (fat) gain, make pharmacokinetics of various drugs complex.[6] The responses to many anesthetic drugs, particularly those employed in some of the unusual situations described in this chapter, are unknown. Caution is therefore in order whenever any agent is used in the pregnant patient.

Fetal Safety

The fetus is potentially at risk by three separate mechanisms: direct effects of anesthetic agents and techniques on fetal cardiorespiratory homeostasis, teratogenic effects of maternally administered drugs, and induction of preterm labor.

Maternal hypoxia and hypotension can adversely affect the fetus. Modest hypoxia is well tolerated by the fetus due to the high concentration of fetal hemoglobin and its affinity for O_2. More severe hypoxia is associated with fetal desaturation and asphyxia. Conversely, hyperoxia does not adversely affect the fetus, owing to high placental shunt flow and the inability of high maternal P_{O_2} to increase maternal oxygen content significantly. High maternal concentrations of oxygen may be given whenever indicated for maternal well-being.[10]

Conversely, the fetus poorly tolerates maternal hypotension if it is severe or prolonged.[11] Uteroplacental blood flow is highly dependent on maternal systemic blood pressure, and decreases in the latter lead to fetal asphyxia. During nonobstetric surgery, causes of maternal hypotension may include hypovolemia, deep general anesthesia, high spinal or epidural anesthesia, aortocaval compression, hemorrhage, positive-pressure hyperventilation, and systemic hypotensive drugs. However, good fetal outcomes have been reported after moderate deliberate hypotension during neurosurgery.[12] Uteroplacental blood flow may also be impaired by systemic agents that produce uterine arterial vasoconstriction or significantly increase myometrial tone.[13] Drugs that may cause these effects include large doses of α-adrenergic agonists, vasopressin, ketamine, and high doses of local anesthetics. In contrast to classic animal studies, however, maternal administration of moderate dose phenylephrine has been associated with normal fetal blood gases at delivery.[14]

Teratogenicity of maternally administered drugs has been extensively reviewed elsewhere, and the reader is referred to these sources for more information. To date, no anesthetic agent has been definitively shown to induce congenital abnormalities in the developing fetus. However, there are a number of associations between anesthetics and either anomalies or abortion strong enough to dictate prudence in their use. Importantly, many drugs found to be teratogenic in earlier animal or uncontrolled human epidemiologic studies have proven safe when using more sophisticated methodology. This includes all commonly used opioids, benzodiazepines, barbiturates, and local anesthetics.[15,16]

Inhalation anesthetics present a more complex picture. In animals, prolonged exposure to more than 50% nitrous oxide (N_2O) induces fetal resorption and skeletal or visceral anomalies, depending on the timing of exposure.[17-19] However, the etiology is complicated and not completely understood. N_2O impairs 1-carbon metabolism via its action on vitamin B_{12}.[20] This cannot explain all of its effects, however, because supplementation with folinic acid or methionine (which should bypass many of the effects of inhibition of methionine synthase on DNA synthesis and methylation reactions) only partially reverses effects on the developing fetus.[21,22] Furthermore, co-administration of isoflurane or halothane blocks many of the effects of N_2O, possibly implicating α-adrenergic uterine vasoconstriction in the pathophysiology of the latter agent's effects.[23] Human epidemiologic studies of healthy women exposed to N_2O in the workplace have yielded conflicting results, and positive studies have shown only a slight increase in spontaneous abortion that may be explained by confounding variables.[24,25] Large epidemiologic investigations have confirmed slight increases in early pregnancy loss and low birth weight but have yielded inconclusive or negative results with regard to congenital anomalies. It is impossible to separate the effect of anesthesia from that of the surgical procedure or underlying disease process requiring surgery in human epidemiologic studies.[3]

Recently, a more ominous and insidious effect of inhalation anesthetics has been suggested and termed *behavioral teratogenicity*. The term refers to behavioral abnormalities occurring in the absence of obvious structural defects. Even relatively brief intrauterine exposure to halogenated anesthetics in rodents has resulted in persistent defects in memory and learning (maze solving).[26,27] Studies in cell culture and pathologic investigation of neonatal brains of rodents exposed in utero to isoflurane have shown widespread apoptosis and, specifically, defects in hippocampal synaptic function, effects that may explain the behavioral phenomena.[26] These results have yet to be confirmed in humans but would suggest caution in blithely exposing the pregnant woman to these agents.

Finally, preterm labor is associated with surgery in pregnancy. Although halogenated anesthetics inhibit uterine contractions, this effect is short lived and does not protect against preterm labor. Intra-abdominal procedures and those occurring during the third trimester are the most likely to be associated with preterm labor. It is not clear from epidemiologic studies whether the surgery itself, or the underlying condition prompting it, is responsible.[28] There is no evidence that any anesthetic technique either increases or decreases the chance of preterm labor. However, tocolytic therapy with magnesium, cyclooxygenase inhibitors, calcium channel blockers, or β-adrenergic agonists can have important anesthetic implications.

Laparoscopic Surgery During Pregnancy

Occasionally, pregnancy can be complicated by acute intra-abdominal pathology, requiring surgical intervention. Laparoscopic surgery is generally preferred to conventional open procedures, and therefore the anesthesiologist must be familiar with the physiologic implications and anesthetic management of pregnant women requiring laparoscopic procedures. In the past decade, laparoscopic procedures have become increasingly popular compared with open procedures, owing to decreased morbidity and convalescence.[29] Although pregnancy was considered a contraindication to laparoscopic cholecystectomy less than a decade ago,[30] it has become the most commonly performed laparoscopic procedure during pregnancy.[31] Other types of laparoscopic surgeries performed safely during pregnancy include appendectomy, ovarian cystectomy,[32] management of adnexal torsion,[33] diagnostic laparoscopies for abdominal pain,[34] splenectomy,[35] heterotopic pregnancies,[36] and adrenal pheochromocytoma.[37]

General Considerations and Effect of Pneumoperitoneum

When faced with providing anesthesia for the pregnant patient undergoing laparoscopic surgery, the anesthesiologist must not only consider the maternal and fetal issues, and prevention of preterm labor, but also pay special attention to patient positioning during surgery and the physiologic and mechanical effects of the CO_2 pneumoperitoneum.

Besides the maternal, fetal, and preterm labor issues, other factors that affect physiologic changes during laparoscopic surgery include pneumoperitoneum and patient positioning. Pneumoperitoneum during laparoscopy can cause cardiovascular and respiratory alterations in nonpregnant patients, and these changes become accentuated in the parturient. Adding pneumoperitoneum to an enlarged uterus further limits diaphragm expansion and is associated with an increase in peak airway pressure, decrease in functional reserve capacity, increased ventilation-perfusion mismatching, increased alveolar-arterial oxygen gradient, decreased thoracic cavity compliance, and increased pleural pressure.[38] Pneumoperitoneum and Trendelenburg positioning moves the carina cephalad, which can convert a low-lying tracheal tube to an endobronchial position. The Trendelenburg position increases intrathoracic pressure and accentuates all the respiratory-related physiologic changes. The combination of pregnancy and CO_2 pneumoperitoneum predisposes the parturient to hypercapnia and hypoxemia. Insufflation of CO_2 results in CO_2 absorption across the peritoneum and into the maternal blood stream. Elimination depends on an increase in minute ventilation; however, mechanical hyperventilation can reduce uteroplacental perfusion, probably owing to decreased venous return.[39] Although end-tidal CO_2 concentrations ($ETCO_2$) correlate well with $PaCO_2$ in healthy patients, they are a poor guide to $PaCO_2$ in sicker patients. Any increase in maternal $PaCO_2$ or decrease in PaO_2 can affect fetal well-being.[38] The cardiovascular changes associated with CO_2 insufflation include reduction in cardiac index and venous return, which can be exacerbated by reverse Trendelenburg positioning.[40] The observed increase in intracardiac filling pressures are probably secondary to an increase in intrathoracic pressure. A combination of reverse Trendelenburg position, general anesthesia, and peritoneal insufflation can decrease the cardiac index by as much as 50%.[41] The hemodynamic effects of aortocaval compression by the gravid uterus could further accentuate the hemodynamic effects of pneumoperitoneum and reverse Trendelenburg positioning, resulting in significant hypotension.[38,42] Steinbrook and Bhavani-Shankar[42] studied the cardiac output changes in four pregnant patients (17 to 24 weeks' gestation) undergoing laparoscopic surgery using thoracic bioimpedance cardiography. Intravenous ephedrine (10 mg) was given if the systolic blood pressure decreased by more than 20% with respect to baseline. The authors noted a 27% decrease in cardiac index after 5 minutes of CO_2 insufflation. Cardiac index remained 21% below baseline after 15 minutes of insufflation. The authors' aggressive management of blood pressures during anesthesia (treating any decrease in blood pressure approaching 20% of baseline measurements with intravenous ephedrine so as to minimize decreases in uterine blood flow) may have resulted in the somewhat smaller reduction in cardiac index during CO_2 insufflation in their patients (27%), as compared with 30% to 50% in nonpregnant subjects in most studies. Mean arterial pressures and systemic vascular resistance increased in these study subjects during CO_2 insufflation, which is similar to that generally observed in nonpregnant subjects laparoscopic surgery.

Monitoring

With the large number of physiologic changes associated with pregnancy, as well as the cardiovascular and pulmonary changes induced by laparoscopic surgery, optimal perioperative monitoring is unclear. The main debate centers on whether perioperative monitoring of arterial blood gases and fetal and uterine activity is necessary in parturients undergoing laparoscopic surgery. The Society of American Gastrointestinal Endoscopic Surgeons (SAGES) published guidelines for laparoscopic surgery during pregnancy that include perioperative monitoring of arterial blood gases, as well as perioperative fetal and uterine monitoring.[43] This belief has been echoed by other authorities.[34,44,45] Amos and colleagues[34] reported four fetal deaths in seven pregnant women who underwent laparoscopic cholecystectomy or appendectomy. During the same period, no fetal deaths occurred in patients who underwent pelvic surgeries by laparotomy. Even though no arterial blood gas data were collected, these authors suggested that the fetal demise could have been due to prolonged respiratory acidosis, despite maintaining $ETCO_2$ in the physiologic range (low to mid 30s mm Hg).[34] These concerns stem from previous studies indicating that elevation in maternal $PaCO_2$ could impair fetal CO_2 excretion across the placenta and could exacerbate fetal acidosis. Other risk factors, however, were present for fetal loss in this series, including perforated appendix and pancreatitis.

Steinbrook and colleagues[38] reported a case series of 10 pregnant women, gestational age 9 to 30 weeks, undergoing laparoscopic cholecystectomy. These authors did not monitor arterial blood gases or perioperative fetal and uterine activity. The patients underwent general anesthesia with controlled ventilation, and the $ETCO_2$ maintained between 32 and 36 mm Hg. Fetal heart rate and uterine activity were assessed preoperatively and immediately postoperatively. All patients had an uneventful recovery and did not need postoperative tocolysis, and no adverse maternal or fetal outcomes were noted. Seven patients were followed to delivery and had normal infants. The authors concluded that standard monitors recommended by the American Society of Anesthesiologists (ASA) are sufficient for the safety and well-being of the parturient and the fetus. Based on a series of 45 laparoscopic cholecystectomies and 22 laparoscopic appendectomies performed during all three trimesters, Affleck and associates[47] supported the use of noninvasive monitors and maintenance of the $ETCO_2$ within the physiologic range. They also recommended preoperative and postoperative fetal heart rate and uterine activity monitoring and no prophylactic tocolysis. In their series there was no fetal loss, nor were there uterine injuries or spontaneous abortions. There was no significant difference in preterm delivery rate, Apgar scores, or birth weights between the open and laparoscopic surgery groups. As in previous reports, the operative groups (both open and laparoscopic appendectomies and cholecystectomies) had a slightly higher rate of preterm labor compared with the general population. Furthermore, multiple case reports have reported successful outcomes with noninvasive monitoring.[48,49] Bhavani-Shankar and coworkers[50] prospectively evaluated the $PaCO_2$-$ETCO_2$ difference in eight parturients undergoing laparoscopic cholecystectomy with CO_2 pneumoperitoneum. The intra-abdominal pressures were maintained around 15 mm Hg. These women underwent surgery with general anesthesia during the second and third trimester of their pregnancies. After adjusting minute ventilation to maintain the $ETCO_2$ at 32 mm Hg, the arterial blood gases (alpha-stat method) were measured at fixed surgical phases: before insufflation, during insufflation, after insufflation, and after completion of surgery. The authors found no significant differences in either mean $PaCO_2$-$ETCO_2$ gradient or $PaCO_2$ and pH during the various phases of laparoscopy. During the surgical phase the maximal $PaCO_2$-$ETCO_2$ difference detected was 3.1 mm Hg (range, 1.1 to 3.1 mm Hg). It appears that $ETCO_2$ correlates well with arterial CO_2, and adjusting ventilation to maintain $ETCO_2$ also maintains optimal maternal arterial CO_2. These results do not support the need for arterial blood gas monitoring during laparoscopy in pregnant patients. Laparoscopic procedures have been performed safely during all trimesters of pregnancy; however, some authors have advocated reserving semi-elective, nonobstetric surgery during pregnancy only during the second trimester. During this period, organogenesis is complete and spontaneous abortions are less common than in the first trimester. Furthermore, procedures during the third trimester have been associated with more preterm labor and potential difficulty in visualization with an enlarged uterus.[31,33,51]

Anesthetic Technique

A summary of recommended anesthetic and surgical interventions for laparoscopy during pregnancy is noted in Table 19-3.[52]

In-Vitro Fertilization

Infertility is defined as 1 year of frequent unprotected sex without achieving a pregnancy and is not an irreversible state. Infertility is becoming more common with the trend for advanced maternal age before conception.[53,54] The prognosis for infertility caused by major causes and tubal and male factors has improved significantly with the introduction of assisted reproductive technologies (ART).[55] ART involves the handling and manipulation of the oocyte and spermatozoa to achieve a successful pregnancy. In-vitro fertilization (IVF), the most common form of ART, was first introduced in 1978[56] and has increased tremendously over the past two decades, with a recent article from North America reporting over 88,077 ART cycles since its inception.[57,58] The majority of these cycles (63,639) consisted of IVF, with a delivery rate per retrieval of 29.8%.[58] Overall, there was an increase of 7.5% and 0.4% for cycles and deliveries per retrieval, respectively. However, the high cost and the 70% failure rate have led reproductive endocrinologists to analyze factors that may affect the outcome of IVF, such as stimulation protocol, embryo factor, physician supervising the cycle, and patient selection.[59,60] As such, close scrutiny of other factors that may affect outcome, including medications and techniques used to provide anesthesia, would be expected.[61]

IVF produces a variable amount of pain that many practitioners consider a significant disadvantage.[62] Abdominal pain levels have been correlated with body mass index, number of follicles, and duration of technique and may

TABLE 19–3   Suggested Anesthetic Plan for Laparoscopic Surgery During Pregnancy

Oral	Left or right uterine displacement
Premedication	Oral sodium citrate, 30 mL; metoclopramide, 10 mg intravenously
Induction	Rapid-sequence sodium pentothal and succinylcholine
Ventilatory adjustments	Keep end-tidal Pco_2 between 32 and 34 mm Hg
Maintenance of anesthesia	Desflurane, fentanyl, oxygen in air, and muscle relaxants (vecuronium)
Positioning	Gradual change to reverse Trendelenburg
Fetal heart rate monitoring	16 weeks, preoperative and immediate postoperative period
Insufflation technique	Open trocar technique
Tocolysis	Terbutaline, 0.25 mg subcutaneous, if needed
Hypotension	Increments of ephedrine
Postoperative period	Left or right uterine displacement, oxygen supplements, fetal heart monitoring

Data from Bhavani-Shankar K: Anesthetic considerations for minimally invasive surgery. In: Current Review of Minimally Invasive Surgery, 2nd ed. Philadelphia, 1998, p 29.

vary between patients. Although conscious sedation remains the most widely used method for pain relief, and is used in 95% of centers in the United States,[63,64] it is rarely effective in preventing ovarian puncture pain. Lack of coverage for IVF by most insurance companies[65] and a concern for a decreased pregnancy rate with anesthetic agents may account for the decreased use of general and regional techniques for IVF.[57] However, recent state laws requiring that insurance companies provide either partial or complete coverage for IVF,[65] and similar embryo implantation and pregnancy rates with the use of local anesthetics and short-acting general anesthetic agents,[57] are likely to increase the use of general and regional anesthesia. Therefore, it is important to understand the implications of anesthetic techniques on IVF as well as the implications of assisted reproductive techniques on regional and general anesthesia (Tables 19-4 and 19-5).

Anesthetic Implications on IVF

Transvaginal ultrasound guided oocyte retrieval (TUGOR) is a relatively short procedure. On average the procedure lasts 10 to 20 minutes and could be performed under conscious sedation, paracervical block, neuraxial blockade, or general anesthesia. Therefore, short-acting agents are desired to minimize the recovery time of patients undergoing this treatment. Monitored anesthesia care or conscious sedation relies on adequate local anesthesia. However, it is inadequate to anesthetize the ovary. Patient discomfort, motion due to pain, and a deep level of conscious sedation leading to airway obstruction are serious risks. In addition, significant discomfort may leave patients with bad memories and may discourage future attempts at IVF. Therefore, we prefer to use neuraxial techniques or intravenous general anesthesia (IVGA).

TABLE 19–4   Different Types of Assisted Reproductive Techniques

	TUGOR	GIFT	ZIFT	PROST	TET
Average Duration	10-20 min	60-90 min	Two different procedures: embryo retrieval (10-20 min) followed by transfer (30-60 min) 24-48 hr after fertilization		
Embryo Transfer	Fertilized oocyte on day 3 or 5	Unfertilized oocyte transferred shortly after retrieval	Fertilized oocyte transferred 24-48 hr after retrieval		
Anesthetic Options	Multiple; general or spinal preferred	Mainly general owing to need for laparoscopy	Two different anesthetics: intravenous general or short-acting spinal preferred for embryo retrieval and general anesthetic preferred for laparoscopy for transfer		

TUGOR, Transvaginal ultrasound-guided oocyte retrieval; GIFT, gamete intrafallopian transfer; ZIFT, zygote intrafallopian transfer; PROST, pronuclear stage tubal transfer; TET, tubal embryo transfer.

<table>
<tr><td></td><td>General Anesthesia</td><td>Neuraxial Blockade</td><td>Paracervical Block</td><td>Conscious Sedation</td></tr>
<tr><td>Benefits</td><td>Fast induction and emergence</td><td>Able to avoid intravenous agents if so desired</td><td colspan="2">Fast induction and emergence without the need for anesthesia personal</td></tr>
<tr><td>Drawbacks</td><td>Conflicting results on the effects of different agents on embryo implantation and pregnancy rates</td><td>Longer induction and recovery times</td><td>Ovaries are not anesthetized; operator dependent; lidocaine appears in the follicular fluid</td><td>Relies on adequate local anesthesia that is difficult to achieve</td></tr>
</table>

TABLE 19–5   Anesthetic Options for Assisted Reproductive Techniques

Embryo transfer (ET) is a simple procedure that occurs on day 3 or 5 after TUGOR, relies on a fertilized oocyte, and rarely requires any anesthetic involvement. After speculum insertion into the vagina and examination of the cervix, a flexible catheter loaded with embryos and culture medium is advanced past the cervical os and injected into the uterus. Conscious sedation or light IVGA may be necessary in cases of significant discomfort with speculum insertion, or when there is difficulty advancing the flexible catheter past the cervical opening.

Gamete intrafallopian transfer (GIFT) is an alternative to IVF-ET that was more common prior to the recent improvement in embryo culture techniques and successful pregnancies with IVF-ET. After hormone stimulation and TUGOR, unfertilized oocytes are mixed with sperm and transferred shortly after retrieval into the fallopian tube. Laparoscopy performed under general anesthesia is preferred so as to have direct visualization of the flexible catheter and fallopian tubes. Although spinal anesthesia is rarely used for laparoscopic procedures because of concerns of shoulder discomfort and difficulty breathing with CO_2, there is a report highlighting the safety of spinal anesthesia for laparoscopic oocyte retrieval.[66] There is another technique performed with a minilaparoscopic approach, allowing for a reduction in intraperitoneal pressure and CO_2, and obviating the need for general anesthesia.[67] Pregnancy rates are similar between IVF-ET and GIFT, and therefore IVF-ET, being less invasive, is more commonly performed. GIFT allows for the oocyte fertilization in vivo and may be acceptable for couples with religious beliefs that preclude IVF. Other transfer options include zygote intrafallopian transfer (ZIFT), pronuclear stage tubal transfer (PROST), and tubal embryo transfer (TET). Although fertilization is confirmed before embryo transfer, all of these techniques require TUGOR to aspirate the follicular fluid and laparoscopically guided transfer into the fallopian tube 24 to 48 hours after fertilization. Similar pregnancy rates, and the need for two different procedures and anesthetics, have led to a marked decline in the performance of these techniques.

Earlier reports of IVF, when the procedure length was significantly longer, reported the use of general endotracheal anesthesia with a combination of inhalation agents, with or without N_2O. General endotracheal anesthesia is now rarely used, except in cases of laparoscopic oocyte retrieval or when dictated by the patient's condition. Concern about the use of N_2O for these procedures originated from earlier reports suggesting that it had a teratogenic effect and caused fetal death in rats when used during organogenesis.[68] In addition, lower DNA and RNA content and morphologic abnormalities have been demonstrated in the embryos of pregnant rats when exposed to N_2O during organogenesis.[69,70] This potential teratogenicity has been attributed, in part, to the inactivation of methionine synthase. Short exposures to clinical concentrations of N_2O, isoflurane, and halothane had no deleterious effect on IVF and early embryonic growth up to the morula stage in the mouse.[71] Despite the deleterious effect of N_2O in some rat studies, no significant differences between rates of fertilization or pregnancy were demonstrated in humans undergoing laparoscopic oocyte retrieval and isoflurane/N_2O or isoflurane/air general anesthesia.[72] Inhaled agents have not been demonstrated to possess a teratogenic or embryo effect.[73] Furthermore, halothane has been demonstrated to protect against N_2O-induced teratogenicity and spontaneous abortions in rats.[23] In addition, greater pregnancy rates have been demonstrated in women undergoing laparoscopic pronuclear stage transfer (PROST) under isoflurane/N_2O when compared with propofol/N_2O anesthesia.[74]

Propofol is an ideal induction and maintenance agent owing to its short-acting half-life and antiemetic properties. There were some reservations regarding the use of this agent, because early reports demonstrated that propofol diffuses into follicular fluid, with greater levels observed with higher doses of propofol.[75,76] Even though follicular fluid concentrations have been demonstrated to be higher in the last follicle when compared with the first follicle, no differences were found in the ratio of mature to immature follicles, or in fertilization, cleavage, or embryo cell number.[76] In addition, a report on the use of propofol for intravenous general anesthesia for TUGOR of donor oocytes demonstrated a lack of negative effect on the oocyte, as evaluated by cumulative embryo scores and rates of implantation and pregnancy.[77] Reports on the use of propofol (propofol, N_2O) for the transfer of fertilized embryos demonstrated fewer pregnancies when compared with an isoflurane, N_2O-based anesthesia.[74] However, higher maternal serum concentrations were needed in this study to provide anesthesia for laparoscopic pronuclear stage transfer when compared with the use of propofol for IVF-ET procedures.[78] Another study on mouse oocytes demonstrated that high levels of propofol in the follicular fluid may affect pregnancy rates.[79] The use of thiopental and thiamylal for laparoscopic egg retrieval has also been associated with accumulation in follicular fluid,[80] and a comparison of thiopental and propofol when used for laparoscopic GIFT demonstrated similar pregnancy rates.[81] A case-controlled study comparing propofol IVGA to paracervical block did not demonstrate any difference between the fertilization rates, embryo cleavage characteristics, or pregnancy rates between the two groups.[82] Neither group received premedication, both groups received 0.5 mg alfentanil at the time of anesthesia induction, and the propofol group received a full induction dose (2 mg/kg), followed by a continuous infusion without any additional anesthetic.[82] The results of this study are compelling, as an IVGA was compared to a local anesthetic group without premedication. In addition, there are no studies demonstrating a teratogenic effect of propofol. Overall, the data support the notion that although propofol, when used for intravenous general anesthesia for brief IVF procedures, may appear in follicular fluid, it does not have an adverse effect on pregnancy rates.

Fentanyl, alfentanil, and midazolam, when used as premedications prior to TUGOR, reach very low intrafollicular levels and have no effect on rates of implantation or pregnancy.[83,84] The absolute concentration of intrafollicular levels is extremely low when compared with plasma levels.[84,85] Alfentanil had the lowest follicular fluid to plasma ratio (1:40) when compared with midazolam (1:20) and fentanyl (1:10).[84] Remifentanil is a relatively new analgesic agent with pharmacokinetic properties, including a fast onset and a very short recovery, suitable for IVF procedures. A comparison of propofol/fentanyl anesthesia to a midazolam/remifentanil technique demonstrated a decreased need for manual ventilation and a faster recovery of function in the latter group. More patients in the former group experienced intraoperative awareness and did not enjoy the anesthetic, but there were no differences in the time to discharge.[86] Other studies have compared a propofol-based anesthetic with a sedative combination of ketamine and midazolam without demonstrating a difference in the recovery profile, embryo transfers, or pregnancy rates.[87] Of note, there are sparse data on the safety of ketamine or remifentanil on ART.

Nonsteroidal anti-inflammatory agents (NSAIDs), such as intravenous ketorolac, would be ideal for the acute visceral pain during and after TUGOR. However, there is reluctance to use them because prostaglandins (PGE_2, $PGF_{2\alpha}$, PGI_2) in the embryo and endometrium are involved in processes that are important for implantation.[88,89] Prostaglandin H synthase, also known as cyclooxygenase, is an essential enzyme in prostaglandin synthesis, is primarily localized in the endometrial epithelium, and is important for embryo implantation.[90] Despite these concerns, there are no animal or human data that demonstrate any changes produced by cyclooxygenase inhibitors on the embryo or on implantation rates. Furthermore, implantation does not occur until 3 to 5 days after egg retrieval. Some centers in the United Kingdom routinely use NSAIDs without any known effects on endometrial lining or implantation rates.[91] We prefer to use NSAIDs for egg donors or for patients with pain refractory to significant doses of opioids until further data are available. Future studies should help to clarify some of these concerns.

Nausea and vomiting are the most common complications of general anesthesia but is reduced with the use of propofol, low doses of opioids, and the avoidance of inhaled anesthetic agents. We prefer to avoid metoclopramide in patients undergoing IVF, as the risk of affecting embryo implantation and a successful pregnancy is greater than its benefit in patients that are not at a significantly high risk for acid aspiration syndrome. Metoclopramide, a dopamine receptor antagonist, causes elevated prolactin levels that may be associated with inhibition of pulsatile gonadotropic releasing hormone secretion, a hypoestrogenic state, and ovulatory dysfunction.[92] Although not helpful for gastric motility, ondansetron use for the treatment or prevention of nausea and vomiting is not contraindicated during IVF. Serotonergic agents, unlike $5-HT_3$ receptor antagonists such as ondansetron, may also cause an elevation of prolactin levels. We prefer to use a neuraxial technique for patients at increased risk for postoperative nausea and vomiting or acid aspiration syndrome.

During TUGOR, a transvaginal approach is utilized to puncture the ovary and aspirate the follicular fluid. Both sympathetic and parasympathetic nerves supply the ovaries. Although most of the sympathetic nerves are derived from the ovarian plexus that accompanies the ovarian vessels, a minority are derived from the plexus that surrounds the ovarian branch of the uterine artery.[93] Acute visceral pain is often diffuse in distribution, vague in location of origin, and referred to remote areas of the body.[94] Paracervical block (PCB) has been utilized with and without conscious sedation for TUGOR to improve pain relief.[63,95,96] It has been postulated that PCB anesthetizes the vaginal mucosa, uterosacral ligaments, and peritoneal membrane over the pouch of Douglas.[95] Although the ovaries are not anesthetized, their pain sensitivity is the lowest when compared with the rest of the internal female genital organs.[94] PCB with 150 mg of lidocaine reduced abdominal pain by one half when compared with placebo.[95] The Visual Analogue Pain Score (VAPS 0-100 mm linear visual analogue scale) decreased from 43.7 to 21.2 mm when evaluated 4 hours after TUGOR.[95] Another study demonstrated no difference in VAPS when 50 mg of lidocaine was compared with 100 and 150 mg for PCB.[96] Assessing VAPS immediately after the procedure demonstrated median abdominal pain levels of 30 to 32 mm. Although small concentrations of lidocaine appear in the follicular fluid and have been shown to have adverse effects in mouse oocyte fertilization and embryo development,[95,97] they do not affect embryo implantation or pregnancy rates.[98] PCB alone is not sufficient to provide complete analgesia, owing to its 10% to 15% failure rate and lack of interference with afferent sensory fibers originating from the ovarian plexus. This finding is reflected in the 2.5 times higher vaginal and abdominal pain levels with PCB alone when compared with PCB with the addition of conscious sedation.[63]

Neuraxial techniques have also been utilized for TUGOR and are more likely to anesthetize the ovary, vaginal mucosa, and peritoneal membrane. A thoracic dermatomal level of T10 or higher is needed to anesthetize the ovaries. Spinal anesthesia is more likely to be beneficial owing to its increased reliability and fast onset. It requires minimal to no conscious sedation for its performance and can be tailored to minimize high sensory levels and motor blockade. The optimal spinal anesthetic should allow adequate surgical anesthesia with minimal side effects, a fast onset, a short recovery time, and a similar rate of successful pregnancies when compared with other anesthetic techniques. Earlier reports described the use of 60 mg of 5% lidocaine for spinal anesthesia,[99] but long recovery times and the finding of transient neurologic symptoms caused some concerns. In an effort to decrease recovery times and keep patients comfortable, Martin and colleagues[100] decreased the dose to 45 mg of lidocaine and evaluated the benefit of adding 10 μg of fentanyl to the spinal anesthetic. A comparison of these studies[99,100] demonstrated decreased times to ambulate, void, and discharge in the lower dose lidocaine group. The addition of fentanyl to the lidocaine resulted in improved analgesia during the procedure and, postoperatively, a decreased opioid consumption and no change in side effects or in the ability to ambulate, void, or be discharged. The addition of increased amounts of fentanyl to the spinal technique, and surgical improvements leading to a shorter duration in egg retrievals, led to a further decrease in the dose of lidocaine to 30 mg. Although we have had a good success with the use of subarachnoid 30 mg of lidocaine combined with fentanyl of 25 μg, controversy due to lidocaine and transient neurologic symptoms led to the evaluation of bupivacaine as an alternative. However, a comparison of 30 mg of lidocaine with equipotent doses of bupivacaine (3.75 mg) demonstrated a longer time to micturition and recovery with bupivacaine.[101] Of note, patients undergoing IVF procedures demonstrate decreased serum albumin and α_1-acid

glycoprotein levels during supraphysiologic estrogen states at the time of oocyte retrieval. This may lead to an increased free fraction of highly protein bound drugs such as bupivacaine.[102] However, this may only be significant when using larger doses of bupivacaine during epidural anesthesia, which is rarely used during IVF. At our institution, spinal anesthesia even with low doses of local anesthetic and opioid is associated with longer times to voiding and discharge when compared with intravenous general anesthesia. This finding and short surgical time led us to use IVGA as our standard anesthetic for TUGOR. Spinal anesthesia with 30 mg of lidocaine and 25 μg of fentanyl is used at the patient's request in patients with significant gastroesophageal reflux disease and/or morbid obesity, in cases where the patient has eaten and the oocytes must be retrieved before spontaneous ovulation occurs, or when indicated because of severe side effects to IVGA, such as postoperative nausea and vomiting.

Male factor is the most common form of infertility.[103] New variations of IVF include direct sperm harvesting and a single sperm injection into the cytoplasm of the oocyte (intracytoplasmic sperm injection [ICSI]). ICSI has markedly increased pregnancy rates in patients with male factor infertility due to low sperm counts and is often combined with direct sperm aspiration from the epididymis or testicular biopsy. Earlier reports described a more invasive microepididymal sperm aspiration (MESA) with an open surgical aspiration of the scrotum.[104] Recent work has pioneered less invasive techniques such as percutaneous epididymal sperm aspiration (PESA) and testicular sperm aspiration (TESA).[104] These two techniques have been reported to be done under local anesthesia of the superior and inferior spermatic nerves and the genital branch of the genitofemoral nerve without any premedication.[104] We prefer to use spinal anesthesia or IVGA for these procedures to minimize patient discomfort and movement.

IVF Implications on Anesthesia

IVF consists of different stages, including suppression therapy, stimulation therapy, trigger or ovulation therapy, egg retrieval, fertilization, postovulation therapy with progesterone, and embryo transfer. Therapy with leuprolide acetate (Lupron), a gonadotropin-releasing hormone agonist, causes suppression of gonadotropins (follicle-stimulating hormone [FSH] and luteinizing hormone [LH]) and results in a lack of production of estrogen and progesterone. Stimulation therapy is conducted with FSH- and LH-containing human menopausal gonadotropin and causes ovarian follicle growth. Human chorionic gonadotropin (hCG) causes ovulation to occur within 36 hours, and TUGOR is performed at this time. Supplemental progesterone is given after embryo transfer.

Stimulation therapy with gonadotropins such as human menopausal gonadotropin or FSH preparations may lead to very high estrogen levels and ovarian hyperstimulation.[105] High estrogen levels place patients at risk for thromboembolic phenomena. In its more severe form, ovarian hyperstimulation syndrome (OHSS) may lead to increased vascular permeability with leaky capillaries and findings such as weight gain, intravascular volume depletion, ascites, pleural effusions, electrolyte changes, and renal dysfunction. These patients usually experience a state of fibrinolysis with higher fibrinogen, plasmin/α_2-antiplasmin, thrombin/antithrombin complexes, and D-dimer levels when compared with women with lower estrogen levels.[106-108] In addition, tissue factor increases markedly with high estrogen levels and is a powerful trigger of the extrinsic pathway of the coagulation cascade.[108,109] Treatment is usually supportive, with intravascular volume expansion, analgesics, bed rest, and thrombosis prophylaxis. More invasive methods, such as paracentesis and thoracentesis, are more helpful for relief of symptoms such as abdominal pain and shortness of breath. Conscious sedation is often required for these procedures and should take into account the increased sensitivity to medications due to intravascular volume contraction. Caution should be approached if regional anesthetic techniques are a consideration for these patients because of the potential for anticoagulation.

The retrieval of oocytes from the follicles is not considered an elective procedure, as failure to retrieve them may lead to spontaneous ovulation and a wasted cycle. In addition, failure to empty the follicles may lead to ovarian hyperstimulation syndrome with all of its known complications. Our preference is to perform TUGOR under spinal anesthesia with minimal sedation under these circumstances. Aspiration prophylaxis is recommended with sodium citrate and metoclopramide, despite the concerns for increased prolactin levels with metoclopramide.

In summary, assisted reproductive techniques have increased tremendously over the past two decades. Although the rate of success continues to increase, there are still a significant number of cycles that do not result in a live birth. Therefore, it is expected that close scrutiny will be paid to variables that may affect oocyte retrieval or embryo transfer. It is essential to understand the impact of different anesthetic techniques and medications on IVF and to read carefully any data that links these factors with implantation or pregnancy rates. Not only may there be an impact of the anesthetic on ART but also one of ART on the anesthetic.

OBSTETRIC ANESTHESIA FOR UNCOMMON CONDITIONS

Morbid Obesity in Pregnant Women

A weight greater than 300 pounds in a gravida at term is considered to be morbidly obese.[110] Pregnancy in obese patients may have four important implications.[111]

First, some of the physiologic changes associated with pregnancy (e.g., increases in blood volume, cardiac output, reduction in functional residual capacity) may further exacerbate deleterious effects produced by pathophysiologic alterations of obesity. Second, there is susceptibility for obese patients to acquire pregnancy-related diseases and complications (e.g., preeclampsia, gestational diabetes). Third, there is an association between increased incidence of obstetric and perinatal complications and morbid obesity. Finally, a combination of these three factors may lead to the fourth implication: an unfavorable outcome of pregnancy.

Obese women should be strongly encouraged to lose weight before conceiving. This will decrease obstetric and perinatal morbidity and mortality. Careful systemic evaluation should be performed at the first opportunity during pregnancy in morbidly obese women to determine the systemic pathophysiologic alterations of obesity. This includes the degree of respiratory impairment resulting in hypoxia, with consequences such as pulmonary hypertension, right ventricular hypertrophy, and right ventricular impairment. The left ventricle undergoes eccentric hypertrophy as a result of increased cardiac output, hypertension, and blood volume. The end result is a biventricular hypertrophy. A bedside method of knowing the degree of hypoxemia is to determine the decreases in oxygen saturation on assuming the supine position from an erect posture. If hypoxia occurs in assuming the supine position, further evaluation should be performed to determine the right ventricular functional changes.[111] Pregnancy in morbidly obese women can exaggerate sleep apnea, resulting in pulmonary hypertension during pregnancy.[112]

Increased body mass index, increased prepregnancy weight, and excessive maternal weight gain increase the risk of cesarean section.[113] Abnormal presentations, fetal macrosomia, and prolonged labor are predisposing factors associated with increased incidence of cesarean delivery among obese women. There is evidence that obese patients are at increased risk for abnormal labor.[114,115] The incidence of cesarean delivery for failure to progress was much higher in the morbidly obese group than in the control group, although the difference was not statistically significant.

There is high incidence of umbilical arterial pH less than 7.10 among obese women, regardless of whether they had a trial of labor or elective cesarean delivery.[116] There is significantly higher incidences of neonates with an Apgar score of less than 5 at 1 minute, Apgar score less than 7 at 5 minutes, birth weight greater than 4500 g, birth weight less than 2500 g, intrauterine growth retardation, and neonatal intensive care unit admissions among infants born to obese parturients, as compared with those in nonobese parturients.[117] There seems to be an association between gravid obesity and congenital anomalies in infants born to gravid obese parturients. Waller and associates found that these infants are at a greater risk for developing neural tube defects and other congenital malformations.[118]

Anesthetic Management

It is strongly recommended that the patient should be seen by an anesthesiologist at around 28 weeks' gestation to determine the effect of pregnancy on various systems (Box 19-1). A multidisciplinary approach should be instituted, depending on the systemic findings. Careful evaluation of airway should be performed, and the anesthetic plan should be formulated well in advance and communicated to the patient, as well as the obstetrician. Regional anesthesia is most appropriate for labor and delivery. An early institutionalization of epidural anesthesia is recommended, which will provide ample time to negate difficulties encountered during epidural placements. Continuous spinal anesthesia is a reasonable alternative. These two techniques provide satisfactory analgesia and anesthesia as needed for cesarean delivery, urgent or otherwise. If general anesthesia is contemplated, a second pair of hands is a boon, and necessary airway backup equipment should be at hand. Difficult intubation should be anticipated, and a contingency backup plan should be set in motion as needed. Great care must be exercised in appropriately positioning morbidly obese pregnant women for cesarean delivery. Hypoxia may occur in the supine position, which may require elevation of the back rest of the operating table. Retraction of the pannus to facilitate surgery can result in exaggerated supine hypotensive syndrome of pregnancy that may occasionally result in cardiac arrest. A multidisciplinary approach is the key to a successful outcome of pregnancy in morbidly obese women.

Amniotic Fluid Embolism

Amniotic fluid embolism is one of the most intriguing complications of pregnancy. Its diagnosis is difficult and uncertain at times, its pathophysiology is debatable, its treatment is difficult and often inadequate and nonspecific, and morbidity and mortality are high. Amniotic fluid or amniotic debris enters the maternal circulation more often than perceived. However, only a few develop full-blown amniotic fluid embolism and what initiates the chain of events remains unclear.

The mortality of amniotic fluid embolism continues to be high for patients who are symptomatic. It varies anywhere from 61% to 86%.[119,120] The classic description of amniotic fluid embolism is profound and unexpected shock, followed by cardiovascular collapse and, in most cases, death.[121] The syndrome was thought most likely to occur in multiparous women who had an unusually strong or rapid labor or who had just followed such a labor.[122] The use of uterine stimulants, meconium staining of the amniotic fluid, or the presence of a large or dead fetus was also believed to increase the risk. However, it has been revealed that there are a number of exceptions to this classic description. There are several case reports of amniotic fluid emboli occurring during cesarean deliveries and therapeutic abortions, as well as occasional cases in the late postpartum period or very rarely in nonlaboring patients.[123-126] Other cases have been associated with abdominal trauma, ruptured uterus, or intrapartum amnioinfusion.[127,128]

It has been postulated that amniotic fluid may be trapped in the uterine veins during contraction of the uterus at delivery, which is then released into the circulation later, during normal postpartum uterine involution.[129] This explains why some cases of amniotic fluid embolism occur in the late postpartum period. Another reason for delayed presentation would be that the initial onset was either transient or subclinical and went unrecognized. This, in turn, could account for the delayed or atypical presentation reported in the literature.

Clinical Presentation

Cardiorespiratory collapse was almost invariably present in most of the cases, as seen in the Morgan series.[119] However, the presenting symptom in 51% of patients was respiratory distress. In the remainder, the first indication of a problem was hypotension in 27%, a coagulopathy in 12%, and seizures in 10%. Clark and coworkers, on the other hand, found that, of those women presenting before delivery, 30% had seizures or seizure-like activity, whereas 27% complained of dyspnea.[120] Fetal bradycardia (17%) and hypotension (13%) were the next most common presenting features. Of the 13 patients who developed symptoms after the delivery of the infant, 7 (54%) presented with an isolated coagulopathy manifested by postpartum hemorrhage. Several additional case reports have suggested that the presentation of amniotic fluid embolus can be quite variable with regard to timing, presenting symptoms, and subsequent course.[128] Therefore,

---

BOX 19–1   Anesthetic Considerations in Morbidly Obese Pregnant Women

- Perform a preanesthetic evaluation during pregnancy.
- Assess airway.
- Evaluate associated cardiorespiratory abnormalities of obesity.
- Perform early epidural placement to ensure a good working catheter.
- Consider continuous spinal technique if epidural anesthesia is unsuccessful and airway is anticipated to be difficult.
- Place several folded bed sheets in a stepwise fashion from the back to the occiput, to attain a good intubating position.
- Know that a large pannus may cause hemodynamic instability after induction of regional anesthesia.

there is a need to consider the differential diagnosis carefully while at the same time maintaining a high index of suspicion for this disorder (Box 19-2).

Etiology

Intact fetal membranes isolate amniotic fluid from the maternal circulation. After delivery, uterine vessels on the raw surface of the endometrium become exposed to amniotic fluid. Normally, uterine contractions are very effective in collapsing these veins. Therefore, in addition to ruptured membranes, for amniotic fluid embolism to occur there must be a pressure gradient favoring the entry of amniotic fluid from the uterus into the maternal circulation.[119] Although the placental implantation site is one potential portal of entry, particularly with partial separation of the placenta, this is otherwise unlikely if the uterus remains well contracted. On the other hand, small tears in the lower uterine segment and endocervix are common during labor and delivery and are now thought to be the most likely entry points.[119,123] In support of this concept, Bastein and associates reported a case of amniotic fluid embolus where postmortem examination revealed marked plugging of both cervical vasculature and the lungs by various amniotic fluid elements.[130]

There is a misconception in the literature that amniotic fluid routinely enters the maternal circulation at delivery. This misconception arose from the belief that the presence of squamous cells in the pulmonary vasculature was a marker signaling the entry of amniotic fluid into the maternal circulation. Studies have now shown that squamous cells can appear in the pulmonary blood of heterogenous populations of both pregnant and nonpregnant patients who have undergone pulmonary artery catheterization.[131,132] The presence of these cells is thought to have resulted from contamination by either exogenous sources during specimen preparation or by

epithelial cells derived from the entry site of the pulmonary artery catheter.[131] Because it is difficult to differentiate adult from fetal epithelial cells, the isolated finding of squamous cells in the pulmonary circulation of pregnant patients without amniotic fluid embolus is most likely a contaminant and not indicative of maternal exposure to amniotic fluid. Furthermore, it was determined that although squamous cells may be present in both groups (clinical evidence with and without amniotic fluid embolus), only the former had evidence of other fetal debris such as mucin, vernix, and lunago. In these patients, squamous cells and other granular debris were frequently coated with leukocytes, suggesting a maternal reaction to foreign material. Where other occasional unidentifiable debris was detected, the authors stated that the material present in the patients who did not have an amniotic fluid embolism was "clearly different" from that seen in the sample.[132] Additional cause for the confusion regarding whether amniotic fluid routinely enters the maternal circulation centers on the importance of trophoblastic embolization to the maternal lung. Trophoblastic cells are normally free floating in the intervillous space and therefore have direct access to the maternal circulation.[119] Hence, their presence in the maternal peripheral or central vascular circulation is neither surprising nor indicative of an amniotic fluid embolus. Further evidence that amniotic fluid does not normally enter the maternal circulation can be found from autopsies of parturients who died of various complications of pregnancy. Roche and Norris compared lung specimens obtained from 20 toxemic patients with an equal number who had clinical evidence of amniotic fluid embolus. Utilizing a specific stain for acid mucopolysaccharide, they were able to confirm the presence of mucin in the lung secretions from all of the amniotic fluid embolism patients. None of the sections from the toxemic patients stained positive.[133]

In summary, the presence of squamous or trophoblastic cells in the maternal pulmonary vasculature must not be equated with the entry of amniotic fluid into the maternal circulation. There is no evidence to suggest or support that amniotic fluid embolus is a common physiologic event.

Pathophysiology

Once the amniotic fluid enters the maternal circulation, a number of physiologic changes occur that contribute to the syndrome that we observe. The pathophysiology is multifactorial, and the clinical presentation will depend on the predominant physiologic aberration.

Hemodynamic Changes

Animal models have suggested that severe pulmonary hypertension was the major pathophysiologic change.[134] This was believed to be either due to critical obstruction of

---

BOX 19–2   Considerations in Amniotic Fluid Embolus

- Cardiorespiratory collapse may be the first sign of amniotic fluid embolism.
- Occasionally, hypotension, seizures, dyspnea, and isolated coagulopathy may be the presenting feature.
- Coagulopathy is an invariable accompaniment of amniotic fluid.
- Presence of squamous cells and other fetal debris (mucin, vernix, lunago) coated with leukocytes in the maternal circulation is the hallmark of amniotic fluid embolism.
- Initial pulmonary hypertension, hypoxia, left ventricular failure, and coagulopathy are the primary events in amniotic fluid embolism.
- Management is basically symptomatic and directed toward the maintenance of oxygenation, circulatory support, and correction of coagulopathy.

the pulmonary vessels by embolic material or to pulmonary vasospasm secondary to the response of the pulmonary vasculature to fetal debris, resulting in acute asphyxiation, cor pulmonale, and, in turn, sudden death or severe neurologic injury.[123,134] However, human hemodynamic data do not support sustained periods of pulmonary hypertension.[135,136] In fact, left ventricular failure seems to be the pathognomonic feature in humans.[128] Clark reviewed the available hemodynamic data from the published cases of amniotic fluid embolus in humans and found only mild to moderate elevations in pulmonary artery pressures, whereas all patients had evidence of severe left ventricular dysfunction. Calculation of pulmonary vascular resistance further revealed that, with one exception, all were either normal or in a range that was reflective of isolated left ventricular failure.[134] In an attempt to reconcile clinical and animal experimental findings, Clark proposed a biphasic model to explain the hemodynamic abnormalities that occur with amniotic fluid embolus.[134] He suggested that acute pulmonary hypertension and vasospasm might be the initial hemodynamic response. The resulting right-sided heart failure and accompanying hypoxia could account for the cases of sudden death or severe neurologic impairment. Those patients who survive the initial phase of pulmonary hypertension, which is transient, proceed to the next stage of left ventricular failure. Several mechanisms contribute to the later phase of left ventricular failure. They include hypoxia, leftward shift of interventricular septum secondary to right-sided heart failure (resulting in an decrease in cardiac output, leading to impaired coronary artery perfusion), and the direct myocardial depressant effect of amniotic fluid itself. Endothelin, which is in amniotic fluid in abundance, has been cited as the cause of left ventricular failure.[137] Several authors have suggested that other humoral factors, including proteolytic enzymes, histamine, serotonin, prostaglandins, and leukotrienes, may contribute to the hemodynamic changes and consumptive coagulopathy associated with amniotic fluid embolism.[128] Because of the clinical resemblance of presentation of amniotic fluid embolus with sepsis and anaphylaxis, Clark suggested that the syndrome of amniotic fluid embolism is due to anaphylactoid reaction to amniotic fluid and named the syndrome "anaphylactoid syndrome of pregnancy."[120] Antigenic potential can vary in individuals and therefore can lead to different grades of the syndrome. For example, women carrying a male fetus are more likely to be affected.[120] Similarly, fluid containing thick meconium may be more toxic than clear amniotic fluid.[120] Human data have shown that, although most patients dying of amniotic fluid emboli have had clear amniotic fluid, there is a shorter time from the initial presentation to cardiac arrest and an increased risk of neurologic damage or death in the presence of meconium or a dead fetus.[120] Further indirect evidence for an immunologic basis is the occurrence of fatal amniotic fluid emboli during first-trimester abortions. This suggests that under the right circumstances, maternal exposure to even small amounts of amniotic fluid can initiate the syndrome.[120] Confirming the theory of "anaphylactoid reaction" to amniotic fluid needs further research using tryptase markers.

Coagulopathy

The association of a consumptive coagulopathy is common with amniotic fluid emboli. In Morgan's review, 12% of patients presented with a bleeding diathesis, with subsequent development of a bleeding diathesis in an additional 37%.[119] More recent reviews, however, found an even higher incidence. Clark reported that 83% of the cases in the national registry had either clinical or laboratory evidence of a consumptive coagulopathy. The remaining 17% died before the clotting status could be assessed by either clinical or laboratory techniques. Similarly, in 15 cases of fatal amniotic fluid emboli associated with induced abortion, two patients presented with coagulopathy and an additional 75% of initial survivors went on to develop disseminated intravascular coagulation (DIC).[138] It now appears that amniotic fluid embolus is almost always associated with some form of DIC, with or without clinically significant bleeding. Isolated DIC causing maternal hemorrhage may be the first indication of the problem in a small number of patients.[139,140] The current laboratory evidence also supports the opinion that amniotic fluid embolus is invariably associated with coagulation changes. Harnett and associates studied the effect of varying concentrations of amniotic fluid (10 to 60 μL added to 330 μL of whole blood) on thromboelastography variables and found amniotic fluid to be procoagulant even with a 10-μL study sample.[141]

The etiology of the coagulopathy remains somewhat obscure. Investigations that have attempted to clarify the mechanism have yielded inconclusive and sometimes contradictory results. Although amniotic fluid contains activated coagulation factors II, VII, and X, their concentrations are well below those found in maternal serum at term.[142] On the other hand, amniotic fluid has been shown to have a direct factor X activating property and thromboplastin-like effect. Both of them increase with gestational age. The thromboplastin-like effect is likely due to substantial quantities of tissue factor in amniotic fluid. Potential sources include sloughed fetal skin and epithelial cells derived from the fetal respiratory, gastrointestinal, and genitourinary tract mucosa. Tissue factor activates the extrinsic pathway by binding with factor VII. This complex, in turn, triggers clotting by activating factor X. Lockwood and colleagues speculated that once clotting was triggered in the pulmonary vasculature, local thrombin generation could then cause vasoconstriction and microvascular thrombosis, as well as secretion of vascular endothelin.[142] This vasoactive peptide can depress both myometrial and myocardial contractility and may primarily or secondarily contribute to the hemodynamic changes and uterine atony that are generally associated with this syndrome.

Diagnosis

There are no diagnostic criteria to confirm the presence of amniotic fluid embolus. The differential diagnosis includes air or thrombotic pulmonary emboli, septic shock, acute myocardial infarction, cardiomyopathy, anaphylaxis, aspiration, placental abruption, eclampsia, uterine rupture, transfusion reaction, and local anesthetic toxicity.[128] In the presence of central venous access, blood from the pulmonary vasculature should be collected using the method described by Masson.[122] He suggested that to minimize the possibility of maternal or exogenous contamination, a more representative sample of the pulmonary microvasculature can be obtained if blood is drawn from the distal lumen of a wedged pulmonary artery catheter. After discarding the first 10 mL of blood, an additional 10 mL is drawn, heparinized, and analyzed utilizing Papanicolaou's method.[143] The presence of components of amniotic fluid, including squamous cells and mucous strands, reinforces the diagnosis. Although pulmonary vasculature preparations may occasionally be contaminated by maternal squames, when squamous cells are found in large numbers in such a sample it is clinically significant and strongly supportive of the diagnosis of amniotic fluid embolus.[143] This is particularly true if the squamous cells are coated with neutrophils, or if other fetal debris, such as mucin or hair, accompanies them. Lee and coworkers suggested that a more reliable method of confirming the diagnosis might center on the identification of other amniotic fluid elements in the maternal pulmonary vasculature, as opposed to squamous cells.[132,144]

Recent progress in the diagnosis of amniotic fluid embolus has centered on the attempt to develop simple, noninvasive, sensitive tests utilizing peripheral maternal blood. Kobayashi and coworkers studied maternal serum sialyl Tn antigen levels in four women with clinical amniotic fluid emboli and compared them to both pregnant and nonpregnant controls.[145] Sialyl is a mucin-type glycoprotein that originates in fetal and adult intestinal and respiratory tracts. It is present in both meconium and in clear amniotic fluid. Using a sensitive antimucin antibody, TKH-2, the authors found no difference in the serum levels of pregnant patients throughout gestation or in the early postpartum period, when compared with healthy nonpregnant controls. However, the antigen levels were elevated in the amniotic fluid embolus group.[145] Nonetheless, this test appears promising, although it needs further evaluation. Kanayama and

colleagues also studied a second marker of diagnosis that involves the measurement of plasma concentrations of zinc coproporphyrin, a characteristic meconium component, and found they were higher in patients with amniotic fluid embolus.[146]

Management

The management of amniotic fluid embolus is basically symptomatic and directed toward the maintenance of oxygenation, circulatory support, and correction of coagulopathy. Depending on the circumstances, full cardiopulmonary resuscitation protocol may be required. If the fetus is sufficiently mature and is undelivered at the time of cardiac arrest, cesarean delivery should be instituted as soon as possible.

Treatment of hemodynamic instability includes optimization of preload with rapid volume infusion. Direct-acting vasopressors may be required in restoring aortic perfusion pressure in the initial stages. Once this is attained, other inotropes such as dopamine and dobutamine can be added to improve myocardial function. When clinically feasible, pulmonary artery catheterization can be instituted to help guide therapy. Diuretics may be required to mobilize pulmonary edema fluid. Treatment of the coagulopathy associated with amniotic fluid embolus involves the administration of blood component therapy. Amniotic fluid embolus is associated frequently with massive hemorrhage, requiring replacement with packed red cells. O-negative or group-specific blood can be used if crossmatched blood is unavailable. Plasma and platelets are given to replace the clotting factors. Ongoing therapy is generally guided by the clinical condition of the patient and laboratory evidence of coagulopathy. Although cryoprecipitate is not first-line therapy for treating coagulopathy, it may be useful in circumstances in which fibrinogen is low and volume overload is a concern. It has also been reported to be useful in a patient with severe acute respiratory distress syndrome secondary to amniotic fluid embolus.[147] After administration of cryoprecipitate, the patient's cardiopulmonary and hematologic status improved dramatically, leading the authors to suggest that it may be useful in cases in which conventional medical therapy appears unsuccessful in maintaining blood pressure, oxygenation, and hemostasis. Their recommendation was based on similar treatment protocols for severely ill patients with multiple trauma, burns, and postoperative sepsis. In these clinical settings, it is believed that there is impairment in the clearance of circulating microaggregates and immune complexes by the reticuloendothelial system, leading to the development of cardiopulmonary insufficiency and DIC. Cryoprecipitate is rich in opsonic α_2 surface-binding glycoprotein, also known as fibronectin, which facilitates the reticuloendothelial system in the filtration of antigenic and toxic particulate matter. Depleted levels of this glycoprotein have been reported in severely ill patients, with marked improvement in the clinical status after repletion of fibronectin levels.[147]

Isolated reports of other modalities of treatment for amniotic fluid emboli exist in the literature. One patient, a serine proteinase inhibitor, FOY, was utilized in the treatment of an associated DIC.[148] Nitric oxide and aerosolized prostacyclin have been used to treat refractory hypoxemia.[149,150] Clark has suggested the use of high-dose corticosteroids and epinephrine as useful therapeutic adjuvants in the light of the similarities of amniotic fluid embolism to anaphylaxis.[120]

Complications of Preeclampsia: Eclampsia, HELLP Syndrome, and Pulmonary Edema

Preeclampsia is not uncommon and complicates 6% to 8% of all pregnancies. In this section we consider three conditions that need special mention, because they are not as common as preeclampsia. However, they may coexist with preeclampsia and contribute to significant morbidity and mortality in pregnant women.

Eclampsia is a life-threatening emergency that occurs suddenly, most commonly in the third trimester near term. Approximately 60% of convulsions/coma precede delivery. Most postpartum cases occur during the first 24 hours, but seizures attributed to eclampsia have been reported as late as 22 days after delivery. Approximately 50% of all patients have evidence of severe preeclampsia. In the remaining, the classic triad of preeclampsia (hypertension, proteinuria, and edema) may be absent or mildly abnormal.[151] There is a wide variation in the incidence of eclampsia in the literature (1 in 100 to 1 in 3448 pregnancies).[151] Eclampsia remains a significant complication of pregnancy in the United States. In a study of 399 consecutive women with eclampsia, the mortality rate was 1% and antepartum onset carried the greatest risk, especially before 32 weeks' gestation. Postpartum eclampsia was, however, more likely to be associated with neurologic deficits.[152] Eclampsia remains a common condition and a leading cause of maternal and perinatal mortality in developing countries.[153] Major maternal complications can follow, including placental abruption, HELLP syndrome, DIC, neurologic deficits, pulmonary aspiration, pulmonary edema, cardiopulmonary arrest, and acute renal failure.[152]

Headache, visual disturbances, and epigastric or right upper quadrant pain are consistent with severe preeclampsia and may forewarn of impending eclampsia. Seizures have an abrupt onset, typically beginning as facial twitching and followed by a tonic phase that persists for 15 to 20 seconds. This progresses to a generalized clonic

phase characterized by apnea, which lasts approximately 1 minute. Breathing resumes with a long stertorous inspiration, and the patient enters a postictal state, with a variable period of coma. Pulmonary aspiration of gastric contents may complicate a seizure. The number of seizures varies from 1 or 2 to as many as 100 in severe, untreated cases. The causes of eclampsia are poorly understood. It is generally believed that cerebral vasospasm and ischemia result in eclampsia. However, cerebral edema, hemorrhage, and hypertensive encephalopathy have also been implicated in its pathogenesis.[154,155]

Until proven otherwise, the occurrence of seizures during pregnancy should be considered eclampsia. Conditions simulating eclampsia should be considered (e.g., encephalitis, epilepsy, meningitis, cerebral tumor, and cerebrovascular accident) only after ruling out eclampsia (Box 19-3).[156] Computed tomography (CT) may be normal, or it may show evidence of cerebral edema, infarction, or hemorrhage. The last complication occurs more frequently in elderly gravidas with preexisting hypertension and may frequently result in death or permanent disability.[156] Other neurologic abnormalities include temporary blindness, retinal detachment, postpartum psychosis, and other transient neurologic deficits.[151] Electroencephalography is also abnormal, showing focal or diffuse slowing, as well as focal or generalized epileptiform activity.[155]

Management of Eclampsia

Supplemental oxygen should be delivered immediately during seizure. A soft nasopharyngeal airway may facilitate oxygenation during seizure. Ventilation may be

---

BOX 19–3   Considerations in Eclampsia

- Eclampsia can occur during prepartum, intrapartum, and postpartum periods.
- Headache, visual disturbances, and epigastric or right upper quadrant pain may forewarn of impending eclampsia.
- Seizures have an abrupt onset beginning as facial twitching followed by a tonic phase and clonic phase.
- CT may be normal, or it may show evidence of cerebral edema, infarction, or hemorrhage.
- Management involves maintenance of airway, oxygenation, and ventilation.
- Thiopentone sodium, midazolam, and succinyl choline may be required to facilitate oxygenation and ventilation.
- Magnesium sulfate is the preferred drug for the definitive treatment of seizures.
- Eclamptic patients should undergo expeditious delivery.
- Regional anesthesia to facilitate labor and delivery can be considered in patients who are seizure free, conscious, and rational in behavior with no evidence of increased intracranial pressure and absence of coagulopathy.

assisted once seizures end. Simultaneously, precautions should be observed to minimize chances of gastric aspiration. Midazolam in incremental doses up to 20 mg may be necessary, either to suppress seizures or facilitate further treatment in a combative patient. Occasionally, thiopentone sodium and succinylcholine may be required to facilitate oxygenation and ventilation. Immediate monitoring should include pulse oximetry, electrocardiogram, and blood pressure recordings. Left uterine displacement should be maintained throughout the resuscitative effort and until delivery of the infant.

Magnesium sulfate is the preferred drug for the definitive treatment of seizures. After an immediate loading dose of 4 to 6 g infused intravenously over 20 to 30 minutes, a maintenance dose of 1 to 2 g/hr is initiated, assuming that the patient has adequate urine output. Hourly monitoring of urine output, regular evaluation of deep tendon reflexes, and observation of respiratory rate should be implemented to guard against magnesium toxicity.

Unless otherwise contraindicated, eclamptic patients should undergo expeditious delivery. The frequent indications of cesarean delivery include fetal distress, placental abruption, prematurity with an unfavorable cervix, persistent seizures, and persistent postictal agitation.

Regional anesthesia to facilitate labor and delivery can be considered in patients who are seizure free, conscious, and rational in behavior with no evidence of increased intracranial pressure and absence of coagulopathy. Moodley and associates found no difference in maternal and neonatal outcomes when comparing epidural anesthesia with general anesthesia for cesarean delivery in conscious women with eclampsia.[157] Unconscious or obtunded patients, or those with evidence of increased intracranial pressure, should have general anesthesia in line with neurosurgical anesthesia recommendations. Hyperventilation can be initiated soon after the delivery of the infant to minimize the effect of low $Paco_2$ on the uterine arteries. The patient can be extubated at the conclusion of surgery if awake and conscious. On the other hand, if general anesthesia was undertaken in a women who was not conscious to begin with, consideration can be given to leaving the patients intubated and transferring them to intensive care for blood pressure control and controlled weaning from assisted ventilation while assessing neurologic recovery. Prolonged unconsciousness should prompt further evaluation with CT. Magnesium should be continued until the blood pressure normalizes and central nervous system hyperexcitability disappears.

HELLP Syndrome

The HELLP syndrome is believed to be a clinical state that may represent an advanced form of preeclampsia (Box 19-4). Hemolysis, Elevated Liver enzymes, and Low Platelets characterize this condition. Based on the platelet count,

---

> **BOX 19–4 Considerations in HELLP Syndrome**
>
> - Hemolysis, Elevated Liver enzymes, and Low Platelets characterize this condition.
> - Classification of HELLP is based on platelet number: class I ($< 50,000/mm^3$), class II $50,000$-$100,000/mm^3$), and class III ($>100,000/mm^3$).
> - Etiology of HELLP still remains elusive.
> - Delivery represents the only definitive treatment of HELLP syndrome and should be undertaken immediately, with few exceptions.
> - Dexamethasone increases the platelet number significantly.

the HELLP syndrome is divided into three classes. Class I patients have a platelet count of less than $50,000/mm^3$, class 2 is defined by a platelet count between $50,000$ and $100,000/mm^3$, and class 3 is defined by a platelet count over $100,000/mm^3$.[158] The etiology of HELLP remains elusive. Its clinical and pathologic manifestations result from an unknown insult that leads to intravascular platelet activation and microvascular endothelial damage. Hemolysis, which is defined as the presence of microangiopathic hemolytic anemia, is the highlight of the disorder. Sibai, after reviewing published reports, noted a lack of consensus regarding the diagnostic features of HELLP syndrome.[159] He suggested the following diagnostic criteria: (1) hemolysis, defined by an abnormal peripheral blood smear and an increased bilirubin level (1.2 mg/dL or greater); (2) elevated liver enzymes, defined as an increased aspartate aminotransferase of at least 70 U/L and a lactate dehydrogenase level greater than 600 U/L; and (3) a low platelet count ($<100,000/mm^3$). A diagnosis of the HELLP syndrome is made only if all three criteria are present. A diagnosis of partial HELLP syndrome is made if only one or two of the three criteria are present, and a diagnosis of severe preeclampsia is made if none is present.[160] Patients with full HELLP syndrome are likely to have a higher incidence of stroke, cardiac arrest, DIC, placental abruption, need for blood transfusion, pleural effusion, acute renal failure, and wound infections.[160] Most cases of HELLP syndrome occur preterm, but 20% may present post partum. Patients who develop HELLP postpartum have a higher incidence of pulmonary edema and renal failure.[161]

A number of studies have demonstrated better maternal outcome with administration of 10 mg of dexamethasone intravenously at 12-hour intervals until disease remission is noted.[162] Dexamethasone therapy is continued until the following occurs: blood pressure is 150/100 mm Hg or less, urine output is at least 30 mL/hr for 2 consecutive hours without a fluid bolus or the use of diuretics, platelet count is greater than $50,000/mm^3$, the lactate dehydrogenase level begins to decline, and the patient appears clinically stable. When these occur, dexamethasone is decreased to 5-mg doses administered intravenously 12 hours apart.[162]

Compensated DIC may be present in all patients with the HELLP syndrome.[163] In addition, patients with this syndrome may experience right upper quadrant pain and neck pain, shoulder pain, or relapsing hypotension due to subcapsular hematoma and intraparenchymal hemorrhage. Because abnormal liver function tests do not accurately reflect the presence of liver hematoma and hemorrhage, this subset of patients, particularly if associated with thrombocytopenia, should undergo CT examination of the liver.[164] An abnormal hepatic imaging finding was noted in 77% of patients with a platelet count of 20,000/mm^3 or less.[164]

Delivery represents the only definitive treatment of the HELLP syndrome and should be undertaken immediately, with few exceptions. Conservative treatment that includes bed rest, antithrombotic agents, and plasma volume expansion is typically unsuccessful and often results in early maternal or fetal deterioration. In the presence of prematurity, corticosteroids may be administered to accelerate lung maturity, followed by delivery 48 hours later. Administration of high doses of corticosteroids may increase platelet numbers to allow placement of a regional anesthetic, especially if a latency of 24 hours is achieved before delivery.[165]

Pulmonary Edema in Preeclampsia

Three percent of women with severe preeclampsia develop pulmonary edema (Box 19-5).[166] Pulmonary edema occurs as a result of low colloid oncotic pressure, increased intravascular hydrostatic pressure, and/or increased pulmonary capillary permeability.[167] Many cases develop 2 to 3 days post partum, and hence there is need to keep patients with preeclampsia under careful surveillance in the immediate postpartum period. The resolution of pulmonary edema requires management of the underlying cause (e.g., overhydration, sepsis, cardiac failure). Echocardiography may be required to exclude cardiogenic causes of pulmonary edema.[168,169] The initial treatment includes administration of supplemental oxygen, fluid restriction, and administration of a diuretic. In a subset of patients, if no resolution of pulmonary edema is in sight, pulmonary artery catheter placement may facilitate further management. This includes vasodilator therapy to reduce preload or afterload and administration of dopamine or dobutamine in women with evidence of left ventricular failure. Colloid administration may prove beneficial if the colloid oncotic pressure-pulmonary capillary wedge pressure gradient is lowered. In rare instances, tracheal intubation and ventilation may be required if respiratory failure complicates refractory pulmonary edema.[170] Adult respiratory distress syndrome can complicate severe preeclampsia, especially if an increase in pulmonary capillary permeability exists.[171]

Abnormal Placentation and Massive Hemorrhage

Despite the overall decrease in maternal mortality during the past decade, peripartum hemorrhage is still a major cause of maternal morbidity and mortality, accounting for around 10% of maternal deaths.[172] Hemorrhage is one of the leading causes of maternal death in the United States and is the leading cause of maternal death in developing countries. There are many conditions that predispose to hemorrhage, and abnormal placentation is one of the major causes, perhaps the one increasing at the fastest rate. An understanding of the risk factors, identification, and obstetric management of abnormal placentation may prove to be lifesaving for the mother and fetus, because unexpected hemorrhage often occurs with little or no warning and may be massive and life threatening. Therefore, proper preparation to manage it may be lifesaving (Table 19-6).

Unlike other places in the body where hemostasis depends on vasospasm and blood clotting, hemostasis at the placental site depends on myometrial contraction and retraction. At term, approximately 600 mL/min of blood flows through the placental site.[173] As the placenta separates, the blood from the implantation site may escape into the vagina immediately (Duncan mechanism) or it may be concealed behind the placenta and membranes (Schultze mechanism) until the placenta is delivered.

BOX 19–5 Pulmonary Edema in Preeclampsia

- Three percent of women with severe preeclampsia develop pulmonary edema.
- Pulmonary edema occurs as a result of low colloid oncotic pressure, increased intravascular hydrostatic pressure, and/or increased pulmonary capillary permeability.
- It is likely to occur 2 to 3 days postpartum.
- Treatment involves management of the underlying cause (overhydration, sepsis, cardiac failure).
- Treatment includes administration of supplemental oxygen, fluid restriction, and administration of diuretic.
- Occasionally, pulmonary artery catheter placement may facilitate further management (vasodilators, inotropes).
- Rarely, tracheal intubation and ventilation may be required if respiratory failure complicates refractory pulmonary edema.

Placenta Accreta

Adherent pieces of placenta prevent effective contraction of the myometrium and may cause bleeding. Placenta

TABLE 19-6 Anesthetic Considerations for Patients with Abnormal Placentation

	General Anesthesia	Regional Anesthesia
Invasive Monitors	Could be inserted after induction when patient unaware	Need for sedation to minimize discomfort
Blood Loss	Controlled hypotension may help minimize blood loss	Sympathectomy likely to decrease blood loss
Comfort	Patient is more comfortable in the setting of blood transfusions and decreased blood pressure	Sedation likely will be needed and there should be a low threshold for general anesthesia
Airway	Protected	Sedation, mental status, and volume resuscitation may compromise airway

accreta describes any placental implantation in which there is abnormally firm adherence to the myometrium of the uterine wall. It is the result of deficient decidual development resulting in implantation of the placenta into the myometrium without intervening decidua basalis. While in placenta accreta the placental villi are attached to the myometrium, in placenta increta the placental villi invade the myometrium, as opposed to placenta percreta, where the placental villi penetrate through the myometrium. The abnormal adherence may involve all or a few of the cotyledons (total vs. partial placenta accreta). The predominant histopathologic feature is the absence of decidua with direct attachment or invasion of the cotyledon into the myometrium. Decidua deficiency is also partly responsible for placenta previa and may account for the high incidence of their coexistence.[174] Other causes of placenta accreta include prior uterine surgery, infection, or trauma, because they could adversely affect the endometrium. Uterine trauma may occur as a result of dilatation and curettage, endometritis, leiomyoma, Asherman's syndrome, or prior pregnancies. The overall incidence of placenta accreta in the obstetric population is 1:2500 but is markedly elevated in those with a history of placenta previa (1:26), a previous cesarean section (1:10), or both.[175] The greater the number of previous cesarean sections, the greater the risk for placenta accreta.

The incidence of placenta accreta ranges from 0.26% in an unscarred uterus to 25% in the presence of placenta previa and three prior cesarean sections, and it has overtaken uterine atony as the most common reason for a postpartum hysterectomy. A high index of suspicion should be raised in the parturient with placenta previa and/or a prior cesarean section, especially with an anterior placenta, because the diagnosis of placenta accreta may be difficult by ultrasound. Modern ultrasonographic techniques and magnetic resonance imaging are providing a more reliable diagnosis of adherent placenta.

The diagnosis should also be suspected during attempts at manual removal of the placenta without success or with continued bleeding. Typical attempts at removal do not usually succeed, because a cleavage plane between the maternal placental surface and the uterine wall cannot be formed, and continued traction on the umbilical cord may lead to uterine inversion and life-threatening hemorrhage. Successful control of the bleeding may be challenging, because the bleeding is unlikely to respond to uterotonic agents or uterine massage because the uterus is unable to contract with retained placental tissue.

Once the level of suspicion is high, exploratory laparotomy should be performed in cases of a vaginal delivery. In both vaginal and cesarean deliveries, prompt hysterectomy is the treatment of choice, because 85% of patients will require a hysterectomy. In those cases in which the diagnosis is made and attempts at removal of the placenta are stopped, the maternal mortality is low (3%), with an average blood loss of approximately 3500 mL. There are several case reports of ligation of hypogastric, uterine, and ovarian arteries. However, all of these techniques have a highly variable success rate, and massive blood loss with potential maternal morbidity and mortality is four times higher if conservative management is employed. Selective transcatheter embolization of the pelvic arteries is an alternative to more invasive procedures and has shown promise as a technique that has the potential to preserve the uterus and fertility.[176] It could be performed prophylactically in cases in which massive hemorrhage is suspected in order to decrease the blood flow to the uterus even when the plan is to perform a hysterectomy. It consists of the preoperative placement of balloon catheters in the internal iliac arteries and is performed in the interventional radiology suite. The balloons are inflated at the time that hemorrhage is expected and should be deflated once hemostasis is achieved, to maximize blood flow to the lower extremities. It could also be utilized as a treatment for unexpected massive hemorrhage in a patient who desires to preserve fertility. When properly utilized, it appears to be safe and effective, is minimally invasive, and has often been beneficial in avoiding hysterectomy.[176] Of note, a low threshold should be utilized in performing a hysterectomy once massive hemorrhage develops.

Massive blood loss is common with placenta accreta. Even though antepartum recognition and elective hysterectomy are likely to decrease blood loss and morbidity, significant hemorrhage may occur as a result of the increased vascularity of the gravid uterus. Two large-bore intravenous lines should be started, crossmatched blood should be available, and consideration should be given to invasive monitoring, including arterial and central venous lines. A regional technique is permissible in a patient requiring gravid hysterectomy, as long as no significant hemorrhage has occurred and adequate volume resuscitation is maintained.[177] The most challenging cases happen with the retention of an adherent placenta after delivery of a neonate in a patient without risk factors for placenta accreta, because sudden massive blood loss can happen with multiple attempts at manual removal of the placenta. The anesthetic technique in this situation is very different, owing to major hemodynamic changes that may be present in the parturient. It is highly recommended to assess the ability of the anesthesiologist to both manage the airway and volume resuscitate the patient simultaneously. We perform epidural anesthesia in parturients at high risk or with known placenta accreta, but we ensure that there is a low likelihood of a difficult airway, that we have adequate intravenous access, and that there is a low threshold to convert to general anesthesia. If hypovolemia is suspected, strong consideration should be given to induce general anesthesia to have earlier control of the airway.[178] Other reasons for conversion to general anesthesia include generalized patient discomfort due to prolonged surgery, difficult operating conditions, and earlier control of the airway before swelling results with massive fluid resuscitation. We have previously reported peripartum airway changes during cesarean hysterectomy and fluid resuscitation that gradually resolved over the following 2 days.[179]

Uterine Rupture

Cesarean delivery is the most common operation performed in the United States, with the most common reason being elective repeat cesarean sections. The increased risks of bleeding, infection, thromboembolism, and cost with cesarean section led to a push to encourage vaginal birth after a cesarean section (VBAC) during the past two decades. This was successful, in part, with an increase in the rate of VBAC from 6.6% in 1985 to 30.3% in 1996. However, this rate has declined over the past 5 years, in part owing to publications demonstrating that major complications such as uterine rupture, hysterectomy, injury to uterine arteries, bladder, and ureter, and neonatal mortality were higher in women attempting VBAC when compared with elective repeat cesarean sections.[180,181] It is well known that uterine rupture may occur at the site of a prior uterine scar, usually a previous

cesarean section scar, and that a classic cesarean section scar goes through uterine muscle and is more likely to dehisce than a low transverse cesarean section scar. It was always believed that the risk of uterine rupture in patients attempting VBAC was under 1%. However, recent publications have demonstrated that this rate may be as high as 1.5% with a low transverse incision and higher with other types of incisions. VBAC is allowed only in cases of a low transverse scar. The American College of Obstetricians and Gynecologists (ACOG) has issued a practice bulletin for VBAC recommending that physicians caring for parturients attempting VBAC should be immediately available to provide emergency care.[182] Not only are these parturients at an increased risk for uterine rupture, but its results may be life threatening. The relative risk of uterine rupture is 3-fold to 5-fold with spontaneous labor and labor induced without prostaglandins but an astonishingly 15-fold when there is induction of labor with prostaglandins when compared with elective repeat cesarean section. The incidence of infant death was increased 10-fold in the presence of uterine rupture.[181] This finding led ACOG to issue a committee opinion discouraging the use of prostaglandins for cervical ripening or for the induction of labor in women attempting VBAC.[183]

Risk factors for rupture of the uterus include a tumultuous labor, prolonged labor, infection, previous uterine manipulations (dilation and curettage or evacuation), midforceps delivery, breech version, and extraction and uterine trauma. Signs and symptoms of uterine rupture include sudden abdominal pain, shock, vaginal bleeding, fetal distress, change of uterine contour, and loss of a uterine contraction pattern. Some obstetric authorities used to discourage epidural analgesia for VBAC because of the concern of masking the abdominal pain. However, only a very high and dense epidural anesthetic such as the one used for a cesarean section would blunt the pain of uterine rupture. Regional anesthesia can be safely employed, and although it does not have an effect on the success rate of a vaginal delivery, it is more likely to encourage parturients to attempt a VBAC. It is best to use dilute solutions of local anesthetic with opioids because a sudden incidence of abdominal pain in an otherwise comfortable patient in labor (VBAC) with a labor epidural should raise the suspicion for uterine rupture. Also, abdominal pain is one of the least reliable signs of uterine rupture, because pain may be minimal, particularly when a previous cesarean section scar dehisces. The best diagnostic signs for uterine rupture are changes in contraction pattern, changes in configuration of the abdomen, and fetal distress. Continuous fetal heart rate monitoring is paramount for its early diagnosis. Rapid recognition and management are necessary to prevent maternal and fetal death. Except in partial rupture of a previous low transverse uterine scar, which can be repaired under a spinal or epidural anesthetic, emergency hysterectomy is usually needed. This is likely to require rapid anesthesia induction, even in the presence of shock, to allow control of the hemorrhage. It is important to mention that spontaneous uterine rupture of an unscarred uterus, although much less common (1 in 15,000) than rupture of a previous uterine scar, is more serious and catastrophic. It results in a high maternal (≥50%) and fetal mortality (up to 80%) with massive blood loss, often exceeding 15 units in severe cases.

Management of Massive Hemorrhage

Adequate surgical hemostasis and careful fluid and blood replacement are essential to achieve good hemodynamic control. Increases in maternal blood volume and coagulation proteins compensate for the average blood loss, and parturients are often able to tolerate 1000 to 1500 mL of blood loss without major hemodynamic changes.[184] However, obstetric hemorrhage can occur rapidly, especially when difficulties in placental separation arise, as 600 to 700 mL of blood flows through the placental intervillous spaces each minute. DIC may occur with little or no warning, in part owing to the mixing of fetal and maternal blood and other cellular products and intensify blood loss.[185] Physiologic changes of pregnancy may allow signs of significant hemorrhage to be concealed until sudden hypotension and tachycardia occur. Urine output, heart rate, and blood pressure assessments are useful in estimating the volume status. Aggressive volume replacement is essential to maintain tissue perfusion and oxygenation. Early consideration should be given to colloids and blood products, along with a request for assistance, a second large-bore intravenous line, and rapid infusion equipment for transfusion. A type and crossmatch for at least 2 to 4 units of packed red blood cells should be considered when the potential for significant blood loss is likely, such as in cases of placenta accreta. Uncrossmatched, type O, Rh-negative blood is rarely necessary if sufficient precautions are taken to order blood products in advance, except in cases where massive hemorrhage is unexpected and happens within a short time period. Other blood products may be necessary but are frequently utilized unnecessarily. The ASA task force on blood component therapy recommends the transfusion of packed red blood cells, platelets, and fibrinogen only after the careful assessment of volume status, surgical conditions, and laboratory monitoring. Transfusion of blood components is rarely necessary unless the hemoglobin is less than 6 g/dL, the platelet count is less than 50/mm^3 or there is evidence of platelet dysfunction and microvascular bleeding, or the fibrinogen concentration is less than 80 to 100 mg/dL in the presence of microvascular bleeding.[186]

There are some modalities for blood conservation that are especially helpful in parturients that are at high risk for hemorrhage, refuse blood products, and are scheduled for a planned procedure. These include autologous donation (parturient's own blood) prior to the scheduled procedure, acute normovolemic hemodilution immediately before the procedure (parturient's own blood is removed and replaced with an equal proportion of crystalloid or colloid), and intraoperative cell salvage. Although there is the potential for re-infusion of blood containing amniotic fluid, intraoperative cell salvage has been safely utilized with leukocyte depletion filtration to remove amniotic fluid.[187,188] These techniques are still in evolution, especially in parturients, and future studies will be needed to validate their utility and safety.[189,190] However, they should always be considered in patients who refuse blood products.

In summary, retention of an adherent placenta and a ruptured uterus could present with little or no warning and should be in the differential diagnosis of postpartum hemorrhage. Massive blood loss is common, and the anesthesiologist should be prepared to provide massive volume resuscitation. Regional anesthesia can be safely and effectively utilized, but some situations warrant general endotracheal anesthesia. Therefore, identification of risk factors, antepartum recognition of the condition and early planning with multidisciplinary teamwork is quite important.

Peripartum Cardiomyopathy

Peripartum cardiomyopathy occurs rarely, with an exact incidence that remains unknown. In part because the definition of the disorder is a matter of some dispute, and perhaps due to reporting bias in different areas of the United States and countries of the world, rates from 1:100 to 1:15,000 live births have been reported.[191] The generally accepted incidence in the United States is 1:3000 to 1:4000.[192] The disease is characterized by onset of cardiac failure occurring late in gestation or, most commonly, in the first few months postpartum. The diagnosis is one of exclusion, because there are no pathognomonic signs or definitive diagnostic tests. Criteria used for establishing the diagnosis were recently formulated by a National Institutes of Health consensus panel and are listed in Table 19-7.[192]

The differential diagnosis includes many other causes of the clinical signs of peripartum cardiomyopathy, such as severe hypertension, diastolic dysfunction, pulmonary or amniotic fluid embolism, exacerbation of valvular heart disease, infection, and toxic/metabolic disorders. A wide variety of "risk factors" have been suggested for the condition, but because it is so rare, few are widely accepted or strongly associated. These include maternal age older than 30 years, black race, multiparity, multiple gestation, family history, long-term tocolysis, preeclampsia, cocaine abuse, malnutrition, and infections.[191] In Africa, some populations demonstrate a much higher incidence

TABLE 19–7   Diagnosis of Peripartum Cardiomyopathy
All of the following must be present:
● Cardiac failure occurring in the last month of pregnancy, or within 5 months post partum
● Absence of an identifiable cause for the cardiac failure
● Absence of heart disease before the last month of pregnancy
● Echocardiographic evidence of left ventricular systolic dysfunction (LVEF < 45%, fractional shortening < 30%, or end-diastolic dimension > 2.7 cm/m²)
Data from Pearson GD, Veille JC, Rahimtoola S, et al: Peripartum cardiomyopathy: National Heart, Lung, and Blood Institute and Office of Rare Diseases (National Institutes of Health) workshop recommendations and review. JAMA 2000;283:1183-1188.

of peripartum cardiomyopathy (1%), apparently associated with peripartum and postpartum consumption of large salt loads and high ambient temperature.[193]

The clinical presentation is similar to other forms of dilated cardiomyopathy. Patients may complain of dyspnea, orthopnea, cough or hemoptysis, generalized fatigue, and chest or abdominal pain. Physical findings include peripheral edema, crackles on pulmonary auscultation, jugular venous distention, a third heart sound, and a mitral regurgitation murmur.[194] Electrocardiography and chest films will show typical signs of cardiomyopathy, including tachycardia, atrial ectopy, cardiomegaly, and pulmonary edema. As noted earlier, echocardiography shows signs of left ventricular systolic dysfunction.

The pathophysiology of peripartum cardiomyopathy remains unknown. One prevailing theory suggests that myocarditis of viral or autoimmune origin is responsible for the ventricular failure. Some series have found a high incidence (nearly 80%) of myocarditis on endomyocardial biopsy,[195] but others found an incidence of less than 10%, similar to age- and sex-matched controls with idiopathic cardiomyopathies.[196] Still others have found the incidence of myocarditis to be greater in peripartum cardiomyopathy than in idiopathic dilated cardiomyopathy (29% vs. 9%).[197] The wide discrepancy in myocarditis may be due to differences in timing of biopsy and criteria for diagnosis.[191] Other hypothesized pathophysiologic mechanisms include abnormal cytokines (e.g., tumor necrosis factor α [TNF-α], interleukin-6, Fas/APO-1), abnormalities of relaxin, selenium deficiency, and genetic factors.[191]

Treatment of peripartum cardiomyopathy is largely supportive and aimed at establishing normal hemodynamics, avoiding further deterioration of cardiac function, and avoiding complications of heart failure, such as thromboembolism. In the minority of cases appearing antepartum, consideration must be given to possible adverse effects on the fetus. Sodium and water restriction and diuresis are initial steps. Digoxin has been shown to improve symptoms and is safe in pregnant patients. β-blockade, especially with vasodilating antagonists (e.g., carvedilol), improves hemodynamics and reduces mortality in idiopathic dilated cardiomyopathy, though efficacy in peripartum cardiomyopathy has not been conclusively demonstrated.[192,198] Recently, Sliwa and associates suggested that the addition of pentoxifylline (which decreases TNF-α) to conventional therapy with diuretics and β blockers significantly improved outcome in patients with peripartum cardiomyopathy.[199] Angiotensin-converting enzyme (ACE) inhibitors are recommended in other dilated cardiomyopathies but cause renal toxicity in the fetus or breastfed newborn. Hydralazine is the vasodilator of choice.[192] Anticoagulation is generally recommended if the left ventricular ejection fraction (LVEF) is markedly decreased. Heparin, low-molecular-weight heparin, and warfarin have been used; warfarin is generally reserved for postpartum patients owing to teratogenic effects in early pregnancy. However, its use in late pregnancy, when peripartum cardiomyopathy occurs, has not been demonstrated to be harmful. All types of anticoagulants may be safely used in postpartum women, including those who are breastfeeding, because none is secreted in breast milk.[192] Other therapies of possible efficacy include maneuvers designed to ameliorate myocarditis, including immunosuppressive drugs such as prednisone and azathioprine[200] or intravenous immunoglobulins.[201] Cardiac transplantation has been described, including the use of left ventricular assist devices (LVAD) as bridges to transplant.[202] Successful pregnancy after transplantation has been reported.[203]

Prognosis is poor unless rapid normalization of LVEF occurs (<6 months). Mortality ranges from 25% to 50%, although more recent series indicate better outcomes than in historical series.[192,204] Survivors whose ventricular function has returned to normal have reduced contractile reserve and experience further deterioration with subsequent pregnancies.[205]

Anesthetic management of an undelivered parturient with initial or recurrent peripartum cardiomyopathy has been described. Most case reports have utilized continuous spinal or combined spinal-epidural analgesia.[206-210] Invasive monitoring with an arterial catheter and a central venous or pulmonary artery catheter has generally been recommended as well.[206-211] Active anticoagulation may contraindicate regional anesthesia. One case report described general anesthesia with target concentration-controlled propofol and remifentanil for emergency cesarean section in a patient with peripartum cardiomyopathy in active labor.[212] Peripartum cardiomyopathy has also first appeared during anesthetic management for cesarean delivery, requiring intraoperative resuscitation.[213,214] The hemodynamic picture should guide the management of patients who have recovered from a previous episode, although the limited cardiac reserve in these patients should be kept in mind.[211]

Cardiac Arrest and Cardiopulmonary Resuscitation in Pregnancy

Cardiac arrest occurs infrequently in pregnancy, at an estimated rate of 1:30,000 late pregnancies.[215] Unfortunately, maternal survival is rare. Causes of cardiac arrest in pregnancy include hemorrhage, embolism (air, amniotic fluid), complications of preeclampsia, peripartum cardiomyopathy, preexisting cardiac disease (e.g., coronary syndromes, valvular disease, congenital defects, dysrthythmias), intracranial hemorrhage, trauma, anaphylaxis, sepsis, local anesthetic toxicity, failed airway management, and hemodynamic effects of spinal and epidural anesthesia. Whereas the most common etiology overall is hemorrhage, the most common conditions producing arrest in late pregnancy are embolism and hypertension.[216] As is the case in any resuscitation situation, the fundamental goals are establishment of an effective airway and circulation (basic cardiopulmonary resuscitation [CPR]), followed by electrical and pharmacologic steps to restore spontaneous circulation. The care of the pregnant patient in cardiac arrest must also include consideration of the physiologic changes of pregnancy (see earlier) and the welfare of the fetus, if of viable gestational age (Table 19-8).

TABLE 19–8   Cardiopulmonary Resuscitation in Pregnancy

Basic Life Support
- No change in technique of chest compressions
- Noninvasive ventilation complicated by anatomic and physiologic changes of pregnancy
- Early intubation recommended
- Left uterine displacement essential (folded clothing, linens, rescuer's knees, Cardiff wedge)

Advanced Cardiac Life Support
- *No change in ACLS protocols*
- No change in defibrillation techniques or voltages
- Caution when using paddle electrodes to avoid shocking rescuers on enlarged breasts
- Obstetric anesthesiologist is logical "code leader"
- Consider open-chest massage or cardiopulmonary bypass for reversible conditions not responding to conventional ACLS

Delivery of infant
- Delivery within 5 minutes enhances intact neonatal survival
- Delivery may improve success of maternal resuscitation
- Incision at 4 minutes of ACLS, delivery at 5 minutes

Basic Life Support

A fundamental principle in resuscitation of the arrested pregnant patient is that the best way to care for both mother and infant is to restore circulation to the mother.[217] Thus, pregnant basic life support (CPR) is essentially nonpregnant basic life support. Mouth-to-mouth, pocket mask, or bag/mask ventilation should be established immediately, followed as soon as possible by endotracheal intubation and ventilation. Noninvasive ventilation is made more difficult and potentially dangerous by the higher oxygen consumption, reduced compliance of the chest, pressure on the diaphragm by the enlarged uterus, enlarged breasts, obesity, and potential for regurgitation of gastric contents all associated with pregnancy.[215] Successful use of the laryngeal mask airway in the setting of failed airway in an obstetric emergency has been described.[218] Chest compressions should begin promptly, followed by advanced cardiac life support (ACLS) techniques, as the clinical situation dictates.

A vital aspect of CPR in pregnancy is the maintenance of uterine displacement to facilitate venous return to the heart. Any convenient soft object (e.g., a blanket, towel, pillow, or clothing) may be used as a wedge, placed under the patient's right flank. Chest compressions have been found to be effective in tilted patients up to 30 degrees.[215] However, CPR is more effective when the patient is on a hard surface. For this reason, some have suggested a purpose-built device known as the Cardiff wedge that tilts the patient on a rigid wooden structure with a lip on the dependent edge to keep her from sliding off.[219] To date, this device is not commercially available. A "human wedge" has also been described in which the patient is tilted over the knees of a kneeling person on the right side of the patient.[220] A chair inverted to rest on the seat and top of the back may also provide a firm, tilted support for the arrested pregnant patient.[217]

Advanced Cardiac Life Support

The American Heart Association (AHA) recommends that *no changes from standard ACLS protocols* be implemented when caring for pregnant patients. The reader is referred to standard texts to review such protocols.[221] A few special considerations are notable. First, there has been theoretical concern regarding the appropriate method for direct-current cardioversion. The enlarged breasts in pregnant patients may make access to the apex of the heart difficult, particularly when the patient is severely wedged. Furthermore, the anatomic and physiologic changes of pregnancy may, in theory, alter the electrical properties of the chest. However, measurements taken in pregnant women have demonstrated normal impedance.[222] However, others have cautioned that care should be taken to ensure that the left breast does not contact the hand of the person administering the shock.[215] There is no known risk to the fetus of direct-current defibrillation or cardioversion. The AHA recommends standard timing and energies for such maneuvers.[221] Similar recommendations have been made for pharmacologic interventions, including large doses of α-adrenergic agonists (epinephrine) to support the maternal circulation, even though these may theoretically decrease uteroplacental blood flow.[221]

A logistical question concerns who should serve as the "code leader" for resuscitative efforts in pregnant patients. Although the availability of various personnel and local customs may dictate otherwise, we believe that a senior anesthesiologist is the most appropriate clinician to fill this role. Anesthesiologists are skilled in airway management, intravenous access techniques, and the pharmacologic interventions of ACLS. Other personnel often present at cardiac arrest situations, including internists and surgeons, may not appreciate the physiologic changes of pregnancy and their impact on resuscitation of the mother to as great an extent as an obstetric anesthesiologist. Finally, the obstetrician should attend to the fetal status and make preparations for possible emergency cesarean delivery.

Delivery of the Infant

Significant controversy surrounds the decision on whether and when to perform an emergency cesarean section during cardiac arrest in pregnant patients. There are two reasons to consider such a drastic intervention. First, there is substantial evidence from retrospective reviews that fetal outcome is markedly improved with cesarean delivery when maternal resuscitative efforts are not rapidly successful. In a review of 61 perimortem cesarean sections performed in the 20th century through the mid 1980s, Katz and coworkers[223] reported 100% of the 42 infants delivered within 5 minutes of maternal arrest survived with no neurologic sequelae. As the interval from arrest to delivery lengthened, the chance of survival decreased and the incidence of severe neurologic damage increased among survivors. When the interval exceeded 15 minutes, intact survival was rare. Although no large series has appeared in the ensuing two decades, most authors continue to advocate early delivery of the viable infant when initial maternal resuscitation is unsuccessful.[224-229] Katz and colleagues[223] and subsequent authors, including the AHA,[217] have recommended that preparations for operation begin immediately, incision occur at 4 minutes of arrest, and delivery be accomplished by 5 minutes.

A second reason to consider emergency cesarean delivery during CPR is to improve the maternal condition.[217,225,227,229] This may be the case even when the fetus is pre-viable, because the mechanism of improvement may be both relief of aortocaval compression and removal of the low-resistance uteroplacental circulation.[217] The AHA

recommends cesarean delivery even for very premature infants if the maternal condition does not appear immediately reversible, so that some chance of fetal survival is preserved and maternal resuscitation is facilitated.[217]

Additional Interventions

Cardiopulmonary arrest during pregnancy is considered one of the possible indications for attempting open chest cardiac massage, although the AHA does not specifically endorse its use.[217] In cases in which anatomic factors limit the success of closed-chest CPR or the etiology of the arrest indicates it (e.g., pulmonary embolus, penetrating chest or abdominal trauma), thoracotomy and open cardiac massage may be considered. Retrospective data suggest invasive CPR is most likely to be successful when initiated relatively early in the resuscitation sequence.

Finally, cardiopulmonary bypass has been successfully employed in selected clinical situations involving pregnant patients in cardiac arrest. This includes hypothermia due to massive transfusion,[230] bupivacaine cardiotoxicity,[231] and pulmonary embolism.[226]

Postresuscitation Considerations

Restoration of spontaneous circulation may be accompanied by other problems, depending on the etiology of the arrest. Liver rupture has been reported after CPR in pregnant patients.[232] Hemostasis during cesarean section in the setting of cardiac arrest may initially be straightforward, owing to shunting of blood away from the uterus, but subsequently cause further hemodynamic compromise after resuscitation.[216] Management of brain-dead mothers with spontaneous circulation and undelivered infants has also been reported.[233]

CONDITIONS COMPLICATING REGIONAL ANESTHESIA

Regional Anesthesia and Anticoagulation

Pregnancy is a prothrombotic state with an increase in most coagulation factors (except factors XI and XIII) and a decrease in clot inhibitors such as protein S. The hypercoagulable state of pregnancy is also characterized by increased platelet hemostatic capacity, despite a decreased platelet count. Fibrinogen increases by as much as 50%.[93] Prothrombin and the thrombin-antithrombin complex are also elevated in normal pregnancies, whereas fibrinolysis is diminished. This is demonstrated by elevated levels of plasminogen activator inhibitor 1 and 2.[234] In addition, the increase in estrogen that accompanies pregnancy is a well-known prothrombotic cause.[235] The tendency toward exaggerated coagulation is further worsened by anatomic factors, such as the decrease of the blood flow in the lower extremities by the gravid uterus, a condition worsened in the supine position, the increased maternal vascular volume, and by a decreased ability to exercise, leading to venous congestion of the lower extremities and an impediment to venous return. Maternal conditions such as preterm labor and placenta previa, in addition to a decreased exercise capacity due to normal physiologic changes, may lead to prolonged periods of bed rest and further predispose the patient to lower extremity venous thrombosis.

Hypercoagulable states are very common in the general population, with some reports demonstrating that 5% of whites are heterozygous for factor V Leiden, a point mutation of factor V that renders it resistant to activated protein C. Other less common but more severe hypercoagulable states include factor V Leiden homozygosity, and deficiencies of protein S, protein C, and antithrombin III.[236] Many of the low-risk thrombophilias, such as being heterozygous for factor V Leiden, are silent until pregnancy, when they may become manifest as a result of the imbalance between the prothrombotic and antithrombotic forces. Initial manifestations of prothrombotic conditions during pregnancy may include the first presentation of deep venous thrombosis, repeated missed abortions, and recurrent late fetal losses.[237-239] Prophylactic anticoagulation may be indicated in some cases to prevent venous or placental thrombosis, because improved placental blood flow is likely to lead to better pregnancy outcomes.

Common anticoagulation options include warfarin, unfractionated heparin, and low-molecular-weight heparin (Table 19-9). It is our belief that knowledge of the pharmacokinetics and pharmacodynamics of these agents is essential for the practitioner involved in the care of parturients, because this will lead to a better understanding of the implications on the obstetric and anesthetic management. Currently accepted guidelines for the use of regional anesthesia and anticoagulation[240,241] are better used to complement rather than to replace the understanding of the pharmacology of commonly utilized anticoagulants during the puerperium.

Warfarin, a competitive inhibitor of vitamin K, is rarely used during pregnancy, because it readily crosses the placenta, is a first-trimester teratogen, and may cause fetal intracranial hemorrhage during the third trimester of pregnancy.[242-244] It is most important to avoid warfarin during weeks 6 to 12, the period of organogenesis, and the last 2 weeks of pregnancy to diminish the risk of warfarin embryopathy and of bleeding in the mother and infant.[244,245] The fetus has a smaller concentration of vitamin K–dependent factors, and, therefore, normal targeted maternal anticoagulation may lead to an exaggerated anticoagulation in the fetus. Nevertheless, warfarin continues to be the anticoagulant of choice in parturients with prosthetic heart valves, as there are no data documenting the benefits of subcutaneous unfractionated or low-molecular-weight heparin in this patient population.[244] There are reported cases of prosthetic heart valve thrombosis and of maternal and fetal deaths with the use of low-molecular-weight heparin.[246,247]

Unfractionated heparin is a strongly acidic, anionic, sulfated mucopolysaccharide with a large molecular weight (3,000 to 30,000 daltons average) that prevents placental passage and makes it, along with other forms of heparin discussed later in the chapter, the anticoagulant of choice during pregnancy.[248,249] It has a unique pentasaccharide sequence (only one third of heparin molecules) that is responsible for the anticoagulation properties by activating a conformational change in antithrombin III (AT III), leading to an accelerated interaction between AT III, thrombin (factor IIa) and factor Xa. Heparin leads to a similar inhibition of factors IIa and X (1:1 ratio). In addition, although to a lesser degree, unfractionated heparin catalyzes the inactivation of factors IIa, IXa, Xa, XIa, and XII. It also indirectly affects the thrombin-mediated activation of factors V and VIII, the end result being a decrease in important cofactors (Va and VIIIa) in the coagulation cascade.

Unfractionated heparin is cleared from the circulation rapidly, because high-molecular-weight species are cleared more rapidly than low-molecular-weight species. It has a

TABLE 19–9 Comparison of Unfractionated Heparin and Low-Molecular-Weight Heparin

	Unfractionated Heparin	Low-Molecular-Weight Heparin
Molecular Weight	3,000-30,000 daltons	1,000 to 10,000 daltons
Placental Passage	None	None
Anti–Factor Xa/Factor IIa Ratio	1:1	Greater than 2:1
Bioavailability	Around 30%	Close to 100%
Half-life	1-2 hr	3-6 hr
Measurement of Activity	Activated plasma thromboplastin time	Anti–factor Xa activity
Clearance	Saturable cellular mechanism; dose dependent	Renal
Protamine Response	Neutralizes activity	Partial reversal due to reduced binding

saturable cellular mechanism of clearance via receptors on endothelial cells and macrophages, having a rapid saturable mechanism with low doses, a combination of rapid saturable and dose-dependent mechanisms with therapeutic doses, and a much slower first-order mechanism via the kidneys that is nonsaturable and dose independent with high doses. This dose-dependent mechanism of clearance leads to nonlinear pharmacodynamic properties that affect the intensity and duration of action of unfractionated heparin, noticed the most when very high doses are used.[250] In addition, the nonlinear pharmacodynamic properties of unfractionated heparin lead to an unpredictable bioavailability when injected subcutaneously, a condition that is easily noticed when low-dose subcutaneous injections are used. Its bioavailability ranges from 30% with low doses to 100% with very high doses (greater than 35,000 U). Although very high doses of subcutaneous unfractionated heparin have a bioavailability that is similar to an intravenous injection with peak levels 3 hours (range, 2 to 4 hours) after injection, its duration of action is much less predictable, with reported durations of greater than 24 hours after injection.[251] Other causes of an exaggerated response to unfractionated heparin include prolonged therapy and its use in debilitated patients. The half-life of intravenous unfractionated heparin is also affected, although to a lesser degree, by its nonlinear pharmacodynamic properties.

A knowledge of the pharmacodynamic properties of unfractionated heparin may be more important than following laboratory tests, as the activated partial thromboplastin time (aPTT) response to heparin during pregnancy is attenuated secondary to increased levels of factor VIII and fibrinogen, despite significantly elevated heparin levels.[250,251] The use of small dose (≤5,000 U) subcutaneous unfractionated heparin for prophylaxis does not usually prolong the aPTT, and blood levels are not typically monitored. The use of subcutaneous unfractionated heparin for more than 5 days may lead to a decrease in the platelet count. However, the aPTT may be a better predictor of unfractionated heparin levels, compared with pharmacodynamic properties, when very high doses of subcutaneous injections are used. It is our recommendation to check the aPTT of a parturient taking high doses of subcutaneous unfractionated heparin on arrival at the labor floor and to wait for the result before performing a neuraxial technique. It has been our experience that the anticoagulant effect of high doses, as reflected by the aPTT, may persist for up to 28 hours after the last injection. In addition, a platelet count is recommended for any parturient who received unfractionated heparin for more than 4 days. It is important to realize that parturients at risk for deep venous or placental thrombosis are maintained on some form of heparin for most of the pregnancy. High doses of unfractionated heparin may be used throughout the pregnancy or, more commonly, after 36 weeks'

gestation at the time when the low-molecular-weight heparin is discontinued.

The American Society of Regional Anesthesia (ASRA) developed guidelines for the performance of neuraxial techniques in the anticoagulated patient in 1996, and these guidelines were updated in 2003.[240] ASRA based these guidelines on the available scientific information, but in some cases this information may be sparse. In addition, guidelines are recommendations and not standards or absolute requirements. They are based on not only scientific information but also on synthesis of expert opinion and clinical feasibility data. Variances from recommendations may be acceptable based on the physician's judgment, and specific outcomes cannot be guaranteed by following these recommendations.[240,241] Moreover, clinical and scientific information and evolving clinical practices may modify these guidelines with time.

The ASRA guidelines for the anesthetic management of the patient receiving unfractionated heparin state that performance of a neuraxial technique should proceed for at least 1 hour before systemic intravenous anticoagulation with unfractionated heparin. Systemic intravenous anticoagulation with unfractionated heparin should be discontinued 2 to 4 hours before a neuraxial technique or epidural catheter manipulation (including removal).[240] In addition, the coagulation status should be evaluated with the aPTT, with a normalization being necessary before epidural catheter insertion or removal. Despite the limited risk for epidural hematoma formation when subcutaneous unfractionated heparin is combined with neuraxial techniques, we prefer to perform this technique either greater than 4 hours after the injection of subcutaneous heparin (half-life of 2 to 4 hours) or before its administration (≥1-hour interval). However, ASRA states that there does not appear to be an increased risk with neuraxial block in the presence of subcutaneous unfractionated heparin. The addition of other medications, such as nonsteroidal anti-inflammatory agents, aspirin, oral anticoagulants, and other forms of heparin that affect the coagulation cascade may increase the risk of epidural hematoma when subcutaneous unfractionated heparin is used concomitantly with a neuraxial technique. Our recommendation for the performance of neuraxial techniques following higher than usual doses or prolonged therapy was outlined previously.

Low-molecular-weight heparin (LMWH) has a molecular weight of 1,000 to 10,000 daltons, does not cross the placenta,[252] is formed by controlled depolymerization of unfractionated heparin, and has the same pentasaccharide sequence (potentiates action of antithrombin), but overall it has a lower number of chains with greater than 18 saccharide units (one half to one fourth of LMWH fragments), providing a greater anti–factor Xa to anti–factor IIa ratio.[251,253] The 18 saccharide units are required for the inhibition of factor IIa but not for that of factor Xa.

Different LMWH have different anti–factor Xa/factor IIa activity (e.g., 2.7:1 for enoxaparin vs. 2.1:1 for dalteparin) but have equivalent anticoagulation on clinical practice.[253,254] Exogenous protamine completely reverses the anti–factor IIa activity of LMWH but only 60% of the anti–factor Xa activity, owing to a reduced binding to its components. There are few trials comparing LMWHs with functional or structural heterogeneity, although there is a report from the orthopedic population, where enoxaparin was similar to tinzaparin for deep venous thrombosis prophylaxis.[254] Enoxaparin is discussed here because it is the most widely used LMWH in the United States, the one referred in most manuscripts, review articles, and published guidelines, and the one that we currently use at our institution and are more familiar with.

LMWH has a lower binding to proteins and endothelial cells and dose-independent clearance compared with unfractionated heparin. The end result is a renal excretion that is dosage independent, a pharmacodynamic effect that is proportional to the dose used and more predictable, and a better bioavailability at low doses. In addition, LMWH has a similar bioavailability after subcutaneous and intravenous injection and is less immunogenic. Its dosage is adapted to body weight, and there is a risk of accumulation with obesity and renal failure.[254] The half-life of LMWH is 3 to 6 hours after subcutaneous injection, is independent of the dose, and is longer than that of unfractionated heparin. LMWH has a peak activity in 3 to 4 hours, low interpatient variability because of its more predictable dose response, and an increased popularity in its use with a once- or twice-a-day dosage that is very convenient for a parturient. LMWH has significant anti–factor Xa levels 12 hours after injection because of its longer half-life. There is a controversy over whether blood level testing with an anti–factor Xa assay is helpful in monitoring the response to LMWH and whether it is helpful prior to performing neuraxial techniques in the parturient anticoagulated with LMWH (see later). It is no surprise that LMWH is slowly replacing unfractionated heparin when prophylactic anticoagulation is needed in a parturient despite their similar efficacy; it is due to its improved bioavailability, longer half-life, more predictable dose response with a greater activity against factor Xa, and lower incidence of bleeding complications.[255]

The safety and efficacy of LMWH in pregnancy is supported by a review of 624 high-risk parturients with a prior incidence of thrombosis receiving enoxaparin prophylaxis.[256,257] This study demonstrated a congenital anomaly rate of 2.5%, which is not greater than that in the general population, and a 1.1% fetal death rate unrelated to enoxaparin. There was only one enoxaparin-related hemorrhage and a 1.3% incidence of recurrent maternal venous thrombotic events, which is very low for this high-risk population. The overall conclusion of this study, supported by an ACOG committee opinion,[257] is that LMWH is safe and efficacious for the prevention of thrombosis in parturients who are at a high risk for this complication.[256,257] Typical prophylactic doses of LMWH during pregnancy are 40 mg subcutaneously (1 mg is equivalent to 100 units) of enoxaparin per day, or 30 mg subcutaneously twice a day. These dosages are used in parturients with a remote history of thrombosis but without a thrombophilia, low-risk thrombophilia, recurrent pregnancy loss, or a history of fetal demise. Prophylactic doses are usually discontinued at 36 weeks' gestation and changed to subcutaneous unfractionated heparin. High-dose therapy typically ranges from 1.0 to 1.5 mg/kg of subcutaneous enoxaparin twice a day and is indicated for the management of acute thrombosis, a remote history of thrombosis, and the presence of antiphospholipid antibodies or a high-risk thrombophilia. High-dose therapy is usually continued until 24 hours before induction of labor or a planned cesarean section.

LMWH does not usually influence the aPTT but has an effect on anti–factor Xa values. An anti–factor Xa chromogenic assay measures the activity against factor Xa but not that against factor IIa.[258] Although minimal anticoagulation is equivalent to values below 0.2 U/mL, prophylactic levels of 0.1 to 0.2 U/mL may suffice.[258] It is not usually measured for prophylactic doses owing to the predictable dose response of LMWH. It may be prudent to check assay values in cases of obesity, low body weight, or renal failure, because LMWH has a renal elimination and is affected by changes in body weight.[258,259] It has been recommended to check anti–factor Xa levels while using high doses during pregnancy owing to increases in glomerular filtration rate, clotting factor concentration, weight, and volume of distribution.[260] Testing may also be useful with prolonged therapy and in parturients at high risk of bleeding or thrombosis.[259] Whether this assay confers any improved efficacy and safety has not been confirmed, and critics point out that there is interassay variability.[261] Further investigation is needed on this topic. The peak activity of LMWH is already reduced by the end of the first trimester, further reduced by the beginning of the third trimester, and returns to normal postpartum.[260] Overall there is a volume expansion as a term pregnancy approaches, leading to subtherapeutic levels. Occasionally, LMWH is changed to intravenous unfractionated heparin in very high risk patients and then discontinued 4 to 6 hours before the time of delivery. This may create a problem if the patient requires a surgical procedure or the placement of a regional anesthetic, because a combination of both agents may result in an unpredictable anti–factor Xa and aPTT response. We recommend to check both tests before a cesarean section or neuraxial technique under this circumstance.

Epidural hematoma is the most feared complication of neuraxial techniques and is much more likely in the setting of an inherited clotting abnormality or the use of anticoagulants while performing these techniques. While a review of the literature in 1994 found 61 cases over an 88-year period, 1906-1994,[262] in 2003 a Food and Drug Administration (FDA) MedWatch found 60 cases over a 9-year period associated with the use of neuraxial anesthesia and LMWH therapy.[263] There was one case of an epidural hematoma in a parturient receiving LMWH. The timing of the administration of LMWH, the removal of the epidural catheter, and the development of the hematoma are unclear, and the patient had a temporary lower extremity motor weakness that resolved spontaneously without any surgical intervention. The 1994 review had only five cases in parturients (8.2% of cases),[262] results that go along with the pregnancy-associated prothrombotic state and its associated resistance to anticoagulation. These factors counteract the epidural venous plexus engorgement, with an increased incidence of intravascular epidural catheters, present during pregnancy. An analysis of the obstetric cases demonstrates that the majority occurred when the anticoagulant dosing was in close proximity to the placement of a neuraxial technique or when patients were taking other medications that alter coagulation. In addition, a review from the United Kingdom found no cases of epidural hematoma in over 9000 epidurals placed in parturients who were taking aspirin as possible prophylactic treatment for preeclampsia. Although aspirin was not found to be beneficial for the prevention of preeclampsia, it was not associated with a significant increase in placental hemorrhages or in bleeding during preparation for epidural anesthesia.[264] Of note, the decreased incidence of epidural hematoma during pregnancy should not modify the recommendations regarding the use of neuraxial techniques in parturients with clotting abnormalities or in those being anticoagulated. In addition, it has been documented that epidural catheter placement is as important as its removal, because both situations could lead to epidural hematoma in the anticoagulated patient.[262]

Epidural hematoma is a very rare complication of neuraxial techniques, with an incidence ranging from 1:220,000 after spinal anesthesia to 1:150,000 after epidural anesthesia.[262] It is more common in the presence of LMWH, with an incidence as high as 1:3,000 after a continuous epidural catheter and 1:40,000 after a spinal anesthetic.[253] It is important to use very low concentrations of local anesthetic to detect any change in the patient's neurologic state. In addition, close follow-up of the neurologic status is essential after the removal of an epidural catheter. Clinical symptoms of epidural hematoma include radicular back pain, bowel or bladder dysfunction, and sensory or motor deficits.[265,266] Interestingly, and different from common wisdom, severe radicular back pain is rarely the presenting symptom. Magnetic resonance imaging is the best diagnostic test for a suspected epidural hematoma, and early decompressive laminectomy is the treatment of choice.

The previously mentioned ASRA guidelines were developed in part because of the increased incidence of epidural hematoma associated with the use of LMWH and neuraxial techniques.[240] These guidelines recommend discontinuing prophylactic doses of LMWH at least 10 to 12 hours before a regional technique, and a single-dose spinal anesthetic is the preferred technique. Therapeutic doses should be discontinued at least 24 hours before a regional technique, and LMWH should not be started until 2 hours after epidural catheter removal. The presence of blood at the time of epidural catheter placement may increase the risk of bleeding into the epidural space and necessitates a delay of 24 hours before LMWH administration. Although epidural catheters are not usually kept for postoperative pain management in parturients, in part because of the excellent and prolonged analgesia with neuraxial morphine, it is important to be careful when these catheters are kept in place in parturients who require LMWH prophylaxis or therapy. Epidural catheters can be safely continued while using prophylactic doses, as long as the LMWH is not started before 6 to 8 hours postoperatively and the catheter is removed 10 to 12 hours after the last LMWH dose. Epidural catheters should be removed in parturients receiving therapeutic doses, and the first dose should not be given earlier than 24 hours postoperatively. ASRA does not recommend the use of the anti–factor Xa assay because, according to the published guidelines, the anti–factor Xa level is not predictive of the risk of bleeding.[240] We consider this item controversial, because it is well known that the anti–factor Xa activity of LMWH is affected by body weight, renal dysfunction, pregnancy, and prolonged therapy.[259,267] We do not routinely check this assay in parturients taking prophylactic doses of LMWH if the last dose was greater than 24 hours before the placement of a neuraxial technique. However, we do measure this test in the presence of therapeutic doses of LMWH, or if the last prophylactic dose of LMWH was less than 24 hours from a regional technique. Our target dose is less than 0.1 U/mL, as this dose is associated with minimal anticoagulation. We are aware that although high levels of this assay would most likely preclude a regional technique, there are no data to support the safety of neuraxial techniques with lower levels. We encourage more senior anesthesiologists to perform the block, and we prefer to use midline neuraxial techniques to minimize the risk of intravascular epidural catheters.

Newer anticoagulants are being compared to traditional anticoagulants, such as unfractionated heparin, and are being used with an increased frequency, in part because of their similar safety profile and ease of administration. Fondaparinux, one of these agents, is a synthetic pentasaccharide that gained FDA approval at the end of 2001. It selectively binds to antithrombin, inducing a conformational change that significantly increases the anti–factor Xa activity without inhibition of factor IIa.[268-270]

It does not cross react with antibodies against heparin/platelet factor 4 complexes and, therefore, is unlikely to lead to thrombocytopenia. It has a very long half-life of about 18 hours, a fact that must be known by practitioners of regional anesthesia. It takes at least 4 days to completely eliminate this agent from the circulation, and regional anesthesia should be avoided during this time period. It may be reasonable to check anti–factor Xa activity before the performance of a neuraxial technique. It may also be reasonable to administer fondaparinux 2 hours after an atraumatic single spinal needle pass or epidural catheter removal.[240] We have already seen a parturient as a high-risk anesthesia consult because she was taking fondaparinux, 2.5 mg/day. She had a history of antiphospholipid antibodies and deep venous thrombosis, requiring thromboprophylaxis during her pregnancy, and was allergic to LMWH. Therapeutic doses range from 5 to 10 mg.[268,269]

In summary, it is important to use appropriate neuraxial techniques, to avoid multiple anticoagulants, and to exercise caution in proper parturient selection. Finally, and perhaps most importantly, a knowledge of the pharmacokinetics and pharmacodynamics of commonly used anticoagulants during pregnancy is essential to avoid the use of neuraxial techniques at a time when a significant anticoagulant effect may still be present. In addition, an understanding of the mechanism of action, side effect profile, and half-life of newer anticoagulants is quite important. The use of guidelines should not be used as a substitute but to complement this knowledge.

Local Anesthetic Allergy

A true IgE-mediated anaphylactic reaction to an anesthetic agent, while often life threatening, is quite rare under anesthesia. The incidence varies between 1:3,500 and 1:20,000, with neuromuscular blocking drugs and latex being the most common offending agents. A recent review on allergic reactions during anesthesia in France during a 2-year period found no cases of local anesthetic allergy.[271] Local anesthetics belong to the ester or amide type. Whereas ester local anesthetics are metabolized to p-aminobenzoic acid (PABA), amide local anesthetics are metabolized in the liver to a variety of compounds. Methylparaben is a preservative that may be present in amide or ester local anesthetics and can have some cross reactivity with PABA. An IgE-mediated reaction to a local anesthetic, most likely due to the PABA metabolite from esters or methylparaben, accounts for less than 1% of all reactions to local anesthetics.[272] Almost all cases of questionable allergic reactions to local anesthetics are due to a vasovagal episode, systemic injection of local anesthetic with central nervous system manifestations, or intravascular injection of epinephrine, with its associated cardiovascular manifestations. Furthermore, most allergic reactions to local anesthetics are due to a type IV delayed hypersensitivity reaction that presents as a contact dermatitis.[272]

Cross reactivity to other local anesthetics should be considered in cases where a true IgE-mediated reaction to an amide or ester group local anesthetic is suspected or confirmed by prior testing. Skin tests should then be conducted, not only for the suspected agent but also for other local anesthetics, including agents of both types, to identify a safe alternative.[273] There is even a report of an IgE-mediated reaction to ropivacaine in a patient with a history of an anaphylactic reaction to other amide local anesthetics, including lidocaine, bupivacaine, and mepivacaine.[273] This particular patient tolerated procaine, an ester local anesthetic, well. Skin tests are conducted by intradermally injecting small quantities of local anesthetic and watching for a wheal and flare response. Should a positive response be observed, then a skin prick test followed by a subcutaneous injection is recommended, because the results are equivocal in many cases.[274] The Chandler methodology for provocative skin testing[275] can be performed over a 1- to 2-hour period by a trained allergist by incrementally performing subcutaneous injections of a local anesthetic while observing the patient closely on a monitored unit for any signs of an allergic reaction.

The history of a local anesthetic allergy in an obstetric patient is more complicated, because skin testing is not recommended during pregnancy unless the results obtained will lead to a significant implication on treatment.[276] Regional anesthesia is much safer in parturients when compared with general anesthesia,[277] and regional analgesia is by far the most effective means of analgesia during labor and delivery. Although the best time to conduct skin testing is before pregnancy, it has been argued that provocative challenge skin testing can be conducted during pregnancy to rule out the possibility of a true local anesthetic allergy.[278,279] The timing of the testing during pregnancy is also controversial, because an allergic reaction due to skin testing before fetal viability may lead to untoward effects on the fetus. Other risks include the possibility of fetal sensitization and the fact that it remains unclear whether a response to skin testing is modified by pregnancy.[280] Therefore, in the event that testing has not been performed during pregnancy, we recommend that a very thorough history be conducted first to rule out other causes of an adverse local anesthetic reaction. In addition, it is important to elicit a family history, as genetic linkage has been postulated.[280] Other options for anesthesia and analgesia should be considered, and a very thorough informed consent process with the patient is strongly recommended while conducting a risk benefit analysis. An awareness of the risks of skin testing during pregnancy should also be discussed with the patient and made only in close collaboration with an allergist and the obstetrician. Should the decision to proceed with skin testing be

BOX 19–6 Differential Diagnosis of Local Anesthetic Allergy

- Vasovagal episode
- Systemic local anesthetic injection
  - Central nervous system
- Systemic epinephrine
  - Cardiac toxicity
- Type IV cell-mediated reaction
  - Contact dermatitis
- Type I cell-mediated reaction
  - Anaphylaxis

made, the timing should be close to the date of delivery to maximize fetal well-being.

In summary, most cases of reactions to local anesthetics are not allergic and should not preclude their use. However, even though a life-threatening anaphylactic reaction to a preservative-free local anesthetic is quite uncommon, it has been reported and should be taken seriously and followed closely if confirmed or strongly suspected (Box 19-6).

CONCLUSION

Pregnancy is a common and nonpathologic condition. However, the altered physiology of pregnancy complicates the anesthetic care of even healthy pregnant patients. When unusual conditions of pregnancy further alter the physiologic state, the anesthesiologist faces additional challenges. Although nearly every disease entity may complicate pregnancy, the scope of this chapter is not sufficient to cover them all. In these situations, basic principles of management of the pregnant patient should apply and have been summarized in this chapter, as well as some of the more important specific conditions specific to pregnant patients.

References

1. Wiesen AR, Gunzenhauser JD: Laboratory-measured pregnancy rates and their determinants in a large, well-described adult cohort. Milit Med 2004;169:518-521.
2. Brodsky JB, Cohen EN, Brown BW Jr, et al: Surgery during pregnancy and fetal outcome. Am J Obstet Gynecol 1980;138:1165-1167.
3. Mazze RI, Kallen B: Reproductive outcome after anesthesia and operation during pregnancy: A registry study of 5405 cases. Am J Obstet Gynecol 1989;161:1178-1185.
4. Manley S, de Kelaita G, Joseph NJ, et al: Preoperative pregnancy testing in ambulatory surgery: Incidence and impact of positive results. Anesthesiology 1995;83:690-693.
5. Farraghar R, Bhavani Shankar K: Obstetric anesthesia. In Healy TEJ, Knight PR (eds): Wylie and Churchill Davidson's: A Practice of Anesthesia, 7th ed. London, Arnold, 2003, pp 923-940.
6. Chang B: Physiological changes of pregnancy. In Chestnut DH C (ed): Obstetric Anesthesia: Principles and Practice. Philadelphia, Elsevier, 2004, pp 15-36.
7. Chan MT, Mainland P, Gin T: Minimum alveolar concentration of halothane and enflurane are decreased in early pregnancy. Anesthesiology 1996;85:782-786.
8. Leighton BL, Cheek TG, Gross JB, et al: Succinylcholine pharmacodynamics in peripartum patients. Anesthesiology 1986;64:202-205.
9. Kussman B, Shorten G, Uppington J, Comunale ME: Administration of magnesium sulphate before rocuronium: Effects on speed of onset and duration of neuromuscular block. Br J Anaesth 1997;79:122-124.
10. Khazin AF, Hon EH, Hehre FW: Effects of maternal hyperoxia on the fetus: I. Oxygen tension. Am J Obstet Gynecol 1971;109:628-637.
11. Brann AW Jr, Myers RE: Central nervous system findings in the newborn monkey following severe in utero partial asphyxia. Neurology 1975;25:327-338.
12. Newman B, Lam AM: Induced hypotension for clipping of a cerebral aneurysm during pregnancy: A case report and brief review. Anesth Analg 1986;65:675-678.
13. Li H, Gudmundsson S, Olofsson P: Acute increase of umbilical artery vascular flow resistance in compromised fetuses provoked by uterine contractions. Early Hum Dev 2003;74:47-56.
14. Lee A, Ngan Kee WD, Gin T: A quantitative, systematic review of randomized controlled trials of ephedrine versus phenylephrine for the management of hypotension during spinal anesthesia for cesarean delivery. Anesth Analg 2002;94:920-926, table of contents.
15. Shepard TH, Lemire RJ: Catalog of Teratogenic Agents, 11th ed. Baltimore, Johns Hopkins University Press, 2004.
16. Teiling AK, Mohammed AK, Minor BG, et al: Lack of effects of prenatal exposure to lidocaine on development of behavior in rats. Anesth Analg 1987;66:533-541.
17. Mazze R I, Wilson AI, Rice SA, Baden JM: Reproduction and fetal development in rats exposed to nitrous oxide. Teratology 1984;30: 259-265.
18. Baden JM, Fujinaga M: Effects of nitrous oxide on day 9 rat embryos grown in culture. Br J Anaesth 1991;66:500-503.
19. Lane GA, Nahrwold ML, Tait AR, et al: Anesthetics as teratogens: Nitrous oxide is fetotoxic, xenon is not. Science 1980;210:899-901.
20. Chanarin I: Cobalamins and nitrous oxide: A review. J Clin Pathol 1980;33:909-916.
21. Keeling PA, Rocke DA, Nunn JF, et al: Folinic acid protection against nitrous oxide teratogenicity in the rat. Br J Anaesth 1986;58:528-534.
22. Fujinaga M, Baden JM: Methionine prevents nitrous oxide-induced teratogenicity in rat embryos grown in culture. Anesthesiology 1994;81:184-189.
23. Mazze RI, Fujinaga M, Baden JM: Halothane prevents nitrous oxide teratogenicity in Sprague-Dawley rats; folinic acid does not. Teratology 1988;38:121-127.
24. Brodsky JB, Cohen EN: Health experiences of operating room personnel. Anesthesiology 1985;63:461-464.
25. Spence AA: Environmental pollution by inhalation anaesthetics. Br J Anaesth 1987;59:96-103.
26. Jevtovic-Todorovic V, Hartman RE, Izumi Y, et al: Early exposure to common anesthetic agents causes widespread neurodegeneration in the developing rat brain and persistent learning deficits. J Neurosci 2003;23:876-882.
27. Levin ED, Bowman RE: Behavioral effects of chronic exposure to low concentrations of halothane during development in rats. Anesth Analg 1986;65:653-659.
28. Mazze RI, Kallen B: Appendectomy during pregnancy: A Swedish registry study of 778 cases. Obstet Gynecol 1991;77:835-840.
29. Cunningham AJ, Brull SJ: Laparoscopic cholecystectomy: Anesthetic implications. Anesth Analg 1993;76:1120-1133.
30. Fitzgibbons R Jr: Laparoscopic cholecystectomy. JAMA 1991;266:269.
31. Lachman E, Schienfeld A, Voss E, et al: Pregnancy and laparoscopic surgery. J Am Assoc Gynecol Laparosc 1999;6:347-351.
32. Andreoli M, Servakov M, Meyers P, Mann WJ Jr: Laparoscopic surgery during pregnancy. J Am Assoc Gynecol Laparosc 1999;6:229-233.
33. Barnard JM, Chaffin D, Droste S, et al: Fetal response to carbon dioxide pneumoperitoneum in the pregnant ewe. Obstet Gynecol 1995;85:669-674.

34. Amos JD, Schorr SJ, Norman PF, et al: Laparoscopic surgery during pregnancy. Am J Surg 1996;171:435-437.

35. Hardwick RH, Slade RR, Smith PA, Thompson MH: Laparoscopic splenectomy in pregnancy. J Laparoendosc Adv Surg Tech A 1999;9:439-440.

36. Wang PH, Chao HT, Tseng JY, et al: Laparoscopic surgery for heterotopic pregnancies: a case report and a brief review. Eur J Obstet Gynecol Reprod Biol 1998;80:267-271.

37. Demeure MJ, Carlsen B, Traul D, et al: Laparoscopic removal of a right adrenal pheochromocytoma in a pregnant woman. J Laparoendosc Adv Surg Tech A 1998;8:315-319.

38. Steinbrook RA, Brooks DC, Datta S: Laparoscopic cholecystectomy during pregnancy: Review of anesthetic management, surgical considerations. Surg Endosc 1996;10:511-515.

39. Levinson G, Shnider SM, DeLorimier AA, Steffenson JL: Effects of maternal hyperventilation on uterine blood flow and fetal oxygenation and acid-base status. Anesthesiology 1974;40:340-347.

40. Wahba RW, Beique F, Kleiman SJ: Cardiopulmonary function and laparoscopic cholecystectomy. Can J Anaesth 1995;42:51-63.

41. Joris JL, Noirot DP, Legrand MJ, et al: Hemodynamic changes during laparoscopic cholecystectomy. Anesth Analg 1993;76:1067-1071.

42. Steinbrook RA, Bhavani-Shankar K: Hemodynamics during laparoscopic surgery in pregnancy. Anesth Analg 2001;93:1570-1571, table of contents.

43. (SAGES) SoAGES: Guidelines for laparoscopic surgery during pregnancy. Surg Endosc 1998;12:189-190.

44. Cruz AM, Southerland LC, Duke T, et al: Intraabdominal carbon dioxide insufflation in the pregnant ewe: Uterine blood flow, intraamniotic pressure, and cardiopulmonary effects. Anesthesiology 1996;85:1395-1402.

45. Hunter JG, Swanstrom L, Thornburg K: Carbon dioxide pneumoperitoneum induces fetal acidosis in a pregnant ewe model. Surg Endosc 1995;9:272-277; discussion 7-9.

46. Shankar KB, Mushlin PS: Arterial to end-tidal gradients in pregnant subjects. Anesthesiology 1997;87:1596.

47. Affleck DG, Handrahan DL, Egger MJ, Price RR: The laparoscopic management of appendicitis and cholelithiasis during pregnancy. Am J Surg 1999;178:523-529.

48. Elerding SC: Laparoscopic cholecystectomy in pregnancy. Am J Surg 1993;165:625-627.

49. Soper NJ, Hunter JG, Petrie RH: Laparoscopic cholecystectomy during pregnancy. Surg Endosc 1992;6:115-117.

50. Bhavani-Shankar K, Steinbrook RA, Brooks DC, Datta S: Arterial to end-tidal carbon dioxide pressure difference during laparoscopic surgery in pregnancy. Anesthesiology 2000;93:370-373.

51. Curet N, Allen D, Josloff R, et al: Laparoscopy during pregnancy. Arch Surg 1996;131:546.

52. Bhavani-Shankar K, Steinbrook RA: Anesthetic considerations for minimally invasive surgery. In Brooks DC (ed): Current Review of Minimally Invasive Surgery, 2nd ed. Philadelphia, Current Medicine, 1998, p 29.

53. Mosher WD, Pratt WF: Fecundity and infertility in the United States: Incidence and trends. Fertil Steril 1991;56:192-3.

54. Collins JA: Unexplained Infertility: Evaluation and Treatment. Philadelphia, WB Saunders, 1995.

55. Meldrum DR: Female reproductive aging—ovarian and uterine factors. Fertil Steril 1993;59:1-5.

56. Steptoe PC, Edwards RG: Birth after the reimplantation of a human embryo. Lancet 1978;2:336.

57. Tsen LC: Darwin to desflurane: Anesthesia for assisted reproductive technologies. Anesth Analg 2002;94S:109-114.

58. Society for Assisted Reproductive Technology in the United States: 1999 results generated from the American Society for Reproductive Medicine/Society for Assisted Reproductive Technology Registry. Fertil Steril 2002;78:918-931.

59. Lu MC: Impact of "non-physician factors" on the "physician factor" of in vitro fertilization success: Is it the broth, the cooks, or the statistics? Fertil Steril 1999;71:998-1000.

60. Karande VC, Morris R, Chapman C, et al: Impact of the "physician factor" on pregnancy rates in a large assisted reproductive technology program: Do too many cooks spoil the broth? Fertil Steril 1999;71:1001-1009.

61. Jennings JC, Moreland K, Peterson CM: In vitro fertilisation: A review of drug therapy and clinical management. Drugs 1996;52:313-343.

62. Awonuga A, Waterstone J, Oyesanya O, et al: A prospective randomized study comparing needles of different diameters for transvaginal ultrasound-directed follicle aspiration. Fertil Steril 1996;65:109-113.

63. Hung Yu Ng E, Kwai Chi Chui D, Shan Tang O, Chung Ho P: Paracervical block with and without conscious sedation: A comparison of the pain levels during egg collection and the postoperative side effects. Fertil Steril 2001;75:711-717.

64. Ditkoff EC, Plumb J, Selick A, Sauer MV: Anesthesia practices in the United States common to in vitro fertilization (IVF) centers. J Assist Reprod Genet 1997;14:145-147.

65. Jain T, Harlow BL, Hornstein MD: Insurance coverage and outcomes of in vitro fertilization. N Engl J Med 2002;347:661-667.

66. Silva PD, Kang SB, Sloane KA: Gamete intrafallopian transfer with spinal anesthesia. Fertil Steril 1993;59:841-843.

67. Pellicano M, Zullo F, Fiorentino A, et al: Conscious sedation versus general anesthesia for minilaparoscopic gamete intra-fallopian transfer: A prospective randomized study. Hum Reprod 2001;16:2295-2297.

68. Lane GA, Nahrwold ML, Tait AR, et al: Anesthetics as teratogens: Nitrous oxide is fetotoxic, xenon is not. Science 1980;210:899-901.

69. Hansen DK, Grafton TF: Effect of nitrous oxide on embryonic macromolecular synthesis and purine levels. Teratog Carcinog Mutagen 1988;8:107-115.

70. Baden JM, Fujinaga M: Effects of nitrous oxide on day 9 rat embryos grown in culture. Br J Anaesth 1991;66:500-503.

71. Lee EJ, Bongso A, Kumar A: Evaluation of inhalational anaesthetics on murine in vitro fertilization. Ann Acad Med Singapore 1994;23:479-485.

72. Rosen MA, Roizen MF, Eger EI, et al: The effect of nitrous oxide on in vitro fertilization success rate. Anesthesiology 1987;67:42-44.

73. Kennedy GL, Smith SH, Keplinger ML, Calandra JC: Reproductive and teratologic studies with isoflurane. Drug Chem Toxicol 1977;1:75-88.

74. Vincent RDJ, Syrop CH, Van Voorhis BJ, et al: An evaluation of the effect of anesthetic technique on reproductive success after laparoscopic pronuclear stage transfer: Propofol/nitrous oxide versus isoflurane/nitrous oxide. Anesthesiology 1995;82:352-358.

75. Coetsier T, Dhont M, De Sutter P, et al: Propofol anaesthesia for ultrasound guided oocyte retrieval: Accumulation of the anaesthetic agent in follicular fluid. Hum Reprod 1992;7:1422-1424.

76. Ben-Shlomo I, Moskovich R, Golan J, et al: The effect of propofol anesthesia on oocyte fertilization and early embryo quality. Hum Reprod 2000;15:2197-2199.

77. Rosenblatt MA, Bradford CN, Bodian CN, Grunfeld L: The effect of a propofol-based sedation technique on cumulative embryo scores, clinical pregnancy rates, and implantation rates in patients undergoing embryo transfers with donor oocytes. J Clin Anesth 1997;9:614-617.

78. Tillman Hein HA, Putman JM: Is propofol a proper proposition for reproductive procedures? J Clin Anesth 1997;9:611-613.

79. Janssenwillen C, Christiaens F, Camu F, Van Steirteghem A: The effect of propofol on pathogenetic activation, in vitro fertilization and early development of mouse oocytes. Fertil Steril 1997;67:769-774.

80. Endler GC, Stout M, Magyar DM, et al: Follicular fluid concentrations of thiopental and thiamylal during laparoscopy for oocyte retrieval. Fertil Steril 1987;48:828-833.

81. Pierce ET, Smalky M, Alper MM, et al: Comparison of pregnancy rates following gamete intrafallopian transfer (GIFT) under general anesthesia with thiopental sodium or propofol. J Clin Anesth 1992;4:394-398.

82. Christiaens F, Janssenwillen C, Van Steirteghem A, et al: Comparison of assisted reproductive technology performance after oocyte retrieval under general anaesthesia (propofol) versus paracervical local anaesthetic block: A case-controlled study. Hum Reprod 1998;13:2456-2460.

83. Chopineau J, Bazin JE, Terrisse MP, et al: Assay for midazolam in liquor folliculi during in vitro fertilization under anesthesia. Clin Pharm 1993;12:770-773.
84. Soussis I, Boyd O, Paraschos T, et al: Follicular fluid levels of midazolam, fentanyl, and alfentanil during transvaginal oocyte retrieval. Fertil Steril 1995;64:1003-7.
85. Shapira SC, Chrubasik S, Hoffmann A, et al: Use of alfentanil for in vitro fertilization oocyte retrieval. J Clin Anesth 1996;8:282-285.
86. Casati A, Valentini G, Zangrillo A, et al: Anaesthesia for ultrasound guided oocyte retrieval: midazolam/remifentanil versus propofol/fentanyl regimens. Eur J Anaesth 1999;16:773-778.
87. Ben-Shlomo I, Moskovich R, Katz Y, Shalev E: Midazolam/ketamine sedative combination compared with fentanyl/propofol/isoflurane anaesthesia for oocyte retrieval. Hum Reprod 1999;7:1757-1759.
88. Marshburn PB, Shabanowitz RB, Clark MR: Immunohistochemical localization of prostaglandin H synthase in the embryo and uterus of the mouse from ovulation through implantation. Mol Reprod Dev 1990;25:309-316.
89. van der Weiden RM, Helmerhorst FM, Keirse MJ: Influence of prostaglandins and platelet activating factor on implantation. Hum Reprod 1991;6:436-442.
90. Van Voorhis BJ, Huettner PC, Clark MR, Hill JA: Immunohistochemical localization of prostaglandin H synthase in the female reproductive tract and endometriosis. Am J Obstet Gynecol 1990;163:57-62.
91. Bokhari A, Pollard BJ: Anaesthesia for assisted conception: A survey of UK practice. Eur J Anaesth 1999;16:225-230.
92. Monroe SE, Levine L, Chang RJ, et al: Prolactin-secreting pituitary adenomas: V. Increased gonadotroph responsivity in hyperprolactinemic women with pituitary adenomas. J Clin Endocrinol Metab 1981;52:1171-1178.
93. Cunningham F, Gant N, Leveno K, et al: Williams Obstetrics, 21st ed. New York, McGraw-Hill, 2001.
94. Koninckx PR, Renaer M: Pain sensitivity of and pain radiation from the internal female genital organs. Hum Reprod 1997;12:1785-1788.
95. Hung Yu Ng E, Shan Tang O, Kwai Chi Chui D, Chung Ho P: A prospective, randomized, double-blind and placebo-controlled study to assess the efficacy of paracervical block in the pain relief during egg collection in IVF. Hum Reprod 1999;14:2783-2787.
96. Hung Yu Ng E, Miao B, Chung Ho P: A randomized double-blind study to compare the effectiveness of three different doses of lignocaine used in paracervical block during oocyte retrieval. J Assist Reprod Genet 2003;20:8-12.
97. Schnell VL, Sacco AG, Savoy-Moore RT, et al: Effects of oocyte exposure to local anesthetics on in vitro fertilization and embryo development in the mouse. Reprod Toxicol 1992;6:323-327.
98. Wikland M, Evers H, Jakobsson AH: The concentration of lidocaine in follicular fluid when used for paracervical block in a human IVF-ET programme. Hum Reprod 1990;5:920-923.
99. Manica VS, Bader AM, Fragneto R, et al: Anesthesia for in vitro fertilization: A comparison of 1.5% and 5% lidocaine for ultrasonically guided oocyte retrieval. Anesth Analg 1993;77:453-456.
100. Martin R, Tsen LC, Tzeng G, et al: Anesthesia for in vitro fertilization: The addition of fentanyl to 1.5% lidocaine. Anesth Analg 1999;88:532-536.
101. Tsen LC, Schultz R, Martin R, et al: Intrathecal-low dose bupivacaine vs. lidocaine for in-vitro fertilization procedures. Reg Anesth Pain Med 2001;26:52-56.
102. Tsen LC, Arthur GR, Datta S, et al: Estrogen-induced changes in protein binding of bupivacaine during in vitro fertilization. Anesthesiology 1997;87:879-883.
103. Hull M, Glazener CM, Kelly NJ, et al: Population study of causes, treatment, and outcome of infertility. BMJ 1985;291:1693-1697.
104. Gorgy A, Meniru GI, Naumann N, et al: The efficacy of local anesthesia for percutaneous epididymal sperm aspiration and testicular sperm aspiration. Hum Reprod 1998;13:646-650.
105. Rein MS, Barbieri RL: The Infertile Couple—Part I, 7th ed. St. Louis, Mosby, 1999.
106. Kodama H, Fukuda J, Karube H, et al: Status of the coagulation and fibrinolytic systems in ovarian hyperstimulation syndrome. Fertil Steril 1996;66:417-424.
107. Kodama H, Fukuda J, Karube H, et al: Characteristics of blood hemostatic markers in a patient with ovarian hyperstimulation syndrome who actually developed thromboembolism. Fertil Steril 1995;64:1207-1209.
108. Magnani B, Tsen LC, Datta A, Bader AM: Do short-term changes in estrogen levels produce increased fibrinolysis? Am J Clin Pathol 1999;112:485-491.
109. Aune B, Oian P, Osterud B: Enhanced sensitivity of the extrinsic coagulation system during ovarian stimulation for in vitro fertilization. Hum Reprod 1993;9:1349-1352.
110. Hood DD, Dewan DM: Anesthetic and obstetric outcome in morbidly obese parturients. Anesthesiology 1993;79:1210-1218.
111. Bhavani Shankar K, Lee-Paritz A: Anesthesia for pregnant obese parturients. In Datta S (ed): Anesthesia and Obstetric Management of High Risk Pregnancy, 3rd ed. New York, Springer, 2003, pp 53-66.
112. Lewis DF, Chesson AL, Edwards MS, et al: Obstructive sleep apnea during pregnancy resulting in pulmonary hypertension. South Med J 1998;91:761-762.
113. Sebire NJ, Jolly M, Harris JP, et al: Maternal obesity and pregnancy outcome: A study of 287,213 pregnancies in London. Int J Obes Relat Metab Disord 2001;25:1175-1182.
114. Johnson JW, Longmate JA, Frentzen B: Excessive maternal weight and pregnancy outcome. Am J Obstet Gynecol 1992;167:353-370; discussion 370-372.
115. Peckham CH, Christianson RE: The relationship between prepregnancy weight and certain obstetric factors. Am J Obstet Gynecol 1971;111:1-7.
116. Chauhan SP, Magann EF, Carroll CS, et al: Mode of delivery for the morbidly obese with prior cesarean delivery: Vaginal versus repeat cesarean section. Am J Obstet Gynecol 2001;185:349-354.
117. Perlow JH, Morgan MA, Montgomery D, et al: Perinatal outcome in pregnancy complicated by massive obesity. Am J Obstet Gynecol 1992;167:958-962.
118. Waller DK, Mills JL, Simpson JL, et al: Are obese women at higher risk for producing malformed offspring? Am J Obstet Gynecol 1994;170:541-548.
119. Morgan M: Amniotic fluid embolism. Anaesthesia 1979;34:20-32.
120. Clark SL, Hankins GD, Dudley DA, et al: Amniotic fluid embolism: Analysis of the national registry. Am J Obstet Gynecol 1995;172:1158-1167; discussion 1167-1169.
121. Steiner PE, Lushbaugh CC: Landmark article, Oct. 1941: Maternal pulmonary embolism by amniotic fluid as a cause of obstetric shock and unexpected deaths in obstetrics. JAMA 1986;255:2187-2203.
122. Masson RG: Amniotic fluid embolism. Clin Chest Med 1992;13:657-665.
123. McDougall RJ, Duke GJ: Amniotic fluid embolism syndrome: Case report and review. Anaesth Intensive Care 1995;23:735-740.
124. Dudney TM, Elliott CG: Pulmonary embolism from amniotic fluid, fat, and air. Prog Cardiovasc Dis 1994;36:447-474.
125. Lawson HW, Atrash HK, Franks AL: Fatal pulmonary embolism during legal induced abortion in the United States from 1972 to 1985. Am J Obstet Gynecol 1990;162:986-990.
126. Sterner S, Campbell B, Davies S: Amniotic fluid embolism. Ann Emerg Med 1984;13:343-345.
127. Maher JE, Wenstrom KD, Hauth JC, Meis PJ: Amniotic fluid embolism after saline amnioinfusion: Two cases and review of the literature. Obstet Gynecol 1994;83:851-854.
128. Davies S: Amniotic fluid embolus: A review of the literature. Can J Anaesth 2001;48:88-98.
129. Courtney LD: Coagulation failure in pregnancy. BMJ 1970;1:691.
130. Bastien JL, Graves JR, Bailey S: Atypical presentation of amniotic fluid embolism. Anesth Analg 1998;87:124-126.
131. Clark SL, Pavlova Z, Greenspoon J, et al: Squamous cells in the maternal pulmonary circulation. Am J Obstet Gynecol 1986;154:104-106.

132. Lee W, Ginsburg KA, Cotton DB, Kaufman RH: Squamous and trophoblastic cells in the maternal pulmonary circulation identified by invasive hemodynamic monitoring during the peripartum period. Am J Obstet Gynecol 1986;155:999-1001.

133. Roche WD Jr, Norris HJ: Detection and significance of maternal pulmonary amniotic fluid embolism. Obstet Gynecol 1974;43:729-731.

134. Clark SL: New concepts of amniotic fluid embolism: A review. Obstet Gynecol Surv 1990;45:360-368.

135. Clark SL, Cotton DB, Gonik B, et al: Central hemodynamic alterations in amniotic fluid embolism. Am J Obstet Gynecol 1988;158:1124-1126.

136. Clark SL, Montz FJ, Phelan JP: Hemodynamic alterations associated with amniotic fluid embolism: A reappraisal. Am J Obstet Gynecol 1985;151:617-621.

137. el Maradny E, Kanayama N, Halim A, et al: Endothelin has a role in early pathogenesis of amniotic fluid embolism. Gynecol Obstet Invest 1995;40:14-18.

138. Guidotti RJ, Grimes DA, Cates W Jr: Fatal amniotic fluid embolism during legally induced abortion, United States, 1972 to 1978. Am J Obstet Gynecol 1981;141:257-261.

139. Choi DM, Duffy BL: Amniotic fluid embolism. Anaesth Intensive Care 1995;23:741-743.

140. Davies S: Amniotic fluid embolism and isolated disseminated intravascular coagulation. Can J Anaesth 1999;46:456-459.

141. Harnett M, Datta S, Bhavani-Shankar K: How does amniotic fluid effect coagulation? Anesthesiology 2001;94:A45.

142. Lockwood CJ, Bach R, Guha A, et al: Amniotic fluid contains tissue factor, a potent initiator of coagulation. Am J Obstet Gynecol 1991;165:1335-1341.

143. Masson RG, Ruggieri J: Pulmonary microvascular cytology: A new diagnostic application of the pulmonary artery catheter. Chest 1985;88:908-914.

144. Lee KR, Catalano PM, Ortiz-Giroux S: Cytologic diagnosis of amniotic fluid embolism: Report of a case with a unique cytologic feature and emphasis on the difficulty of eliminating squamous contamination. Acta Cytol 1986;30:177-182.

145. Kobayashi H, Ohi H, Terao T: A simple, noninvasive, sensitive method for diagnosis of amniotic fluid embolism by monoclonal antibody TKH-2 that recognizes NeuAc alpha 2-6GalNAc. Am J Obstet Gynecol 1993;168:848-853.

146. Kanayama N, Yamazaki T, Naruse H, et al: Determining zinc coproporphyrin in maternal plasma—a new method for diagnosing amniotic fluid embolism. Clin Chem 1992;38:526-529.

147. Rodgers GP, Heymach GJ 3rd: Cryoprecipitate therapy in amniotic fluid embolization. Am J Med 1984;76:916-920.

148. Taenaka N, Shimada Y, Kawai M, et al: Survival from DIC following amniotic fluid embolism: Successful treatment with a serine proteinase inhibitor; FOY. Anaesthesia 1981;36:389-393.

149. Van Heerden PV, Webb SA, Hee G, et al: Inhaled aerosolized prostacyclin as a selective pulmonary vasodilator for the treatment of severe hypoxaemia. Anaesth Intensive Care 1996;24:87-90.

150. Capellier G, Jacques T, Balvay P, et al: Inhaled nitric oxide in patients with pulmonary embolism. Intensive Care Med 1997;23:1089-1092.

151. Gambling D: Hypertensive disorders. In Chestnut D (ed): Obstetric Anesthesia: Principles and Practice. Philadelphia, Elsevier, 2004, pp 794-835.

152. Mattar F, Sibai BM: Eclampsia: VIII. Risk factors for maternal morbidity. Am J Obstet Gynecol 2000;182:307-312.

153. Usta IM, Sibai BM: Emergent management of puerperal eclampsia. Obstet Gynecol Clin North Am 1995;22:315-335.

154. Barton JR, Sibai BM: Cerebral pathology in eclampsia. Clin Perinatol 1991;18:891-910.

155. Kaplan PW, Repke JT: Eclampsia. Neurol Clin 1994;12:565-582.

156. Witlin AG, Friedman SA, Egerman RS, et al: Cerebrovascular disorders complicating pregnancy—beyond eclampsia. Am J Obstet Gynecol 1997;176:1139-1145; discussion 45-48.

157. Moodley J, Jjuuko G, Rout C: Epidural compared with general anaesthesia for caesarean delivery in conscious women with eclampsia. Br J Obstet Gynecol 2001;108:378-382.

158. Martin JN Jr, Rinehart BK, May WL, et al: The spectrum of severe preeclampsia: Comparative analysis by HELLP (hemolysis, elevated liver enzyme levels, and low platelet count) syndrome classification. Am J Obstet Gynecol 1999;180:1373-1384.

159. Sibai BM: The HELLP syndrome (hemolysis, elevated liver enzymes, and low platelets): Much ado about nothing? Am J Obstet Gynecol 1990;162:311-316.

160. Audibert F, Friedman SA, Frangieh AY, Sibai BM: Clinical utility of strict diagnostic criteria for the HELLP (hemolysis, elevated liver enzymes, and low platelets) syndrome. Am J Obstet Gynecol 1996;175:460-464.

161. Sibai BM, Ramadan MK, Chari RS, Friedman SA: Pregnancies complicated by HELLP syndrome (hemolysis, elevated liver enzymes, and low platelets): Subsequent pregnancy outcome and long-term prognosis. Am J Obstet Gynecol 1995;172:125-129.

162. Magann EF, Martin JN Jr: Critical care of HELLP syndrome with corticosteroids. Am J Perinatol 2000;17:417-422.

163. de Boer K, Buller HR, ten Cate JW, Treffers PE: Coagulation studies in the syndrome of haemolysis, elevated liver enzymes and low platelets. Br J Obstet Gynaecol 1991;98:42-47.

164. Barton JR, Sibai BM: Hepatic imaging in HELLP syndrome (hemolysis, elevated liver enzymes, and low platelet count). Am J Obstet Gynecol 1996;174:1820-1825; discussion 1825-1827.

165. O'Brien JM, Shumate SA, Satchwell SL, et al: Maternal benefit of corticosteroid therapy in patients with HELLP (hemolysis, elevated liver enzymes, and low platelet count) syndrome: Impact on the rate of regional anesthesia. Am J Obstet Gynecol 2002;186:475-479.

166. Fox DB, Troiano NH, Graves CR: Use of the pulmonary artery catheter in severe preeclampsia: A review. Obstet Gynecol Surv 1996;51:684-695.

167. Benedetti TJ, Kates R, Williams V: Hemodynamic observations in severe preeclampsia complicated by pulmonary edema. Am J Obstet Gynecol 1985;152:330-334.

168. Desai DK, Moodley J, Naidoo DP, Bhorat I: Cardiac abnormalities in pulmonary oedema associated with hypertensive crises in pregnancy. Br J Obstet Gynaecol 1996;103:523-528.

169. Mabie WC, Hackman BB, Sibai BM: Pulmonary edema associated with pregnancy: Echocardiographic insights and implications for treatment. Obstet Gynecol 1993;81:227-234.

170. Dildy GA 3rd, Cotton DB: Management of severe preeclampsia and eclampsia. Crit Care Clin 1991;7:829-850.

171. Catanzarite V, Willms D, Wong D, et al: Acute respiratory distress syndrome in pregnancy and the puerperium: Causes, courses, and outcomes. Obstet Gynecol 2001;97:760-764.

172. Chichakli LO, Atrash HK, MacKay A, et al: Pregnancy-related mortality in the United States due to hemorrhage: 1979-1992. Obstet Gynecol 1999;94:721-725.

173. Hepner DL, Gaiser RR: The patient with retained placenta. Anesthesiol News 1997;23:20-29.

174. Breen JL, Neubecker R, Gregori CA, Franklin JE: Placenta accreta, increta, and percreta: A survey of 40 cases. Obstet Gynecol 1977;49:43-47.

175. Clark SL, Koonings PP, Phelan JP: Placenta previa/accreta and prior cesarean section. Obstet Gynecol 1985;66:89-92.

176. Ornan D, White R, Pollak J, Tal M: Pelvic embolization for intractable postpartum hemorrhage: Long-term follow-up and implications for fertility. Obstet Gynecol 2003;102:904-910.

177. Chestnut DH, Dewan DM, Redick LF, et al: Anesthetic management for obstetric hysterectomy: A multi-institutional study. Anesthesiology 1989;70:607-610.

178. Kamani AA, Gambling DR, Christilaw J, Flanagan ML: Anaesthetic management of patients with placenta accreta. Can J Anaesth 1987;34:613-617.

179. Bhavani-Shankar K, Lynch EP, Datta S: Airway changes during cesarean hysterectomy. Can J Anaesth 2000;47:338-341.

180. McMahon MJ, Luther ER, Bowes WA, Olshan AF: Comparison of a trial of labor with an elective second cesarean section. N Engl J Med 1996;335:689-695.

181. Lydon-Rochelle M, Holt VL, Easterling TR, Martin DP: Risk of uterine rupture during labor among women with a prior cesarean delivery. N Engl J Med 2001;345:3-8.

182. ACOG: ACOG practice bulletin: Vaginal birth after previous cesarean delivery. Number 5, July 1999 (replaces practice bulletin number 2, October 1998). Clinical management guidelines for obstetrician-gynecologists. American College of Obstetricians and Gynecologists. Int J Gynaecol Obstet 1999;66:197-204.

183. ACOG: Induction of labor for vaginal birth after cesarean delivery. ACOG Committee Opinion No. 271. American College of Obstetricians and Gynecologists. Obstet Gynecol 2002;99:679-680.

184. Hepner DL, Gutsche BB: Obstetric hemorrhage. Curr Rev Clin Anesth 1998;22:213-224.

185. Azeez Pasha SA, Kooheji AJ, Azeez A: Anesthetic management of peripartum hemorrhage. Sem Anesth Periop Med Pain 2000;19:225-236.

186. Stehling LC, Doherty DC, Faust RJ, et al: Practice Guidelines for Blood Component Therapy: A Report by the American Society of Anesthesiologists Task Force on Blood Component Therapy. Anesthesiology 1996;84:732-747.

187. Waters JH, Biscotti C, Potter PS, Philipson E: Amniotic fluid removal during cell-salvage in the cesarean section patient. Anesthesiology 2000;92:1531-1536.

188. Catling SJ, Williams S, Fielding AM: Cell salvage in obstetrics: An evaluation of the ability of cell salvage combined with leucocyte depletion filtration to remove amniotic fluid from operative blood loss at caesarean section. Int J Obstet Anesth 1999;8:79-84.

189. Weiskopf RB: Erythrocyte salvage during cesarean section (editorial). Anesthesiology 2000;92:1519-1521.

190. Camann WC: Cell salvage during cesarean delivery: Is it safe and valuable? Maybe, maybe not! (editorial). Int J Obstet Anesth 1999;8:75-76.

191. de Beus E, van Mook WN, Ramsay G, et al: Peripartum cardiomyopathy: A condition intensivists should be aware of. Intensive Care Med 2003;29:167-174.

192. Pearson GD, Veille JC, Rahimtoola S, et al: Peripartum cardiomyopathy: National Heart, Lung, and Blood Institute and Office of Rare Diseases (National Institutes of Health) workshop recommendations and review. JAMA 2000;283:1183-1188.

193. Boomsma LJ: Peripartum cardiomyopathy in a rural Nigerian hospital. Trop Geogr Med 1989;41:197-200.

194. Lee W, Cotton DB: Peripartum cardiomyopathy: Current concepts and clinical management. Clin Obstet Gynecol 1989;32:54-67.

195. Sanderson JE, Olsen EG, Gatei D: Peripartum heart disease: An endomyocardial biopsy study. Br Heart J 1986;56:285-291.

196. Rizeq MN, Rickenbacher PR, Fowler MB, Billingham ME: Incidence of myocarditis in peripartum cardiomyopathy. Am J Cardiol 1994;74:474-477.

197. O'Connell JB, Costanzo-Nordin MR, Subramanian R, et al: Peripartum cardiomyopathy: Clinical, hemodynamic, histologic and prognostic characteristics. J Am Coll Cardiol 1986;8:52-56.

198. Sliwa K, Skudicky D, Bergemann A, et al: Peripartum cardiomyopathy: Analysis of clinical outcome, left ventricular function, plasma levels of cytokines and Fas/APO-1. J Am Coll Cardiol 2000;35:701-705.

199. Sliwa K, Skudicky D, Candy G, et al: The addition of pentoxifylline to conventional therapy improves outcome in patients with peripartum cardiomyopathy. Eur J Heart Fail 2002;4:305-309.

200. Midei MG, DeMent SH, Feldman AM, et al: Peripartum myocarditis and cardiomyopathy. Circulation 1990;81:922-928.

201. Bozkurt B, Villanueva FS, Holubkov R, et al: Intravenous immune globulin in the therapy of peripartum cardiomyopathy. J Am Coll Cardiol 1999;34:177-180.

202. Lewis R, Mabie WC, Burlew B, Sibai BM: Biventricular assist device as a bridge to cardiac transplantation in the treatment of peripartum cardiomyopathy. South Med J 1997;90:955-958.

203. Carvalho AC, Almeida D, Cohen M, et al: Successful pregnancy, delivery and puerperium in a heart transplant patient with previous peripartum cardiomyopathy. Eur Heart J 1992;13:1589-1591.

204. Felker GM, Jaeger CJ, Klodas E, et al: Myocarditis and long-term survival in peripartum cardiomyopathy. Am Heart J 2000;140:785-791.

205. Sliwa K, Forster O, Zhanje F, et al: Outcome of subsequent pregnancy in patients with documented peripartum cardiomyopathy. Am J Cardiol 2004;93:1441-1443, A10.

206. Velickovic IA, Leicht CH: Continuous spinal anesthesia for cesarean section in a parturient with severe recurrent peripartum cardiomyopathy. Int J Obstet Anesth 2004;13:40-43.

207. Connelly NR, Chin MT, Parker RK, et al: Pregnancy and delivery in a patient with recent peripartum cardiomyopathy. Int J Obstet Anesth 1998;7:38-41.

208. Velickovic IA, Leicht CH: Peripartum cardiomyopathy and cesarean section: Report of two cases and literature review. Arch Gynecol Obstet 2004;270:307-310.

209. Kaufman I, Bondy R, Benjamin A: Peripartum cardiomyopathy and thromboembolism; Anesthetic management and clinical course of an obese, diabetic patient. Can J Anaesth 2003;50:161-165.

210. Shnaider R, Ezri T, Szmuk P, et al: Combined spinal-epidural anesthesia for Cesarean section in a patient with peripartum dilated cardiomyopathy. Can J Anaesth 2001;48:681-683.

211. Gambling DR, Flanagan ML, Huckell VF, et al: Anaesthetic management and non-invasive monitoring for caesarean section in a patient with cardiomyopathy. Can J Anaesth 1987;34:505-508.

212. McCarroll CP, Paxton LD, Elliott P, Wilson DB: Use of remifentanil in a patient with peripartum cardiomyopathy requiring Caesarean section. Br J Anaesth 2001;86:135-138.

213. Wake K, Takanishi T, Kitajima T, et al: [Cardiac arrest during emergency cesarean section due to peripartum cardiomyopathy—a case report]. Masui 2003;52:1089-1091. Japanese.

214. Malinow AM, Butterworth JF, Johnson MD, et al: Peripartum cardiomyopathy presenting at cesarean delivery. Anesthesiology 1985;63:545-547.

215. Morris S, Stacey M: Resuscitation in pregnancy. BMJ 2003;327:1277-1279.

216. Luppi CJ: Cardiopulmonary resuscitation in pregnancy: What all nurses caring for childbearing women need to know. AWHONN Lifelines 1999;3:41-45.

217. Guidelines 2000 for Cardiopulmonary Resuscitation and Emergency Cardiovascular Care: VIII. Advanced challenges in resuscitation: Section 3: special challenges in ECC. The American Heart Association in collaboration with the International Liaison Committee on Resuscitation. Circulation 2000;102(8 Suppl):I247-I249.

218. Keller C, Brimacombe J, Lirk P, Puhringer F: Failed obstetric tracheal intubation and postoperative respiratory support with the ProSeal laryngeal mask airway. Anesth Analg 2004;98:1467-1470, table of contents.

219. Rees GA, Willis BA: Resuscitation in late pregnancy. Anaesthesia 1988;43:347-349.

220. Goodwin AP, Pearce AJ: The human wedge: A manoeuvre to relieve aortocaval compression during resuscitation in late pregnancy. Anaesthesia 1992;47:433-434.

221. Hazinski MF, Cummins RO, Field JM, American Heart Association: 2000 Handbook of Emergency Cardiovascular Care for Healthcare Providers. Dallas, American Heart Association, 2000.

222. Nanson J, Elcock D, Williams M, Deakin CD: Do physiological changes in pregnancy change defibrillation energy requirements? Br J Anaesth 2001;87:237-239.

223. Katz VL, Dotters DJ, Droegemueller W: Perimortem cesarean delivery. Obstet Gynecol 1986;68:571-576.

224. Finegold H, Darwich A, Romeo R, et al: Successful resuscitation after maternal cardiac arrest by immediate cesarean section in the labor room. Anesthesiology 2002;96:1278.

225. Baraka A, Kawkabani N, Haroun-Bizri S: Hemodynamic deterioration after cardiopulmonary bypass during pregnancy: Resuscitation by

postoperative emergency Cesarean section. J Cardiothorac Vasc Anesth 2000;14:314-315.

226. Ilsaas C, Husby P, Koller ME, et al: Cardiac arrest due to massive pulmonary embolism following caesarean section: Successful resuscitation and pulmonary embolectomy. Acta Anaesthesiol Scand 1998;42:264-266.

227. Parker J, Balis N, Chester S, Adey D: Cardiopulmonary arrest in pregnancy: Successful resuscitation of mother and infant following immediate caesarean section in labour ward. Aust N Z J Obstet Gynaecol 1996;36:207-210.

228. Awwad JT, Azar GB, Aouad AT, et al: Postmortem cesarean section following maternal blast injury: Case report. J Trauma 1994;36:260-261.

229. Cordero DR, Toffle RC, McCauley CS: Cardiopulmonary arrest in pregnancy: The role of caesarean section in the resuscitative protocol. WV Med J 1992;88:402-403.

230. Litwin MS, Loughlin KR, Benson CB, et al: Placenta percreta invading the urinary bladder. Br J Urol 1989;64:283-286.

231. Long WB, Rosenblum S, Grady IP: Successful resuscitation of bupivacaine-induced cardiac arrest using cardiopulmonary bypass. Anesth Analg 1989;69:403-406.

232. Lau G: A case of sudden maternal death associated with resuscitative liver injury. Forensic Sci Int 1994;67:127-132.

233. Mallampalli A, Powner DJ, Gardner MO: Cardiopulmonary resuscitation and somatic support of the pregnant patient. Crit Care Clin 2004;20:747-761, x.

234. Suzuki S, Morishita S: Platelet hemostatic capacity (PHC) and fibrinolytic inhibitors during pregnancy. Semin Thromb Hemost 1998;24:449-451.

235. Carr BR, Ory H: Estrogen and progestin components of oral contraceptives: Relationship to vascular disease. Contraception 1997;55:267-272.

236. Heijboer H, Brandjes DP, Buller HR, et al: Deficiencies of coagulation-inhibiting and fibrinolytic proteins in outpatients with deep-vein thrombosis. N Engl J Med 1990;323:1512-1516.

237. Bare SN, Poka R, Balogh I, Ajzner E: Factor V Leiden as a risk factor for miscarriage and reduced fertility. Aust N Z J Obstet Gynaecol 2000;40:186-190.

238. Ray JG, Laskin CA: Folic acid and homocyst(e)ine metabolic defects and the risk of placental abruption, pre-eclampsia and spontaneous pregnancy loss: A systematic review. Placenta 1999;20:519-529.

239. Ridker PM, Miletich JP, Buring JE, et al: Factor V Leiden mutation as a risk factor for recurrent pregnancy loss. Ann Intern Med 1998;128:1000-1003.

240. Horlocker TT, Wedel DJ, Benzon H, et al: Regional anesthesia in the anticoagulated patient: Defining the risks (the second ASRA Consensus Conference on Neuraxial Anesthesia and Anticoagulation. Reg Anesth Pain Med 2003;28:172-197.

241. Bergqvist D, Wu CL, Neal JM: Anticoagulation and neuraxial regional anesthesia: perspectives (editorial). Reg Anesth Pain Med 2003;28:163-166.

242. Ginsberg JS, Chan WS, Bates SM, Kaatz S: Anticoagulation of pregnant women with mechanical heart valves. Arch Intern Med 2003;163:694-698.

243. Chan WS, Anand S, Ginsberg JS: Anticoagulation of pregnant women with mechanical heart valves: A systematic review of the literature. Arch Intern Med 2000;160:191-196.

244. Hung L, Rahimtoola SH: Prosthetic heart valves and pregnancy. Circulation 2003;107:1240-1246.

245. Ginsberg JS, Hirsh J: Use of antithrombotic agents during pregnancy. Chest 1998;114:524S-530S.

246. Rowan JA, McCowan LM, Raudkivi PJ, North RA: Enoxaparin treatment in women with mechanical heart valves during pregnancy. Am J Obstet Gynecol 2001;185:633-637.

247. Lev-Ran O, Kramer A, Gurevitch J, et al: Low-molecular-weight heparin for prosthetic heart valves: Treatment failure. Ann Thorac Surg 2000;69:264-265.

248. Ginsberg JS, Greer I, Hirsh J: Use of antithrombotic agents during pregnancy. Chest 2001;119:122S-1231S.

249. Nelson-Piercy C, Letsky EA, de Swiet M: Low-molecular-weight heparin for obstetric thromboprophylaxis: Experience of sixty-nine pregnancies in sixty-one women at high risk. Am J Obstet Gynecol 1997;176:1062-1068.

250. Morris TA: Heparin and low molecular weight heparin: Background and pharmacology. Clin Chest Med 2003;24:39-47.

251. Hirsh J, Warkentin TE, Shaughnessy SG, et al. Heparin and low-molecular-weight heparin: Mechanism of action, pharmacokinetics, dosing, monitoring, efficacy, and safety. Chest 2001;119:64S-94S.

252. Dimitrakakis C, Papageorgiou P, Papageorgiou I, et al: Absence of transplacental passage of low molecular weight heparin enoxaparin. Haemostasis 2000;30:243-248.

253. Horlocker TT, Heit JA: Low molecular weight heparin: Biochemistry, pharmacology, perioperative prophylaxis regimens, and guidelines for regional anesthetic management. Anesth Analg 1997;85:874-885.

254. White RH, Ginsberg JS: Low-molecular-weight heparins: Are they all the same? Br J Haematol 2003;121:12-20.

255. Lensing AW, Prins MH, Davidson BL, Hirsh J: Treatment of deep venous thrombosis with low-molecular weight heparins: A metaanalysis. Arch Intern Med 1995;1555:601-607.

256. Lepercq J, Conard J, Borel-Derlon A, et al. Venous thromboembolism during pregnancy: A retrospective study of enoxaparin safety in 624 pregnancies. Br J Obstet Gynecol 2001;108:1134-1140.

257. ACOG: Safety of lovenox in pregnancy. Committee opinion No. 276. American College of Obstetricians and Gynecologists. Obstet Gynecol 2002;100:845-846.

258. Aguilar D, Goldhaber SZ: Clinical uses of low-molecular-weight heparins. Chest 1999;115:1418-1423.

259. Laposata M, Green D, Van Cott EM, et al: College of American Pathologists Conference XXXI on laboratory monitoring of anticoagulant therapy: The clinical use and laboratory monitoring of low-molecular-weight heparin, danaparoid, hirudin and related compounds, and argatroban. Arch Pathol Lab Med 1998;122:799-807.

260. Casele HL, Laifer SA, Woelkers DA, Venkataramanan R: Changes in the pharmacokinetics of the low-molecular-weight heparin enoxaparin sodium during pregnancy. Am J Obstet Gynecol 1999;181:1113-1117.

261. Kitchen S: Problems in laboratory monitoring of heparin dosage. Br J Haematol 2000;111:397-406.

262. Vandermeulen EP, Van Aken H, Vermylen J: Anticoagulants and spinal-epidural anesthesia. Anesth Analg 1994;79:1165-1177.

263. Wedel DJ: Anticoagulation and regional anesthesia. Anesth Analg 2003;96:114S-1147S.

264. CLASP: A randomised trial of low-dose aspirin for the prevention and treatment of pre-eclampsia among 9364 pregnant women. CLASP (Collaborative Low-dose Aspirin Study in Pregnancy) Collaborative Group. Lancet 1994;343:619-629.

265. Horlocker TT: Complications of regional anesthesia. Anesth Analg 2004;98:S56-S63.

266. Horlocker TT, Wedel DJ: Neurologic complications of spinal and epidural anesthesia. Reg Anesth Pain Med 2000;25:83-98.

267. Sephton V, Farquharson RG, Topping J, et al: A longitudinal study of maternal dose response to low molecular weight heparin in pregnancy. Obstet Gynecol 2003;101:1307-1311.

268. Buller HR, Davidson BL, Decousus H, et al: Subcutaneous fondaparinux versus intravenous unfractionated heparin in the initial treatment of pulmonary embolism. N Engl J Med 2003;349:1695-1702.

269. Treatment of proximal deep vein thrombosis with a novel synthetic compound (SR90107A/ORG31540) with pure anti–factor Xa activity: A phase II evaluation. The Rembrandt Investigators. Circulation 2000;102:2726-2731.

270. Diuguid DL: Choosing a parenteral anticoagulant agent. N Engl J Med 2001;345:1340-1342.

271. Mertes PM, Laxenaire MC, Alla F, Groupe d'Etudes des Reactions Anaphylactoides: Anaphylactic and anaphylactoid reactions occurring during anesthesia in France in 1999-2000. Anesthesiology 2003;99:536-545.

272. Hepner DL, Castells MC: Anaphylaxis during the perioperative period. Anesth Analg 2003;97:1381-1395.

273. Morais-Almeida M, Gaspar A, Marinho S, Rosado-Pinto J: Allergy to local anesthetics of the amide group with tolerance to procaine. Allergy 2003;58:827-828.

274. Finucane BT: Allergies to local anesthetics—the real truth. Can J Anaesth 2003;50:869-874.

275. Chandler MJ, Grammer LC, Patterson R: Provocative challenge with local anesthetics in patients with a prior history of reaction. J Allergy Clin Immunol 1987;79:883-886.

276. Bernstein IL, Storms WW: Practice parameters for allergy diagnostic testing. Joint Task Force on Practice Parameters for the Diagnosis and Treatment of Asthma. The American Academy of Allergy, Asthma and Immunology and the American College of Allergy, Asthma and Immunology. Ann Allergy Asthma Immunol 1995;75:543-625.

277. Hawkins JL, Koonin LM, Palmer SK, Gibbs CP: Anesthesia-related deaths during obstetric delivery in the United States, 1979-1990. Anesthesiology 1997;86:277-284.

278. Palmer CM, Voulgaropoulos D: Management of the parturient with a history of local anesthetic allergy. Anesth Analg 1993;77:625-628.

279. Balestrieri PJ, Ferguson JE 2nd: Management of a parturient with a history of local anesthetic allergy. Anesth Analg 2003;96:1489-1490.

280. Hepner DL, Castells MC, Tsen LC: Should local anesthetic allergy testing be routinely performed during pregnancy? Anesth Analg 2003;97:1853-1854.

20 The Geriatric Patient

FREDERICK E. SIEBER, MD, and JIAN HANG, MD, PHD

Poliomyelitis

Huntington's Chorea (Huntington's Disease)

Zenker's Diverticulum

Amyloidosis

Acute Mesenteric Ischemia

Idiopathic Pulmonary Fibrosis

Polycythemia Vera

Essential Thrombocythemia

Myeloid Metaplasia with Myelofibrosis

Elderly surgical patients are subject to many of the same rare diseases seen in younger populations. The focus in this chapter is on several uncommon diseases that are more unique to aged individuals.

POLIOMYELITIS

Poliomyelitis was common in the western world until the early 1960s. The disease has three distinct stages: acute poliomyelitis, recovery period, and stable disability. The acute disease is no longer a threat to most countries of the world thanks to the effort for worldwide eradication initiated by the World Health Organization (WHO) in 1988. The number of cases of poliomyelitis worldwide has dropped drastically from more than 350,000 per year in over 125 countries in 1988 to affecting fewer than 1,000 children in three countries in 2003. Currently, the epidemic areas are limited to five regions in India, Nigeria, and Pakistan. The Americas have been polio free since 1991. It is estimated, however, that there are 250,000[1] to 300,000[2] survivors of poliomyelitis in the United States. The long-term effects and late sequelae of poliomyelitis have attracted attention recently as new-onset muscle weakness has been reported in survivors of polio many years after their initial illness.

Pathophysiology. Acute poliomyelitis (infantile paralysis) is a viral infection caused by poliovirus, a positive single-stranded RNA enterovirus (picornavirus) that is transmitted via the orofecal route. The virus has a predilection for the motor neurons of the anterior horn gray matter in the cervical and lumbar spinal cord, which can result in neuron injury or death. The damage or death of the motor neurons in the spinal cord results in wallerian degeneration of the axons and myelin. The associated muscle fibers become denervated and paralyzed, resulting in acute paralytic poliomyelitis. Worldwide vaccination efforts with oral polio vaccine (OPV) have drastically decreased the number of acute paralytic poliomyelitis cases.

History and Physical Findings Consistent with Diagnosis. The vast majority of infected individuals remain asymptomatic or experience a self-limited illness. The clinical features of acute polio are listed in Table 20-1. The muscles may be tender to palpation; tremors and muscle weakness may appear. Paralysis can occur at any time during the febrile period if the virus crosses the blood-brain barrier, attacking neurons in the brain, brainstem, and spinal cord.

Paralytic polio is classified into two forms: spinal polio and bulbar polio (Table 20-2). Spinal polio is the most common type and involves damage to the motor neurons of the spinal cord. It is characterized by asymmetrical, flaccid paralysis of muscles, primarily in the lower limbs. Bulbar polio involves damage to neurons in the reticular formation and the nuclei of cranial nerves in the brain stem. Life-threatening respiratory failure, autonomic dysfunction, and cardiac arrhythmias may occur when bulbar polio involves the autonomic nuclei of the respiratory center.

Recovery Period from Acute Poliomyelitis. In those patients who survive the acute illness, slow partial recovery of muscle strength occurs as a result of several physiologic processes, including terminal sprouting, myofiber hypertrophy, fiber type transformation, and ongoing denervation and reinnervation. The process can last over several months to years. The muscle may regain up to 80% of its strength in

TABLE 20–1   Acute Poliomyelitis

Clinical Features

Fever
Headache
Vomiting
Lethargy
Irritability
Neck, back, abdominal and extremity pain
Muscle spasm

Residual Complications

Muscle paresis and paralysis
Skeletal deformities
Joint contractures
Movement disability
Growth retardation of affected limb
Osteoporosis and pain from wear and tear
Compression neuropathy
Venous stasis
Chronic colonic distention
Respiratory insufficiency
Cold intolerance

TABLE 20–2   Classification of Paralytic Poliomyelitis

Spinal Poliomyelitis

Most common
Spinal motor neurons
Asymmetrical flaccid paralysis of extremity muscles, more
  commonly of the lower limbs than upper limbs and trunk

Bulbar Poliomyelitis

Less common
Reticular formation
The nuclei of cranial nerves
Facial weakness
Weakness of the sternocleidomastoid and trapezius muscles
Pharyngolaryngeal airway muscles
Dysphagia, dysphonia, nasal voice, regurgitation
Difficulty in chewing and inability to swallow or expel saliva
  and secretion
Involvement of autonomic nuclei
Respiratory failure
Autonomic dysfunction
Cardiac arrhythmia

the first 6 months, and further improvement may continue over the next 2 years. There are many possible residual complications of acute poliomyelitis (see Table 20-1).

The Late Effects of Poliomyelitis. Paralytic poliomyelitis has been eradicated from the western world for decades. Only polio survivors with late effects might be encountered in our practice. Numerous risk factors are associated with the development of late effects (Table 20-3). There is no consensus on specific diagnostic criteria for this disease entity. Late effects of poliomyelitis refer to a diffuse group of symptoms (see Table 20-3).[3] The diagnosis is generally considered in paralytic polio survivors of many years who develop new-onset cluster of symptoms consistent with the disease after excluding relevant medical, orthopedic, and neurologic conditions.[4]

Preoperative Preparation. Polio survivors should be specifically questioned concerning any new onset or increased muscle weakness, muscle pain, or fatigue. New weakness has been reported to occur in 20% to 60% of polio survivors. The time period between acute polio and the onset of late effects has ranged from 8 to 71 years, with an average interval of 35 years. Patients with a history of polio who appear normal with good muscle strength clinically may have significant underlying denervation when tested with electromyography, which should be considered in all patients with prior history of polio to determine the severity of denervation.

Scoliosis, thoracic kyphosis, and deformed thoracic cage, along with muscle weakness, are very common in polio patients. New respiratory difficulties have been reported in 27% to 58% of subjects in surveys of late effects

of poliomyelitis. Thus, comprehensive pulmonary evaluation, optimization of pulmonary function, and treatment of any pulmonary infections should be accomplished before surgery. Post-polio patients have a high incidence of sleep disturbances such as obstructive sleep apnea and/or central sleep apnea. Pulmonary hypertension may also exist secondary to chronic hypoxemia, hypercapnia, or obstructive sleep apnea.

Polio survivors may have increasing difficulty performing their daily activities as the result of respiratory insufficiency, muscle weakness and pain, deformity, and/or coexisting cardiac diseases. In addition, information concerning chronic use of pain medicines should be sought.

Preoperative assessment of cognitive function in people with a history of polio is important. Cognitive problems reported by polio survivors suggest that the fatigue experienced cannot be explained merely by damage to the anterior horn motor neurons but may be related to changes and loss of brain activating system neurons that survive the acute polio infection.

Perioperative Considerations. A potentially difficult airway should be anticipated, especially in patients with chest deformity, scoliosis, thoracic kyphosis, or obstructive sleep apnea. Respiratory insufficiency and secondary muscle weakness, along with difficulty in clearing secretions, will make respiratory management challenging. Cautious extubation should be practiced in patients with obstructive or central sleep apnea. If a prior polio patient suffered cardiac disease, whether it is primary or secondary to polio, appropriate anesthetic techniques should be employed based on the cardiac status.

TABLE 20–3   Late Effects of Poliomyelitis
Risk Factors
Age at onset
Severity of paralysis
Use of ventilator
Hospitalization
Years of acute polio infection
Gender
Polio to post-polio interval
Current age
Functional recovery
Residual impairment
Weight gain
Presence of muscle pain associated with exercise
Signs and Symptoms
Muscle pain, weakness, and atrophy
Joint pain
Musculoskeletal imbalance
Skeletal deformities
Growth retardation
Compression neuropathy
Degenerative arthritis
Repetitive motion problems
Respiratory insufficiency
Dysphagia
Speech difficulty
Fatigue
Sleep impairment
Cold intolerance
Difficulties with activities of daily living

Affected muscles have varying degrees of denervation. Therefore, succinylcholine should be used with caution because of the risk of massive potassium release after depolarization. The pharmacology of nondepolarizing muscle relaxants may be unpredictable owing to neuromuscular junction transmission defects and muscle atrophy. Nondepolarizing muscle relaxants appear to have increased potency in poliomyelitis survivors.[5]

Prior polio patients often suffer cold intolerance. Vigilant efforts should be made to preserve heat and maintain patient's body temperature, especially during general anesthesia.

HUNTINGTON'S CHOREA (HUNTINGTON'S DISEASE)

Huntington's chorea is a rare, autosomal dominant, inherited degenerative disorder of the nervous system. It was first described by George Huntington in 1872. Its incidence is 5 to 10/100,000. It is characterized by the clinical hallmarks of progressive chorea and dementia. The onset is usually in the fourth or fifth decade of life, but there is a wide range in age at onset, from childhood to late life (>75 years). Symptoms appear to progressively worsen with age.

Pathophysiology. Huntington's disease is an autosomal dominant disorder with complete penetrance. The Huntington's disease gene, *IT15,* is located on chromosome 4p, contains CAG-trinucleotide repeats, and codes for a protein called huntingtin. The protein is found in neurons throughout the brain; its normal function is unknown. Transgenic mice with an expanded CAG repeat in the Huntington's disease gene develop a progressive movement disorder.

Huntington's disease is a basal ganglia disease, with caudate and putamen being the regions most severely affected. The most significant neuropathologic change is a preferential loss of medium spiny neurons in the neostriatum. Neurochemically, there is a marked decrease of γ-aminobutyric acid (GABA) and its synthetic enzyme glutamic acid decarboxylase throughout the basal ganglia, as well as reductions of other neurotransmitters such as substance P and enkephalin. The movement disorder is slowly progressive and may eventually become disabling.

Diagnosis. The DNA repeat expansion forms the basis of a diagnostic blood test for the disease gene. Persons having 38 or more CAG repeats in the Huntington's disease gene have inherited the disease mutation and will eventually develop symptoms if they live to an advanced age. Each of their children has a 50% risk of also inheriting the abnormal gene. There is a rough correlation between a larger number of repeats and an earlier age at onset.

Huntington's can also be diagnosed by caudate atrophy on magnetic resonance imaging in the context of an appropriate clinical history.

Differential Diagnosis. Differential diagnosis of Huntington's disease includes other choreas, hepatocerebral degeneration, schizophrenia with tardive dyskinesia, Parkinson's disease, Alzheimer's disease, and other primary dementias and drug reactions.

Preoperative Preparation. Even though memory in patients suffering from Huntington's disease is frequently not impaired until late in the disease, attention, judgment, awareness, and executive functions may be seriously deficient at an early stage. Depression, apathy, social withdrawal, irritability, fidgeting, and intermittent disinhibition are common. Delusions and obsessive-compulsive behavior may occur. These signs, along with poor articulation of speech, make preoperative evaluation and obtaining consent arduous tasks. Characteristic choreoathetoid movements, plus frequent, irregular, sudden jerks and movements of any of the limbs or trunk make physical examination, as well as regional anesthesia, difficult to perform.

Cachexia and frailty may be observed in the elderly Huntington's patient. Pharyngeal muscle involvement leads to dysphagia and makes these patients susceptible to pulmonary aspiration.[6] Before elective surgery, it is important to rule out ongoing aspiration pneumonitis or pneumonia by careful physical examination and chest radiography.

Chronic Medications for Condition. There is no specific treatment to stop progression of the disease, but the movements and behavioral changes may partially respond to phenothiazines, haloperidol, benzodiazepines, or olanzapine. Selective serotonin reuptake inhibitors may help with associated depression.

Perioperative Considerations. Major concerns in anesthetic management of Huntington's disease are potential difficult airway, sleep apnea, risk of aspiration, and altered reactions to various drugs. A difficult airway may result from a rigid, stiff, unstable posture with hyperextension of the neck. Sleep apnea may also be present.

It is controversial whether the pharmacology of anesthetic agents is altered in Huntington's disease. Authors have reported a decrease in plasma cholinesterase activity and a prolonged effect of succinylcholine.[7] In addition, there may be an exaggerated response to sodium thiopental[8] or midazolam.[9] On the other hand, both thiopental[10] and succinylcholine[10,11] have been used safely in Huntington's patients. Other agents that have been used safely include propofol[12] and sevoflurane.[10] The safety profile and pharmacokinetics of the nondepolarizing muscle relaxants mivacurium and rocuronium are similar to those in patients without Huntington's disease.[10,13,14]

It is generally recommended that rapid-sequence or modified rapid-sequence induction with cricoid pressure be used for induction of general anesthesia in these patients. Other authors suggested using a total intravenous anesthesia technique to reduce the risk of postoperative shivering related to inhalational agents so as to avoid the precipitation of generalized tonic spasms.

Summary. Huntington's chorea is an inherited disease characterized by choreoathetosis, rigidity, and dementia that is most commonly seen in late life. Patients suffering from Huntington's disease are at higher risk of intraoperative complications, including pulmonary aspiration, altered anesthetic pharmacology, and worsening generalized tonic spasms. Rapid-sequence induction with cricoid pressure is recommended for induction of general anesthesia in these patients.

ZENKER'S DIVERTICULUM

Zenker's diverticulum is an outpouching of the pharyngoesophageal mucosa in the natural zone of weakness of the posterior hypopharyngeal wall (Killian's triangle), between the inferior pharyngeal constrictor muscle and the cricopharyngeus muscle (upper esophageal sphincter). It always occurs above and never below the cricopharyngeus muscle. Its incidence is estimated to range from 0.01% to 0.11% of the population. Zenker's diverticulum is rare in patients younger than 30 years of age, with a peak incidence in the seventh to ninth decades. The prevalence is similar in Europe and the United States. It is rarely reported in the Middle and Far East.

Pathophysiology. The etiology of Zenker's diverticulum is not completely understood. The formation of pharyngoesophageal mucosa is thought to result from asynchronous coordination of the cricopharyngeus muscle during swallowing. Over time, the increased pressure causes herniation of the mucosa posteriorly through the single sheet of the thyropharyngeus (the dehiscence of Killian) between thyropharyngeus muscle and cricopharyngeus muscle.

Diagnosis/Differential Diagnosis. The signs and symptoms of Zenker's diverticulum are shown in Table 20-4. Most patients (98%) present with some degree of dysphagia, combined with regurgitation of undigested food particles. In this clinical context the differential diagnosis is mainly limited to Zenker's diverticulum and achalasia. Although the diverticulum can reach a size of 15 cm or more, it is rarely palpable. The diagnostic procedure of choice is barium swallow. Endoscopy is indicated to exclude neoplasia if the contrast study shows esophageal mucosal irregularities. Coexistent hiatal hernia, esophageal spasm, achalasia, and esophagogastroduodenal ulceration are common.

Perioperative Considerations. The surgical procedure of choice in patients with symptomatic Zenker's diverticulum is cricopharyngeus myotomy. The surgery for Zenker's diverticulum can be done under general anesthesia as well as local or regional anesthesia. Local or regional anesthesia may facilitate the identification of the diverticulum intraoperatively and may reduce the mean postoperative stay, although no statistical difference has been demonstrated between different anesthetic techniques.[15]

The most important anesthetic complication that occurs in these patients is pulmonary aspiration.[16,17] Preoperative fasting is important, although it does not

TABLE 20-4   Signs and Symptoms of Zenker's Diverticulum
Dysphagia
Odynophagia
Halitosis and regurgitation of undigested food
Noisy deglutition
Weight loss
Poor nutrition
Pulmonary complications, such as aspiration and pneumonia

guarantee an empty pouch. Surgery should be delayed if foreign bodies, food, or barium is known to be present in the diverticulum, and a reasonable time should be allowed for the material to be expelled. Oral premedication should be avoided. Because the contents of the pouch have an alkaline pH, the use of antacids or H2 blockers, such as sodium citrate or ranitidine, have no value. Manually emptying the contents of the diverticulum by exerting external pressure over the pouch before induction is the most important and effective maneuver to ensure decreased pressure within the pouch. Inserting a gastric tube should probably be avoided, because it may lead to the perforation of the diverticulum.

Patients with Zenker's diverticulum should be placed in a head-up position of 10 to 30 degrees to decrease the likelihood of regurgitation. Rapid-sequence induction *without* cricoid pressure should be used. Cricoid pressure during induction may not prevent regurgitation of diverticular contents and may even promote regurgitation because the diverticulum is above the cricopharyngeus muscle whereas the cricoid ring is below the neck of the diverticulum.[18] Intraoperatively, a moist gauze pack may be placed around the endotracheal tube to prevent aspiration.

Aspiration may still happen postoperatively,[18] and caution should be taken to maintain minimal sedation and a semi-sitting position when nursing the patient.

Summary. Zenker's diverticulum carries a high risk of aspiration during surgical correction. Manual emptying of the sac is an important preoperative maneuver in these patients. General anesthesia should be induced using a rapid-sequence intubation without cricoid pressure, with the patient positioned in a head-up tilt of 10 to 30 degrees. Aspiration precautions should also be taken postoperatively.

AMYLOIDOSIS

Amyloidosis results from the deposition of insoluble, fibrillar proteins (amyloid), mainly in the extracellular spaces of organs and tissues in amounts sufficient to impair normal function. Amyloid fibrils can be deposited locally or may involve virtually every organ system of the body. Symptoms and signs depend on the organs and tissues involved.

Pathophysiology. The cause of amyloid production and its deposition in tissues is unknown. All amyloid fibrils share an identical secondary structure, the β-pleated sheet conformation. The polypeptide backbone of these protein precursors assume similar fibrillar morphologies that render them resistant to proteolysis. The amyloidoses have been classified into 18 subtypes[19] based on the amyloid protein involved. The name of the amyloidosis subtype uses the capital letter A as the first letter of designation and is followed by the protein designation. Three major types of amyloid and several less common forms have been defined biochemically.

Whether an amyloidosis is systemic or localized (organ limited) depends on the biochemical structure of the amyloid protein. Systemic amyloidoses include biochemically distinct forms that are neoplastic, inflammatory, genetic, or iatrogenic, whereas localized or organ-limited amyloidoses are associated with aging and diabetes and occur in isolated organs, often endocrine, without evidence of systemic involvement. Despite their biochemical differences, the various amyloidoses share common pathophysiologic features (Table 20-5).

Three major systemic clinical forms are currently recognized: primary or idiopathic (AL), secondary amyloidosis (AA), and hereditary amyloidosis (Table 20-6). The most common form of systemic amyloidosis seen in current clinical practice is AL (light-chain amyloidosis, primary idiopathic amyloidosis, or that associated with multiple myeloma).

Diagnosis/Differential Diagnosis. Symptoms and signs vary depending on the involved systems and organs. The nephritic syndrome is the most striking early manifestation. The renal lesion is usually not reversible and progressively leads to azotemia and death.

Regardless of etiology, the clinical diagnosis of amyloidosis is usually not made until the disease is far advanced because of nonspecific symptoms and signs of the disease. The diagnosis is made by identification of amyloid fibrils in biopsy or necropsy tissue sections using Congo red stain. A unique protein (member of the pentraxin family of proteins) called AP (or serum AP) is universally associated with all forms of amyloid and forms the basis of a diagnostic test. Once amyloidosis is diagnosed, it can be further classified by genomic DNA, protein, and immunohistochemical studies; the relationship of immunoglobulin-related amyloid to multiple myeloma should be confirmed by electrophoretic and immunoelectrophoretic studies.

Preoperative Preparation. A comprehensive survey of all systems should be performed, focusing on the most frequently involved organs. Careful evaluation for systemic involvement of amyloidosis or associated disease is important even in apparently isolated tumorous amyloidosis (Table 20-7).

Chronic Medications/Treatment for Condition. Treatment of localized amyloid tumors is surgical excision. However, there is no effective treatment of systemic amyloidosis. Current care is generally supportive, and therapy is directed at reducing production and promoting lysis of amyloid fibrils. Hemodialysis and immunosuppressive therapy may be useful. Current treatment of primary amyloidosis

---

TABLE 20–5   Amyloidosis: Multisystem Involvement and Clinical Manifestations

System	Clinical Features
Nervous System	
Polyneuropathy	Sensory loss; carpal tunnel syndrome; myopathy; myelopathy; vitreous opacities
Autonomic neuropathy	Postural hypotension; inability to sweat; sphincter incompetence
Respiratory System	
Upper respiratory tract	Localized tumor can be found in respiratory tracts and lungs
Nasal sinuses, larynx, and trachea	Tracheobronchial lesions, or diffuse alveolar deposits
Tongue	Macroglossia
Lower respiratory tract and lung parenchyma	Accumulation of amyloid which block the ducts; may resemble a neoplasm
Heart	
Conduction system	Arrhythmia, heart block
Endocardium and valves	Valvular diseases
Myocardium	Cardiomyopathy: dilated, restrictive and obstructive forms, congestive heart failure
Pericardium	Pericarditis
Gastrointestinal System	
Liver	Hepatomegaly; abnormal liver functions; portal hypertension
Gastrointestinal tract	Unexplained gastrointestinal diseases, malabsorption; unexplained diarrhea or constipation; obstruction, ulceration and protein loss; esophageal motility disorders
Kidney	Nephrotic syndrome, proteinuria, renal failure; renal tubular acidosis or renal vein thrombosis
Spleen	Spleen enlargement; not associated with leukopenia and anemia
Musculoskeletal System	Pseudomyopathy; cystic bone lesions
Endocrine System	
Thyroid gland	Hypothyroidism; full-blown myxedema (almost invariably accompanies medullary carcinoma of thyroid)
Adrenal gland	Type II diabetes
Pituitary gland, pancreas	Other endocrine abnormalities
Skin	Lichen amyloidosis; papules; plaques; ecchymoses
Hematologic System	Fibrinogenopenia including fibrinolysis
Endothelial damage	Selective deficiency of clotting factors (factor X) Clotting abnormalities, abnormal bleeding time
Other	Rheumatoid arthritis, chronic inflammation and infection

---

includes a program of prednisone/melphalan or prednisone/melphalan/colchicine. Liver transplantation, kidney transplantation, and stem cell transplants have yielded some promising results. In certain heredofamilial amyloidoses, genetic counseling is an important aspect of treatment. Ultimately some people with amyloidosis continue to deteriorate. The major causes of death are heart disease and renal failure. Sudden death, presumably due to arrhythmias, is common.

Perioperative Considerations. Localized amyloid deposition has been reported at various sites. Amyloid in the tongue can cause macroglossia to a degree requiring glossectomy.[20] In addition, amyloid macroglossia may be associated with coexisting hypothyroidism.[21] Laryngeal amyloidosis is fragile and carries the risk of spontaneous massive hemorrhage

even without manipulation.[22] The airway tumor should be assessed by noninvasive imaging, such as computed tomography (CT) or magnetic resonance imaging. Prior to intubation, preparations should be made for both difficult airway and massive hemorrhage.

A smaller endotracheal tube may be considered. In addition, direct laryngoscopy monitored by a fiberscope-video system, rather than blind insertion of the endotracheal tube through vocal cords over a fiberoptic bronchoscope,[23] has been advocated.

It is controversial whether depolarizing muscle relaxants should be administered to patients with amyloidosis, especially those with cardiac involvement. Patients with familial amyloid polyneuropathy have a high incidence of cardiac arrhythmias during anesthesia. It has been hypothesized that exaggerated elevations in potassium

TABLE 20–6	Major Systemic Amyloidosis: Clinical Features and Diagnosis		
Type	**Primary (AL) (or Idiopathic)**	**Secondary (AA) (or Secondary, Acquired, Reactive)**	**Hereditary**
Commonly Involved Organs	Localized amyloid tumors may be found in the respiratory tract. Vascular system, especially the heart, is involved frequently. Other organs may also involved: tongue, thyroid gland, heart, lung, liver, intestinal tract, spleen, kidney and skin.	Spleen, liver, kidney, adrenal glands, lymph nodes and vascular involvement occurs. No organ is spared, but significant involvement of the heart is rare.	Peripheral sensory and motor neuropathy, often autonomic neuropathy Carpal tunnel syndrome Vitreous abnormalities Cardiovascular and renal amyloid
Associated Diseases	Multiple myeloma	Infection (tuberculosis, bronchiectasis, osteomyelitis, leprosy) Inflammation (rheumatoid arthritis, granulomatous ileitis) Familial Mediterranean fever Tumors such as Hodgkin's disease	
Diagnosis	Monoclonal immunoglobulin in urine or serum plus any of the following: macroglossia; cardiomyopathy; hepatomegaly; malabsorption or unexplained diarrhea or constipation; unexplained nephrotic syndrome; carpal tunnel syndrome; or peripheral neuropathy	Chronic infection (osteomyelitis, tuberculosis), chronic inflammation (rheumatoid arthritis, granulomatous ileitis) plus any of the following: hepatomegaly, unexplained gastrointestinal disease, or proteinuria	Family history of neuropathy plus any of the following: early sensorimotor disassociation, vitreous opacities, cardiovascular disease, gastrointestinal disease, autonomic neuropathy, or renal disease

concentrations occur after succinylcholine administration and may be a contributing factor.[24] However, Viana and associates[25] reported that the average increase in plasma potassium concentrations after succinylcholine administration in patients with familial amyloid polyneuropathy was similar to the increase observed in a normal population by others. However, the authors could not exclude that a dangerous rise in serum potassium concentration might not occur in a certain percentage of patients with familial amyloid after administration of succinylcholine. This may also be true in patients with amyloidosis who also suffer from long-standing polyneuropathy.[26] Thus, it may be prudent to avoid administration of depolarizing muscle relaxants in patients with amyloidosis, especially in the presence of coexisting polyneuropathy and/or cardiac disease.

Autonomic dysfunction secondary to amyloidosis has dramatic perioperative ramifications.[25] In particular, the administration of anesthetic drugs to patients with amyloidotic polyneuropathy presents a risk of significant hypotension (even use of ketamine does not prevent hypotension). Patients with decreased preload are especially sensitive. In addition, hypotension is frequent even in patients with adequate preload as a result of low systemic vascular resistance. Given these observations, one should consider using invasive blood pressure monitoring and preparation of a vasoconstrictor infusion for effective anesthetic management of these patients.

ACUTE MESENTERIC ISCHEMIA

Acute mesenteric ischemia primarily results from reduction of arterial blood supply and carries with it a high morbidity and mortality. Table 20-8 shows the subclassifications of this disease. Occlusion accounts for about 75% of acute mesenteric ischemia, which is a disease of the elderly; the median age of patients presenting with mesenteric arterial embolism is 70 years. The exact etiology of nonocclusive mesenteric ischemia is unclear. However, splanchnic vasoconstriction and reduced blood flow to the splanchnic bed have been proposed as possible mechanisms after initial insults such as shock, sepsis, hemorrhage, cardiac decompensation, or other conditions with profound physiologic stress (Table 20-9). Mesenteric venous thrombosis is seen primarily in younger patients.

Diagnosis. Early diagnosis is often difficult because symptoms and signs are few, nonspecific, and unreliable and the

TABLE 20–7   Amyloidosis: Preoperative Assessment and Workup

Nervous System	Peripheral neuropathy: document preexisting peripheral neurologic symptoms Autonomic neuropathy: orthostatic blood pressure, etc.
Airway	Macroglossia
Pulmonary	Diffuse dysfunction: pulmonary function tests
Cardiac	Arrhythmia, cardiomyopathy, and valvular involvement: cardiac function echocardiogram and electrocardiogram
Gastrointestinal	Esophageal motility abnormality, intestinal obstruction
Liver	Liver function tests
Kidney	Abnormal renal function: electrolytes, renal function tests
Hematology	Enlarged spleen, check complete blood cell count: red blood cells, platelet, coagulation coagulopathy, and factor deficiency
Endocrine	Pancreatic or adrenal gland involvement; thyroid function test to rule out hypothyroidism

severity of the objective findings is disproportionate to patient symptoms.

In addition, the differential diagnosis encompasses many acute abdominal processes. Definitive diagnosis is made by angiography in suspected patients presenting with sudden onset of severe, poorly localized periumbilical pain associated with fever, nausea, vomiting, and diarrhea.

Treatment. Early operative treatment to reestablish blood flow by removing the embolus, bypassing the thrombosis, and resecting nonviable intestine is the key to a successful outcome. Many patients are poor surgical candidates owing to advanced age, hemodynamic instability, metabolic derangement, and sepsis. Angiography has been used as a therapeutic maneuver. Papaverine, a potent local vasodilator, can be selectively infused as a temporizing measure while surgical decisions are being deliberated.

The primary treatment of nonocclusive mesenteric ischemia is pharmacologic. Most experience has been reported with papaverine delivered by selective catheter placed by an interventional radiologist.

Preoperative Preparation. Acute mesenteric ischemia is a true medical and surgical emergency and requires vigorous resuscitation. Patients with acute mesenteric ischemia lose substantial amounts of protein-rich fluid into the gut. Aggressive fluid resuscitation should be ongoing and guided by urine output, central venous pressure, and pulmonary artery catheter in the setting of a history of cardiac disease. Invasive blood pressure monitoring is indicated for hemodynamic instability.

The goal of fluid resuscitation is to maintain blood pressure without pharmacologic support, because many vasopressors further aggravate mesenteric ischemia. Norepinephrine and phenylephrine are particularly deleterious. Dopamine may act as a mesenteric vasodilator at low doses and produce less severe mesenteric vasoconstriction. Digitalis is also a well-recognized mesenteric vasoconstrictor. The stomach should be decompressed via nasogastric tube to promote intestinal perfusion and minimize risk of aspiration. Anticoagulation should be stopped preoperatively.

Perioperative Management. Vigorous fluid resuscitation should be continued intraoperatively, including use of blood products and electrolyte-rich fluid. Metabolic abnormalities should be corrected and arrhythmias treated accordingly.

Sepsis is common in patients with acute mesenteric ischemia, and broad-spectrum antibiotics should be continued intraoperatively. One must be on the alert for the development of multiple organ system failure (see Table 20-9).

If appropriate, total parenteral nutrition should be initiated as soon as possible postoperatively. Despite aggressive surgical and medical treatment, acute mesenteric ischemia has an overall mortality rate in excess of 60%.[27]

IDIOPATHIC PULMONARY FIBROSIS

Idiopathic pulmonary fibrosis is also known as fibrosing alveolitis, alveolocapillary block, cryptogenic fibrosing alveolitis, diffuse fibrosing alveolitis, Hamman-Rich syndrome, or interstitial diffuse pulmonary fibrosis.

Pathophysiology. The pathophysiology of idiopathic pulmonary fibrosis is not currently understood. It may represent a model of chronic dysregulated repair and lung remodeling, resulting from an epithelial/endothelial insult and persistent inflammatory cell activation.[28] The initial injury event remains undefined. However, evidence has suggested that viral infections or environmental factors may provide mediating events. Interestingly, a majority of patients with idiopathic pulmonary fibrosis have a smoking history. Current theories suggest that ongoing epithelial cell damage and/or inflammation produces abnormal mesenchymal cell activation. With activation, the phenotype of mesenchymal cells may be altered, for example from fibroblast to myofibroblast. In addition, activation of mesenchymal cells leads to enhanced matrix production and deposition. The end stage of pulmonary fibrosis is the culmination of this abnormal wound healing process

TABLE 20–8	Acute Mesenteric Ischemia: Clinical Profile			
	Incidence (%)	Age	Risk Factors	Mortality
Occlusive mesenteric ischemia				
Thrombosis	50	Elderly	Systemic atherosclerosis Malignancy Coagulation disorders	Very high
Embolism	25	Elderly	Recent myocardial infarction Congestive heart failure Arrhythmias Rheumatic fever Valvular diseases	High
Nonocclusive mesenteric ischemia	20	Elderly	Hospitalization Cardiogenic shock Hypotension Congestive heart failure Hemorrhage Cardiopulmonary bypass Sepsis Burns Pancreatitis Vasopressors and digitalis	Highest
Mesenteric venous thrombosis	5	Younger	Hypercoagulability Portal hypertension Inflammation Prior surgery Trauma	Lowest

involving an ongoing interaction between epithelium and mesenchymal cells.

History and Physical Findings Consistent with Diagnosis.
Symptoms associated with idiopathic pulmonary fibrosis (Table 20-10) include breathlessness, fatigue, weight loss, and a chronic dry cough. On physical examination dry "Velcro" crackles may be heard throughout the lung fields. Cyanosis and clubbing may also be observed. As the disease progresses, signs of pulmonary hypertension and right-sided heart failure (loud S2 heart sound, right ventricular heave, or pedal edema) may be present.

Laboratory tests are important in making a diagnosis. A chest radiograph may show interstitial infiltrates in the lung bases. CT is more sensitive than a chest radiograph for detecting disease early. Typically, CT shows a pattern of patchy white lines in the lower lungs. In areas of more severe involvement, the thick scarring often creates a honeycombing appearance. Pulmonary function tests show a restrictive pattern. Arterial blood gas analysis may show hypoxemia with minimal exercise and, as the disease progresses, even at rest. However, the definitive test to confirm diagnosis is lung biopsy.

Differential Diagnosis. The diagnosis of idiopathic pulmonary fibrosis should be reserved for patients with a specific type of fibrosing interstitial pneumonia known as usual interstitial pneumonia. Foremost in the differential diagnosis is to distinguish usual interstitial pneumonia from other idiopathic interstitial pneumonias. This distinction is made on a pathologic basis.[29]

Numerous other disease processes may lead to pulmonary fibrosis and should be ruled out as diagnoses. Fibroses may occur as a result of occupational or environmental exposure to toxic substances, lung infection, drug exposure, connective tissue disease, and sarcoidosis.

Comorbidities Commonly Seen with Condition. Idiopathic pulmonary fibrosis may be associated with respiratory failure and chronic hypoxemia in the later stages of the disease. Polycythemia also occurs in this context. Cor pulmonale should be specifically sought for in evaluation of these patients. There is an increased incidence of bronchogenic carcinoma with this disease.

Critical Questions to Ask Patient and/or Primary Care Physician. The critical questions to ask the patient and/or family doctor should be focused on determining how advanced the disease has become and how much pulmonary reserve is present (see Table 20-10). In appropriate patients, one should assess for the long-term complications of corticosteroid administration.

TABLE 20–9 Acute Mesenteric Ischemia

Contributing Factors	*Occlusive mesenteric ischemia:* advancing age, hypertension, peripheral vascular disease, recent myocardial infarction, congestive heart failure, low flow states, atrial fibrillation *Nonocclusive mesenteric ischemia:* congestive heart failure, systemic hypotension, hemorrhagic blood loss, sepsis and endotoxemia, digitalis and pressor use, dehydration can be contributing factors.
Differential Diagnosis	Primary gastrointestinal disease (peptic ulcer disease, bowel obstruction, diverticulitis, colon cancer, appendicitis, hernia) Hepatic diseases Biliary (cholecystitis) Pancreas (pancreatitis) Renal (pyelonephritis) Urinary (cystitis, bladder obstruction) Vascular emergency (leaking aneurysm) Other (psoas abscess, abdominal wall hematoma)
Preoperative Preparation	Perform aggressive fluid resuscitation. Establish hemodynamic monitoring and intravenous access. Wean off aggravating pressors (e.g., norepinephrine and phenylephrine). Switch to less offensive pressor such as dopamine. Discontinue digitalis. Decompress intestinal tract by placement of nasogastric tube. Initiate broad-spectrum antibiotics.
Multisystem Failure in Severe Acute Mesenteric Ischemia	Cardiac (myocardial infarction, congestive heart failure, arrhythmia) Pulmonary (respiratory failure, pneumonia, acute respiratory distress syndrome) Liver (hepatic dysfunction) Renal (renal failure) Gastrointestinal (recurrent ischemia, bleeding) Coagulation (coagulopathy)

List of Chronic Medications for Condition. At present, the therapeutic options available to treat idiopathic pulmonary fibrosis are limited (see Table 20-10). Many patients receive corticosteroids or immunosuppressants despite the fact that no studies have clearly documented their efficacy. The same is true of colchicine. Many patients require home oxygen.

Perioperative Considerations. Typical surgical procedures where one may encounter idiopathic pulmonary fibrosis include open or thoracoscopic lung biopsy and lung transplantation. In these procedures, one-lung ventilation is often required. Therefore, the major anesthetic consideration is the inability to tolerate one-lung ventilation secondary to hypoxemia or the generation of high airway pressures.[30] In addition, hypercapnia may occur in these patients during one-lung ventilation.[31] An arterial catheter is indicated when anesthetizing these patients, because frequent blood gas studies may be required. In addition, central venous access should be strongly considered.

These patients may generate large negative intrathoracic pressures during spontaneous ventilation. Therefore, special care must be taken to prevent air emboli during placement of the central line. Access to inhaled nitric oxide should be available for patients with cor pulmonale.[32]

In patients with limited pulmonary reserve, regional or local anesthesia should be considered if the surgical procedure permits.

Summary. Idiopathic pulmonary fibrosis is characterized by an exaggerated fibroproliferative response, ultimately leading to the end point of pulmonary fibrosis. Symptoms associated with idiopathic pulmonary fibrosis include breathlessness, fatigue, weight loss, and a chronic dry cough. A chest radiograph may show interstitial infiltrates in the lung bases. Pulmonary function tests show a restrictive pattern. Arterial blood gas analysis may show hypoxemia with minimal exercise and, as the disease progresses, even when the person is resting. Anesthetic evaluation and plan should be focused on determining how advanced the disease has become and how much pulmonary reserve is present.

POLYCYTHEMIA VERA

Pathophysiology. Polycythemia vera is a clonal stem cell disorder in which all three myeloid components are involved. Erythrocytosis is the foremost expression of the disease. Studies suggest that impaired signaling of hematopoietic growth factors may be an underlying pathophysiologic mechanism of polycythemia vera.

TABLE 20–10	Idiopathic Pulmonary Fibrosis
Symptoms	Breathlessness; dry cough; weight loss; fatigue
Physical Findings	Change in shape of fingers and toenails (clubbing); cyanosis (late stages of disease); dry "Velcro" crackles throughout lung fields on auscultation
Differential Diagnosis	Pathologic distinction from other types of fibrosing interstitial pneumonia—desquamative interstitial pneumonia (respiratory bronchitis, interstitial lung disease); acute interstitial pneumonia; nonspecific interstitial pneumonia; cryptogenic organizing pneumonia (bronchiolitis obliterans, organizing pneumonia) Pulmonary fibrosis resulting from occupational or environmental exposure—asbestosis; silicosis; farmer's lung; bird breeder's lung; exposure to metal, dust, bacteria, fumes, animals, dust, gases Fibrosis resulting from infection—tuberculosis; pneumococcus; *Pneumocystis carinii*; bacterial, fungal, viral pneumonia Drug exposure—bleomycin Connective tissue disease—rheumatoid arthritis; systemic sclerosis Sarcoidosis
Comorbidities	Respiratory failure; chronic hypoxemia; cor pulmonale; polycythemia; increased incidence of lung cancer
Critical Questions Influencing Patient Care	Is the patient approaching end-stage disease? Is there a history of respiratory failure? Is there a need for home oxygen? Are there any signs and symptoms of chronic hypoxemia? Is there any evidence of cor pulmonale?
Chronic Medications	Corticosteroids; cyclophosphamide (Cytoxan); oxygen; colchicine

This hypothesis is based on several findings. For instance, erythropoietin levels are lower in polycythemia vera than in any other disease, and in vitro erythroid colony formation can occur independently of erythropoietin.[33] In addition, erythroid precursors have shown both hypersensitivity to growth factors as well as increased expression of anti-apoptotic proteins.[34]

Patients with polycythemia vera are prone to both thrombotic and hemorrhagic events. The mechanisms underlying thrombotic complications may be related to the increased red cell mass.[35] An elevated hematocrit increases both blood viscosity and red cell aggregation, inducing a hypercoagulable state.[34] Hemorrhagic events are associated with elevations in the absolute platelet count. Defects in platelet function have been reported in polycythemia vera. In addition, an acquired von Willebrand's disease occurs with elevated platelet counts in myeloproliferative syndromes. This acquired von Willebrand's disease is characterized by decreased large von Willebrand multimers and increased cleavage products.[35]

History and Physical Findings Consistent with Diagnosis. Polycythemia can evoke both general symptoms or those secondary to underlying thrombotic or hemorrhagic pathologic processes. General symptoms include bone pain and tingling or burning of the hands and feet (Table 20-11). In addition, exposure to warm water may provoke an intense pruritus. Patients may initially present with ischemic or thrombotic vascular symptoms, including stroke, intermittent claudication, or angina. Signs of a bleeding diathesis can also be present, such as epistaxis or gastrointestinal bleeding.

On physical examination a ruddy complexion or plethora may be noted. Polycythemia vera is also associated with hypertension. Patients may complain of visual changes, and retinal vein engorgement may be noted. Hepatomegaly and splenomegaly occur late in the course of the disease.

Differential Diagnosis. Alternative conditions that should be considered when presented with a polycythemic patient include any underlying mechanism that decreases blood oxygenation. Second, aberrant erythropoietin production may cause polycythemia. Third, polycythemia may result from hemoconcentration (see Table 20-11).

Comorbidities Commonly Seen with the Condition. The comorbidities observed with polycythemia vera may be of a hemorrhagic or thrombotic nature (see Table 20-11). In addition, gout commonly occurs in these patients.

Preoperative Preparation. Before surgery it is important to ascertain how the elevated red cell mass has been treated, if at all. There is strong evidence that phlebotomy is the most effective remedy for the hypercoagulability observed with polycythemia vera. A recommended therapeutic end point is a hematocrit less than 42% in women and 45% in men.[36] Optimally, the hematocrit should be normalized 2 to 4 months before elective surgery. Patients who are older than 60 years or who have had a previous thrombotic episode are defined as high risk. These individuals may also receive cytoreductive treatment in an attempt to aggressively treat the disease. Perioperative risk of thrombotic or hemorrhagic events is influenced by how aggressively the polycythemia has been treated. Thus, it is important to obtain a history of the platelet counts and hematocrit values to determine past treatment of the disease.

Coagulation studies, including bleeding time, should be obtained before surgery.

Chronic Medications for Condition. Cytoreductive agents are administered in high-risk patients. Aspirin is often used as adjunctive therapy, even in low-risk individuals. Patients with severe pruritus may be treated with interferon alfa or paroxetine (see Table 20-11).

Perioperative Considerations. Uncontrolled polycythemia vera is associated with a high risk of perioperative bleeding and postoperative thrombosis. Control of the disease before surgery will reduce the incidence of these complications.

It is important to ensure adequate vascular access in case bleeding occurs. In addition, the ready availability of platelet transfusion should be ensured in larger blood loss cases. At the present time there is insufficient evidence to determine whether antiplatelet drugs are contraindicated during the perioperative management of the polycythemic patient.

The use of regional versus general anesthesia is controversial. Both techniques have been used successfully in patients with polycythemia vera. Studies suggest a lower incidence of deep vein thrombosis with regional techniques. However, this moderate effect must be weighed against the risk of epidural or subarachnoid hemorrhage in a patient who may be predisposed toward bleeding events.

Summary. Uncontrolled polycythemia vera is associated with a high risk of perioperative bleeding and postoperative thrombosis. Aggressive control of the disease before surgery will reduce the incidence of these complications.

TABLE 20–11	Polycythemia Vera
Symptoms	*General:* headaches, tinnitus, fatigue, shortness of breath, pruritus (aquagenic), tingling or burning of hands and feet, visual changes, bone pain, weight loss, night sweats, vertigo *Thrombotic:* stroke, myocardial infarction, angina, intermittent claudication *Hemorrhagic:* bleeding diathesis, gastrointestinal bleeding, unusual bleeding from minor cuts, epistaxis
Physical Findings	Splenomegaly (later stages), hepatomegaly, retinal vein engorgement, ruddy complexion, hypertension
Differential Diagnosis	Is there an underlying decrease in tissue oxygenation secondary to lung disease, high altitude, intracardiac shunt, hypoventilation syndromes, abnormal hemoglobin, smoking, or carbon monoxide poisoning? Is there aberrant erythroprotein production secondary to tumors (brain, liver, uterus) or cysts (especially renal)? Has hemoconcentration occurred secondary to diuretics, burns, diarrhea, or stress?
Comorbid Conditions	*Hemorrhagic:* gastric ulcer; epistaxis *Thrombotic:* Budd-Chiari syndrome; cerebral, coronary, mesenteric, or pulmonary thrombosis *Other:* gout
Critical Questions Influencing Perioperative Care	Does the patient undergo phlebotomy? Is the patient on myelosuppressive therapy? What is the most recent hematocrit and platelet count? What are the results of the most recent coagulation studies?
Chronic Medications	Cytoreductive drugs including ^{32}P Alkylating agents (chlorambucil, busulfan) Hydroxyurea Interferon-α Paroxetine Aspirin
Intraoperative Management	Ensure adequate access and availability of blood products, including platelets. Use of regional techniques is controversial.

ESSENTIAL THROMBOCYTHEMIA

The World Health Organization has defined essential thrombocythemia as a sustained platelet count of greater than 600,000 with a bone marrow biopsy showing mainly proliferation of the megakaryocytic lineage. In addition, patients must show no evidence of polycythemia vera, chronic myeloid leukemia, idiopathic myelofibrosis, myelodysplastic syndrome, or reactive thrombocytosis.[37]

Pathophysiology. The principal feature of essential thrombocythemia is an increase in megakaryocytes and platelets. Disease pathogenesis more than likely involves alterations in the signaling pathways that regulate thrombopoiesis (Fig. 20-1). Alterations in several regulatory proteins, including thrombopoietin, the thrombopoietin receptor c-Mpl, and transforming growth factor-β have been suggested as possible candidates. Currently, none of these proteins has panned out as the precise molecular mechanism behind alterations in platelet number. Other possible contributing factors may include modifications in the sensitivity of megakaryocytes to certain cytokine regulators as well as accessory cell defects.

The principal pathophysiologic features of essential thrombocytosis are thrombosis and hemorrhage. Thrombosis may involve the microcirculation or large vessel occlusions, predominantly of the arteries. The incidence rate is approximately 8.0% per patient year in untreated patients.[38] Hemorrhagic complications only occur with very high platelet counts and may be associated with decreases in von Willebrand's ristocetin cofactor activity, as well as decreased high-molecular-weight von Willebrand's multimers.[39]

History and Physical Findings Consistent with Diagnosis. Symptoms of essential thrombocythemia are associated with vasomotor changes in the cerebral and peripheral circulation. These may include headache, transient ischemic attacks, or migraines (Table 20-12).

The principal clinical features of essential thrombocythemia are thrombosis affecting the arterial more frequently than venous circulation and hemorrhage. Major arterial thrombosis may include both stroke and peripheral arterial occlusion. The most common presentation of bleeding involves the gastrointestinal tract, although bleeding may occur from the skin, gums, and nose.

Patients may present with splenomegaly and/or hepatomegaly secondary to extramedullary hematopoiesis. In the peripheral circulation acrocyanosis and erythromelalgia are common complaints. Erythromelalgia is characterized by burning pain and erythema of the digits, especially of the lower extremity. Of note, the pain associated with this condition increases with heat and improves with cold. Likewise, pruritus may occur in the extremities when exposed to warmth but improves with colder temperatures.

Differential Diagnosis. In particular, two differential diagnoses should be considered when encountering a patient with essential thrombocytosis (see Table 20-12). First, essential thrombocytosis may represent part of a continuum of the myeloproliferative disorders. Over the course of time patients with essential thrombocytosis may develop myelofibrosis, myelodysplastic syndrome, or acute myelocytic leukemia. In addition, both polycythemia vera and myelofibrosis may present as thrombocytosis. Second, reactive thrombocytosis must be ruled out. Numerous conditions, both acute and chronic, may produce thrombocytosis.

Comorbidities Commonly Seen with Condition. The comorbidities of interest to the anesthesiologist that occur with essential thrombocytosis are associated with the complications of hemorrhage and thrombosis.

Critical Questions to Ask Patient and/or Primary Care Physician. One must first assess a patient's risk of thrombosis (see Table 20-12). Several studies have shown that the primary risk factors for a thrombotic event are history of previous thrombosis and age. Other less significant risk factors include a history of smoking and obesity. Retrospective studies have shown that the incidence of thrombotic events per year is 1.7%, 6.3%, and 15.1%, at younger than 40 years, 40 to 60 years, and older than 60 years of age, respectively.[40] In addition, the incidence rate of thrombosis has been reported at 31.4% and 3.4% per year in patients with and without a history of previous

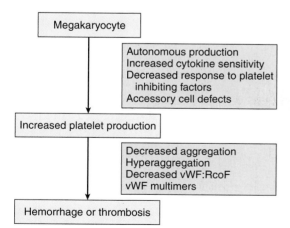

FIGURE 20-1 Pathophysiology of essential thrombocytosis. Increased platelet production from megakaryocytes occurs as a result of several hypothesized mechanisms, including autonomous production, increased sensitivity to cytokines, decreased sensitivity to platelet-inhibiting factors, and accessory cell defects. The resulting thrombosis and hemorrhage may occur secondary to hyperaggregation, decreased platelet aggregation, decreased von Willebrand's ristocetin cofactor activity (vWF:RcoF), and decreased high-molecular-weight von Willebrand's (vWF) multimers.

TABLE 20–12	Essential Thrombocythemia
Signs	Splenomegaly; digital pain that increases with heat, improves with cold; sweating; pruritus; low-grade fever; hepatomegaly; bleeding from skin, gums, nose
Symptoms	*Vasomotor symptoms of cerebral circulation:* headache; dizziness; visual disturbance; transient ischemic attacks; migraines *Vasomotor symptoms of peripheral circulation:* paresthesias; acrocyanosis; erythromelalgia *Thrombotic symptoms:* venous thrombotic events; superficial thrombophlebitis; deep venous thrombosis; portal or splenic venous thrombosis; major arterial thrombosis, including stroke *Hemorrhagic symptoms:* bleeding diathesis, especially gastrointestinal bleeding
Differential Diagnosis	*Clonal thrombocytosis:* associated with other chronic myeloproliferative disorders *Reactive thrombocytosis:* acute bleeding; hemolysis; iron deficiency anemia; acute and chronic inflammatory conditions such as arthritis; stress or surgery; osteoporosis; metastatic cancer; severe trauma; splenectomy; medication
Critical Questions Influencing Perioperative Care	Does the patient have a history of previous thrombosis? Platelet count? Obesity? Smoking? Age? Any evidence of ongoing bleeding? How has the platelet count been managed?
Chronic Medications	Cytoreductive drugs, including hydroxyurea, anagrelide, interferon-α, or ^{32}P Low-dose aspirin
Perioperative Management	Platelet counts should be normalized before surgery. Consider plateletpheresis in emergency situations to achieve a rapid decrease in platelet count. Administer cytoreductive therapy to decrease platelet count before surgery.

thrombosis.[40] The absolute platelet count cannot provide a definitive assessment of thrombotic risk. Thrombotic events have been reported with platelet counts in the range of 400,000 to 600,000/mm³.[41] Although the platelet count does not necessarily predict the risk of thrombosis, evidence suggests that controlling the platelet count does decrease the incidence of thrombosis. Prospective studies comparing long-term risk of thrombosis in patients treated with myelosuppressive therapy versus those without found incidence rates of 8.0% versus 1.5% per patient year in untreated and treated patients, respectively.[38] Hence, the degree of controlling the platelet count assumes importance in assessing thrombotic risk. The main risk factor for hemorrhage is a platelet count greater than 1.5 million.[36]

List of Chronic Medications for Condition.
Treatment of essential thrombocytosis consists of myelosuppressive drugs. These are administered on a chronic basis to manage the platelet count in high-risk individuals. Antiplatelet drugs may also be included in the regimen. Low-dose aspirin has been shown to be efficacious in managing both erythromelalgia and transient ischemic attacks associated with essential thrombocytosis.[42]

Perioperative Considerations. The most important issue in perioperative management of the patient with essential thrombocythemia is whether to normalize the platelet count before surgery. There are no clear guidelines as to which patients should be aggressively normalized preoperatively, and consultation with a hematologist should be pursued. However, suffice it to say that elderly patients with consistently elevated platelet counts and a history of prior thrombosis represent a high-risk group requiring aggressive management. Elective surgical patients may have adequate time to undergo cytoreductive therapy preoperatively. In the case of urgent or emergency surgery the use of plateletpheresis may be considered.

Summary. Essential thrombocytosis is a myeloproliferative disorder characterized by chronic elevation of the platelet count. Thrombosis and hemorrhagic events are frequent with this disorder. Patients at high risk for these complications include the elderly and those with a prior history of a thrombotic event. The most important issue in perioperative management of the patient with essential thrombocythemia is whether to normalize the platelet count before surgery.

MYELOID METAPLASIA WITH MYELOFIBROSIS

Pathophysiology. The intrinsic characteristics of this disease include both myeloproliferation and myelofibrosis (Fig. 20-2). There is tri-lineage myeloproliferation (granulocytic, erythroid, and megakaryocytic) that results from a clonal amplification of primitive progenitor cells.[43] However, the fibroblast proliferation of myelofibrosis appears to be polyclonal, suggesting that myelofibrosis is a reactive process. It is currently hypothesized that the stromal reaction of the bone marrow occurs as a result of elevations in cytokines produced by the cells involved in clonal myeloproliferation. Evidence suggests that cytokines produced by megakaryocytes and monocytes enhance fibroblast proliferation (platelet-derived growth factor, calmodulin), collagen synthesis (transforming growth factor-β), angiogenesis (vascular endothelial growth factor, basic fibroblast growth factor), and osteogenesis (transforming growth factor-β, basic fibroblast growth factor).

Physical Findings Consistent with Diagnosis. Myeloid metaplasia with myelofibrosis may present in a variety of ways. Constitutional symptoms may relate to the catabolic aspects of this disease and include cachexia, fatigue, weight loss, low-grade fever, and night sweats (Table 20-13).

Extramedullary hematopoiesis may evoke a constellation of symptoms and signs. The most common presenting feature is hypersplenism. Extramedullary hematopoiesis may also occur in other organ systems such that lymphadenopathy, acute cardiac tamponade, hematuria, papular skin nodes, pleural effusion, pulmonary hypertension, and spinal cord compression may be observed. Of note, pulmonary hypertension has a poor prognosis.

TABLE 20–13	Myeloid Metaplasia with Myelofibrosis
History	Constitutional symptoms, including weight loss, night sweats, low-grade fever
Physical Findings	Splenomegaly; anemia; pallor; petechiae and ecchymosis; gout
Findings Related to Extramedullary Hematopoiesis	Acute cardiac tamponade; hematuria; lymphadenopathy; papular skin nodes; pleural effusion; spinal cord compression
Laboratory Findings	Anemia; white blood cell count increased or decreased; platelet count increased or decreased; myelophthisis
Differential Diagnosis	Malignancies that may display bone marrow fibrosis Essential thrombocythemia Granulomatous involvement of bone marrow such as histoplasmosis, tuberculosis
Associated Conditions	Portal hypertension Splenic infarction Complications related to extramedullary hematopoiesis
Perioperative Management	Obtain complete blood cell count and platelet count Consider cytoreductive therapy in patients without significant thrombocytopenia Bleeding may require platelet transfusion or cryoprecipitate Obtain disseminated intravascular coagulation panel

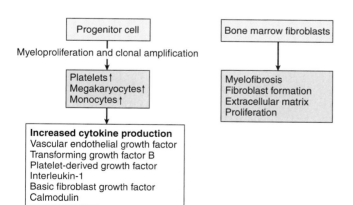

FIGURE 20-2 Proposed pathophysiology of myeloid metaplasia with myelofibrosis. Primitive progenitor cells undergo clonal amplification resulting in tri-lineage myeloproliferation with increases in platelets, megakaryocytes, and monocytes. Increased production of cytokines by megakaryocytes and monocytes is thought to mediate fibroblast proliferation and myelofibrosis.

Fifty to 75 percent of patients are anemic at diagnosis, whereas the white blood cell count and platelet count initially may be either increased or decreased. An early finding on peripheral blood smear is myelophthisis. Myelophthisis is characterized by teardrop-shaped red blood cells, immature granulocytes, and nucleated red cells.

Differential Diagnosis. Several disorders are also associated with myelophthisis and possible myelofibrosis (see Table 20-13). Therefore, the differential diagnosis must include other malignancies such as chronic myeloid leukemia, myelodysplastic syndrome, metastatic cancer, lymphoma, Hodgkin's disease, and plasma cell dyscrasia. Granulomatous involvement of the bone marrow may cause myelofibrosis. Thus, tuberculosis and histoplasmosis must also be entertained as possible diagnoses. In patients presenting with elevated platelet counts and minimal myelofibrosis it may be difficult to exclude the diagnosis of essential thrombocythemia.

Comorbidities Commonly Seen with Condition. The conditions commonly associated with myelofibrosis and myeloid metaplasia result from the underlying pathophysiology (see Table 20-13). Portal hypertension may result from either increased portal flow secondary to splenomegaly or thrombotic obstruction of small hepatic veins. The complications of extramedullary hematopoiesis have been discussed previously.

Perioperative Considerations. The greatest experience in perioperative management of myelofibrosis and myeloid metaplasia has occurred with splenectomy. Indications for splenectomy include splenomegaly refractory to chemotherapy, portal hypertension, or progressive anemia. Morbidity and mortality after this procedure have been reported at 30.5% and 9%, respectively.[44] Significant perioperative complications after splenectomy include hemorrhage (14.8%), infection (8.5%), and thrombosis (7.5%).[44] The primary cause of death includes hemorrhage (4.5%), infection (2.7%), and thrombosis (1.3%).[44] The only preoperative variable that correlates with increased hemorrhage or thrombosis is a platelet count of less than 100,000.[44] With the above in mind, the critical information and/or interventions before surgery would include a complete blood cell count and platelet count. In patients without thrombocytopenia, prophylactic cytoreductive therapy should be considered to reduce the risk of perioperative thrombosis. Adequate blood products should be available before surgery, including access to platelets and cryoprecipitate. Occult disseminated intravascular coagulation (DIC) has been associated with perioperative bleeding.[43] Therefore, a preoperative DIC panel should be performed. Splenectomy should be postponed in patients with D-dimer levels greater than 0.5 μg/mL.[44]

Summary. The intrinsic characteristics of myeloid metaplasia with myelofibrosis include both myeloproliferation and myelofibrosis. Extramedullary hematopoiesis occurs in this disease and may evoke a constellation of symptoms, signs, and complications. The greatest experience of perioperative management of patients with myelofibrosis and myeloid metaplasia has occurred with splenectomy, where complications included hemorrhage (14.8%), infection (8.5%), and thrombosis (7.5%). Perioperative management of this disease should include careful management of the platelet count as well as attention to the ability to adequately treat hemorrhagic complications.

Referecnces

1. Driscoll BP, Gracco C, Coelho C, et al: Laryngeal function in postpolio patients. Laryngoscope 1995;105:35-41.
2. Dalakas MC, Elder G, Hallett M, et al: A long-term follow-up study of patients with post-poliomyelitis neuromuscular symptoms. N Engl J Med 1986;314:959-963.
3. Cosgrove JL, Alexander MA, Kitts EL, et al: Late effects of poliomyelitis. Arch Phys Med Rehabil 1987;68:4-7.
4. Dalakas MC: The post-polio syndrome as an evolved clinical entity: Definition and clinical description. Ann NY Acad Sci 1995;753: 68-80.
5. Gyermek L: Increased potency of nondepolarizing relaxants after poliomyelitis. J Clin Pharmacol 1990;30:170-173.
6. Cangemi CF Jr, Miller RJ: Huntington's disease: Review and anesthetic case management. Anesth Prog 1998;45:150-153.
7. Propert DN: Pseudocholinesterase activity and phenotypes in mentally ill patients. Br J Psychiatry 1979;134:477-481.
8. Davies DD: Abnormal response to anaesthesia in a case of Huntington's chorea. Br J Anaesth 1966;38:490-491.
9. Rodrigo MR: Huntington's chorea: Midazolam, a suitable induction agent? Br J Anaesth 1987;59:388-389.
10. Nagele P, Hammerle AF: Sevoflurane and mivacurium in a patient with Huntington's chorea. Br J Anaesth 2000;85:320-321.
11. Costarino A, Gross JB: Patients with Huntington's chorea may respond normally to succinylcholine. Anesthesiology 1985;63:570.
12. Kaufman MA, Erb T: Propofol for patients with Huntington's chorea? Anaesthesia 1990;45:889-890.
13. Lowry DW, Carroll MT, Mirakhur RK, et al: Comparison of sevoflurane and propofol with rocuronium for modified rapid-sequence induction of anaesthesia. Anaesthesia 1999;54:247-252.
14. Kulemeka G, Mendonca C: Huntington's chorea: Use of rocuronium. Anaesthesia 2001;56:1019.
15. Ochando Cerdan F, Moreno Gonzalez E, Hernandez Garcia D, et al: Diagnostic and treatment of Zenker's diverticulum: Review of our series pharyngo-esophageal diverticula. Hepatogastroenterology 1998;45:447-450.
16. Cope R, Spargo P: Anesthesia for Zenker's diverticulum. Anesth Analg 1990;71:312.
17. Thiagarajah S, Lear E, Keh M: Anesthetic implications of Zenker's diverticulum. Anesth Analg 1990;70:109-111.
18. Aouad MT, Berzina CE, Baraka AS: Aspiration pneumonia after anesthesia in a patient with a Zenker diverticulum. Anesthesiology 2000;92:1837-1839.
19. Westermark P, Araki S, Benson MD, et al: Nomenclature of amyloid fibril proteins. Report from the meeting of the International Nomenclature Committee on Amyloidosis, August 8-9, 1998. Part 1. Amyloid 1999;6:63-66.
20. Seguin P, Freidel M, Perpoint B: Amyloid disease and extreme macroglossia: Apropos of a case. Rev Stomatol Chir Maxillofac 1994;95:339-342.
21. Weiss LS, White JA: Macroglossia: A review. J La State Med Soc 1990;142:13-16.
22. Chow LT, Chow WH, Shum BS: Fatal massive upper respiratory tract haemorrhage: An unusual complication of localized amyloidosis of the larynx. J Laryngol Otol 1993;107:51-53.
23. Noguchi T, Minami K, Iwagaki T, et al: Anesthetic management of a patient with laryngeal amyloidosis. J Clin Anesth 1999;11: 339-341.
24. Eriksson P, Boman K, Jacobsson B, et al: Cardiac arrhythmias in familial amyloid polyneuropathy during anaesthesia. Acta Anaesthesiol Scand 1986;30:317-320.
25. Viana JS, Neves S, Vieira H, et al: Serum potassium concentrations after suxamethonium in patients with familial amyloid polyneuropathy type I. Acta Anaesthesiol Scand 1997;41: 750-753.
26. Silverman DG: Nerve injury, burns, and trauma. In Silverman DG (eds): Neuromuscular Block in Perioperative and Intensive Care. Philadelphia, JB Lippincott, 1994, pp 332-348.
27. Sternbach Y, Perler BA: Acute mesenteric ischemia. In Zuidema GD, Yeo CJ (eds): Shackelford's Surgery of the Alimentary Tract. Philadelphia, WB Saunders, 2001, pp 17-31.
28. Strieter RM: Mechanisms of pulmonary fibrosis: conference summary. Chest 2001;120:77S-85S.
29. Gross TJ, Hunninghake GW: Idiopathic pulmonary fibrosis. N Engl J Med 2001;345:517-525.
30. Collard HR, King TE Jr: Demystifying idiopathic interstitial pneumonia. Arch Intern Med 2003;163:17-29.

31. Conacher ID, Dark J, Hilton CJ, et al: Isolated lung transplantation for pulmonary fibrosis. Anaesthesia 1990;45:971-975.

32. Maruyama K, Kobayasi H, Taguchi O, et al: Higher doses of inhaled nitric oxide might be less effective in improving oxygenation in a patient with interstitial pulmonary fibrosis. Anesth Analg 1995;81:210-211.

33. Prchal JF, Axelrad AA: Letter: Bone-marrow responses in polycythemia vera. N Engl J Med 1974;290:1382.

34. Spivak JL: Polycythemia vera: Myths, mechanisms, and management. Blood 2002;100:4272-4290.

35. Tefferi A: Polycythemia vera: A comprehensive review and clinical recommendations. Mayo Clin Proc 2003;78:174-194.

36. Solberg LA Jr: Therapeutic options for essential thrombocythemia and polycythemia vera. Semin Oncol 2002;29:10-15.

37. Harrison CN, Green AR: Essential thrombocythemia. Hematol Oncol Clin North Am 2003;17:1175-1190.

38. Finazzi G, Ruggeri M, Rodeghiero F, et al: Second malignancies in patients with essential thrombocythaemia treated with busulphan and hydroxyurea: Long-term follow-up of a randomized clinical trial. Br J Haematol 2000;110:577-583.

39. Budde U, Schaefer G, Mueller N, et al: Acquired von Willebrand's disease in the myeloproliferative syndrome. Blood 1984;64:981-985.

40. Cortelazzo S, Viero P, Finazzi G, et al: Incidence and risk factors for thrombotic complications in a historical cohort of 100 patients with essential thrombocythemia. J Clin Oncol 1990;8:556-562.

41. Regev A, Stark P, Blickstein D, et al: Thrombotic complications in essential thrombocythemia with relatively low platelet counts. Am J Hematol 1997;56:168-172.

42. Griesshammer M, Bangerter M, van Vliet HH, et al: Aspirin in essential thrombocythemia: Status quo and quo vadis. Semin Thromb Hemost 1997;23:371-377.

43. Tefferi A: Myelofibrosis with myeloid metaplasia. N Engl J Med 2000;342:1255-1265.

44. Tefferi A, Mesa RA, Nagorney DM, et al: Splenectomy in myelofibrosis with myeloid metaplasia: A single-institution experience with 223 patients. Blood 2000;95:2226-2233.

21 The Pediatric Patient

Doreen Soliman, MD, Franklyn Cladis, MD,
and Peter Davis, MD

For neonates to survive in the extrauterine environment, a series of adaptations must occur. These adaptations or physiologic transitions have profound implications. These adaptations are interdependent on each other and include (1) conversion of the cardiovascular circulation from a parallel circulation to one in series; (2) establishment of a functional residual capacity and maintenance of an air exchange; (3) regulation of fluid and electrolytes in the presence of an immature kidney and the absence of a placenta; and (4) temperature homeostasis in an organism easily overwhelmed by its environment. All of these physiologic or transitional tasks can be further compromised by the presence of surgical or medical diseases. The transition from neonate to infant is characterized by maturation of all of its organ systems and occurs over weeks to months. However, the relative immaturity of these organ systems in infants, compared with adults, creates challenges for the anesthesiologist. To understand how best to approach uncommon diseases of the infant, a basic understanding of normal physiology is required.

PHYSIOLOGY

Cardiac Physiology

*Transitional Circulation/
Pulmonary Vascular Resistance*

The transition from fetal to neonatal circulation is characterized by a change from parallel circulation (cardiac output contributes to both pulmonary and systemic perfusion, simultaneously allowing mixing of oxygenated and deoxygenated blood) to one that occurs in series (cardiac output contributes to either pulmonary or systemic perfusion with minimal admixture). High pulmonary vascular resistance (PVR) and relatively low systemic vascular resistance (SVR) also characterize fetal circulation. In utero, oxygenated blood from the placenta is transported to the fetus via the umbilical vein (Fig. 21-1). Blood from the gastrointestinal tract combines with the umbilical vein to become the ductus venosus, which drains into the

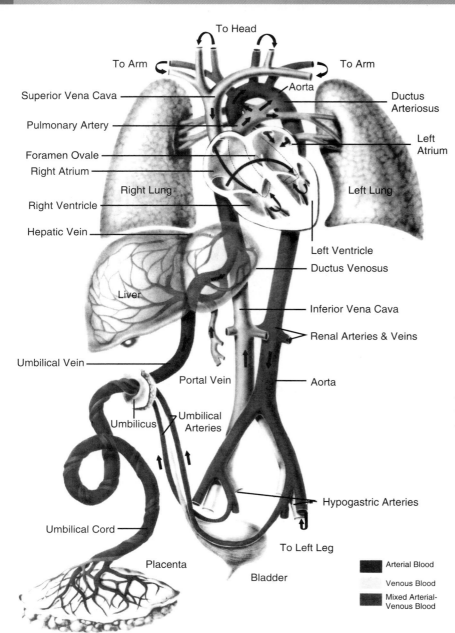

FIGURE 21–1 Course of the fetal circulation in late gestation. Note the selective blood flow patterns across the foramen ovale and the ductus arteriosus. *(From Greeley WJ, Steven JM, Nicolson SC: Anesthesia for pediatric cardiac surgery. In Miller RD [ed]: Miller's Anesthesia, 6th ed. Philadelphia, Churchill Livingstone, 2005, p 2007, with permission.)*

inferior vena cava (IVC). Blood from the IVC enters the right atrium and preferentially crosses the foramen ovale to the left atrium and left ventricle, thereby providing slightly more oxygenated blood for cerebral circulation. The superior vena cava (SVC) drains into the right atrium and is pumped primarily to the systemic circulation via the ductus arteriosus. Less than 10 percent of combined ventricular output contributes to pulmonary flow.[1] A series of events occur at birth that change fetal (parallel) circulation into neonatal circulation (series).

During delivery PVR decreases and SVR increases, allowing for a significant increase in pulmonary blood flow. The increase in SVR occurs secondary to separation from the placenta. The decrease in PVR occurs for several reasons. With the onset of lung ventilation, there is a decrease in the mechanical compression of the alveoli and an increase

in P_{O_2}.[2,3] At birth, the mechanical distention of the alveoli coupled with the increased oxygen tension results in a precipitous decrease in PVR. The changes in PVR are mediated by biochemical factors, including nitric oxide and prostaglandin. In the newborn period, the pulmonary vessels exhibit a highly reactive tone. Maintenance of an elevated PVR is lethal to the neonate. Pulmonary vasoconstriction with right-to-left shunting in response to hypoxia, hypercarbia, sepsis, and acidosis can cause severe hypoxemia and death.

With a decrease in PVR, pulmonary blood flow and venous return to the left atrium increase. The increase in left atrial pressure and flow closes the foramen ovale. Over the next few months of life, PVR decreases even further. Hypoxemia and acidosis are two important factors that affect PVR. An increase in PVR can lead to right-to-left shunting across the foramen ovale and ductus arteriosus. This persistence of an elevated PVR can lead to further hypoxemia and tissue acidosis. Thus, hypoxemia and acidosis can lead to a vicious cycle of increased PVR, increased right-to-left shunting, increased hypoxemia, increased tissue acidosis, and further increase in PVR and shunting.

The neonatal myocardium is immature and continues its development after birth. Many functional differences between the neonatal and adult myocardium are directly related to the immaturity of the neonatal tissue components.[4] At delivery and extending into the neonatal period, there are fewer contractile elements and there is less elastin in the newborn's myocardium, resulting in a decreased contractile capacity and decreased ventricular compliance, respectively. Fetal myocardium has limited ability to generate the equivalent contractile force as the adult myocardium throughout the entire range of the length-tension curve. The consequence is a reduced capacity to adapt to increases in preload or afterload.[5,6] This does not mean the stroke volume is fixed. There is echocardiographic evidence that the immature heart, while limited, is able to increase stroke volume.[7] Because of this immaturity, the neonatal heart has a diminished capacity to handle significant volume loads and more easily develops ventricular overload and failure.

Respiratory Physiology

A significant difference between neonatal and adult respiration is oxygen consumption. Neonatal oxygen consumption is two to three times greater than that of the adult (5 to 8 mL/kg/min vs. 2 to 3 mL/kg/min).[8] This contributes to the rapid oxygen desaturation observed in infants during periods of apnea or hypoventilation.

The neonatal/infant lung is less compliant than the adult lung. The immature lung in the pediatric patient is characterized by small and poorly developed alveoli with thickened walls and decreased elastin. The amount of elastin in the lung continues to increase until late adolescence.[9] Before and after late adolescence, pulmonary elastin is decreased. Elastin provides elasticity to the lung, without which there is airway collapse. Because infants and older adults have less elastin, they are prone to alveolar collapse.[9,10] The closing capacity, the lung volume at which there is airway collapse, occurs at a larger lung volume in the very young and the very old (Fig. 21-2). In the infant, airway closure can occur before end exhalation, resulting in atelectasis and right-to-left transpulmonary shunting. In contrast to the pediatric lung, the pediatric chest wall is more compliant than the adult chest wall. The increased amount of cartilage in pediatric ribs accounts for this. This increased chest wall compliance may help contribute to airway collapse because negative intrathoracic pressure can result in chest wall collapse.

Temperature Regulation

Neonates and infants are at increased risk of thermoregulatory instability because they are more prone to heat loss and they have a decreased ability to produce heat. They are at increased risk of heat loss because of their large surface area to volume ratio.[11] They also have decreased ability to restrict heat loss secondary to limited vasoconstriction compared with adults.[12] The primary method of heat production in the neonate and infant consists of nonshivering thermogenesis. This compensates poorly for heat loss. Nonshivering thermogenesis occurs primarily in brown fat, which may be decreased in premature neonates. This mechanism can also be inhibited by inhalational agents.[13,14] Nonshivering thermogenesis is mediated by norepinephrine. Norepinephrine is a potent pulmonary vasoconstrictor. Consequently cold stresses can cause elevations to PVR and provide a mechanism for right-to-left shunting. Shivering thermogenesis assumes a less significant role in infants. Temperature stability can be ensured by using neonatal warming lights, forced warm air blankets,

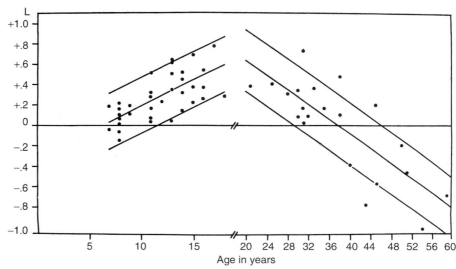

FIGURE 21–2 Closing capacity in relation to age. The difference between functional residual capacity (FRC) and closing capacity is charted against age. Note that closing capacity is greater than FRC in children younger than 5 years old and adults older than 45 years old. *(From Mansell A, Bryan C, Levison H: Airway closure in children. J Appl Physiol 1972;33: 771-774, with permission.)*

intravenous fluid warmers (if large amounts of fluids or blood products are given) increasing the ambient temperature of the operating room and keeping the infant covered.

Renal Physiology

In the first few days of life a major physiologic priority of the neonate is to lose weight as a result of a reduction in extracellular body water. This physiologic weight loss usually is a function of an isotonic contraction of body fluids. Perturbations of this process can affect infant morbidity and mortality.

The neonatal kidney develops its full complement of nephrons by 36 weeks' gestation. The glomerular filtration rate is lower in the neonate (approximately 25% of adult value) and achieves adult values within the first few years of life. Tubular function in the neonate is also limited; consequently, a glomerular to tubular imbalance is present in the first few years of life as well.

Neonates have limited capacity to concentrate their urine. When challenged, term infants can concentrate to 800 mOsm/kg of plasma water, whereas preterm infants can concentrate to 600 mOsm/kg of plasma water. Neonates have diminished end organ responsiveness to vasopressin, whereas fluid-challenged term infants and premature infants can dilute their urine to 50 and 70 mOsm/kg of plasma water, respectively. Thus, excessive fluid restriction and overhydration can result in dehydration and intravascular volume overload. Renal sodium losses are inversely related to gestational age and disease states (hypoxia, respiratory distress, acute tubular necrosis, and hyperbilirubinemia can exacerbate these losses).

Pain and Perioperative Stress Response

Pain and stress have been shown to induce significant physiologic and behavioral consequences. Newborns and infants are capable of mounting a hormonal response to the stress of their illness.[15,16] A better understanding of the causes, mechanisms, and treatments of pain during development has provided clinicians with a wide array of techniques to safely manage procedural and postoperative pain.[17-19] The nervous system at birth displays hypersensitivity to sensory stimuli in comparison to that of the nervous system of the mature adult. In neonates, thresholds of response to mechanical and thermal stimulation are reduced and further sensitization can occur with sustained or repetitive stimulation, which is different from the mature nervous system.[20] Structural and functional changes in the peripheral and central nervous systems that take place in the postnatal period involve alterations in expression, distribution, and function of receptors, ion channels, and neurotransmittors.[21] These changes can profoundly affect the character of nociceptive responses at different stages of development. Perinatal brain plasticity is affected by this sensitization and increases the vulnerability of the neonatal brain to early adverse experiences. These adverse experiences lead to abnormal neurologic development and behavior.[22,23]

A multimodal approach to pain management is necessary and may involve pharmacologic and nonpharmacologic methods.[24] The use of nonopioid analgesics (acetaminophen, nonsteroidal anti-inflammatory drugs), opioids, local anesthetics, and regional techniques provides a balanced analgesic approach to pain management.

NERVOUS SYSTEM

Meningomyelocele

Meningomyelocele (MMC) is a defect of neural tube development occurring around the fourth week of gestation. The incidence of MMC is 0.5 to 1.0 per 1,000 live births. The etiology is multifactorial but may occur secondary to folate deficiency, exposure to toxins (valproic acid, carbamazepine), and genetic disorders (trisomy 13 and 18). This is the most common neural tube defect and is characterized by lack of development of the layers that naturally cover and protect the spinal cord, resulting in protrusion of the meninges through the bony defect overlying the cord. The sac created by the protruding meninges may (MMC) or may not (meningocele) contain nerve tissue. The defect may occur anywhere along the spinal cord, but the lumbosacral region is the most common site. Defects at the thoracic and cervical region occur rarely. MMC results in neurologic injury below the level of the lesion. The neurologic injuries can include paraplegia, urinary and fecal incontinence, and sexual dysfunction; however, there is considerable clinical variation.

Associated Anomalies. The most common associated neurologic anomaly is the Chiari 2 malformation, which is characterized by downward herniation of the cerebellar vermis and the fourth ventricle. Infants with Chiari 2 malformations can present with clinical evidence of brain stem compression, resulting in a weak cry, poor swallowing, poor feeding, aspiration, apnea, and opisthotonus (Fig. 21-3). Older children may present with neurologic symptoms involving the upper extremity. Hydrocephalus can occur in as many as 85% of patients with lumbar MMC. The etiology of the hydrocephalus is not clear but may occur secondary to anatomic abnormalities associated with the Chiari malformation and/or abnormal cerebrospinal fluid (CSF) absorption.[25] Other associated anomalies include clubfeet, Klippel-Feil syndrome, hydronephrosis, exstrophy of the bladder, and congenital heart defects.

Pathophysiology. Most children with MMC survive into early adulthood.[26] Thirty percent of the deaths in the first two decades of life are secondary to respiratory complications. These complications are largely attributable to

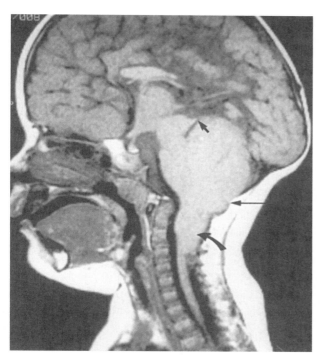

FIGURE 21–3 MR image of a patient with Chiari II malformation. Note the upward herniation of the cerebellum as indicated by the *short arrow*. The *curved arrow* indicates downward herniation of the brainstem through the foramen magnum. The *thin long arrow* marks the foramen magnum.

hydrocephalus and Chiari 2 malformation.[27] In the first few weeks of life, infants with MMC require immediate repair to prevent infection, further neurologic injury, and dehydration.

Anesthetic Considerations (Preoperative). Infants with MMC present to the operating room for primary repair of their MMC. Later in life they present for ventriculoperitoneal shunts (VPS), VPS revisions, tethered cord repairs, and posterior spine fusions.

The anesthetic management of the infant with MMC begins with a complete preoperative assessment. Infants with Chiari 2 malformations may be at risk for apnea and aspiration. Preoperative echocardiography and renal ultrasound may be part of the evaluation to rule out congenital heart defects and hydronephrosis. Examination of the neck may reveal decreased range of motion secondary to Chiari 2 malformation and/or Klippel-Feil sequence. An assessment of the patient's volume status is important, given the risk of significant intraoperative third space losses from the open skin defect. Laboratory data can be tailored to the needs of the infant, but at least a blood glucose value should be checked. Bleeding can occur secondary to tissue dissection. A hemoglobin/hematocrit type and screen may be performed preoperatively (Table 21-1).

Induction. Anesthesia can be induced with intravenous induction agents or a standard inhalational agent. Standard intravenous induction agents include atropine,

---

TABLE 21–1 Anesthetic Considerations with Meningomyelocele and Occipital and Nasal Encephalocele

Pathology	Associated Anomalies	Anesthetic Issues
Meningocele	Chiari 2 malformation Apnea	*Preoperative labs:* blood glucose, hemoglobin, type and screen
Meningomyelocele	Hydrocephalus: VPS Congenital cardiac defects Genitourinary Klippel-Feil	*Preoperative labs:* blood glucose, hemoglobin, type and screen, and renal ultrasound, echocardiogram *Airway management:* possible decreased neck extension from Chiari 2 and Klippel-Feil (rare), intubation may be lateral decubitus to protect neural elements *Hypothermia risk:* full access heating blanket, neonatal warming lights *Latex precautions* *Postoperative apnea*
Occipital encephalocele	As above	*Preoperative labs:* blood glucose, hemoglobin, type and screen *Airway management:* head positioning for mask ventilation and intubation may be more difficult secondary to location of neural elements
Nasal encephalocele	As above	*Preoperative labs:* blood glucose, hemoglobin, type and screen *Airway management:* may be difficult to mask ventilate secondary to nasal defect *Craniotomy:* consider an arterial catheter. *Positioning:* may be positioned head up or sitting; consider a central venous catheter. Postoperative ventilation may be required secondary to airway edema or blood in the upper airway.

sodium pentothal, or propofol and a neuromuscular blocking agent. Succinylcholine has been administered to patients with MMC without any reported increase in serum potassium levels.[28] Airway management may be more challenging in the infant with MMC because of associated neck pathology (Chiari malformation, Klippel-Feil), positioning, and increased association with short tracheas.[29] Positioning during airway management and laryngoscopy is critical to avoid pressure and subsequent injury to the neural placode. The infant can be induced and intubated on the side or supine, provided there is appropriate support to the back to protect the neural elements. Towels can be rolled and used to support the infant when supine. The neural cord defect can also be placed in a donut-shaped small gel head ring to allow the infant to be supine without causing pressure to be placed on the neural elements. The trachea may be short in infants with MMC.[29] Attention must be paid to identifying the carina and properly positioning the endotracheal tube to prevent endobronchial intubation.

Maintenance. Anesthesia can be maintained with an inhalational agent and nitrous oxide. Remifentanil may be advantageous given its rapid clearance, short terminal half-life, and nonaccumulating properties.[30] Subsequent use of intraoperative neuromuscular blocking agents is not recommended because nerve stimulation by the neurosurgeons is sometimes performed to identify neural tissue. The open skin defect can occupy a large portion of surface area and can result in significant third space fluid losses. These infants are also at risk for hypothermia because of the relatively large area of exposed skin and may require resuscitation with room temperature fluids. Maintaining a warm room and using a full access forced warm air blanket can reduce this risk. Because the patient is positioned prone for the primary closure, the face, eyes, and extremities must be appropriately padded and protected.

Regional Anesthesia. Spinal anesthesia has been reported for the primary repair of lumbosacral MMCs. Infants with thoracic lesions were excluded. The initial introduction of intrathecal local anesthetic was by the anesthesiologists. The dural puncture was performed at the most caudad region of the defect, with a hyperbaric mixture of tetracaine. The block was supplemented by the neurosurgeons, if needed, and a pacifier along with intravenous midazolam was provided for those infants who remained unsettled after supplementation. Fourteen infants were successfully anesthetized and surgically corrected. Half required supplementation of local anesthetic. Two of the 14 had postoperative apnea, and no new neurologic events were noted immediately after surgery.[31]

Latex Precautions. Latex sensitization is increased in children with myelodysplasia. Pittman and colleagues studied the prevalence of latex specific IgE among children

with MMC: 47% of the children with MMC had antibodies against latex, compared with 15% of the chronically ill control group, and 3.8% of the medical control group.[32] Using epicutaneous skin testing, Shah and colleagues demonstrated latex sensitization in 44% of children and adolescents with MMC: 21% of these children had a history of clinical latex allergy. Age and number of surgical procedures were significantly correlated with latex sensitization.[33] Patients with latex allergies often have additional allergies. Most commonly these are secondary to repeated antibiotic exposure, but reports of sensitization to opioids and neuromuscular blocking agents have been reported.[34]

Postoperative Considerations. Infants with meningomyelocele may be at increased risk of postoperative apnea. Extubation after primary repair of the defect may take place in hemodynamically stable infants who are awake and can maintain their airway. Infants should recover in a monitored setting with respiratory and cardiac monitors.

Fetal Surgery. Prenatal intervention had been proposed, initially in an attempt to improve neurologic and urologic function. Earlier animal studies suggested an improvement in postnatal function. However, in humans there was no significant improvement in lower leg function. It appears that the benefit derived from early fetal intervention may be a reduction in hindbrain herniation and shunt-dependent hydrocephalus.[35]

OTOLARYNGOLOGY

Congenital Laryngeal Webs and Atresia

Congenital laryngeal webs are uncommon and have an estimated incidence of 1 in 10,000 births. Most laryngeal webs are glottic with extension into the subglottic area. The laryngeal web is a result of a failure to recanalize the laryngeal inlet at about 10 weeks' gestation. The symptoms vary according to the location of the web and the degree of involvement (Fig. 21-4; Table 21-2). Symptoms are related to vocal cord dysfunction and range from mild hoarseness to aphonia. Most webs involve the anterior glottis and are generally thin and associated with mild hoarseness and minimal airway obstruction. With laryngoscopy the vocal folds are visible. Subglottic webs are infrequent, and supraglottic webs are rare. Complete congenital laryngeal atresia is incompatible with life unless an emergency tracheotomy is carried out in the delivery room. Complete congenital atresia is associated with tracheal and esophageal anomalies (Fig. 21-5).[36]

Diagnosis/Differential Diagnosis. Signs and symptoms of infants with congenital laryngeal webs include disorders of phonation, stridor, and airway obstruction. Table 21-3

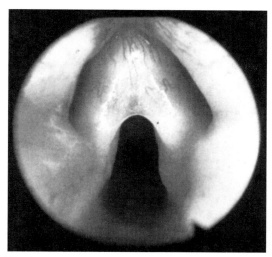

FIGURE 21–4   Medium congenital glottic web. This is a medium-sized, thicker congenital anterior glottic web. (*Courtesy of Charles Bluestone, MD.*)

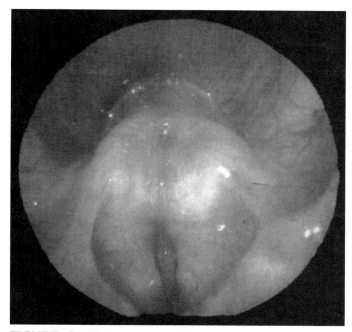

FIGURE 21–5   Laryngeal atresia. (*Courtesy of Charles Bluestone, MD.*)

outlines the different pathologic processes that may mimic the symptoms of congenital laryngeal webs.

Treatment. Thin anterior webs and webs in the glottic area may require incision and dilatation. If the web involves the subglottic larynx, the anterior cricoid plate is usually abnormal. In these instances treatment requires an external approach with division of the web and the cricoid plate and the use of cartilage grafting.[37]

Anesthetic Management (Table 21-4). A systematic approach to evaluation of the airway is essential. Flexible fiberoptic nasopharyngolaryngoscopy and rigid laryngoscopy and bronchoscopy are needed to fully assess the airway. Because anesthetic agents can affect vocal cord motion, flexible fiberoptic nasopharyngolaryngoscopy is used to assess vocal cord mobility with the patient awake or lightly sedated.

An experienced endoscopist and anesthesiologist should provide the care for these infants, in an operating room fully equipped for managing pediatric airway emergencies. Communication between the surgeon and the anesthesiologist is of paramount importance.[38] Intravenous access can be established after the induction of general anesthesia using inhalational agents. Sevoflurane or halothane can be used, although the former has been associated with fewer side effects.[39] Anticholinergic agents are recommended for rigid bronchoscopy to decrease secretions and minimize the risk of bradycardia. Topical anesthesia of the vocal cords and the trachea is used as an adjunct. Lidocaine 1% has a short duration of action (10 minutes).[40]

Total intravenous anesthesia, including remifentanil and propofol, can be used for maintenance of anesthesia.[41] The choice of spontaneous or controlled ventilation depends on the severity of airway obstruction.[42] Spontaneous ventilation is probably the ventilation mode of choice in patients with severe airway compromise. Intravenous dexamethasone, 0.5 to 1.0 mg/kg, should be administered to treat potential airway edema. In cases of severe stenosis, cricotracheal resection requires postoperative nasotracheal

TABLE 21–2   Signs and Symptoms of Congenital Laryngeal Webs
Phonatory abnormalities: A high-pitched or absent cry occurs with glottic anomalies. A muffled cry is characteristic of supraglottic obstruction.
Stridor
Severe airway obstruction that is associated with increased work of breathing (retractions), tachypnea, apnea, and cyanosis.

From Gerber ME, Holinger LD: Congenital laryngeal anomalies. In Bluestone CD, Stool SE, Alper CM, et al (eds): Pediatric Otolaryngology, 4th ed. Philadelphia, Elsevier, 2003, vol 2, pp 1460-1472.

TABLE 21–3   Disorders that Mimic Laryngeal Webs
Laryngomalacia
Congenital subglottic stenosis
Laryngeal and laryngotracheoesophageal clefts
Vascular anomalies (hemangiomas)
Vocal cord paralysis

TABLE 21–4   Anesthetic Management of Laryngeal Web

Experienced anesthesiologist and ear nose and throat surgeon
Operating room equipped with airway emergency equipment
Careful communication with the surgeon and anesthesiologist
Fasting protocols observed except for emergencies
Anticholinergics: glycopyrrolate, 5 to 10 μg/kg, or atropine, 10 mcg/kg
Topical anesthesia with lidocaine 1%
Dexamethasone, 0.5 to 1 mg/kg
Postoperative care: humidified oxygen therapy

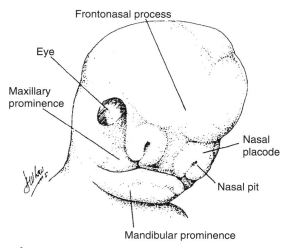

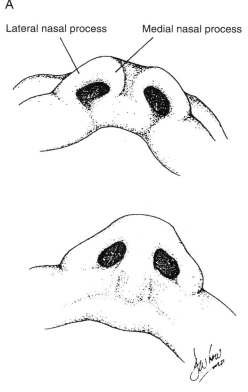

FIGURE 21–6 A, The five facial prominences: frontonasal process, paired mandibular processes, and paired maxillary processes. **B,** Fusion of the medial and lateral nasal processes. *(From Losee JE, Kirschner RE, Whitaker LA, Bartlett SP: Congenital nasal anomalies: A classification scheme. Plast Reconstr Surg 2004;113:676-689, with permission.)*

intubation and mechanical ventilation for 5 to 14 days. This postoperative care requires the use of sedation, neuromuscular blockade, and intensive care monitoring to avoid accidental endotracheal extubation. Prolonged use of neuromuscular blockade can result in residual muscle weakness, which may compromise or delay planned extubation.[43]

Choanal Atresia

Choanal atreasia occurs in approximately 1 in 7,000 live births. Ninety percent of the atresias are bony, and 10% are membranous. Abnormal embryogenesis of neuroectodermal cell lines may explain choanal atresia. The primitive face develops from five facial prominences (Fig. 21-6). The frontonasal prominence is responsible for nasal development from week 3 to 10 of gestation. Migrating neural crest cells form the nasal or olfactory placode, which are convex thickenings on the frontonasal prominence. The primitive nasal pit is formed from a central depression in these placodes. Mesenchymal proliferation around the nasal placode allows horseshoe-shaped medial and lateral prominences to develop and fuse to form the nostril. The nasal pits grow backward.[44]

Choanal atresia is thought to result from the persistence of bucconasal and buccopharyngeal membranes or an insufficient excavation of the nasal pits. Postnasal cavity outlet obstruction is more common. Fifty percent of patients with choanal atresia have other congenital anomalies.[45] Choanal atresia may be partial or one of a constellation of congenital abnormalities known as the CHARGE association (*c*oloboma, *h*eart disease, *a*tresia [choanal], *r*etarded growth, *g*enital abnormalities, *e*ar deformity). Choanal atresia can be unilateral or bilateral. Because neonates are obligate nose breathers, bilateral choanal atresia frequently presents as immediate onset of respiratory distress. Obstruction of the nasal cavity can present with apneic episodes and "cyclic" cyanosis, which are exacerbated by feeding and improved with crying.[46]

The initial presentation of the newborn with bilateral choanal atresia is the immediate onset of respiratory distress. The relationship between the neonatal tongue and the palate perpetuates this obstruction. The use of an oral airway or McGovern nipple (a nipple modified with enlarged perforations at the tip) acts as an alternative temporary airway. Unilateral choanal atresia is usually asymptomatic, except for unilateral mucoid discharges.

TABLE 21–5 Craniofacial Associations with Choanal Atresia

CHARGE association (coloboma, heart defects, atresia of choanae, retarded growth or development of the central nervous system, genitourinary ear anomalies, or deafness)
Apert syndrome: craniosynostosis, syndactylism, difficult airway
Fraser syndrome: laryngeal/tracheal stenosis, congenital heart disease, genitourinary anomalies, renal agenesis/hypoplasia

From Papay FA, McCarthy VP, Eliachar I, et al: Laryngotracheal anomalies in children with craniofacial syndromes. J Craniofacial Surg 2002;13:351-364.

Diagnosis. Inability to pass a 6-Fr catheter through the nasal cavity to more than 32 mm, coupled with an endoscopic examination, verifies the suspected diagnosis. Axial computed tomography (CT) remains the study of choice to delineate the type of atresia and aid with operative planning (transpalatal vs. transnasal approach). Adequate preparation of the patient before scanning by aspirating secretions and the use of decongestant drops helps ensure the best quality radiographic result. Associated craniofacial syndromes can be found in Table 21-5.

Treatment. Ninety percent of patients have bone involvement, whereas in 10% the obstruction is membranous. For bilateral choanal atresia surgical correction occurs in the neonatal period and involves a transnasal correction using CO_2 or neodymium:yttrium-aluminum-garnet (Nd:YAG) lasers. The nasal passage is stented open for 3 to 5 weeks to improve airway patency. The surgical technique generally involves an endoscopic approach where a vertical mucosal incision is made in the posterior bony septum and a perforation within the atresia plate is created (Fig. 21-7). This perforation is then amenable to serial dilatation.[47]

A transpalatal approach has also been used for bony and bilateral atresia. However, the disadvantages of the transpalatal approach are the procedure's long operative time and large blood loss. Additionally, malocclusion occurs in 50% of patients and oronasal fistulas are not uncommon. In patients with unilateral choanal atresia surgical treatment is usually carried out at any time during childhood. The surgical approach can be transnasal or transpalatal.[48]

Anesthetic Considerations. Anesthetic concerns for infants undergoing choanal surgery involve age-appropriate concerns as well as management of a difficult airway. In addition, for infants having the CHARGE association any underlying cardiac issue must be addressed. The airway is secured with an oral RAE tube after an inhalational or intravenous induction. The anesthetic agent is titrated to allow the patient to be extubated as awake as possible with the patient's airway reflexes intact. However, if the procedure has been lengthy, airway edema is present, or hemodynamic instability is present, then the patient should remain intubated until these issues have resolved.

Cystic Hygroma

Cystic hygroma is a congenital cystic lymphatic malformation. It is caused by congenital dysplasia of lymphatics but may be secondary to hamartoma or true neoplasm. The lesion is rare, occurring in 1 in 12,000. Clinically, a cystic hygroma occurs most often (60% to 70%) in the neck (Fig. 21-8). Typically, the neck mass develops in the posterior triangle. If it develops higher in the neck (suprahyoid), it can occupy the anterior triangle and may be associated with intraoral lesions. Suprahyoid lymphangiomas

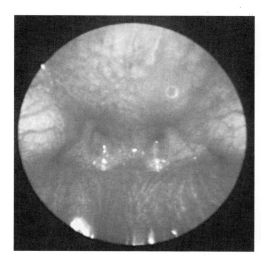
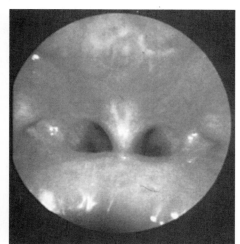

FIGURE 21–7 Choanal atresia. **A,** Choanal atresia in a neonate. The atresia plate on the right side has just been perforated. **B,** The situation after the opening in the atresia plate has been enlarged. *(Courtesy of Charles Bluestone, MD.)*

A   B

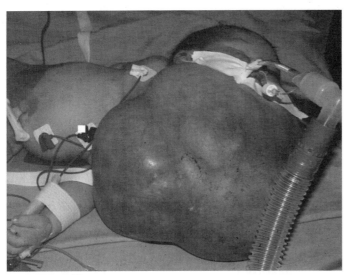

FIGURE 21–8 Neonate with a large neck mass consistent with cystic hygroma. *(From Zitelli BJ, Davis HW: Atlas of Pediatric Physical Diagnosis, 4th ed. St. Louis, Mosby, 2002, p 560, with permission.)*

are more likely to involve the mouth and cause feeding problems and airway obstruction.[49] Infection or hemorrhage into the cyst can also cause acute airway compromise. Twenty percent of cystic hygromas occur below the clavicles in the axillae or the mediastinum. Mediastinal extension can cause respiratory symptoms. Usually, cystic hygromas are diagnosed at birth; however, many are diagnosed during prenatal ultrasound.

Anesthetic Management. During the preoperative evaluation, infants with feeding difficulties should be suspected of having intraoral lesions. Those with respiratory symptoms or coughing should be evaluated for mediastinal involvement with a chest radiograph or CT. Delay in the evaluation should be minimized because the lesions can grow rapidly. The primary anesthetic concern during induction is airway management. Inhalational induction can be performed, but difficulty with both ventilation and intubation has been described.[50] A nasopharyngeal airway may help open the airway and restore ventilation. If preoperative examination suggests difficulty with both ventilation and intubation, consideration should be given to performing an awake or a sedated fiberoptic nasal intubation. Other options include sedated placement of a laryngeal mask airway (LMA) with subsequent fiberoptic intubation, blind nasotracheal intubation, or a sedated tracheostomy.

The surgical resection of a cystic hygroma can be associated with significant blood loss. Intraoperative management should focus on maintaining normovolemia and normothermia. Intravascular access with two large intravenous catheters and an arterial catheter may be required to manage the resuscitation. Central venous access from the neck or chest may not be possible depending on the location of the lymphangioma. Femoral venous cannulation should be considered as an alternative. Fluid shifts and third space fluid losses may be significant. Maintenance of body temperature can be achieved with warming lights, fluid warmers, and forced warm air blankets. Surgical resection may involve manipulation of the vagal nerve, which can result in bradycardia. Evaluation at the end of surgery will determine the feasibility of early extubation. Infants with difficult intubation, significant fluid shifts, or hemodynamic instability should remain intubated and undergo recovery in the intensive care unit. Vocal cord dysfunction can occur secondary to nerve injury from the surgical dissection and should be considered if acute airway obstruction occurs after extubation.

Management of prenatally diagnosed cystic hygromas may involve delivery via the EXIT (ex-utero intrapartum treatment) procedure. During the EXIT procedure the head and torso of the fetus are delivered and the airway is secured while uteroplacental support is maintained.[51,52] Intubation can be achieved with direct laryngoscopy. If this is impossible because of the anatomy, rigid bronchoscopy or tracheostomy can be performed (Fig. 21-9). Tracheostomy may be very difficult if the mass repositions or covers the trachea.

CRANIOFACIAL ANOMALIES

Craniofacial anomalies are characterized by congenital or acquired deformities of the cranial and/or facial skeleton. Craniofacial anomalies, although rare, make up a considerably diverse group of defects. The incidence of all of the anomalies may be difficult to determine because they include only those defects that are well defined. An estimated 1200 persons per year are born with these defects. In the past 2 decades the surgical repairs have advanced significantly and now include the surgical expertise from multiple fields. These specialties include plastic surgery, neurosurgery, oral maxillofacial surgery, otorhinolaryngology, dentistry, orthodontics, speech pathology, genetics, and anesthesiology. The goal of surgical intervention is to restore both form and function.

The classification of craniofacial anomalies is very difficult because of their variability, rarity, and degree of severity and lack of understanding of the etiology and pathogenesis. The Committee on Nomenclature and Classification of Craniofacial Anomalies of the American Cleft Palate Association has proposed the following classification: (1) clefts, (2) synostosis, (3) hypoplasia, (4) hyperplasia, and (5) unclassified.[53]

Clefts

Craniofacial clefts involve a defect of the underlying cranial and/or facial skeleton. This group of deformities has been

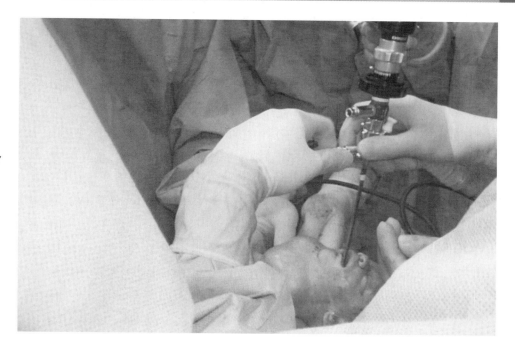

FIGURE 21–9 Rigid bronchoscopy performed during the EXIT procedure on a neonate with cystic hygroma. (Courtesy of Laura Myers, MD.)

best classified by Tessier, who uses the orbit as the center of the defect from which the clefts radiate like the spokes of a wheel (Fig. 21-10). Cleft lip and palate are the more commonly recognized examples of craniofacial clefts. Treacher Collins syndrome, which is also known as mandibulofacial dysostosis, is an example of a craniofacial cleft that involves clefts 6, 7, and 8 (see Figs. 21-10 and 21-11).

Treacher Collins syndrome was first described in 1846 by Thompson and was further elaborated by Treacher Collins. This is a rare syndrome of facial clefting and is transmitted in an autosomal dominant pattern. The syndrome is characterized by poorly developed supraorbital ridges, aplastic/hypoplastic zygomas, ear deformities, cleft palate (in one third), and mandibular and midface hypoplasia (Fig. 21-11). From birth, issues of airway adequacy take priority. The hypoplastic maxillae and mandible along with choanal atresia and glossoptosis all contribute to varying degrees of airway obstruction. Tracheostomy may be required during infancy for those at highest risk of obstructive sleep apnea and sudden infant death syndrome (SIDS).[54] Aside from cleft lip and palate repair, the timing of major reconstruction typically occurs during childhood or adolescence when the cranio-orbital-zygomatic bony development is nearly complete. Infants and children with Treacher Collins syndrome can have congenital cardiac defects.

Anesthetic Considerations. Anesthetic concerns specific to this syndrome primarily involve the airway. Infants and children with Treacher Collins syndrome may be very difficult or impossible to mask ventilate and/or intubate, and this airway difficulty may increase with age.[55] Several techniques have been successfully used to safely manage the airway in these infants. The LMA has been used to successfully ventilate a newborn with Treacher Collins syndrome for an extended period of time.[56] Direct laryngoscopy, regardless of the blade used, may be difficult. The Bullard laryngoscope has been used successfully.[57] The LMA has also been used to assist in the intubation of these children.[58,59] Given the potential for difficult mask ventilation and intubation, this population may be best managed with a sedated fiberoptic intubation or a sedated tracheostomy. Another concern for the anesthesiologist is protecting the patient's eyes. Because of the maxillary and zygomatic hypoplasia, prone positioning may increase the risk of orbital compression and perioperative blindness.

Synostosis

Craniosynostosis is defined as a premature closure of one or more of the cranial sutures. This results in abnormalities in the size and shape of the calvarium, cranial base, and orbits and constitutes a diverse group of deformities. The craniosynostoses not only affect cosmetic appearance but also can affect brain growth, intracranial pressure (ICP), and vision, resulting in developmental delay, increased ICP, and visual loss. The synostoses are classified based on head shape, not the involved suture (Fig. 21-12).

Craniosynostosis can occur by itself (simple) or as a major component of a syndrome (complex or syndromic). Five syndromes are associated with craniosynostosis. They include Apert, Pfeiffer, Saethre-Chotzen, Carpenter, and Crouzon syndromes. Table 21-6 lists the various syndromes and their associated anomalies and anesthetic concerns. Four of the five are categorized as acrocephalosyndactylies because they involve deformities of the

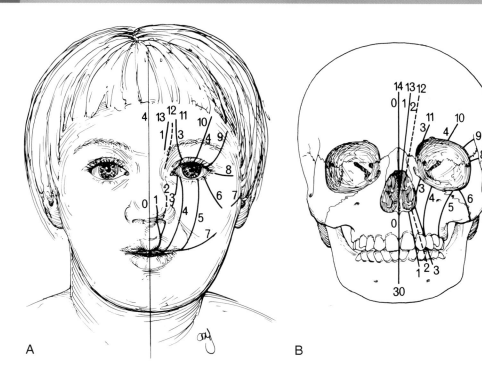

FIGURE 21–10 Tessier classification of rare craniofacial clefts. Using orbit as center of reference, clefts are oriented like spokes of wheel, with those caudad to the orbit considered facial and those cephalad considered cranial. For descriptive purposes, those clefts involving two regions are designated by two numbers (e.g., 4, 10), the sum of which is typically 14. Bony clefts (**B**) are usually reflected in soft tissue (**A**). *(From Whitaker LA, Bartlett SP: Craniofacial anomalies. In Jurkiewicz J, Krizek T, Mathes S, Ariyan S [eds]: Plastic Surgery: Principles and Practice. St. Louis, Mosby, 1990, p 109, with permission.)*

head *(cephalo)* and extremities *(syndactaly)*. Crouzon's syndrome does not have musculoskeletal anomalies as part of the syndrome. Infants and children with synostosis present to the operating room for cranial vault remodeling to reduce ICP, prevent brain injury, and enhance appearance. Repair of syndromic craniosynostosis may be more complicated and appears to be associated with increased blood loss. The etiology of the increased bleeding is unclear, but it might be related to the length of surgery.[60]

Apert syndrome is part of a group of craniofacial disorders, referred to as acrocephalosyndactylies, that are characterized by craniofacial and extremity anomalies. There is an autosomal dominant pattern of inheritance. The etiology of the syndrome is from a mutation with the fibroblast growth factor receptor-2 gene *(FGFR2)*.[61] The characteristic features of Apert's syndrome include turribrachycephaly (high steep flat forehead and occiput), midface hypoplasia, and orbital hypertelorism (Fig. 21-13). Cleft palate occurs in approximately 30%. Choanal atresia and occasionally tracheal stenosis have been reported and can cause airway obstruction. Congenital cardiac disease is one of the more common associated visceral anomalies, occurring in approximately 10%. Genitourinary anomalies (hydronephrosis, cryptorchidism) also occur in 10% of patients with Apert's syndrome.[62] Severe synostosis can result in increased ICP and, if uncorrected, developmental delay. Syndactyly of the hands and feet often present as the fusion of digits 2 to 4, which can make intravenous access difficult. Cervical spine fusion has been reported in Apert's syndrome and may make endotracheal intubation even more challenging if there is decreased neck mobility.[63] Many children with Apert's syndrome have been intubated

uneventfully. However, suboptimal laryngoscopic views secondary to abnormal anatomy may require flexible fiberoptic intubation. The LMA may also be a reasonable adjunct in those patients who are difficult to ventilate or intubate. However, to date there are no reported cases of their use in infants and children with Apert's syndrome. The clinical features and the anesthetic implications of Apert's syndrome and the other acrocephalosyndactylies are outlined in Table 21-6. Unlike Apert's syndrome, the other acrocephalosyndactylies are not typically associated with difficult airways. However, midface hypoplasia is common in these infants and may cause significant upper airway obstruction intraoperatively and postoperatively.[64]

Crouzon's disease, also known as craniofacial dysostosis, is also part of the syndromic craniosynostosis. These infants present with craniofacial anomalies without visceral or extremity involvement. The anomalies can result in significant airway obstruction that may require early tracheostomy. Crouzon's disease results from a mutation in the *FGFR2*, the same gene that causes Apert's syndrome. Table 21-6 outlines the main clinical features and anesthetic issues. During infancy these patients may present to the operating room for tracheostomy and/or cranial vault remodeling.

Hypoplasia

Hypoplasia of the craniofacial skeleton is a category of craniofacial anomalies characterized by hypoplasia or atrophy of a portion of the craniofacial soft tissue and skeleton. Pierre Robin sequence and hemifacial microsomia

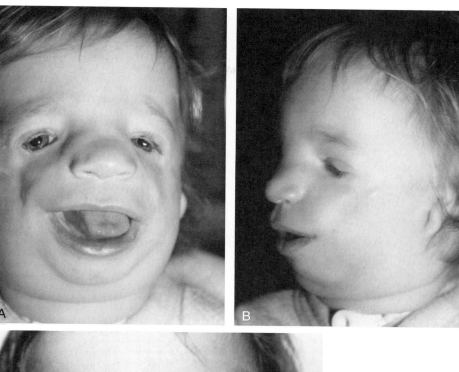

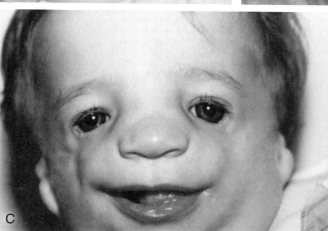

FIGURE 21–11   Child with Treacher Collins syndrome. *(From Losee JE, Bartlett SP: Treacher Collins syndrome. In Lin KY, Ogle RC, Jane JA [eds]: Craniofacial Surgery: Science and Surgical Technique. Philadelphia, WB Saunders, 2001, pp 288-308, with permission.)*

(including Goldenhar's syndrome) are examples of these anomalies.

Pierre Robin sequence is characterized by retrognathia, glossoptosis (tongue falling to the back of the throat), and airway obstruction and probably occurs secondary to a fixed fetal position in utero that inhibits mandibular growth. Management of this sequence is dependent on the severity of respiratory distress and airway obstruction. Those infants with mild obstruction and minimal respiratory distress who can continue to feed may require prone positioning only or no intervention at all. For more severe respiratory distress, the tongue can be surgically attached to the lower lip (tongue lip adhesion) to decrease airway obstruction and allow time for the mandible to grow.

Anesthetic Management. Airway management in the infant with Pierre Robin sequence can be very challenging because of difficulty with mask ventilation and intubation. The LMA has been successfully used to ventilate and to assist in the intubation of these patients.[65] Nasal intubation with the flexible fiberoptic scope has also been described.[66] In infants who present with significant difficulty with ventilation or intubation, aside from oral pharyngeal and nasal airways, a suture (0-silk) can be placed at the base of the tongue to displace the tongue anteriorly to assist with ventilation or intubation.

Hemifacial microsomia is characterized by unilateral or asymmetrical development of the facial bones and muscles and frequently involves the ear. This manifests as hypoplasia of the malar-maxillary-mandibular region and

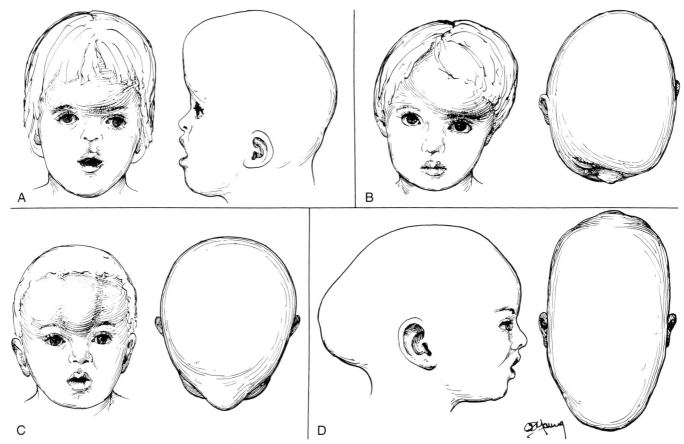

FIGURE 21–12 Typical patterns of craniofacial morphology associated with craniosynostosis. **A,** Turribrachycephaly. **B,** Plagiocephaly. **C,** Trigonocephaly. **D,** Scaphocephaly. *(From Whitaker LA, Bartlett SP: Craniofacial anomalies. In Jurkiewicz J, Krizek T, Mathes S, Ariyan S [eds]: Plastic Surgery: Principles and Practice. St. Louis, Mosby, 1990, p 119, with permission.)*

usually involves the temporomandibular joint. The defect occurs from an anomaly of the first and second branchial arches and is believed to be secondary to a fetal vascular accident. Goldenhar's syndrome is a subset of hemifacial microsomia and is composed of hemifacial microsomia, epibulbar dermoid, and/or rib or vertebral, anomalies. The vertebral pathology can involve the cervical vertebrae and can significantly reduce the cervical range of motion. Other associated anomalies of hemifacial microsomia include cardiac (ventricular septal defect, tetralogy of Fallot, coarctation), renal, and neurologic defects (hydrocephalus). Patients with hemifacial microsomia can have significant upper airway obstruction and obstructive sleep apnea.

Anesthetic Management. Airway management is a major concern in these patients. Mask ventilation may be difficult because of the facial asymmetry. Intubation is more challenging because of micrognathia, asymmetrical mandibular hypoplasia, and potentially from decreased cervical range of motion. This difficulty may decrease with age but may increase after surgical reconstruction. Successful ventilation and intubation of an infant with Goldenhar's syndrome

has been reported with an LMA and flexible fiberoptic scope.[67]

Surgical Correction of Craniofacial Anomalies

Surgical correction of these anomalies is performed to improve form and function and to minimize disability. Airway obstruction, increased ICP, developmental delay, and visual loss are some of the pathologic processes that may be corrected or prevented with appropriate surgical intervention. Several procedures are performed to correct these deformities. They include strip craniectomy, cranial vault remodeling, frontal-orbital advancement, midface advancement (Le Fort I, Le Fort III, monoblock advancement), and distraction osteogenesis. Strip craniectomy, cranial vault remodeling, and frontal-orbital advancement are surgical approaches to correct craniosynostosis. The goal is to release the synostotic sutures and open up the cranium to allow brain growth and development. Strip craniectomy involves less blood loss but because of premature refusion is usually reserved only for patients

TABLE 21–6 Anesthetic Considerations with Craniofacial Syndromes

Syndrome	Affected Suture	Clinical Features	Anesthetic Issues
Apert syndrome	Coronal	*HEENT:* turribrachycephaly, midface hypoplasia, orbital hypertelorism, cleft palate in 30%, occasional choanal atresia and tracheal stenosis, airway obstruction *Cardiac:* congenital heart disease occurs in 10%; may include ventricular septal defect, pulmonary stenosis *Genitourinary:* hydronephrosis in 3%, cryptorchidism in 4.5% *Musculoskeletal:* syndactyly of the hands and feet, fusion of digits 2 to 4, fusion of the cervical vertebrae can occur *Neurologic:* mental retardation common, may have elevated intracranial pressure *Dermatologic:* acne vulgaris common	*Preoperative labs:* hematocrit, type and screen *Airway management:* may be very difficult mask ventilation because of midface hypoplasia, choanal atresia, and tracheal stenosis; may be difficult intubation secondary to facial anomalies and decreased neck mobility *Cardiac:* emphasis on balancing pulmonary and systemic blood flow, de-air intravenous lines, endocarditis prophylaxis *Musculoskeletal:* cervical fusion may decrease neck extension; syndactyly may make vascular access difficult *Neurologic:* caution with premedication if elevated intracranial pressure
Pfeiffer syndrome	Coronal and occasionally sagittal	*HEENT:* tower skull, midface hypoplasia, orbital hypertelorism, proptosis, choanal atresia uncommon *Pulmonary:* obstructive sleep apnea *Cardiac:* may have cardiac defects *Musculoskeletal:* usually mild syndactyly involving broad thumbs and great toes; rarely ankylosis of the elbow occurs; fusion of cervical vertebrae reported *Neurologic:* generally normal but mild developmental delay can occur; may have increased intracranial pressure	*Preoperative labs:* hematocrit, type and screen *Airway management:* no reported cases of difficult intubation; airway obstruction may occur intraoperatively or postoperatively *Cardiac:* emphasis on balancing pulmonary and systemic blood flow, de-air intravenous lines, endocarditis prophylaxis *Musculoskeletal:* cervical fusion may decrease neck extension; syndactyly may make vascular access difficult *Neurologic:* caution with premedication if elevated intracranial pressure; eyes require protection if ocular proptosis present
Saethre-Chotzen syndrome	Coronal and others	*HEENT:* brachycephaly, maxillary hypoplasia, orbital hypertelorism, beaked nose, occasional cleft palate *Genitourinary:* renal anomalies and cryptorchidism *Musculoskeletal:* short stature, mild syndactyly; cervical fusion possible *Neurologic:* mild developmental delay; rare increased intracranial pressure	*Preoperative labs:* hematocrit, type and screen *Airway management:* no reported cases of difficulty with ventilation or intubation *Musculoskeletal:* cervical fusion may decrease neck extension; syndactyly may make vascular access difficult *Neurologic:* caution with premedication if elevated intracranial pressure
Carpenter syndrome	Coronal and others	*HEENT:* tower skull, down-thrust eyes, orbital hypertelorism, low-set ears, small mandible *Cardiac:* cardiac defects common (ventricular and atrial septal defects) *Genitourinary:* hypogonadism *Musculoskeletal:* syndactyly of hands and feet *Neurologic:* developmental delay common but variable, may have increased intracranial pressure *Other:* obesity	*Preoperative labs:* hematocrit, type and screen *Airway management:* small mandible may make intubation difficult; obesity may make ventilation difficult *Musculoskeletal:* syndactyly may make intravenous access difficult *Neurologic:* caution with premedication if elevated intracranial pressure

TABLE 21-6	Anesthetic Considerations with Craniofacial Syndromes—cont'd		
Syndrome	Affected Suture	Clinical Features	Anesthetic Issues
Crouzon Syndrome	Coronal, lambdoid, others	*HEENT:* frontal bossing, tower skull, midface hypoplasia, beaked nose, hypertelorism, ocular proptosis, airway obstruction can occur *Neurologic:* occasional mild developmental delay, may have increased intracranial pressure	*Preoperative labs:* hematocrit, type and screen *Airway management:* may be a difficult intubation; may have airway obstruction during awake or sleep states; caution with premedication *Neurologic:* caution with premedication if elevated intracranial pressure; eyes require protection if ocular proptosis present

with sagittal synostosis. The surgical approach for these three procedures is through a bicoronal incision. Subperiosteal dissection allows access to the upper facial skeleton for surgical manipulation (Fig. 21-14). These procedures are performed during the first year of life. They can involve significant blood loss, and preparations to ensure patient safety include adequate intravenous access and availability of blood products.

Mandibular advancement procedures are frequently performed to correct appearance, malocclusion, and airway obstruction. These procedures are not routinely performed in the infant. Generally these surgeries take place during early to late childhood.

Distraction osteogenesis is a technique that was developed to create bone elongation by creating a bone cut (osteotomy) and distracting the two ends. It was first developed and utilized by orthopedic surgeons but was not used for craniofacial surgery until 1992 when McCarthy described distraction osteogenesis to lengthen the human mandible.[68] This technique has now been used in many children to distract the mandible and midface (Fig. 21-15). Distraction of the mandible and midface can be used to correct appearance and to correct upper airway obstruction. Airway obstruction has been corrected using distraction osteogenesis in infants as young as 14 weeks old.[69]

Anesthetic Management. The anesthetic management of infants with craniofacial anomalies begins with a complete preoperative evaluation. The history should define the anomaly and identify if there is an associated syndrome. Infants and children with syndromes may have more difficult airways, other organ involvement, and more complicated surgical repair with more bleeding. Associated anomalies that can present a challenge to the anesthesiologist include facial and airway features that make mask ventilation and intubation difficult. Airway pathology can also cause obstruction, and some of these children have obstructive sleep apnea. History of fatigue or sweating with feedings, cyanosis, and syncope are suggestive of an underlying cardiac anomaly. Cardiac pathology is associated with some of the syndromes (e.g., Treacher Collins, Apert, Pfeiffer, Carpenter, and hemifacial microsomia). Some of these infants and children may have increased ICP. This may manifest as headaches, vomiting, and somnolence.

A thorough airway examination may be difficult to perform on an infant. Features that may predict difficulty with mask ventilation include midface hypoplasia and enlarged tongues. In addition, a small mandibular space, decreased jaw opening and translocation, and decreased neck flexion and extension predict difficult intubation. The rest of the examination should focus on identifying heart murmurs. In infants with syndactyly, identifying potential intravenous and arterial access sites is critical. For reconstructions that involve significant blood loss a preoperative hematocrit and type and crossmatch should be performed. Former premature infants and infants younger than 1 month old should have their glucose level monitored. Premedication can be performed for most

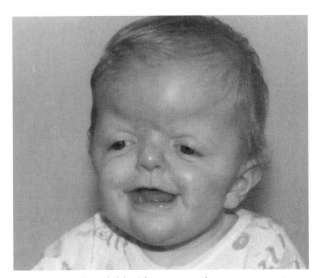

FIGURE 21-13 Child with Apert syndrome. *(From Buchman SR, Muraszko KM: Syndromic craniosynostosis. In Lin KY, Ogle RC, Jane JA [eds]: Craniofacial Surgery: Science and Surgical Technique. Philadelphia, WB Saunders, 2001, pp 252-271, with permission.)*

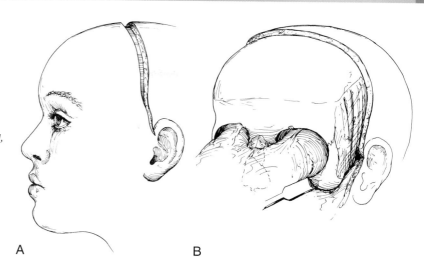

FIGURE 21–14 Bicoronal incision (**A**) with extensive subperiosteal dissection (**B**) provides access for surgical manipulation of upper facial skeleton. *(From Whitaker LA, Bartlett SP: Craniofacial anomalies. In Jurkiewicz J, Krizek T, Mathes S, Ariyan S [eds]: Plastic Surgery: Principles and Practice. St. Louis, Mosby, 1990, p 107, with permission.)*

A   B

children older than the age of 1 but is rarely necessary in those younger than 10 months old. Children with evidence of airway obstruction or increased ICP should not receive a premedicant. Endocarditis prophylaxis should be considered in those patients with congenital heart disease.

Airway management in these patients may be very challenging. As previously stated, the difficulty may present during attempts at ventilation, intubation, or both. Fortunately, difficult airways are not common. However, the incidence is higher in those patients with congenital syndromes and in those patients who have had previous reconstruction. Many techniques have been successfully described in infants; these include using the Bullard laryngoscope, LMA, flexible fiberoptic scope, and retrograde intubation.[57,66,70] A combination of techniques may be required to secure the airway. For example, the LMA has been used to facilitate the passage of the fiberoptic scope and endotracheal tube.[58] Some infants with craniofacial anomalies require tracheostomy because of significant upper airway obstruction.[64,71] Adequate preparation entails having all of the necessary equipment available and having personnel who are trained and experienced to use these airway instruments. It may also mean having a pediatric otorhinolaryngologist immediately available.

Several intraoperative considerations exist when managing the anesthetic for craniofacial repairs. Often these procedures are long and expose infants to the risks of hypovolemia, hypothermia, blood loss, and venous air emboli. The craniofacial procedures performed during the first year of life include cranial vault remodeling, fronto-orbital advancement, strip craniectomy, and distraction osteogenesis. The cranial-based procedures can involve significant blood loss because of the duration of the procedure and also because of complications such as entering the sagittal sinus. Nearly 90% to 100% of the infants undergoing these procedures will require a blood transfusion.[72] Even the strip craniectomy, which is typically performed to correct sagittal synostosis and results in less blood loss, can still produce significant hemorrhage. Infants are particularly at risk of being exposed to transfusions because they can present to the operating room at the nadir of their physiologic anemia (2 to 3 months of age). Preparation for these procedures requires a baseline hematocrit and a type and crossmatch. Adequate intravenous access needs to be obtained for resuscitation. In an infant, at least two large-bore (22 to 18 gauge) peripheral intravenous catheters should provide adequate access.

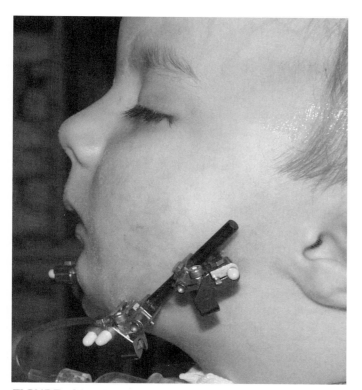

FIGURE 21–15 Mandibular distractor in an infant with Pierre Robin sequence. *(Courtesy of Joseph E. Losee.)*

Arterial pressure monitoring is recommended for beat-to-beat analysis of blood pressure and intravascular volume status, as well as for blood gas monitoring.

Techniques to minimize blood loss have been proposed and include preoperative recombinant erythropoietin, acute normovolemic hemodilution, induced hypotension, electrocautery, aprotinin, and use of a cell saver. Preoperatively, recombinant erythropoietin may decrease the transfusion requirements in infants having craniosynostosis repair. The reported dose of erythropoietin is 300 to 600 units/kg given subcutaneously one to three times per week, along with oral iron supplementation. Erythropoietin is started three weeks before surgery. A prospective study of once-weekly dosing decreased the incidence of transfusion in infants having craniosynostosis repair from 93% to 57%.[60]

Aprotinin, a serine protease inhibitor, may also decrease perioperative blood loss and transfusion requirements during craniofacial procedures. In a prospective randomized and blinded placebo-controlled study evaluating the effect of aprotinin in infants and children having cranial vault remodeling and frontal orbital advancements, D'Errico and coworkers noted a reduction in the amount of packed red blood cells being transfused intraoperatively and postoperatively in those receiving aprotinin. However, the number of patients requiring transfusion was not reduced.[73] No adverse events were reported.

In the past, the use of cell saver has been reported as being impractical for small pediatric patients because of the size of the receptacle.[74] Recently, the cell saver reservoirs are available in sizes as small as 55 mL. This technology may reduce the rate of autogenous blood transfusion in infants having craniofacial surgery. In a prospective analysis evaluating the use of cell saver with a 55-mL pediatric bowl in patients pretreated with erythropoietin, only 30% of those infants having cranial vault remodeling required allogenic blood.[75]

Venous air embolism (VAE) is a potential complication of craniofacial and neurosurgical procedures. It can present as hemodynamic instability and can result in death. VAE can occur commonly in pediatric patients having cranial-based procedures. A prospective study using a precordial Doppler in infants and children having craniosynostosis repair detected VAE in 82% of the patients. Thirty-one percent developed hypotension secondary to VAE, but none developed cardiovascular collapse.[76] This is higher than the previously reported incidence of 66%.[77] Infants may be at increased risk of VAE because they can hemorrhage significantly during cranial vault remodeling, resulting in low central venous pressures. In addition, the relatively large size of the infant head may raise the surgical site above the level of the heart, thereby increasing the pressure gradient for air entrainment. Some advocate the placement of central venous catheters to monitor the trend of central

venous pressures and minimize the risk of air embolism. However, there are no data that suggest central venous pressure monitoring decreases the risk of VAE. Management of VAE begins with preventing hypovolemic states by providing adequate volume resuscitation and using a precordial Doppler for early detection of VAE. Lowering the head of the bed, flooding the surgical field with saline, applying bone wax, discontinuing nitrous oxide, and providing inotropic support are all measures that have been utilized to acutely manage VAE.

Craniofacial procedures can be very long, lasting several hours. Complications resulting from long surgical procedures include skin breakdown, neuropathic injury, and hypothermia. Attention must be paid to the initial setup to ensure adequate positioning and padding to minimize these intraoperative injuries. Infants having cranial vault remodeling may be positioned prone, and attention to protecting the face and eyes is important. Patients with syndromes that alter the architecture of the midface may present a challenge when placed prone because adequately protecting the face and eyes may be more difficult. An example of the initial setup is shown in Figure 21-16. The infant is placed on a full access Bair hugger to minimize hypothermia, and the surgical site (head) is then isolated from the body using plastic drapes. This not only minimizes convective and radiant heat losses but also prevents conductive heat loss to a wet bed from irrigation and blood. Blood products should be warmed through a fluid warmer before administration (except for platelets).

Postoperative Management. The postoperative management of infants having craniofacial surgery depends on coexisting morbidities and the procedure performed. Infants who have had distractors placed may have a more difficult airway after extubation because of location of the device. Mask ventilation can be very difficult with mandibular distractors. Airway equipment, including appropriately sized LMAs, should be available after extubation. External maxillary distractors are not typically placed in infants. However, their use in older children can make access to the airway more challenging, and personnel and equipment to remove part of the device are important in the operating room.[78] Infants having cranial vault remodeling and frontal orbital advancements can experience significant blood loss intraoperatively. Providing these patients are adequately resuscitated and are hemodynamically stable, they can often be extubated in the operating room. Infants with difficult airway, significant airway obstruction, or who have experienced intraoperative complications may benefit from delayed extubation in the intensive care unit/operating room after their condition has stabilized. Ongoing blood loss is common after major craniofacial surgery, and infants may require repeat transfusions in the immediate postoperative setting. Other complications include cerebral edema,[79] visual changes,[80] CSF leak,[81]

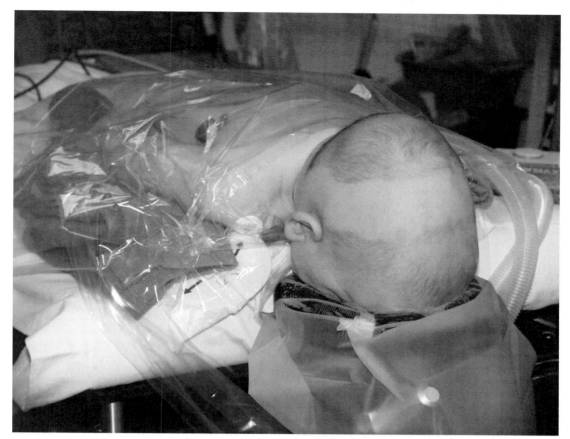

FIGURE 21–16 Operating room setup for posterior cranial vault remodeling. Note application of forced warm air plastic sheets to separate the head from the body. This creates a barrier to fluids (blood, prep solution, irrigation). Special attention to avoid ocular pressure is essential. *(Courtesy of Joseph E. Losee.)*

infection,[82] electrolyte abnormalities (hyponatremia),[79] metabolic acidosis, and transfusion reactions.

MEDIASTINAL MASSES

Mediastinal masses in infants and children present a diagnostic and therapeutic dilemma to the medical team caring for them. Careful communication between the oncologists, pediatric surgeons, anesthesiologists, radiologists, and intensivists is important for a favorable outcome. An understanding of the pathology, clinical presentation, diagnosis, imaging, and treatment is instrumental in the efficient and safe care of these children with mediastinal masses.

Anatomic Considerations. A classification of mediastinal masses based on location is presented in Table 21-7. The anterior mediastinum is the zone posterior to the sternum, anterior to the pericardium, superior to the diaphragm, and inferior to the plane through the sternomanubrial junction. Anterior mediastinal masses are common in children. The most common anterior mediastinal masses are teratomas, thymomas, and lymphomas (Hodgkin's and

non-Hodgkin's lymphoma). They account for approximately 40% of the tumors. The middle mediastinum is defined by the pericardium and origins of the great vessels. The posterior mediastinum is outlined by the pericardium and great vessels anteriorly, the vertebral column posteriorly, and the parietal pleurae laterally. Generally, neurogenic tumors occur in the posterior mediastinum, of which neuroblastoma is the most common.[83]

Pathology. Anterior mediastinal masses have been reported mostly in older children, but there are several cases reported in infants.[84-86] Most masses in children younger than 2 years of age are benign. Malignant masses are more frequently found in older children and are mostly lymphomas, Hodgkin's and non-Hodgkin's, as well as neurogenic tumors.[87,88]

Masses of the mediastinum surround the large airways, heart, and great vessels. Compression of the airways and great vessels can result in respiratory and cardiovascular symptoms.

Clinical Presentation. The signs and symptoms depend on the size and location of the mediastinal mass and on the

TABLE 21–7 Mediastinal Tumors

	Benign	Malignant
Anterior	Thymoma Thymic cyst Thymolipoma Thymic hyperplasia Thyroid Cystic hygroma Parathyroid adenoma Foramen of Morgagni hernia	Thymic carcinoma Thyroid carcinoma Seminoma Mixed germ cell Lymphoma Thymic carcinoid
Middle	Benign adenopathy Cysts Esophageal Hiatal hernia Cardiac and vascular structures Lipomatosis Cardiac and vascular structures Cardiophrenic fat pad Foramen of morgagni hernia Ectopic thyroid	Lymphoma Metastases Esophageal cancer Thyroid carcinoma
Posterior	Neurofibroma Schwannoma Foramen of Bochdalek hernia Meningocele	Neuroblastoma

From Yoneda KY, Louie S, Shelton DK: Mediastinal tumors. Curr Opin Pulm Med 2001;7:226-233.

extent of compression of the tracheobronchial tree and the cardiovascular system.[89] Symptoms related to compression of the tracheobronchial tree include cough, dyspnea, and orthopnea. The symptoms are generally exacerbated when the child is in the supine position. Signs of respiratory compromise include stridor, cyanosis, wheezing, and decreased breath sounds. Compression of the cardiovascular system manifests as fatigue, headaches, fainting spells, and orthopnea and may cause SVC obstruction or SVC syndrome (edema of the head and neck; distended neck veins and collateral veins on the chest wall; plethora; cyanosis of the face, neck, and arms; proptosis; and

TABLE 21–8 Clinical Findings in Patients with Mediastinal Masses

History	Physical Examination	Laboratory
Airway		

Cough
Cyanosis
Dyspnea
Orthopnea
	Decreased breath sounds
	Wheezing
	Stridor
	Cyanosis
		Chest radiograph (posteroanterior and
		  lateral to look for tracheal deviation or
		  compression)
		Flow-volume loops supine and sitting

Cardiovascular		

Fatigue
Faintness
Headache
Shortness of
  breath and
  orthopnea
Cough
	Neck or facial edema
	Jugular distention
	Papilledema
	Blood pressure changes or changes
	  in pallor with postural changes
	
	Pulsus paradoxus
		Chest radiographic changes in cardiac
		  silhouette
		Echocardiogram done supine and sitting

From Pulleritz J, Holzman RS: Anaesthesia for patients with mediastinal masses. Can Anaesth Soc J 1989;36:681-688.

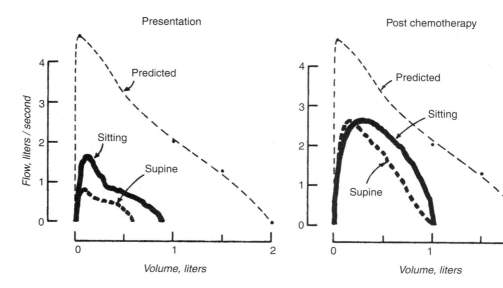

Horner's syndrome.[90] Symptoms of cerebral edema from venous hypertension can occur with SVC obstruction and include headaches, syncope, and lethargy (Table 21-8).

Diagnosis. Procurement of tissue for diagnosis of mediastinal masses can be achieved by several methods. Fine-needle aspiration biopsy can be performed by experienced interventional radiologists. However, this procedure carries a 15% inconclusive result.[91] This requires surgical biopsy to ascertain the diagnosis. Surgical approaches depend on the location of the mass. Consideration should always be given to collecting tissue from a remote location, such as a cervical lymph node or pleural fluid, under local anesthesia. If these sites are not possible then a tissue sample will need to be collected from the mediastinum. Anterior mediastinotomy (Chamberlain procedure), in which the second or third interspace is incised for exposure, allows access to the anterior mediastinum, right paratracheal, and aortopulmonary areas.[91,91a] Mediastinoscopy and thoracoscopy with video assistance have become widely accepted for the diagnosis and management of mediastinal disease. If local anesthetic techniques are not possible and the patient is considered at high anesthetic risk, empirical therapy with irradiation or corticosteroids may be considered. A brief preoperative course of radiation has been described in patients believed to be at highest risk of perioperative complications. Anesthesia was safely provided to all of the patients, and the tissue sample was still adequate to make a diagnosis.[92] Limiting the duration of treatment or shielding an area of the tumor from the radiation may improve the chances of a tissue diagnosis. However, empirical therapy can alter the tissue and should be considered as a last resort.

Preanesthetic Evaluation. Many mediastinal tumors are asymptomatic and are first noted on routine chest radiography. In some studies only 30% of children with Hodgkin's disease demonstrated symptoms.[93] Chest CT with iodinated contrast is the study of choice to determine the location and extent of compression of adjacent structures in the chest. Magnetic resonance imaging (MRI) is superior to CT for imaging nerve plexus and blood vessels. MRI is useful when iodinated contrast is contraindicated or in the diagnosis of thyroid masses.[94] When cardiovascular structures are involved, echocardiography, contrast medium–enhanced CT, or cardiac MRI is essential. Echocardiography may provide dynamic information regarding ventricular compression and performance. Pulmonary function testing in the supine and sitting position is important in determining the extent of airway compromise. The supine position tends to exacerbate the respiratory compromise. Intrathoracic obstruction causes distortion of the maximal expiratory flow rate, whereas extrathoracic obstruction causes distortion of the inspiratory flow rate. An equal reduction of both inspiratory and expiratory flow rates is affected by fixed lesions. In patients with mediastinal masses pulmonary function testing reveals both an obstructive and a restrictive impairment (Fig. 21-17).[95]

The essential component of the preanesthetic evaluation is to identify those patients at highest risk of perioperative respiratory and cardiovascular complications. One study suggests that the narrowing of the trachea and bronchi to less than 50% predicted on CT indicates an increase in anesthetic risk.[96] In another study all children with anterior mediastinal masses who demonstrated tracheal cross-sectional areas greater than 50% predicted or a peak expiratory flow rate greater than 50% predicted underwent uneventful general anesthesia.[95] The only symptom that appears to correlate with cross-sectional area of the airway is orthopnea. In the previous study, no patients with a cross-sectional area of the airway greater than 50% demonstrated orthopnea; and in several cases, orthopnea was the only symptom that consistently preceded

FIGURE 21–17 Expiratory flow volume loops in an 8-year old with an anterior mediastinal mass. Note the reduction in maximum flows that improves after 4 days of chemotherapy. *(From Shamberger RC, Holzman RS, Griscom NT, et al: CT quantitation of tracheal cross-sectional area as a guide to the surgical and anesthetic management of children with anterior mediastinal masses. J Pediatr Surg 1991;26: 138-142.)*

respiratory collapse on induction of anesthesia.[86,96,97] In adults it appears that those with cardiorespiratory signs and symptoms, both obstructive and restrictive abnormalities on pulmonary function tests, and those with tracheal compression greater than 50% are at greatest risk of having early postoperative life-threatening complications.[98]

Anesthetic Management. Several reports have described the risk of life-threatening airway obstruction and cardiovascular collapse during general anesthesia in patients with mediastinal masses.[86,97,99] These catastrophic outcomes occur because of the physiologic changes that occur during general anesthesia. During general anesthesia, lung volume is reduced owing to loss of inspiratory muscle tone, as well as to the loss of the tethering effect that the expanded lung has on the airway. The normal transpleural pressure gradient that distends the airway during inspiration is diminished, and this further compromises the airway caliber. During spontaneous ventilation, the diaphragm moves caudad. While the patient is paralyzed with neuromuscular blocking agents the diaphragm shifts cephalad at the end of expiration.[100] This change further compromises the airway. The size of the infant may magnify the physiologic consequences of anterior mediastinal masses. The increased cartilaginous component of the ribs increases the compliance of the thoracic wall, making it less likely to support the weight of a tumor. Also, a reduction in an already small airway will significantly increase airway resistance (the Poiseuille equation demonstrates that the resistance of laminar flow in a tube is inversely proportional to the fourth power of the radius).

Laminar gas flow through a narrow airway is best maintained with spontaneous ventilation.[100] Positive-pressure ventilation and airway obstruction disrupt laminar flow and increase the resistance to gas flow in the airways. An inspired mixture of helium and oxygen decreases resistance to gas flow through the airways because of helium's lower density compared with oxygen.[101] During turbulent flow, the pressure gradient required to produce a given gas flow becomes directly proportional to the density of the gas. Also helium's lower density increases the likelihood of laminar flow, thus reducing resistance further.[101] Heliox (helium-oxygen) has been described in a 3-year-old patient with a large symptomatic anterior mediastinal mass who underwent general anesthesia with an LMA.[102]

For patients undergoing diagnostic procedures or catheter placement, an effort should be made to perform the procedure under local anesthesia with sedation. General anesthesia can be performed safely; however, there needs to be a high index of suspicion for respiratory and cardiovascular complications. The induction of anesthesia can be achieved with either intravenous or inhalational techniques. The emphasis should be on maintaining spontaneous ventilation. Airway management with mask, LMA, and endotracheal tube has been described.[102,103]

Reinforced armor tubes have also been described to help maintain airway patency, and rigid bronchoscopy may become necessary should complete airway collapse occur.[84,85,104] In older children who require intubation but are clinically too tenuous for general anesthesia, a fiberoptic intubation can be accomplished with sedation and topical anesthesia of the airway. The Chamberlain approach has been performed under sedation with local anesthetic infiltration in children and should be considered for those at greatest risk of complications. In patients with respiratory compromise, intravenous access should be secured before the start of anesthesia and in patients with SVC syndrome intravenous access should be secured in the lower extremities. Because the supine position during induction of anesthesia may compromise an already tenuous airway, patients with mediastinal masses should be positioned in a semi-sitting position. If severe airway obstruction develops, the patient should be placed in the prone or lateral position. Patients who are believed to be at greatest risk of cardiovascular collapse should be considered preoperatively for cardiopulmonary bypass (Fig. 21-18, Table 21-9).

CONGENITAL MALFORMATION OF THE LUNG

Bronchogenic and Pulmonary Cysts

Bronchogenic cysts occur from abnormal budding of bronchial tissue. The cysts may occur anywhere from the mediastinum to the periphery, depending on when they separate during embryogenesis. They can be classified as mediastinal (central) or pulmonary (peripheral). Mediastinal cysts are more common and are usually located in the paratracheal and paraesophageal area, with the majority occurring between the trachea and the esophagus. The majority of pulmonary (peripheral) cysts occur in the lower lobes. Bronchogenic cysts may be filled with air or mucoid or serous fluid.[105,106] Although unlikely, they may communicate with the tracheobronchial tree. Most patients are asymptomatic, but if symptoms do occur they are related to airway, respiratory, and cardiovascular compromise from cyst enlargement or from infection. Infection may present as chronic cough, fever, and recurrent pneumonia.[107] Diagnosis is made with chest radiography and chest CT. The management of symptomatic patients is surgical resection (Table 21-10).

Anesthetic Management. Concerns regarding the anesthetic management include respiratory compromise secondary to cyst expansion from positive-pressure ventilation and/or nitrous oxide and spillage of cyst contents into the airway. A review of the anesthetic management of 24 cases of bronchogenic cysts indicated that these complications do not occur as commonly as previously thought. All of

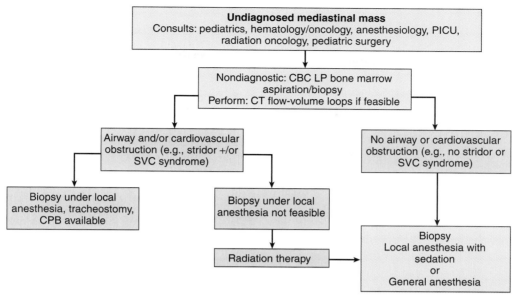

FIGURE 21–18 Algorithm for anesthetic management of the child with an anterior mediastinal mass. CBC, complete blood count; CPB, cardiopulmonary bypass; CT, computed tomography; CXR, chest radiograph; LP, lumbar puncture; PICU, pediatric intensive care unit; SVC, superior vena cava. *(Adapted from Hammer GB: Anaesthetic management for the child with a mediastinal mass. Pediatr Anesth 2004;14: 95-97, with permission.)*

the patients in this case series received muscle relaxation and positive-pressure ventilation intraoperatively, and no problems were encountered. There were three reports of excessive tracheal secretions that may have been related to drainage of fluid-filled cysts. Repeated suctioning was required, but no airway compromise was reported. The use of one lung ventilation was not described.[107] Spillage of cyst fluid in the airway with transient oxygen desaturation has been reported after induction of anesthesia. Lung isolation was also not employed in this case.[108] During the anesthetic management of bronchogenic cysts, lung isolation techniques may be advantageous, particularly with the manipulation of fluid-filled cysts. Whereas positive-pressure ventilation and the use of nitrous oxide appear to be reasonably well tolerated, it is unclear just how much risk they present.

Congenital Cystic Adenomatous Malformation

Congenital cystic adenomatoid malformation (CCAM) occurs secondary to an abnormal overgrowth of terminal bronchioles with a lack of mature alveoli, bronchial glands, and cartilage.[109] They are rare and occur at an estimated incidence of 1:25,000 to 1:35,000.[110] These cysts communicate with the tracheobronchial tree. CCAMs may be made up of a solid mass or a cystic structure that may consist of a single large dominant cyst or multiple cysts. Stocker classified CCAMs into three groups based on size and the histology of the cyst lining. Associated anomalies include renal agenesis and dysgenesis and prune belly syndrome. Clinical signs and symptoms at presentation depend largely on the size of the mass. The cystic lesions communicate with the tracheobronchial tree and

---

TABLE 21–9 Anesthetic Considerations for Management of Mediastinal Masses

Evaluate with computed tomography, echocardiography, pulmonary function tests, chest radiography.

Attain intravenous access in the lower extremity if superior vena cava syndrome is present.

Prepare to change position lateral or prone.

Maintain spontaneous ventilation.

Have rigid bronchoscope available.

Have cardiopulmonary bypass on standby.

TABLE 21–10 Anesthetic Management of Bronchogenic Cysts

Preoperative Evaluation of Bronchogenic Cysts

History: may have respiratory symptoms, cough, fever, recurrent lung infections
Chest radiography/computed tomography: evaluate location and size of cyst, evaluate for cardiac compression
Laboratory: hematocrit, type and screen, oxygen saturation

Anesthetic Management

Consider single lung ventilation if fluid-filled cyst.
Consider avoiding nitrous oxide.

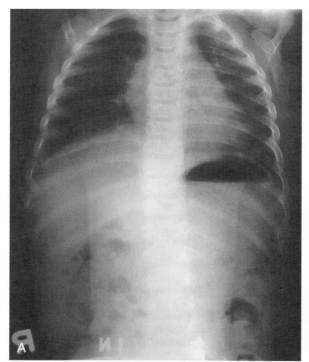

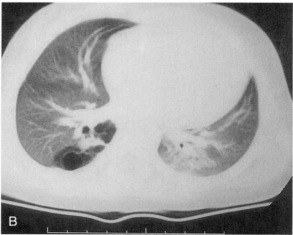

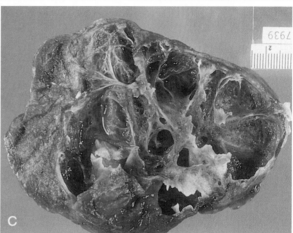

FIGURE 21–19 Microcystic adenomatoid malformation seen on plain film (**A**), CT (**B**), and surgical specimen (**C**). *(From Zitelli BJ, Davis HW: Atlas of Pediatric Physical Diagnosis, 4th ed. St. Louis, Mosby, 2002, p 565, with permission.)*

may behave like a ball-valve effect, becoming distended secondary to gas trapping. In-utero compromise with anasarca and ascites may occur if the lesion is large enough to impair fetal circulation. Compression of surrounding structures can result in lung hypoplasia. Neonates and infants may present with significant respiratory distress, requiring immediate resection. Patients presenting after the neonatal period often develop recurrent pulmonary infections localized to one lobe.[111] Diagnosis is made by clinical symptoms, chest radiography, and chest CT (Fig. 21-19). In-utero diagnosis is made during prenatal ultrasound. Definitive treatment is surgical removal of the affected lobe (Table 21-11).

Anesthetic Management. Communication of the CCAM with the tracheobronchial tree potentially increases the anesthetic risk. Positive-pressure ventilation and nitrous oxide may expand the lesion and cause cardiovascular and respiratory compromise. Spillage of cyst contents during anesthesia and obstruction of the endotracheal tube have also been reported.[108] Induction of anesthesia

---

TABLE 21–11   Anesthetic Management of Congenital Cystic Adenomatous Malformation (CCAM)

Preoperative Evaluation

History: symptoms depend on size of mass, respiratory distress (may be severe), recurrent lung infection
Chest radiography/computed tomography: evaluate location and size of CCAM
Laboratory: hematocrit, type and screen, oxygen saturation

Associated Anomalies

Renal agenesis or dysgenesis
Prune belly syndrome

Anesthetic Management

Spillage of CCAM contents can occur into airway; consider single-lung ventilation.
CCAM can expand; consider avoiding nitrous oxide; consider single-lung ventilation.

by an inhalational anesthetic with spontaneous ventilation may be preferential, but maintaining spontaneous ventilation during thoracotomy or thoracoscopy is very difficult and not feasible. Lung isolation may be ideal because it not only minimizes the risk of cyst overinflation during positive-pressure ventilation but also minimizes the risk of exposure to cyst contents should it rupture. Lung isolation in neonates and infants can be achieved either with purposeful mainstem intubation of the right or left bronchus or with placement of a 5-Fr bronchial blocker. The advantage of the bronchial blocker is that it may allow better protection from drainage of cyst contents into the contralateral lung. However, neither option for lung isolation allows suctioning, oxygenation, or continuous positive airway pressure (CPAP) to the isolated lung.

Standard surgical exposure is achieved via a thoracotomy. However, the development of smaller equipment has allowed this procedure to occur less invasively via a thorascopic approach. The potential advantages include less pain and faster recovery, with potentially shorter hospital stays. Lung isolation may facilitate the surgeon's exposure, and some centers routinely employ this technique. The CCAM has also been removed while the fetus is on uteroplacental support during the EXIT procedure.[112]

Pulmonary Sequestration

Pulmonary sequestration is characterized by a segment of lung tissue that is ectopic and serves no ventilatory function. It does, however, have its own vascular supply that typically arises from the thoracic or abdominal aorta.[113] Venous drainage has been reported through the pulmonary, azygous, or portal veins. Unlike the cystic malformations of the lung, sequestrations have no tracheobronchial communications and are not at risk of spillage of contents or expansion. There are two types of pulmonary sequestrations: intralobar and extralobar. The intralobar or intrapulmonary sequestration is located within a lobe and has no distinct pleural covering. Extralobar sequestrations have their own pleural covering and are associated with other congenital anomalies in 50% of cases. Some of these anomalies include communication with the gastrointestinal tract, duplication of the colon and ileum, cervical vertebral anomalies, pulmonary hypoplasia, diaphragmatic defects, and bronchial atresia of right upper lobe with anomalous pulmonary venous drainage. Sequestration with anomalous pulmonary venous drainage has the characteristic appearance of a wedge shape along the right heart border resembling a scimitar on chest radiography (Fig. 21-20).[113]

Clinically, these two types of sequestrations present differently. Often intralobar sequestrations are asymptomatic and may not present until later childhood or adolescence.[114] Extralobar sequestrations usually present before the age of 2. Symptoms include cough, pneumonia, and failure to thrive. Plain radiographs will identify

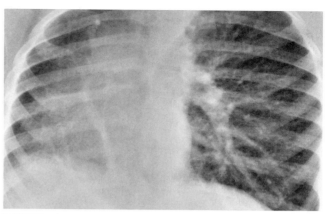

FIGURE 21–20 Chest radiograph demonstrating scimitar syndrome in a child with pulmonary sequestration. *(From Zitelli BJ, Davis HW: Atlas of Pediatric Physical Diagnosis, 4th ed. St. Louis, Mosby, 2002, p 134, with permission.)*

sequestrations but are unable to discern between intralobar and extralobar sequestrations. Angiography provides definitive diagnosis and identifies the arterial supply and venous drainage. MRI and angiography (MRA) may provide high-definition images and may replace the need for angiography.[115]

Surgical resection is the treatment of choice for symptomatic sequestration. Asymptomatic patients may also benefit from resection to prevent the occurrence of infection. Because of its separate pleural covering, removal of extralobar sequestrations can be performed without sacrificing surrounding lung tissue. Lobectomy, however, is usually required to resect intralobar sequestrations because of the intimate relationship with normal lung.[116]

Congenital Lobar Emphysema

Congenital lobar emphysema is characterized by overinflation of a pulmonary lobe secondary to an in-utero bronchial ball-valve obstruction. The bronchial obstruction may occur because of intrinsic or extrinsic compression. Defects of the bronchial wall cause the intrinsic obstruction. This defect usually occurs in the upper lobes and is caused by a deficiency in the quantity or quality of the cartilage in the bronchial wall.[117] Extrinsic compression is usually from cardiac or vascular abnormalities. These abnormalities may include tetralogy of Fallot, patent ductus arteriosus, and vascular rings or slings. Other causes of extrinsic obstruction include intrathoracic masses (teratoma), enlarged lymph nodes, and bronchogenic cysts.[117] Congenital cardiac deformities occur in approximately 15% of patients with congenital lobar emphysema[118] (Table 21-12).

Most cases of congenital lobar emphysema are diagnosed by 6 months of age. Thirty-three percent are diagnosed at birth and 50% are diagnosed by 1 month.[119] Respiratory distress and cyanosis are the most common

TABLE 21–12   Anesthetic Management of Congenital Lobar Emphysema

Preoperative Evaluation

Signs and symptoms: respiratory distress, cyanosis
Computed tomography: rule out vascular rings and slings, intrathoracic masses
Chest radiography: evaluate size and location of emphysematous lobe
Laboratory: hematocrit, type and screen, oxygen saturation

Associated Anomalies

Cardiac: congenital heart disease 15%

Differential Diagnosis

Tension pneumothorax
Bronchial obstruction: foreign body, mucus plug

Anesthetic Management

Maintain spontaneous ventilation; consider lung isolation.
Avoid nitrous oxide.

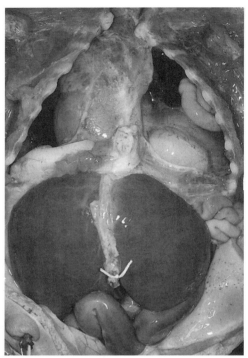

FIGURE 21–21   Congenital diaphragmatic hernia at postmortem showing obliteration of the left pleural cavity and severe compression of the right heart and lung. *(From Zitelli BJ, Davis HW: Atlas of Pediatric Physical Diagnosis, 4th ed. St. Louis, Mosby, 2002, p 563, with permission.)*

presenting symptoms. Chest radiography reveals a large emphysematous lobe with ipsilateral atelectasis. These findings may be misinterpreted as a tension pneumothorax.[120] The differential diagnosis also includes bronchial obstruction from a foreign body or mucus plug. Accurate diagnosis is important because surgical management of a foreign body or mucus plug would be bronchoscopy, not thoracic surgery.

Anesthetic Management. Definitive treatment for congenital lobar emphysema is lobectomy and is usually performed in patients with hypoxemia ($PaO_2 < 50$ mm Hg), despite supplemental oxygen.[119] Rarely, cases have been described that have resolved spontaneously.[121] The primary concern during the anesthetic management of these patients is the deleterious effects of positive-pressure ventilation. Positive-pressure ventilation may expand the emphysematous lobe and cause respiratory and cardiovascular collapse. Maintaining spontaneous ventilation when feasible and employing lung isolation techniques may minimize this risk. Nitrous oxide is also contraindicated because of the risk of expansion of the emphysematous lobe.

Congenital Diaphragmatic Hernia

Congenital diaphragmatic hernia (CDH) is characterized by a defect in the diaphragm that allows the herniation of abdominal contents into the thoracic cavity. The defect occurs on the left in about 85% of cases, and the most common form is the herniation through a left posterolateral defect or foramen of Bochdalek. Herniation through the anterior foramen of Morgagni occurs in only 2%. The incidence of CDH is approximately 1 in 3000 to 5000 births (Fig. 21-21).[130] A typical chest radiographic finding of bowel content herniation into the left thorax is demonstrated in Figure 21-22.

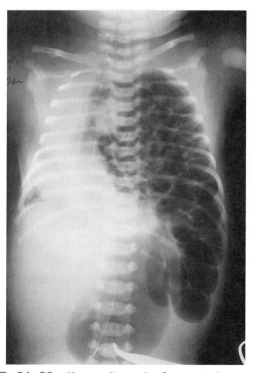

FIGURE 21–22   Chest radiograph of congenital diaphragmatic hernia. *(From Zitelli BJ, Davis HW: Atlas of Pediatric Physical Diagnosis, 4th ed. St. Louis, Mosby, 2002, p 563, with permission.)*

The severity of disease correlates with the timing of the diagnosis, the size of the defect, and the associated anomalies. Diagnosis prior to 25 weeks' gestation and large defects (lung to head ratio < 1 and liver herniation into the thorax) have been correlated with increased mortality.[122,123] Associated anomalies can occur in as many as 40% to 50% of cases of CDH.[124] The most common of these involve the central nervous system and the cardiac system. Congenital cardiac defects may include ventricular outflow tract obstructions (hypoplastic left heart syndrome, tetralogy, coarctation) as well as atrial and ventricular septal defects.[125] Genitourinary, gastrointestinal, and chromosomal abnormalities also occur in 23%, 17%, and 10%, respectively (Table 21-13).[126,127]

The failure of the fusion of the pleuroperitoneal membrane allows the abdominal contents to enter the thoracic cavity during the 10th week of gestation. This in-utero compression prevents lung development and causes alveolar and vascular hypoplasia. The degree of pulmonary hypoplasia depends on the size of the defect and the duration of the compression. Typically, both lungs are involved, even though the defect is unilateral. A controversial theory regarding the embryology of CDH states that the initial defect is primary pulmonary hypoplasia with secondary diaphragmatic defect.[128] Regardless of the etiology, the result is alveolar and vascular hypoplasia. Medial thickening occurs in the preacinar and intra-acinar arterioles, causing an increase in pulmonary vascular resistance, which ultimately contributes to persistent pulmonary hypertension. Pulmonary hypertension is a significant determinant of mortality in neonates with CDH.

Other entities may mimic CDH (Table 21-14), such as a large CCAM near the diaphragm. Abdominal ultrasound or a CT can help determine the integrity of the diaphragm. Diaphragmatic eventration may occur secondary to birth trauma or anterior horn cell neuropathy (Werdnig-Hoffman disease) and can be diagnosed by demonstrating paradoxical diaphragmatic excursion on ultrasonography or fluoroscopy.[129]

Medical Management. The goal of medical management consists primarily of maintaining adequate oxygenation

and ventilation, but most important, it is to avoid iatrogenic barotrauma from mechanical ventilation (Table 21-15). At the time of delivery, the patient should be endotracheally intubated. An effort should be made to minimize bag-mask ventilation before intubation to reduce the risk of gastric expansion. Immediately after intubation, the gut should be decompressed and vascular access should be obtained. The umbilical vein and artery may be utilized or a right radial arterial catheter (for preductal arterial blood gas analysis) and a central venous catheter may be placed. Preductal and postductal measurement of oxygenation should be performed to assess the degree of right-to-left shunting, a surrogate marker of pulmonary hypertension. Shunting through the ductus arteriosus is suggested if the preductal Pao_2 is 15 to 20 mm Hg higher than the postductal Pao_2. Shunting at the level of the foramen ovale will decrease the predicted value of the preductal Pao_2 and will not produce a gradient when compared with the postductal Pao_2. Preductal saturation also reflects cerebral oxygenation. The ventilatory strategy should achieve a preductal oxygen saturation of greater than 85%, while maintaining a $Paco_2$ of 45 to 55 mm Hg and a pH greater than 7.3, with peak inspiratory pressures less than or equal to 25 cm H_2O.[130] Neonates who require peak pressures greater than

TABLE 21-13 Anomalies Associated with Congenital Diaphragmatic Hernia

Central nervous system (meningomyelocele, hydrocephalus)
Congenital heart disease (atrial and ventricular septal defects, coarctation, tetralogy of Fallot)
Gastrointestinal (malrotation, atresia)
Genitourinary (hypospadias)

From David TJ, Illingworth CA: Diaphragmatic hernia in the southwest of England. J Med Genet 1976;13:253.

TABLE 21-14 Differential Diagnosis of Congenital Diaphragmatic Hernia

Congenital cystic adenomatous malformation
Diaphragmatic eventration (trauma, Werdnig-Hoffman disease)

TABLE 21-15 Medical Management of Congenital Diaphragmatic Hernia

Airway
Endotracheal intubation
Breathing
Decompress stomach.
Ventilation goal: positive inspiratory pressure < 25 cm H_2O, preductal Sao_2 > 85%, $Paco_2$ 45-55 mm Hg
pH > 7.3
Consider high-frequency oscillatory ventilation if unable to oxygenate with pressures < 25 cm H_2O.
Circulation
Cardiac echocardiography to:
Exclude congenital heart disease
Assess right ventricular function
Assess pulmonary hypertension
Assess right-to-left shunting at ductal level

25 cm H_2O for adequate oxygenation may need to be ventilated with high-frequency oscillatory ventilation (HFOV) to minimize the risk of ventilator-associated barotrauma.

Permissive hypercarbia was first proposed by Wung in 1985 for infants with persistent fetal circulation. In many centers this strategy has been adopted for neonates with CDH.[131] Hypercarbia and ductal shunting may be tolerated by the neonates with CDH, provided there is adequate right-sided heart function and systemic perfusion. Adequate right-sided heart function can be evaluated with echocardiography, and adequate systemic perfusion can be demonstrated with normal lactate levels, mixed venous saturation greater than 70%, and the absence of a metabolic acidosis. Patients with evidence of persistent pulmonary hypertension with elevated right ventricular pressures, or preductal oxygen saturation less than 85%, may require a trial of nitric oxide (iNO). Although there may be a response to iNO in neonates with CDH, there are no clear data that this impacts on survival.[132] Neonates with right ventricular dysfunction and low systemic pressures may require intravenous fluids and inotropic support. Predictors of outcome during the initial resuscitation are inexact. The inability to achieve a preductal PaO_2 greater than 100 mm Hg predicted 100% mortality in one study.[133] Apgar scores and birth weight have also been described to predict mortality in neonates with CDH.[134]

The benefit of extracorporeal membrane oxygenation (ECMO) on the morbidity and mortality of CDH is controversial. Some centers reported significant improvement in survival with the introduction of ECMO.[135] This has to be tempered with the fact that some centers have experienced the same survival statistics without the use of ECMO.[136] There is also significant morbidity associated with the use of ECMO. Anticoagulation with heparin to prevent clot formation in the ECMO circuit and platelet activation and consumption increase the risk of bleeding. Bleeding may cause significant morbidity if this occurs in the central nervous system, and bleeding may complicate attempts at surgical correction while on ECMO. Inclusion criteria for ECMO include gestational age greater 34 weeks, weight greater than 2 kg, presence of reversible disease, and predicted mortality of greater than 80%. Neonates with an oxygenation index (OI = FIO_2 × mean airway pressure × $100/PaO_2$) greater than 40 to 50 may represent those at greatest risk (>80%) of mortality. Intraventricular hemorrhage more than grade II or those with another life-threatening congenital anomaly should be excluded from ECMO.[137] ECMO is considered in neonates with progressive hypoxia, hypercarbia, and persistent pulmonary hypertension who have failed other attempts at medical correction, including iNO, inotropic support, or opening the ductus with prostaglandin E_1.[130] A review of all of the published data has indicated that there may be a short-term benefit with the use of ECMO but there may not be a long-term benefit because of the associated morbidity.[138]

Surgical Management. In the past it was believed that CDH represented a neonatal emergency requiring immediate surgical decompression of the thorax. Postoperatively, patients experienced a "honeymoon" period of brief improved oxygenation. This was soon followed by worsening hypoxia secondary to increased pulmonary vascular resistance and increased right-to-left shunting.[139] The poor outcomes with immediate repair raised the question of whether these patients should be stabilized preoperatively before surgical repair. To date there are no clear data to support delayed repair over early surgical intervention. A prospective randomized trial evaluated the importance of timing on survival and incidence of ECMO between early (6 hours) versus late (96+ hours) surgery and found no difference between the groups.[139a] All of the existing published data were reanalyzed in a Cochrane Database Systematic review in 2003 and again there was no clear advantage demonstrated with delayed surgical repair after medical stabilization.[139b]

Most often the surgical approach is through a subcostal incision. The majority of the repairs take place through a left-sided incision. After the abdominal contents are removed from the thoracic cavity, the bowel is eviscerated from the abdominal cavity to expose the defect. The diaphragmatic defect may be closed primarily or with a Gore-Tex patch. After the abdominal contents are replaced, there may be a significant elevation in abdominal pressure with surgical wound closure.[139] A silo may be required to gradually reintroduce the abdominal contents.

Fetal surgery for CDH was initiated after animal models demonstrated a reversal of lung hypoplasia when diaphragmatic hernias were corrected in utero.[140] Fetal repair in humans was first described in 1990.[141] Overall success of the open fetal approach was limited by maternal morbidity, which included premature rupture of membranes and preterm labor. Fetal intervention was only considered for those fetuses at highest risk of mortality. Research during the late 1970s introduced the concept of tracheal occlusion to reverse the lung pathophysiology from diaphragmatic herniation. This concept resulted in a fetal strategy in humans to temporarily occlude the trachea in utero until birth (PLUG—Plug the Lung Until it Grows).[142-144] However, this strategy and variations of this strategy have not demonstrated any survival advantage over standard postnatal medical management.[145]

Anesthetic Management (Table 21-16). Preoperative assessment of the neonate with CDH should begin with an evaluation of the degree of respiratory compromise and pulmonary hypertension. Attention to the type of ventilatory support and associated blood gas values is important. Consideration should be given to using the newborn intensive care unit ventilator or HFOV if there is any concern about achieving adequate ventilation. Cardiovascular evaluation should focus on identifying any congenital

TABLE 21-16 Anesthetic Management of Congenital Diaphragmatic Hernia

Preoperative Evaluation

Place oral or nasogastric tube.

Evaluate severity of pulmonary hypoplasia and pulmonary hypertension.

Ventilation: what ventilation requirements exist? Preductal saturation < 85%? Right ventricular strain on echocardiography?

Echocardiography: to evaluate right ventricular function, right-to-left shunting, and pulmonary hypertension

Chest radiography: evaluate size of hernia

Laboratory: arterial blood gas analysis, hematocrit, type and screen, preductal and postductal oxygen saturation, vitamin K given? Hypokalemia from diuretics?

Anesthetic Management

Monitors: arterial catheter, preductal and postductal pulse oximeter, precordial on contralateral chest

Avoid nitrous oxide.

Decompress stomach.

Use endotracheal intubation.

Ventilation goal: positive inspiratory pressure < 25 cm H_2O, preductal SaO_2 > 85%, $PaCO_2$ 45-55 mm Hg, pH > 7.3

Maintain normothermia.

Administer bicarbonate to maintain normal pH.

Continue inhalational nitric oxide if used preoperatively.

Administer dextrose intravenous solution.

Opioid-based anesthetic; consider epidural analgesia.

Consider contralateral pneumothorax if clinical deterioration occurs.

---

heart defects and the degree of right-to-left shunting, pulmonary hypertension, and right ventricular performance. Severe pulmonary hypertension can result in severe hypoxia, decreased cardiac output, and metabolic acidosis. This information can be provided from echocardiography and preductal and postductal blood gas analysis. Associated neurologic findings include MMC and hydrocephalus. Premature neonates are at risk for the development of intraventricular hemorrhages. This will exclude them from ECMO because of the anticoagulation. Head ultrasounds are routinely performed in this population and should be performed before ECMO cannulation. Hematologic issues require maintaining an adequate hemoglobin (approximately 12 mg/dL) and checking for vitamin K administration at birth. Some of these patients may be on diuretics. An electrolyte panel should be performed to evaluate for hypokalemia. The neonate will already have a nasogastric or orogastric tube in place. If not, this should be placed to decompress the stomach.

Intraoperative management consists of first ensuring adequate room temperature and utilizing either warming lights or a forced warm air blanket to maintain normothermia. Induction of anesthesia has been described using both intravenous and inhalation techniques. Given the risk of aspiration and the resulting injury to already immature lungs, a rapid-sequence intubation may be preferred after the gastric tube is suctioned and the neonate is preoxygenated. If there appear to be any barriers to safe intubation such as a difficult airway, then an awake intubation may be safest. Positive-pressure mask ventilation should be minimized to prevent gaseous distention of the stomach.

In addition to the standard monitors, a preductal arterial catheter should be placed, but an umbilical artery catheter may also be used. Both preductal and postductal pulse oximeters should be placed, and a precordial stethoscope on the contralateral chest can be used to identify a pneumothorax. If central venous access is attempted, consideration should be given to avoid the internal jugular veins, because these may be future cannulation sites for ECMO.

The hallmark of medical management of these patients is to minimize the risk of iatrogenic ventilatory injury. Peak pressures should not exceed 25 to 30 cm H_2O. An opioid-based anesthetic has been described and may minimize the surgical stress and pulmonary vascular lability.[146] Muscle relaxation is typically employed to facilitate surgical exposure and abdominal closure. Nitrous oxide is not used because of the risk of bowel distention. This could impair ventilation while the bowel is in the thoracic cavity and may impede abdominal closure once the abdominal contents are replaced in the abdominal cavity. Nitrous oxide can also accelerate the onset of a pneumothorax. Contralateral pneumothorax is a potential intraoperative complication and needs to be considered if there is an acute clinical deterioration. Pulmonary hypertension can be managed by maintaining a normal pH, PaO_2, and $PaCO_2$ and minimizing hypothermia and surgical stress. Sodium bicarbonate may need to be administered to treat acidosis and/or to alkalinize the blood and thereby treat pulmonary hypertension. If iNO is used preoperatively, it should be continued in the operating room. Epidural analgesia has been described in the anesthetic management of neonates with CDH. This option for intraoperative and postoperative management may best be suited in those with smaller defects who likely will not require prolonged ventilation or anticoagulation for ECMO.[147]

Despite the advances in the medical and surgical care of fetuses and neonates with CDH, the mortality still remains significant. Delayed surgery, HFOV, iNO, ECMO, and fetoscopic surgery have not been proven to significantly improve the overall mortality. A recent outcome study demonstrated a mortality of 62% that did not vary statistically despite the introduction of ECMO, iNO, surfactant, and delayed surgery.[140] The concept of permissive hypercarbia and gentle ventilation may have had the most significant impact on survival in neonates with CDH.

Some centers have observed an improvement in survival from 50% to 75% to 90%, with the introduction of this ventilation strategy.[130,148]

Tracheoesophageal Fistula

Tracheoesophageal fistula (TEF) is a generalized term for a condition characterized by esophageal atresia with or without a communication (fistula) between the esophagus and the trachea. There are several anatomic variations that cannot all be described by one definition. Esophageal atresia is the most common esophageal anomaly, occurring in approximately 1 in 2000 to 1 in 5000 live births. Prematurity and polyhydramnios are associated with TEF. The inability to swallow amniotic fluid in utero results in polyhydramnios. Associated anomalies occur in 30% to 50%. Mortality varies from 5% to 60%. Recent analysis indicates a survival rate of approximately 95%.[149] Morbidity and mortality are increased in infants with severe coexisting congenital anomalies and prematurity. Cardiac and pulmonary anomalies appear to be the most significant with those children, with severe congenital cardiac anomalies and respiratory complications requiring mechanical ventilation at highest risk.

Classification. Gross created a classification system in 1953.[150] This classification outlines five types of esophageal atresia with and without fistula (types A to F) (Fig. 21-23)

A—Esophageal atresia without fistula
B—Esophageal atresia with communication of the upper esophageal segment to the trachea
C—Esophageal atresia with communication of the lower esophageal segment to the trachea
D—Esophageal atresia with both upper and lower esophageal segments communicating with the trachea
E—No esophageal atresia but there is a tracheoesophageal fistula
F—Esophageal stenois without fistula

Type C is the most common, occurring in approximately 85% of TEFs.

Infants with esophageal atresia are unable to manage their oral secretions and present with excessive oral and nasal salivation, choking, coughing, and regurgitation with first feeding. The tracheoesophageal communication results in gastric dilatation and aspiration of gastric contents. Pneumonia (of the right upper lung) and pneumonitis can occur, as well as respiratory compromise from gastric dilatation. These patients can present with cyanosis and apnea. Tracheomalacia can also occur, resulting in a barking cough.[151]

Associated Anomalies. Associated anomalies occur in 30% to 50% of patients with TEF. A common association is the VATER complex.[152] This mnemonic leaves out cardiac anomalies. A more appropriate complex name would be VACTERL.

Vertebral anomalies
Anorectal/intestinal anomalies (atresia)
Cardiac anomalies: incidence of 14% to 24%. The most common lesions are ventricular septal defect, coarctation, tetralogy of Fallot, and atrial septal defect.
Tracheoesophageal fistula
Esophageal atresia
Renal and radial anomalies
Limb

Diagnosis of TEF is based on clinical signs and symptoms. The inability to pass an orogastric catheter into the stomach and a chest radiograph showing the catheter in the proximal esophageal pouch confirms the diagnosis. Gastric air may or may not be present, depending on the anatomy of the lesion.

Surgical Management. Surgical management consists of identifying and ligating the TEF and then anastomosing the atretic esophagus. If the gap between the esophageal segments is large enough to prevent a primary anastomosis,

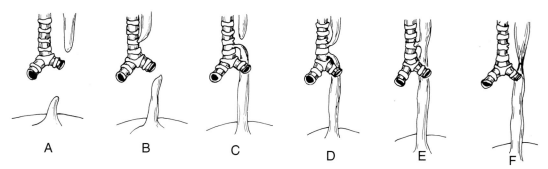

FIGURE 21–23 Gross's classification of esophageal atresia without fistula (**A**), esophageal atresia with proximal fistula (**B**), esophageal atresia with distal fistula (**C**), esophageal atresia with proximal and distal fistula (**D**), tracheoesophageal fistula without atresia (**E**), and esophageal stenosis (**F**). *(From Ulma G, Geiduschek JM, Zimmerman AA, Morray JP: Anesthesia for thoracic surgery. In Gregory GA [ed]: Pediatric Anesthesia, 4th ed. Philadelphia, Churchill Livingstone, 2002, p 440, with permission.)*

a staged repair is performed. This may consist of interposing a segment of colon or upward movement of the stomach.[153]

The primary goal in the preoperative period is to prevent pulmonary complications. These infants should be kept NPO. Prone or lateral positioning with the head of the bed at 30 degrees may reduce the risk of aspiration. A nasoesophageal catheter should be attached to suction. Pneumonia should be treated, and a gastrostomy to vent the stomach should only be considered in the infant with immature lungs or respiratory distress syndrome. Intubation is avoided, if possible, to minimize gastric distention. Metabolic acidosis should be treated before surgical repair. Lastly, associated anomalies need to be identified and evaluated. This evaluation may include echocardiography, abdominal ultrasound, and radiographs of the spine and extremities. These infants may already have central intravenous access for total parenteral nutrition. Routine preoperative blood work should include a hemoglobin, type and crossmatch, and glucose determination.

Anesthetic Management. The principal issues that dictate anesthetic management include the risk of aspiration, negative effects of positive-pressure ventilation before ligation of the fistula, management of associated anomalies, including prematurity, and surgical technique (thoracotomy) (Table 21-17).

Standard monitoring includes electrocardiography, pulse oximetry, noninvasive blood pressure, temperature, and capnography. An arterial catheter may be beneficial in the infant with significant pulmonary disease and/or cardiac disease. An esophageal stethoscope placed over the left chest will facilitate the detection of endotracheal tube migration into the right mainstem bronchus. Positioning for definitive surgical repair requires left lateral positioning for a right thoracotomy.

Aspiration and gastric distention with respiratory embarrassment are the initial concerns during induction of anesthesia. In medically unstable infants, a gastrostomy may be required before induction to relieve gastric distention, and an awake intubation may be considered. In patients who are stable, an intravenous or mask induction can be performed. Positive-pressure ventilation should be minimized to small tidal volumes, or spontaneous ventilation should be maintained if possible. Presence of a gastrostomy may slow mask inductions, requiring transient partial clamping of the tube. Endotracheal tube positioning is important to minimize gastric distention. Usually the fistula inserts along the posterior aspect of the trachea just above the carina. Proper positioning can be achieved by purposefully placing the endotracheal tube into the right mainstem bronchus and then slowly withdrawing until breath sounds are just heard at the left axillae. Placement can also be confirmed with a fiberoptic bronchoscope. Other options for minimizing gastric

TABLE 21–17 Anesthetic Management of Tracheoesophageal Fistula

Tracheoesophageal Fistula

Signs and symptoms: respiratory distress, coughing, choking, unable to pass oral catheter into stomach; pneumonia, pneumonitis
Radiographs of spine and upper extremities: evaluate vertebral and radial anomalies
Chest radiography: radiopaque oral catheter in proximal esophagus, gastric gas pattern
Echocardiography: evaluate cardiac defects
Imaging: renal ultrasound
Laboratory: hematocrit, type and screen, oxygen saturation, glucose

Associated Anomalies

VACTER association:
  Vertebral anomalies
  Anal atresia
  Cardiac defects
  Tracheoesophageal fistula
  Radial/renal anomalies

Anesthetic Management

Preoperative management: oral esophageal suctioning, maintain NPO, gastrostomy tube for respiratory distress syndrome or immature lungs; may require endotracheal intubation; treat metabolic acidosis
Monitoring: arterial catheter
Induction: maintain spontaneous ventilation until fistula is isolated (mainstem intubation, bronchial blocker)

Complications

Obstruction of endotracheal from secretions, purulent drainage, blood, or mechanical bend
Atelectasis

distention include placement of a balloon-tipped catheter (Fogarty, 2 to 3 Fr) into the fistula, either from above (through the trachea, next to endotracheal tube) or from below via the gastrostomy (5 Fr). The Fogarty catheter can be placed from above during bronchoscopy by the surgeon to evaluate the location of the fistula and other anatomic anomalies.[154] Occasionally massive gastric distention can occur, resulting in respiratory compromise and cardiovascular collapse, requiring an emergency gastrostomy. The risk of gastric distention increases with the size of the fistula. Muscle relaxation has been described successfully in the anesthetic management of TEF in those with smaller fistulas.[155] Fistulas that are large or are located near the carina may benefit from isolation with a Fogarty catheter.

Once the fistula is isolated, muscle relaxation and controlled ventilation can be used. A frequently occurring problem is hypoxemia. Hypoxemia can occur secondary to right mainstem intubation, ETT obstruction from secretions, drainage from lung infections, and bleeding. In addition, kinking of the bronchus or even the trachea by surgical manipulation can occur, as well as atelectasis of the retracted lung during surgical exposure. Recruitment maneuvers to reexpand the lungs may be necessary to improve intraoperative oxygenation. A forced air heating blanket is used to prevent hypothermia. Dextrose-containing intravenous solution is provided to prevent hypoglycemia. Extubation at the end of surgery may minimize manipulation of the anastomosis from the ETT, but respiratory distress syndrome or pneumonias may require prolonged intubation. Intravenous opioids are effective for intraoperative and postoperative pain management, but regional anesthesia is advantageous to avoid opioids and the risk of postoperative respiratory depression. Providing there are no significant vertebral anomalies, a caudal catheter can be placed and threaded to the thoracic region. The catheter's position can be confirmed by injecting low ionic strength contrast medium (0.5 mL Omnipaque 180).[156]

Postoperative Considerations. Postoperative concerns include the management of an orogastric tube that will be marked to the level of the esophageal anastomosis. There should be no suctioning beyond this point to prevent disruption of the anastomosis. Also, head extension can put tension on the anastomosis and should be minimized.

Postoperative complications include anastomotic leak, tracheomalacia or bronchomalacia, stricture, pneumonia, and pneumothorax.[157] Complications can also occur secondary to underlying medical conditions and result in significant morbidity and mortality. All patients who have undergone TEF repair are considered to have esophageal dysmotility and gastroesophageal reflux.

ABDOMINAL WALL DEFECTS

Omphalocele, gastroschisis, and bladder and cloacal exstrophy are various forms of congenital abdominal wall defects. Congenital abdominal wall defects present a peculiar challenge to neonatologists, surgeons, and anesthesiologists. The optimal management of neonates with anterior wall defects depends on the careful prenatal assessment of these patients, as well as the experience and knowledge of the defect's natural history. A multidisciplinary approach can improve neonatal outcome.

Omphalocele and Gastroschisis

Gastroschisis and omphalocele are congenital defects of the anterior abdominal wall that differ in many aspects. The diagnostic distribution between the two entities is important because of the associated abnormalities. Omphaloceles have a much higher incidence of associated abnormalities (Fig. 21-24). Omphaloceles have associated cardiac, neurologic, genitourinary, skeletal, or chromosomal abnormalities in two thirds of patients. In addition, gastrointestinal anomalies are frequent. Prematurity occurs in 60% of patients with abdominal wall defects (Table 21-18).

Anatomy and Embryology. These defects are thought to result from an imbalance between cell proliferation and apoptotic cell death. The apoptotic cell death in the region of the umbilical ring results in relative growth delay in that region, whereas rapid development of the foregut causes herniation of the bowel through the umbilical stalk.

In gastroschisis, the abdominal wall forms in a dysplastic fashion owing to decreased cell deposition or vascular abnormality. This results in the formation of a thin area in the abdominal wall to the right of the umbilicus. This area ruptures from increased intra-abdominal pressure. Another explanation is that gastroschisis represents a rupture of the hernia of the umbilical cord that occurs at the weakest point of the hernia sac, the site where the right umbilical vein involutes. Patients with omphalocele present with a central defect of the umbilical lining, and the abdominal contents are contained within a sac.[158]

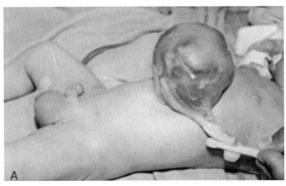
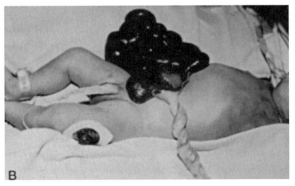

FIGURE 21–24 **A,** Infant with an omphalocele. Note how abdominal wall contents are enclosed in a sac-like structure that is related to the umbilical cord. **B,** Infant with gastroschisis. Note the thickened abdominal viscera and the position of the umbilical cord. *(From Keljo DJ, Gariepy CE: Anatomy, histology, embryology, and developmental anomalies of the small and large intestine. In Feldman M, Friedman LS, Sleisenger MH [eds]: Sleisenger & Fordtran's Gastrointestinal and Liver Disease, 7th ed, 2002, p 1651, with permission.)*

TABLE 21–18   Comparison of Gastroschisis and Omphalocele

	Gastroschisis	Omphalocele
Incidence	1: 10,000 Intact umbilical cord and evisceration of bowel through a defect in the abdominal wall right of the cord	1: 4,000-7,000 Herniation of bowel and liver thorough umbilical wall covered by membranes unless ruptured liver and other organs
Sac	No membrane covering (sac absent)	Present
Associated Organs	No	
Associated Anomalies	Intestinal atresia 25% Cryptorchidism 31%	Chromosomal anomalies Trisomy 18, 13, 15, and 21 Beckwith-Wiedemann syndrome Pentalogy of Cantrell Prune belly syndrome
Maternal Age	<25 yr	Older
Smoking and Alcohol Use	Yes	No
Teratogens	Acetaminophen, aspirin, pseudoephedrine use in pregnancy: Yes	No
Congenital Heart Disease	12%	24%
Prematurity	40%-67%	10%-23%

Clinical Management. Prognosis for the infant with gastroschisis is determined by the condition of exteriorized bowel. Elective cesarean section, especially for gastroschisis, was advocated to prevent bowel trauma. However, data from 15 publications dealing with the mode of delivery were analyzed and it was concluded that cesarean section had no distinct advantage over vaginal delivery with regard to neonatal outcome.[158] Bowel damage has been attributed to exposure to amniotic fluid and constriction at the abdominal wall defect. Preterm delivery may be advisable for patients with increasing bowel distention. The risk of prematurity should be weighed against the potential advantage of preterm delivery to salvage the bowel.

Surgical Repair. Initial management for neonates with abdominal wall defects is focused on newborn resuscitation, fluid and electrolyte maintenance, temperature homeostasis, and protection of the eviscerated organs. After the infant is stabilized, which includes administration of broad-spectrum antibiotics, protection of the eviscerated organs with wrapped fluids, impermeable dressings, and intravenous hydration, the neonate is brought to the operating room for either a primary closure or a staged repair.

Anesthesia is induced with intravenous agents, and the patient's trachea is intubated. The major intraoperative concerns include (1) fluid requirements, (2) temperature regulation, (3) cardiovascular stability, and (4) increased intra-abdominal pressure. Large third space losses can be associated with anterior wall defects, in both the preoperative and intraoperative period. Hypothermia is a frequent complication and is multifactorial. The infant's ongoing fluid requirements, increased evaporative water loss, and increased radiant heat loss are all major contributing factors. Cardiovascular instability can result from both the ongoing water and heat losses, as well as the instability associated with the normal changes that occur with the transition from a fetal- to an adult-type circulation. In addition, cardiovascular compromise can occur from the increase in intra-abdominal pressure that occurs with the reduction of the eviscerated organs.

The surgical approach to treatment involves decompressing the intestines, nasogastric suction, and anorectal irrigation. The goal of surgical management is reduction of abdominal contents and the approximation of the fascial edges and skin coverage. Primary closure is attempted if abdominal pressure does not impair ventilation, venous return, cardiac output, or perfusion to the gut, kidneys, and lower extremities. Because the reduction of the intestinal contents can create a high increased intra-abdominal pressure, compromise to the organs, as well as compromise of the inferior vena cava, blood return can occur. Monitoring of gastric pressure, bladder pressure, and arterial venous pressure has been advocated.[159,160] If primary repair is not feasible, then a staged repair with a silo is placed. A prosthetic silo is sutured to the fascial edges of the defect, and in days to weeks the abdominal contents are reduced back into the abdomen. At completion, the silo is removed and the ventral hernia or abdominal wall defect is repaired. In the postoperative period the major concerns center on nutrition, sepsis, and intestinal obstruction.

Anesthetic management of patients with abdominal wall defects involves the use of intravenous and/or inhalational anesthetic agents. Increased intra-abdominal pressure can result in reduced drug clearance;

consequently, infusions of fentanyl and sufentanil can lead to drug accumulation and prolonged drug effect. Remifentanil, an opioid that is metabolized by plasma and tissue esterases and has an ultrashort duration of action, can be an ideal anesthetic agent for neonates. Muscle relaxants should be used to help facilitate abdominal closure. In those patients in whom primary closure cannot be achieved, postoperative ventilation may be necessary. During abdominal closure monitoring of the patient's airway pressure and blood pressure help to determine whether a primary repair or staged repair is necessary. In addition, central venous pressure monitoring can also be used to detect caval compression and increased intra-abdominal pressure.

Postoperative management is a function of the surgical procedure and any associated congenital abnormality. In infants with large intraoperative fluid requirements or infants suspected of having elevated intra-abdominal pressures, mechanical ventilation should continue until diuresis has occurred or until the increased intra-abdominal pressure resolves.

Prune Belly Syndrome

Prune belly syndrome (PBS, triad syndrome, Eagle-Barrett syndrome, abdominal muscular deficiency) presents with a lax, wrinkled abdominal wall.[161] PBS is a specific constellation of anomalies that involve an abdominal wall deficient in muscular tissue, dilated urinary tracts, bilateral cryptorchidism, pulmonary hypoplasia due to in-utero impaired drainage of the bladder and oligohydramnios, gastrointestinal abnormalities, and orthopedic (musculoskeletal) disorders (congenital dislocation of the hip, scoliosis, pectus excavatum, clubfeet, congenital muscular torticollis, renal osteodystrophy).[162] The pathogenesis of PBS arises from the effects of intrauterine urethral obstruction associated with olighydramnios.[163] Oligohydramnios produces limited intrauterine space leading to fetal compression and resultant deformities. Clinically, patients with PBS vary widely. They can have significant respiratory compromise secondary to pulmonary hypoplasia and a decreased ability to cough. There is evidence that they can also develop restrictive lung disease secondary to the absence of abdominal musculature.[164] Because of these defects, they may have recurrent respiratory tract infections and may be more prone to postoperative respiratory complications.[165,166] In severe forms death occurs in the neonatal period. Some patients may have no pulmonary hypoplasia but significant renal involvement and failure to thrive. Other patients may have an abnormally appearing urinary tract but normal renal function. Anesthetic management is determined by the patient's underlying pulmonary and renal status.

In patients with impaired renal function, selection of anesthetic agents is important. Although renal insufficiency has no effect on the choice of inhaled anesthetic agents, renal insufficiency can alter a patient's response to muscle relaxants and intravenous opioids. The kidneys have a minor role in the elimination of most opioids. Fentanyl has been administered to anephric patients without untoward effects. Alfentanil kinetics are variable in patients with renal failure.[167]

Morphine kinetics are unchanged in patients with renal failure; however, its metabolites, morphine-3-glucuronide and morphine-6-glucuronide, are significantly prolonged. Because the 6-glucuronide is pharmacologically active, it can lead to respiratory depression. Meperidine is mainly metabolized by the liver, but its principal metabolite, normeperidine, is pharmacologically active, causes CNS excitability (tremors, myoclonus, and seizures), and is excreted by the kidney. The elimination half-life is double in patients with renal failure. Although renal excretion of meperidine plays a minor role in adults, Chan and colleagues noted that patients with renal disease had higher plasma concentrations, longer elimination half-lives, decreased protein binding, and large volumes of distribution.[168]

Neuromuscular blocking agents are generally excreted in the urine and bile. In patients with renal failure, the sensitivity of the neuromuscular junction does not appear to be affected. Atracurium and cisatracurium, which undergo Hoffman elimination and enzymatic hydrolysis, are not affected by patients with renal disease. Vecuronium and rocuronium clearance can be prolonged in patients with renal failure. In patients with renal failure and low levels of plasma pseudocholinesterase, mivacurium administration may result in a prolonged effect. Pancuronium elimination, half-life, and duration of action are also prolonged in patients with renal disease.

The depolarizing drug succinylcholine is relatively contraindicated in patients with renal failure. Because serum potassium level increases in patients after its administration, acute life-threatening hyperkalemia can occur in patients with an elevated serum potassium concentration.

The use of sevoflurane in patients with renal failure does not appear to be unsafe. Sevoflurane is metabolized in vivo to inorganic fluoride and hexafluoroisopropanol, whereas in vitro sevoflurane is degraded by soda lime or Baralyme to compound A. Both intravenous fluoride levels and compound A have been associated with nephrotoxicity.[169] However, nephrotoxicity does not appear to occur in humans.[170] Reasons for this lack of nephrotoxicity may be related to sevoflurane's low solubility, its rapid elimination, and the small amount of intrarenal metabolism that sevoflurane undergoes.[171] Compound A is a product of sevoflurane degradation produced by alkaline hydrolysis in the presence of soda lime or Baralyme. Although compound A has produced histologic changes in rats, a nephrotoxic effect of compound A in humans is lacking. Although preexisting renal insufficiency is a risk factor for postoperative renal dysfunction, neither high-flow nor low-flow sevoflurane anesthesia in patients with preexisting renal disease appears to alter renal function compared with isoflurane.[172,173]

Bladder and Cloacal Exstrophy

Bladder and cloacal exstrophy are rare but devastating anomalies. Bladder exstrophy is a developmental defect seen in 1 in 40,000 live births, whereas cloacal exstrophy is found in about 1 in 200,000 births.

Embryology. Bladder exstrophy is a defect of the caudal fold of the anterior abdominal wall. It results from persistence of the cloacal membrane, preventing cephalad migration of the mesoderm to the midline during development. When the cloacal membrane eventually degenerates, it leaves behind a midline defect.

A small defect may cause epispadias alone, whereas a large defect leads to exposure of the posterior bladder wall.[174] Classic exstrophy is characterized by wide pubic separation and an exposed bladder. Cloacal exstrophy involves the urinary and gastrointestinal tract. OEIS refers to the association of bladder exstrophy with omphalocele, exstrophy of the bladder, imperforate anus, and spinal defects such as myelomeningocele.[175] Diastasis of the pubis and absence of the genitalia are frequent findings in

TABLE 21–19   Anesthetic Considerations for Bladder and Cloacal Exstrophy

Care of the newborn
    Prevention of heat loss: fluid warmers, forced air blankets
    Glucose management: check blood glucose level
    Fluid management for third space losses

Evaluation of other associated congenital anomalies
Regional anesthesia
Latex precautions

patients with cloacal exstrophy, neural tube defects are present in 50% of infants, and congenital short bowel syndromes occur in 20% (Fig. 21-25).[176]

Diagnosis. Prenatal sonographic diagnosis reveals absence of the bladder as well as associated genitourinary anomalies.[177] Cloacal exstrophy has been identified due to associated neural tube defects, omphalocele, or splaying of the pubic rami. Prenatal diagnosis of bladder or cloacal exstrophy should be followed by a careful search for other chromosomal and structural anomalies. Parental counseling by a multidisciplinary team should address issues of continence and possible sex reassignment.

Treatment. Reconstruction involves several surgical procedures. These include urologic and orthopedic surgeries. A three-stage approach is commonly used to repair the exstrophy complex. The first procedure is performed in the neonatal period and involves bladder closure, pubic symphysis approximation, and abdominal wall closure. The second-stage procedure later in infancy involves epispadias repair. The final procedure involves bladder neck reconstruction and is generally performed at the age when toilet training is begun.[178] Osteotomies are performed to allow approximation of the pubic symphysis to facilitate midline repair. This is followed by pelvic stabilization with traction and external fixation or with plate fixation.

Anesthetic Considerations. Bladder and cloacal exstrophy repair need to be addressed at birth. The newborn will undergo the initial repair, and anesthetic considerations for the care of the newborn should be observed (Table 21-19). Regional anesthesia can be utilized for intraoperative and postoperative pain management with a single shot caudal with injection of local anesthetic (bupivacaine 0.125% or ropivacaine 0.1%) with Duramorph (20 µg/kg). A catheter threaded to the lumbar level is another option for continuous epidural analgesia. A combined general and regional technique allows for the use of fewer inhalational agents and early extubation of the neonate. With the use of epidural narcotics the neonate needs to undergo recovery in a

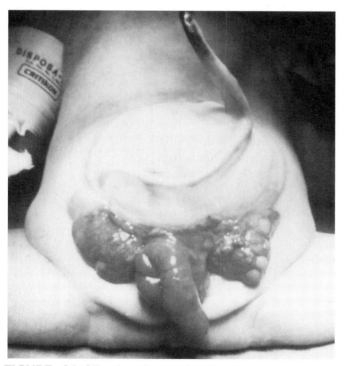

FIGURE 21–25 Cloacal exstrophy. Female newborn showing omphalocele, prolapsed ileocecal valve, and symmetrical bladder halves. *(From Gearhart JP: Exstrophy, epispadias, and other bladder anomalies. In Walsh PC [ed]: Campbell's Urology, 8th ed. Philadelphia, WB Saunders, 2002, p 2177.)*

monitored environment. Spina bifida associated with cloacal exstrophy may be a contraindication for regional techniques.[179] Latex precautions should be observed in this patient population because 75% of children with bladder exstrophy are sensitized to natural rubber latex and develop a latex allergy.[180,181]

References

1. Rudolph AM: Congenital Diseases of the Heart. Chicago, Year Book Medical Publishers, 1974.
2. Teitel DF, Iwamoto HS, Rudolph AM: Effects of birth related events on central blood flow patterns. Pediatric Res 1987;22:557-566.
3. Cassin S, Dawes GS, Mott JC, et al: The vascular resistance of the foetal and newly ventilated lung of the lamb. J Physiol 1964;171: 61-79.
4. Baum VC, Palmisano BW: The immature heart and anesthesia. Anesthesiology 87:1529-1548, 1997.
5. Berman W, Musselman J: Myocardial performance in the newborn lamb. Am J Physiol 1979;237:H66-H70.
6. Friedman WF: Intrinsic physiologic properties of the newborn heart. Prog Cardiovasc Dis 1972;15:87-111.
7. Kenny J, Plappert T, Doubilet P, et al: Effects of heart rate on ventricular size, stroke volume, and output in the normal human fetus: A prospective Doppler echocardiographic study. Circulation 1987;76:52-58.
8. Polgar G, Weng TR: The functional development of the respiratory system: From the period of gestation to adulthood. Am Rev Respir Dis 1979;120:625-695.
9. Peirce J, Hobcott J: Studies on the collagen and elastin content of the human lung. J Clin Invest 1960;39:8.
10. Mansell A, Bryan C, Levison H: Airway closure in children. J Appl Physiol 1972;33:771.
11. Hurgoiu V: Thermal regulation in preterm infants. Early Human Dev 1992;28:1-5.
12. Jahnukainen T, Van Ravensswaaij-Arts C, Jalonen J, et al: Dynamics of vasomotor thermoregulation of the skin in term and preterm neonates. Early Hum Dev 1993;33:133-143.
13. Dicker A, Ohlson KB, Johnson L, et al: Halothane selectively inhibits nonshivering thermogenesis: Possible implications for thermoregulation during anesthesia of infants. Anesthesiology 1995;82:491-501.
14. Ohlson KB, Mohell N, Cannon B, et al: Thermogenesis in brown fat adipocytes is inhibited by volatile anesthetics: A factor contributing to hypothermia in infants. Anesthesiology 1994;81:176-183.
15. Anand KJ, Sippell WG, Aynsley-Green A: Randomised trial of fentanyl anaesthesia in preterm babies undergoing surgery: Effects on the stress response. Lancet 1987;10;1:62-66.
16. Anand KJ, Hickey PR: Halothane-morphine compared with high-dose sufentanil for anesthesia and postoperative analgesia in neonatal cardiac surgery. N Engl J Med 1992;326:1-9.
17. Howard RF: Current status of pain management in children. JAMA 2003;290:2464-2469.
18. Eland JM, Anderson JE: The experience of pain in children. In Jacox A (ed): Pain: A Source Book for Nurses and Other Health Professionals. Boston, Little, Brown, 1977, pp 453-473.
19. Schechter NL, Allen DA, Hanson K: Status of pediatric pain control: A comparison of hospital analgesic usage in children and adults. Pediatrics 1986;77:11-15.
20. Fitzgerald M, Beggs S: The neurobiology of pain: Developmental aspects. Neuroscientist 2001;7:246-257.
21. Alvares D, Fitzgerald M: Building blocks of pain: The regulation of key molecules in spinal sensory neurons during development and following peripheral axotomy. Pain 1999;Suppl 6:S71-S85.
22. Anand KJ, Scalzo FM: Can adverse neonatal experiences alter brain development and subsequent behavior? Biol Neonate 2000;77:69-82.
23. Evans DJ, MacGregor RJ, Dean HG, et al: Neonatal catecholamine levels and neurodevelopmental outcome: A cohort study. Arch Dis Child Fetal Neonatal Ed 2001;84:F49-F52.
24. Johr M: Postoperative pain management in infants and children: New developments. Curr Opin Anaesthesiol 2000;13:285-289.
25. Gilbert JN, Jones KL, Rorke LB, et al: Central nervous system anomalies associated with meningomyelocele, hydrocephalus, and the Arnold-Chiari malformation: Reappraisal of theories regarding the pathogenesis of posterior neural tube closure defects. Neurosurgery 1986;18:559-564.
26. Bowman RM, McLone DG, Grant JA, et al: Spina bifida outcome: A 25-year prospective. Pediatr Neurosurg 2001;34:114-120.
27. McLone DG: Continuing concepts in the management of spina bifida. Pediatr Neurosurg 1992;18:254-256.
28. Dierdorf SF, McNiece WL, Rao CC, et al: Failure of succinylcholine to alter plasma potassium in children with myelomeningocoele. Anesthesiology 1986;64:272-273.
29. Wells TR, Jacobs RA, Senac MO, Landing BH: Incidence of short trachea in patients with myelomeningocele. Pediatr Neurol 1990;6:109-111.
30. Ross AK, Davis PJ, DeLDear G, et al: Pharmacokinetics of remifentanil in anesthetized pediatric patients undergoing elective surgery or diagnostic procedures. Anesth Analg 2001;93:1393-1401.
31. Viscomi CM, Abajian JC, Wald SL, et al: Spinal anesthesia for repair of meningomyelocele in neonates. Anesth Analg 1995;81:492-495.
32. Pittman T, Kiburz J, Gabriel K, et al: Latex allergy in children with spina bifida. Pediatr Neurosurg 1995;22:96-100.
33. Shah S, Cawley M, Gleeson R, et al: Latex allergy and latex sensitization in children and adolescents with meningomyelocele. J Allergy Clin Immunol 1998;101:741-746.
34. Holzman RS: Clinical management of latex-allergic children. Anesth Analg 1997;85:529-533.
35. Tulipan N, Bruner JP, Hernanz-Schulman M, et al: Effect of intrauterine myelomeningocele repair on central nervous system structure and function. Pediatr Neurosurg 1999;31:183-188.
36. Gerber ME, Holinger LD: Congenital laryngeal anomalies. In Bluestone CD, Stool SE, Alper CM, et al (eds): Pediatric Otolaryngology, 4th ed. Philadelphia, Elsevier, 2003, vol 2, pp 1460-1472.
37. Biavati M, Wood WE, Kearns DB, Smith RJ: One stage repair of congenital laryngeal webs. Otolaryngol Head Neck Surg 1995;112:447.
38. Farrell PT: Rigid bronchoscopy for foreign body removal: Anesthesia and ventilation. Paediatr Anesth 2004;14:84-89.
39. Brown K, Aun C, Stocks J, et al: A comparison of the respiratory effects of sevoflurane and halothane in infants and young children. Anesthesiology 1998;89:86-92.
40. Whittet HB, Hayward AW, Battersby E: Plasma lignocaine levels during paediatric endoscopy of the upper respiratory tract: Relationship with mucosal moistness. Anaesthesia 1988;43:439-442.
41. Berkenbosch JW, Graff GR, Stark JM, et al: Use of a remifentanil-propofol mixture for pediatric flexible fiberoptic bronchoscopy sedation. Paediatr Anesth 2004;14:941-946.
42. Soodan A, Pawar D, Subramanium R: Anesthesia for removal of inhaled foreign bodies in children. Paediatr Anesth 2004;14:947-952.
43. Yellon RF: Prevention and management of complications of airway surgery in children. Paediatr Anesth 2004;14:107-111.
44. Losee JE, et al: Congenital nasal anomalies: A classification scheme. Plast Reconstr Surg 2004;113:676-689.
45. Hengerer AS, Wein RO: Congenital malformations of the nose and the paranasal sinuses. In Bluestone CD, Stool SE, Alper CM, et al (ed): Pediatric Otolaryngology, 4th ed. Philadelphia, Elsevier, 2003, pp 979-994.
46. Derkay CS, Grundfast KM: Airway compromise from nasal obstruction in neonates and infants. Int J Pediar Otorhinolaryngol 1990;155:345.
47. Stankiewicz JA: The endoscopic repair of choanal atresia. Otolaryngol Head Neck Surg 1990;103:931.
48. Park AH, Brockenbrough J, Stankiewicz J: Endoscopic versus traditional approaches to choanal atresia. Otolaryngol Clin North Am 2000;33:77.

49. Ricciardelli EJ, Richardson MA: Cervicofacial cystic hygroma: Patterns of recurrence and management of the difficult case. Arch Otolaryngol Head Neck Surg 1991;117:546-553.

50. Sharma SS, Aminuldin AG, Azlan W: Cystic hygroma: Anesthetic considerations and review. Singapore Med J 1994;35:529-531.

51. Liechty KW, Crombleholme TM, Flake AW, et al: Intrapartum management for giant neck masses: The EXIT procedure. Am J Obstet Gynecol 1997;177:870-874.

52. Mychaliska GB, Bealer JF, Graf JL, et al: Operating on placental support: The ex utero intrapartum treatment procedure. J Pediatr Surg 1997;32:227-230.

53. Whitaker LA, Bartlett SP: Craniofacial anomalies. Congenital and Developmental Anomalies. In: Jurkiewicz J, Krizek T, Mathes S, Ariyan S (eds): Plastic Surgery Principles and Practice. St. Louis, CV Mosby, 1990, pp 99-136.

54. Losee JE, Bartlett SP: Treacher Collins. In Lin KY, Ogle RC, Jane JA (eds): Craniofacial Surgery: Science and Surgical Technique. Philadelphia, WB Saunders, 2002, pp 288-308.

55. Nargozian C: The airway in patients with craniofacial abnormalities. Paediatr Anesth 2004;14:53-59.

56. Bucx MJ, Grohman W, Kruisinga FH, et al: The prolonged use of the laryngeal mask airway in a neonate with airway obstruction and Treacher Collins syndrome. Paediatr Anaesth 2003;13;530-533.

57. Brown RE, Vollers JM, Rader GR, et al: Nasotracheal intubation in a child with Treacher Collins syndrome using the Bullard intubating laryngoscope. J Clin Anesth 1993;5:492-493.

58. Inada T, Fujise K, Kazuya T, et al: Orotracheal intubation through the laryngeal mask airway in paediatric patients with Treacher Collins syndrome. Paediatr Anesth 1995;5:129-132.

59. Ebata T, Nishiki S, Masuda A, Amaha K: Anaesthesia for Treacher Collins syndrome using a laryngeal mask airway. Can J Anaesth 1991;38:1043-1045.

60. Fearon JA, Weinthal J: The use of recombinant erythropoietin in the reduction of blood transfusion rates in craniosynostosis repair in infants and children. Plast Reconstr Surg 2001;109:2190-2196.

61. Wilkie AOM, Slanley SF, Oldridge M: Apert syndrome results from localized mutations of *FGFR2* and is allelic with Crouzon syndrome. Nat Genet 1995;9:165-172.

62. Cohen MM, Kreiborg S: Visceral anomalies in the Apert syndrome. Am J Genet 1993;45:758-760.

63. Kreiborg S, Barr M, Cohen MM: Cervical spine in the Apert syndrome. Am J Med Genet 1992;43:704-708.

64. Perkins JA: Airway management in children with craniofacial anomalies. Cleft Craniofacial J 1997;34:135-140.

65. Markakis DA, Sayson SC, Schreiner MS: Insertion of the laryngeal mask airway in awake infants with the Robin sequence. Anesth Analg 1992;75:822-824.

66. Blanco G, Melman E, Cuairan V, et al: Fiberoptic nasal intubation in children with anticipated and unanticipated difficult intubation. Paediatr Anesth 2001;11:49-53.

67. Johnson CM, Sims C: Awake fiberoptic intubation via a laryngeal mask airway in an infant with Goldenhar syndrome. Anaesth Intensive Care 1994;22:194-197.

68. McCarthy JG, Schreiber J, Karp N, et al: Lengthening the human mandible by gradual distraction. Plast Reconstr Surg 1992;89:1.

69. Cohen SR, Simms C, Burstein FD: Mandibular distraction osteogenesis in the treatment of upper airway obstruction in children with craniofacial deformities. Plast Reconstr Surg 1998;101:312.

70. Cooper CM, Murray-Wilson A: Retrograde intubation: Management of a 4.8 kg, 5 month old. Anesthesia 1987;42:1197-1200.

71. Sculerati N, Gottlieb MD, Zimbler MS: Airway management in children with major craniofacial anomalies. Laryngoscope 1998;108;1806-1812.

72. Faberowski LW, Black S, Mickle JP: Blood loss and transfusion practice in the perioperative management of craniosynostosis repair. J Neurosurg Anesthesiol 1999;11:167.

73. D'errico CC, Hamish MM, Buchman SR, et al: Efficacy of aprotinin in children undergoing craniofacial surgery. J Neurosurg 2003;99; 287-290.

74. De Ville A: Editorial: Blood saving in pediatric patients. Paediatr Anaesth 1997;7;181-182.

75. Fearon JA: Reducing allogenic blood transfusions during cranial vault surgical procedures: A prospective analysis of blood recycling. Plast Reconstr Surg 2004;113;1126-1130.

76. Faberowski LW, Black S, Mickle JP: Incidence of venous air embolism during craniectomy for craniosynostosis repair. Anesthesiology 2000;92;20-23.

77. Harris MM, Davidson A, Straffors MA, et al: Venous air embolism during craniectomy in supine infants. Anesthesiology 1987;67; 816-819.

78. Wong GB, Nargozian C, Padwa BL: Anesthetic concerns of external maxillary distraction osteogenesis. J Craniofacial Surg 2004;15;78-82.

79. Levine JP, Stelnicki E, Weiner HL, et al: Hyponatremia in the postoperative craniofacial pediatric patient population: A connection to cerebral salt wasting syndrome and management of the disorder. Plast Reconstr Surg 2001;108:1501-1508.

80. Lo LJ, Hung KF, Chen YR: Blindness as a complication of Le Fort I osteotomy for maxillary distraction. Plast Reconstr Surg 2002;109: 688-698; discussion 699-700.

81. Fearon JA: Rigid fixation of the calvaria in craniosynostosis without using "rigid" fixation. Plast Reconstr Surg 2003;111:27-38; discussion 39.

82. Fialkov JA, Holy C, Forrest CR, et al: Postoperative infections in craniofacial reconstructive procedures. J Craniofac Surg 2001;12:362-368.

83. Saenz NC, Shamberger RC: Posterior mediastinal masses. J Pediatr Surg 1993;28:172-176.

84. Lam JC, Chui CH, Jacobsen AS, et al: When is a mediastinal mass critical in a child? An analysis of 29 patients. Pedatr Surg Int 2004;20:180-184.

85. Vas L, Naregal F, Naik V, et al: Anaesthetic management of an infant with an anterior mediastinal mass. Paediatr Anaesth 1999;9:439-443.

86. Azizkhan RG, Dudgeon DL, Buck JR, et al: Life threatening airway obstruction as a complication to the management of mediastinal masses in children. J Pediatr Surg 1985;20:816-822.

87. Freud E, Ben-Ari J, Schonfeld T: Mediastinal tumors in children: A single institution experience. Clin Pediatr 2002;41:219-223.

88. King RM, Telander RL, Smithson WA, et al: Primary mediastinal tumors in children. J Pediatr Surg 1982;17:512-520.

89. Pulleritz J, Holzman RS: Anaesthesia for patients with mediastinal masses. Can Anaesth Soc J 1989;36:681-688.

90. Dilworth KE, McHugh, K, Stacey S, et al: Mediastinal mass obscured by a large pericardial effusion in a child: A potential cause of serious anaesthetic morbidity. Paediatr Anaesth 2001;11:479-482.

91. Yang SC: Biopsy of mediastinal tumors: Needle biopsy versus mediastinoscopy. J Bronchol 2001;8:139-143.

91a. Shamberger RC. Preanesthetic evaluation of children with anterior mediastinal masses. Semin Pediatr Surg 1999;8(2):61-68.

92. Foley RW, Rodriguez MI: Preoperative irradiation of selected mediastinal masses. J Cardiovasc Surg 2001;42:695-697.

93. King DR, Patrick LE, Ginn-Pease ME, et al: Pulmonary function is compromised in children with mediastinal lymphoma. J Pediatr Surg 1997;32:294-299.

94. Yoneda KY, Louie S, Shelton, DK: Mediastinal tumors. Curr Opin Pulm Med 2001;7:226-233.

95. Shamberger RC, Holzman RS, Griscom NT, et al: Prospective evaluation by CT and pulmonary function tests of children with mediastinal masses. Surgery 1995;118:468-471.

96. Shamberger RC, Holzman RS, Griscom NT, et al: CT quantitation of tracheal cross-sectional area as a guide to the surgical and anesthetic management of children with anterior mediastinal masses. J Pediatr Surg 1991;26:138-142.

97. Keon TP: Death on induction of anesthesia for cervical node biopsy. Anesthesiology 1981;55:471-472.

98. Bechard P, Letourneau L, Lacasse Y, et al: Perioperative cardiorespiratory complications in adults with mediastinal masses: Incidence and risk. Anesthesiology 2004;100:826-834.

99. Piro AH, Weiss DR, Hellman S: Mediastinal Hodgkin's disease: A possible danger for intubation anesthesia. Int J Radiat Oncol Biol Phys 1976;1:415-419.

100. Sibert KS, Biondi JW, Hirsch NP: Spontaneous respiration during thoracotomy in a patient with a mediastinal mass. Anesth Analg 1987;66:904-907.

101. Barnett TB: Effects of helium and oxygen mixtures on pulmonary mechanics during airway constriction. J Appl Physiol 1967;22:707-713.

102. Polaner DM: The use of heliox and laryngeal mask airway in a child with anterior mediastinal mass. Anesth Analg 1996;82:208-210.

103. Ferrari LR, Bedford RF: General anesthesia prior to treatment of anterior mediastinal masses in pediatric cancer patients. Anesthesiology 1990;72:991-995.

104. Hammer GB: Anaesthetic management for the child with a mediastinal mass. Paediatr Anaesth 2004;14:95-97.

105. Ramenofsky ML, Leape LL, McCauley RGK: Bronchogenic cyst. J Pediatr Surg 1979;14:219-224.

106. St-Georges R, Deslauriers J, Duranceau A: Clinical spectrum of bronchogenic cysts of the mediastinum and lung in the adult. Ann Thorac Surg 1991;52:6-13.

107. Birmingham PK, Uejima T, Luck SR: Anesthetic management of the patient with a bronchogenic cyst: A review of 24 cases. Anesth Analg 1993;76:879-883.

108. Politis GD, Baumann R, Hubbard AM: Spillage of cystic pulmonary masses into the airway during anesthesia. Anesthesiology 1997;87:693-696.

109. Kravitz RM: Congenital malformations of the lung. Pediatr Clin North Am 1994;41:453-472.

110. Laberge JM, Flageole H, Pugash D, et al: Outcome of the prenatally diagnosed congenital cystic adenomatoid lung malformation: A Canadian experience. Fetal Diag Ther 2001;16:178-186.

111. Nishibayashi SW, Andrassy RJ, Woolley MM: Congenital cystic adenomatoid malformation: A 30 year experience. J Pediatr Surg 1981;16:704-706.

112. Bouchard S, Johnson MP, Flake AW, et al: The EXIT procedure: Experience and outcome in 31 cases. J Pediatr Surg 2002;37:418-426.

113. Savic B, Birtel FJ, Tholen W, et al: Lung sequestration: Report of seven cases and review of 540 published cases. Thorax 1979;34:96-101.

114. Collin JP, Desjardins JG, Khan AH: Pulmonary sequestration. J Pediatr Surg 1987;22:750-753.

115. Vegunta RK, Teach S: Preoperative diagnosis of extralobar pulmonary sequestration with unusual vasculature: A case report. J Pediatr Surg 1999;34:1307-1308.

116. Piccione W, Burt ME: Pulmonary sequestration of the newborn. Chest 1990;97:244-246.

117. Berlinger NT, Porto DP, Thompson TR: Infantile lobar emphysema. Ann Otol Rhinol Laryngol 1987;96:106-111.

118. Lincoln JC, Stark J, Subramanian S, et al: Congenital lobar emphysema. Ann Surg 1971;173:55-62.

119. Karnak I, Senocak ME, Ciftci AO, et al: Congenital lobar emphysema: Diagnostic and therapeutic considerations. J Pediatr Surg 1999;34:1347-1351.

120. Kennedy CD, Habibi P, Matthew DJ, et al: Lobar emphysema: Long-term imaging follow up. Radiology 1991;180:189-193.

121. Eigen H, Lemen RJ, Waring WW: Congenital lobar emphysema: Long-term evaluation of surgically and conservatively treated children. Am Rev Respir Dis 1976;113:823-831.

122. Adzick NS, Harrison MR, Glick PL, et al: Diaphragmatic hernia in the fetus: Prenatal diagnosis and outcome in 94 cases. J Pediatr Surg 1985;20:357-361.

123. Flake AW, Crombleholme TM, Johnson MP, et al: Treatment of severe congenital diaphragmatic hernia by fetal tracheal occlusion: Clinical experience with fifteen cases. Am J Obstet Gynecol 2000;183:1059-1066.

124. Tibboel D, Gaag AV: Etiologic and genetic factors in congenital diaphragmatic hernia. Clin Perinatol 1996;23:689-699.

125. Greenwood RD, Rosenthal A, Nadas AS: Cardiovascular abnormalities associated with congenital diaphragmatic hernia. Pediatrics 1976;57:92-97.

126. David TJ, Illingworth CA: Diaphragmatic hernia in the Southwest of England. J Med Genet 1976;13:253.

127. Fauza DO, Wilson JM: Congenital diaphragmatic hernia and associated anomalies: Their incidence, identification, and impact on prognosis. J Pediatr Surg 1994;29:1113-1117.

128. Iriani I: Experimental study on the embryogenesis of congenital diaphragmatic hernia. Anat Embryol 1984;169:133.

129. Skarsgard ED, Harrison MR: Congenital diaphragmatic hernia: The surgeon's perspective. Neo Reviews, October 1999, pp 71-78.

130. Bohn D: Congenital diaphragmatic hernia. Am J Respir Crit Care Med 2002;166:911-915.

131. Wung JT, James LS, Kilchevsky E, James E: Management of infants with severe respiratory failure and persistence of fetal circulation, without hyperventilation. Pediatrics 1985;76:488-494.

132. Neonatal inhaled nitric oxide study group (NINOS): Inhaled nitric oxide and hypoxic respiratory failure in infants with congenital diaphragmatic hernia. Pediatrics 1997;99:838-845.

133. Stolar C, Dillon P, Reyes C: Selective use of extracorporeal membrane oxygenation in the management of congenital diaphragmatic hernia. J Pediatr Surg 1988;23:207-211.

134. Congenital diaphragmatic hernia study group: Estimating disease severity of CDH in the first five minutes of life. J Pediatr Surg 2001;36:141-145.

135. Semakula N, Stewart DL, Goldsmith LJ, et al: Survival of patients with congenital diaphragmatic hernia during the ECMO era: An 11-year experience. J Pediatr Surg 1997;32:1683-1689.

136. Al-Shanafey S, Giacomantonio M, Henteleff H: Congenital diaphragmatic hernia: Experience without extracorporeal membrane oxygenation. Pediatr Surg Int 2002;18:28-31.

137. Stolar CJ, Snedecor SS, Bartlett RH: Extracorporeal membrane oxygenation and neonatal respiratory failure: Experience from the extracorporeal life support organization. J Pediatr Surg 1991;26:563.

138. Elbourne D, Field D, Mugford M: Extracorporeal membrane oxygenation for severe respiratory failure in newborn infants: Cochrane review. Cochrane Database Syst Rev 2002;1;CD001340

139. Sakai H, Tamura M, Hosokawa Y, et al: Effect of surgical repair on respiratory mechanics in congenital diaphragmatic hernia. J Pediatr 1987;111;731-734.

139a. Nio M, Haase G, Kennaugh J, et al: A prospective randomized trial of delayed versus immediate repair of congenital diaphragmatic hernia. J Pediatr Surg 1994;29(5):618-621.

139b. Moyer V, Moya F, Tibboel R, et al: Late versus early surgical correction for congenital diaphragmatic hernia in newborn infants. Cochrane Database Syst Rev 2002(3):CD001695.

140. Adzick NS, Outwater KM, Harrison MR, et al: Correction of congenital diaphragmatic hernia in utero: IV. An early gestational fetal lamb model for pulmonary vascular morphometric analysis. J Pediatr Surg 1985;20:673-680.

141. Harrison MR, Adzick NS, Longaker MT, et al: Successful repair in utero of a fetal diaphragmatic hernia after removal of herniated viscera from the left thorax. N Engl J Med 1990;322:1582-1584.

142. Hedrick MH, Estes JM, Sullivan KM, et al: Plug the Lung Until it Grows (PLUG): A new method to treat congenital diaphragmatic hernia in utero. J Pediatr Surg 1994;29:612-617.

143. Albanese CT, Jennings RW, Filly RA, et al: Endoscopic fetal tracheal occlusion: Evolution of techniques. Pediatr Endosurg Innovative Tech 1998;2:47-55.

144. Vanderwall KJ, Skarsgard ED, Filly RA, et al: Fetendo-clip: A fetal endoscopic tracheal clip procedure in a human fetus. J Pediatr Surg 1997;32:970-972.

145. Harrison MR, Keller MD, Hawgood SB, Kitterman JA, et al: A randomized trial of fetal endoscopic tracheal occlusion for severe fetal congenital diaphragmatic hernia. N Engl J Med 2003;349:1916-1924.

146. Vacanti JP, Crone JD, Murphy JD, et al: The pulmonary hemodynamic response to perioperative anesthesia in the treatment of high risk

infants with congenital diaphragmatic hernia. J Pediatr Surg 1984;19:672-679.

147. Hodgson RE, Bosenberg AT, Hadley LG: Congenital diaphragmatic hernia repair—impact of delayed surgery and epidural analgesia. S Afr J Surg 2000;38:31-35.

148. Bagolan P, Casaccia F, Crescenzi A, et al: Impact of a current treatment protocol on outcome of high risk congenital diaphragmatic hernia. J Pediatr Surg 2004;39:313-318.

149. Engum SA, Grosfeld JL, West KW, et al: Analysis of morbidity and mortality in 227 cases of esophageal atresia and/or tracheoesophageal fistula over two decades. Arch Surg 1995;130:502-508; discussion 508-509.

150. Gross RE: The Surgery of Infancy and Childhood. Philadelphia, WB Saunders, 1953, p 76.

151. Kovesi T, Rubin S: Long-term complications of congenital esophageal atresia and/or tracheoesophageal fistula. Chest 2004;126:915-925.

152. Quan L, Smith DW: The VATER association, vertebral defects, anal atresia, TE fistula with esophageal atresia, radial and renal dysplasia: A spectrum of associated defects. J Pediatr Surg 1973;82:104.

153. Richardson JV, Heintz SE, Rossi NP, et al: Esophageal atresia and tracheoesophageal fistula. Ann Thorac Surg 1980;29:364-368.

154. Reeves ST, Burt N, Smith CD: Is it time to reevaluate the airway management of tracheoesophageal fistula? Anesth Analg 1995;81:866-869.

155. Andropoulos DB, Rowe RW, Betts JM: Anaesthetic and surgical airway management during tracheo-oesophageal fistula repair. Paediatr Anaesth 1998;8:313-319.

156. Vas L, Kulkarni V, Mali M, Bagry H: Spread of radiopaque dye in the epidural space in infants. Paediatr Anaesth 2003;13:233-243.

157. Konkin DE, O'hali WA, Webber EM, Blair GK: Outcomes in esophageal atresia and tracheoesophageal fistula. J Pediatr Surg 2003;38:1726-1729.

158. Langer JC: Abdominal wall defects. World J Surg 2003;27:117-124.

159. Lacey SR, Carris LA, Beyer AJ, Azizkhan RG: Bladder pressure monitoring significantly enhances care of infants with abdominal wall defects: A prospective clinical study. J Pediatr Surg 1993;28:1370.

160. Yaster M, Buck JR, Dudgeon DL, et al: Hemodynamic effects of primary closure of omphalocele/gastroschisis in human newborns. Anesthesiology 1988;69:84-88.

161. Jennings RW: Prune belly syndrome. Semin Pediatr Surg 2000;9:115-120.

162. Brinker MR, Palutsis RS, Sarwark JF: The orthopedic manifestations of prune belly syndrome. J Bone Joint Surg Am 1995;77:251-257.

163. Stephens FD, Gupta D: Pathogenesis of the prune belly syndrome. J Urol 1994;152:2328-2331.

164. Crompton CH, MacLusky IB, Geary DF: Respiratory function in the prune belly. Arch Dis Child 1993;68:505-506.

165. Henderson AM, Vallis CJ, Sumner E: Anaesthesia in the prune belly syndrome: A review of 36 cases. Anaesthesia 1987;42:54-60.

166. Soylu H, Kutlu N, Sonmezgoz E, et al: Prune belly syndrome and pulmonary hypoplasia: A potential cause of death. Pediatr Int 2001;43:172-175.

167. Corall IM, et al: Plasma concentrations of fentanyl in normal surgical patients and those with severe renal and hepatic disease. Br J Anesth 1980;52:101P.

168. Chan K, Tse J, Jennings F, Orme ML: Pharmacokinetics of low dose pethidine in patients with renal dysfunction. J Clin Pharmacol 1987;27:516-522.

169. Gonsowski CT, Laster MJ, Eger EI II, et al: Toxicity of compound A in rats: Effect of a 3-hour administration. Anesthesiology 1994;80:556.

170. Nishiyama T, Aibiki M, Hanoka K: Inorganic fluoride kinetics and renal tubular function after sevoflurane anesthesia in chronic renal failure patients receiving hemodialysis. Anesth Analg 1996;83:574-577.

171. Tsukamoto N, Hirabayashi Y, Shimizu R, Mitsuhata H: The effects of sevoflurane and isoflurane anesthesia on renal tubular function in patients with moderately impaired renal function. Anesth Analg 1996;82:909-913.

172. Conzen PF, Kharasch ED, Czerner SF, et al: Low-flow sevoflurane compared with low-flow isoflurane anesthesia in patients with stable renal insufficiency. Anesthesiology 2002;97:578-584.

173. Mazze RI, Callan CM, Galvez ST, et al: The effects of sevoflurane on serum creatinine and blood urea nitrogen concentrations: A retrospective, twenty-two-center, comparative evaluation of renal function in adult surgical patients. Anesth Analg 2000;90:683-688.

174. Sponseller PD, Bisson LJ, Gearhart JP, et al: The anatomy of the pelvis in the exstrophy complex. J Bone Joint Surg Am 1995;77:177-189.

175. Kutzner DK, Wilson WG, Hogge WA: OEIS complex (cloacal exstrophy): Prenatal diagnosis in the second trimester. Prenat Diagn 1988;8:247.

176. Molenaar JC: Cloacal extrophy. Semin Pediatr Surg 1996;5:133.

177. Mirk P, Calisti A, Fileni A: Prenatal sonographic diagnosis of bladder exstrophy. J Ultrasound Med 1986;5:291.

178. Okubadejo GO, Sponseller PD, Gearhart JP: Complications in orthopedic management of exstrophy. J Pediatr Orthop 2003;23:522-528.

179. Aram L, Krane EJ, Kozloski LJ, et al: Tunneled epidural catheters for prolonged analgesia in pediatric patients. Anesth Analg 2001;92:1432-1438.

180. Nieto A, Estornell F, Mazon A, et al: Allergy to latex in spina bifida: A multi-variate study of associated factors in 100 consecutive patients. J Allergy Clin Immunol 1996;98:501-507.

181. Ricci G, Gentili A, di Lorenzo F, et al: Latex allergy in subjects who had undergone multiple surgical procedures for bladder extrophy: Relationship with clinical intervention and atopic diseases. BJU Int 1999;84:1058-1062.

Index

Note: Page numbers followed by the letter b refer to boxed material; those followed by the letter f refer to figures, and by the letter t refer to tables.

A

Abciximab, in glycoprotein IIbIIIa receptor inhibition, 370
Abdominal compartment syndrome, 245
Abdominal surgery, in HIV/AIDS patients, 393
Abdominal wall defects, in pediatric patient, 632-636. See also specific defect.
Abscess
  appendiceal, 398
  diverticular, 399
  liver
    amebic, 397
    pyogenic, 396, 396t
  splenic, 398
Abuse, substance-related, 484-485
Acetaminophen, for burn patients, 540
  pediatric, 543
Achondroplasia
  anesthetic management issues in, 329, 329t
  cervical spine abnormalities in, 292t
  comorbidities associated with, 328t
  differential diagnosis of, 327-328, 328t
  intraoperative considerations in, 328-329
  pathophysiology of, 327
  preoperative issues in, 328, 328t
Acidosis, renal tubular, 235
Acquired immunodeficiency syndrome. See HIV/AIDS.
Acromegaly, 21-22, 429
  anesthetic concerns in, 22, 22t
Actinomycosis
  aortic stenosis in, 59t
  cardiomyopathy in, 32t
Activated partial thromboplastin time (aPTT) response, to heparin, 571
Acute intermittent porphyria, 171-172, 172t
Acute respiratory distress syndrome, 141-142, 141t
Acute tubular necrosis, 180, 242. See also Renal failure, acute.
Acyl-coenzyme A dehydrogenase deficiency, 316
Addison's disease, 426, 437
Adenoma
  adrenal, 436
  parathyroid, 414
  pituitary, 21, 429
Adenosine, for ventricular failure, 53t
Adenosine triphosphate synthesis, mitochondria in, 455, 456f
Adrenal cortex, 433-440
  androgens of, 434-435
  glucocorticoids of, 433-434, 434t
    control of secretion of, 434
    hypersecretion of, 435-436, 436t
    hyposecretion of, 437-438

Adrenal cortex (Continued)
  mineralocorticoids of, 434
    hypersecretion of, 437
    hyposecretion of, 438
  physiology of, 433-435
  response of, to prescribed corticosteroids, 438-439
  sex hormone–secreting tumors of, 435
Adrenal insufficiency
  laboratory tests for, 416t
  primary (Addison's disease), 426, 437
  secondary, 437
Adrenal medulla, 440-443
  pheochromocytoma of. See Pheochromocytoma.
  physiology of, 440-441
Adrenal virilizing tumors, 435
Adrenalectomy, bilateral, for Cushing's syndrome, 436
β-Adrenergic receptor blockers
  for hypertension, 423
  for pheochromocytoma, 442
Adrenocorticotropic hormone, 427, 428
  deficiency of, 437
  secretion of, 434
Adrenocorticotropic hormone stimulation test, 438-439
Advanced cardiac life support, in pregnancy, 568-569
Aggressive behavior, in elderly, 488-489
Agonist stimulus, platelet response test to, 373
Air embolism, as complication of craniofacial surgery, 618
Airway(s)
  assessment of, in neurofibromatosis, type 1, 285-286
  compromised, in HIV/AIDS patients, 391, 392t
  diseases of, 127-147. See also Respiratory disease.
  edema of, dexamethasone for, 607
  inhalation injury to, 537-538
  obesity and, 205
    perioperative concerns associated with, 208-209, 209f, 210f
  stabilization of, in resuscitation for septic shock, 382-383
Airway management
  in craniofacial correction surgery, 617
  in Klippel-Feil syndrome, 295
  of burn patient, 539-540
  of trauma patient, 504-510
    anesthetic considerations in, 508-510, 509t, 510f
    evaluation of injury in, 507-508, 507t
    medications in, 509t
    pathophysiology of injury in, 506-507, 507t
    preoperative preparation in, 508, 508f

Alagille syndrome (arteriohepatic dysplasia), 164-165
Albumin, in liver disease, 158t, 159
Alcohol abuse, 484
Alcohol Use Disorders Identification Test (AUDIT), 484
Alcoholism, cardiomyopathy in, 33
Aldolase deficiency (type XII), 313
Aldosterone, 434
Alfentanil, in in-vitro fertilization, 554
Alkaline phosphatase, in liver disease, 158t, 159
Allergy, anesthetic
  differential diagnosis of, 575b
  in obstetric patient, 574-575
  skin tests for, 574
Alpha cells, of pancreas, 443
Alternative medicine, 501, 502f
Alveolar proteinosis, pulmonary, 137-138
Alveolitis, fibrosing, cryptogenic, 140-141, 141t
Alzheimer's disease, 263t
Amanita mushrooms, toxicity of, 175
Amebic liver abscess, 397
American College of Obstetricians and Gynecologists (ACOG) bulletin, on vaginal birth after cesarean section, 565
American Society of Anesthesiologist (ASA) guidelines, for care of patients with tuberculosis, 395t
γ-Aminobutyric acid, 181
Aminoglycosides
  deafness caused by, 459t
  toxicity of, 254
    vs. botulism, 409t
Aminotransaminase, in hepatic injury, 159-160
Aminotransferases, in hepatic disease, 158t
Ammonia
  in hepatic clearance, 158
  in hepatic encephalopathy, 181
Amniotic fluid embolism
  clinical presentation of, 557, 558b
  consumptive coagulopathy associated with, 559
  diagnosis of, 559-560
  etiology of, 557-558
  hemodynamic changes in, 558-559
  management of, 560
  pathophysiology of, 558
Amyloidosis
  aortic insufficiency in, 62t
  aortic stenosis in, 59t
  cardiomyopathy with, 34t, 41t
  clinical features of, 589t
  diagnosis of, 587
  hypothyroidism with, 425
  in geriatric patient, 587-589
  mitral regurgitation in, 66t
  mitral stenosis in, 65t

Marasmus, 214, 216f
  clinical implications of, 215-216
  vs. kwashiorkor, 218t
Marble bone disease, 343-344
Marfan's syndrome
  anesthetic concerns in, 7, 7t
  aortic insufficiency in, 62t
  early manifestations of, 6-7
  mitral regurgitation in, 66t
  ocular manifestations of, 6
Maroteaux-Lamy syndrome, 275t
Massage therapy, 501, 502f
Mast cell mediators, 337t
Mastocytosis, 337-338, 337t, 338t
Maternal safety, during nonobstetric surgery,
    548-549, 548t
McArdle's disease, 312
Mechanical ventilation, for burn patients, 540
Mediastinal masses
  anatomic considerations in, 619, 620t
  anesthetic management of, 622, 623f, 623t
  clinical presentation of, 619-621
  diagnosis of, 621
  in pediatric patient, 619-622
  pathology of, 619, 620t
  preanesthetic evaluation of, 621-622, 621f
Mediastinal tumors, pulmonic stenosis with, 60t
Medullary carcinoma, of thyroid, 426
Megaloblastic anemia, 361-362
Melioidosis, cardiomyopathy with, 32t
Memory enhancers, 487t
Meningocele, in pediatric patient, anesthetic
    considerations for, 605t
Meningococcemia, antibiotics for, 387
Meningococcus, cardiomyopathy with, 32t
Meningomyelocele, in pediatric patient, 604-606
  anesthetic considerations for, 605, 605t
  anesthetic induction and maintenance with,
    605-606
  anomalies associated with, 604-605, 605f
  latex sensitivity and, 606
  pathophysiology of, 605
Mental disorders. See also specific disorder.
  characterization of, 471
  epidemiology of, 470-471
  preoperative evaluation of, 471
Mental retardation, 488
Mental status, impaired, in trauma patient, 507
Mesenteric ischemia, acute, in geriatric patient,
    589-590, 591t, 592t
Mesocardia, 78, 78f
Metabolic disorders
  cardiomyopathy with, 34t
  corneal pathology with, 3, 3t
  of fatty acids, 315-316, 316f
  of pyruvate, 316
Metabolism
  bilirubin, 156-157
  burn-induced changes in, 536-537
  carbohydrate, 153-155, 154f
  copper, 173
  iron, anemia and, 361t
  lipid, 155, 156f
Metapyrone test, of pituitary-adrenal axis, 428-429
Methadone, for burn patients, 540
Methimazole, for euthyroidism, 424
Methoxyflurane, altered renal function
    due to, 253
Methylprednisolone, potency of, 434t
Methysergide
  aortic insufficiency associated with, 62t
  aortic stenosis associated with, 59t
  mitral stenosis associated with, 65t
  tricuspid stenosis associated with, 65t
Metoclopramide, avoidance of, in in-vitro
    fertilization procedures, 554

Metronidazole, for amebic liver abscess, 397
Microcirculatory failure, in sepsis, 381
Microminerals, 223t
Microsomia, hemifacial, 613-614
Midazolam
  dosage of, 215t
  for seizures, in eclampsia, 561
  in emergency airway management, 509t
  in in-vitro fertilization, 554
  sedation with, 85
Midface fractures, 521
Milk-alkali syndrome, hypercalcemia with,
    415, 416t
Milrinone, for ventricular failure, 53t
Minacurium, dosage of, 215t
Mineralocorticoids, 434
  hypersecretion of, 437
  hyposecretion of, 438
Minerals, 222, 223t, 224
Mitochondria
  effect of anesthetics on, 456-457, 457t
  in adenosine triphosphate synthesis, 455, 456f
  self-destruction of, 462
Mitochondrial disorders, 455-465
  adult-onset, 458-462
    acquired, 460-461
      gradual onset of, 461-462, 462f
    inherited, 458-460, 460f
  anesthetic management of, 464-465, 464t, 465f
  background in, 455-456, 456f
  childhood onset of, 457-458, 458t, 459t
  heteroplasmy in, 456
  preoperative evaluation of, 463, 463t, 464t
Mitochondrial encephalopathy, lactic acidosis,
    and stroke-like episodes (MELAS), 458, 459t
Mitochondrial neurogastrointestinal
    encephalomyopathy (MNGIE), 458
Mitral valve
  prolapse of, 67
  regurgitation of, 64-67, 66t
    in dilated cardiomyopathy, 36
  stenosis of, 64, 65t
Monamine oxidase (MAO) inhibitors
  anesthetic interactions with, 483t
  for depression, 473t, 475
Mönckeberg sclerosis, aortic stenosis with, 59t
Mononucleosis, infectious, cardiomyopathy
    with, 32t
Monosomy, in congenital heart disease, 83t
Mood disorders, 472-479
  bipolar, 476-479, 477t
  depression in, 472-476
  dysthymic, 476
Morbid obesity, in pregnancy, 556-557
Morphine, in emergency airway
    management, 509t
Morquio's syndrome, 275t, 338, 338t
  aortic insufficiency in, 62t
  cervical spine abnormalities in, 292t
Motor evoked potential (MEP) monitoring, of
    spinal trauma, 145
Motor neuron degeneration, 265-267, 266t
Movement dysfunction disorders, 263t. See also
    specific disorder, e.g., Parkinson's disease.
MtDNA depletion syndrome (MDS), 458
Mucocutaneous lymph node syndrome, 46
Mucopolysaccharidoses, 169-170, 338-340, 338t
  anesthetic issues in, 339, 340t
  cervical spine abnormalities in, 292t
  classification of, 275t
  comorbidities associated with, 339t
  pathophysiology and diagnosis of, 275
  perioperative considerations in, 275-276
  preoperative issues in, 339, 339t
Multiple endocrine adenoma, types IIa and IIb,
    440-441

Multiple endocrine adenomatosis syndrome, 429
Multiple myeloma, 365-366
Multiple organ dysfunction syndrome,
    381-382, 382f
  definition of, 378t
Multiple sclerosis, 273-274
  perioperative considerations in, 274
Multiple system atrophy, 283-284
  differential diagnosis of, 283t
Mumps, cardiomyopathy with, 32t
Muscle(s)
  periodic paralysis of
    hyperkalemic, 318-319
    hypokalemic, 319
  tone of, definition of, 261
Muscle disease(s), 303-323. See also Muscular
    dystrophy; Myopathy; Myotonia entries.
  in fatty acid metabolism, 315-316, 315f
  in glycogen storage disease. See Glycogen
    storage disease.
  in malignant hyperthermia, 316-318
  in oxidative phosphorylation, 314-315
  in pyruvate metabolism, 316
  myasthenic, 319-322, 320f
Muscle lactate dehydrogenase deficiency
    (type XI), 313
Muscle phosphofructokinase deficiency, type VII
    (Tauri's disease), 312-313
Muscle relaxants
  in muscular dystrophy, 308t
  in noncardiac surgery of CHD patient, 93-94
  in ocular trauma, 520
  in renal disease, 252-253
Muscular dystrophy, 304-309, 304f
  anesthetic considerations in, 307-309, 308t
  congenital, 307t
  diagnosis of, 305
  differential diagnosis of, 305, 306t-307t
  Duchenne
    cardiomyopathy with, 34t
    pathophysiology of, 304-305
  oculopharyngeal, 307t
Musculoskeletal system
  anomalies of, in congenital heart disease,
    82-83
  pregnancy-induced changes of, 529t
Mustard procedure, for transposition of great
    arteries, 112, 112f
Mutant DNA, in mitochondria, 456
Myasthenia gravis, 320-322, 320t
  anesthetic considerations in, 322
  classification of, 321t
  diagnosis of, 321
  differential diagnosis of, 321t
  secondary causes of, 321t
  therapeutic options for, 321-322
  vs. botulism, 409
Myasthenic crisis, intubation after, risk factors
    associated with, 320t
Mycobacterium tuberculosis, 394. See also
    Tuberculosis.
Mycotic infections, in myocarditis, 31, 32t
Myelodysplastic syndrome, 366
Myelofibrosis, myeloid metaplasia with, in
    geriatric patient, 597-598, 597f, 597t
Myeloid metaplasia, with myelofibrosis, in
    geriatric patient, 597-598, 597f, 597t
Myeloma
  laboratory tests for, 416t
  multiple, 365-366
Myeloproliferative disease, chronic, 366
Myocardial ischemia, 43-48. See also Heart
    disease, ischemic.
Myocarditis, 31, 32t-33t, 33
  bacterial, 32t
  end-stage, 41t

Optic nerve hypoplasia, 2
Orbital blowout fractures, 519, 522t
Organophosphate poisoning, 407t
  vs. botulism, 409t
Orthopedic injury, 524-528
  evaluation of, 525-526
  intraoperative consideration(s) in, 526-528
    deep venous thrombosis as, 527-528, 528t
    fat embolism as, 527
    positioning as, 526
    temperature as, 526-527
    tourniquet problems as, 527
  pathophysiology of, 525, 525t
  preoperative preparation in, 526
Osmolarity, calculation of, 431
Osmotic diuretics, for traumatic brain injury, 517
Osteogenesis, distraction, in craniofacial
    correction, 616, 617f
Osteogenesis imperfecta
  aortic insufficiency with, 62t
  clinical manifestations of, 341-342, 341t
  intraoperative management in, 342-343
  mitral regurgitation with, 66t
  preoperative issues in, 342, 342t
Osteomalacia, 343
Osteopetrosis, 343-344, 344t
Osteoporosis, 343
  of skull, 345
Ostium primum, 94, 94f
Ostium secundum, 94-95, 94f
Otolaryngeal disorders, in pediatric patient,
    606-610. See also specific anomaly.
Ovarian hyperstimulation syndrome, 556
Overlap syndromes, 323
Overweight. See also Obesity.
  prevalence of
    age-adjusted, 204f
    by ethnicity, 204f
    in children and adolescents, 205t
Oxidative phosphorylation, disorders of, 314-315
Oximetry, pulse, in congenital heart disease,
    87-88
Oxygen
  for seizures, in eclampsia, 561
  supply-demand balance of, in coronary artery
      disease, 44-45, 45f
Oxygen delivery, 359
  calculation of, 360b
Oxygen saturation monitoring, arterial, in
    congenital heart disease, 88, 88f

P

Paget's disease, 345-346
  aortic stenosis in, 59t
  comorbidity associated with, 345t
  laboratory tests for, 416t
  perioperative issues in, 346, 346t
Pain
  congenital insensitivity to, with anhidrosis,
      277t, 281-282
  in Paget's disease, 345
  management of
    after in-vitro fertilization, 554
    in burn patients, 540
    pediatric, 543
  response to, in pediatric patient, 604
Pancreas, 443-451
  cells of, 443
  disorders of. See Diabetes mellitus;
      Hypoglycemia.
  insulin storage in, 443
  islet cell tumors of, 443-444
  physiology of, 443
Pancreatitis, laboratory tests for, 419t

Pancuronium
  dosage of, 215t
  for renal patients, 252
Panic attacks, 480-481
Panniculitis, 346-347, 347t
  α-antitrypsin deficiency and, 347
Pantothenic acid, 222
Papillomatosis, recurrent respiratory, 17-20, 18t
Paracervical blockade, in in-vitro fertilization,
    553t, 554-555
Paralysis, tick-borne, 35t
  vs. botulism, 409t
Parathyroid glands, 413-420. See also
    Hyperparathyroidism; Hypoparathyroidism.
  adenoma of, 414
  cancer of, 414, 415, 416t
  physiology of, 413-414
Parathyroid hormone, 413-414
  ectopic production of, laboratory tests for, 416t
  excessive secretion of, 418
Parkinson's disease, 262, 263t, 264
  differential diagnosis of, 283t
Patent ductus arteriosus, 98-99, 98f
Patent foramen ovale, 94, 94f
Patient-initiated movement, impairment in, 261
Pediatric patient, 601-636
  abdominal wall defects in, 632-636. See also
      specific defect.
  burns in, 541-543, 542t
    procedural sedation for, 542-543
  cardiac physiology in, 601-603, 602f
  central venous catheter in, recommended
      length of, 88t
  choanal atresia in, 608-609, 608f-609f, 609t
  congenital lung anomalies in, 622-632. See also
      specific anomaly.
  craniofacial anomalies in, 610-619. See also
      specific anomaly.
    surgical correction of, 614, 616-619,
        617f, 619f
  cystic hygroma in, 609-610, 610f-611f
  laryngeal webs in, 606-608, 607f, 607t, 608t
  mediastinal masses in, 619-622, 620t, 621f,
      623f, 623t
  meningomyelocele in, 604-606, 605f, 605t
  mitochondrial disorders in, 457-458, 458t, 459t
  obesity in, 203
  pain and stress responses in, 604
  protein-energy malnutrition disorders in,
      214-216
  refeeding syndrome in, 214-215, 217t
  renal physiology in, 604
  respiratory physiology in, 603, 603f
  temperature regulation in, 603-604
Pelvic fracture, 525
Pemphigoid, 347-348, 348t
Pemphigus, 347-348
Penetrating trauma, 523-524
  to face, 521
D-Penicillamine, for Wilson's disease, 174
Pentobarbital, sedation with, 85
Periarteritis nodosa, cardiomyopathy with, 35t
Pericardiectomy, bleeding with, 58
Pericarditis, constrictive, 52, 55
  anesthetic considerations in, 56-58, 57f
  characteristic hemodynamic features of, 55
  conditions producing, 54t
  pulmonic stenosis in, 60t
Peripheral neuropathy, 267, 268t, 269-270
  hereditary, 276-282, 277t. See also specific
      neuropathy, e.g., Charcot-Marie-Tooth
      disease.
Peritoneal dialysis, 248
Pfeiffer's syndrome, anesthetic considerations in,
    615
Phenothiazines, anesthetic interactions with, 483t

Phenoxybenzamine, in pheochromocytoma, 442
Phentolamine, in ventricular failure, 53t
Phenylephrine
  in septic shock, 385t, 386
  in ventricular failure, 53t
Phenytoin, in myotonic dystrophy, 310
Pheochromocytoma, 440-443
  anesthetic considerations in, 441-443, 441t
  cardiac manifestations of, 43
  diagnosis of, 441
  hypertension in, 440
  optimal preoperative conditions for, 442
  physiology of, 440-441
  resection of, perioperative mortality in, 441t
Phobia, social, 479
Phosphoglycerate kinase deficiency (type IX), 313
Phosphoglycerate mutase deficiency (type X), 313
Phosphorus, 223t
Phosphorus intoxication, cardiomyopathy
    with, 35t
Phosphorylase B kinase deficiency (type XI), 313
Phosphorylation, oxidative, disorders of, 314-315
Pickwickian syndrome, 213
Pierre Robin sequence, 613
  mandibular distractor for, 616, 617f
Pituitary gland, 427-433
  adenoma of, 21, 429
  anterior, 427
    disorders of, 428-430
      anesthetic considerations in, 429-430
    hyperfunction of, 429
    hypofunction of, 428-429
    physiology of, 427-428, 428f
  posterior, 427
    disorders of, 430-432, 430t
      anesthetic considerations in, 432-433
  tumors of, 429, 436
Placenta accreta, 563-565, 563b, 564t
  blood loss in, 565
  hysterectomy for, 564
  incidence of, 564
Placentation, abnormal, 563-566
  anesthetic considerations in, 564t
Plagiocephaly, 614f
Plague, 405, 407
  differential diagnosis of, 403t, 406t
  infection control issues for, 404t
Platelet(s)
  abnormal, screening for, 367
  circulating, 366
  disorders of, 366-373
    drug-induced, 368t, 370
    in Bernard-Soulier syndrome, 368t, 369
    in Glanzmann's thrombasthenia, 368t, 369
    in idiopathic thrombocytopenic
        purpura, 367
    in impaired coagulation, 371
    in thrombasthenic syndromes, 367-371, 368t
    in thrombotic disorders, 371-372
    in thrombotic thrombocytopenic
        purpura, 367
    in von Willebrand's disease, 368-369, 368t
    testing modalities for, 368t
  transfusion of, for burn patient, 541
Platelet aggregometry, 373
Platelet count
  diminished, after burns, 537
  normal, 366-367
Platelet function monitoring, 372-373
Platelet response test, to agonist stimulus, 373
Platelet sequestration, 367
Pneumonia
  community-acquired, antibiotics for, 386
  eosinophilic, 136
Pneumonic plague, 403t, 404t, 405, 407
Pneumoperitoneum, during laparoscopy, 550